McGraw-Hill Education Specialty Board Review

PEDIATRICS EXAMINATION AND BOARD REVIEW

McGraw-Hill Education Specialty Board Review

PEDIATRICS EXAMINATION AND BOARD REVIEW

Edited by

Andrew R. Peterson, MD, MSPH
Clinical Associate Professor
Stead Family Department of Pediatrics
Carver College of Medicine
University of Iowa
Iowa City, Iowa

Kelly E. Wood, MD
Clinical Assistant Professor
Stead Family Department of Pediatrics
Carver College of Medicine
University of Iowa
Iowa City, Iowa

Mc Graw Hill Education

New York / Chicago / San Francisco / Athens / London / Madrid / Mexico City
Milan / New Delhi / Singapore / Sydney / Toronto

McGraw-Hill Education Specialty Board Review: Pediatrics Examination and Board Review

1 2 3 4 5 6 7 8 9 DSS 21 20 19 18 17 16

ISBN 978-0-07-184768-1
MHID 0-07-184768-5

Notice

Medicine is an ever-changing science. As new research and clinical experience broaden our knowledge, changes in treatment and drug therapy are required. The authors and the publisher of this work have checked with sources believed to be reliable in their efforts to provide information that is complete and generally in accord with the standards accepted at the time of publication. However, in view of the possibility of human error or changes in medical sciences, neither the authors nor the publisher nor any other party who has been involved in the preparation or publication of this work warrants that the information contained herein is in every respect accurate or complete, and they disclaim all responsibility for any errors or omissions or for the results obtained from use of the information contained in this work. Readers are encouraged to confirm the information contained herein with other sources. For example and in particular, readers are advised to check the product information sheet included in the package of each drug they plan to administer to be certain that the information contained in this work is accurate and that changes have not been made in the recommended dose or in the contraindications for administration. This recommendation is of particular importance in connection with new or infrequently used drugs.

This book was set in Minion Pro by Cenveo® Publisher Services.
The editors were Andrew Moyer and Christie Naglieri.
The production supervisor was Catherine Saggese.
Project Management was provided by Yashmita Hota, Cenveo Publisher Services.
Cover Photo: JGI/Tom Grill/Getty Images.
RR Donnelley was printer and binder.

This book is printed on acid-free paper.

Library of Congress Cataloging-in-Publication Data

Pediatrics (Peterson)
    Pediatrics / edited by Andrew R. Peterson, Kelly E. Wood.—1ed.
          p. ; cm.—(McGraw-Hill Education specialty board review)
    Includes index.
    ISBN 978-0-07-184768-1 (pbk. : alk. paper)—ISBN 0-07-184768-5 (pbk. : alk. paper)
    I. Peterson, Andrew R., editor.   II. Wood, Kelly E., editor.   III. Title. IV.
    Series: McGraw-Hill specialty board review.
    [DNLM: 1.   Pediatrics—Examination Questions.   WS 18.2]
    RJ48.2
    618.9200076—dc23
                                                    2015034899

Contents

Contributors

Dina Al-Zubeidi, MD
Clinical Assistant Professor of Pediatrics
Division of Gastroenterology
Stead Family Department of Pediatrics,
  Carver College of Medicine
University of Iowa
Iowa City, Iowa [16]

William Aughenbaugh, MD
Associate Professor and Program Director
Department of Dermatology
Vice Chair of Education in the Department of Dermatology
  and Director of Specialty Clinical Medical Education and
  Residency Preparation
University of Wisconsin
Madison, Wisconsin [33]

LaTisha L. Bader, PhD, LP, LAC,CC-AASP
Center for Dependence, Addiction and Rehabilitation
  (CeDAR)
University of Colorado Hospital
Aurora, Colorado [35]

Rebecca Benson, MD, PhD
Medical Director, Pediatric Pain and Palliative Care Program
Medical Director for Clinical Ethics and Director,
  Ethics Consult Service
Stead Family Department of Pediatrics
University of Iowa Children's Hospital,
  University of Iowa Hospitals and Clinics
Iowa City, Iowa [12]

James D. Burkhalter, LISW
Director of DBT Programming
Social Work Specialist, Department of Psychiatry
University of Iowa Hospitals and Clinics
Iowa City, Iowa [29]

Gayathri Chelvakumar, MD, MPH
Nationwide Children's Hospital
Section of Adolescent Medicine
Columbus, Ohio [1]

Paula Cody, MD, MPH
Assistant Professor
Department of Pediatrics
University of Wisconsin School of Medicine
  and Public Health
Madison, Wisconsin [1]

Cassandra J. Collins, BSW, LISW
Clinical Social Worker
Department of Social Service
University of Iowa Hospitals & Clinics
Iowa City, Iowa [29]

Amy L. Conrad, PhD
Assistant Professor
The Stead Family Department of Pediatrics
University of Iowa Children's Hospital
Iowa City, Iowa [6]

Linda J. Cooper-Brown, PhD
Clinical Associate Professor
Stead Family Department of Pediatrics,
  Division of Pediatric Psychology
The University of Iowa
Iowa City, Iowa [3]

Vanessa A. Curtis, MD
Clinical Assistant Professor
Department of Pediatrics
Division of Endocrinology and Diabetes
University of Iowa Carver College of Medicine
Iowa City, Iowa [11]

Anthony J. Fischer, MD, PhD
Assistant Professor
Department of Pediatrics
Division of Allergy, Pulmonology, and Immunology
University of Iowa Children's Hospital
Iowa City, Iowa [32]

Chris Hogrefe, MD, FACEP
Assistant Professor
Department of Medicine—Sports Medicine
Department of Emergency Medicine
Department of Orthopaedic Surgery—Sports Medicine
Northwestern Medicine
Northwestern University Feinberg School of Medicine
Chicago, Illinois [27]

Sandy D. Hong, MS, MD
Assistant Clinical Professor
Division of Rheumatology
Department of Pediatrics
University of Iowa Children's Hospital
Iowa City, Iowa [7]

Erin Howe, MD
University of Iowa Stead Family
Department of Pediatrics
Iowa City, Iowa [19]

Jennifer G. Jetton, MD
Clinical Assistant Professor
Division of Pediatric Nephrology, Dialysis and Transplantation
Stead Family Department of Pediatrics
University of Iowa Children's Hospital
Iowa City, Iowa [31]

Kathleen Kieran, MD, MS
Associate Professor of Urology
Department of Urology
University of Washington/Seattle Children's Hospital
Seattle, Washington [18]

Todd Kopelman, PhD, BCBA
Clinical Assistant Professor
Department of Psychiatry
University of Iowa Hospitals and Clinics
Iowa City, Iowa [6]

Kathy Lee-Son, MD, MHSc
Clinical Assistant Professor
Pediatric Nephrology Department
Stead Family University of Iowa Children's Hospital
Iowa City, Iowa [31]

Ashley Loomis, MD
Assistant Professor, Pediatric Critical Care
University of Minnesota
Minneapolis, Minnesota [8]

Rebecca L. Lozman-Oxman, DNP, APRN, MSN, BSN, MPH
Pediatric Nurse Practitioner
Pediatrics, New London Hospital/Newport
  Health Center
New London, New Hampshire [28]

Elizabeth H. Mack, MD, MS
Associate Professor of Pediatrics
Division of Pediatric Critical Care
Medical University of South Carolina
Charleston, South Carolina [25]

Jessie Marks, MD, FAAP
Clinical Assistant Professor
University of Iowa Carver College of Medicine
Stead Family Department of Pediatrics,
  University of Iowa Children's Hospital
Iowa City, Iowa [14]

Ross Mathiasen, MD
Department of Emergency Medicine
Department of Family Medicine
Institute for Orthopaedics, Sports Medicine, and Rehabilitation
The University of Iowa Carver College of Medicine
Iowa City, Iowa [35]

Satsuki Matsumoto, MD
Associate of Pediatrics
Department of Pediatrics, Division of Neurology and
  Developmental and Behavioral Pediatrics
Roy J. and Lucille A. Carver College of Medicine
University of Iowa
Iowa City, Iowa [23]

Jennifer McWilliams, MD
Child and Adolescent Psychiatrist
Department of Behavioral Health
Children's Hospital and Medical Center
Omaha, Nebraska [3]

Gary Milavetz, Pharm D, FCCP, FAPhA
Associate Professor and Division Head
The University of Iowa College of Pharmacy
Department of Pharmacy Practice and Science
Division of Applied Clinical Sciences
Iowa City, Iowa [26]

Sarah L. Miller, MD
Clinical Assistant Professor
Department of Emergency Medicine
University of Iowa Hospitals and Clinics
Iowa City, Iowa [10]

Ashley A. Miller, MD, FAAP
Pediatrician
Pediatrics
Geisel School of Medicine at Dartmouth
Hanover, New Hampshire [28]

Lisa K. Muchard, MD
Assistant Clinical Professor
Department of Dermatology
University of Wisconsin
Madison, Wisconsin [33]

Blaise Nemeth, MD, MS
Associate Professor (CHS)
Pediatric Orthopedics, American Family
  Children's Hospital
Department of Orthopedics and Rehabilitation
University of Wisconsin School of
  Medicine and Public Health
Madison, Wisconsin [22]

Benton Ng, MD
Pediatric Cardiologist
Pediatrics, All Children's Hospital
St. Petersburg, Florida [5]

Erin A. Osterholm, MD
Assistant Professor of Pediatrics
Department of Pediatrics, Division of Neonatology
University of Minnesota
Minneapolis, Minnesota [14]

Niyati Patel, MD
Assistant Professor, Pediatric Critical Care
University of Minnesota
Minneapolis, Minnesota [8]

Andrew R. Peterson, MD, MSPH
Clinical Associate Professor
Stead Family Department of Pediatrics,
  Carver College of Medicine
University of Iowa
Iowa City, Iowa [30, 34]

Catherina Pinnaro, MD
Pediatrics Resident, Department of Pediatrics
University of Iowa
Iowa City, Iowa [12]

Nathan Price, MD
Clinical Assistant Professor
Pediatric Infectious Diseases
Stead Family Department of Pediatrics
Iowa City, Iowa [20]

Gregory M. Rice, MD
Associate Professor of Pediatrics, Division of Genetics
  and Metabolism
Co-Director, WSLH Biochemical Genetics Laboratory;
  Director, Medical Genetics Residency Program
University of Wisconsin School of Medicine and Public Health
Madison, Wisconsin [17]

Eric T. Rush, MD, FAAP, FACMG
Departments of Pediatrics and Internal Medicine
University of Nebraska Medical Center
  and Children's Hospital and Medical Center
Omaha, Nebraska [21]

Judith Regine Sabah, MD, PhD, MBA
Ophthalmologist—Comprehensive
  and Pediatric/Adult Strabismus
Operative Care, Eugene VA Healthcare System
Eugene, Oregon [13]

Melanie A. Schmitt, MD
Assistant Professor of Pediatric Ophthalmology
  and Director of Ophthalmic Genetics
Department of Ophthalmology and Visual Sciences
University of Wisconsin-Madison
Madison, Wisconsin [13]

Laura Steinauer, Pharm D Candidate
Student Pharmacist
The University of Iowa College of Pharmacy
Iowa City, Iowa [26]

Natalie Stork, MD
Assistant Professor
University of Missouri-Kansas City School of Medicine
Department of Orthopedic Surgery
  and Department of Pediatrics
The Children's Mercy Hospital, Division of Orthopedics
Section of Sports Medicine
Kansas City, Missouri [22]

Alex Thomas, MD
Allergist/Immunologist
Internal Medicine/Pediatrics
Presence Sts. Mary and Elizabeth Medical Center,
  Advocate Children's Hospital
Chicago, Illinois [2]

Amy O. Thomas, MD
Allergist/Immunologist
Allergy and Immunology Department
Dreyer Medical Clinic- Advocate Hospital System
Aurora, Illinois [2]

Elizabeth C. Utterson, MD
Assistant Professor of Pediatrics
Division of Pediatric Gastroenterology,
  Hepatology and Nutrition
Washington University
St. Louis, Missouri [16]

Jeffrey Robert Van Blarcom, MD
Assistant Professor
Department of Pediatrics, Division of Inpatient Medicine
University of Utah
Salt Lake City, Utah [15, 26]

Susan S. Vos, PharmD, BCPS, FAPhA
Clinical Associate Professor
The University of Iowa College of Pharmacy
Department of Pharmacy Practice and Science
Division of Applied Clinical Sciences
Iowa City, Iowa [26]

Tammy L. Wilgenbusch, PhD
Clinical Assistant Professor
Stead Family Department of Pediatrics,
    Division of Psychology
University of Iowa Children's Hospital
Iowa City, Iowa [6]

Adam D. Wolfe, MD, PhD
Assistant Professor of Pediatric Hematology-Oncology
Baylor College of Medicine
Children's Hospital of San Antonio
San Antonio, Texas [4]

Kelly E. Wood, MD
Clinical Assistant Professor
Stead Family Department of Pediatrics
Carver College of Medicine
University of Iowa
Iowa City, Iowa [24, 29]

Leah Zhorne, MD
Clinical Assistant Professor
Department of Pediatrics, Division of Neurology and
    Developmental and Behavioral Pediatrics
Roy J. and Lucille A. Carver College of Medicine
University of Iowa
Iowa City, Iowa [23]

Derek Zhorne, MD
Clinical Assistant Professor of Pediatrics
Division of General Pediatrics and Adolescent Medicine
Stead Family Department of Pediatrics
Iowa City, Iowa [9]

Preface

Welcome to the *Pediatrics Examination and Board Review* book. This is a comprehensive board review designed to help the reader study for the general pediatrics board examination.

This text covers all the content that the American Board of Pediatrics (ABP) says you need to know for the board exam. The 35 chapters in this text correspond to the 35 sections of the ABP content specifications and are written by specialists in the topic areas. The majority of the content is presented as cases followed by question/answer/discussion. The discussions are in depth but written in an informal manner to avoid the feeling that you are reading a textbook. For visual learners, we have included tables, figures, and photos. The goal of this book is to make studying for the boards more engaging.

Each chapter is meant to stand alone, allowing you to focus on challenging content areas or those where you may need to spend more time. A final exam is included at the end to help you test what you have learned. Each question is referenced in the book so you can go back and review what you may have missed.

Pediatricians trying to pass a national board exam are not the only ones who might benefit from this book. Anyone wanting to learn more about pediatric medicine should read this book. It provides a broad overview perfect for both early and seasoned learners.

We are very proud of the final product and believe it provides the reader with an exceptional resource to cover the entire breadth of pediatric medicine.

We would like to thank all of the authors who contributed to this book. Without their hard work, this book would have never come together. We would also like to thank Christie Naglieri, Andrew Moyer, Alyssa Fried, and Samantha Williams at McGraw-Hill for their help and guidance throughout. But most of all, we would like thank our friends, family, and coworkers for their love, understanding, and support during the final push to complete this project.

Andrew R. Peterson, MD, MSPH
Kelly E. Wood, MD

Adolescent Medicine and Gynecology

1

Gayathri Chelvakumar and Paula Cody

A 14-year-old boy presents to your office with concerns of delayed puberty. The patient is shorter than most of his classmates. He is active in basketball and is worried that his lack of height will affect his ability to play. His mother is 5 feet, 7 inches tall and had her first menses at age 14 years. His father is 6 feet, 4 inches tall and reports that he was a "late bloomer" and attained most of his adult height in college. The patient is otherwise healthy, developmentally appropriate, and not on any medications. On physical exam he is a well-appearing, well-nourished young male. He has mild acne, his testes are descended bilaterally and 3 mL in volume, and there is scant pubic hair and minimal penile development. He has grown 5 cm in the last year. (See Figure 1–1.)

Question 1-1

Which of the following tests will most likely establish the diagnosis for this patient?
A) CBC.
B) Calculation of midparental height.
C) Bone age.
D) Growth hormone levels.
E) Thyroid studies.

Discussion 1-1

The correct answer is "C." The age at which puberty is considered delayed is 14 years in boys and 13 years in girls. Constitutional delay of puberty is the most common cause, especially in boys. This patient most likely has a constitutional delay of puberty—short but normal growth rate and a positive family history. The best test to establish the diagnosis would be a bone age. Delayed puberty in boys is defined as lack of pubertal testicular development (sexual maturity rating [SMR] 2) by age 14 years in boys. (See Table 1–1 for details.) SMR is also known as Tanner

staging, after the pediatrician who first described the sequence of secondary sexual characteristics. (See Figures 1–2 and 1–3.) The delay leads to a comparative decrease in growth velocity compared to age-matched peers, leading to short stature as the primary complaint in most patients. Prepubertal growth velocity is typically 4 to 6 cm/y in adolescent boys and increases to a peak velocity of approximately 9.5 cm/y at SMR 3 to 4. Most delayed puberty in boys is due to a constitutional delay from delayed activation of the hypothalamic-pituitary-gonadal axis. Once puberty begins patients generally have catch-up growth and attain a normal adult height. Often there is a family history of "late bloomers" or other family members with constitutional delay of puberty. Delayed puberty and short stature can have significant effects on self-esteem, particularly in boys, and short courses of androgen replacement therapy may be indicated. (Think back to junior high when the girls towered over the boys.) Underlying metabolic, endocrine, or systemic disorders are an unlikely cause of delayed puberty in this patient given his previous normal growth velocity and development and otherwise healthy state. A bone age test will help establish the diagnosis. In constitutional delay of puberty bone age will be decreased compared with chronological age as it is more closely related to skeletal maturity and pubertal stage. A normal bone age would be seen with familial short stature and Turner syndrome. An advanced bone age is seen with precocious puberty for which early closure of the growth plates will result in a short adult unless treated.

> **Helpful Tip**
> Calculation of a midparental height can help determine a child's genetic height potential.
> For girls: (Mother's height in cm + Father's height in cm)/2 − 6.5 cm
> For boys: (Mother's height in cm + Father's height in cm)/2 + 6.5 cm

2 to 20 years: Boys
Stature-for-age and Weight-for-age percentiles

NAME _____

RECORD # _____

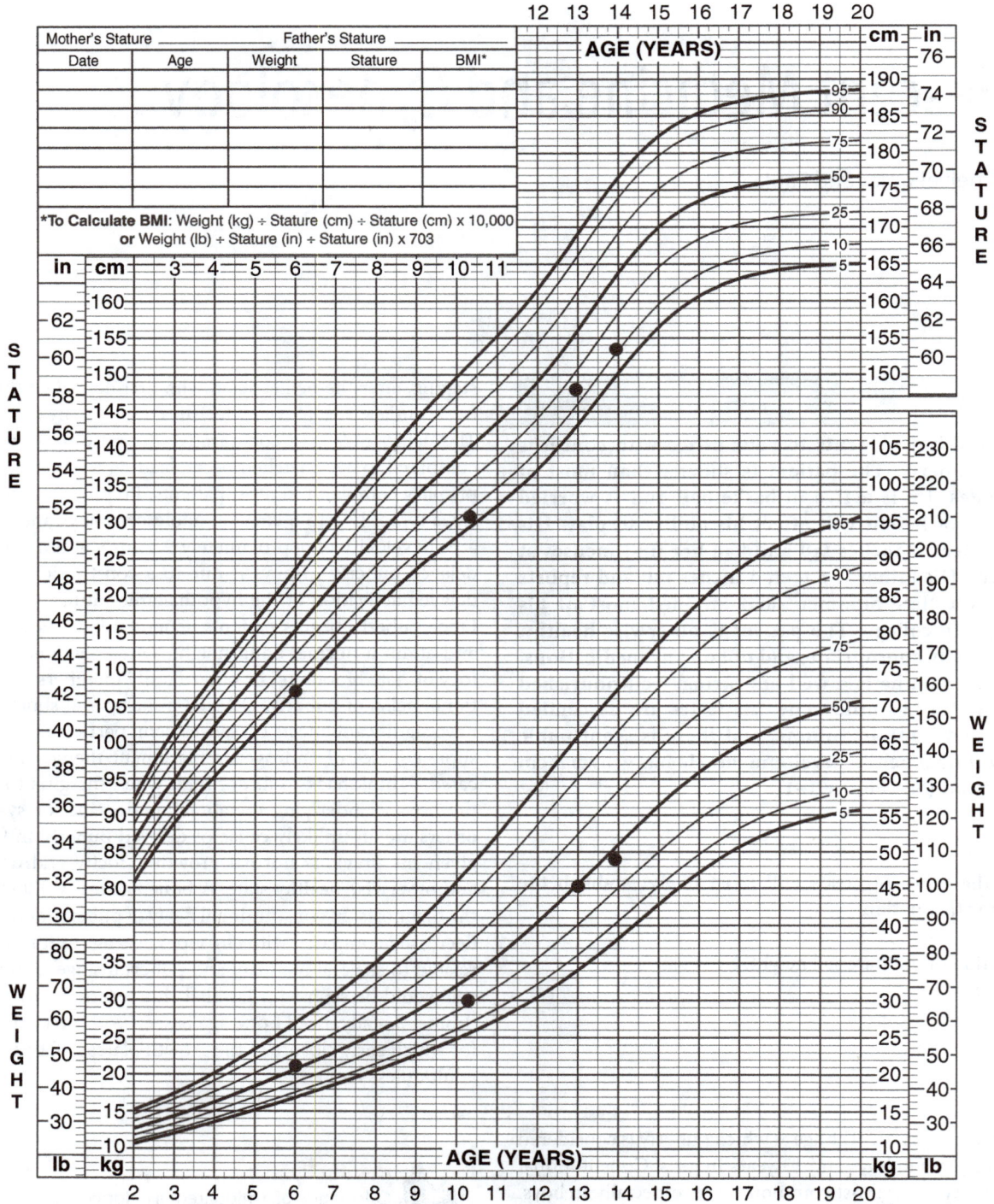

FIGURE 1–1. Growth chart of boy in Case 1. (Reproduced with permission from the National Center for Health Statistics in collaboration with the National Center for Chronic Disease Prevention and Health Promotion [2000]. http://www.cdc.gov/growthcharts.)

TABLE 1–1   SEXUAL MATURITY RATING (SMR) IN MALES

SMR in Males	Pubic Hair Development	Testicular Development	Penile Development
1	No pubic hair	Prepubertal genitalia	Prepubertal genitalia
2	Sparse, downy hair at base of penis	Enlargement of testis (volume > 4 mL), scrotal sac enlarges, redder in appearance	No change
3	Hair becomes thicker, longer, and curlier, still in limited midline distribution	Continued enlargement of testes and scrotum	Penis begins to grow in length first, then diameter
4	Adult type hair in quality but limited distribution	Thickening and darkening of scrotal sac with continued growth of testes	Continued growth of penis, enlargement of glans
5	Adult quality hair with spread to medial thighs	Adult appearance, adult testicular volume of 12–27 mL	Adult appearance

Data from Bordini B, Rosenfield R. Normal pubertal development part II: Clinical aspects of puberty. *Pediatr Rev*. 2011;32(7):281–292; and Neinstein LS, ed. *Handbook of Adolescent Healthcare*. Philadelphia, PA: Lippincott Williams & Wilkins; 2009.

▶ **CASE 2**

Your next patient is a 13-year-old boy who is distressed because he reports that he is developing breasts. On exam you note that he has a firm, rubbery, mobile, and tender 0.5 cm mass under both nipples. His testicular exam reveals testicular volume of 6 mL and no masses. The remainder of his exam is normal, his growth and development is otherwise normal, and he is not on any medications.

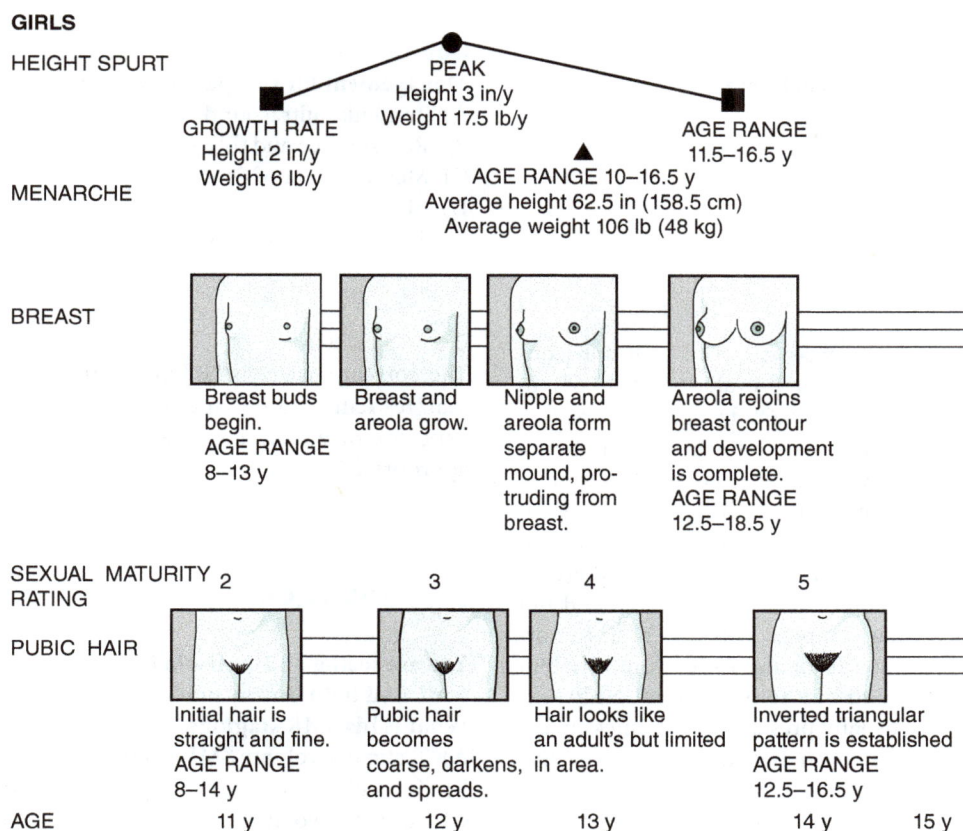

FIGURE 1–2. Adolescent female sexual maturation and growth. (Reproduced with permission from Hay WW, Levin MJ, Deterding RR, Abzug MJ, eds. *Current Diagnosis and Treatment Pediatrics*. 22nd ed. New York, NY: McGraw-Hill Education, Inc., 2014; Fig. 4–4.)

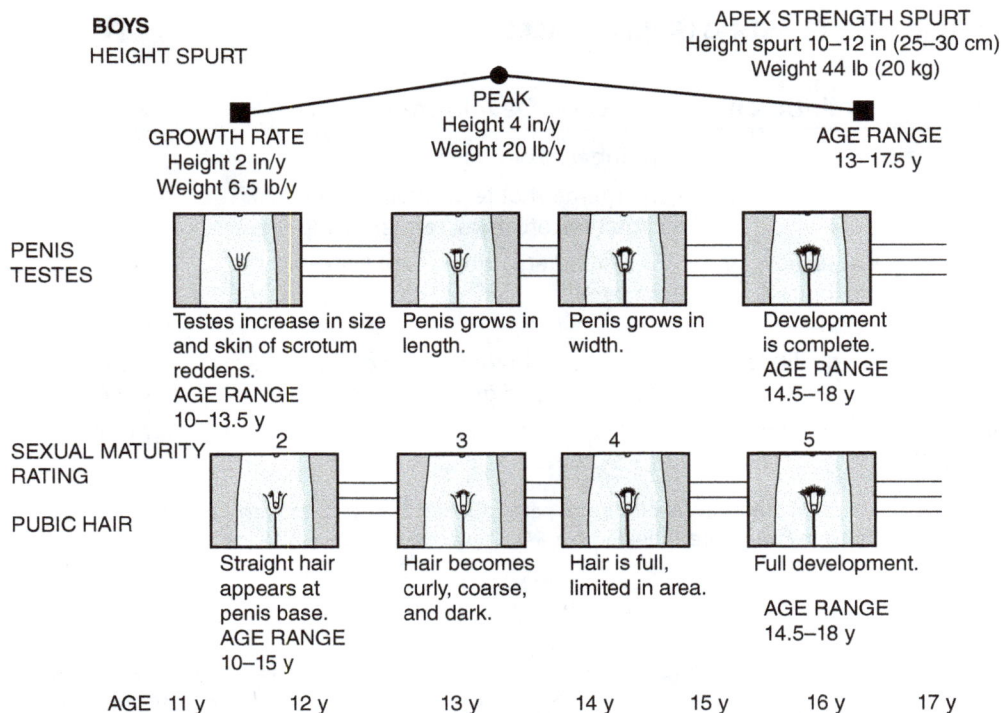

FIGURE 1–3. Adolescent male sexual maturation and growth. (Reproduced with permission from Hay WW, Levin MJ, Deterding RR, Abzug MJ, eds. *Current Diagnosis and Treatment Pediatrics*. 22nd ed. New York, NY: McGraw-Hill Education, Inc., 2014; Fig. 4–3.)

Question 2-1

The most likely diagnosis for this patient is:

A) Pseudogynecomastia.
B) Testicular tumor.
C) Gynecomastia.
D) Normal puberty.
E) Phytoestrogen consumption.

Question 2-2

Management for this patient would include:

A) Testicular ultrasound.
B) Reassurance and follow-up exam in 6 months.
C) Measurement of gonadotropins.
D) Measurement of prolactin.
E) Testosterone injections.

Discussion 2-1

The correct answer is "C." Gynecomastia is a common condition in adolescent males with a prevalence of 19.6% in 10.5-year-old males, increasing to 64.6% by age 14 years. It is caused by an imbalance of estrogen to testosterone in pubertal males. The relative increased estrogen leads to proliferation of glandular breast tissue. It is important to differentiate gynecomastia from pseudogynecomastia, which results from excess fat deposition as opposed to glandular tissue. In pseudogynecomastia, tissue tends to be more widely distributed and not localized to the nipple areolar complex. This patient has a normal testicular exam, making a testicular cancer unlikely. But take the opportunity to remind him to perform monthly self-exams as testicular cancer usually presents as a painless mass. Soy products contain phytoestrogen, but eating tofu won't give you breasts. Have you ever seen an orchidometer? To avoid confusion, be sure to explain that it is standard practice to compare the patient's testicles to wooden beads on a string to determine the testicular volume.

Discussion 2-2

The correct answer is "B." Given that this patient has a normal testicular exam and no signs of exogenous estrogen exposure or underlying disease, reassurance and follow up is appropriate.

⌛ QUICK QUIZ

You are seeing a 13-year-old boy who has testicular volume of 6 mL and light downy pubic hair.

What is his SMR staging?

A) Testicular volume SMR 2; pubic hair SMR 2.
B) Testicular volume SMR 1; pubic hair SMR 2.
C) Testicular volume SMR 2; pubic hair SMR 3.
D) Testicular volume SMR 3; pubic hair SMR 3.
E) Testicular volume SMR 2; pubic hair SMR 1.

Discussion

The correct answer is "A."

> **Helpful Tip**
>
> The average age of menarche in the United States is 12.6 years, with range of 11.0 to 14.1. Menarche occurs earlier in African American and Mexican American girls.

QUICK QUIZ

What is the most common breast mass in adolescent females?
A) Fibroadenoma.
B) Fibrocystic changes.
C) Rhabdomyosarcoma.
D) Hemangioma.
E) Galactocele.

Discussion

The correct answer is "A". Most breast masses in adolescent girls are benign. A fibroadenoma feels like a rubbery, smooth, mobile, round mass. It is nontender and usually located in the upper outer quadrant of the breast. Other common benign masses include fibrocystic changes, cysts, abscesses, and fat necrosis from trauma. Options "D" and "E" are less common benign causes. Malignancy such as option "C" is a rare cause. Before a nipple is pierced or a hair is plucked, remember to counsel that both can cause an abscess.

► CASE 3

You are seeing a 14-year-old girl in your office for her annual exam. When speaking with you confidentially, she mentions that she is concerned that she has not yet started her period like all of her friends. She reports breast development starting approximately 1 year ago. On exam she has palpable breast tissue extending just beyond her areola and pubic hair that is thick and curly and primarily midline in distribution.

Question 3-1

Which of the following most accurately describes her SMR staging?
A) Breast SMR 1; pubic hair SMR 2.
B) Breast SMR 3; pubic hair SMR 2.
C) Breast SMR 1; pubic hair SMR 4.
D) Breast SMR 3; pubic hair SMR 3.
E) Breast SMR 5; pubic hair SMR 5.

Discussion 3-1

The correct answer is "D." The patient described in the vignette has breast and pubic hair development consistent with SMR 3. (See Table 1–2 for details.)

TABLE 1–2 SEXUAL MATURITY RATING (SMR) IN FEMALES

SMR in Females	Pubic Hair Development	Breast Development
1	No pubic hair	Prepubertal breasts
2	Sparse, downy hair	Formation of breast bud, glandular tissue palpable under areola; areola is slightly widened and projects as a small mound
3	Hair becomes thicker, longer, and curlier, still in limited midline distribution	Enlargement of breast with elevation of breast contour and enlargement of areola
4	Adult type hair in quality but limited distribution	Areola forms a secondary mound over contour of breast
5	Adult quality hair with spread to medial thighs	Fully mature breast with continuous contour between areola and breast

Data from Bordini B, Rosenfield R. Normal pubertal development part II: Clinical aspects of puberty. *Pediatr Rev*. 2011;32(7):281–292; and Neinstein LS, ed. *Handbook of Adolescent Healthcare*. Philadelphia, PA: Lippincott Williams & Wilkins; 2009.

Question 3-2

The first sign of puberty in females is typically:
A) Breast development.
B) Development of pubic hair.
C) Menses.
D) Body odor.
E) Acne.

Discussion 3-2

The correct answer is "A." Breast development (thelarche) is typically the first sign of puberty in girls and typically occurs between age 8 and 13 years (see Figure 1–2). Breast development typically precedes pubarche (pubic hair development) though in some girls pubarche may occur first or simultaneously. Pubarche typically occurs 1 to 1.5 years after breast development. Menarche occurs approximately 2.5 years after thelarche at an average age of 12.6 years in Caucasians and earlier in African Americans and Mexican Americans. Girls reach their peak height velocity of 8.25 cm/y earlier than boys at approximately SMR 3. Peak height velocity in girls always precedes menarche. Peak height velocity occurs at approximately SMR 4 to 5 in boys.

Helpful Tip

The first stage of puberty for males is testicular enlargement, defined as a testis volume of 4 mL or greater, or 2.5 cm in diameter. For girls, it is the appearance of breast buds.

QUICK QUIZ

Which of the following is correct?
A) Adrenarche results from testosterone secretion by the gonads.
B) Activation of the hypothalamic-pituitary-gonadal axis (HPA) causes gonadarche and adrenarche.
C) Estrogen secretion causes armpit hair development.
D) All of the above.
E) None of the above.

Discussion

The correct answer is "E." Puberty encompasses gonadarche and adrenarche. Both are separate events, but the timing typically overlaps. Gonadarche, growth and maturation of the gonads (testes, ovaries), is under the control of the HPA secretion of gonadotropin-releasing hormone (GnRH). Before puberty, release of GnRH from the hypothalamus is inhibited. Adrenal androgen secretion (dehydroepiandrosterone [DHEA] and androstenedione) causes pubic and axillary hair development, acne, and body odor (adrenarche).

Helpful Tip

Detection of nocturnal luteinizing hormone (LH) pulses is the first hormonal sign that puberty has started. At puberty, the hypothalamus is no longer inhibited and releases GnRH in a pulsatile fashion. GnRH stimulates the anterior pituitary to secrete gonadotropins—LH first, then follicle-stimulating hormone (FSH). FSH and LH stimulate the gonads to produce gametes (eggs or sperm) and sex hormones (estradiol or testosterone).

Question 3-3

What is the next step in management of this patient?
A) Bone age.
B) Measurement of gonadotropins.
C) Reassurance and follow up in 6 months to a year if no menses.
D) Thyroid studies.
E) CBC.

Discussion 3-3

The correct answer is "C." This patient is progressing through the stages of puberty and will likely attain menarche in the next 6 months to 1 year. If no menses occur by age 16 further workup would be warranted.

Helpful Tip

Don't forget that isolated GnRH deficiency has been associated with both Kallman syndrome and anosmia.

► CASE 4

A mother brings her 17-year-old son for his annual health maintenance exam. When you ask if she has any concerns about him, she mentions that he sleeps all the time. She also states that he was always a happy child but recently has become more withdrawn and always seems tired. She reports that his grades have been declining, and he does not seem to enjoy activities he previously enjoyed, such as playing soccer and video games with friends.

Question 4-1

The next step in diagnosing this patient is:
A) Obtaining a CBC and iron studies.
B) Obtaining a complete psychosocial history from the patient.
C) Thyroid testing.
D) Intelligence testing.
E) Completion of Vanderbilt forms by parents and teachers.

Discussion 4-1

The correct answer is "B." Adolescence is time of rapid growth and development. It can be a stressful time, manifesting as anxiety, withdrawal, aggression, somatic complaints, depression, or poor coping skills such as using drugs. The most common causes of morbidity and mortality in adolescence are related to the risk-taking behavior and experimentation that is a normal part of adolescent development. Obtaining a thorough psychosocial history is important in screening for these risk-taking behaviors and identifying protective factors. The symptoms the mother has described raise concern about depression in this patient. A thorough psychosocial assessment using the HEADSSS screening tool with a follow-up depression screen will likely reveal the cause of his symptoms. How many knew that Vanderbilt scales assess for attention deficit hyperactivity disorder (ADHD)?

Helpful Tip

HEADSSS was developed as a psychosocial screening tool.

H – Home (Who lives with the teen? How does the teen get along with family?)

E – Education (Is the teen in school? How is he or she performing in school? School performance can be an important indication of how a teen is functioning.)

E – Eating (meal consistency; body image)

A – Activities

D – Drugs (alcohol, tobacco, marijuana, and other drug use, including prescription and over-the-counter)

S – Sexuality (Sexual attraction: Are you attracted to males, females, both, neither? Sexual behavior: Have you ever had sex, how many partners, history of sexually transmitted infection diagnosis and testing, condom use, contraceptive use, last sexual activity, history of forced sex?)

S – Suicide/Depression

S – Safety (Does the teen feel safe at home or school? What is his or her exposure to violence?)

Through the HEADDSS assessment you learn that the patient is attracted to males and recently entered a relationship with a boy at school. He wrote a letter to the boy which another student found and shared with the whole class. Since then the patient reports that he is teased by many of his classmates and has been skipping classes to avoid being teased. His depression screen is positive for sadness, anhedonia (no pleasure in activities), excessive sleeping, and feelings of guilt. He denies any thoughts of self-harm or suicidality.

Question 4-2

Adolescents who identify as lesbian, gay, or bisexual are at increased risk for which of the following?
A) Eating disorders.
B) Substance abuse.
C) Depression.
D) Bullying.
E) All of the above.

Discussion 4-2

The correct answer is "E." Sexual development is one part of adolescent development. During *early* adolescence pubertal development is just beginning. At this stage of development adolescents are very focused on changes occurring in their bodies and questioning whether they are normal. Adolescents may begin to experience sexual fantasies and experience sexual pleasure through masturbation. Sexual intercourse at this stage is uncommon, but may occur. Adolescents often experience crushes, which may be same sex or opposite sex. These patterns of attraction may or may not persist into future stages. In *middle* adolescence physical development is nearing completion; at this stage adolescents are forming their sexual orientation and identity. Sexual experimentation is common at this stage and many adolescents may have intercourse for the first time. By *late* adolescence the goal is to become a sexually healthy adult with the ability to form long-lasting relationships. Sexual orientation refers to an individual's pattern of physical and emotional attractions to others and involves complex components such as fantasies and feelings. Personal, family, cultural, developmental, and social factors can affect an individual's ability to identify, accept, and act on his or her attractions. Adolescents who identify as lesbian, gay, or bisexual are at an increased risk for a number of conditions, including eating disorders, substance abuse, and mental health illnesses, particularly depression and anxiety.

The patient has questions about how to stay safe when he does become sexually active with his partner.

Question 4-3

Which of the following is true about sexually transmitted infection (STI) transmission?
A) HIV transmission rates are low with receptive anal intercourse.
B) STIs cannot be transmitted through oral sex.
C) Women who have sex with women are at a low risk for STIs.
D) Condoms are effective at reducing STI transmission.

Discussion 4-3

The correct answer is "D." HIV transmission rates are high with receptive anal intercourse due to microtrauma during intercourse. STIs can be transmitted through oral sex, and it is important to educate patients to use condoms when having oral sex to reduce the risk of contracting an STI. Studies have shown that women who have sex with women are at an increased risk of contracting human papillomavirus (HPV), trichomoniasis, and HIV. Condoms are an effective method of STI prevention and when properly used have been shown to reduce rates of transmission of HIV, gonorrhea, chlamydia, trichomonas, and hepatitis B. They can also be effective at preventing STIs transmitted by skin-to-skin or mucosal contact, such as herpes simplex virus (HSV), syphilis, and HPV, but only if the affected area is covered by the condom. Equally important is making sure adolescents know how to put on a condom. Pregame practice is a good idea.

Question 4-4

You also counsel the patient that the most common cause of mortality in the adolescent population is:
A) Cardiac disease.
B) Unintentional injuries.
C) Suicide.
D) Homicide.
E) Cancer.

Discussion 4-4

The correct answer is "B." The leading cause of death in the adolescent population is unintentional injuries, with motor vehicle collisions being the most frequent cause of such injury in this population. (See Figure 1–4.) Homicide is the second leading cause of death, followed closely by suicide. Organic disease is a less frequent cause of mortality in this age group. Screening for risk factors such as substance use, mental illness, and exposure to violence is important in this population to address the leading causes of mortality. Good driving habits, including no texting while driving, should be discussed.

⏳ QUICK QUIZ

Which of the following is a risk factor for suicide?
A) Bullying.
B) Witnessing violence.
C) Social isolation.
D) Mental illness.
E) All of the above.

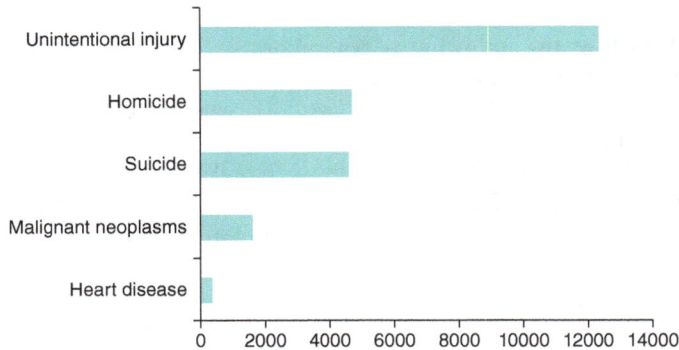

FIGURE 1–4. 2010 Leading causes of death in youth ages 15 to 24 years of age in the United States. (Reproduced with permission from the Centers for Disease Control and Prevention, National Center for Injury Prevention and Control, Web-based Injury Statistics Query and Reporting System (WISQARS). Accessed January 28, 2015 from http://www.cdc.gov/injury/wisqars/.)

Discussion

The correct answer is "E." Additional risk factors include family history of suicide, history of abuse, previous attempt, access to means such as firearms, alcohol and drug use, stressful events, and sexual identification other than heterosexuality.

The patient's mother mentions that she recently caught him smoking pot in the garage with some friends. She is requesting that you drug test him without letting him know.

Question 4-5

Your next step is to:
A) Do as the mother requests.
B) Notify the patient and perform testing regardless of his wishes.
C) Notify the patient and perform the testing if he agrees.
D) Refuse to perform drug testing.
E) Reassure the mother that catching him guarantees he will stop using.

Discussion 4-5

The correct answer is "C." Recreational drug use is an under-recognized cause of morbidity and mortality in adolescents. Indications for drug testing in the acute care setting include acute presentation with altered mental status, suicide attempt, unexplained seizures, syncope, arrhythmias, or the presence of toxidromal signs. In the primary care setting voluntary drug testing can be helpful for assessment, therapy, and monitoring. The American Academy of Pediatrics (AAP) currently cautions against involuntary drug testing of adolescents in nonemergent settings. Testing of competent adolescents without their knowledge is unethical and illegal, and without their consent is impractical. If a pediatrician suspects that a patient is abusing drugs and the patient refuses drug testing, documentation of the refusal and referral to a mental health or addiction specialist may be warranted. Given the limitations of currently available drug tests, a thorough substance abuse history often provides more useful information on drug abuse/use than a drug test.

► CASE 5

A 16-year-old girl and her mother present to your office with concerns about irregular periods. The patient had her first menses at 12 years of age and had regular monthly periods until 6 months ago when her periods stopped. She has had an accompanying 50-pound weight loss over the past 6 months. When asked further about the weight loss, she reports that she has been working on more healthful eating, has cut all desserts and junk foods out of her diet, and eats a low-fat and low-carb diet. In addition she has started running 3 miles a day in order to "get healthy." On physical exam her vital signs are temperature 36.4°C (97.5°F), heart rate 44 beats per minute, blood pressure 96/60 mm Hg, and respirations 16 breaths per minute. She appears thin, with sallow-looking skin and dry hair. She is bradycardic on exam, with no murmurs and a regular rhythm. Her heart rate increases by 19 beats during positional changes from sitting to standing, with minimal change in her blood pressure. Her pulses are strong and symmetric while her fingers and toes are cool to touch.

Question 5-1

Which of the following is the most likely cause of this patient's symptoms?
A) Thyroid disease.
B) Anorexia nervosa.
C) Bulimia nervosa.
D) Diabetes mellitus.
E) Coarctation of the aorta.

Discussion 5-1

The correct answer is "B." Eating disorders are a common but often underdiagnosed condition in the pediatric population. The 12-month prevalence of anorexia nervosa among young females in approximately 0.4%, the prevalence of bulimia nervosa is approximately 1% to 1.5%. Anorexia nervosa has a mortality rate of 5% to 6%, the highest of any psychiatric illness. Patients with anorexia nervosa generally present with rapid weight loss secondary to caloric restriction, which may present as elimination of "junk food" from the diet; avoidance of certain food groups, such as carbohydrates and fats; or changing to a restrictive vegan or vegetarian diet. Patients may also try and reduce weight by over-exercising or purging through self-induced vomiting or use of diuretics and laxatives. In contrast, patients with bulimia nervosa typically present with cycles of binging that trigger purging or inappropriate compensatory behaviors. Compensatory behaviors could include self-induced vomiting, use of diuretics, use of laxatives, fasting, or over-exercising. Patients with bulimia nervosa are typically of normal weight or overweight. Patients with anorexia nervosa often present with signs of malnutrition (eg, bradycardia); hair, skin, and nail changes, often manifesting as dry and brittle hair, nails, and skin; menstrual irregularities (eg, amenorrhea and oligomenorrhea); orthostatic vital sign changes; cold intolerance; acrocyanosis; mood changes; and fatigue. The DSM is revised periodically and eating disorder diagnostic criteria often change. Due to copyright restrictions, we are unable to print the DSM-5 diagnostic criteria for anorexia and bulimia.

TABLE 1–3 COMMON FEATURES OF ANOREXIA NERVOSA

- Restricted eating
- Low body weight for age and sex
- Fear of gaining weight or becoming fat
- Behaviors that interfere with gaining weight
- Disturbance of body image
- Excessive influence of body weight or shape on self-evaluation
- Lack of recognition of the seriousness of low body weight

Summaries of their common features are included in Tables 1–3 and 1–4. But the reader should make themselves familiar with the current DSM criteria for both conditions.

Question 5-2

Which of the following would be a reason for inpatient hospitalization for this patient?
A) Hypertension.
B) Bradycardia.
C) Hypokalemia.
D) Rapid weight loss.
E) Amenorrhea.

Discussion 5-2

The correct answer is "B." The AAP suggests that the following signs and symptoms warrant inpatient hospitalization:

For anorexia nervosa:

- Bradycardia (<45 bpm daytime or <45 bpm nighttime)
- Hypotension (<90 mmHg systolic)
- Arrhythmia
- Hypothermia
- Weight <75% ideal body weight
- Body Fat < 10%
- Refusal to eat
- Failure of outpatient treatment

TABLE 1–4 COMMON FEATURES OF BULIMIA NERVOSA (MUST BE PRESENT AT LEAST ONCE A WEEK FOR 3 MONTHS)

- Eating a large amount of food over a short amount of time
- Lack of control during the episode—feels as though one cannot stop eating
- Behaviors to compensate for episodes of binge eating.
- Excessive influence of body weight or shape on self-evaluation
- Diagnosis is not better explained by a diagnosis of anorexia nervosa

For bulimia nervosa:

- Syncope
- Hypokalemia
- Severe hypochloremia (<88 mmol/L)
- Esophageal tears
- Arrhythmia
- Hypothermia
- Suicidality
- Intractable vomiting
- Hematemesis
- Failure of outpatient treatment

This patient warrants inpatient treatment due to her bradycardia. Note that the AAP endorses electrolyte abnormalities as admission criteria for bulimia, but not anorexia. In reality, a patient with anorexia and severe electrolyte abnormalities would also likely be admitted to the hospital. Also of interest is that hypothermia is defined for one but not both disorders. The goal in hospital admission is medical stabilization, which is usually achieved through nutritional rehabilitation and correction of any underlying electrolyte abnormalities. Fluid and electrolyte shifts can occur with the reintroduction of nutrition in a patient who has been malnourished. This is called *refeeding syndrome* and most typically manifests as decrease in phosphate, magnesium, and potassium, as well as an increase in extracellular volume causing peripheral edema or congestive heart failure, or both. These fluid and electrolyte shifts can lead to cardiac arrhythmias; thus monitoring of cardiac status, electrolytes, and fluid status is important in the inpatient setting.

Question 5-3

Which of the following will likely NOT be a part of this patient's treatment?
A) Nutritional rehabilitation.
B) Psychotherapy.
C) Medical monitoring for complications of illness.
D) Use of an appetite stimulant.
E) Family therapy.

Discussion 5-3

The correct answer is "D." Treatment of eating disorders is multidisciplinary and includes medical monitoring for complications of the illness such as refeeding syndrome; psychotherapy to address eating disorder thoughts and body image concerns; and nutritional rehabilitation, which involves reintroducing meals and snacks in a stepwise fashion with a goal of restoring body weight. The use of appetite stimulants is not recommended as this does not address the disordered thoughts and behaviors that are a part of the eating disorder. Treatment goals include medical stabilization; nutritional rehabilitation as measured by restoration of body weight, usually at a rate of 0.25 to 1 kg per week in the outpatient setting; decrease in eating disorder thoughts and behaviors; and improvement in body image. Healthy family involvement is always good.

> **Helpful Tip**
>
> Anorexic patients are at risk for refeeding syndrome. Hypophosphatemia is the hallmark and the primary culprit of refeeding syndrome.

Question 5-4

Which of the following laboratory findings would NOT be expected in a patient with anorexia nervosa?

A) Hyperkalemia.
B) Leukopenia.
C) Normal laboratory results.
D) Hypoglycemia.
E) Elevated liver enzymes.

Discussion 5-4

The correct answer is "A." Most patients with eating disorders have normal laboratory findings. General laboratory workup includes a CBC with white blood cell count differential; full chemistry panel, including liver and renal studies; thyroid studies; nutritional markers, such as vitamin D and prealbumin; and coagulation studies. Don't forget an ECG. Technically it isn't a lab test but we needed to include it somewhere! Additional testing may be indicated to exclude alternative diagnoses. Common laboratory abnormalities that may be seen in patients with anorexia include *hypokalemia* (not hyperkalemia) and hypochloremic metabolic alkalosis secondary to purging. Hypoglycemia can be seen secondary to malnutrition. Hyponatremia may be seen as a sign of water-loading or excessive water intake. Leukopenia can be seen, and in severe cases pancytopenia. Mild elevation of liver enzymes can also be seen secondary to malnutrition.

QUICK QUIZ

What is NOT a complication of anorexia nervosa?

A) Diarrhea.
B) Gastroparesis.
C) Osteopenia.
D) Brain atrophy.
E) Pericardial effusion.

Discussion

The correct answer is "A." Anorexia causes constipation, not diarrhea (unless the patient is taking laxatives).

▶ CASE 6

A 16-year-old Caucasian girl comes to the adolescent clinic for the first time because she has never had a menstrual period. She is a runner on her school's cross-country team and recently was diagnosed with a stress fracture. Although she has had to sit out practice and competitions for the past few weeks, she has kept active by riding a stationary bike and swimming. She is otherwise healthy and takes no medication. The patient's breast development began at about 12 years of age and pubic hair 2 years ago. Her brother has insulin-dependent diabetes mellitus and her mother has hypertension. The mother states that her own menses started at 14 years of age. The patient is a sophomore in high school and is getting straight A's. She has a boyfriend but denies sexual activity. She denies all substance use. Review of systems is negative for headaches, nausea, vomiting, abdominal pain, constipation, diarrhea, or vaginal discharge. On physical exam she is 5 feet, 6 inches tall and weighs 110 pounds, with a heart rate of 56 bpm and a blood pressure of 110/70 mm Hg. She is SMR 3 for breasts and pubic hair. The rest of her exam is normal.

Question 6-1

The definition of primary amenorrhea includes absence of menses by what age, assuming normal secondary sexual development?

A) 12 years.
B) 14 years.
C) 16 years.
D) 18 years.

Discussion 6-1

The correct answer is "C." Primary amenorrhea refers to the absence of menses (1) by age 16 years with normal secondary sexual development; (2) by age 14 years in the absence of any breast maturation; or (3) despite having attained SMR 5 for 1 year or more, or despite the onset of thelarche 4 years previously. Focus on remembering the first and second criteria.

Question 6-2

The most likely cause of primary amenorrhea in this patient is:

A) Hypothalamic amenorrhea.
B) Hypothyroidism.
C) Hyperprolactinemia.
D) Hypopituitarism.
E) Imperforate hymen.

Discussion 6-2

The correct answer is "A." Causes of primary amenorrhea include conditions resulting from central dysfunction (hypothalamic or pituitary), ovarian dysfunction, or anatomic abnormalities of the genital tract. Given this patient's clinical presentation, the most likely diagnosis would be functional hypothalamic amenorrhea, due to partial or complete inhibition of GnRH release. This inhibition can be due to nutritional deficiencies, cystic fibrosis, eating disorders, excessive exercise, stress, or severe or prolonged illness. Excessive exercise is to blame in this teenage girl. She has developed a stress fracture from excessive running. Signs and symptoms of hypothyroidism include constipation, dry skin, weight gain, and increased sensitivity to cold. When hypothyroidism is present in children and teens, one may also see delayed puberty and poor growth, resulting in short stature. Hyperprolactinemia is usually due to a prolactin-secreting adenoma that also may cause headaches, visual changes (bitemporal hemianopsia), and galactorrhea. Hyperprolactinemia can also be caused by physiologic hypersecretion of prolactin (pregnancy), hypothalamic-pituitary stalk damage, certain systemic disorders, or drug-induced hypersecretion (eg, risperidone). With hypopituitarism, the pituitary gland fails to produce or does not produce enough of one or more of its hormones, and multiple body functions can be affected. If the complaint relates to menstruation, always make sure everything is anatomically correct. Young women need "girl parts" to have periods and an open outflow path (eg, no imperforate hymen).

Question 6-3

If this patient lacked breast development, which of the following would be included in the diagnosis?
A) Agenesis of müllerian structures.
B) Complete androgen insensitivity syndrome.
C) Asherman syndrome.
D) Pure gonadal dysgenesis (46,XX with streak gonads).

Discussion 6-3

The correct answer is "D." With pure gonadal dysgenesis, the streak gonads are unable to produce sex hormones. In a female with pure gonadal dysgenesis, the ovaries do not produce estrogen, resulting in absence of breast development. Agenesis of müllerian structures impacts the formation of the internal reproductive tract (uterus, fallopian tubes, and upper third of the vagina), not the ovaries, and has no effect on breast development. Individuals with complete androgen insensitivity syndrome are resistant to testosterone due to defective androgen receptors. They do not develop testosterone-dependent male sexual characteristics, and the testosterone produced by the testes is aromatized into estrogen, leading to phenotypically female appearance with normal breast development. Their genotype is male (46,XY) but their external genitalia look female. Internal female structures such as a uterus are not present as the testes make müllerian-inhibiting substance. Asherman syndrome occurs when uterine synechiae or adhesions obstruct or obliterate the uterine cavity, leading to amenorrhea. Adhesions may develop after uterine infection or other disruption. Breast development is not affected.

⏳ QUICK QUIZ

Which of the following clinical characteristics would NOT be seen in a patient with complete androgen insensitivity syndrome?
A) Absent menses.
B) Normal breast development.
C) Tanner 3 pubic hair.
D) Normal linear growth.

Discussion

The correct answer is "C." Patients with complete androgen insensitivity syndrome are (46,XY) and have a defect in androgen receptors. Thus they do not develop testosterone-dependent male sexual characteristics, such as pubic and axillary hair.

Question 6-4

What tests should you order to assess primary amenorrhea in this patient in order to confirm your diagnosis?
A) Pregnancy test.
B) Follicle-stimulating hormone (FSH) and luteinizing hormone (LH).
C) Prolactin.
D) Thyroid-stimulating hormone (TSH).
E) All of the above.

Discussion 6-4

The correct answer is "E." Pregnancy should always be excluded, even in patients who deny sexual activity. It is useful to obtain FSH and LH levels to differentiate between hypothalamic (low or normal LH and FSH) and ovarian insufficiency (elevated LH and FSH). A prolactin level would confirm the presence of a pituitary microadenoma, which might (or might not) also cause headache, galactorrhea, and bitemporal hemianopsia (decreased vision in the outer half). TSH level is used to diagnose thyroid abnormalities, which may impact menses. Even though you suspect hypothalamic amenorrhea (suppression from excessive exercise), you should rule out both hyperprolactinemia and thyroid abnormalities.

Question 6-5

Which of the following would make Turner syndrome an unlikely diagnosis in a patient with amenorrhea?
A) Short stature.
B) Hypogonadotropic hypogonadism.
C) Hypergonadotropic hypogonadism.
D) Webbed neck.
E) Widely spaced nipples.

Discussion 6-5

The correct answer is "B." Tuner syndrome (45,XO) is the most common cause of primary gonadal failure (primary hypogonadism) in adolescent girls and is characterized by ovarian dysgenesis (accelerated stromal fibrosis and decreased or absent oocyte production), short stature, and a wide variety of phenotypical abnormalities (widely spaced nipples, webbed neck, coarctation of the aorta, lymphedema), and elevated gonadotropins. The hypothalamus and pituitary function normally but the ovary does not, so FSH and LH are elevated. Most women with Turner syndrome do not develop breasts or have periods (primary amenorrhea) but some develop normally with secondary amenorrhea as their presenting symptom. Short stature is a big clue.

Helpful Tip

To differentiate between primary and secondary hypogonadism, use FSH and LH to guide your thinking. In *hypo*gonadotropic hypogonadism, the problem is central (hypothalamus or pituitary, or both) and FSH and LH levels will be low or normal. In *hyper*gonadotropic hypogonadism, the problem is the gonads (testes or ovaries) and FSH and LH will be elevated.

You decide to proceed with a progesterone challenge in your patient, which does NOT result in a withdrawal bleed.

Question 6-6

Which of the following are possible causes for failure of a progesterone challenge?
A) Elevated estrogen level.
B) Ovarian cyst.
C) Transverse vaginal septum.
D) Septate hymen.
E) Bicornate uterus.

Discussion 6-6

The correct answer is "C." A progesterone challenge helps determines the level of endogenous estrogen and confirm the patency of the outflow tract. If no bleeding occurs after a progesterone challenge, either the anatomy is disrupted (imperforate hymen, vaginal atresia, vaginal septum, müllerian agenesis, absent uterus) or there is not enough circulating estrogen. Estrogen stimulates buildup of the uterine lining, which is shed in the progesterone challenge. A transverse vaginal septum is a thin horizontal membrane in the vagina that may cause obstruction. A septate hymen has an extra band of tissue in the middle that causes two vaginal openings but not obstruction. A bicornate uterus is just shaped funny.

▶ CASE 7

A 17-year-old girl presents to the adolescent clinic complaining of irregular periods for the past 6 months. Menarche was at 11 years of age. Menses have been regular, coming every month and lasting 5 days for the past 4 years until 6 months ago. In the past 6 months, she has had only 2 periods, the last one was 2 weeks ago and lasted 10 days. She has gained 25 pounds in the past year (current BMI is 33 kg/m²). She has noticed increasing acne and dark, velvety skin in her neck and axilla. She is sexually active with boyfriend of 1 year and uses condoms consistently. The last sexual activity was about 3 weeks ago.

Question 7-1

Which of the following qualifies as dysfunctional uterine bleeding?
A) Menstrual cycles occurring 19 days apart.
B) Menstrual cycles occurring 35 days apart.

C) Menstrual cycles lasting 7 days.
D) Menstrual cycles resulting in blood loss of 60 mL.

Discussion 7-1

The correct answer is "A." Dysfunctional uterine bleeding (DUB), also known as *anovulatory abnormal uterine bleeding*, is defined as menstrual cycles occurring less than 20 days or more than 45 days apart, and lasting longer than 8 days, or menstrual cycles resulting in blood loss of greater than 80 mL. DUB is characterized as (1) oligomenorrhea—too few periods (> 45 days apart), (2) polymenorrhea—too many periods (< 20 days apart), (3) metrorrhagia—too-frequent bleeding irregularly or between periods, (4) menorrhagia—too-heavy blood loss (> 80 mL or lasting > 7 days), and (5) menometrorrhagia—too-frequent and heavy blood loss. Anovulation is a common cause of DUB in adolescents. Without ovulation, progesterone secretion is disrupted, resulting in estrogen-induced overgrowth of the endometrial lining. The thickened lining outgrows it blood supply and then is shed irregularly.

Helpful Tip

Anovulatory cycles are common in early menstrual cycles and are characterized by large variations in estrogen levels and lack of progesterone. During the first 2 years following menarche, anovulation is associated with 50% to 80% of bleeding episodes. Two to 4 years after menarche, anovulation is associated with 30% to 55% of bleeding episodes. Four to 5 years after menarche, 20% of bleeding episodes are anovulatory.

Helpful Tip

The female athlete triad includes osteoporosis, amenorrhea, and disorders of nutritional intake.

A urine pregnancy test was negative. Based on the clinical picture, you suspect polycystic ovary syndrome (PCOS).

Question 7-2

What test should you order to help confirm the diagnosis?
A) CBC.
B) Estradiol level.
C) Total and free testosterone.
D) FSH level.
E) Ovarian ultrasound.

Discussion 7-2

The correct answer is "C." Obesity, acanthosis nigricans (see Figure 1–5), and menstrual irregularities suggest PCOS. There are several diagnostic criteria for PCOS. Essentially, there needs to be evidence of ovulatory dysfunction and clinical or biochemical

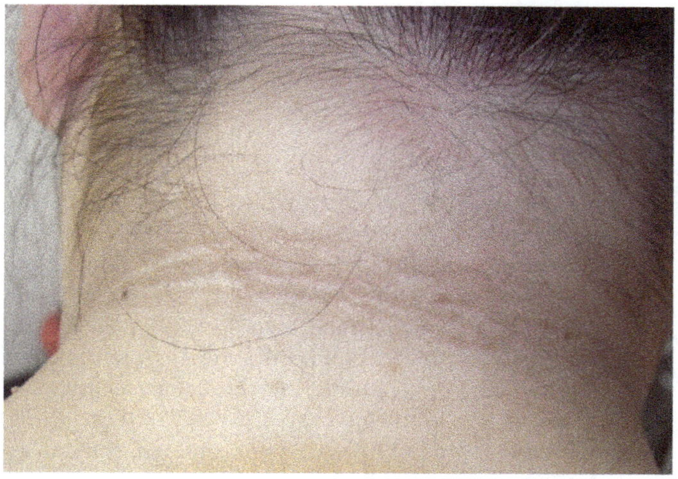

FIGURE 1–5. Acanthosis nigricans on the back of the neck. (Reproduced with permission from Hoffman BL, Schorge JO, Schaffer JI, Halvorson LM, Bradshaw KD, Cunningham FG, Calver LE, eds. *William's Gynecology*. 2nd ed. New York, NY: McGraw-Hill Education, Inc., 2012; Fig. 17–6.)

signs of androgen excess. Ultrasound evidence of polycystic ovaries is suggestive but not required for the diagnosis. Women with PCOS often have an increased level of both total testosterone and free testosterone. FSH level will not be helpful on its own; however, in combination with LH level it may be helpful as half of patients with PCOS have an LH:FSH ratio of 2.5:1. Most women with PCOS have normal estradiol levels.

Question 7-3

Additional laboratory studies that should be ordered in patients with PCOS include:
A) Glucose.
B) Lipid panel.
C) Insulin.
D) Glucose tolerance test.
E) All of the above.

Discussion 7-3

The correct answer is "D." PCOS patients are at higher risk for impaired glucose tolerance and insulin resistance, as well as metabolic syndrome, which is a group of cardiovascular risk factors that include dyslipidemia, type 2 diabetes mellitus, hypertension, and obesity.

Question 7-4

The type of cancer that people with PCOS are at risk for includes:
A) Endometrial cancer.
B) Ovarian cancer.
C) Breast cancer.
D) Cervical cancer.
E) None of the above.

Discussion 7-4

The correct answer is "A." Women with PCOS have an increased risk of developing endometrial cancer. A major factor for this increased malignancy risk is the prolonged exposure of the endometrium to unopposed estrogen that results from anovulation. Women with PCOS are not at increased risk of ovarian, breast, or cervical cancer.

Question 7-5

Other conditions that may show evidence of excess androgen include:
A) Adrenal tumor.
B) Late-onset congenital adrenal hyperplasia.
C) Anabolic steroid use.
D) All of the above.

Discussion 7-5

The correct answer is "D." Adrenal tumors can manifest as virilization and can be diagnosed by means of an elevated dehydroepiandrosterone sulfate (DHEA-S) level. Late-onset congenital adrenal hyperplasia may become apparent during mid-childhood and can lead to early pubic hair, accelerated bone age, hirsutism, and possible mild clitoral enlargement. This can be diagnosed based on elevated serum 17-hydroxyprogesterone. Anabolic steroids have effects similar to testosterone in the body.

⧗ QUICK QUIZ

Which is a clinical feature of PCOS?
A) Acanthosis nigricans.
B) Hirsutism.
C) Acne.
D) Obesity.
E) All of the above.

Discussion

The correct answer is "E." Obesity, menstrual irregularities, and infertility are common. Hirsutism, male pattern alopecia, and acne result from androgen excess. Acanthosis nigricans, as seen in the patient in this case, is a manifestation of insulin resistance.

▶ CASE 8

The mother of a 14-year-old girl calls the clinic stating that her daughter's first period began 2 weeks ago and she continues to bleed heavily. Her daughter is complaining of feeling increasingly tired. Review of the girl's chart shows that the 14-year-old was previously healthy. She has never had any surgical procedures. The family history indicates that both the mother and maternal grandmother had hysterectomies in their 30s due to heavy menstrual bleeding. You tell the mother to bring her daughter to the clinic. At arrival, the girl's vital signs are heart rate of 120 bpm and blood pressure of 100/70 mm Hg. On exam, her skin is pale and vaginal exam shows active bleeding from the cervix.

Question 8-1

Which of the following conditions would be an unlikely cause of abnormal vaginal bleeding in this patient?

A) Endometrial cancer.
B) Pregnancy-related condition.
C) Sexually transmitted infections.
D) Anovulatory cycle.
E) Bleeding disorder.

Discussion 8-1

The correct answer is "A." Most cases of abnormal vaginal bleeding in adolescence are secondary to dysfunctional uterine bleeding from anovulatory cycles. Genital cancers are very rare in young adolescents. The differential diagnosis includes:

- Pregnancy-related conditions (intrauterine or ectopic pregnancy, spontaneous abortion, and molar-trophoblastic disease)
- Infections (vaginitis, cervicitis, endometritis, salpingitis, and pelvic inflammatory disease)
- Other gynecologic conditions (ovarian cyst, genital cancers, breakthrough bleeding associated with contraceptive use, ovulation bleeding, polyps, endometriosis)
- Systemic disease (renal and liver failure)
- Bleeding disorders
- Direct trauma and foreign body
- Medications (anticoagulants and platelet inhibitors)

Question 8-2

The following tests should be included in the workup of this patient:

A) Pregnancy test.
B) Hemoglobin/hematocrit.
C) Coagulation studies.
D) Nucleic acid amplification testing (NAAT) for gonorrhea and chlamydia.
E) All of the above.

Discussion 8-2

The correct answer is "E." A pregnancy test is essential to exclude complications of pregnancy. Hemoglobin and hematocrit values will help determine the magnitude of bleeding. Coagulation studies may reveal coagulopathies or blood dyscrasias, particularly in this case of heavy bleeding since onset of menarche and a family history of abnormal vaginal bleeding. STIs such as gonorrhea and chlamydia are common causes of prolonged or irregular vaginal bleeding. Other causes to consider include endocrine abnormalities such as hypothyroidism.

The pregnancy test was negative. Her hemoglobin is 8.5 g/dL.

Question 8-3

What is the next appropriate step?

A) Reassurance.
B) Start a multivitamin with iron.
C) Start a combined oral contraceptive pill daily.
D) Admit to hospital for higher doses of estrogen and possible blood transfusion.
E) Uterine dilational and curettage.

Discussion 8-3

The correct answer is "D." Treatment of abnormal uterine bleeding depends on the severity of the bleeding, hemoglobin level, and degree of associated hemodynamic changes. Mild cases associated with a hemoglobin level of 12g/dL or higher require only reassurance, a multivitamin with iron, and close follow up. Individuals with a hemoglobin level of 10 to 12 g/dL should take a combined oral contraceptive pill (OCP) every 6 to 12 hours for 24 to 48 hours until the bleeding stops, taper to one pill per day, and then continue daily OCPs for 3 to 6 months. Patients with a hemoglobin level of less than 10 g/dL may require hospitalization and initial treatment of higher doses of estrogen if hemodynamically unstable. This patient has anemia and is subsequently tachycardic. She needs aggressive management.

Question 8-4

The most common inherited bleeding disorder, which often presents as menorrhagia in adolescent females is:

A) Factor VIII deficiency.
B) Factor IX deficiency.
C) von Willebrand disease.
D) Protein C deficiency.
E) Antiphospholipid syndrome.

Discussion 8-4

The correct answer is "C." The most common inherited bleeding disorder in the United States population is von Willebrand disease, with an estimated prevalence of 1% to 2%. The prevalence of von Willebrand disease rises in studies involving women with menorrhagia, with estimates ranging as high as 10% to 20% in Caucasian women, and 1% to 2% among African American women. Von Willebrand factor helps with formation of the initial blood clot (binds platelets and factor VIII). Other bleeding disorders seen in adolescents with menorrhagia are disorders of inherited platelet dysfunction, clotting factor deficiencies, thrombocytopenia, and disorders of the fibrinolytic pathway. People with antiphospholipid syndrome and protein C and S deficiencies are at increased risk for thromboembolism, not menorrhagia.

▶ **CASE 9**

A 16-year-old girl comes to your clinic requesting birth control. She just started having sexual intercourse with her boyfriend of 1 year. They have used condoms with each episode of vaginal intercourse. Menarche was at 12 years of age. Menses occurs every month, lasts for 5 days, and is associated with mild cramps. Her past medical history consists of well-controlled absence seizures diagnosed at 16 years of age for which she takes a medication. She had an appendectomy in the past year; imaging during the diagnostic evaluation showed a left ovarian cyst measuring 1.6 × 2 × 1.8 cm. Her mother takes medication for high blood pressure and her father has high cholesterol.

Question 9-1

Which of the following contraceptive options has the lowest failure rate during typical use in adolescence?
A) Male condom.
B) Combined OCPs.
C) Implantable etonogestrel rod.
D) Injectable depo-medroxyprogesterone.
E) Progestin-only pills.

Discussion 9-1

The correct answer is "C." See Table 1–5 for failure rates of different methods of contraception. With so many choices, why aren't all sexually active adolescents using contraception and STI protection? Perhaps the adolescent has difficulty planning ahead, fails to recognize potential consequences, lives in the moment, fears a pelvic exam or side effects, or has concerns over confidentiality.

TABLE 1–5 FAILURE RATES WITH PERFECT USE AND TYPICAL USE OF DIFFERENT CONTRACEPTIVE METHODS

Contraceptive	Failure Rate	
	With Perfect Use (%)	With Typical Use (%)
Withdrawal method	4	22
Rhythm method/ periodic abstinence	5	24
Male condom	2	18
Female condom	5	21
Combined OCPs	0.3	9
Combined transdermal patch	0.3	8
Combined vaginal ring	0.3	8
Progestin-only pill	0.3	9
Injectable DMPA	0.2	6
Implantable etonogestrel rod	0.05	0.05
Levonorgestrel IUD	0.2	0.2
Copper IUD	0.6	0.8

DMPA, depot medroxyprogesterone acetate; IUD, intrauterine device; OCP, oral contraceptive pill.

Data from Hatcher RA, Trussell J, Nelson AL, et al. *Contraceptive Technology*. 20th rev ed. New York, NY: Ardent Media; 2011.

Question 9-2

Combined OCPs can safely be used by an adolescent with any of the following conditions EXCEPT:
A) Migraine with aura.
B) Blood pressure of 135/80 mm Hg.
C) Hypothyroidism.
D) History of ovarian torsion.
E) Asthma.

Discussion 8-2

The correct answer is "A." According to the Centers for Disease Control and Prevention's (CDC) US Medical Eligibility Criteria for Contraceptive Use, absolute (level 4) contraindications to combined OCP use include current breast cancer or estrogen-dependent tumor, thromboembolic disease or high risk for thromboembolism (thrombogenic mutation, antiphospholipid antibody), migraine with aura, blood pressure of 160/100 mm Hg or higher, cardiovascular disease, liver disease, and cerebrovascular events.

⧗ QUICK QUIZ

Which is a noncontraceptive benefit of estrogen–progestin–containing birth control?
A) Increased risk of ovarian cancer.
B) Increased acne.
C) Worsening menstrual cramps.
D) Decreased bone density.
E) Prevents menstrual migraines without aura.

Discussion

The correct answer is "E". Combined hormone–containing pills, patch, and vaginal ring improve bone density and decrease (1) risk of ovarian and endometrial cancer; (2) menstrual cycle disorders, including menorrhagia and dysmenorrhea; (3) acne; and (4) pelvic pain from endometriosis.

Question 9-3

Which of the following antibiotics interferes with the contraceptive effectiveness of the OCP?
A) Amoxicillin.
B) Rifampin.
C) Cephalosporin.
D) Sulfonamides.

Discussion 9-3

The correct answer is "B." Rifampin is the only antibiotic proven to decrease the contraceptive effectiveness of the pill. Amoxicillin, cephalosporins, and sulfonamides do not affect birth control effectiveness. Griseofulvin, an antifungal medication used to treat tinea infections, also speeds up metabolism of OCPs, decreasing their effectiveness.

Question 9-4

Which of the following antiseizure medications decreases the contraceptive effectiveness of the OCP?
A) Gabapentin.
B) Phenobarbital.
C) Valproate.
D) Levetiracetam.
E) All of the above.

Discussion 9-4

The correct answer is "B." Antiepileptics that induce the cytochrome P450 system (increasing metabolism), and therefore make the birth control pill less effective, include carbamazepine, felbamate, phenobarbital, phenytoin, primidone, and topiramate. Lamotrigine clearance is increased in presence of estrogen-containing birth control options, meaning the effectiveness of the seizure medication is decreased.

Your patient does not think she would remember to take a birth control pill every day and would like to hear about the other options.

Question 9-5

Which of the following correctly matches the contraceptive with its duration of action?
A) Transdermal patch; 3 weeks.
B) Vaginal ring; 3 months.
C) Levonorgestrel intrauterine device (IUD); 10 years.
D) Copper IUD; 10 years.
E) None of the above.

Discussion 8-5

The correct answer is "D." The birth control patch needs to be changed weekly. The birth control ring is typically replaced after 3 weeks. There are two different levonorgestrel IUDs; one lasts for 3 years and the other for 5 years. The copper IUD is replaced every 10 years.

She returns 6 months later and tells you that she is pregnant.

Question 9-6

Which of the following would put her at higher risk for an ectopic pregnancy?
A) Prior episode of pelvic inflammatory disease.
B) History of OCP use.
C) History of labial adhesions requiring estrogen cream.
D) Frequent yeast infections.
E) All of the above.

Discussion 9-6

The correct answer is "A." Risk factors for ectopic pregnancies include previous ectopic pregnancy; infection of the uterus, fallopian tubes, or ovaries (pelvic inflammatory disease); pregnancy when an IUD is in place; or pregnancy after tubal ligation.

She hasn't told anyone about her pregnancy. Upon further questioning, she discloses that she was sexually assaulted by a classmate while at a party 3 months ago. She has not told anyone about the assault and still sees the person who assaulted her at school. She does not want to report the incidence because she doesn't want her boyfriend to know that he may not be the father of her child.

Question 9-7

Legally, you:
A) Agree to her wishes to not disclose the assault.
B) Arrange for her boyfriend to undergo paternity testing.
C) Inform her that it is your legal obligation to report the assault to the authorities because she is a minor.
D) Inform her that you are going to tell her parents.

Discussion 9-7

The correct answer is "C." All sexual assaults involving a minor must be reported to authorities, even if the minor does not want the assault disclosed.

⏳ QUICK QUIZ

True or false: Pregnancy related risks in adolescents are age dependent.
A) True.
B) False.

Discussion

The correct answer is "A." Younger adolescents are at increased risk for pregnancy complications, including poor weight gain, anemia, pregnancy-induced hypertension, and poor prenatal care; are less likely to finish high school; and are more likely to be single parents. They may lack the maturity to care for an infant. Infants of adolescent mothers are at increased risk for prematurity and low birth weight. Pregnant adolescents are more likely to live in poverty, not finish high school and require governmental assistance. Care should be multidisciplinary, involve community resources, stress the importance of school, and provide positive reinforcement for successes.

▶ CASE 10

A 16-year-old girl presents to clinic with dysuria and vaginal discharge. She has had four sexual partners in her lifetime: three male and one female. She started having sex at 12 years of age. The pH of the vaginal discharge obtained during saline mount (wet prep) collection is 7.

Question 10-1

Which of the following is an unlikely cause of the vaginal discharge?
A) Bacterial vaginosis.
B) Trichomoniasis.

C) Vaginal candidiasis.
D) *Gardnerella vaginalis*.
E) None of the above.

Discussion 10-1

The correct answer is "C." The pH for yeast infection is less than 4.5 (acidic), and budding yeast or pseudohyphae can be seen on KOH prep. The pH for bacterial vaginosis (caused by *Gardnerella vaginalis*) and trichomoniasis is greater than 4.5.

On speculum exam, you see a red and friable cervix and white, frothy discharge in the cul-de-sac.

Question 10-2

On the wet mount, you are likely to find:
A) Trichomonads.
B) Budding yeast.
C) Pseudohyphae.
D) Clue cells.
E) No-clue cells.

Discussion 10-2

The correct answer is "A." The clinical appearance of the discharge provides important clues to the diagnosis. Gray, frothy discharge is consistent with trichomoniasis (along with the appearance of the red, friable cervix, or "strawberry cervix"). The discharge associated with yeast infections is usually described as thick and curdlike, and adheres to vaginal walls. The discharge associated with BV is usually described as thin, grayish, and foul smelling. With BV, clue cells are present on wet prep and the whiff test is positive. No one likes a fishy odor. If you chose option "E," it suggests that you were clueless about this question.

Question 10-3

What additional diagnostic tests should you order?
A) Urine pregnancy test.
B) NAAT for gonorrhea.
C) NAAT for chlamydia.
D) HIV.
E) All of the above.

Discussion 10-3

The correct answer is "E." The patient admits to having unprotected sex and already has been diagnosed with one STI (trichomonas). She is at risk for other infections as well as pregnancy. The CDC's STI screening guidelines for sexually active adolescents include (1) annual *Chlamydia trachomatis* screening for all females younger than 25 years old, (2) *C. trachomatis* screening of males in certain settings, and (3) annual *Neisseria gonorrhoeae* screening in all at-risk females. HIV screening should be discussed and encouraged for sexually active adolescents and those who use injection drugs. Screening for certain STIs in asymptomatic adolescents (eg, syphilis, trichomoniasis, hepatitis B) is not recommended.

QUICK QUIZ

Which is NOT an indication for a pelvic exam?
A) Amenorrhea.
B) Pregnancy.
C) Yearly checkup.
D) Persistent vaginal discharge.
E) Dysuria in a sexually active female.

Discussion

The correct answer is "C". The guidelines for Papanicolaou (Pap) testing have changed and noninvasive STI testing is available, so fewer adolescents need pelvic exams. (See Table 1–6.) A Pap smear and pelvic exam are no longer required at the onset of sexual activity or before prescribing birth control. Current guidelines recommend performing the first Pap test at age 21 years, with these exceptions: (1) immunocompromised (includes HIV) adolescents need annual tests once sexually active, and (2) adolescents who have already been found to have cervical intraepithelial neoplasia (CIN) 2 or 3 or carcinoma need periodic screening and, in the case of CIN 3, treatment.

> **Helpful Tip**
> Consider acute retroviral syndrome in any sexually active adolescent with nonspecific viral symptoms, including fever, malaise, lymphadenopathy, and skin rash. The syndrome occurs in the first few weeks of infection, before antibody testing is confirmed as positive. The test to order for acute retroviral syndrome is an HIV PCR-DNA or HIV plasma RNA. Acutely infected patients are highly contagious during this stage.

The patient does not want her parents to know that she is being tested for STIs.

TABLE 1–6 INDICATIONS FOR PELVIC EXAMINATION

Persistent vaginal discharge	Sexually active with dysuria or urinary tract symptoms
Dysmenorrhea not helped by NSAIDs	Amenorrhea
Abnormal vaginal bleeding	Lower abdominal pain
IUD or diaphragm contraceptive counseling	Perform Pap test
Suspected or reported /rape or sexual abuse	Pregnancy

IUD, intrauterine device; NSAID, nonsteroidal anti-inflammatory drug.

Question 10-4

You tell her:
A) Minors can consent to STI testing without parental notification.
B) Minors require parent or guardian consent for STI testing.
C) Minors can consent to STI testing but parents must be notified.
D) None of the above.

Discussion 10-4

The correct answer is "A." All 50 states and the District of Columbia allow minors to consent to STI services without parental notification. Eighteen states allow, but do not require, a physician to inform a minor's parents that he or she is seeking or receiving STI services when the physician deems it in the minor's best interests. A key consideration is that you can't control what is on the insurance claims.

The patient wants to know what type of complications could occur if she was exposed to gonorrhea.

Question 10-5

You explain that gonorrhea can cause all of the following EXCEPT:
A) Rash.
B) Arthritis.
C) Pelvic inflammatory disease.
D) Painless ulcer.
E) Perihepatitis.

Discussion 10-5

The correct answer is "D." Gonorrhea infection can cause mucopurulent cervicitis, intermenstrual bleeding, and pelvic inflammatory disease. Disseminated gonococcal infection occurs in 1% to 3% of individuals with gonorrhea. It can present as petechial or pustular skin lesion, tenosynovitis, septic arthritis, and perihepatitis (Fitz-Hugh-Curtis syndrome). A painless ulcer is indicative of primary syphilis (chancre), granuloma inguinale, or lymphogranuloma venereum.

The patient's boyfriend has a history of chlamydia, which was picked up on routine screening.

Question 10-6

What is the treatment of chlamydial infections in men?
A) Azithromycin.
B) Ceftriaxone.
C) Penicillin.
D) Metronidazole.
E) Fluconazole.

Discussion 10-6

The correct answer is "A." The preferred treatment of chlamydia consists of a single 1 g oral dose of azithromycin or a 1-week course of doxycycline (100 mg twice daily). Those who test positive for chlamydia or gonorrhea should have a test of cure

3 months after treatment. Reinfection rates are high, especially if partners are not treated.

> **Helpful Tip**
> Empiric antibiotic prophylaxis after possible STI exposure includes ceftriaxone (250 mg intramuscular injection) for gonorrhea, azithromycin (1 g orally) or doxycycline (100 mg twice daily for 7 days) for chlamydia, and metronidazole (2 g orally) for trichomoniasis.

The patient is seen in the emergency department 2 months later with a 3-day history of fever and abdominal pain, but no dysuria, vomiting, or diarrhea. She states that a new vaginal discharge developed 1 week ago. She continues to be sexually active with sporadic use of condoms and has had one new male sexual partner. Her last episode of unprotected sex was 2 weeks ago. On exam, she is febrile to 38.5°C (101.3°F) and has pain and rebound tenderness in the left lower quadrant. On pelvic exam, her SMR is 5 with normal external genitalia. On speculum exam, there is discharge coming from the cervical os. On bimanual exam, cervical motion tenderness and fullness of the left adnexa are present.

Question 10-7

Which is NOT a diagnostic criterion for her acute condition?
A) Uterine tenderness.
B) Adnexal tenderness.
C) Lower abdominal pain.
D) History of sexual activity.
E) Positive result for *Neisseria gonorrhoeae*.

Discussion 10-7

The correct answer is "E." Pelvic inflammatory disease (PID) is an infection of the upper reproductive tract, including endometritis, salpingitis, tubo-ovarian abscess, and pelvic peritonitis. Adolescent girls are disproportionately affected. Infection occurs when lower genital tract (vagina, cervix) bacteria move into the upper genital organs. Symptoms range from mild to severe. The CDC recommends treatment for presumed PID in a sexually active woman at risk for STIs presenting with the minimum clinical criteria of (1) lower abdominal or pelvic pain *and* (2) uterine, adnexal, or cervical motion tenderness. Supportive criteria include fever (> 38.3°C [100.9°F]), mucopurulent discharge (vaginal, cervix), white blood cells on saline microscopy, elevated inflammatory markers, and known positivity for *N. gonorrhoeae* or *C. trachomatis*. Don't forget you have to rule out alternative causes first. (See Table 1–7.)

Question 10-8

Which is a bacterial cause of PID?
A) *Neisseria gonorrhea*.
B) *Chlamydia trachomatis*.
C) *Ureaplasma urealyticum*.
D) *Haemophilus influenzae*.
E) All of these bacteria can cause PID.

TABLE 1–7 CAUSES OF ACUTE PELVIC PAIN

Urinary	Urinary tract infection
	Pyelonephritis
	Nephrolithiasis
	Urolithiasis
Gastrointestinal	Appendicitis
	Cholecystitis
	Mesenteric lymphadenitis
	Inflammatory bowel disease
	Gastroenteritis
Gynecologic	Ovarian torsion, cyst, or tumor
	Pelvic inflammatory disease
	Ectopic pregnancy
	Intrauterine pregnancy
	Endometriosis
	Hematometrocolpos
Musculoskeletal	Psoas muscle abscess
	Pelvic osteomyelitis

Discussion 10-8
The correct answer is "E." Multiple bacteria can cause PID, including STIs, genital flora, respiratory pathogens, and enteric organisms. PID is considered a polymicrobial infection and a causative agent is not always found.

Question 10-9
Which is NOT a complication of PID?
A) Tubo-ovarian abscess.
B) Infertility.
C) Renal abscess.
D) Ectopic pregnancy.
E) Peritonitis.

Discussion 10-9
The correct answer is "C." Short-term complications include tubo-ovarian abscess, perihepatitis, and periappendicitis. Long-term problems include infertility from tubal scarring, ectopic pregnancy, and chronic pelvic pain.

Her pregnancy test is negative. Saline mount (wet prep) reveals many white blood cells. KOH testing is negative. Endocervical specimens are sent for *N. gonorrhea* and *C. trachomatis* testing. Urinalysis and urine culture are normal.

Question 10-10
What should be done next?
A) Order an abdominal ultrasound.
B) Admit to the hospital.
C) Administer intravenous antibiotics.
D) Consult a surgeon.
E) All of the above.

Discussion 10-10
The correct answer is "E". She has a tubo-ovarian abscess, which can be diagnosed by ultrasound. All girls with PID need treatment with broad-spectrum antibiotics. Hospitalization is indicated for surgical emergencies, pregnancy, failed outpatient treatment, severe illness, or tubo-ovarian abscess. The latter may require surgical drainage.

Her male sexual partner is contacted and he agrees to be evaluated. He reports burning with urination and penile discharge for the last week. On exam, he is afebrile, SMR 5, and has erythema at the urethral meatus but no lesions. Purulent discharge is seen after stripping the urethra.

Question 10-11
What do you tell him?
A) He has an STI.
B) He does not require treatment.
C) He can continue to have sex as long as he wears a condom.
D) He should avoid spermicides.
E) He does not need more testing.

Discussion 10-11
The correct answer is "A". Urethritis is most commonly caused by STIs bacteria, including *N. gonorrhoeae* or *C. trachomatis*. Other causes include *Ureaplasma urealyticum, Trichomonas vaginalis,* and herpes simplex virus. Noninfectious causes include trauma, chemical irritation, Stevens-Johnson syndrome, Kawasaki disease, and Reiter syndrome. Pyuria, white blood cells on Gram stain of a urethral swab, or mucopurulent discharge on exam confirm the diagnosis. He should be tested for gonorrhea, chlamydia, and HIV. If Gram stain of a urethral swab is suggestive of gonorrhea, he should be treated with ceftriaxone and azithromycin or doxycycline. If gonococci are not present, only azithromycin or doxycycline is needed. He should not have sex for 1 week after treatment to prevent transmission. Spermicides can cause chemical irritation, but he has an STI. Fill his pockets with condoms before he leaves.

► CASE 11

An adolescent girl comes to the clinic for her yearly checkup. Her major complaint is acne. She wants a cream to make it go away. She reports feeling less attractive than her classmates. She says that all the girls in her class get to go out on school nights but her mom won't let her, which means she will never be popular. When asked, she understands that her mother doesn't want her to be too tired for school.

Question 11-1
Which period of adolescence best describes this girl?
A) Early adolescence.
B) Middle adolescence.
C) Late adolescence.
D) None of the above.
E) Adolescence has too many stages.

TABLE 1–8 CHARACTERISTICS OF EARLY, MIDDLE, AND LATE ADOLESCENCE

	Early Adolescence (11–14 years)	Middle Adolescence (15–17 years)	Late Adolescence (18–21 years)
Physical	Growth spurt Secondary sex characteristics	Puberty completed Growth slows Acne and odor	Physically mature Growth complete
Cognitive	Concrete thinking Poor problem solving Lack impulse control	Abstract thinking Struggles with decision making in times of stress Feelings of omnipotence and invincibility	Future oriented Understands future consequences of decisions Able to compromise and set limits
Emotional	Self-conscious about body image Struggles with sense of identity	Self-centered Attractiveness concerns Mood swings Intense emotions	Strong personal identity Increased emotional stability
Social/Peers	Same-sex relationships	Strong peer influence Looks up to peers Peers are role models Risk-taking behaviors	Less influenced by peers Seeks more intimate relationships
Family	Desires privacy Less interest in family activities	Peaked conflict with parents	Accepts parental advice
Sexual	Preoccupied with changes in genitals	Questions sexual orientation Dating Sexual activity	Establishing sexual identity

Discussion 11-1

The correct answer is "B." Adolescence is a time of many changes and consists of three distinct periods: early, middle, and late. (See Table 1–8.) The body is maturing and changing. Rapid body changes may make an adolescent feel self-conscious or awkward. Socially peers take on a larger role. Separation from family occurs. Thinking moves from concrete to abstract. The adolescent is determining who he or she is (self-identity). Middle adolescence is a time of acne, concerns over attractiveness, stereotypical behaviors, increased role of peers, the start of abstract thinking and struggles with family for autonomy.

....

The mother is frustrated with her daughter's attitude. They are arguing more lately. What is especially trying is the adolescent will "blow up" then go to her room to be alone. Mom is worried that the girl is spending too much time texting friends on her cell phone. The mother wants to know if these behaviors are normal.

Question 11-2

What do you tell her?

A) Recommend drug testing without telling her daughter.
B) Spending more time with peers is normal.
C) Mood swings are uncommon during adolescence.

D) Peers do not have a strong influence on likes, dislikes, choices, and behaviors.
E) She should take away her daughter's cell phone when she "blows up."

Discussion 11-2

The correct answer is "B." Emotional and physical separation from family is a normal part of adolescent development. Seeking autonomy, being argumentative, and demanding privacy are normal behaviors. Adolescents will spend more time with peers. Peers or an adult outside the family (ie, coach) will be sought for advice, emotional support, or both. Parents must adapt their parenting style based on the teen's developmental ability to think through problems, assess consequences, and problem solve. Negotiation works better than being authoritative. Parents need to stay involved and supportive as connectedness protects against risk-taking behaviors. Adolescents should be interviewed alone, allowing the opportunity to talk freely. The discussion is confidential and information should be shared with the parents only if it is life threatening. The AAP discourages drug testing without consent except when the adolescent lacks decision-making capacity or there is strong suspicion of drug abuse from the history or exam. Issues surrounding minors and consent are variable. If in doubt look it up on the Guttmacher Institute's website. In general, the adolescent should be given the opportunity to consent.

⌛ QUICK QUIZ

Concrete thinking is characteristic of which stage of adolescence?
A) Early.
B) Middle.
C) Late.

Discussion

The correct answer is "A." Concrete thinking is typically seen in early adolescence (see Table 1–8). It is important to remember that physical, cognitive, and social development may not be synchronous. For example, a 14-year-old patient who has almost completed puberty would be classified as being in middle to late adolescence based on secondary sex characteristics and physical development, but may still have very concrete thinking and be classified as being in early adolescence in terms of cognitive development.

> **Helpful Tip**
> The CRAFFT screening tool for substance abuse is a useful tool for screening for high risk alcohol and substance use disorders in adolescents. The interviewer first asks an opening question asking if a patient has drunk any alcohol (more than a few sips), smoked any marijuana, or used anything else to get high. If the answer to all these questions is no, then only the first question of the CRAFFT screen is asked; if the answer is yes, then all six questions are asked. The screening tool consists of six questions:
>
> **C** –Have you ever ridden in a CAR driven by someone (including yourself) who was "high" or had been using alcohol or drugs?
>
> **R** –Do you ever use alcohol or drugs to RELAX, feel better about yourself, or fit in?
>
> **A** –Do you ever use alcohol/drugs while you are by yourself, ALONE?
>
> **F** –Do you ever FORGET things you did while using alcohol or drugs?
>
> **F** –Do your family or FRIENDS ever tell you that you should cut down on your drinking or drug use?
>
> **T** –Have you gotten into TROUBLE while you were using alcohol or drugs?

▶ CASE 12

A mother brings her 14-year-old daughter to your clinic with complaints of abdominal pain during her menstrual cycles. The pain typically occurs in her lower abdomen and starts the day before her cycle, lasting 2 to 3 days. She has missed 6 days of school in the past 6 months due to the pain. She has tried acetaminophen at home with minimal relief. Menses started at age 12, currently occur monthly, and last 5 to 6 days, with moderate flow requiring her to change her pad/tampon every 4 to 6 hours. She reports that she is attracted to boys and, when asked confidentially, that she has never been sexually active.

Question 12-1

What is the most likely cause of her abdominal pain?
A) Ovarian cyst.
B) Endometriosis.
C) Primary dysmenorrhea.
D) Pelvic infection.
E) Endometrial polyp.

Discussion 12-1

The correct answer is "C." Dysmenorrhea or pain with menses is a common complaint in menstruating adolescents. Studies estimate that more than 50% of adolescents experience dysmenorrhea. Primary dysmenorrhea is lower abdominal or pelvic pain with menses that is not secondary to pelvic pathology. Pain is typically described as crampy, begins 1 to 2 days before menses and may continue for 1 to 3 days into menses. Associated symptoms include low back pain, nausea or vomiting, diarrhea, fatigue, dizziness, and headaches. Dysmenorrhea symptoms typically appear 1 to 3 years after menarche when regular ovulatory cycles have been established. The mechanism of primary dysmenorrhea is prostaglandin formation from the endometrial lining with ovulatory cycles. The differential diagnosis for primary dysmenorrhea includes all causes of secondary dysmenorrhea. Gynecologic causes of pelvic pain include endometriosis, adenomyosis, fibroids, ovarian cysts, chronic PID, obstructive endometrial polyps, congenital obstructive müllerian malformations, cervical stenosis, and pelvic congestion syndrome. Nongynecologic causes include inflammatory bowel disease, irritable bowel syndrome, and psychogenic disorders. Patients with a typical history of dysmenorrhea as described above and a normal pelvic exam can be diagnosed with primary dysmenorrhea. Atypical elements of the history that may indicate an underlying cause of dysmenorrhea include pain that begins at onset of menarche, which could be related to müllerian duct or hymenal abnormalities; menstrual pain that becomes progressively worse over time, which could be associated with endometriosis; or a history of STIs, which may be related to intrauterine or pelvic adhesions.

> **Helpful Tip**
> Menses typically begin between ages 12 and 13 years in well-nourished American teens. Cycles can be irregular in the first few years of menses due to anovulation, with typical cycle intervals ranging from 21 to 45 days. Length of menstrual flow is typically 2 to 7 days. Typical menstrual product use is 3 to 6 pads or tampons a day.

Question 12-2

What would be the most appropriate first line therapy for management of these symptoms?
A) Fluoxetine.
B) Naproxen sodium.
C) Tramadol.
D) Antibiotics.
E) Laparoscopy.

Discussion 12-2

The correct answer is "B." Nonsteroidal anti-inflammatory drugs (NSAIDs) are considered first-line treatment for dysmenorrhea. Patients should be told to take the medication at the first sign of cramps and continue to take it as scheduled through the first 1 to 2 days of the cycle. Appropriate dosing should be reviewed with the patient. Naproxen sodium is often preferable to ibuprofen due to ease of dosing. Tramadol can be used in patients who have a contraindication to NSAIDs but is not typically considered a first-line agent. Exercise and other interventions to reduce stress can also be helpful. Adolescents should be evaluated within 3 to 4 months to evaluate the effectiveness of the medication.

The patient returns to the clinic 3 months later for follow up. Her pain is improved but continues to limit her activities 1 day a month.

Question 12-3

What is the most appropriate next step in management?
A) Referral to a gastroenterologist.
B) Laparoscopy.
C) Combination OCPs.
D) Pelvic ultrasound.

Discussion 12-3

The correct answer is "C." If a patient continues to have symptoms after a trial of NSAIDs, or if a patient needs contraception, combination OCPs can be started. OCPs work by suppressing ovulation, which leads to a thinner endometrial lining with decreased prostaglandin production and bleeding. If symptoms continue after 3 to 4 months on OCPs, laparoscopy and a pelvic ultrasound should be considered to evaluate for causes of secondary dysmenorrhea.

BIBLIOGRAPHY

American Academy of Pediatrics, Committee on Adolescence and Committee on Early Childhood and Adoption, and Dependent Care. American Academy of Pediatrics: Care of adolescent parents and their children. *Pediatrics.* 2001;107(2):429–434.

American Academy of Pediatrics Committee on Substance Abuse. Testing for drugs of abuse in children and adolescents. *Pediatrics.* 1996;98:305–307.

American Psychiatric Association. *Diagnostic and Statistical Manual of Mental Disorders.* 5th ed. Washington, DC: American Psychiatric Association; 2013.

Bordini B, Rosenfield R. Normal pubertal development part II: Clinical aspects of puberty. *Pediatr Rev.* 2011;32(7):281–292.

Campbell MA, McGrath PJ. Use of medication by adolescents for the management of menstrual discomfort. *Arch Pediatr Adolesc Med.* 1997;151:905.

Centers for Disease Control and Prevention. Sexually transmitted disease guidelines, 2010. *MMWR Morb Mortal Wkly Rep.* 2010;59(RR-12):1–116.

Centers for Disease Control and Prevention. US medical eligibility criteria for contraceptive use, 2010. *MMWR Morb Mortal Wkly Rep.* 2010;59(RR-4):1–88.

Diamant AL, Schuster MA, McGuigan K, et al. Lesbians' sexual history with men: Implications for taking a sexual history. *Arch Intern Med.* 1999;159(22):2730–2736.

Dickey RP. *Managing Contraceptive Pill Patients.* 12th ed. New Orleans, LA: Emis Medical Publishers; 2004.

Emans SJ. Amenorrhea in the adolescent. In: Emans SJ, Laufer MR, Goldstein DP, eds. *Pediatric & Adolescent Gynecology.* 5th ed. Philadelphia, PA: Lippincott Williams & Wilkins; 2005:214–269.

Emans SJ. Delayed puberty. In: Emans SJ, Laufer MR, Goldstein DP, eds. *Pediatric & Adolescent Gynecology.* 5th ed. Philadelphia, PA: Lippincott Williams & Wilkins; 2005:181–213.

Emans SJ. Dysfunctional uterine bleeding. In: Emans SJ, Laufer MR, Goldstein DP, eds. *Pediatric & Adolescent Gynecology.* 5th ed. Philadelphia, PA: Lippincott Williams & Wilkins; 2005:270-286.

Fankowski B. Sexual orientation and adolescents. *Pediatrics.* 2004;113(6):1827–1832.

Fleishman A, Gordon CM, Neinstein LS. Menstrual disorders: Amenorrhea and polycystic ovary syndrome. In: Neinstein LS, ed. *Handbook of Adolescent Healthcare.* Philadelphia, PA: Lippincott Williams & Wilkins; 2009:470–478.

Garofalo R, Katz E. Health care issues of gay and lesbian youth. *Curr Opin Pediatr.* 2001;13(4):298–302.

Garofalo R, Wolf RC, Kessel S, et al. The association between health risk behaviors and sexual orientation among a school-based sample of adolescents. *Pediatrics.* 1998;101(5):895–902.

Gray SH. Menstrual disorders. *Pediatr Rev.* 2013;34(1):6–18.

Guttmacher Institute. State policies in brief: Minors' access to STI services, as of October 1, 2015. Accessed October 2, 2015 from http://www.guttmacher.org/statecenter/spibs/

Hatcher RA, Trussell J, Nelson AL, et al. *Contraceptive Technology.* 20th rev ed. New York NY: Ardent Media; 2011.

Hwang LY, Shafer M. Vaginitis and vaginosis. In: Neinstein LS, ed. *Handbook of Adolescent Healthcare.* Philadelphia, PA: Lippincott Williams & Wilkins; 2009:491–498.

Joffe A: Gynecomastia. In: Neinstein LS, ed. *Handbook of Adolescent Healthcare.* Philadelphia, PA: Lippincott Williams & Wilkins; 2009:108–111.

Kaplowitz PB. Delayed puberty. *Pediatr Rev.* 2010;31(5):5189–5195.

Klein JR, Litt IF: Epidemiology of adolescent dysmenorrhea. *Pediatrics.* 1981;68:661.

Levy S, Siqueira LM. Testing for drugs of abuse in children and adolescents. *Pediatrics*. 2014;133(6):e1798–1807.

Marrazzo JM, Koutsky LA, Kiviat NB, et al. Papanicolaou test screening and prevalence of genital human papillomavirus among women who have sex with women. *Am J Public Health*. 2001;91(6):947–952.

Master-Hunter T, Heiman DL. Amenorrhea: Evaluation and treatment. *Am Fam Physician*. 2006;73(8):1374–1382.

Nicoletti AM. Teen pregnancy. In: Emans SJ, Laufer MR, Goldstein DP, eds. *Pediatric & Adolescent Gynecology*. 5th ed. Philadelphia, PA: Lippincott Williams & Wilkins; 2005:844–878.

Reddy DS. Clinical pharmacokinetic interactions between antiepileptic drugs and hormonal contraceptives. *Expert Rev Clin Pharmacol*. 2010;3(2):183–192.

Rodeghiero F, Castaman G, Dini E. Epidemiological investigation of the prevalence of von Willebrand's disease. *Blood*. 1987;69(2):454–459.

Rosen DS. Identification and management of eating disorders in children and adolescents. *Pediatrics*. 2010;126(6):1240–1253.

Rosenfield RL, Lipton RB, Drum ML. Thelarche, pubarche, and menarche attainment in children with normal and elevated body mass index. *Pediatrics*. 2009;123:84–88

Trent M. Pelvic inflammatory disease. *Pediatr Rev*. 2013;34(4):163–172.

Wilson CA, Keye WR: A survey of adolescent dysmenorrhea and premenstrual symptom frequency. A model program for prevention, detection, and treatment. *J Adolesc Health Care*. 1989;10:317.

Allergic and Immunologic Disorders

2

Amy O. Thomas and Alex Thomas

► CASE 1

A newborn boy is delivered at 38 weeks' gestation after an uncomplicated pregnancy and delivery. He is discharged home from the hospital on day of life 2. You are contacted by the lab after it was noted that the newborn screen revealed a T-cell receptor excision circle (TREC) of 0.

Question 1-1

What diagnosis should you be concerned of with this finding?

A) Severe combined immunodeficiency (SCID).
B) Complete DiGeorge syndrome.
C) Bruton's X-linked agammaglobulinemia (XLA).
D) Transient hypogammaglobulinemia of infancy (THI).
E) A and B only.
F) All of the above.

Discussion 1-1

The correct answer is "E." TRECs serve as a biomarker for naïve T-cell production. They are found in 70% of naïve T cells. They have served as a rapid DNA-based newborn screening tool for disorders of the immune system manifesting with T-cell lymphopenia, such as cases of SCID, ataxia-telangiectasia, or complete DiGeorge syndrome with athymia. T-cell lymphopenia has also been noted in some cases of trisomy 21 and preterm birth with very low birth weight (< 800 g), but counts should not be completely absent. XLA will manifest with absent mature B cells due to arrest in the pre–B-cell stage of development. This will show with absent circulating immunoglobulins of all classes. THI is due to prolongation of the normal physiologic nadir of immunoglobulin G (IgG) production that occurs in most infants between 4 and 6 months of age, following a drop in circulating maternal IgG. Typically, this is outgrown by 3 to 4 years of age, with few children requiring immunoglobulin replacement. IgM is typically normal in these infants.

Question 1-2

What should be the next step in confirming diagnosis?

A) Arrange for flow cytometry to enumerate B-, T-, and NK-cell populations.
B) Obtain an echocardiogram.
C) Obtain quantitative immunoglobulins.
D) Watch and wait for development of any clinical signs of infection.

Discussion 1-2

The correct answer is "A." SCID is defined by severely diminished T-cell function and abnormal B-cell function. It affects between 1 in 50,000 and 1 in 70,000 births. SCID is a medical emergency and requires careful but prompt diagnosis once suspected. Flow cytometry looks at cell counts identified by cell surface markers. Both SCID and DiGeorge syndrome results in deficient T-cell development. DiGeorge syndrome develops from a mutation on the long arm of chromosome 22, and patients often have characteristic morphologic findings, cardiac abnormalities, and hypoparathyroidism. In patients with complete DiGeorge, the immune dysfunction results in absent T cells and nonfunctioning B cells, with consequences similar to SCID. Thymic transplant is curative. For partial DiGeorge, as the name implies, the immune defect is less severe, with some functional T- and B-cell capabilities that often improve over time. Do you remember or have you heard of the boy in the bubble? A boy from Texas with X-linked SCID lived for 12 years in a plastic, germ-free bubble. His story brought national attention to SCID.

> **Helpful Tip**
> A low lymphocyte count is a tipoff to a T-cell problem as the majority of circulating lymphocytes (60% to 70%) are T cells. Flow cytometry can identify more specifically the subpopulations using cell surface markers of B (CD19, CD20), T (CD3CD4, CD3CD8), and NK (CD16, CD56) cell lines.

► CASE 2

You are starting in a new pediatric practice in the rural outskirts of a small town in Pennsylvania. Your first patient of the day is an 18-month-old boy who is presenting with a 4-week history of a persistent dry cough now progressing to dyspnea. On review of the history with parents, they state he was born full term without issue, via a home delivery. He was treated for four episodes of otitis media in his first year of life, most of which required back-to-back courses of antibiotics to clear. At 9 months he was hospitalized for pneumonia and dehydration secondary to diarrhea. As you piece through the remainder of his chart, you note there has been no weight gain for the past 4 months and he has now dropped several percentiles on his growth chart. Currently, he is tachypneic with rales and rhonchi noted. He is slightly tachycardic with a temperature of 37.3°C (99.2°F). You note the oral cavity has what appears to be several white patches with surrounding erythema and nearly absent tonsils. His oxygen saturation is 88% on room air in the office.

Question 2-1

In addition to acute management of this patient, what diagnosis must you consider and address urgently?
A) Selective antibody deficiency.
B) Enlarged adenoids.
C) SCID.
D) None of the above; this is a normal infection history for a child his age.

Discussion 2-1

The correct answer is "C." Look for the history of immune deficiency that may have escaped detection on a newborn screen (see Case 1). In the current case, the history of a "home birth" should be followed with questions of whether a newborn screen was submitted. SCID will most often present in the first few months of life with chronic lung infections, diarrhea, thrush, and failure to thrive. With T- and B-cell deficiencies, lymphoid tissue (lymph nodes, tonsils, adenoids, thymus) may be absent or reduced in size. Thrush outside of the infancy period is atypical and should not be dismissed as normal. Possible causes include a primary or secondary cellular immunodeficiency, use of inhaled corticosteroids, chemotherapy, and antibiotics.

He is admitted to the hospital for further care. On arrival, a chest x-ray reveals bilateral pneumonia and an absent thymic shadow, prompting the start of empiric antibiotics and further immunology evaluation. A sputum culture reveals respiratory syncytial virus and adenovirus. A peripheral CBC shows a WBC of 4000 cells/μL, with noted lymphopenia (absolute lymphocyte count of 400 cells/μL). A quick glance at the family history shows he has a 5-year-old sister and an 8-year-old sister, both of whom are healthy. A maternal uncle died in early childhood of overwhelming infection, but there is little other available information about his cause of death. The results of flow cytometry return, and you note absent T cells, absent NK cells, but normal circulating numbers of B cells. Alarmed, you send off further immune studies, including quantitative immunoglobulins, which are found to be universally low. Mitogen proliferation studies show an absent response to phytohemagglutinin, pokeweed mitogen, and candida.

Question 2-2

What is the likely defect causing his condition?
A) Adenosine deaminase (ADA) deficiency.
B) Common gamma chain mutation.
C) *Recombination-activating gene 1 (RAG1)* deficiency.
D) gp91phox mutation in the nicotinamide adenine dinucleotide phosphate (NADPH) oxidase complex.

Discussion 2-2

The correct answer is "B." X-linked SCID is the most common cause of SCID (~50% of cases) and is caused by a defect in the common gamma chain, a key protein involved in the signaling cascade used in lymphocyte maturation and proliferation. With X-linked recessive inheritance, only males are affected. The common gamma chain is shared by several key signaling receptors and pathways including interleukin-2 receptor (IL2R), IL4R, IL7R, IL9R, IL15R, and IL21R and the associated downstream Janus kinase 3 (JAK3) signaling protein. In X-linked SCID, T and NK cells are typically low or absent, but B cell numbers can be normal (T-B+NK- SCID). However, B cells cannot properly function without help from T cells, so even if B cells are not directly affected by a mutation, they will be rendered nonfunctional. Deficiency of JAK3 due to a mutation in the *JAK3* gene will also cause T-B+NK- SCID but is inherited in an autosomal recessive mode. In the case of your 18-month-old patient, both the flow cytometry profile as well as family history of normal females but affected males on the maternal lineage suggests X-linked SCID as the diagnosis. Among autosomal recessive forms of SCID, ADA deficiency (leading to toxic buildup of metabolites in T and B cells) and *RAG* mutations (leading to impaired somatic gene recombination necessary for B- and T-cell receptor synthesis) are among the most common. Both of these mutations will lead to absent B and T cells (T-B-NK- SCID) on flow analysis. Chronic granulomatous disease is associated with errors in the assembly of the NADPH oxidase complex, of which gp91phox is a major protein. B and T cells are not directly affected by this mutation. (See Table 2–1.)

> **Helpful Tip**
>
> In an immunosuppressed patient presenting with history of persistent cough or dyspnea, concern must be raised for infection with opportunistic infections such as *Pneumocystis jiroveci* (formerly *Pneumocystis carinii*). In immunocompromised patients, look for a history of atypical or severe infections such as pneumocystis, cytomegalovirus, rotavirus, mycobacteria, and aspergillus.

TABLE 2–1 SEVERE COMBINED IMMUNODEFICIENCY (SCID) PHENOTYPES

Abnormality	SCID Mutation
T-B-NK-	ADA deficiency
T-B-NK+	RAG, Omenn syndrome
T-B+NK-	Common gamma chain, JAK3, PNP
T-B+NK+	CD3, IL7R
T+B+NK+	Zap70

ADA, adenosine deaminase deficiency; PNP, purine nucleoside phosphorylase; RAG, recombinant activating genes; SCID, severe combined immunodeficiency.

Helpful Tip

SCID patients are almost always lymphopenic; however, recall that age-adjusted normal ranges are available for children. Normal infant lymphocyte counts are generally higher than those for older children and adults.

Question 2-3

What additional steps should be taken in his care?

A) Start intravenous immunoglobulin (IVIG) for immunoglobulin replacement.
B) Place him on prophylactic antifungal and antiviral medications to prevent the development of opportunistic infections.
C) Begin HLA typing for bone marrow transplantation.
D) Avoid live viral vaccines and nonirradiated blood products.
E) All of the above.

Discussion 2-3

The correct answer is "E." B cells require T cells to assist in normal development and production of functional antibodies. Therefore this patient will need supplemental IVIG to supplement his humoral response and prophylactic antifungals and antivirals to protect against opportunistic infections from the deficient cellular immunity. Early bone marrow transplantation is the preferred method of treatment for SCID, ideally before any major infections have occurred. While bone marrow transplantation will restore T-cell function, B-cell function typically remains abnormal, and thus IVIG must often be continued indefinitely. Attenuated live virus vaccines must be avoided, and any blood products used must be irradiated. Nonirradiated blood products contain T cells which could lead to development of graft-versus-host disease.

Helpful Tip

Omenn syndrome (a form of SCID) is a variant of RAG deficiency (partial inactivation), manifesting with erythroderma, hepatosplenomegaly, chronic diarrhea, failure to thrive, eosinophilia, and elevated IgE levels.

QUICK QUIZ

Which is not a potential clinical indicator of an immunodeficiency?

A) Measles after receiving the MMR vaccine.
B) Recurrent thrush.
C) Chronic diarrhea.
D) Liver abscess.
E) Recurrent self-limited viral upper respiratory tract infections in a child in daycare.

Discussion

The correct answer is "E." The average child can have several "illnesses" in the span of a year without concern for underlying immune deficiency. In fact, infants and children may have 8 to 10 respiratory infections in a year with symptoms lasting at least 1 week per infection. However, a history of recurrent deep-seated infections or abscesses, antibiotic usage with little effect or requirement for multiple back to back courses, and failure to thrive or loss of linear growth should all prompt further workup for primary immune deficiency. In addition to recurrent infection, patients with immune deficiency are at increased risk for development of autoimmune disease and malignancy. (See Table 2–2.) Signs of a cellular immunodeficiency include recurrent viral, fungal, or mycobacterium infections; chronic diarrhea; failure to thrive; and reaction to live viral vaccines. Symptoms may present early

TABLE 2–2 RED FLAGS FOR AN IMMUNODEFICIENCY

Family history of an immunodeficiency

Failure to thrive

Chronic diarrhea

Infections requiring intravenous antibiotics

Severe or life-threatening infections

Recurrent abscesses, especially those involving solid organs (eg, liver)

Recurrent sinusitis, pneumonia, or otitis media

Infection with opportunistic or atypical organisms (eg, *Burkholderia*, *Pneumocystis jiroveci*)

Recurrent candidiasis

Poor wound healing

Granulomas

Lymphoma in infancy

Complications from live viral vaccines (vaccine-associated infection)

Lymphopenia

Eosinophilia

Vaccine unresponsiveness

Delayed hypersensitivity skin responses (low sensitivity)

Rheumatologic disorders

in infancy. Signs of a humoral immunodeficiency include recurrent bacterial infections (eg, sinopulmonary, otitis), infections with encapsulated bacteria, and enterovirus infections. Humoral immunodeficiencies present later in infancy (> 4 months) or beyond due to maternal transplacentally acquired IgG.

Complement deficiency can be due to a deficiency in the alternative or classical pathway. Overwhelming *Neisseria* sepsis is a clue to an underlying complement deficiency. Most of these are inherited in an autosomal recessive fashion. Classically patients with complement deficiencies present with severe or recurrent *Neisseria* infections such as meningococcemia or meningococcal meningitis.

▶ CASE 3

A 3-year-old boy presents to your office with his sixth ear infection this year. He has concurrent purulent nasal drainage and his parents feel he is "always congested" despite being on antibiotics as recently as 2 weeks ago. He was treated for pneumonia confirmed on chest X-ray at 21 months of age. Last year, he developed osteomyelitis of the tibia after a fall at the playground, requiring a 4-week course of intravenous antibiotics. He has had few to no issues with viral or fungal infections. He is growing and developing normally and has had no issues with excessive bleeding or bruising. There is no history of recurrent rashes. On close examination, you note the absence of tonsils.

Question 3-1

In addition to treating the current infection, what diagnosis should you consider?

A) None; this is a typical infection pattern for a child of his age.
B) Bruton's agammaglobulinemia.
C) SCID.
D) Complement deficiency.
E) Wiskott-Aldrich syndrome.

Discussion 3-1

The correct answer is "B." X-linked agammaglobulinemia (XLA), also known as Bruton's agammaglobulinemia, occurs due to a mutation in the *Bruton tyrosine kinase* (*btk*) gene (responsible for a tyrosine kinase protein), causing arrest of B cells in the pre–B-cell stage. Prevention of B-cell maturation leads to absence of plasma cells and the inability to produce circulating immunoglobulins. Lymphoid tissues where B cells are often found concentrated, such as the tonsils, adenoids, spleen, and lymph nodes, are often atrophic on physical exam. The T-cell count is paradoxically often noted to be elevated. The absence of humoral immunity leads to increased infection with encapsulated organisms such as *Streptococcus pneumoniae*, *Pseudomonas* species, or *Haemophilus influenzae* type B. Enterovirus is also common in humoral deficiency. As implied in the name, it is inherited in an X-linked recessive fashion, thus only affecting males. Female carriers are asymptomatic. Diagnosis is made with screening for low or absent immunoglobulin levels (IgG, IgM, IgA). Confirmation is made through flow cytometry with noted absent B-cell profile (look for low markers of CD19, CD20). Treatment is with immunoglobulin replacement (IVIG). SCID would place a child at increased risk of fungal and viral infections with impaired cellular immunity. Wiskott-Aldrich syndrome (WAS) is an X-linked recessive disease with characteristic severe eczema, thrombocytopenia, and immunodeficiency (cellular and humoral) due to mutations in the *WAS* gene which encodes for the Wiskott-Aldrich syndrome protein (WASp). Small platelets are noted on blood smear.

▶ CASE 4

An 18-year-old boy presents to the emergency department with abdominal pain, shortness of breath, and cough. He reports that symptoms began approximately 3 weeks ago but have progressively worsened in the past 48 hours. He notes that he has been treated for pneumonia once or twice per year for the last 5 years. He has several scarred areas on his arms where he states previous skin infections "healed funny." A poorly healing ulcer is noted on his lower leg that he said developed after being scraped while helping to clear shrubbery on his father's farm. Chest X-ray shows "cotton ball densities" in both lungs. A fine needle aspiration of the lung lesions is obtained and shows *Aspergillus fumigatus*. Abdominal CT shows a multicentric liver abscess that contains *Serratia marcescens*. IV antibiotics and antifungal medications are started and he is admitted to the hospital for further care. He has a mildly elevated WBC of 14,000 with slight predominance of neutrophils (75%). Quantitative immunoglobulin levels are normal.

Question 4-1

Based on his presentation and infection history, what is the most likely underlying diagnosis?

A) Common variable immunodeficiency (CVID).
B) Severe combined immunodeficiency (SCID).
C) Kostmann syndrome.
D) Chronic granulomatous disease (CGD).

Discussion 4-1

The correct answer is "D." CGD is characterized by defective intracellular killing of bacterial and fungal infections by phagocytes (neutrophils, macrophages, monocytes). Commonly, CGD patients have infections with catalase positive organisms such as *Staphylococcus aureus*, *S. marcescens*, and *Burkholderia cepacia* complex, as well as fungal organisms such as *Aspergillus*. The disease results from a mutation in the NADPH oxidase complex, leading to failed production of superoxide by the phagosome (respiratory burst) and ineffective killing and clearance of intracellular organisms. Neutrophil numbers can be normal or elevated; however, their function is impaired. Severe congenital neutropenia (Kostmann syndrome) is due to a mutation in the *HAX1* gene leading to chronic neutropenia (not seen in this patient). CVID is the most common primary immunodeficiency. B cells fail to fully differentiate into plasma cells, leading to a deficiency in some (IgG, IgM, IgA) or all of the immunoglobulin subtypes as well as poor vaccine responses. There is an increased risk of autoimmunity and malignancy in patients with CVID. IVIG is required for long-term immunoglobulin replacement. For diagnosis, look for absent or low levels of class-switched memory B cells in CVID patients (IgM−IgD−CD27+CD19+).

Question 4-2

What test should be ordered to confirm your suspicion?
A) Vaccine titers and mitogen proliferation studies.
B) CD11, CD18 markers on flow cytometry.
C) Dihydrorhodamine 123 fluorescence assay.
D) HIV viral load, as an antibody test would be unreliable in this patient.

Discussion 4-2

The correct answer is "C." Diagnosis of suspected CGD is made through use of dihydrorhodamine (DHR) assay. DHR is a non-fluorescent dye used to stain whole blood phagocytes, which are then stimulated with phorbol myristate acetate (PMA). Normal phagocytes are able to oxidize the dye, causing increased fluorescence, through production of superoxide. The fraction of fluorescent cells is measured by use of a fluorescence-activated cell-sorting machine (FACS). Older techniques employed used of nitroblue tetrazolium (NBT), a dye that turned from yellow to blue when reduced by superoxide. DHR is thought to be a more accurate measurement and allows for distinction between X-linked recessive and autosomal recessive forms of the disease.

Question 4-3

In addition to the identified pathogens, which other pathogen is commonly associated with the type of immunodeficiency seen in this patient?
A) *Salmonella typhimurium*.
B) *Chromobacterium violaceum*.
C) *Actinomyces* species.
D) *Nocardia* species.
E) All of the above.

Discussion 4-3

The correct answer is "E."

> **Helpful Tip**
> Infections with catalase-positive bacteria and fungi are characteristic of CGD. The most common pathogen is *Staphylococcus aureus*.

You tell the patient he has an immunodeficiency disease, explaining that certain cells in his body are unable to kill bacteria and fungi. He wants to know what type of infections he is susceptible to as a result of his disease.

Question 4-4

Which of the following is associated with CGD?
A) Pneumonia.
B) Colitis.
C) Liver abscess.
D) Recurrent skin abscesses.
E) All of the above.

Discussion 4-4

The correct answer is "E." Common infections in CGD include pneumonia, lymphadenitis, skin abscess, liver abscess, perianal abscess, and osteomyelitis. Staphylococcal liver abscesses are strongly associated with CGD. Additionally, granulomas (collection of inflammatory cells) are common, which may obstruct the urinary or gastrointestinal tract. Some patients develop Crohn-like inflammatory bowel disease.

⌛ QUICK QUIZ

A 3-year-old boy has had three episodes of cellulitis and two episodes of pneumonia in the last year. Both were caused by *Staphylococcus aureus*. His gums bleed chronically, especially with brushing his teeth. On exam, he has mouth ulcers, inflamed gingiva with areas of bleeding, and a few nonhealing wounds on his legs and arms.

Which of the following immunodeficiencies is included in the differential diagnosis for this child?
A) Leukocyte adhesion deficiency.
B) Chédiak-Higashi syndrome.
C) Hyperimmunoglobulin E syndrome.
D) Chronic granulomatous disease.
E) All of above are possible diagnoses.

Discussion

The correct answer is "E." This case screams that the neutrophils are not working or not present. Phagocytes include neutrophils, monocytes, and macrophages and are part of the innate immune system. Primary phagocytic disorders present with recurrent bacterial (staphylococci) and fungal (aspergilli, candida) infections of the respiratory tract and skin. Mucositis (mouth ulcers), gingivitis, and poor wound healing may also occur. Neutropenia has multiple causes that may be congenital or acquired. Chédiak-Higashi syndrome, an autosomal recessive condition, is associated with skin and eye albinism, mild coagulopathy, neutropenia, and neurologic problems (nystagmus, ataxia, neuropathies). Characteristic large azurophil granules are seen in neutrophils and other granulocytes. Leukocyte adhesion deficiencies result in the inability of neutrophils to undergo chemotaxis from the bloodstream to the site of infection; therefore, pus is not made and blood neutrophil counts are elevated. With infection, neutrophil counts may reach 100,000 cells/mm³. A classic clue is delayed separation of the umbilical cord (> 1 month). Autosomal dominant hyper-IgE syndrome (HIES), as known as Job syndrome, is characterized by recurrent abscesses from *S. aureus*, coarse facies, and severe eczema-like rash. Abscesses may be "cold" or not appear inflamed. Serum IgE levels are elevated and eosinophilia is present. Pneumonia may lead to abscess and pneumatocele formation. Other characteristics include retained primary teeth and skeletal fractures from minor trauma.

▶ CASE 5

An 8-year-old boy is new to your practice. You note as he enters the room with his mother that he seems somewhat "off balance" to which his mom replies that she had noted changes in his gait for the last 3 to 4 years, but thought he was just "clumsy." You are reviewing his medical history and find that he has been treated for recurrent otitis media and sinusitis despite having three sets of tympanostomy tubes since age 2. On examination, you note several superficial blood vessels apparent in the eyes and on the pinna of the ear. Concerned with the history and examination findings, you order a CBC that demonstrates profound lymphopenia as well as quantitative immunoglobulin levels and vaccine titers to pneumococcus and tetanus, all of which are low.

Question 5-1

What diagnosis are you most concerned with based on the constellation of symptoms?
A) Neuroblastoma.
B) Chédiak-Higashi syndrome.
C) WHIM syndrome.
D) Ataxia-telangiectasia.
E) Hyper-IgM syndrome.

Discussion 5-1

The correct answer is "D." Ataxia-telangiectasia (AT) is caused by a defect in ATM repair gene, which leads to a combined B- and T-cell defect. Low immunoglobulin levels and lymphopenia will be noted on screening labs. Progressive cerebellar ataxia and neuron loss occur with age. Ataxia is the earliest clinical manifestation, with initial symptoms beginning around 2 to 3 years of age. Telangiectasias of the bulbar conjunctiva and skin typically manifest with disease progression. AT is inherited in an autosomal recessive pattern. Serum alpha fetoprotein is often elevated in AT. WHIM (warts, hypogammaglobulinemia, infections, and myelokathexis) syndrome and Chédiak-Higashi syndrome are associated with neutropenia. Hyper-IgM syndrome is characterized by elevated IgM, low IgG and IgA, and decreased T-cell response to antigens. Affected individuals have recurrent infections similar to other conditions with combined impaired B- and T-cell function.

Question 5-2

What should be avoided in this patient?
A) DTaP vaccine.
B) Pneumococcal vaccine.
C) X-rays.
D) Irradiated blood products.

Discussion 5-2

The correct answer is "C." With a defect in the DNA repair machinery, ionizing radiation must be avoided as it increases strand breakage and malignancy risk. Live attenuated viral vaccines should be deferred in any patient with a suspicion of cellular immunodeficiency. Irradiated blood products should be given to patients with a T-cell immunodeficiency requiring transfusion to prevent the development of graft-versus-host disease.

Helpful Tip
Live viral vaccines should be avoided in patients with cellular (T-cell) immunodeficiencies. If given, the virus may cause infection in the patient.

⏳ QUICK QUIZ

Which immunodeficiency is not correctly matched with its mode of inheritance?
A) Chronic granulomatous disease—X-linked recessive and autosomal recessive.
B) Ataxia-telangiectasia (AT)—autosomal dominant.
C) X-linked agammaglobulinemia—X-linked recessive.
D) Severe combined immunodeficiency (SCID)—X-linked recessive and autosomal recessive.
E) Wiskott-Aldrich syndrome—X-linked recessive.

Discussion

The correct answer is "B." AT is an autosomal recessive condition.

▶ CASE 6

An 18-year-old girl injured her knee after waterskiing at her family's lake house. She saw her primary care physician who advised rest and icing, as well as ibuprofen if needed for pain. Thirty minutes after taking 400 mg of ibuprofen, she develops diffuse hives and swelling of her lips and eyelids. Alarmed, her family rushes her to the emergency department, where on arrival she vomits, feels short of breath, and is lightheaded.

Question 6-1

What medication should be administered first to this patient?
A) Epinephrine.
B) Benadryl.
C) Normal saline intravenous fluid bolus.
D) Steroids.

Discussion 6-1

The correct answer is "A." Anaphylaxis is a type 1 hypersensitivity reaction with IgE-mediated mast cell degranulation involving multiorgan systems. First-line treatment for anaphylaxis is epinephrine—every time. If the first round of epinephrine is ineffective at fully reversing symptoms, a second round of epinephrine should be administered. Dosing for epinephrine is 0.01 mg/kg intramuscular of a 1:1000 solution. Early administration of epinephrine reduces mortality associated with anaphylaxis. Epinephrine should be given intramuscularly rather than subcutaneously.

Helpful Tip
General rule of thumb for epinephrine dosing:
- For children < 25 kg, give 0.15 mg in an epinephrine autoinjector
- For children and adults > 25 kg, give the standard dose of 0.3 mg in an epinephrine autoinjector

Being the astute ED physician of the day, you decide to administer epinephrine. After 10 minutes, you note her symptoms persist and she is now becoming hypotensive. Her father tells you that she was recently started on a beta-blocker medication as a form of migraine prophylaxis.

Question 6-2

In addition to establishing an IV, what is the next step in her care?
A) Repeat epinephrine.
B) Glucagon.
C) "Stress-dose" steroids, as the hypotension is secondary to adrenal insufficiency.
D) Vasopressor infusion.

Discussion 6-2

The correct answer is "A." The treatment of choice is epinephrine. Beta-blocker medications increase the risk of a more severe reaction and treatment-resistant anaphylaxis. Between 15% and 30% of reactions may require a second dose of epinephrine. Epinephrine causes both alpha- and beta-adrenergic effects, leading to vasoconstriction, tachycardia, bronchial relaxation, and increased vascular permeability. This effect can sometimes be blunted in patients taking beta-blockers. If two to three rounds of epinephrine are ineffective at fully reversing the reaction, glucagon should be administered to patients taking a beta-blocker medication. Glucagon has both positive inotropic and chronotropic effects on the heart. It does not involve catecholamines, and therefore is unaffected by beta blockade. In patients with prolonged hypotension from recalcitrant anaphylaxis, adrenal hemorrhage and resulting insufficiency has been described. Consider this when hypotension is persistent with an appropriate clinical history. Second-line therapies sometimes used include antihistamines (H$_1$ and H$_2$), bronchodilators, and corticosteroids. Antihistamines treat itching, angioedema, and hives but are not lifesaving and do not treat airway obstruction or shock. Corticosteroids have a delayed onset of action and had traditionally been given to treat protracted anaphylaxis and prevent biphasic reactions though this has not been supported by the literature. Biphasic reactions occur in a small percentage of patients. Symptoms reoccur typically within 8 to 10 hours despite no repeat exposure to the trigger.

Question 6-3

Anaphylactic shock is typically characterized as what kind of shock?
A) Cardiogenic shock.
B) Neurogenic shock.
C) Hypovolemic-distributive shock.
D) Nephrogenic shock.

Discussion 6-3

The correct answer is "C." Physiologic changes in anaphylaxis include vasodilation and loss of intravascular fluid from increased vascular permeability, followed by vasoconstriction and myocardial depression with reduced cardiac output. There

is a transient increase in pulmonary vascular resistance. Sitting upright has been associated with fatal anaphylaxis due to pulseless electrical activity cardiac arrest presumably due to inadequate cardiac filling from severe hypotension with decreased venous blood return, therefore; patients with anaphylaxis should be placed supine with their legs elevated.

> **Helpful Tip**
> In anaphylaxis, position the patient supine with his or her legs elevated. This will help preserve intravascular volume and venous return to the heart to prevent empty ventricle syndrome, which may result in cardiac arrest and sudden death.

She improves after two rounds of epinephrine. She is alert, talkative, and has normal vital signs. Her rash and facial swelling have resolved. She is admitted to monitor for the return of signs or symptoms of anaphylaxis.

Question 6-4

Which is NOT a sign or symptom of anaphylaxis?
A) Periorbital edema.
B) Clinging to parents.
C) Targetoid skin lesions.
D) Throat tightness.

Discussion 6-4

The correct answer is "C." Mast cell and basophil degranulation with the release of histamine and other mediators is responsible for the local and systemic manifestations of anaphylaxis (immunologic and nonimmunologic). Anaphylaxis is a clinical diagnosis. Symptoms may onset in minutes to several hours. Clinicians must remain aware that symptoms may be delayed as to avoid missing the diagnosis and delaying treatment with epinephrine. Infants cannot describe their symptoms and may exhibit nonspecific behavioral changes such as crying, fussing, clinging to parents, and irritability. (See Table 2–3.)

After speaking with the girl, you find out she ate cashews 1 hour before she broke out in hives. She eats cashews infrequently and thinks her throat may have felt scratchy the last time she ate them, but nothing like this has happened before.

Question 6-5

Which is NOT a trigger for anaphylaxis?
A) Egg.
B) Nonsteroidal anti-inflammatory medications.
C) Latex.
D) Mosquito bites.
E) Bee stings.

Discussion 6-5

The correct answer is "D." Foods, insect stings (*Hymenoptera* insects), and medications—especially antibiotics—are common

TABLE 2-3 CLINICAL SIGNS AND SYMPTOMS OF ANAPHYLAXIS

Clinical Signs	Symptoms
Urticaria (hives)	Pruritus
Flushing	Nasal congestion, rhinorrhea
Angioedema (face, lips, tongue)	Itching of oropharynx (lips, throat, tongue)
Bronchospasm (wheezing)	Dyspnea
Stridor	Cough
Hypoxia	Vomiting
Respiratory arrest	Abdominal pain
Hypotension	Diarrhea
Tachycardia	Palpitations
Arrhythmias	Chest pain, tightness
Cardiac arrest	Syncope
Conjunctival injection	Sense of impending doom
Tearing	Feeling anxious

causes of IgE-dependent reactions. No trigger may be found in some cases. Milk, soy, egg, peanuts, tree nuts (eg, cashews), shellfish, fish, and wheat are the primary food triggers.

Helpful Tip

Foods are the most common trigger of anaphylaxis in children and adolescents.

⏳ QUICK QUIZ

Which of the following are risk factors for anaphylaxis?
A) Age.
B) Gender.
C) Atopy.
D) Geography.
E) Socioeconomic status.
F) All of the above.

Discussion

The correct answer is "F." Lifetime risk of anaphylaxis is 0.5% to 2%. Atopy is an increased risk for idiopathic, exercise-induced, food, radiocontrast, and latex anaphylaxis. *It is not a risk factor for anaphylaxis to medications.* Anaphylaxis is more common in males until age 15, and in adult females. More cases involve children. More epinephrine pens are prescribed in the northern United States than in the southern counterpart. Higher income also seems to be a risk factor. Exercise, acute infection, fever, and emotional stress are examples of co-factors that may amplify the anaphylactic reaction.

Helpful Tip

Anaphylaxis with exercise may occur upon eating certain foods before exercising. Anaphylaxis does not occur if the food is eaten without exercising. This is called food-dependent, exercise-induced anaphylaxis.

⏳ QUICK QUIZ

Hypersensitivity reactions to radiocontrast media are due to what mechanism?
A) Immunologic anaphylaxis.
B) Nonimmunologic anaphylaxis.
C) Secondary to shellfish allergy.

Discussion

The correct answer is "B." Immunologic anaphylaxis is an IgE-mediated systemic reaction to an allergen. Nonimmunologic (formerly known as anaphylactoid) reactions are non–IgE-mediated. Contrast allergy is secondary to rapid shifts in osmolality with fluid changes causing physical degranulation of mast cells and basophils. Pretreatment with steroids and antihistamines in the hours leading up to contrast administration can often blunt or prevent this response. There is no association between contrast reactions and shellfish/iodine content. Other examples of non-immunologic anaphylaxis (direct mast cell activation) include exercise, cold exposure, and opioid medications.

Helpful Tip

Tryptase is a subgroup of serine peptidases found in mast cells (and to a lesser degree basophils). It is released into the serum following mast cell degranulation. Plasma tryptase levels peak at 60 to 90 minutes after onset of anaphylaxis and persist up to 5 hours after the event. Tryptase is often not elevated in food-induced anaphylaxis.

▶ CASE 7

On a chilly December afternoon, a 12-year-old girl, presents to your office with hives and swelling on her face and hands. She noted them after walking home from the bus stop. Alarmed, her mother rushed her to your office. En route, the girl had mentioned eating a peanut butter candy on the bus that a friend had given her to try. She has no personal history of known food allergy. Other than feeling "itchy" from the hives, she denies any abdominal pain, nausea, chest tightness, or feelings of lightheadedness. On further history, it is noted that she has experienced hives on and off over the past 3 years, mostly in the winter months. She has never had issues during the summer. An episode last year prompted epinephrine administration in the emergency department when she developed full body hives, wheezing, and hypotension after participating in the local "polar plunge" into a partially frozen lake. The family was told to "see an allergist" for further workup but failed to keep the appointment.

Question 7-1

What is the best test to confirm your suspected diagnosis?
A) Ice cube test.
B) Autologous sweat test.
C) Serum-specific IgE to peanut.
D) 24-hour urine histamine collection.
E) C1 inhibitor level and functional assessment (C1 INH).

Discussion 7-1

The correct answer is "A." Cold-induced urticaria is a type of physical urticaria associated with rapid-onset pruritus, erythema, and swelling after exposure to a cold stimulus. Symptoms are often maximal after the area is rewarmed. Massive mediator release can be found when the cold is immersive, such as swimming in cold bodies of water, and may manifest with hypotension. The disease can begin at any age. An ice cube test (placing an ice cube on the arm for 4 minutes, followed by 10 minutes of observation) is diagnostic. Treatment is with antihistamines, with cyproheptadine being preferred in this type of physical urticaria. The problem may resolve spontaneously or persist for several years. Cholinergic urticaria is defined by acute onset of small, punctate wheals and flares associated with exercise, hot showers, sweating, and anxiety. It is diagnosed by an autologous sweat test. Looking for food allergy should be considered in any patient presenting with acute urticaria and angioedema but does not explain the history of hive development outside of this instance. A 24-hour urine histamine collection is helpful in diagnosis of anaphylaxis or suspected mast cell disorders; however, it would not be the best choice in this patient. A C1 INH level and functional assessment are used in the diagnosis of hereditary angioedema. This condition is secondary to a defect in bradykinin metabolism leading to recurrent episodes of angioedema typically with an absence of urticaria.

> **Helpful Tip**
> Physical urticaria comes in various forms, including cold induced, heat induced, cholinergic, pressure, vibration, solar, or aquagenic. A careful history and clinical reproducibility are diagnostic.

QUICK QUIZ

What is the most common cause of acute urticaria in children?
A) Viral illness.
B) Antibiotics.
C) Pet dander.
D) Venom hypersensitivity.

Discussion

The correct answer is "A." Urticaria are transient, raised, blanching, erythematous, pruritic lesions that come and go over the course of several hours to days secondary to released mediators (eg, histamine, leukotriene, prostaglandin, anaphylatoxins such as C5a, etc). These mediators lead to changes in vascular permeability. Acute urticaria is common and thought to affect as many as 20% of people. The most common cause of acute urticaria (hives lasting less than 6 weeks) in children is a recent viral infection. The hives may precede, follow, or occur concurrent to the illness, which often leads to confusion about the diagnosis. Food and drugs are other causes of acute hives. Chronic urticaria (lasting more than 6 weeks) is less common, seen in 1% of the population. Despite common belief, it is rarely associated with food. If persistent, chronic hives should prompt workup for underlying inflammatory conditions such as infection, neoplasm, or autoimmunity. Treatment of acute urticaria is with oral antihistamines, and in severe cases, a short course of oral steroids may be warranted. For chronic urticaria management, a stepwise approach is used to suppress symptoms with a slow wean looking for recurrence. Second-generation H_1 blockade with a nonsedating antihistamines up to four times typical dosing may be used. If hives persist, addition of H_2 blockade and leukotriene receptor blockade may be necessary. For resistant cases, immunomodulators (eg, cyclosporine and mycophenolate) as well as omalizumab (anti-IgE monoclonal antibody) may be appropriate for long-term control.

▶ CASE 8

You are seeing a 5-year-old girl for her springtime well-child check. Mom states her daughter has been doing great overall; however, over the past 1 to 2 years she has noted the child seems to have chronic nasal congestion and pruritus. She will go into "sneezing fits" when she awakes in the morning. Last year, she developed hives along her back and legs after rolling in the grass. You examine the child and note pale, boggy nasal turbinates.

Question 8-1

What would the most effective medicine be in treating her symptoms?
A) Nasal antihistamines.
B) Antileukotriene therapy.
C) Nasal corticosteroids.
D) Oral antihistamines.

Discussion 8-1

The correct answer is "C." Intranasal steroids are the most effective medication for treatment of allergic rhinitis. Allergic rhinitis is commonly noted in older children (must be older than age 3) with primary symptoms of rhinorrhea, nasal or ocular pruritus (or both), eyelid edema, and tearing. It is an IgE-mediated disease associated with other atopic conditions. Its lifetime prevalence is 25%, with 80% of cases developing in childhood. Allergic rhinitis occurs frequently in times of high allergic exposure. For children with tree and grass pollen allergy, this is commonly in the spring (March through June in the northern hemisphere). The fall allergy season is predominantly mold, ragweed, and weeds spanning from mid-August to early frost. Perennial allergens, such as dust mites and animal dander, may lead to year-round symptoms. Allergic rhinitis is uncommon in children younger than age 3, therefore; alternative diagnoses should be considered, including foreign bodies and infectious rhinitis, especially if occurring in the winter months. If the rhinorrhea and congestion is not associated with pruritus and is triggered by strong odors, changes in temperature, foods, emotions, or changes in humidity, it is more likely to be vasomotor rhinitis. This type of nasal symptom responds well to nasal antihistamine sprays. If symptoms are poorly controlled with intranasal corticosteroids an additional agent (options A, B, or D) should be added.

You continue to treat the girl for her allergies for the next several years, but her symptoms are becoming more difficult to adequately control with medications. She was treated for sinusitis twice in the fall during ragweed season. Her mom would like to consider starting her on allergen immunotherapy.

Question 8-2

What is true about allergen immunotherapy?

A) In monosensitized children, allergen immunotherapy can reduce the rate of development of new allergen sensitivities.

B) Immunotherapy is protective against the development of asthma in patients being treated for rhinitis only.

C) Therapy for 3 to 5 years may provide long-lasting remission of symptoms in a third of patients.

D) Immunotherapy causes several changes to the immune system, including induction of T regulatory cells and IgG_4 (blocking antibodies) production, as well as down-regulation of allergen-specific IgE.

E) All of the above.

Discussion 8-2

The correct answer is "E." Children or adolescents not improving with medications and allergen avoidance should be referred to a specialist for allergy testing and consideration of immunotherapy (subcutaneous "allergy shots" or sublingual). The US Food and Drug Administration (FDA) recently approved 3 allergy tablets (sublingual therapy), two for grass pollens and one for ragweed. Immunotherapy involves the repeated exposure to escalating doses of a specific allergen. The child or adolescent must have a documented allergy (history, allergy testing). The goal is to increase immune tolerance to the antigen. Immunotherapy is effective treatment for allergic rhinitis, allergic conjunctivitis, allergic asthma and venom hypersensitivity. Severe or poorly controlled asthma is a contraindication to immunotherapy as it may induce bronchospasm. Subcutaneous therapy may cause anaphylaxis and should be given in a medical setting. Sublingual therapy is safer, has fewer allergic reactions, and may be given at home after the first dose. Currently, immunotherapy is not recommended for food allergies.

Helpful Tip

Consider the evaluation of allergies in children manifesting with recurrent sinusitis or otitis media. When allergies have been excluded, anatomic obstructions preventing normal drainage should be suspected.

Helpful Tip

Nonallergic rhinitis with eosinophilia syndrome (NARES) can present similar to allergic rhinitis, with eosinophils noted on nasal smear cytology, however will have negative skin testing and serum allergen specific IgE. It is thought to be localized mucosal allergy, though the mechanism is poorly understood. It is typically seen in adults and is treated with nasal steroids.

▶ CASE 9

A 13-month-old is brought into your office after developing hives 10 minutes after ingestion of scrambled egg yesterday morning. This was her second exposure to scrambled eggs. Mom immediately gave her diphenhydramine, and the hives resolved shortly thereafter without progression of symptoms. Mom brings her in today and states she wants her "tested for everything!"

Question 9-1

What is the appropriate test to perform in this patient?

A) Skin prick testing for egg.

B) Serum IgE testing for egg.

C) Intradermal testing for egg to overcome the recent antihistamine use.

D) Panel scratch testing for multiple foods, including those currently in her diet.

Discussion 9-1

The correct answer is "B." Skin testing identifies positive IgE sensitization and is thought to be the most sensitive test for detecting allergy. It is measuring released histamine in response to tested allergens, and therefore patients must be off antihistamine medications prior to testing. A general rule of thumb is that long-acting antihistamines (eg, cetirizine, fexofenadine, and loratadine) must be stopped 5 days prior to testing, and shorter acting antihistamines (eg, diphenhydramine) stopped 48 to 72 hours prior to testing. If the response to the histamine control is blunted during testing and the patient has been off oral antihistamines, you must review the medication list to evaluate whether other classes of medications (eg, antidepressants) are leading to antihistaminergic effects. Serum-specific IgE testing (formerly known as RAST testing) measures the amount of allergen-specific IgE produced and circulated in the serum. A patient may remain on antihistamines for this type of testing. It is helpful when skin prick testing cannot be performed (severe atopic dermatitis with poor surface area for testing) or insufficient time has passed since stopping antihistamines. Panel testing for foods is not recommended as there is a high rate of false positives detecting sensitization but not clinical allergy. Intradermal testing to foods is never indicated as it is associated with increased risk of anaphylaxis. Among skin testing techniques, percutaneous (prick/puncture) testing is generally preferred over intradermal testing and can be performed in infants as young as 1 month of age.

> **Helpful Tip**
> A positive skin test or serum IgE for an allergen indicates sensitization. A child is considered allergic if he or she has a concurrent clinical history of symptoms after exposure to the particular allergen.

Question 9-2

What listed factor should not affect validity of allergen skin prick testing?
A) Body area used in testing.
B) Age.
C) Medications.
D) Gender.

Discussion 9-2

The correct answer is "D." Gender does not affect skin testing accuracy or reliability. Skin reactivity can differ depending on where the test is applied, with upper back and forearm thought to be more reliable than areas around the wrist. Infants and elderly patients can have a smaller wheal on testing than those in the second and third decade of life. Antihistamines are obvious contraindications for a histamine-based scratch test; however, other medications such as tricyclic antidepressants and omalizumab can also suppress results. Leukotriene receptor antagonists and oral corticosteroids will not affect results.

QUICK QUIZ

Which is NOT a contraindication for allergy skin testing?
A) Dermatographism.
B) Sunburn.
C) Poorly controlled asthma.
D) Recent anaphylaxis.

Discussion

The correct answer is "B." Limitations of skin testing include the following: (1) it may induce anaphylaxis; (2) it is contraindicated in cases of severe or poorly controlled asthma; (3) it cannot be performed on children with dermatographism, urticaria, and cutaneous mastocytosis (false positive results); (4) it should be avoided in patients with severe eczema; and (5) it is suppressed by certain medications. In cases where skin testing is unable to be performed, serum levels of allergen-specific IgE should be measured.

► CASE 10

A 13-month-old boy is brought to your office by his mother. It seems each time he has a viral upper respiratory tract infection, he develops a cough and wheeze that only resolve with nebulized albuterol. His mother smoked while pregnant, his father has a history of asthma, and the mother is also concerned her baby may have a ragweed allergy. His mother wonders what risk factors may have predisposed him to having these wheezing episodes with upper respiratory tract infections.

Question 10-1

Which of the following is a risk factor for early-onset wheezing?
A) Maternal smoking during pregnancy.
B) Family history of asthma.
C) Ragweed allergy.
D) All of the above.

Discussion 10-1

The correct answer is "A." Transient early wheezing is characterized by repeated episodes of wheezing associated with viral respiratory illnesses occurring in infants up to 2 to 3 years old and resolving thereafter. This is not the same as asthma. The predictor of these wheezing illnesses is premorbid reduced lung function before the development of wheezing. Decreases in lung function are in part determined by passive smoke exposure in utero and result in airway obstruction when infants are infected with respiratory viruses. Atopy and family history of asthma do not influence the incidence of this phenotype. Older children (> 2 to 3 years of age) who wheeze with viral infections are more likely predisposed to asthma. A subset of recurrent wheezers (four or more episodes per year) younger than 3 years of age will go on to have persistent asthma. Risk factors include having a parent with asthma, atopic dermatitis, sensitization to aeroallergens and food (IgE to allergen present, not always symptomatic), eosinophilia (blood), and wheezing without viral respiratory infections. Onset of asthma in children younger than age 3 has been shown in studies to be associated with reduced lung function and growth over time.

> **Helpful Tip**
> Passive smoke exposure including in utero is associated with recurrent wheezing in children younger than 2 years of age.

Question 10-2

What are the three hallmark characteristics of asthma?
A) Fixed airflow obstruction, bronchial hyperresponsiveness, and chronic airway inflammation.
B) Variable airflow obstruction, bronchial hyperresponsiveness, and chronic airway inflammation.
C) Variable airflow obstruction, bronchial hyporesponsiveness, and chronic airway inflammation.
D) Variable airflow obstruction, bronchial hyperresponsiveness, and chronic airway scarring.

Discussion 10-2

The correct answer is "B." Asthma is characterized by variable airflow obstruction, bronchial hyperresponsiveness, and chronic airway inflammation, all of which are likely intertwined and interdependent. It develops in genetically susceptible individuals after environmental exposures such as viral respiratory tract infections, allergens, air pollutants including tobacco smoke, or a combination of these factors. The immune processes involved in the development of these characteristics in asthma are complex, redundant, and interactive, making it difficult to specifically define which factor, or factors, are the principal contributors to these processes and the eventual pathophysiology of asthma. This provides an explanation for the multiple phenotypes of asthma in which the clinical profiles and patterns of inflammation have distinct though overlapping characteristics. Asthma is a disease in which adaptive and innate immunity play major roles. Airway inflammation may result from an imbalanace between proinflammatory cytokines (helper T-cell type 2 response) and protective cytokines (helper T-cell type 1 response).

The mother of the 13-month-old also wonders if where her son was born could have had an effect on his chances of developing asthma. She recalls hearing that the prevalence of asthma varies in different parts of the country, and the world.

Question 10-3

In what region is asthma prevalence generally higher?
A) Urban North America.
B) Rural Africa.
C) Rural Asia.
D) Rural Europe.
E) None of the above.

Discussion 10-3

The correct answer is "A." Large variations in the prevalence of childhood asthma have been reported. Affluent, urbanized centers generally have higher prevalence than poorer centers. Lower levels are seen in rural areas of Africa, Asia, and among farmer's children in Europe. Numerous environmental factors have been examined, but no conclusive explanation for these trends has been found. The "hygiene hypothesis" proposes that the higher prevalence of asthma in Western countries is related to decreased exposure to infections, increased antibiotic use, and decreased exposure to other children (eg, daycare). It is thought that infections early in life cause the immune system to develop along a nonallergic pathway, decreasing the risk of asthma and allergic diseases.

Taking a family history, it is discovered that the 13-month-old has an 8-year-old brother with a history of cat and dust mite allergies and recurrent wheezing. The mother asks if the 8-year-old will wheeze for the rest of his life.

Question 10-4

Which factors would predispose him NOT to outgrow symptoms by adolescence?
A) Frequency of ear infections.
B) Sensitization to allergens.
C) His younger sibling's history of wheezing.
D) Exercise-induced symptoms.
E) None of the above.

Discussion 10-4

The correct answer is "B." Wheezing among school-aged children can be classified into atopic and nonatopic phenotypes. Nonatopic wheezers outgrow symptoms and retain lung function. In atopic wheezers, the timing of atopic sensitization and severity of airway responsiveness determines the progression of this phenotype to asthma from childhood to adolescence. Most epidemiologic studies have used cross-sectional designs and do not allow differentiation between these wheezing phenotypes. Only prospective studies following infants from birth through adolescence will identify different wheezing phenotypes and enable analysis of risk factors for certain wheezing phenotypes.

When the 8-year-old child is exposed to cats, he immediately develops wheezing, itchy watery eyes, and nasal congestion. He notes that a day after exposure, his exercise-induced respiratory symptoms (ie, cough, wheeze) and cold air–induced respiratory symptoms can be worse.

Question 10-5

What is responsible for his early reaction and for his later response to cat dander?
A) Early—eosinophil; late—histamine.
B) Early—T cell; late—B cell.
C) Early—IgE; late—IgG.
D) Early—mast cell; late—eosinophil.
E) All of the above.

Discussion 10-5

The correct answer is "D." During the allergen sensitization phase, IgE-bearing immune cells are established in the nasal and bronchial mucosa. With subsequent allergen exposure, the antigen binds to the two adjacent IgE antibodies on a mast cell or basophil (receptor crosslinking). This leads to degranulation and release of proinflammatory mediators such as histamine, tryptase, leukotrienes, and prostaglandins. These mediators are responsible for the symptoms of an immediate allergic reaction. The late phase reactions occur 4 to 8 hours after an immediate response. Mast cell–derived mediators cause endothelial cells to recruit eosinophils, basophils, and lymphocytes. In addition, tryptase may increase vascular permeability. These leukocytes are then drawn to the airways where they release cytokines and tissue-damaging proteases that contribute to the late-phase response. In allergic rhinitis the late phase response can be congestion and in asthma it can be renewed bronchoconstriction. This chronic inflammation eventually produces airway hyperresponsiveness.

⏳ QUICK QUIZ

True or false: The prevalence of asthma is greater in males than females in all age groups.
A) True.
B) False.

Discussion

The correct answer is "B." In the first decade of life, boys with asthma outnumber girls by 2.5:1. In contrast, adolescence is a dynamic time for the inception and regression of asthma: the prevalence tends to decrease in boys while the incidence increases in girls. In adults, asthma is slightly more common in females, but more importantly, the disease tends to be more severe in female patients.

▶ CASE 11

A 13-year-old comes to your office complaining of shortness of breath since starting a running unit in her gym class. Her symptoms usually start after she has been running for 20 minutes and completely resolve within 5 minutes once she stops to catch her breath. She otherwise has no previous history of asthma or atopic disease. There is no family history of asthma. Her parents wonder if she has exercise-induced asthma.

Question 11-1

What would you tell her parents regarding her respiratory symptoms?
A) Her symptoms are diagnostic of exercise-induced asthma and she should start a daily inhaled corticosteroid.
B) Her symptoms are diagnostic of exercise-induced asthma and she should start albuterol as needed.
C) Her symptoms are not diagnostic of exercise-induced asthma and further evaluation is needed.
D) Her symptoms are diagnostic of persistent asthma and she should start albuterol as needed.

Discussion 11-1

The correct answer is "C." Exercise-induced asthma is acute bronchospasm that is caused by a loss of heat, water, or both from the lung during exercise because of hyperventilation of air that is cooler and dryer than the air in the lungs. Release of inflammatory mediators is also likely involved in the etiology of exercise-induced asthma. Exercise-induced asthma usually occurs during or minutes after vigorous activity, reaches its peak 5 to 10 minutes after stopping the activity, and resolves in another 20 to 30 minutes. The adolescent's timing of symptoms are not diagnostic of exercise-induced asthma and could be related more to deconditioning rather than underlying asthma. Further evaluation is needed. (See Figure 2–1.)

She is seen by an allergist and is later diagnosed with exercise-induced asthma.

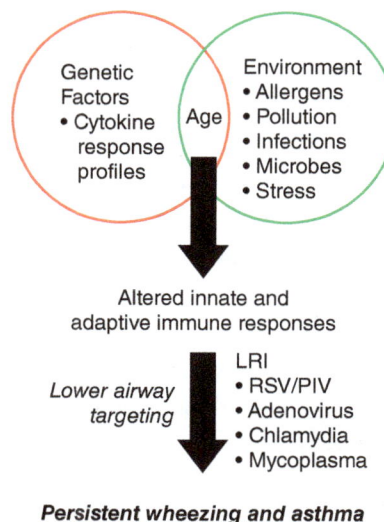

Host factors and environmental exposures

FIGURE 2–1. Host factor and environmental exposures in asthma. LRI, lower respiratory illnesses; PIV, parainfluenza virus; RSV, respiratory syncytial virus. (Reproduced with permission from the National Education and Prevention Program, Expert Panel 3. *Guidelines for the Diagnosis and Management of Asthma*. NIH Publication Number 08-5846. Bethesda, MD: National Institute of Health, October 2007.)

Question 11-2

What recommendations should be made for her as she goes to school?
A) She should use albuterol as needed for shortness of breath from exercise.
B) She should not participate in activities that involve running or other aerobic activity.
C) She should use albuterol 10 to 15 minutes before exercise.
D) She should use albuterol 10 to 15 minutes before exercise and as needed for shortness of breath from exercise.
E) None of the above.

Discussion 11-2

The correct answer is "D." Inhaled beta$_2$-agonists (bronchodilator) will prevent exercise-induced bronchospasm in more than 80% of patients. Inhaled beta$_2$-agonists used 10 to 15 minutes before exercise may be helpful for 2 to 3 hours. An important dimension of adequate asthma control is a patient's ability to participate in any activity he or she chooses without experiencing asthma symptoms. Exercise-induced asthma should not limit either participation or success in vigorous activities. Experts recommend that teachers and coaches be notified that a child or adolescent has exercise-induced asthma, that the child or adolescent should be able to participate in activities, and that the child or adolescent may need inhaled medication before activity.

▶ CASE 12

A new mother is very vigilant about her newborn being exposed to sick contacts. She has also tried to keep her infant away from animal dander and cigarette smoke. She and her husband both have a history of atopic disease.

Question 12-1

Exposure to what viral infection is most likely to affect the possibility of her newborn developing childhood asthma?

A) Human rhinovirus (HRV).
B) Respiratory syncytial virus (RSV).
C) Influenza A virus.
D) Influenza B virus.
E) None of the above; viral illnesses do not affect the development of asthma.

Discussion 12-1

The correct answer is "A." Asthma, the most common chronic disease of childhood, often presents during the preschool years (> 2 years of age) with wheezing viral respiratory infections. Viral wheezing illnesses during childhood are pervasive, with up to 50% of children having at least one episode of wheezing prior to school age. Improvements in molecular diagnostic techniques, through the advent of PCR, have enhanced our ability to recognize novel species and types of viruses previously undocumented or underestimated in the wheezing child, with viral pathogens detected in up to 90% of acute wheezing episodes within the first 3 years of life. HRV, RSV, parainfluenza, coronavirus, influenza, adenovirus, bocavirus, and human metapneumovirus (hMPV) have all been identified in wheezing children, along with bacteria including non-typeable *Haemophilus influenza*, *Streptococcus pneumoniae*, *Moraxella catarrhalis*, *Mycoplasma pneumoniae*, and *Chlamydia pneumoniae*. RSV and HRV are common causes of wheezing respiratory tract infections (bronchiolitis) in infants. In older children and adolescents, rhinovirus is more common. Both are associated with recurrent wheezing but the risk of developing asthma is much higher after HRV infection. The previously difficult to culture HRV-C species has now been identified, with data indicating that this particular virus may be intrinsically more virulent and likely to incite wheezing. It is unclear if infection causes asthma or unmasks asthma in a predisposed child. (See Figure 2–2.)

> **Helpful Tip**
> Rhinovirus and RSV lower respiratory tract infection during infancy and toddlerhood is a risk factor for developing asthma later in childhood.

Question 12-2

In what way could recurrent respiratory infections in infancy lead to asthma?

A) Respiratory epithelium injury.
B) Generation of inflammatory mediators.
C) Activation of inflammatory cells.
D) Abnormal epithelium repair.
E) All of the above.

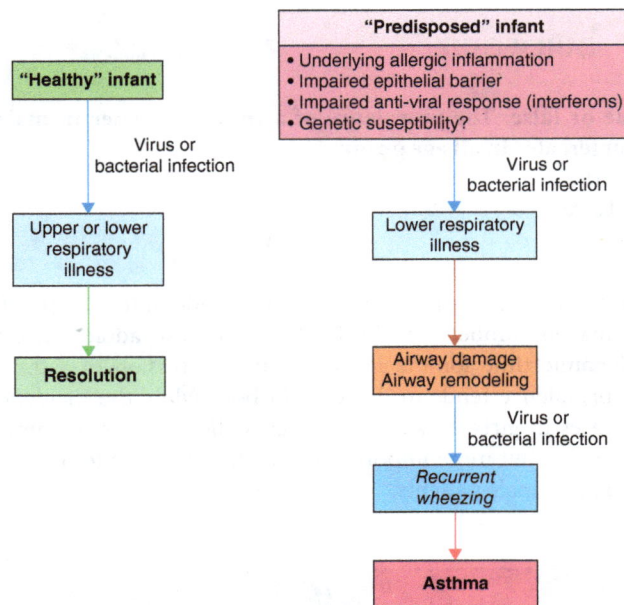

FIGURE 2–2. Pathogenesis of asthma inception. (Reproduced with pemission from Jackson DJ, Lemanske RF Jr: The role of respiratory virus infections in childhood asthma inception, *Immunol Allergy Clin North Am* 2010 Nov;30(4):513–522.)

Discussion 12-2

The correct answer is "E." The epithelium lining cells of the airway is critically involved in asthma. The generation of inflammatory mediators, recruitment and activation of inflammatory cells, and infection by respiratory viruses can cause epithelial cells to produce more inflammatory mediators or injure the epithelium itself. Following injury to the epithelium, the repair process may be abnormal in asthma, and can worsen the obstructive lesions that occur in asthma.

> **Helpful Tip**
> Atelectasis in a person with asthma is not necessarily a sign of pneumonia. The edematous inflammatory response in the airways in asthma can lead to air trapping, hyperinflation, tachypnea, wheezing, and atelectasis

▶ CASE 13

A 14-year-old boy with seasonal allergies and asthma is accompanied by his father for an evaluation in your office. He has symptoms once daily and 2 times per week. He is using albuterol to relieve symptoms once per day. He is not using any other asthma medications.

Question 13-1

What is the initial classification of his asthma severity?

A) Intermittent.
B) Mild intermittent.
C) Mild persistent.
D) Moderate persistent.
E) Severe persistent.

Discussion 13-1

The correct answer is "D." At diagnosis, asthma severity should be classified and triggers and comorbidities identified. Note that asthma care including diagnosis and treatment is divided by age group into 0 to 4 years, 5 to 12 years, and older than 12 years of age. Severity is separated into present impairment (current symptoms, quality of life) and future risk (exacerbations, lung function loss). Impairment is measured based on symptoms and lung function/spirometry (for children 5 years of age or older).

Patients with asthma who have daytime symptoms and use a short-acting beta$_2$-agonist (SABA) less than 2 days per week, nighttime symptoms less than 2 days per month, normal lung function, up to one exacerbation requiring a systemic corticosteroid per year, and no interference with daily activities have intermittent asthma, the least severe classification of the disease. Patients whose symptoms are not controlled by intermittent SABA therapy, leading to daytime symptoms more than 2 days per week, nighttime symptoms more than 2 days per month, worsening lung function, greater than 2 exacerbations requiring systemic corticosteroids per year, and limitations of daily activities have persistent asthma. (See Figure 2–3.) The severity classifications within persistent asthma—mild, moderate, and severe—are based on degree of the intensity of the above-mentioned impairments. An adolescent with moderate persistent asthma would have daily symptoms, nighttime awakenings from asthma more than once per week but not nightly, daily use of albuterol, some limitation to normal activities, and an FEV$_1$ greater than 60% but less than 80% of predicted. (See Tables 2–4 and 2–5.)

Helpful Tip

The term *mild intermittent asthma* is no longer preferred and has been replaced with *intermittent asthma*. This is because the frequency and severity of exacerbations are highly variable among those with asthma. The severity of the disease *does not* always correlate with the frequency or intensity of exacerbations. For example, even those with "intermittent asthma" can have severe exacerbations. This distinction led to reclassification of "mild intermittent asthma" to "intermittent asthma" in the latest asthma guidelines to indicate that these patients cannot be excluded from the risk of severe exacerbations.

Components of severity		Classification of asthma severity (age ≥ 12 years)			
		Intermittent	Persistent		
			Mild	Moderate	Severe
Impairment Normal FEV$_1$/FVC: 8–19 yr - 85% 20–39 yr - 80% 40–59 yr - 75% 60–80 yr - 70%	Symptoms	≤ 2 days/week	> 2 days/week not daily	Daily	Throughout the day
	Nightime awakenings	≤ 2x/month	3-4x/month	> 1x/week but not nightly	7x/week
	SABA use for symptom control	≤ 2 days/week	> 2 days/week but not > 1x/day	Daily	Several time per day
	Interference with normal activity	None	Minor limitation	Some limitation	Extremely limited
	Lung function	Normal FEV$_1$ between exacerbations FEV$_1$ > 80% predicted FEV$_1$/FVC normal	FEV$_1$ ≥ 80% predicted FEV$_1$/FVC normal	FEV$_1$ > 60% but < 80% predicted FEV$_1$/FVC reduced 5%	FEV$_1$ < 60% predicted FEV$_1$/FVC reduced > 5%
Risk	Exacerbations requiring oral systemic corticosteroids	0–1/year	≥ 2/year		
		← Consider severity and interval since last exacerbation. → Frequency and severity may fluctuate over time for patients in any severity category. Relative annual risk of exacerbations may be related to FEV$_1$.			
Recommended step for initiating treatment		Step 1	Step 2	Step 3	Step 4 or 5
				Consider short course of oral corticosteroids	
		In 2–6 weeks, evaluate level of control that is achieved and adjust therapy accordingly			

FIGURE 2–3. Classification of asthma severity. (Reproduced with permission from the National Education and Prevention Program, Expert Panel 3. *Guidelines for the Diagnosis and Management of Asthma.* NIH Publication Number 08-5846. Bethesda, MD: National Institute of Health, October 2007.)

TABLE 2–4 CLASSIFICATION OF ASTHMA SEVERITY IN CHILDREN 0 TO 4 YEARS OF AGE

	Intermittent	Persistent		
		Mild	Moderate	Severe
Daytime symptoms	≤ 2 days/week	> 2 days/week	Daily	Continuous
Nighttime symptoms	None	≤ 2 nights/month	> 2 nights/month	Weekly
SABA use[a]	≤ 2 days/week	> 2 days/week	Daily	Multiple times per day
Activity limitations	None	Minor	Some	Very
Lung function	N/A	N/A	N/A	N/A
Courses of oral corticosteroids	0–1/year	≥ 2/6 months		

[a]Short-acting beta$_2$-agonist (SABA) use for acute symptoms not before exercise

Helpful Tip

When assessing asthma symptoms to determine severity or control, think of the number 2. In general, values ≤ 2 = intermittent or well-controlled asthma (see below). Values > 2 = persistent or poorly controlled asthma.

Daytime symptoms ≤ 2 days per week

Use of relief inhaler (SABA) ≤ 2 times per week

Nighttime symptoms ≤ 2 nights per month

Exacerbations needing oral corticosteroids < 2 per year

Question 13-2

What would the appropriate initial therapy be based on this patient's level of asthma severity?

A) Low-dose inhaled corticosteroid (ICS).
B) Leukotriene receptor antagonist (montelukast).
C) Low-dose ICS + long-acting beta$_2$-agonist (LABA) combination medication.
D) High-dose ICS + LABA combination medication.
E) Monoclonal antibody therapy (omalizumab).

Discussion 13-2

The correct answer is "C." Asthma medications are classified as controllers (taken daily) or quick relief (taken as needed for

TABLE 2–5 CLASSIFICATION OF ASTHMA SEVERITY IN CHILDREN 5 TO 19 YEARS OF AGE

	Intermittent	Persistent		
		Mild	Moderate	Severe
Daytime symptoms	≤ 2 days/week	> 2 days/week	Daily	Continuous
Nighttime symptoms	≤ 2 nights/month	> 2 nights/month	Weekly	Nightly
SABA use[a]	≤ 2 days/week	> 2 days/week	Daily	Multiple times per day
Activity limitations	None	Minor	Some	Very
Lung function 5–11 years	Normal FEV$_1$ between exacerbations FEV$_1$ > 80% FEV$_1$/FVC > 85%	FEV$_1$ ≥ 80% FEV$_1$/FVC > 80%	FEV$_1$ 60–80% FEV$_1$/FVC 75–80%	FEV$_1$ < 60% FEV$_1$/FVC < 75%
Lung function 12–19 years	Normal FEV$_1$ between exacerbations FEV$_1$ > 80% FEV$_1$/FVC normal	FEV$_1$ ≥ 80% FEV$_1$/FVC normal	FEV$_1$ 60–80% FEV$_1$/FVC > 80%	FEV$_1$ < 60% FEV$_1$/FVC < 80%
Courses of oral corticosteroids	0–1/year	≥ 2/year		

[a]Short-acting beta$_2$-agonist (SABA) use for acute symptoms not before exercise.

acute symptoms). Persistent asthma should be treated with a daily controller medication. In all age groups, ICS are the preferred choice when starting a controller. Asthma is treated in a stepwise approach: step 1, intermittent; step 2, mild persistent; step 3, moderate persistent; and step 4, severe persistent; with escalation to steps 5 and 6 if needed. Treatment can be "stepped up" or "stepped down" based on symptoms and lung function. Please refer to the asthma stepwise management figures in the National Asthma Education and Prevention Program Expert Panel Report 3 (ECR-3), *Guidelines for the Diagnosis and Management of Asthma*, published by the National Institute of Health in 2007. (See Figure 2–4.) Based on the adolescent's moderate persistent asthma severity classification, the recommended step for initiating care is step 3. For step 3 care, current guidelines suggest two preferred options, starting a long-acting beta₂-agonist (LABA) in addition to a low-dose ICS, or simply increasing the dose of ICS alone to medium-dose range. Previously, inhaled glucocorticoids alone were considered the first-line treatment for patients

with moderate to severe persistent asthma. The results of the Formoterol and Corticosteroid Establishing Therapy (FACET) study in 1997 supported two components of the stepwise approach to asthma: First, that the addition of a LABA to low-dose ICS in patients with persistent symptoms despite a daily low-dose ICS leads to greater control; and second, that a step up in maintenance dose of ICS may be more appropriate in patients with repeated severe exacerbations of asthma. An alternative therapy option would be to add a leukotriene receptor antagonists (LTRAs) to a low-dose ICS. Omalizumab, anti-IgE, is not indicated in this scenario. It may be used in cases of moderate to severe persistent asthma not controlled by high doses of ICS with LABA when the child has concurrent allergies. It is important to regularly monitor the child's response to medication and make appropriate adjustments as not all children respond the same to medications. In the event that a child is not responding to a specific step 3 therapy, rather than escalate to step 4 therapies, alternative step 3 treatments should be considered.

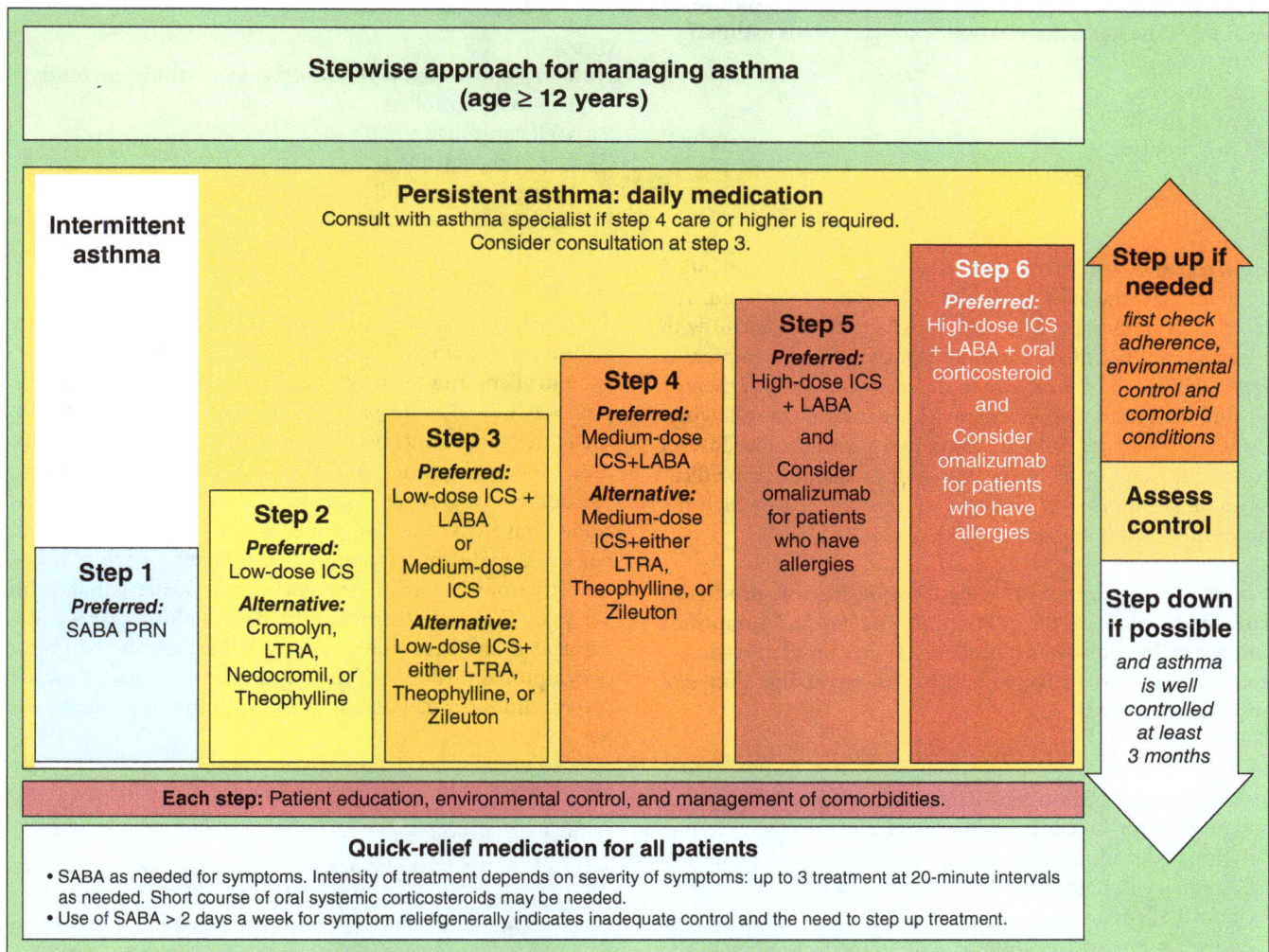

FIGURE 2–4. Stepwise approach for managing asthma. ICS, inhaled corticosteroid; LABA, long-acting beta₂-agonist; LTRA, leukotriene receptor antagonist; SABA, short-acting beta₂-agonist. (Reproduced with permission from the National Education and Prevention Program, Expert Panel 3. *Guidelines for the Diagnosis and Management of Asthma.* NIH Publication Number 08-5846. Bethesda, MD: National Institute of Health, October 2007.)

> **Helpful Tip**
>
> In persistent asthma, ICS are the most effective long-term controller medication and the preferred choice in all age groups. To minimize adverse effects, the lowest ICS dose necessary to maintain control should be used.

> **Helpful Tip**
>
> A LABA such as salmeterol should not be used as a quick-relief medication or monotherapy for long-term control. As a controller medication, a LABA is combined with inhaled corticosteroids to treat moderate to severe persistent asthma.

He is started on a low-dose ICS/LABA combination.

Question 13-3

What is the appropriate time for him to be seen in follow-up to evaluate if he has achieved better control of his asthma?
A) 2 to 5 days.
B) 2 to 6 weeks.
C) 9 to 12 weeks.
D) 3 to 6 months.
E) No follow up is necessary.

Discussion 13-3

The correct answer is "B." Two to 6 weeks is the recommended time to evaluate the level of control that has been achieved. The goal of asthma therapy is to maintain long-term control with the least amount of medication. Responsiveness to treatment is variable with each patient, and to determine if goals of therapy are being met, follow-up assessments are critical. At follow-up, decisions to increase or decrease (when possible) the dose of medication, number of medications, or frequency of medication administration is determined by the degree to which the goals of therapy are being met (level of control).

He returns for a follow-up evaluation on his low-dose ICS/LABA medication. In the past month, he has had symptoms throughout the night, has nighttime awakenings from wheezing every night of the week, and is also requiring albuterol several times per day.

Question 13-4

In addition to prescribing medications, what else is helpful in managing his asthma as an outpatient?
A) Asthma education and creating an asthma action plan.
B) Pulmonary function testing (PFTs).
C) Control of environmental factors.
D) Assessing appropriate compliance and medication administration technique.
E) All of the above.

Discussion 13-4

The correct answer is "E." The ECR-3 asthma guidelines outline four major components of asthma management: (1) objective measurement of lung function (spirometry, exam, history) to assess severity and monitor control, (2) patient and family education, (3) elimination of environmental factors that cause symptoms or exacerbations, and (4) pharmacologic therapy for both maintenance and exacerbations. Spirometry is recommended for all children 5 years of age or older for diagnosing and managing asthma. To properly understand whether pharmacologic therapy is working, it is necessary to confirm good compliance and appropriate medication administration technique.

> **Helpful Tip**
>
> In children, FEV_1/FVC is a more sensitive measurement for classifying asthma severity and monitoring control than FEV_1.

Question 13-5

How well controlled is the adolescent's asthma currently?
A) Too well controlled.
B) Well controlled.
C) Not well controlled.
D) Very poorly controlled.
E) It is too early to make an appropriate assessment.

Discussion 13-5

The correct answer is "D." Once diagnosed, the focus of asthma management depends on whether or not the disease is controlled. The terms used to describe disease control are *well*, *not well*, or *very poorly* controlled. Control is based on the same components used to classify asthma severity. In addition, loss of lung function and adverse effects of treatment are considered. In general, patients with asthma that is well controlled have daytime symptoms or SABA use 2 days or more per week, nighttime symptoms 2 nights per month or less, and exacerbations requiring oral corticosteroids less than 2 times per year. The main distinction between asthma that is not well controlled and very poorly controlled asthma is the presence of symptoms throughout the day, nightly, the use of albuterol several times per day, and an extreme limitation to daily activities. (See Figure 2–5.)

> **Helpful Tip**
>
> At the time of diagnosis and start of therapy, asthma is classified by severity (ie, persistent or intermittent). Afterward the focus is on the degree of control, which will guide clinical management, including medication adjustment.

Components of control		Classification of asthma control (age ≥ 12 years)		
		Well controlled	**Not well controlled**	**Very poorly controlled**
Impairment	Symptoms	≤ 2 days/week	> 2 days/week not daily	Throughout the day
	Nightime awakenings	≤ 2x/month	3–4x/month	7x/week
	Interference with normal activity	None	Minor limitation	Extremely limited
	SABA use for symptom control	≤ 2 days/week	> 2 days/week	Several time per day
	FEV$_1$ or peak flow	> 80% predicted/ personal best	60–80% predicted/ personal best	<60% predicted/ personal best
	Validated questionnaires			
	ATAQ	0	1–2	1–2
	ACQ	≤ 0.75	≥ 1.5	N/A
	ACT	≥ 20	16–19	≤ 15
Risk	Exacerbations requiring oral systemic corticosteroids	0–1/year	◄———— ≥ 2/year ————►	
	Progressive loss of function	◄—— Consider severity and interval since last exacerbation ——►		
		Evaluation requires long-term followup care		
	Treatment-related adverse effects	Medication side effects can vary in intensity from none to very troublesome and worrisome. The level of intensity dose not correlate to specific levels of control but should be considered in the overall assessment of risk.		
Recommended action for treatment		Maintain current step Regular followups every 1–6 months to maintain control Consider step down if well controlled for atleast 3 months	Step up 1 step and reevaluate in 2–6 weeks For side effects, consider alternative treatment options.	Consider short course of oral systemic corticosteroids. Step up 1–2 step, and reevaluate in 2 weeks. For side effects, consider alternative treatment options.

FIGURE 2–5. Classification of asthma control. SABA, short-acting beta$_2$-agonist. (Adapted with permission from the National Education and Prevention Program, Expert Panel 3. *Guidelines for the Diagnosis and Management of Asthma*. NIH Publication Number 08-5846. Bethesda, MD: National Institute of Health, October 2007.)

Question 13-6

With his current symptoms and loss of asthma control, what would be the next appropriate step to manage this patient's symptoms?

A) Advising him to use his albuterol more often.
B) Telling him to allow more time for his low-dose ICS/LABA medication to work.
C) Beginning a short course of oral corticosteroids.
D) Changing his low-dose ICS/LABA to a medium-dose ICS medication alone.
E) None of the above.

Discussion 13-6

The correct answer is "C." Given his very poorly controlled asthma, asthma guidelines recommend a short course (burst) of oral corticosteroids. A short course is recommended when

necessary, because of well-documented risk for side effects from chronic systemic therapy, including adrenal suppression, linear growth suppression, hypertension, development of cushingoid facies, immunosuppression, cataracts, muscle weakness, and decreased bone mineral density.

Question 13-7

Moving forward in his treatment regimen, what would be an appropriate the next step in therapy to consider for the adolescent based on his level of asthma control?

A) Changing to a leukotriene receptor antagonist (montelukast).
B) Changing to a low-dose ICS.
C) Changing to a medium-dose ICS.
D) Changing to a high-dose ICS.
E) Changing to a high-dose ICS + LABA.

Discussion 13-7

The correct answer is "E." In patients with very poorly controlled asthma, guidelines recommend a step-up of one to two steps and a reevaluation in 2 weeks. The adolescent is currently being treated with a low-dose ICS and LABA (step 3). For step 5, high-dose ICS and LABA is the preferred treatment. Omalizumab (monoclonal anti-IgE antibody) may be considered at this step for patients who have sensitivity to relevant perennial allergens (eg, dust mites, cockroach, cat, or dog). Consultation with an asthma specialist is recommended for patients who require this step of therapy.

The adolescent's father, alarmed by his son's recent worsening of asthma symptoms is concerned about his son having "asthma attacks" and wants guidance on when he should take his son to the emergency department for treatment.

Question 13-8

What symptoms would indicate more urgent symptoms that would require the adolescent to seek immediate medical care?
A) Intercostal retractions.
B) Increased exercise-induced symptoms.
C) Dyspnea with speaking.
D) Both A and B.
E) Both A and C.

Discussion 13-8

The correct answer is "E." Asthma exacerbations can be acute or subacute, consisting of worsening shortness of breath, cough, wheezing, and chest tightness. The most common trigger is a viral respiratory tract infection. Milder exacerbations in response to dyspnea with activity can usually be managed at home with use of a SABA as needed for symptoms and close follow-up. More severe exacerbations require medical attention, possible hospital admission, and treatment with a short course of oral corticosteroids to decrease airway inflammation. The most severe exacerbations may require admission to the intensive care unit (ICU). Signs and symptoms of a serious exacerbation include dyspnea at rest or interfering with activities, inability to speak due to dyspnea, tachypnea, intercostal retractions, use of accessory muscles, inspiratory and expiratory wheezing, and hypoxia.

⏳ QUICK QUIZ

What of the following has been identified as a risk factor for death from asthma?
A) Requiring intubation during a previous severe asthma exacerbation.
B) Lower socioeconomic status.
C) Hospitalization or emergency department (ED) visit for asthma in the past month.
D) Poor perception of asthma symptoms or severity of exacerbations.
E) All of the above are risk factors.

Discussion

The correct answer is "E." The following have all been identified as risk factors for death from asthma: prior severe exacerbation requiring intubation or ICU admission, two or more asthma-related hospitalizations in the past year, three or more asthma-related ED visits in the past year, asthma-related hospitalization or ED visit in the past month, using more than two canisters of SABA per month, difficulty recognizing asthma symptoms or severity of exacerbations, lower socioeconomic status or inner-city residence, psychiatric illness, and illicit drug use. Reduced FEV_1 and use of more than SABA canister every 1 to 2 months are associated with increased risk of a severe exacerbation and hospital admission.

The patient later develops a severe exacerbation at night and is taken to the ED. There, he is given two doses of nebulized albuterol with some improvement but he continues to have difficultly speaking, is tachypneic, and his oxygen saturation on room air is 88%.

Question 13-9

In addition to a SABA, what else could be given in the emergency department to provide bronchodilation quickly?
A) Inhaled ipratropium bromide.
B) Inhaled corticosteroid.
C) Theophylline.
D) Chest physiotherapy.

Discussion 13–9

The correct answer is "A." Adding ipratropium bromide (0.25 to 0.5 mg nebulizer solution or 4 to 8 puffs by metered dose inhaler [MDI] every 20 minutes as needed) to albuterol produces additional bronchodilation. In the ED, concurrent use of ipratropium is recommended for severe exacerbations and decreases the rates of hospitalization. During hospitalization, it has not been shown to be beneficial and is not recommended. Doubling the dose of the patient's ICS is no longer recommended to treat acute exacerbations. Methylxanthines (theophylline, aminophylline) are not recommended for the treatment of acute exacerbations. For most asthma exacerbations, chest physiotherapy is not helpful and can be stressful to a patient who is acutely short of breath.

He is receiving a combination nebulization treatment containing albuterol and ipratropium. He continues to have wheezing and retractions but is slightly improved.

Question 13-10

What therapy should he receive next?
A) Magnesium sulfate.
B) Systemic corticosteroids.
C) Terbutaline.
D) Antibiotics.

Discussion 13-10

The correct answer is "B." In an asthma exacerbation, patients should receive an inhaled SABA such as albuterol. SABAs are the most effective agents at relieving acute bronchospasm. Repeated doses or continuous administration may be needed for those who do not improve with initial treatment. Systemic corticosteroids (oral, intravenous, intramuscular) should be given for moderate to severe exacerbations. Some mild exacerbations may require treatment with corticosteroids. Oral administration of steroids is as effective as intravenous administration. If the patient fails to improve, additional treatment options, including magnesium sulfate (smooth muscle relaxant), terbutaline (intravenous beta-agonist), and heliox, may be given to try to prevent intubation. These therapies should be administered in an ICU setting. Antibiotics should be given only if a bacterial infection is documented. When using beta-agonists, inhalation has faster onset, fewer adverse effects, and is more effective than intravenous therapy. Oral beta$_2$-agonists are not recommended.

He is admitted to the hospital and placed on continuous albuterol therapy. In the morning, he is improved but is experiencing adverse effects from albuterol, including tachycardia, tremors, and nausea.

Question 13-11
Which of the following is a sign of toxicity from albuterol?
A) Hyperkalemia and hyperglycemia.
B) Hypokalemia and hyperglycemia.
C) Hyperkalemia and hypoglycemia.
D) Hypokalemia and hypoglycemia.
E) None of the above.

Discussion 13-11
The correct answer is "B." Metabolic disturbances, such as hyperglycemia and hypokalemia have been reported as a form of beta-agonist toxicity. Other side effects include tremor, tachycardia, palpitations, nausea, and vomiting. Serious toxicity is rare and generally seen with systemic therapy (ie, intravenous). Levalbuterol (pure R-isomer of albuterol) produces similar side effects as albuterol (racemic mixture of R- and S-isomers).

⧖ QUICK QUIZ

Which is NOT a risk factor for developing asthma?
A) Parent with asthma.
B) Atopic dermatitis.
C) Dust mite allergy.
D) Elevated serum IgE.
E) All of the above.

Discussion
The correct answer is "E." Asthma has a familial component especially if the mother or father is affected. Atopic dermatitis and allergic rhinitis are associated with asthma. Other risk factors include recurrent wheezing and wheezing with viral respiratory tract infections, sensitization to indoor allergens (dust mite, cockroach, *Alternaria*), obesity, and tobacco smoke exposure. Atopy, IgE production in response to allergens, is the strongest risk factor for developing asthma.

▶ CASE 14

A mother brings her 12-month-old son to the office for a follow-up visit after he developed hives from eating his first bite of peanut butter. He was seen by an allergist and was diagnosed with a peanut allergy. His mother is very concerned that he may be allergic to other foods.

Question 14-1
What are the most common foods that cause allergic reactions in childhood?
A) Peanuts, apples, kiwi, and banana.
B) Crab, lobster, shrimp, and oyster.
C) Milk, egg, peanut, tree nuts, wheat, soy, and fish.
D) Gluten and lactose.
E) None of the above.

Discussion 14-1
The correct answer is "C." The most common foods causing allergy in childhood in descending order are milk > egg > peanut > tree nuts > shellfish > fish > wheat > soy. It is important to tell patients and families that similar foods may cross-react. For example, a child with a cashew allergy may be allergic to other tree nuts. Testing for allergies to similar foods may be indicated before these foods are introduced into the diet.

> **Helpful Tip**
> In oral allergy syndrome or pollen-food allergy, symptoms of throat itching and angioedema of lips occur after eating certain raw fruits (eg, apple, kiwi) and vegetables (eg, potato, carrot) in individuals with pollen allergies. The food antigens cross-react with pollen antigens, causing localized symptoms. Cooked or baked forms of the food may be tolerated as the causative proteins are heat labile.

The mother has been eliminating peanuts and peanut butter from her son's diet, but she has questions about other foods that may contain peanut oil.

Question 14-2
What would you tell the mother about exposure to peanut oil?
A) Hot pressed peanut oil typically does not cause reactions in peanut-allergic children.
B) Cold pressed peanut oil typically does not cause reactions in peanut-allergic children.
C) Hot pressed peanut oil can potentially trigger reactions, and should be avoided in peanut-allergic children.
D) All peanut oil should be avoided completely in any peanut-allergic child.

Discussion 14-2

The correct answer is "A." Hot pressed peanut oil typically does not cause reactions in peanut-allergic children as there is insufficient protein to bind mast cell–bound peanut-specific IgE. Cold compressed oils, however, allow enough protein through the refining process to potentially trigger reactions, and thus should be avoided.

> **Helpful Tip**
> In general, delayed introduction (after 4 to 6 months of age) of highly allergenic foods is not recommended and may increase the risk of allergy development. Infants with atopic disease may benefit from testing or allergist evaluation prior to the introduction of certain foods.

The infant is brought back to your office a few months later with concerns that he had an anaphylactic reaction to another food. The previous week, the family was eating at a picnic for lunch. The picnic consisted of potato salad and hotdogs. Later that night (8 hours later), he began to have vomiting and diarrhea that persisted for 3 days. His mother is concerned that he had an anaphylactic reaction and is allergic to potatoes.

Question 14-3

What additional information would speak against the possibility of his symptoms being caused by anaphylaxis?
A) He had eaten both of those foods previously and tolerated them well.
B) Others in the family had similar symptoms.
C) The timing of onset and duration of gastrointestinal symptoms.
D) The absence of other systemic symptoms.
E) All of the above.

Discussion 14-3

The correct answer is "E." All of the above choices support a diagnosis of food poisoning rather than anaphylaxis. Anaphylaxis is a potentially life-threatening reaction that can affect breathing and send the body into shock. Typically, these reactions simultaneously affect different parts of the body (eg, vomiting and diarrhea accompanied by hives). Most food-related anaphylaxis symptoms occur within 2 hours of ingestion; often they start within minutes. Typically symptoms do not occur in foods that were previously tolerated. Symptoms typically resolve within 24 hours of onset. Other family members having similar symptoms would support the possibility of food poisoning.

The mother asks if her son will outgrow his peanut allergy as he gets older. You tell her that it is a possibility but unlikely.

Question 14-4

Which food allergy is a child LEAST likely to outgrow?
A) Almond.
B) Soy.
C) Wheat.
D) Milk.
E) Egg.

Discussion 14-4

The correct answer is "A." Children are most likely to outgrow their allergic reactions to milk, wheat, soy, and eggs, with some studies indicating between 65% and 80% remittance. Peanut, tree nut, shellfish, and fish allergies are likely to persist. Roughly 1 in 5 children will outgrow peanut allergy, with 1 in 10 outgrowing tree nut allergy.

Over the next year, he has increasing problems with atopic dermatitis. You have prescribed him topical emollients and high-dose topical steroids without good control of symptoms. His typical daily diet consists of eggs, milk, wheat, and soy. He infrequently eats apples, melon, broccoli, tomato, chicken, and beef. He continues to avoid peanuts.

Question 14-5

Of the foods below, what could be the most likely to contribute to his persistent moderate to severe atopic dermatitis?
A) Peanut.
B) Chicken.
C) Egg.
D) Broccoli.
E) Tree nuts.

Discussion 14-5

The correct answer is "C." Food allergy can be a contributor to moderate to severe atopic dermatitis. Between 50% and 60% of children with moderate to severe atopic dermatitis have IgE-mediated food allergy. Unlike the immediate IgE-mediated reactions of hives and anaphylaxis with foods, children with atopic dermatitis and food allergy may have a delayed reaction presenting as an acute flare or worsening of their skin disease. It is recommended that children younger than 5 years of age who have moderate to severe atopic dermatitis be evaluated for milk, egg, peanut, wheat, and soy allergies if the child continues to have atopic dermatitis even after treatment. Empiric elimination without evidence of IgE-mediated allergy is not recommended.

QUICK QUIZ

Which is NOT a method for diagnosing an IgE-mediated food allergy?
A) Intradermal (intracutaneous) skin testing
B) Skin prick testing.
C) Serum allergen IgE testing.
D) Oral food challenges.

Discussion

The correct answer is "A." Useful tools to diagnosis an IgE-mediated food allergy include skin prick testing and serum allergen

IgE testing. Remember to diagnosis an allergy the child must have evidence of sensitization (positive test result) and clinical symptoms when the food is ingested. Intradermal testing is not recommended for food allergies. Panel testing for a large number of foods should be avoided. Remember only a small number of foods cause the majority of IgE-mediated reactions, therefore; testing should focus on the suspected food(s) or the most common triggering foods (eg, peanut, milk, egg). If testing is negative but suspicion remains high or the history is uncertain, an oral food challenge should be performed. Oral food challenges are also helpful to determine whether or not an allergy has resolved.

► CASE 15

You are treating an 8-year-old girl with recurrent acute otitis media for an ear infection. She is typically treated successfully with amoxicillin or amoxicillin/clavulanate (Augmentin). On day 7 of her 10-day course of amoxicillin, she develops hives. You advise her mother to stop giving her this medication immediately. The hives continue for 8 days before resolving. In a follow-up call the mother reports that her daughter has no arthritis symptoms, other nonurticarial rashes, angioedema, or respiratory symptoms.

Question 15-1

What type of hypersensitivity reaction is she having?
A) Type I IgE-mediated mast cell degranulation to amoxicillin.
B) Type II cytotoxic antibody (IgG) formation to amoxicillin.

C) Type III immune complex formation and deposition in response to amoxicillin.
D) Type IV delayed type hypersensitivity reaction to amoxicillin.
E) None of the above; this reaction is not likely due to amoxicillin.

Discussion 15-1

The correct answer is "E." The fact that the medication has been previously tolerated on multiple occasions, the onset was after 7 days of use, and resolution came 8 days after stopping the medication make the possibility of this being an IgE-mediated allergic reaction less likely. A type I IgE-mediated hypersensitivity reaction to a medication typically occurs within the first few exposures to a new medication. The onset of symptoms is also typically during the first few doses of the medication. Symptoms typically resolve within 1 to 2 days of discontinuation of the medication. Her symptoms are also not consistent with a type II, type III, or type IV hypersensitivity reaction. Examples of such reactions would be: type II reaction—new anemia while on a medication; type III—fever, arthritis, lymphadenopathy, and hives after taking the medication for more than 1 week; and type IV—macular rash several days after starting the medication. However, rather than a reaction to the medication itself, the girl's hives are most likely related to the underlying infection. Hives in response to infections are the most common identifiable cause of hives in children. In children infections were identified in 57% of acute urticaria cases with viral upper respiratory tract or digestive infections being the most common. As a virus stimulates the immune system, mast cells can be triggered to degranulate and cause hives. This is usually self-limited process that is well controlled with higher doses of nonsedating antihistamines. (See Table 2–6.)

TABLE 2–6 COOMBS AND GELL CLASSIFICATION OF HYPERSENSITIVITY REACTIONS

	Mechanism	Example	Description
Type I	IgE-mediated mast cell or basophil degranulation	Anaphylaxis, urticaria	Free antigens cross-link the IgE on mast cells and basophils, which causes release of vasoactive biomolecules Onset: minutes to hours Must have prior exposure to antigen (sensitization)
Type II	Cytotoxic antibody formation	Autoimmune hemolytic anemia, Goodpasture syndrome, drug-induced thrombocytopenia	IgM or IgG bind to antigen on a target host cell that is perceived by immune system as foreign, leading to cellular destruction Onset: minutes to hours
Type III	Immune complex formation and deposition leading to complement activation	Serum sickness, postinfectious glomerulonephritis	Antibody (IgG) binds to soluble antigen, forming circulating immune complexes that are deposited in blood vessel walls (endothelium), tissues, or both, initiating a local inflammatory reaction Onset: hours
Type IV	Delayed hypersensitivity	Contact dermatitis, positive tuberculin skin test	Helper T cells are activated by an antigen-presenting cell; when the antigen is presented again in the future, memory T cells activate macrophages, causing an inflammatory response; this ultimately can lead to tissue damage Occurs over 1–2 days

► CASE 16

A 5-year-old develops diffuse hives and swelling 15 minutes after his second dose of a sulfonamide-containing antibiotic. His symptoms resolve completely after taking diphenhydramine. He has not taken any more doses of this medication. One week later, his mother brings him to your office and asks you if he is allergic to "sulfa drugs."

Question 16-1

How should a drug allergy be diagnosed in this patient?
A) Skin testing.
B) Blood testing (specific IgE).
C) Patch testing.
D) Oral challenge.
E) The diagnosis can be made by history alone.

Discussion 16-1

The correct answer is "E." Allergy testing by skin or blood test to most drugs is not standardized and has very little data to support interpretations of results. Penicillin is the only drug for which a validated IgE skin test can be performed. However, his symptoms are very suggestive of an IgE-mediated type 1 hypersensitivity reaction. An oral challenge may cause an anaphylactic reaction and is not recommended. Based on his history and description of symptoms, he should be considered to have an allergy to sulfonamide-containing medications. Patch testing is used to identify contact allergens.

QUICK QUIZ

Which drug is NOT capable of causing direct mast cell degranulation?
A) Vancomycin.
B) Opioids.
C) Fluoroquinolones.
D) Penicillin.

Discussion

The correct answer is "D." In a penicillin allergy, mast cell degranulation is IgE-mediated (type 1 hypersensitivity reaction). The other choices cause direct mast cell degranulation (non–IgE-mediated reaction). Radiocontrast dye, mannitol, intravenous iron, N-acetylcysteine, corticosteroids, blood products, and some chemotherapy agents may also cause direct mast cell degranulation. This type of reaction was formerly called an anaphylactoid reaction and is not a true allergy.

► CASE 17

A 3-year-old boy is brought for evaluation of a chronic rash that has been intermittently flaring in the past year. The rash was worse in the winter months. It is dry, pruritic, and patchy and is most severe on his popliteal fossa and antecubital fossa bilaterally.

Question 17-1

What is the most likely cause of his symptoms?
A) Urticaria.
B) Psoriasis.
C) Atopic dermatitis.
D) Molluscum contagiosum.
E) Pityriasis rosea.

Discussion 17-1

The correct answer is "C." Atopic dermatitis or eczema is an inflammatory skin condition characterized by erythema, pruritus, and scaly rashes. It often appears on the arms, legs, hands, and face. The severe pruritus of atopic dermatitis can often disturb sleep. Excessive scratching and excoriation of the skin can lead to superinfection. Approximately 60% of patients develop atopic dermatitis by age 1, and another 30% experience symptoms by age 5. Children born into families that have a history of atopic diseases (eg, asthma or allergic rhinitis) are at an increased risk for developing eczema. Atopic dermatitis is considered to be part of the "atopic march," which involves the development of atopic dermatitis, food allergy, allergic rhinitis, and asthma, usually in that sequential order.

QUICK QUIZ

Which of the following is/are true regarding the pathogenesis of atopic dermatitis?
A) Impaired skin barrier function.
B) Increased skin transepidermal water loss.
C) Increased skin entry of allergens, antigens, and environmental chemicals.
D) All of the above.

Discussion

The correct answer is "D." An intact, healthy skin barrier is a critical first line of defense against various microbes, irritants, and allergens. The epidermis of atopic dermatitis patients is characterized by significant barrier disruption, which leads to increase transepidermal water loss. This may also be why symptoms are worse in the winter months when the climate is drier. Patients with atopic dermatitis also have an increased susceptibility to allergic sensitization as well as microbial colonization and infections.

Question 17-2

What is the best initial treatment for the child's symptoms?
A) Topical antihistamine cream.
B) Oral antihistamine medications.
C) Topical emollients and topical corticosteroids.
D) Topical emollients and oral corticosteroids.
E) Topical corticosteroid only.

Discussion 17-2

The correct answer is "C." A topical emollient (or moisturizer) helps repair the skin barrier and prevent water loss. Ointments or creams (not lotions) are preferred. The emollient should be applied immediately after bathing while the skin is still wet, to help lock moisture in the skin. The topical corticosteroid treats the underlying inflammatory process of atopic dermatitis, reducing inflammation, easing irritation, and reducing pruritus.

You see him for a follow-up visit. While his lower extremity atopic dermatitis has improved, he continues to have persistent cracked, excoriated, dry patches on his antecubital fossa bilaterally. He had food allergy testing that revealed no underlying food allergies.

Question 17-3

What is another recommended treatment for his severe atopic dermatitis?
A) Continue his current medication regimen and add the application of wet bandages on his affected skin patches.
B) Continue his current medication regimen and add the use of calamine lotion.
C) Discontinuing the topical corticosteroid and double the dose of his daily emollient.
D) Continue his current medication regimen and start an empiric egg elimination diet.
E) None of the above.

Discussion 17-3

The correct answer is "A." The use of wet bandages or wet wraps has been proven to be an effective treatment in severe atopic dermatitis. Wet wraps serve a few different functions. As water gradually evaporates from the bandages this cooling of the skin and helps relieve inflammation, itching, and soreness. Emollients applied to the skin and then wrapped with wet bandages are deeply absorbed into the skin to provide a longer lasting moisturizing effect. In a similar manner, there is an enhanced absorption of topical steroid molecules into both the superficial and deeper layers of skin where inflammation is present. The bandages provide protection from the itching and scratching cycle so that skin gets a chance to heal properly. This has been proven to control signs and symptoms within hours to days of application. Wet wrapping can be done at home, but if the area of application is large, it is sometimes it is done in a hospital because it can be labor intensive and require nursing expertise.

The mother is concerned about the long-term complications of her son's atopic dermatitis if it persists.

Question 17-4

Which of the following are potential complications of poorly controlled atopic dermatitis?
A) Sleep problems.
B) Lichen simplex chronicus.
C) Skin infections.
D) Allergic contact dermatitis.
E) All of the above.

Discussion 17-4

The correct answer is "E." All of the listed options can be potential complications of atopic dermatitis. Lichen simplex chronicus (or neurodermatitis) is a skin condition caused by chronic scratching of the skin. This condition can cause the affected skin to become discolored, thick, and leathery. Repeated scratching that breaks the skin can cause open sores and cracks. These increase the risk of infection from bacteria and viruses. Allergic contact dermatitis is common in patients with atopic dermatitis. This may be related to a compromised skin barrier. The itch-scratch cycle can cause children to awaken repeatedly at night and decrease the quality of sleep.

BIBLIOGRAPHY

Bernstein IL, Li JT, Bernstein DI, et al. Allergy diagnostic testing: An updated practice parameter. *Ann Allergy Asthma Immunol.* 2008;100(3 suppl 3):S1–148.

Boguniewicz M, Leung DY. Atopic dermatitis: A disease of altered skin barrier and immune dysregulation. *Immunol Rev.* 2011;242(1):233–246.

Buckley RH. Primary immunodeficiency diseases. In: Adkinson N, Busse W, Bochner B, et al, eds, *Middleton's Allergy: Principles and Practice.* 7th ed. Philadelphia, PA: Mosby; 2008: 801–829.

Cox L, Nelson H, Lockey R, et al. Allergen immunotherapy: A practice parameter third update. *J Allergy Clin Immunol.* 2011;127(1 suppl):S1–55. doi: 10.1016/j.jaci.2010.09.034.

Dezateux C, Stocks J, Dundas I, et al. Impaired airway function and wheezing in infancy: The influence of maternal smoking and genetic predisposition to asthma. *Am J Respir Crit Care Med.* 1999;159:403–410.

Expert Panel Report 3 (EPR-3). *Guidelines for the Diagnosis and Management of Asthma—Full Report 2007.* NIH publication No. 08-5846. Bethesda, MD: US Department of Health and Human Services; National Institutes of Health; National Heart, Lung, and Blood Institute; National Asthma Education and Prevention Program; 2007.

Frew AJ. Allergen immunotherapy. *J Allergy Clin Immunol.* 2010;125:S306–S313.

Geha R, Notarangelo L. *Case Studies in Immunology: A Clinical Companion.* 6th ed. New York, NY: Garland Science; 2011.

Gell PGH, Coombs RRA, eds. *Clinical Aspects of Immunology.* Oxford, England: Blackwell; 1963.

Holt PG, Macaubas C, Stumbles PA, et al. The role of allergy in the development of asthma. *Nature.* 1999;402:B12–B17.

Illi S, von Mutius E, Lau S, et al. Perennial allergen sensitization early in life and chronic asthma in children: A birth cohort study. *Lancet.* 2006;368:763–770.

Jackson DJ, Lemanske RF Jr. The role of respiratory infections in childhood asthma inception. *Immunol Allergy Clin North Am.* 2010;30:513–522.

Johnston SL, Pattemore PK, Sanderson G, et al. Community study of role of viral infections in exacerbations of asthma in 9-11 year old children. *BMJ.* 1995;310:1225–1229.

Kaplan AP. Urticaria and angioedema. In: Adkinson N, Busse W, Bochner B, et al, eds. *Middleton's Allergy:*

Principles and Practice. 7th ed. Philadelphia, PA: Mosby; 2008:1063–1081.

Kelso JM. A second dose of epinephrine for anaphylaxis: Epinephrine for anaphylaxis: How often needed and how to carry? *J Allergy Clin Immunol.* 2006;117:464–465.

Korenblatt P, Lundie MJ, Dankner RE, et al. A retrospective study of epinephrine administration for anaphylaxis: How many doses are needed? *Allergy Asthma Proc.* 1999;20:383–386.

Kuyper LM, Pare PD, Hogg JC, et al. Characterization of airway plugging in fatal asthma. *Am J Med.* 2003;115(1):6–11.

Lieberman PL. Anaphylaxis. In: Adkinson N, Busse W, Bochner B, et al, eds. *Middleton's Allergy: Principles and Practice.* 7th ed. Philadelphia, PA: Mosby; 2008:1027–1049.

Miller EK, Edwards KM, Weinberg GA, et al. A novel group of rhinoviruses is associated with asthma hospitalizations. *J Allergy Clin Immunol.* 2009;123:98–104.

Morgan WJ, Stern DA, Sherrill DL, et al. Outcome of asthma and wheezing in the first 6 years of life: follow-up through adolescence. *Am J Respir Crit Care Med.* 2005;172:1253–1258.

Nelson HS. Immunotherapy for inhalant allergens. In: Adkinson N, Busse W, Bochner B, et al, eds. *Middleton's Allergy: Principles and Practice.* 7th ed. Philadelphia, PA: Mosby, 2008: 1657–1677.

Parameswaran K, Belda J, Rowe BH. Addition of intravenous aminophylline to beta2-agonists in adults with acute asthma. *Cochrane Database Syst Rev.* 2000;(4):CD002742.

Pauwels RA, Lofdahl CG, Postma DS, et al. Effect of inhaled formoterol and budesonide on exacerbations of asthma. *N Engl J Med.* 1997;337:1405–1411.

Platts-Mills TA. The role of immunoglobulin E in allergy and asthma. Am J Respir Crit Care Med. 2001;164:S1–S5.

Plotnick LH, Ducharme FM. Combined inhaled anticholinergics and beta2-agonists for initial treatment of acute asthma in children. *Cochrane Database Syst Rev.* 2000;(4):CD000060.

Polito AJ, Proud D. Epithelia cells as regulators of airway inflammation. *J Allergy Clin Immunol.* 1998;102(5): 714–718. Review.

Sampson HA, Aceves S, Bock SA, et al. Food allergy: A practice parameter update—2014. *J Allergy Clin Immunol.* 2014;134(5), 1016-1025.e1043. doi: 10.1016/j.jaci.2014.05.013.

Sampson HA, Burks WA. Adverse reactions to foods. In: Adkinson N, Busse W, Bochner B, et al, eds. *Middleton's Allergy: Principles and Practice.* 7th ed. Philadelphia, PA: Mosby; 2008:1139–1167.

Seidman MD, Gurgel RK, Lin SY, et al. Clinical practice guideline: Allergic rhinitis. *Otolaryngology Head Neck Surg.* 2015;152(1 suppl):S1–S43. doi: 10.1177/0194599814561600

Simons FE, Ardusso LR, Bilo MB, et al. World allergy organization guidelines for the assessment and management of anaphylaxis. *World Allergy Organ J.* 2011;4(2):13–37. doi: 10.1097/WOX.0b013e318211496c.

Spahn JD, Covar R, Szefer SJ. Glucocorticoids: B. Clinical science. In: Adkinson NJ, Bochner BS, Busse WW, et al, eds. *Middleton's Allergy: Principles and Practice.* 6th ed. Philadelphia: Mosby; 2003:887–913.

Tager IB, Ngo L, Hanrahan JP. Maternal smoking during pregnancy: Effects on lung function during the first 18 months of life. *Am J Respir Crit Care Med.* 1995;152:977–983.

Thomas A, Lemanske RF, Jackson DJ. Approaches to stepping up and stepping down care in asthmatic patients. *J Allergy Clin Immunol.* 2011;128:915–924.

Thomas AO, Lemanske RF Jr, Jackson DJ. Infections and their role in childhood asthma inception. *Pediatr Allergy Immunol.* 2014;25:122–128.

TREC screening can show newborn's T cells are low. July 2013. American Academy of Allergy Asthma and Immunology website. http://www.aaaai.org/global/latest-research-summaries/Current-JACI-Research/TREC-screening. aspx. Accessed October 5, 2015.

Uekert SJ, Akan G, Evans MD, et al. Gender related differences in immune development and the expression of atopy in early childhood. *J Allergy Clin Immunol.* 2006;118(6):1375–1381.

von Mutius E. Paediatric origins of adults lung disease. *Thorax.* 2001;56:153–157.

Wardlaw AJ, Brightling C, Green R, et al. Eosinophils in asthma and other allergic diseases. *Br Med Bull.* 2000;56:985–1003.

Wedi B, Raap U, Wieczorek D, Kapp A. Urticaria and infections. *Allergy Asthma Clin Immunol.* 2009;5(1):10.

Behavioral and Mental Health Issues 3

Linda J. Cooper-Brown and Jennifer Mc Williams

This chapter is meant to cover the behavior and mental health material that could be tested on the Pediatrics Board Exam. However, due to copyright issues, we are not able to share the diagnostic criteria tables from the *Diagnostic and Statistical Manual of Mental Disorders,* Fifth Edition *(DSM-5).* Summaries are provided, but we would encourage the reader to seek out and review the *DSM-5* diagnostic criteria tables for the following disorders:

- Conduct disorder
- Oppositional defiant disorder
- Major depressive disorder
- Depressive disorder severity
- Attention deficit hyperactivity disorder

▶ CASE 1

The father of a 5-year-old child is concerned that his son still sucks his thumb. This behavior is most common when they read a book together at night, while watching television, or when in the car.

Question 1-1
What should this parent do?
A) Point out to the child whenever he is seen sucking his thumb so he knows when it is occurring.
B) Put a bitter substance on the thumb to make thumb sucking aversive.
C) Have the child wear a glove to make it less appealing to suck his thumb.
D) Identify triggers and provide alternative behaviors the child can use.
E) Tell the child that his thumb might fall off if he continues to suck it.

Discussion 1-1
The best answer is "D." Thumb sucking is a common habit among children. Babies have natural rooting and sucking reflexes, and some can even be seen with their thumbs in their mouths in ultrasound images before birth. Babies often develop thumb (or finger) sucking to comfort or soothe themselves.

As children grow older, they often develop other coping skills to use when upset, anxious, or tired. Most children stop sucking their thumbs on their own, usually between 2 and 4 years of age. Thumb sucking usually is not a concern until a child's permanent teeth come in. Because it is most likely a self-soothing activity, children will be more successful at stopping if taught alternative ways to calm or soothe themselves rather than being punished or prevented from sucking. In this case, the child could hold the book or engage his hands when the parent is reading, or the parent could give the child a stuffed animal, Koosh ball, or other "fidget" toy while watching television and during or car rides. The parent should involve the child in helping to identify things to hold or do that would provide comfort at the times most likely to be associated with thumb sucking.

▶ CASE 2

A mother brings her 3-year-old son to the clinic for a well-child visit. He is growing and developing within normal limits; however, the mother states that he is a very "picky" eater, preferring to eat certain foods and refusing to try new foods. She asks you if she should be concerned and what to do.

Question 2-1

What percentage of toddlers are described as picky eaters by their parents?
A) Less than 2%.
B) Less than 10%.
C) Up to 50%.
D) Up to 75%.
E) Close to 100%.

Discussion 2-1

The correct answer is "C." Variation occurs in reporting among studies, but up to 50% of toddlers are described by parents as "picky," meaning the child eats a limited amount or variety of food, is unwilling to try new foods, and has strong food preferences. If the child is growing appropriately, he or she is getting adequate calories. Reassurance and mealtime recommendations may help prevent the need for further intervention.

⌛ QUICK QUIZ

Which is NOT a helpful tip to prevent feeding problems from becoming major problems?
A) Set a schedule for three meals and one or two snacks per day.
B) Establish a routine of what meals and snacks look like. Eat at a dinner table and not on the run.
C) Do not feel pressured to try the new foods being served to the child.
D) Offer a new food many times as it may take 10 to 20 attempts before the child will accept it.
E) Offer new foods at the start of a meal when the child may be hungriest.

Discussion

The correct answer is "C". Other helpful tips include the following: (1) Establish mealtime rituals (sit together, pass dishes, practice manners and etiquette, avoid distractions, and so on). (2) Do not let the child graze on food or dinks throughout the day. The child will not be as likely to eat or try new foods if he or she is full all the time. (3) Establish a routine of what meals and snacks look like. (4) Remember that parents or caregivers serve as role models. You can't expect the child to eat something you won't eat yourself. If you want your child to eat certain foods, you have to eat them, too.

▶ CASE 3

Parents bring their 4-year-old son to the clinic for concerns related to poor eating. They report that the child is willing to eat just about every food offered, but only eats a few bites during meals and then says he is done.

Question 3-1

What would you do?
A) Investigate possible constipation.
B) Identify how much fluid the child is drinking during the day.
C) Ask what happens between these meals related to offering food.
D) All of the above.
E) None of the above.

Discussion 3-1

The correct answer is "D." These are fairly common and relatively easy-to-treat issues that can contribute to a lack of appetite. If the child is constipated, he may not be hungry. Likewise, if the child is drinking excessive amounts of fluid this can curb his appetite. Identify how much fluid is needed for daily intake. Finally, eating (and drinking) throughout the day, especially close to a meal, contribute to reduced hunger. Consistent use of a treatment for constipation, scheduled meals and snacks, and discontinuing fluid intake at least 1 hour before a meal or snack can positively affect food intake.

▶ CASE 4

A 2-year-old girl is brought to the clinic because her mother is worried that she is not yet toilet trained. The child is inconsistently dry after naps and kicks and screams every time a parent tries to have her sit on the potty seat. Grandmother told the mother that her own children were trained well before age 2 years, which has the mother especially worried. Should she be concerned?

Question 4-1

What factors contribute to toilet training readiness? The child:
A) Shows interest in using a potty chair or toilet and may complain about wet or dirty diapers.
B) Stays dry for 2 hours or longer during the day.
C) Can follow basic directions such as "sit down" or "follow me."
D) Can communicate through words, expressions, or posture when needing to go.
E) All of the above.

Discussion 4-1

The correct answer is "E." When it comes to potty training, parents often have unrealistic expectations. Although the mother may have been ready and trained before 2 years of age, this child is not yet ready. The American Academy of Pediatrics (AAP) recommends starting potty training once the child is developmentally ready and shows signs of readiness or interest (see Table 3–1).

> **Helpful Tip**
> Remember, toileting accidents are common when a child is stressed.

▶ CASE 5

A mother brings her 4-year-old son to the clinic. She is frustrated because the child is not yet consistently having bowel movements in the toilet, although he urinates in the toilet.

TABLE 3–1 SIGNS OF READINESS THAT IT IS TIME TO TOILET TRAIN

Can walk to the toilet

Can sit on the toilet

Can stay dry for several hours

Can follow one- and two-step commands

Can communicate the need to use the toilet through words or gestures

Wants to please caregivers

Wants independence

The mother is concerned because he will be starting school soon. She wants to know if this is normal for his age.

Question 5-1

Regarding bowel and bladder control, which of the follow statements is (are) correct?
A) Bowel control is typically achieved before bladder control.
B) Daytime bladder control should be achieved by age 4.
C) Twenty percent of 5-year-olds and 10% of 6-year-olds have primary nocturnal enuresis.
D) Persistent nocturnal stooling in an older child suggests encopresis.
E) All of the above.

Discussion 5-1

The correct answer is "E". The child already uses the toilet successfully for urination and he is older than would be expected to achieve bowel control. He should be assessed for developmental delay, genitourinary abnormalities or constipation. If all is reassuring, you may want to suggest specific strategies for delayed toileting:

- Scheduled toilet-sitting times about 20 minutes after eating.
- Make sure the child has his feet securely positioned on a step stool or the floor to permit adequate "pushing" or bearing down.
- Provide small rewards for "trying" to have a bowel movement and bigger rewards for successes.
- Do not use rewards for an absence of accidents or the child may learn to withhold even more.

> **Helpful Tip**
> If the child has a history of constipation, he or she may not be motivated to use the toilet due to fear of hard stools. Make sure the stool is easy to pass for toilet training success.

> **Helpful Tip**
> The best rewards are often highly preferred activities rather than food. Advise parents to set these activities aside and use them only for toileting times so they remain effective. The rewards may need to be changed weekly to keep the child motivated.

▶ CASE 6

The parents of a 1½-year-old girl express concern that their daughter is biting at home and in a daycare setting. Parents and staff cannot figure out a reason for her behavior, which occurs whether she is happy or upset. They tell her "no" every time it happens, but it continues to occur.

Question 6-1

What is (are) the most likely reason(s) she is biting? She is biting because:
A) She lacks alternative language skills to express herself.
B) She is not getting enough attention during the day.
C) She is not getting enough oral stimulation.
D) She gets a reaction from adults or peers.
E) Both A and D.

Discussion 6-1

The correct answer is "E." Biting is very common in children. Approximately 10% of children younger than 4 years of age have bitten another child at least once. Some are wild animals needing socialization. During infancy children explore their environment using all of their senses. Anything near an infant's mouth is a candidate for mouthing or biting. Biting in infancy is often an experiential occurrence. By 18 months to 2 years, children learn that their behavior leads to desired outcomes and bite because it results in attention or toys. It is not usually the case that the child does not have enough of something. It is more likely that the child has learned (over time) that biting produces the outcome more immediately. For example, a toy that another child is holding is released right away, the child who is biting gets picked up quickly, or she is offered many alternatives after being told "no."

> **Helpful Tip**
> As the child learns more appropriate ways to express wants and needs, and how to wait, biting should decrease. Parents and other adults can help by teaching age-appropriate language skills and rewarding the child (with the desired attention and toys) for using words instead of biting. If biting continues to occur beyond 3½ years of age, a referral to experts such as behavioral psychologists may be helpful.

▶ CASE 7

At a well-child check, the mother of a 5-year-old mentions that her son won't listen to her when she asks a question. He continues to engage in whatever he is doing. She has to ask the question repeatedly and finally get his attention by turning his face toward her. She has tried time-outs, ultimatums, taking things away, and yelling. Nothing works.

Question 7-1

What advice regarding limit setting should you give her?
A) Increase the length of time he sits in time-out.
B) Stop asking him questions if he isn't going to answer.
C) Take notice when he does listen and praise him for the good behavior.
D) Your efforts will be futile no matter what method is used.
E) Long discussions about why his behavior is undesirable are helpful.

Discussion 7-1

The correct answer is "C." Children are not miniature adults. Although they may act as though they want to be in control, they need parents to provide limits and consistent rules. These provide children with a greater sense of security and help them to learn how to get along with others and, eventually, how to discipline themselves.

> **Helpful Tip**
> Top 10 Tips for Discipline and Limit Setting:
> 1. Be consistent. "Yes" means "yes" and "no" means "no."
> 2. Make it short and sweet. Provide concrete one-step directions: "Put the cars in the bin," "put your clothes in this drawer," rather than "Put your toys and clothes away."
> 3. Remember to "catch" your child being good and praise often. Don't take good for granted.
> 4. Provide lots of chances to teach the correct behavior. Don't assume your children know how to be good. Show them.
> 5. Respond quickly to good and bad. Immediacy is important.
> 6. Phrase your request as a statement, not a question. A question implies a choice. For example, "It is time for bed," not "Are you ready for bed?"
> 7. Be patient. Behaviors take time to change. It can take at least a week to change problem behavior for every month it has occurred.
> 8. Be prepared for an increase in problems when trying to change behaviors. Behavior often gets worse before they get better as the child is learning the rules.
> 9. Be united as parents across time and households.
> 10. Pick and choose battles. Not making a request because you are tired is better than making a request and giving in because you cannot follow through on the request.

▶ CASE 8

A mother brings her 3-year-old son to you because she is convinced there is something wrong with him. He just had a birthday and received many new toys, but when they were

TABLE 3–2 COMMON TRIGGERS AND INTERVENTIONS FOR BEHAVIOR PROBLEMS

Trigger	Intervention
Desire to gain access to something such as a toy, activity, or attention ("I want it now")	• Place child in safe area to prevent injury during tantrum • Time-out from reinforcement • Do not give in to tantrum
Desire to avoid or escape unpleasant or nonpreferred activities or tasks ("I don't want to do it")	• Place child in safe area to prevent injury during tantrum • Time-out from reinforcement • Do not give up on original request
Frustration, difficulty communicating	• Ignore until calm (may need to place in safe area to prevent injury during tantrum) • Offer to help after child calms

recently at the store he saw something he wanted and had a major meltdown that included banging his head when told "no." The mother has ignored his screaming, but head banging is a new behavior. She wonders why he would try to hurt himself.

Question 8-1

You tell her that head banging:
A) Is a behavior that suggests deeper mental health issues.
B) Is another form of tantrum behavior.
C) Suggest the need for medical testing.
D) Suggests he has a high pain tolerance.
E) Is caused by a headache.

Discussion 8-1

The correct answer is "B." Tantrums can include behaviors that range from whining, crying, and screaming to hitting, kicking, stomping, and head banging. The causes are varied, and the behaviors can happen anywhere (see Table 3–2). Children often escalate to more severe behaviors when more minor ones do not provide the desired outcome. No matter how smart a child appears, toddlers are not very good at verbally communicating feelings, wants, or needs. As vocabulary and language skills improve, tantrums generally decrease. Identifying the triggers for tantrums leads to intervention strategies. (Would the same strategies work for adult tantrums? If so, reality television might no longer exist.)

The mother is captivated. She has tried time-outs but isn't sure how to use this method of discipline successfully.

Question 8-2

What do you tell her?
A) Time-outs should always last 2 minutes.
B) Time-outs should always last 5 minutes.

C) Time-outs should last until the child has calmed down.
D) The child should be allowed to read a book or other quiet activity while in time-out.
E) A special time-out stool is needed to reinforce the concept to the child.

Discussion 8-2

The correct answer is "C." There are many ways to implement time-out. Some of the key components include the following:

- Time-out needs to last long enough to get the child's attention and convey that negative behaviors result in negative consequences, or put another way, negative behaviors never result in desired outcomes. It does not have to last for a set number of minutes and should last until the child has calmed. It should never end when the child is still having a tantrum.

- Time-out does not have to involve a special location. It should occur away from any action and fun activities. It could mean simply walking away from the child or it could mean removing the child to a carpeted, safe area. Nothing should occur while the child is in time-out.

- For time-out to work there has to be a "time-in" environment. Time-out is actually time out from reinforcement and time-in is all the fun and positive things, including positive attention from parents. First, throughout the day parents should acknowledge positive behavior and not take it for granted. Second, when a child has calmed after time-out, parents should let the child know what kinds of behaviors will work to get the desired outcomes.

▶ CASE 9

A 3-year-old girl attends daycare all day while her parents work. When the family arrives home, is time to fix dinner and do chores. The girl often behaves well at daycare but has tantrums at home. Her parents wonder if she is not getting enough attention from them and if one of them should quit work.

Question 9-1

What do you suggest?
A) The mother should quit her job as daughters respond better to female caregivers.
B) The father should quit his job as daughters respond better to male caregivers.
C) She is not getting adequate sleep and should have an earlier bedtime.
D) The parents should ignore the tantrums and hope they will cease with time.
E) The parents should find time each evening to engage in a fun activity with her.

Discussion 9-1

The correct answer is "E." It is hard to comment about whether one parent should quit work, but because the daughter seems to have the most difficulties at home, it is likely that she has learned that a tantrum is the quickest way to get a parent's attention. This is likely a case of too little "time-in." Her parents are probably busy upon arriving home and ignore her until she engages in a tantrum. Finding times to provide even intermittent attention upon arrival home may reduce some of the tantrums. Advise parents to help the child get started with a fun activity and provide some positive attention as they prepare dinner. Spending 5 minutes with her before starting dinner, and interspersing attention may go a long way in decreasing the unwanted behaviors.

▶ CASE 10

The parent of a 16-month-old girl describes a recent episode in which the child became upset at the park, started crying, stopped suddenly, turned slightly blue around the lips, and then stopped breathing, went limp, and fell to the ground. Less than a minute later the child recovered and returned to normal breathing and activity. The parent is convinced that the child had a seizure and is reluctant to let the child have a tantrum for fear of causing additional seizures.

Question 10-1

What most likely occurred?
A) The child held her breath to upset the parent when she could not get her way.
B) The child had a breath-holding spell beyond her control.
C) The child had a seizure.
D) The child had an episode of supraventricular tachycardia.
E) The child has amazing acting skills.

Discussion 10-1

The correct answer is "B." It is most likely a breath-holding spell. Breath-holding spells typically occur in children starting at 6 to 18 months of age and usually stop by the time the child is 7 years old. Such episodes can be upsetting to parents and others who see them. These are not seizures and do not harm the child, although a child may have a secondary anoxic seizure. Furthermore, the child is not holding his or her breath on purpose to be able to pass out. The episodes can be triggered by fear, pain, anger, or frustration. Typically the child starts to cry and then no further sound is heard but the child still appears to be crying. This is different than voluntarily holding one's breath, which occurs when an individual deeply inhales and then holds his or her breath. Breath-holding spells are sometimes classified into two types of episodes: pallid and cyanotic (see Table 3–3). Breath-holding spells may run in families and are more common in children with iron deficiency. Treatment involves reassuring the parents of the benign nature of the episodes and providing iron supplementation for those who are deficient.

TABLE 3-3 BREATH-HOLDING SPELLS

	Pallid Episodes	Cyanotic Episodes
Trigger	Fear, pain	Frustration, anger
Onset	Gasp, cry	Vigorous crying
Course	• Becomes pale, loses consciousness, goes limp • May become sweaty, stiffen, jerk • Lasts less than 1 minute • Regains consciousness and may appear tired	• Rapidly turns bluish, especially around lips, loses consciousness • May stiffen, arch back • Lasts less than 1 minute • Regains consciousness and returns to normal

Helpful Tip

Although breath-holding spells are triggered when the child becomes upset, they do not represent a behavior problem and most children who have episodes of breath-holding spells are otherwise healthy. The natural tendency would be for the parent to pick up and hold the child, but this position may prolong the event. The best intervention is to leave the child lying on the ground, positioned on his or her side. No other intervention is needed as the child will resume breathing in less than 1 minute. When a child is known to have breath-holding spells, a parent may avoid allowing the child to become upset by giving in to tantrums. However, the spells generally decrease and stop by 7 to 8 years of age. Giving in to crying episodes and tantrums to prevent the child from becoming upset will only create behavior problems. The child will learn quite quickly to start crying to obtain desired outcomes.

QUICK QUIZ

Which strategy is NOT recommended as a way to help a child adjust to the arrival of a baby sibling?
A) Allow the child to help care for the baby.
B) Spend a short amount of time each day with the child.
C) Allow the child to have increased screen time while he or she adjusts.
D) Show the child his or her own baby pictures.
E) Have patience and understand that this is a big adjustment for the child.

Discussion

The correct answer is "C." Tips for helping a child prepare and for and welcome a new sibling include the following:

- The child can be allowed to have a role in preparing the home.
- The parent can have the child help care for the baby by bringing a diaper or selecting an outfit.
- Have the parent schedule special time with each sibling. To do this, the parent sets aside a short time each day (eg, when the baby is napping or another adult is available to care for the baby) to do an activity of the child's choice.
- The parent should share special baby memories with the child as a reminder of how important he or she is to the family.

► CASE 11

A parent comes to the clinic with 5- and 6-year-old siblings for their well-child checks. While in the clinic the children fight over the parent's cell phone, each demanding a turn. One of the children sits in the only small chair in the room, but whenever the child gets up, the other child quickly takes over the chair creating a physical battle and tattling. The parent says it is like this at home, but doesn't know what to do.

Question 11-1

What do you suggest?
A) Remind the parent that all siblings have some rivalry and it will go away someday.
B) Have the parent encourage the children to work out their differences but assist as needed.
C) Suggest the parent ground the children from video time at home and any other fun activities for today.
D) Have the parent listen to each child's story and pick a side.
E) Ignore the behavior even if the children get physical as long as no one gets injured.

Discussion 11-1

The best answer is "B." It is not uncommon for siblings to engage in problem behaviors with each other, but reassurance alone will not help the parent. The children should be given an opportunity to find a way to work out their differences. However, if the children get physical with each other, the parent must step in and make it clear that it is never acceptable to hit, pinch, bite, punch, shove, and so on. These behaviors may require a time-out. The parent's focus should be on teaching appropriate ways to handle differences rather than doling out punishment, such as groundings or removal of activities, for conflicts. Tips for reducing sibling conflicts include the following:

- If the siblings cannot figure out a way to play together, a timer can be used to teach them how to share a desired toy or activity. This is especially useful for very young toddlers who want items immediately and have no concept of sharing. The timer signals the beginning and end of each child's turn with the toy.
- The parent should use an "in/out" rule for tattling: Have the child think about why he or she wants to tell on a sibling. If it is to get someone "in" trouble, the child should not tattle

and the parent will not listen. If it is to keep the sibling from getting hurt or "out" of trouble, the child should let the parent know right away.

- Encourage the parent to show appreciation for each child's uniqueness and avoid comparisons. Rivalry often occurs when comparisons are made. Help the parent focus on each child's unique personality, ability, and temperament, and give compliments whenever possible.
- Remind the parent to "catch" the children playing well together and praise them for following the rules.

For the time in your office, you may want to suggest using a timer for turns with the small chair and other items such as the cell phone. It is also acceptable to put the cell phone in time-out and focus on turns with other items in the office.

► CASE 12

Parents bring their 2½-year-old son to clinic and are concerned that he has started awakening at night and screaming. His eyes are open and he seems awake, but does not react to their attempts to calm him. They want to know what to do.

Question 12-1

What do you tell them?
A) He is having a seizure.
B) He is acting out trying to get his parents' attention.
C) He has no memory of these events.
D) He is hallucinating.
E) He needs to consume less sugar.

Discussion 12-1

The correct answer is "C." The child is having night terrors (see Table 3–4).

► CASE 13

The parents of a 4-year-old boy both work and need a good night's sleep. Their son often has a hard time going to sleep, taking several hours to fall asleep because he needs water, to tell them something, or has other requests. When he doesn't fall asleep he may start crying and want to come to their room. The parents ask if you can prescribe medications to help their son fall asleep and stay asleep.

Question 13-1

Is medication appropriate for this child and, if so, what medication?
A) Yes.
B) No.

Discussion 13-1

The correct answer is "B." The difficultly this child has in initiating sleep is behavioral. The parents need to establish good sleep hygiene habits and a consistent bedtime routine. Consistency is key.

You counsel the parents that even if medication is prescribed, it is important to have good sleep hygiene. The parents look confused.

Questions 13-2

Which strategy is a component of good sleep hygiene?
A) Have a television or other electronic device in the child's bedroom that he can play with or watch until sleepy enough to fall asleep.
B) Have a consistent bedtime routine but vary the actual time the child goes to bed.
C) Minimize late afternoon napping so the child is tired at bedtime.
D) Allow the child to do whatever he wants as long as he stays in his bedroom.
E) Eat a late night sugary snack as a treat to get the child to go to bed.

TABLE 3–4 NIGHTMARES VERSUS NIGHT TERRORS

	Nightmare	Night Terror
What is the child doing?	Eyes open, awake and alert, frightened, breathing fast, aware of parent presence	Appears awake but confused, crying uncontrollably, shaky, breathing fast, glazed look, does not recognize parent
When?	Second half of night when dreaming intense	Early in night when deepest stages of sleep
Is the child awake?	Yes	No
Will the child remember the event?	Yes	No
Will the child return to peaceful sleep?	Maybe	Yes
Best parent response	Immediate comfort and reassurance; when calm help put child back to bed	Prevent child from hurting self; wait for child to calm; do not discuss in the morning

Discussion 13-2

The correct answer is "C." Sleep hygiene refers to good habits and routines that help a child learn to fall asleep and remain sleeping. Tips for establishing good sleep hygiene include the following:

- Set a consistent bedtime. Determine the amount of sleep the child needs and time he or she must awaken in the morning to set the bedtime.
- Develop a consistent routine (eg, taking bath, putting on pajamas, brushing teeth, reading a book), and end with being in bed and turning off the lights.
- Allow for wind down time before sleep time.
- Adjust naps to prevent late sleeping during the day.
- Remove electronic gadgets from the bedroom. These tend to entertain and prevent sleep.

....

The parents seem to be onboard thus far but want to know what you recommend when he keeps waking up. They have not been successful in dealing with this behavior.

Question 13-3

What do you tell the parents about managing the child's frequent nighttime awakening?
A) Briefly check on the child if he is in his bed and provide reassurance.
B) Install a lock on the outside of the door so the child cannot leave his room upon awakening.
C) Allow the child to enter the parent's room as long as he sleeps on the floor and not in the bed.
D) Ignore the child unless he becomes distraught.
E) Alternate one parent lying down with the child until he falls asleep.

Discussion 13-3

The correct answer is "A." Children typically call out or seek out a parent because they want something—usually attention. They often escalate their behavior until the parent gives in to let others in the household sleep. Several strategies can be suggested. Advise parents to do a quick check: Parents tell the child they will come to his room to check on him as long as he is in bed. Check-in should occur for only a matter of seconds and involve looking into the room. Parents determine the timing of these check-ins and how often they occur during a night, gradually lengthening the time between check-ins. In handling problems, parents should:

- Make sure the child is safe but ignore the child's behavior, regardless of how intense or loud.
- Expect sleep-deprived nights.
- If the child leaves the room, return her without discussion or attention.

Bedtime tickets or passes can be used:

- The child is provided a set number of tickets each night to use in requesting a drink, hug, to tell the parent one last thing, and so forth, but without leaving his or her room.

TABLE 3–5 NORMAL SLEEP PATTERNS BY AGE	
Infants (1–2 months)	• 10–18 hours/day • Sleep around the clock • Sleep/wake cycle interacts with need to be fed, changed, held
Infants (3–11 months)	• 9–12 hours/day • About 75% sleep through the night by 9 months of age • One to four naps per day lasting 30 minutes to 2 hours
Toddlers (1–3 years)	• 12–14 hours/day • By 18 months, most nap once per day lasting 1–3 hours
Preschoolers (3–5 years)	• 11–13 hours/day • Most do not nap by 5 years of age
School-aged (5–12 years)	• 10–11 hours/day • May get less than optimal sleep due to scheduled activities or competing attention from electronic gadgets

- Every time the child calls to the parent, the parent enters the room to assist, but removes a ticket.
- When tickets are gone, all behavior must be ignored.
- Any unused tickets are collected in the morning. If any tickets remain, the parent can provide a reward in the morning.

Normal sleep patterns by age are listed in Table 3–5.

⧗ QUICK QUIZ

Which statement does NOT describe parent–infant attachment?
A) It is an emotional relationship between the infant and parent.
B) It is based upon the parent's response to the infant.
C) It involves nonverbal actions.
D) It provides the infant with a sense of security.
E) It is the same as bonding.

Discussion

The correct answer is "E." Attachment is an aspect of the parent-child relationship that contributes to making the child feel safe, secure, and protected. It is not the same as bonding. A simple example can illustrate this process. A family's cat bats their infant son on the head, frightening him. The infant crawls crying to his father and is calmed after he is picked up. The father is viewed as a protector, having conveyed nonverbally that the infant is safe. Factors influencing parent–infant attachment include:

- The parent's response to the infant when he or she is hurt, frightened or upset.
- The amount of care (physical and emotional) provided by the parent.

► CASE 14

The mother of a 6-week-old boy is distraught. She tells you her baby never stops crying. It started 1 month ago and has been getting worse. It always seems to happen in the early evening. The infant will cry uncontrollably for hours. She has tried baths, car rides, stroller rides, carrying him in a sling, feeding, changing his diaper, gripe water, music, and even letting him "cry it out." She reluctantly admits that she has found herself overly frustrated at times and doesn't want to hurt the baby.

Question 14-1

What do you tell her?
A) Colic begins at 2 weeks of age.
B) Colic equally affects breastfed and formula fed babies.
C) An infant cries 2.2 hours per day on average.

Discussion 14-1

The correct answer is "A." Between 10% and 26% of infants are colicky. The etiology of colic is unclear. Colic was defined in a 1954 article as crying more than 3 hours per day, more than 3 days per week, and more than 3 weeks in duration. It usually starts at 2 weeks, peaks at 6 weeks, and resolves by 12 to 16 weeks of age. Babies with colic are more difficult to console.

Question 14-2

How is colic diagnosed?
A) History and physical examination.
B) Elevated creatine kinase level related to tensing of muscles during crying episodes.
C) Elevated amylase level related to excess secretions during crying episodes.
D) An abdominal radiograph showing large amounts of gas.
E) All of the above.

Discussion 14-2

The correct answer is "A." Colic is a diagnosis of exclusion based on history and physical examination. An organic cause is found in less than 5% of infants evaluated for colic.

Question 14-3

What do you NOT offer the mother as a management suggestion?
A) Swaddle the baby in a sleep sack.
B) Ask others to help watch the baby during crying episodes.
C) Change to a soy formula.
D) Develop a safety plan for use when she is feeling frustrated.
E) Use a white noise machine or fan.

Discussion 14-3

The correct answer is "C." Treatment includes parental support, reassurance, and education. Parents should identify other caregivers who would be willing to help. Interventions for the baby include swaddling, minimizing stimulations, white noise, and rocking. It is important to remind parents to never shake a baby! Soy and lactose-free formulas have not been shown to be beneficial although many parents have already tried dietary changes. Simethicone is safe but ineffective. The limited current data do not support the use of complementary and alternative treatments, including probiotics, chiropractic treatment, and massage. (Really? The infants didn't like massage?)

► CASE 15

A mother calls the office after hours, crying. She needs advice on dealing with her 11-year-old son. This year at school he has been caught lying, stealing, and cheating on multiple occasions. He has lost school privileges and had to stay after school but the behaviors continue. The father is not concerned as he feels "boys will be boys". Today the mother was called into the principal's office because her son was caught stealing candy from a school fundraiser.

Question 15-1

What do you recommend?
A) She should have spanked the child more as a toddler.
B) She should send him to a boarding school.
C) He should visit a juvenile detention center for a day to "scare him straight."
D) He should have his cell phone taken away for a short period of time.
E) She should not worry as the child will outgrow the behavior on his own.

Discussion 15-1

The correct answer is "D." Lying and stealing fall under the category of undesirable behaviors. There are two main strategies for dealing with such behavior: removing the positive reinforcement for the behavior and providing a negative reinforcement. Both can be used to take away the positive reinforcement of the behavior. The privilege that is removed must be important to the child in order for this strategy to work. Punishment uses a negative action to reduce the behavior. Punishment may involve verbal reprimands or corporal punishment (inflicting physical pain). If used frequently verbal reprimands lose effectiveness. Spanking has been used by more than 90% of American families to stop undesirable behaviors. Spanking has negative long-term consequences and is less effective than time-out or removal of privileges; therefore, the AAP recommends that physicians help parents develop alternative methods of discipline.

► CASE 16

A 2-year-old girl is brought by her mother for a well-child check. The toddler begins to sob and throw a tantrum when her mother steps out of the exam room to sign some paperwork, leaving her with the nurse. When she returns, the mother apologizes profusely and states that she would like some advice on how to handle her daughter's tantrums as they have increased in intensity to the point that the mother is unable to leave her with anyone else.

Question 16-1

How would you treat the toddler's tantrums?

A) Prescribe fluoxetine for separation anxiety.
B) Refer the child and her mother for therapy with a psychologist who specializes in early childhood disorders.
C) Reassure the mother that the child's behavior is normal for her age.
D) Recommend a multimodal treatment plan including both medication and therapy.

Discussion 16-1

The correct answer is "C." Separation anxiety is normal for children between the ages of 6 and 30 months. While it may be beneficial to counsel parents on how to respond to their child's anxiety, neither medication nor therapy is recommended for this age group.

► CASE 17

An 8-year-old girl is brought to the clinic. The mother says her daughter will not leave her side out of fear that something horrible will happen to the mother. It has gotten so bad the child must sleep with the door open so she can see her parents' room. She hasn't been to school for 2 weeks.

Question 17-1

What do you tell the mother?

A) The child's behavior is normal and often seen at this age.
B) The child may have separation anxiety disorder.
C) The child is likely being bullied at school.
D) The behavior is a ploy by the child to avoid going to school.
E) The child should be allowed to stay home from school.

Discussion 17-1

The correct answer is "B." According to the *DSM-5,* separation anxiety disorder (SAD) is diagnosed when the child has "developmentally inappropriate and excessive anxiety concerning separation" from home or the primary caregiver(s). Typically onset of SAD is between 7 and 9 years of age. In SAD, the child becomes anxious at the thought of being separated from caregivers out fear that something bad will happen to them. Everyone experiences anxiety now and then. (Are you apprehensive about a little thing called boards? If so, congratulations you are anxious!) Anxiety becomes a disorder or disease when it consumes and interferes with life. Separation anxiety is very common and part of normal development. Think of a 2-year-old crying and clinging to a parent at the daycare drop-off. When such anxiety becomes obsessive or persists into childhood, then there is a problem. For example, a fourth grader may be tearful when first dropped off at a sleepover but quickly able to join the fun. Had the child stayed in the corner crying and obsessing, that would be SAD.

Helpful Tip

Anxiety disorders are the leading psychiatric disorders diagnosed in children.

In talking with the mother, you learn that the father was recently diagnosed with cancer. He is undergoing treatment, and doctors are optimistic that his cancer is curable. The mother tells you that the child was sometimes homesick in the past and occasionally had to leave sleepovers when she was younger, but this had improved. She emphasize that the child's behaviors were never this extreme before.

Question 17-2

Which life event is NOT associated with the development of SAD?

A) Death.
B) Divorce.
C) Illness.
D) New baby.
E) All of the above.

Discussion 17-2

The correct answer is "D." Signs of SAD may first appear after the child's home life is disturbed. Examples include divorce of parents, parental illness, death of a family member, financial issues affecting the home, and or a move to a new location.

Question 17-3

Which of the following is a symptom of SAD?

A) School refusal.
B) Headaches.
C) Fear the parent will be harmed.
D) Inability to be separated from the parent for even a short time.
E) All of the above are symptoms of SAD.

Discussion 17-3

The correct answer is "E." Like everything in pediatrics, symptoms vary by age. It is common for teens to worry about school performance or social interactions but these concerns resolve as the adolescent matures. Refusal to go to school out of fear of being separated from a parent is a red flag. Truancy is different. It is a deliberate avoidance of school for no good reason.

You diagnose the child with SAD and have a long discussion with the mother. You provide information and support services. You refer the child to a psychiatrist but it will take a month to get an appointment. She needs help now.

Question 17-4

Which of the following measures is (are) appropriate for SAD?

A) Selective serotonin reuptake inhibitor.
B) Cognitive behavioral therapy.
C) Educating parents to stop enabling the child.
D) Return to school.
E) All of the above.

Discussion 17-4

The correct answer is "E." SAD should not be chalked up to poor coping skills. It is often a gateway to future mental illness. A multimodal treatment plan, including parent psychoeducation, a selective serotonin reuptake inhibitor, and cognitive behavioral therapy, is recommended. Parents need to be assertive, and the child needs to go to school.

► CASE 18

A ninth grader is brought for evaluation by his mother. He has missed 20 days of school this year because of various headaches, stomach aches, and other complaints. No physical causes have been determined despite an extensive workup. When the possibility that he is trying to avoid school is brought up, his mother reports that it has been hard to make him go to school since his dad moved out last year. In addition, she knows there is a "bully problem" at the high school, and she is concerned he is being picked on.

Question 18-1

What is the best next step?
A) Contact the school counselor, after obtaining a release of information form from the mother, and ask about the adolescent's social interactions and academic performance.
B) Refer the adolescent to a psychologist who specializes in anxiety disorders.
C) Suggest to the mother that she call the school's truant officer next time the adolescent refuses to go to school.
D) All of the above.

Discussion 18-1

The correct answer is "A." Children and adolescents with school refusal are a heterogeneous group and the evaluation should include a variety of components. Collateral information from school personnel is very important to help identify psychological factors such as depression and anxiety, social factors such as bullying and peer influences, and academic factors such as learning difficulties. In addition, the evaluation may include a clinical interview or semistructured diagnostic interview with the patient; collateral information from parents regarding psychological, social, and academic factors; and a psychoeducational evaluation to assess for learning disorders. If, after a thorough evaluation has been completed, anxiety is felt to be the primary component of the etiology, then psychotherapy would be vital. If, on the other hand, a disruptive behavior disorder such as conduct disorder is determined to be the primary cause, then involvement of the legal system may be necessary. Often a multimodal treatment plan involving, parents, school officials, psychotherapy, and possibly medication is needed. Regardless, the cause of the school refusal must be fully evaluated first (see Table 3–6).

TABLE 3–6 SCHOOL REFUSAL

Type of School Refusal	Prevalence (%)	Mean Age of Onset (years)	Percentage of Males
Anxious	1.6	10.9	47.9
Truants	5.8	13.1	65.1
Mixed	0.5	—	51.9

► CASE 19

At a 2-year well-child check, you ask if there are any other concerns. The father looks at the floor, then sheepishly mentions that his son likes to touch himself in public. The parents have tried telling him "you shouldn't touch your wee-wee," "that's not nice," and even "good boys don't do that." The grandmother told the father that this is abnormal behavior and there must be something wrong. She actually wondered if the babysitter is touching him. The father asks for advice.

Question 19-1

What do you tell him?
A) Male infants may have erections.
B) It is normal for toddlers to masturbate.
C) Using nicknames for genitalia is not recommended.
D) Children should not be punished for normal sexual behaviors.
E) All of the above.

Discussion 19-1

The correct answer is "E." Normal versus abnormal sexual behaviors are differentiated based on cultural and societal beliefs. Masturbation and sexual exploration are part of normal development that begins in infancy (see Table 3–7). Since this behavior is normal, parents should be reassured and children allowed to explore without reprimand. Early in life, these behaviors occur in public. As the child gets older, privacy becomes important. Parents should be encouraged to use proper anatomical terms for genitalia instead of nicknames, which may cause confusion.

⧗ QUICK QUIZ

Which of the following is NOT a characteristic of a resilient child?
A) Becomes angry when faced with a challenge.
B) Has a strong connection to the community.
C) Knows he or she is loved unconditionally.
D) Recognizes that his or her actions affect outcomes.
E) Able to maintain perspective when dealing with problems.

TABLE 3–7 NORMAL SEXUAL BEHAVIORS BY AGE AND DEVELOPMENTAL STAGE

0–12 months	Masturbation
Infancy	Explore genital area during diaper changes and baths
	Erections
1–4 years	Masturbation (public)
Toddler	Touch mother's body parts (eg, breasts)
	Take clothes off
	Expose genitalia to others
5–11 years	Masturbation (private)
Children	Ask or talk about sex
	Dress up as opposite sex
	Play "doctor" (explore peers' genitalia)
12–18 years	Masturbation
Adolescents	Explore sexual intimacy with others
	Questioning or awareness of sexual orientation
	Sexually active

Discussion

The correct answer is "A." Resiliency allows a child to deal with the ups and downs of life. To be resilient, a child needs to know that an adult believes in and loves him or her unconditionally. Parents can provide their children with the tools they need to become resilient. In 2006, the AAP published a book that identified "7 Cs" of resilience (see Table 3–8).

TABLE 3–8 BUILDING RESILIENCY: THE 7 CS YOU NEED

Key Behavior	Actions for Caregivers
Competence: *Knowing how to handle a situation effectively*	Encourage children to make decisions
	Focus on a child's strengths
Confidence: *Believing in one's abilities* *Gives courage to face difficult situations*	Recognize and compliment when the child has done well
Connection: *Building relationships with others to provide a sense of support and security that leads to the development of strong values*	Provide emotional security at home
	Encourage children to reach out during tough times
Character: *Developing a set of values and morals* *Learning right from wrong behaviors*	Point out how behaviors affect others
	Help the child see himself as a caring person
Contribution: *Experiencing the joy of helping others*	Model generosity
	Point out those who are less fortunate
Coping: *Learning to handle stress*	Model positive coping strategies
Control: *Learning to make wise choices* *Recognizing cause and effect*	Point out how the child's choices contributed to the outcome

► CASE 20

A 16-year-old boy has recently been expelled from school for starting a fistfight with a peer for the fourth time this school year. School personnel are also concerned that he has "conned" a couple of girls into doing his homework each day by lying to them about a fictitious diagnosis of dyslexia. His mother sent him to live with his uncle 6 months ago because she was tired of "constantly arguing with him." He had also run away from home repeatedly for 2 to 3 days at time. She suspects he might be using drugs. His uncle has noted that the adolescent has a very short fuse and gets angry easily. He was arrested and placed on probation earlier this year for shoplifting cough medicine from a local drugstore, but has not had any run-ins with authorities in the last few months.

Question 20-1

What is the adolescent's diagnosis?

A) Oppositional defiant disorder.
B) Bipolar disorder.
C) Conduct disorder.
D) Delinquency.
E) Substance use disorder.

Discussion 20-1

The correct answer is "C." He has met the criteria for conduct disorder by displaying at least three criteria over the course of the last year, with at least one criterion in the last 6 months. He has initiated physical fights, has lied to obtain favors, has stolen items of nontrivial value, and has run away from home overnight. While one could make the argument that the adolescent meets the general description of oppositional defiant disorder (ODD) given his frequent disregard for authority figures, loss of his temper, and argumentativeness, meeting the criteria for conduct disorder is an exclusion criteria for ODD. While many children and adolescents with bipolar disorder display disruptive behavior, the behavior is noted, by those who have regular contact with the child, as being episodic. Bipolar disorder is characterized by several days to weeks of manic behavior that alternates with several day to weeks of depressed behavior. A manic episode is characterized by a mood changes (elevated, irritable), increased energy, decreased need for sleep, pressured excessive speech, inflated self-esteem, flight of ideas, and distractibility. Delinquency is considered a legal term, not a medical diagnosis. While substance abuse may certainly be playing a role in the patient's presentation, there is not enough information to make a diagnosis of a substance use disorder or identify it as the causative factor of the patient's behavior.

> **Helpful Tip**
> People with conduct disorder are mean. They are aggressive toward people and animals, destroy property, lie, steal, and break rules. They violate the basic rights of others and do not respect age-appropriate societal norms.

> **Helpful Tip**
> People with ODD are difficult. They are frequently in an angry/irritable mood and display argumentative or defiant behavior. They are also spiteful or vindictive. They often lose their temper, are easily annoyed, and will argue with authority figures over requests or rules. Note that this is different from conduct disorder. People with ODD fight other people. People with conduct disorder hurt other people.

Question 20-2

What would you recommend to the adolescent's family for treatment?
A) Admission to a "boot camp" residential treatment facility.
B) Admission to a substance abuse treatment facility.
C) A combination of risperidone and methylphenidate.
D) Development of an individual treatment plan involving school, juvenile justice, and mental health professionals, as well as caregivers.

Discussion 20-2

The correct answer is "D." Conduct disorder requires a multimodal treatment plan that accounts for the heterogeneous nature of its etiology. Treatment is the most effective when multiple agencies are involved so that care is coordinated and consistent through each aspect of the patient's life. Family-based programs, such as functional family therapy and multisystemic therapy, can be very effective. Problem-solving and skills training also can be beneficial. Currently, there is no evidence supporting medication as the primary treatment for ODD or conduct disorder. However, medication can be helpful in treating comorbid conditions such as attention deficit hyperactivity disorder (ADHD).

> ► **CASE 21**

A 10-year-old girl has been having difficulty sleeping for the last several months. Her mother reports that she is anxious all the time, but has particular difficulty at night and will lay in bed for hours worrying about things. She worries about doing well in school, her parents getting into car accidents, tornados, and Ebola as a few examples. The mother mentions that as her daughter's list of concerns has gotten longer and her sleep has worsened, she has also become more irritable and withdrawn.

Question 21-1

What is the prevalence of her disorder?
A) 0.5–1%.
B) 3–5%.
C) 10–15%.
D) > 20%.

Discussion 21-1

The correct answer is "B." Anxiety disorders are chronic and reoccurring. All are characterized by uneasiness, rumination, and frequently associated with somatic complaints (see Table 3–9). Younger children may express anxiety as crying, tantrums, clinging, or outbursts of anger. Genetics play a role and frequently there is a family history of anxiety disorders. This patient has generalized anxiety disorder (GAD). Anxiety is very common and normal for children and adolescents and can be protective and beneficial. Anxiety becomes a disorder, however, when it begins to impair an individual's ability to function. Children and adolescents with GAD have chronic, excessive worry in multiple areas of their lives—schoolwork, family, world events—and a minimum of one associated somatic complaint (headache, abdominal pain). People affected by GAD tend to be perfectionists. GAD is estimated to occur in 3% to 5% of children and adolescents. Specific phobias can occur in up to 10% of children. Estimates of the incidence of social anxiety disorder vary widely but have been reported to be as high as 15%.

Question 21-2

What would you recommend as treatment?
A) Prescribe citalopram and alprazolam.
B) Refer her to a therapist who specializes in cognitive behavioral therapy and prescribe citalopram.
C) Refer her to a therapist who specializes in cognitive behavioral therapy and prescribe alprazolam.
D) Reassure her mother that the anxiety will resolve as her daughter gets older.

Discussion 21-2

The correct answer is "B." Psychotherapy is recommended for children with mild to moderate anxiety disorders (eg, GAD, specific phobia, panic disorder). For children with moderate to severe anxiety, or children who do not respond to psychotherapy, the addition of a selective serotonin reuptake inhibitor (eg, citalopram) is recommended. Benzodiazepines (eg, alprazolam)

TABLE 3–9 MAJOR ANXIETY DISORDERS

Disorder	Description	Symptoms	Comorbidities
Generalized anxiety disorder (GAD)	Excessive, chronic worry Interferes with daily function	Somatic complaints Constant worry	Depression ADHD Other anxiety disorders
Separation anxiety disorder (SAD)	Excessive, developmentally inappropriate fear over separation from home or caregivers	Somatic complaints Unable to sleep alone Nightmares about separation School refusal	Depression ADHD Other anxiety disorders Social phobia
Social phobia	Scared or uncomfortable in social settings or performance situations	Difficulty speaking in school, reading aloud, talking with new people, attending parties	Substance abuse Depression Other anxiety disorders
Specific phobia	Excessive, unreasonable fear of a specific thing or situation despite awareness that the fear is unreasonable	Avoids fearful object or situation Distressed if must deal with fearful object or situation	Separation anxiety disorder Substance abuse Depression OCD
Panic disorder	Recurrent, unexpected episodes of fear with physiologic symptoms Fear and avoidance of places or situations where escape is difficult or would draw unwanted attention (eg, agoraphobia)	Heart racing Sweating Shaking Nausea Chills Chest pain Sensation of choking	Depression ADHD Other anxiety disorders Substance abuse

ADHD, attention deficit hyperactivity disorder; OCD, obsessive compulsive disorder; SSRI, selective serotonin reuptake inhibitor.

are generally not recommended for children. While the symptoms of GAD may wax and wane, the course of the disorder is frequently lifelong.

> ▶ **CASE 22**

A 9-year-old girl is new to your practice. She has an existing diagnosis of obsessive compulsive disorder (OCD). Prior to treatment with a combination of a selective serotonin reuptake inhibitor (SSRI) and psychotherapy, she had persistent and intrusive worries about coming in contact with germs and becoming ill. She had developed an intricate ritual of washing her hands a certain way several times a day and never eating in public to keep these worries at bay.

Question 22-1

What comorbidity should you be most concerned about monitoring her for?

A) Tourette's disorder.
B) Schizophrenia.
C) Generalized anxiety disorder.
D) Oppositional defiant disorder.

Discussion 22-1

The correct answer is "C." Obsessions are reoccurring or persistent thoughts or urges that drive compulsions. A compulsion is a repetitive act (ritual) or mental act done in response to an obsession or need to rigidly follow the rules. The features of OCD are unwanted and interfere with the child's and or adolescent's life. Examples of compulsions include hand washing, counting, and checking. A child with OCD may fear an intruder entering the house (obsession), and will check the locks over and over (compulsion) to make sure the house is safe. Over 50% of children with OCD have a comorbid psychiatric diagnosis. Another anxiety disorder is the most common comorbidity. ADHD is also a common comorbidity. Tourette's disorder is often associated with OCD but is less prevalent than ADHD or another anxiety disorder. Disruptive behavior disorders, such as ODD can occur as well, but less frequently than the others. Concurrent psychotic disorders are very rare.

Helpful Tip

Psychiatric disorders frequently occur with other psychiatric disorders. It is important to treat the primary disorder and comorbidities.

▶ CASE 23

During a well-child visit, the father of a 7-year-old boy expresses concern about his son's fear of elevators. His son avoids getting in elevators at all costs: It can take more than 30 minutes to convince him to get into one. When forced to ride in an elevator, he becomes very distressed and often starts crying. As an aside, the father mentions that boy's mother has an intense fear of spiders.

Question 23-1

What do you tell the father?
A) The child has panic disorder.
B) The child has a specific phobia.
C) The child has panic attacks.
D) The child has agoraphobia

Discussion 23-1

The correct answer is "B." The child specifically is scared of elevators. A specific fear becomes a specific phobia when it causes great distress, impairment, or both. A phobia may be tied to a prior traumatic event involving the object or situation. Common phobias include animals, insects, heights, water, blood, needles, airplanes, or clowns. Risk of developing a specific phobia is increased if a first-degree relative is affected. Agoraphobia is a generalized fear of situations or places in which escape would be difficult. Agoraphobia may be present with panic disorder. Panic disorder is characterized by recurrent, unexpected panic attacks. A panic attack is the sudden onset of fear and feeling of impending doom without any real danger; it may be unexpected or triggered by certain situations. Exposure to the specific phobia may trigger a panic attack such as in the patient described.

▶ CASE 24

A 17-year-old girl is evaluated for recurrent episodes in which she relives the car crash in which she was a passenger 6 months ago. Her mother speaks for her. The adolescent's friend was killed in the crash. Going by the accident site or hearing the song that was playing on the radio just before the crash causes her to freeze and the memories flood her mind. Afterward, she has difficulty falling asleep and is irritable. When asked about the events, the adolescent avoids the conversation.

Question 24-1

Regarding her disorder, which of the following is true?
A) Reminders of the event do not cue strong emotions or distress.
B) Patients of all ages present with "flashbacks."
C) Difficultly sleeping or concentrating may persist for prolonged periods after the event.
D) Stimuli and reminders of the event are calming.

Discussion 24-1

The correct answer is "C." Posttraumatic stress disorder (PTSD) develops after a traumatic event associated with real harm, near or actual death, or injury. The traumatic event is recurrently reexperienced. Reminders are avoided and cause significant distress. Avoidance behaviors include unwillingness to talk about the trauma, feeling detached from others, decreased interest in related activities, inability to recall event details, and avoidance of stimuli associated with the trauma. Presentation varies by age. Preverbal children may be clingy, irritable, refuse to explore their environment, aggressive, disrupted sleep, or hard to soothe. Verbal children may rapidly cycle through emotions or reenact the event. Adolescents may experience flashbacks or heightened arousal (insomnia, hypervigilance, angry outbursts, poor concentration) when reminded of the event. Symptoms must be present for more than 1 month for diagnosis of PTSD.

Helpful Tip
Many psychiatric disorders are extensions of normal behaviors and emotions except more intense, and cause impaired functioning in one or more areas of life.

▶ CASE 25

A 14-year-old boy is brought to the clinic by his family because they are concerned about his behavior. For the last 2 months he has been very irritable. He has not been sleeping well and complains that it takes several hours each night before he is finally able to doze off. He has been going to school, but his grades have started to slide and he states he "just can't concentrate." Although he has always been social and outgoing, lately he has preferred to stay home playing video games online. This has been a source of multiple arguments with his father. His mother recently discovered he has been cutting his upper arm with a razor. When she confronted him about this, he became agitated and insisted that he was not suicidal.

Question 25-1

What is the best diagnosis?
A) Major depressive disorder.
B) Bipolar disorder.
C) Borderline personality disorder.
D) Oppositional defiant disorder.

Discussion 25-1

The correct answer is "A." Children and adolescents with depression often present with symptoms of increased irritability rather than sadness. This adolescent's sleep difficulties, poor concentration, and social withdrawal are commonly seen in pediatric depression, as well. While patients with bipolar disorder who are experiencing a manic episode frequently have a decreased need for sleep, they generally do not complain about their limited sleep and instead describe having a great deal of energy and feeling very motivated. Cutting can be a symptom of borderline personality disorder, but adolescents with a variety of psychiatric disorders engage in this behavior. In addition, personality disorders are not diagnosed in children and adolescents because their personalities are not completely developed. Adolescents with depression can display oppositional and defiant behavior, but a diagnosis of ODD cannot be made if this behavior only occurs in the context of a mood disorder.

The family listens intently as you discuss your concerns that their son may have major depressive disorder. The family asks, "How do you know he isn't just in a funk and isn't a normal moody teenager?"

Question 25-2

What should you tell the family?

A) Mood swings are common in adolescents.
B) Mood swings do not interfere with daily life functions.
C) Mood swings are not associated with depressive symptoms (weight changes, concentration problems).
D) Mood swings are not associated with cutting behaviors.
E) All of the above.

Discussion 25-2

The correct answer is "E." Adolescents may experience mood swings and argue frequently with parents but life should not be disrupted nor should depressive symptoms of sleep disturbances, lack of energy, and so forth, be present. Depressive disorders include major depressive disorder (MDD), persistent depressive disorder (formerly dysthymia), disruptive mood dysregulation disorder (DMDD), and premenstrual dysphoric disorder. For diagnosis of MDD, symptoms must be present for 2 weeks, impair functioning, and must include either a depressed or irritable mood, or loss of interest and pleasure in activities.

> **Helpful Tip**
>
> Major depressive disorder is more than just being sad. In order to be diagnosed with MDD, the person must have 2 weeks of symptoms, one of which is either depressed mood or loss of pleasure in normally pleasurable activities. At least five of the following nine symptoms must be present:
> - Depressed mood
> - Loss of interest or pleasure
> - Weight loss
> - Sleeping more or less than usual
> - Psychomotor agitation or retardation (observable, not just subjective)
> - Fatigue or low energy
> - Feelings of worthlessness or guilt
> - Difficulty thinking clearly
> - Thoughts of death or suicide.

Question 25-3

How should you manage the adolescent's depressive symptoms?

A) Prescribe citalopram.
B) Refer him for psychotherapy.
C) Refer him for psychotherapy and prescribe citalopram.
D) Provide reassurance and schedule frequent follow-up.

Discussion 25-3

The correct answer is "C." It is important provide education and engage the family and school. Mild to moderate symptoms may be treated with an initial trial of psychotherapy. If no or minimal response, a selective serotonin reuptake inhibitor (SSRI; eg, citalopram) should be prescribed. For moderate to severe symptoms, psychotherapy and an SSRI should be prescribed. Frequent follow-up is important, but his symptoms require treatment; therefore, reassurance would be inappropriate. It is important to recognize and treat comorbid conditions. As many as 90% of children and adolescents with depression have an additional psychiatric disorder, most frequently anxiety disorders, disruptive disorders (eg, conduct disorder), ADHD, or substance abuse.

> **Helpful Tip**
>
> Major depressive disorder is characterized as mild, moderate, or severe. If you have the bare minimum of symptoms to make the diagnosis, it is mild depression. If you have substantial excess number of symptoms AND the intensity of the symptoms is seriously distressing or unmanageable, it is severe depression. Somewhere in the middle lies moderate depression.

> **Helpful Tip**
>
> Suicide risk may increase after starting a SSRI medication in a depressed adolescent, therefore; close monitoring is warranted.

> **Helpful Tip**
>
> It is important to recognize and treat comorbid conditions. As many as 90% of children and adolescents with depression have an additional psychiatric disorder, most frequently anxiety disorders, disruptive disorders (eg, conduct disorder), ADHD, or substance abuse.

⌛ QUICK QUIZ

Which of the following is NOT a risk factor for developing major depressive disorder?

A) Good coping skills.
B) Difficulties with academics.

C) Bullying.
D) Neglect.

Discussion

The correct answer is "A." MDD is often a familial disorder as are many other psychiatric disorders including anxiety disorders and bipolar disorder. The most predictive risk factor is a family history of depression or anxiety. Other risk factors include abuse, family dysfunction, neglect, loss of a loved one, bullying, poor coping skills, social stressors, presence of comorbid psychiatric disorder, and chronic medical illness.

The adolescent is prescribed an SSRI and referred to psychotherapy. At follow-up, he admits to thinking about suicide and feeling hopeless. He stays in his room the majority of the time avoiding others. You recognize he is at increased risk for suicide.

Question 25-4

What is the strongest predictor of whether he will commit suicide?
A) His diagnosis of depression.
B) His cutting behavior.
C) The absence of guns in the home.
D) The fact that he has never made an attempt before.

Discussion 25-4

The correct answer is "D." The strongest predictor of future suicidal behavior is past suicide attempts. His depression diagnosis and cutting do put him at slightly higher risk. Nearly 90% of children and adolescents who commit suicide had a psychiatric diagnosis. Having guns in the home significantly increases the risk of completing suicide as well. Rates of completed suicide are higher after puberty. Females are more likely to attempt suicide, but males are more likely to complete suicide.

Question 25-5

What is NOT a concerning sign that a child or adolescent is suicidal?
A) Talking about suicide.
B) Feeling hopeless.
C) Feeling he or she has no purpose in life.
D) Difficulty sleeping.

Discussion 25-5

The correct answer is "D." Difficultly sleeping is a symptom of depression but not necessary a red flag for suicide. Suicide is the third leading cause of death for adolescents. Talking or asking about suicide does not cause suicidal actions or ideations in children or adolescents. Primary care providers should ask about suicide as part of routine adolescent health screening. Any patient who threatens suicide, talks about hurting himself or herself, or has a plan or is looking for ways to kill himself or herself should be emergently referred to a mental health provider or emergency department. The American Association

of Suicidology created a helpful mnemonic to remember the warning signs of suicide: "Is (the) path warm?"

I – Ideation
S – Substance abuse
P – Purposelessness
A – Anxiety
T – Trapped
H – Hopelessness
W – Withdrawal
A – Anger
R – Recklessness
M – Mood changes

⏳ QUICK QUIZ

Which of the following is NOT a protective risk factor for suicide?
A) Supportive family members.
B) Good grades.
C) An established relationship with a therapist.
D) Passing a firearms safety course.

Discussion

The correct answer is "D." Having an understanding about the risks and safety measures with firearms is not a protective factor and, in fact, easy access to firearms is a significant risk factor. Protective risk factors include having good community and family support, and access to effective care for mental health, physical health, and substance abuse concerns. Risk factors associated with suicide include a history of previous suicide attempts, a family history of suicide, untreated mental health problems or chronic illness, substance abuse, isolation, or access to lethal means. (See Table 3–10.)

> **Helpful Tip**
> Confidentiality is important and laws vary by state. Exceptions to confidentiality include suspected or reported child abuse, suicidal or homicidal thoughts, and violent behaviors. Abuse must be reported to the state. The others should be reported to the legal guardians.

▶ CASE 26

A 17-year-old is brought to the emergency department by her family. She won't sit down to be interviewed, but instead paces back and forth. Her speech is rapid and you struggle to break into her rambling monolog to ask questions. She admits she has slept only 1 to 2 hours a night for the last week, but states this isn't a problem and has allowed her to dedicate

TABLE 3–10 PROTECTIVE AND RISK FACTORS FOR SUICIDE

Risk Factors	Protective Factors
Previous suicide attempts	Family support
Family history of suicide	Community support
History of abuse or neglect	Access to effective mental health care
Mental health diagnosis	Access to effective physical health care
Alcohol and substance abuse	Access to effective substance abuse care
Impulsive or aggressive tendencies	Skills in problem solving and conflict resolution
Cultural beliefs that suicide is a noble resolution	Cultural and beliefs that discourage suicide and violence
Isolation	Personal satisfaction and areas of achievement
Chronic Illness	
Easy access to lethal means	
Barriers to mental health treatment	

more time to her artwork. She has been painting everything in her bedroom purple and even tried to paint the family dog when he made the mistake of entering her room. She tells you proudly that "monochrome is the next big thing" in interior decorating and she's convinced she is starting a new trend that will "spread like wildfire!"

Question 26-1
How would you treat this adolescent?
A) Start fluoxetine.
B) Start lamotrigine.
C) Start lisdexamfetamine.
D) Start risperidone.

Discussion 26-1
The correct answer is "D." She is clearly experiencing a manic episode. While lithium and anticonvulsants have been well studied as mood stabilizers for adults with mania, the atypical antipsychotics (eg, risperidone) have been the most researched in children and adolescents with mania. Some patients with bipolar disorder require a combination of a mood stabilizer for their manic symptoms and an antidepressant such as an SSRI (eg, fluoxetine) for their depressive symptoms. However, this combination is typically not started at the same time. The mood stabilizer is usually initiated first and then the antidepressant is added cautiously

once the patient's mania is under control. Antidepressants should be used with caution in the absence of a mood stabilizer as they can exacerbate manic symptoms. Lamotrigine is used as a mood stabilizer but is not indicated to reduce mania. It is effective in treating depressive symptoms for patients with bipolar disorder. Lisdexamfetamine is a stimulant used for ADHD. Some of this adolescent's behaviors are similar to hyperactivity; however, it is unlikely that she has suddenly developed ADHD in late adolescence. Stimulants should be used with caution in patients with mania as they can exacerbate manic symptoms.

▶ CASE 27

A 16-year-old girl was admitted for evaluation of seizures. She was monitored by video electroencephalogram (EEG) for 2 days. Although several episodes of seizure-like body movements were recorded on the video, her EEG remained essentially normal throughout her evaluation. An extensive workup was completed and no other physical cause for her movements could be found. Her mother notes that the problem began 2 weeks after one of her friends was sexually assaulted at a party. She had left the party early without her friend and has been feeling guilty about it. The mother worries that someone might have slipped something into her daughter's soda and that has caused the seizures.

Question 27-1
What is the diagnosis?
A) Hypochondriasis.
B) Conversion disorder.
C) Malingering.
D) Factitious disorder.

Discussion 27-1
The correct answer is "B." The definition of conversion disorder is the presentation of a neurologic impairment (eg, nonepileptic seizures, weakness, vision changes) that cannot be explained by any medical cause. The symptoms are produced subconsciously and the patient does not believe he or she has control over them. Frequently the onset is associated with a psychological stressor. Hypochondriasis is the fear of having an illness and is not necessarily associated with the development of symptoms. Malingering and factitious disorder are diagnosed when the symptoms are produced consciously by the patient (ie, "faked"). In factitious disorder, the patient is seeking primary gain; that is, he or she receives psychological benefit from assuming the sick role. In malingering, the patient is seeking secondary gain, attempting to get out of something (eg, school) or gain something (eg, money).

▶ CASE 28

A 14-year-old boy is referred to your clinic with a 2-year history of abdominal pain. He cannot describe the pain well. It does not awaken him from sleep nor does it interfere with activities. He has had no fevers, diarrhea, vomiting, or weight loss. On examination, he is at a proper weight and height, and appears well. The exam findings, including vital signs, are normal. You review a 4-inch stack of records to find that among the hundreds of tests that have been performed all are normal except the serum vitamin D level, which is low. You suspect his symptoms are psychological.

Question 28-1

Which of the following should NOT be used to manage the adolescent?
A) Education.
B) Referral for a second opinion with a gastroenterologist.
C) Psychotherapy.
D) Pharmacotherapy.

Discussion 28-1

The correct answer is "B." Psychosomatic disorders are physical manifestations of emotional stress. The clinical symptoms are not due to an underlying medical illness. Patients may present with various physical complaints, including chest pain, abdominal pain, and headache. They are often diagnoses of exclusion but extensive medical evaluations may reenforce the thought that an undiagnosed medical illness is present. A thorough history and physical exam may help identify red flags that would warrant a diagnostic evaluation. Clues include vague, inconsistent, and multiple symptoms present at the same time. Patients are in good health and have benign physical exams. Education is key and should focus on coping skills. Unnecessary medical evaluation should be avoided. Comorbid psychiatric conditions should be treated. Frequent office visits may be helpful. Psychotherapy, antidepressants (SSRI), or a combination are useful treatments.

▶ CASE 29

A healthy 8-year-old boy has been struggling in school. After completing a thorough clinical interview and obtaining rating scales from his parents and his teachers, you diagnose him with ADHD and prescribe 5 mg of methylphenidate each morning. At his follow-up appointment 2 weeks later, his parents report no change in his behavior and his teacher's rating scales show that he is doing worse.

Question 29-1

What is the best next step?
A) Refer him for neuropsychological testing to evaluate for learning disorders.
B) Switch him to an amphetamine-based stimulant
C) Increase his methylphenidate dose.
D) Refer him to a psychologist who specializes in social skills training.

Discussion 29-1

The best answer is C. According to the American Academy of Child and Adolescent Psychiatry and Texas Children's Medication Algorithm Project, an adequate trial with a methylphenidate-based stimulant, an amphetamine-based stimulant, or atomoxetine is the first step in treating ADHD. He is on a low dose of methylphenidate and the dose-response relationship has been established as a linear response. Before switching to an alternative medication, the next step is to try to optimize the current medication. If he is given a trial of a higher dose and still does not respond, the next step in the algorithm is to switch to a different stimulant. If he does not respond to a second trial or it is determined that he only has difficulty in certain subjects, assessing for learning disorders can be helpful. Psychotherapy has been found to be beneficial for children with comorbid anxiety, mood, or disruptive behavior disorders. Common comorbidities include ODD, conduct disorder, substance abuse issues, learning disability, depression, and anxiety disorders.

You review the patient's original presenting symptoms, which were reported 9 months before your evaluation. He was described then as "spacey," forgetful, and careless. His mother constantly had to bring his schoolwork or lunch box to school as he would forget it. Last year, he lost his lunch card three times and his mother paid for a new one each time. He dislikes playing board games as he says they require too much focus. His mother can't understand why his room is such a mess and he can't organize it. When ask to feed the dog, he will sometimes leave the bag of food next to the empty bowl.

Question 29-2

What was his initial presentation of ADHD?
A) Combined presentation.
B) Predominately inattentive.
C) Predominately hyperactive-impulsive.
D) He did not qualify for the diagnosis of ADHD.

Discussion 29-2

The correct answer is "B." ADHD is characterized by hyperactivity, impulsivity, inattention, or a combination. The pathogenesis of ADHD is unknown but thought to be related to catecholamine metabolism (deficient dopamine activity) in the brain. A number of genes associated with ADHD have been identified, supporting a genetic component. Imaging and testing suggests impaired executive function due to abnormalities in the prefrontal cerebral cortex and basal ganglia. The brain matures normally but at a delayed rate. ADHD is subdivided as predominately inattentive (meets symptom criteria for inattentive only), predominantly hyperactive-impulsive (meets symptom criteria for hyperactive-impulsive only), or combined presentation (meets symptom criteria for both). Symptoms must be present for 6 months, inappropriate for developmental level, cause impairment, onset during childhood, and occur in two or more settings.

Helpful Tip

HEY LOOK! A SQUIRREL! Still reading? Then you probably don't have attention deficit hyperactivity disorder. Or at least not the inattentive type. However, if you are running around a child's playground and blurting out the answers before you even finish reading the question, then you might have the hyperactive-impulsive type.

Helpful Tip

At least six of the following nine symptoms must be present to diagnose inattentive-type ADHD:
- Poor attention to detail
- Difficulty sustaining attention
- Does not seem to listen
- Does not follow through on instructions
- Difficulty organizing tasks
- Avoids or dislikes tasks that require sustained mental effort
- Loses things
- Easily distracted
- Forgetful

Helpful Tip

At least six of the following eight symptoms must be present to diagnose hyperactivity- and impulsivity-type ADHD:
- Fidgets or squirms
- Leaves seat inappropriately
- Runs about or climbs when not appropriate
- Cannot sustain quiet play
- "On the go" or "driven by a motor"
- Talks excessively
- Blurts out answers before the question is completed
- Difficulty waiting for his or her turn

Question 29-3

What is an appropriate diagnostic evaluation for ADHD?

A) ADHD checklist completed by parent and teacher.
B) Brain MRI.
C) EEG.
D) Urine drug screen.

Discussion 29-3

The correct answer is "A." The ADHD checklist should be completed by the parent and teacher. Medical testing such as thyroid function tests or lead level should be obtained as clinically indicated.

QUICK QUIZ

Which is a true fact about ADHD?

A) Males are more frequently affected than females.
B) ADHD is familial.
C) Symptoms may persist into adulthood.
D) All of the above.

Discussion

The correct answer is "D." The male-to-female ratio is 3:1. ADHD tends to run in families. A genetic basis exists as studies have shown ADHD to be strongly inherited, with up to 76% heritance. Most children with ADHD have symptoms into adolescence and some continue to have problems into adulthood that may require treatment.

▶ CASE 30

A 9-year-old boy is referred to your clinic from his school due to concerns about aggressive behaviors. He is easily angered and, when angry, lashes out. He has kicked and punched objects, and broken things. He will grit his teeth, tense up his face and body, and scream. Most recently another child was using a green marker, which he wanted. When he couldn't have it he kicked the wall.

Question 30-1

Regarding his aggressive behaviors, what do you not tell the school?

A) His response is developmentally inappropriate.
B) He has not developed proper problem-solving skills and self-control.
C) He has not developed proper social skills.
D) Children do not outgrow their aggression until junior high.

Discussion 30-1

The correct answer is "D." Aggression and anger in response to frustration is normal in young children. As the child learns social skills, conflict resolution, problem solving, and self-control these behaviors subside. Aggression becomes problematic when it persists, is severe, or happens frequently. For example, a toddler whose stuffed animal is taken away by his sister may respond by hitting her. The toddler has not learned how to handle his emotions. However, a 9-year-old should be able to work out conflict without resorting to physical aggression. Have you ever heard parents tell their child, "use your words"? The parents are trying to develop coping skills in their child. Some children have a genetic or psychological predisposition to aggression. Children who witness aggression by others, including role models and parents, are more likely to be aggressive themselves. Aggressive children may have problems processing and interpreting social cues.

▶ CASE 31

A 13-year-old girl comes into the clinic for a sore throat. During casual conversation, you ask about school. She won't make eye contact. When she finally answers, she tells you that the popular girls are spreading rumors about her and trying to make others not want to be her friend. You recognize she is the victim of bullying.

Question 31-1

Which is NOT an example of bullying?
A) The fastest child in class making fun of the slowest child.
B) The science nerd and math geek getting into a fistfight.
C) The high school heartthrob making fun of the class nerd.
D) The leader of the popular clique of girls spreading rumors about a new girl in school.

Discussion 31-1

The correct answer is "B." To constitute bullying, the two individuals involved cannot be on equal footing. One must be younger, smaller, or less powerful. Bullying is a form of aggression toward peers. It is a repetitive event with the intent is to harm another person physically or socially. There is an imbalance of power. The bully has either more physical or more psychological power than the victim. If two lightweights get into a fight, it isn't bullying. But a heavyweight taking on a lightweight is bullying. Aggression displayed by boys is typically overt and physical. Aggression by girls is more likely to be covert and relational, focusing on damaging someone's social status by spreading rumors, gossiping, or excluding others.

Question 31-2

Which is a management strategy for victims of bullying?
A) Avoid hot spots where bullying occurs.
B) When hot spots are unavoidable, travel with a friend who isn't bullied.
C) Identify a trusted adult at school to turn to when problems arise.
D) At recess, join structured activities such as a game of soccer or tag.
E) All of the above.

Discussion 31-2

The correct answer is "E." Options A through D are all correct.

Helpful Tip
Cyberbullying involves inflicting harm using electronic media, including computers, social networks, and cell phones. In contrast to traditional bullying, it does not involve a power imbalance and is not always repetitive.

▶ CASE 32

A 16-year-old male is brought to the emergency department by his mother for odd behaviors. He reports seeing unicorns. He talks about the troll god's secret plot to steal the unicorn. He has come up with a plan to save the unicorn. As part of his plan, he was going to paint the unicorn,

TABLE 3–11 CAUSES OF PSYCHOSIS

Drug overdose or abuse
- Anticholinergics
- Stimulants (eg, amphetamines, MDMA)
- Hallucinogens (eg, PCP, LSD)

Drug-induced psychosis
- Steroids
- Isoniazid
- Anticonvulsants

Drug-related syndromes
- Serotonin syndrome
- Withdrawal
- Neuroleptic malignant syndrome

Central nervous system masses
- Tumor
- Hydrocephalus
- Abscess

Intracranial injury
- Epidural hematoma
- Subdural hemorrhage

Stroke

Seizure

Migraine

Meningitis or encephalitis

Systemic lupus erythematosus

Metabolic or endocrine disorders
- Urea cycle defects
- Thyroid storm
- Hypothyroidism
- Hashimoto encephalopathy
- Adrenal insufficiency
- Uremia
- Hyperammonemia

Electrolyte abnormalities
- Hypoglycemia
- Hyperglycemia
- Hyponatremia

Menstrual psychosis

Postpartum psychosis

Psychiatric disorders
- Schizophrenia
- Depression
- Bipolar disorder

LSD, lysergic acid diethylamide; MDMA, 3,4-methylenedioxymethamphetamine; PCP, phencyclidine.

disguising it as a horse with a horn. His mother found him rummaging through the paint collection and brought him in for evaluation.

Question 32-1

Which of the following is NOT a possible cause of his psychosis?
A) Substance abuse.
B) Electrolyte derangement.
C) Stroke.
D) Conduct disorder.

Discussion 32-1

The correct answer is "D." Psychosis is defined as disrupted thinking with delusions or hallucinations. Delusions are fixed, false beliefs. Patients who have hallucinations see or hear things that aren't present. The differential diagnosis for acute psychosis is lengthy (see Table 3–11). Identifying whether the symptoms are acute or chronic is helpful in narrowing the differential. Acute onset suggests a medical etiology. Chronic symptoms suggest a psychiatric cause. Before diagnosing a psychiatric disorder, other medical causes must be ruled out. Management includes ensuring the patient's safety (may require restraints), treating reversible conditions, and completion of a diagnostic evaluation to identify the underlying etiology.

> **Helpful Tip**
> Most children with hallucinations do not have schizophrenia and many do not have a psychiatric disorder.

BIBLIOGRAPHY

American Academy of Pediatrics. Building resilience in children. https://www.healthychildren.org/English/healthy-living/emotional-wellness/Building-Resilience/Pages/Building-Resilience-in-Children.aspx. Accessed June 10, 2015.

American Association of Suicidology. Know the warning signs of suicide. http://www.suicidology.org/resources/warning-signs. Accessed June 30, 2015.

American Psychiatric Association. *Diagnostic and Statistical Manual of Mental Disorders: DSM-5.* Washington, DC: American Psychiatric Association; 2013.

Brill SR, Patel DR, MacDonald E. Psychosomatic disorders in pediatrics. *Indian J Pediatr.* 2001;68(7):597–603.

Carruth BR, Ziegler PJ, Gordon A, Barr SI. Prevalence of picky eaters among infants and toddlers and their caregivers' decisions about offering a new food. *J Am Diet Assoc* 2004;104:S57–S64.

Centers for Disease Control and Prevention. Attention-deficit/hyperactivity disorder (ADHD). http://www.cdc.gov/ncbddd/adhd/diagnosis.html. Accessed June 30, 2015.

Cohen GM, Albertini LW. Colic. *Pediatr Rev.* 2012;33(7):332–333. doi: 10.1542/pir.33-7-332.

Cohen JA, Bukstein O, Walter H, et al. Practice parameter for the assessment and treatment of children and adolescents with posttraumatic stress disorder. *J Am Acad Child Adolesc Psychiatry.* 2010;49(4):414–430.

Committee on Psychosocial Aspects of Child and Family Health. Guidance for effective discipline. *Pediatrics.* 1998;101(4):723–728.

Connolly SD, Berstein GA. Practice parameter for the assessment and treatment of children and adolescents with anxiety disorders. *J Am Acad Child Adolesc Psychiatry.* 2007;46(2):267–283.

Dulcan M, ed. *Dulcan's Textbook of Child and Adolescent Psychiatry.* Washington, DC: American Psychiatric Publishing; 2010.

Egger HL, Costello EJ, Angold A. School refusal and psychiatric disorders: A community study. *J Am Acad Child Adolesc Psychiatry.* 2003;42:797–807.

Findling R, ed. *Clinical Manual of Child and Adolescent Psychopharmacology.* Washington, DC: American Psychiatric Publishing; 2008.

Fisher WW, Piazza CC, Roane HS, eds. *Handbook of Applied Behavior Analysis.* New York, NY: Guilford Press; 2013.

Ginsburg KR. *Resilience in Children and Teens: Giving Kids Roots and Wings.* Elk Grove Village, IL: American Academy of Pediatrics; 2006.

Michel RS. Toilet training. *Pediatr Rev.* 1999;20(7):240–245. doi: 10.1542/pir.20-7-240.

Practice parameter for the assessment and treatment of children and adolescents with attention-deficit/hyperactivity disorder. *J Am Acad Child Adolesc Psychiatry.* 2007;46(7):894–921.

Practice parameter for the assessment and treatment of children and adolescents with bipolar disorder. *J Am Acad Child Adolesc Psychiatry.* 2007;46(1):107–125.

Practice parameter for the assessment and treatment of children and adolescents with depressive disorders. *J Am Acad Child Adolesc Psychiatry.* 2007;46(11):1503–1526.

Practice parameter for the assessment and treatment of children and adolescents with obsessive-compulsive disorders. *J Am Acad Child Adolesc Psychiatry.* 2012;51(1):98–113.

Reimers TM. *Help! There's a toddler in the house!* Boystown, NE: Boystown Press; 2011.

Roberts DM, Ostapchuk M, O'Brien JG. Infantile colic. *Am Fam Physician.* 2004;70(4):735–740.

Shetgiri R. Bullying and victimization among children. *Adv Pediatr.* 2013;60(1):33–51. doi: 10.1016/j.yapd.2013.04.004.

Williams KE, Gibbons BG, Schreck KA. Comparing selective eaters with and without developmental disabilities. *J Dev Physical Disabil.* 2005;17:299–309.

Blood and Neoplastic Disorders

4

Adam D. Wolfe

▶ CASE 1

A 12-month-old boy presents to your clinic for his health supervision visit. He is growing and developing normally. His diet consists of approximately 30 ounces of cow's milk daily, as well as mixed table foods. His heart rate is 122 beats per minute. Physical exam reveals gingival and conjunctival pallor and a grade I/VI systolic ejection murmur heard over the left sternal border.

Question 1-1

Which of the following laboratory values is likely to be elevated in this patient?

A) Ferritin.
B) Haptoglobin.
C) Hemoglobin.
D) Mean corpuscular volume.
E) Platelet count.

Discussion 1-1

The correct answer is "E." This patient's age, history, and physical exam findings are most consistent with iron deficiency anemia (IDA). A CBC performed in a patient with IDA would confirm decreased hemoglobin (making option "C" incorrect) and abnormal red cell indices including microcytosis (making option "D" incorrect), and an increased red cell distribution width, reflective of insufficient iron for the construction of hemoglobin and red cells in the bone marrow. Children with IDA often have a reactive thrombocytosis, which is due to cross-reactivity of erythropoietin, elevated in the anemic state, with the megakaryocyte-stimulating thrombopoietin receptor. The blood smear should reveal red cell microcytosis, hypochromia, and anisocytosis. (See Figure 4–1.) Laboratory evaluation of iron may include serum ferritin, which reflects hepatic iron stores and is therefore typically low in IDA (making option "A" incorrect). Serum iron is also likely to be low, while total iron-binding capacity, reflective of hepatic transferrin production in an effort to scavenge additional iron, is likely

to be elevated. Serum haptoglobin is not routinely checked in cases of suspected iron deficiency, in which it would not likely be affected (making option "B" incorrect); haptoglobin is often decreased in patients with hemolytic anemias. IDA is the most common hematologic condition in pediatrics, affecting an estimated 3% to 7% of toddlers and up to 9% of menstruating young women. Toddler-aged children are at greatest risk of IDA when consuming large amounts of cow's milk, as milk interferes with intestinal absorption of dietary iron. Data suggest that children with iron deficiency, even in the absence of anemia, are at increased risk of neurocognitive deficits, lower IQ, behavior problems, and cardiovascular changes, presumably due to altered function of nonhematopoietic enzymatic processes that depend on iron.

▶ CASE 2

A 12-year-old girl with no past medical history presents to the emergency department after suffering a brief syncopal episode in her bathroom at home. Her history is remarkable for an influenza-like febrile illness last month, followed by lingering fatigue and daytime sleepiness. There is no personal or family history of symptoms like these. She has normal vital signs apart from heart rate of 112 beats per minute. Physical exam reveals an awake and alert girl lying in bed, who answers questions appropriately. She has marked facial, conjunctival, and gingival pallor, and scleral icterus. Cardiovascular exam reveals a grade II/VI systolic ejection murmur, capillary refill of less than 3 seconds, and 2+ peripheral pulses in all extremities. Laboratory evaluation includes hemoglobin 5.3 g/dL, white blood cell count $11.9 \times 10^3/mm^3$, and platelets $502 \times 10^3/mm^3$. White cell differential includes 30% neutrophils and 60% lymphocytes. Evaluation of the blood smear reveals normocytosis and normochromia, occasional spherocytes, and no schistocytes. Serum total bilirubin and lactate dehydrogenase (LDH) are both elevated.

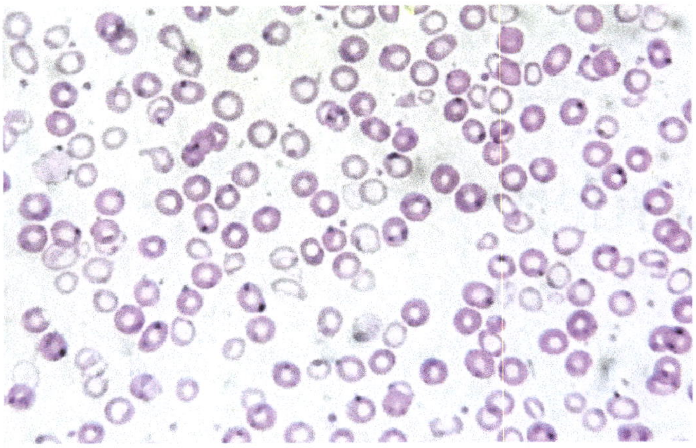

FIGURE 4–1. Peripheral blood smear from a patient with iron deficiency anemia. The red blood cells exhibit marked hypochromia (ie, severe pallor). There is also substantial variation in cell size, or anisocytosis. (Used with permission from Adam D. Wolfe, MD, PhD.)

Question 2-1

Which of the following evaluations is most likely to yield this patient's diagnosis?

A) Glucose-6-phosphate dehydrogenase (G6PD) enzyme activity.
B) Direct antiglobulin (Coombs) test.
C) Ferritin, serum iron, total iron binding capacity.
D) Erythrocyte osmotic fragility test.
E) Bone marrow aspiration and biopsy.

Discussion 2-1

The correct answer is "B." This patient presents with progressive symptoms of anemia, including fatigue, pallor, tachycardia, and ejection murmur, with jaundice, hyperbilirubinemia, and elevated LDH that suggest a hemolytic mechanism. Hemolytic anemias, in contrast to most nutritional anemias, typically exhibit normocytosis and normochromia on the CBC and smear. The onset of new symptoms abruptly following an acute viral illness make it probable that this patient has autoimmune hemolytic anemia (AIHA), and therefore a direct antiglobulin test is most likely to yield a diagnosis. This test will reveal the presence of antibodies directed against red cell membrane antigens. Because the mechanism of red cell depletion involves clearance of antibody-coated cells by the spleen, this is a largely extravascular hemolysis that is unlikely to be accompanied by fragmented red cells as might be seen with intravascular hemolysis. The presence of occasional spherocytes is consistent with deformation of antibody-coated cells. AIHA may occur as an isolated event, or it may be associated with other immune cytopenias, such as thrombocytopenia (seen together in Evans syndrome) or neutropenia. The presence of autoimmune cytopenias in an adolescent patient should raise suspicion for the presence of other autoimmune disorders, and a thorough autoimmune family history and review of systems is appropriate. Further screening for thyroid dysfunction, systemic lupus erythematosus, and inflammatory bowel diseases may then be warranted. Management is generally aimed at quelling inflammation, starting with corticosteroids. Once in remission, AIHA may remain so following a taper of immune suppressive therapy, although recurrence is common. G6PD deficiency (option "A") is an inherited enzymopathy that can present with severe hemolytic anemia in the setting of acute illness, but it is inherited in an X-linked fashion, making it unlikely in this female patient without a family history. The timing of this patient's anemia after antecedent illness, jaundice, and normocytosis are inconsistent with a diagnosis of iron deficiency anemia (option "C"). Despite the presence of occasional spherocytes, explained above, this patient's history of not having jaundice or other hematologic problems until this illness make this less likely to be hereditary spherocytosis, and osmotic fragility testing (option "D") is therefore not expected to be helpful. Finally, while acute leukemias are always in the differential diagnosis for an ill-appearing child with cytopenia, the history and lab findings are more consistent with a nonmalignant process. Should the patient have presented with multiple cytopenias, significant leukocytosis, or blasts on the blood smear, evaluation for leukemia with bone marrow assessment (option "E") would be urgently warranted.

> **Helpful Tip**
> The presence of spherocytes on a peripheral blood smear may be noted in hereditary spherocytosis or autoimmune hemolytic anemia. Order a direct antiglobulin test.

► CASE 3

You are seeing a 6-month-old baby girl for sudden onset of jaundice. Her mother reports that the patient was healthy until 2 days ago, when she developed fever, cough, congestion, and irritability. Last night, her skin appeared yellow, and this has worsened today. Mom reports that she underwent splenectomy when she was 6 years old because of "a problem with her blood," and the infant's maternal grandmother underwent splenectomy and cholecystectomy while in middle school. The exam is remarkable for a crying but nontoxic infant with temperature 38.5°C (101.3°F), scleral icterus, diffuse jaundice, grade II/VI systolic ejection murmur, and spleen palpable 3 cm below the left costal margin. Lab work on the baby reveals white blood cell count of $14.6 \times 10^3/mm^3$ with normal differential, platelets of $457 \times 10^3/mm^3$, hemoglobin 7.3 g/dL, mean corpuscular volume 95 fL, reticulocytes 12%, and indirect bilirubin 6.6 mg/dL.

Question 3-1

Which of the following tests is most likely to establish the diagnosis in this patient?

A) Bone marrow aspirate and biopsy.
B) Direct antiglobulin (Coombs) test.
C) Erythrocyte osmotic fragility test.
D) Glucose-6-phosphate dehydrogenase enzyme activity.
E) Hemoglobin electrophoresis.

Discussion 3-1

The correct answer is "C." This baby exhibits an onset of acute, symptomatic anemia in the setting of a febrile illness; the presence of jaundice suggests a hemolytic process, most likely hereditary spherocytosis (HS). This is suggested by the splenomegaly and mild macrocytosis, as well as by an autosomal dominant inheritance pattern indicated on family history. HS is caused by defects in structural red blood cell transmembrane proteins responsible for vertical interactions that link the cytoskeleton to the cell membrane. Mutations in genes coding for spectrin and ankyrin are most commonly associated with HS, and in some cases mutations in Protein 4.2 and Band 3 are also causative. While HS is inherited in an autosomal dominant fashion, an estimated one third of cases appear to be due to sporadic mutation. The management of HS is supportive and based on clinical severity, which can vary substantially between cases. Some neonates with more severe phenotypes exhibit symptomatic anemia brought about by the physiologic stress of birth and continue to have hemolytic episodes throughout infancy during acute illnesses. Infants with severe HS may also exhibit an exaggerated physiologic nadir within the first 2 months after birth. Infants requiring blood transfusions for HS-associated hemolytic episodes are the most likely to require splenectomy to control their disease at early ages. Note that splenectomy is discouraged in children younger than 6 years due to infection risk. At the other end of the spectrum, at least a quarter of children with HS may have only mild hemolysis, for which they adequately compensate, and develop no clinical problems. In general, individuals with HS are at increased risk of biliary sludging due to chronic red cell turnover and hyperbilirubinemia, and often undergo cholecystectomy at early ages. Diagnosis of HS may be suspected based on red cell indices. Red cells of children with suspected HS are often subjected to osmotic fragility testing, in which the cells are incubated in solutions of increasing tonicity; the weakened red cells of HS will exhibit increased hemolysis at relatively higher tonicity than control cells. Performance of this test is usually deferred until children are at least 6 months of age; therefore, this is an appropriate confirmatory test for the patient in the vignette. Because the patient is exhibiting an appropriate reticulocyte response, has no other cell lines down, and has evidence of hemolysis, a bone marrow failure syndrome or malignancy is unlikely to be causing the anemia (making option "A" less helpful). The relative macrocytosis and the family history make autoimmune hemolytic anemia less likely, and while a direct antiglobulin test might be performed early in this patient's workup, it is expected to be negative (option "B"). Glucose-6-phosphate dehydrogenase (G6PD, option "D") deficiency could cause a clinical picture such as this patient exhibits, particularly with stress-induced hemolysis, but this condition is inherited in an X-linked recessive fashion; the female patient plus family history in the vignette are therefore not suggestive of this diagnosis. Hemolysis may be seen in cases of certain hemoglobinopathies (investigated by option "E"), such as patients with acute exacerbation of sickle cell disease, untreated thalassemia major, or those with (very rare) unstable hemoglobins, but the laboratory findings in the vignette do not indicate any sickling or red cell inclusions to indicate this etiology.

> **Helpful Tip**
> An infection with parvovirus B19 may cause an acute aplastic crisis from transient bone marrow suppression in children with hereditary spherocytosis or other hemoglobinopathy.

⧗ QUICK QUIZ

Which is not a laboratory test finding in a child with hereditary spherocytosis?
A) Spherocytes.
B) Anemia.
C) Low mean corpuscular hemoglobin concentration.
D) Elevated mean corpuscular volume.
E) Elevated lactate dehydrogenase.

Discussion

The correct answer is "E." In hereditary spherocytosis, the anemia is typically normocytic to slightly macrocytic, and the mean corpuscular hemoglobin concentration (MCHC) is often elevated due to dehydration experienced by the red cells.

▶ CASE 4

A 2-year-old boy is brought to your clinic for evaluation after an episode of painless gross hematuria. His mother reports that he had a red-tinged void in his diaper last night, although his void this morning was normal colored. The patient is otherwise healthy, on no medications, and appears to be in no pain. His physical examination reveals a painless, left-sided abdominal mass palpated toward the flank, which does not move with respiration. Urinalysis in clinic today reveals trace heme and no red blood cells. You decide to order an abdominal ultrasound to evaluate the mass further.

Question 4-1

Which is the most likely diagnosis?
A) Wilms tumor.
B) Neuroblastoma.
C) Splenomegaly.
D) Pyelonephritis.
E) Rhabdomyosarcoma.

Discussion 4-1

The correct answer is "A." Painless gross hematuria in a toddler or preschool-aged child, even when intermittent, is highly suspicious for Wilms tumor (WT). A newly-identified abdominal

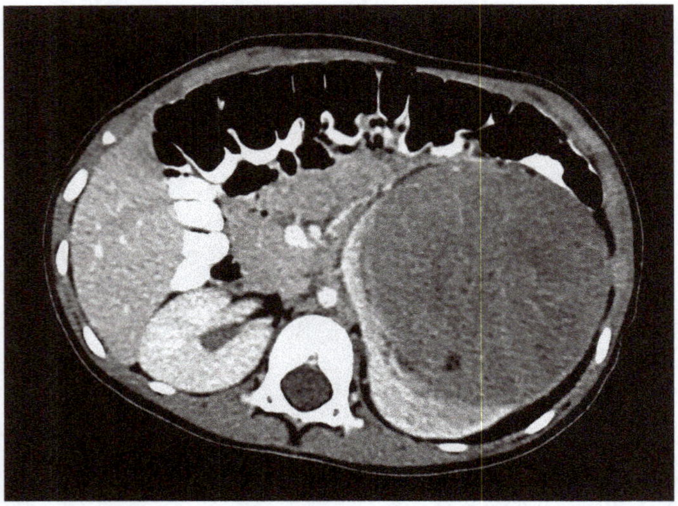

FIGURE 4–2. Wilms tumor. In this axial computed tomography image of the abdomen, there is a large encapsulated mass noted within the lower pole of the left kidney. The mass has no evidence of local infiltration or calcifications. Renal parenchyma, shown by contrast uptake, is pushed aside by the tumor, suggesting an intrinsic renal process. The left kidney remnant appears to be grasping or engulfing the lower-attenuation tumor, a finding sometimes described as a "claw sign." (Used with permission from Adam D. Wolfe, MD, PhD.)

mass is often palpated, and sometimes is the only finding, incidental on a well-child visit, that identifies this tumor. Because the tumor is not adjacent to the diaphragm, it does not move with respirations as an enlarged spleen does (making option "C" incorrect). Associated symptoms for WT are based on mass effect and may include constipation (constant or intermittent) and bladder dysfunction. Staging workup includes CT scan of the chest, abdomen, and pelvis; local extension and distant metastasis—often to the lungs—are both hallmarks of this disease. Therapy includes upfront resection of the affected kidney, followed by chemotherapy and radiation therapy dictated by stage. Cure rates for the most common forms of WT are excellent, well above 90%. Distinguishing WT from neuroblastoma (option "B"), another frequently encountered abdominopelvic tumor in the same age range, is not reliably done by physical exam or ultrasound. CT scan may be helpful, as neuroblastoma tends to exhibit calcifications, while WT arises within the kidney and pushes renal parenchyma toward the capsule. (See Figure 4–2.) Tissue diagnosis is required to be certain. Rhabdomyosarcoma (RMS; option "E") is a soft tissue sarcoma that may arise in nearly any tissue of the body. In boys, it is frequently found arising from the prostate or bladder, which would be unexpected to exhibit a flank mass if involving the midline urogenital system. RMS is also less common overall than WT. Finally, while pyelonephritis (option "D") may exhibit renal complications, the overall well appearance of the child and presence of a mass are not consistent with this diagnosis.

Question 4-2

What is a potential complication of Wilms tumor?

A) Tumor rupture with internal hemorrhage.
B) Hypercalcemia.

C) Tumor lysis syndrome.
D) Adrenal insufficiency.
E) Thrombocytopenia.

Discussion 4-2

The correct answer is "A." Because WT arises within the kidney capsule, as it grows the risk of tumor rupture increases. Rupture may be caused by minimal trauma, such as falling forward while running, as toddlers often do. Ruptured WT may become a life-threatening condition due to internal blood loss, although these tumors often bleed into the retroperitoneum and auto-tamponade limits the quantity of blood loss. Nevertheless, this presents a significantly greater surgical bleeding risk when the tumor is resected. Tumor rupture also seeds the abdomen, which upstages the cancer and leads to therapy with more intensive chemotherapy and a wider radiation field.

▶ CASE 5

A 14-month-old boy is brought to your clinic for rash. His father reports that he has a rash on his neck, elbows and legs, consisting of tiny flat red dots. He has also had increased bruising over the past week on his extremities. He is otherwise healthy, although 2 weeks ago, he had nasal congestion, cough, and diarrhea lasting for 3 days. The patient has not had nosebleeds, bleeding gums, or blood in his urine or stool. He was circumcised at birth, without unusual bleeding. Family history is negative for easy bleeding or bruising. The patient appears very well on exam and is actively playing, running, and smiling. He has several violaceous bruises ranging in size from 2 to 10 cm diameter on his extremities and trunk, and scattered petechiae in the distribution reported for the rash above. A CBC is performed, revealing a platelet count of 9 ×10³/mm³; all other parameters are normal.

Question 5-1

Which of the following is the best initial management for this patient's condition?

A) Splenectomy.
B) Anti-D immune globulin 75 mcg/kg × 1 dose.
C) Prednisolone 1 to 2 mg/kg/day orally for 2 weeks.
D) Anticipatory guidance and observation.
E) Intravenous immunoglobulin (IVIG) 0.8 g/kg × 1 dose.

Discussion 5-1

The correct answer is "D." This patient, who has isolated thrombocytopenia after an acute viral illness, cutaneous bruising, and no other systemic symptoms, most likely has immune thrombocytopenia (ITP—note that the previous name of immune thrombocytopenic purpura has been changed to exclude "purpura" in recent years). ITP commonly presents in the toddler period, and due to an autoimmune response following acute viral infection, or in up to 10% of ITP cases, following vaccination for measles, mumps, and rubella (MMR). Note that no other vaccinations have been associated with this condition. ITP is most commonly

TABLE 4–1 SUMMARY OF FIRST-LINE THERAPIES FOR IMMUNE THROMBOCYTOPENIA (ITP)

Therapy	Dose	Time to Initial Response	Adverse Effects and Comments
Observation	N/A	Weeks	Risk of bleeding, although severe bleeding is rare
Intravenous immunoglobulin (IVIG)	0.8 g/kg IV × 1, may repeat if no response	1–3 days	Infusion reaction including fever, vomiting, pruritus, myalgias; delayed headache; rare hemolytic reactions
Anti-D immune globulin	50–75 mcg/kg IV × 1	1–3 days	Only for patients with Rh+ blood type; often causes 1–2 g/dL drop in hemoglobin; black box warning requires monitoring for 8 hours for development severe hemolysis (rare)
Corticosteroid (eg, prednisone)	Prednisone 1–2 mg/kg/day PO × 1–2 weeks, taper up to several weeks more	4–14 days	No data support a specific dose, duration, or taper, and practice varies significantly; secondary adrenal insufficiency, hypertension, hyperglycemia, and growth concerns limit long-term use

Data from Neunert C, Lim W, Crowther M, et al; American Society of Hematology. The American Society of Hematology 2011 evidence-based practice guideline for immune thrombocytopenia. *Blood*. 2011;117(16):4190–4207.

a self-limited condition, and current evidence-based guidelines indicate that observation alone is adequate management for uncomplicated ITP such as described in the vignette; platelet counts should be expected to correct over the ensuing weeks to months following diagnosis. The most worrisome complication of thrombocytopenia in a toddler is intracranial hemorrhage (ICH), although the incidence of spontaneous ICH associated with ITP is unknown. Treated and untreated patients appear to have similar risk of ICH, up to 0.2%. Parents should be educated to seek immediate medical attention if the child suffers a head injury, or exhibits gastrointestinal bleeding symptoms, although again these are fairly rare complications. Patients with expanding hematoma or mucosal bleeding symptoms, such as prolonged epistaxis or gingival bleeding, may warrant treatment to hasten the recovery of platelets. The current frontline therapies recommended for such patients are IVIG (option "E"), anti-D immune globulin for Rh-positive individuals (option "B"), and corticosteroids (option "C"); each of these has an approximately 70% likelihood of increasing platelet counts in treated children with ITP. See Table 4–1 for a summary of these modalities. In refractory or severe cases, splenectomy (choice A) is also a consideration, but this is discouraged as upfront therapy, especially in children younger than 6 years of age because of the increased risk of infection with encapsulated organisms in asplenic individuals.

Question 5-2

What is NOT a typical test ordered as part of the initial diagnostic workup for suspected ITP?
A) Complete blood count.
B) Coagulopathy panel.
C) Bone marrow aspiration.

D) White cell differential.
E) Peripheral blood smear.

Discussion 5-2

The correct answer is "C." One cohort of 328 children with typical ITP features underwent bone marrow aspiration for evaluation of leukemia, with 0 of them having malignancy; therefore, children with typical ITP are not recommended to undergo bone marrow evaluation to "rule out" leukemia. Atypical features include symptoms such as fevers, weight loss, fatigue, irritability, or pain, and objective findings such as lymphadenopathy, organomegaly, or multiple abnormal cell lines on the blood count; these findings raise suspicion for non-ITP hematologic or oncologic diagnoses. Under these circumstances, evaluation by a hematologist is recommended prior to initiation of therapy.

▶ CASE 6

A 16-year-old adolescent girl initially presented to your clinic with cough, generalized lymphadenopathy, and fever. Onset of symptoms was 6 months ago, with increasing pruritus, flushing, and night sweats. She occasionally felt increasing pressure in her chest while lying down, and was having difficulty taking deep breaths. Physical examination was remarkable for posterior cervical lymphadenopathy, 10 cm on the right and 5 cm on the left. Coarse crackles were appreciated in the lower lung fields bilaterally. Saturation of peripheral hemoglobin by oxygen (SpO$_2$) was 86% on room air. A CBC revealed hemoglobin of 10.6 g/dL, white blood cell count (WBC) 15 ×10^3/mm^3 (differential: neutrophils 15%, lymphocytes 73%, monocytes 8%, eosinophils 4%), and platelets

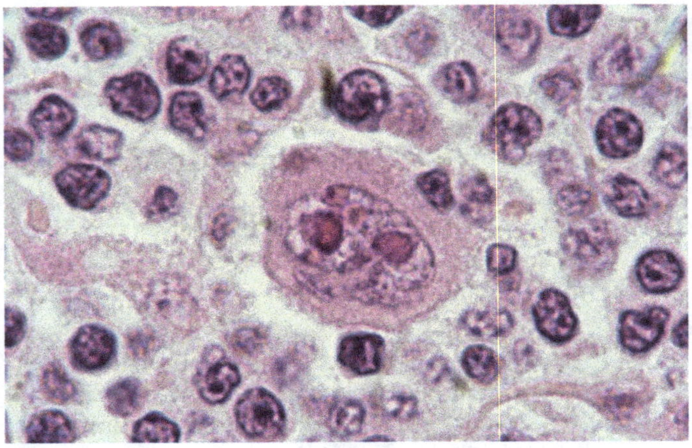

is more common in adolescents and young adults. Hodgkin lymphoma is curable with chemotherapy. In the past, patients with splenic involvement have undergone splenectomy as part of their therapy, although this is not commonly recommended for pediatric patients. Asplenic patients are at increased risk of infection with encapsulated organisms; it is recommended that splenectomy be delayed until 23-valent pneumococcal and meningococcal vaccinations can be administered. Prompt attention to fevers in splenectomized patients, with blood culture and empiric antibiotic therapy during a 48-hour sepsis rule-out, is recommended.

Helpful Tip

A mediastinal mass is never normal and may be caused by leukemia or lymphoma. Orthopnea may be a symptom of a chest mass.

FIGURE 4–3. This finding was noted on excisional biopsy of the patient's enlarged lymph node (Case 6). (Reproduced with permission from Kaushansky K, Lichtman MA, KBeutler E, et al: *Williams Hematology*, 8ed. McGraw-Hill Education, Inc., 2010. Fig 98-34.)

$382 \times 10^3/mm^3$. An excisional lymph node biopsy reveals the finding shown in Figure 4–3.

Question 6-1

Of the following, the most likely diagnosis is:
A) Acute lymphoblastic leukemia.
B) Hodgkin lymphoma.
C) Infectious mononucleosis.
D) Diffuse large B-cell lymphoma.
E) Systemic lupus erythematosus.

Discussion 6-1

The correct answer is "B." Figure 4–3 exhibits a classic binucleate Reed-Sternberg cell, with the typical "owl's eyes" appearance to the nucleoli. It is pathognomonic for Hodgkin lymphoma (HL), although not all HL will present with this finding on biopsy [7]. In a patient with lymphadenopathy that is worrisome for malignancy, such as the patient in the vignette, note that consultation with a pediatric surgeon is recommended to ensure that excisional biopsy is obtained; the sampling error associated with needle core biopsy increases the chance of false-negative results, need for re-biopsy, and delay in diagnosis and treatment. Apart from this piece of data, this is a teenage patient with several months of lymphadenopathy, fever, and cough, with other chest symptoms suggestive of a chest mass. The quality of symptoms may overlap with those of infectious mononucleosis (option "C"), but the duration is atypical, and the CBC did not report atypical lymphocytes that would be suspicious for Epstein-Barr virus infection. Similarly, the largely normal CBC does not raise suspicion for acute lymphoblastic leukemia (ALL, option "A"); one should expect ALL to exhibit marked cytopenias and possibly leukocytosis. The biopsy result is inconsistent with lupus (option "E"). The age of the patient, with constitutional illness and symptoms consistent with a chest mass, should be clues for HL. Non-Hodgkin lymphomas (NHL, option "D") might also have similar presenting findings, although among pediatric patients, NHL is more common in younger children and HL

CASE 7

A 3-year-old boy presents with 4 months of diarrhea, irritability, anorexia, and progressive fatigue. Exam shows an ill-appearing child. Vital signs include temperature 37.2°C (98.9°F), blood pressure 130/80 mm Hg, heart rate 140 beats per minute, respiratory rate 30 breaths per minute. On physical exam, he has periorbital ecchymoses with proptosis, matted firm nonmobile lymph nodes in his left anterior cervical chain, distended abdomen, firm mass in the abdominal right upper quadrant extending to the pelvis, and bilateral inguinal adenopathy. He is pale and has bruises over his lower extremities. Labs show elevated lactate dehydrogenase of 980 units/L, hemoglobin 7.4 g/dL, platelets $650 \times 10^3/mm^3$, and WBC $4.5 \times 10^3/mm^3$ with a normal differential. His albumin is 1.9 g/dL and creatinine is 0.7 mg/dL.

Question 7-1

Which of the following next steps is most likely to yield a diagnosis for this patient?
A) Blood culture.
B) Coagulopathy panel.
C) Manual blood smear evaluation.
D) Serum alkaline phosphatase.
E) Urine catecholamines.

Discussion 7-1

The correct answer is "E." This patient has findings consistent with neuroblastoma. The hypertension, tachycardia, diffuse lymphadenopathy, and abdominal mass, with low albumin and hemoglobin, are all worrisome for this diagnosis and suggest widespread disease. The nearly normal white blood cell count with normal differential, in the context of a large abdominal mass, reduces suspicion for leukemia (making option "C" less helpful). This presentation is less likely to be infection than malignancy, given the presence of a primary abdominal tumor (making option "A" less helpful). While some patients with malignancy can present with disseminated intravascular coagulation (DIC), the presence of a coagulopathy would not establish the underlying diagnosis (making option "B" incorrect). Similarly, while alkaline phosphatase may be elevated in the setting of malignancy, this is often the case with tumors involving bone and is not sufficiently specific to yield this patient's diagnosis (making option "D" incorrect). The most specific study from the answer choices that is likely to yield a diagnosis is the urine catecholamines, which would be expected to be elevated in approximately 90% of neuroblastoma. Staging and risk-stratifying this tumor will require surgical biopsy; imaging with CT chest, abdomen, and pelvis; tumor-specific nuclear medicine imaging; and bone marrow aspiration and biopsy. Neuroblastic tumors can be solitary primary tumors amenable to surgical resection only, or present with widespread metastatic disease, such as described in the vignette. These patients require aggressive, multimodal therapy with chemotherapy, surgical resection, radiation therapy, autologous stem cell transplantation, and immunotherapy. The patient in this vignette has "raccoon eyes," suggestive of periorbital involvement. This is a finding often associated with neuroblastoma despite its relative rarity in clinical practice. Another clinical finding associated with metastatic neuroblastoma is opsoclonus-myoclonus syndrome, a paraneoplastic process associated with irregular, saccading eye movements and myoclonic movements. Both of these clinical findings are suggestive of advanced stage disease, and therefore poorer prognosis.

> **Helpful Tip**
> Neuroblastoma is a malignant tumor of the sympathetic ganglia. Urinary homovanillic acid (HVA) and vanillylmandelic acid (VMA) (catecholamines) are elevated.

▶ CASE 8

A 16-year-old adolescent girl is being seen for a health supervision visit. She is a former 27-week premature infant, who suffered severe necrotizing enterocolitis in early infancy, and underwent surgical resection of necrotic terminal ileum as a result. She was followed in the surgical short gut clinic to support her nutritional needs, but you note that she has not been seen there for over 3 years. Over the past year, the patient reports becoming progressively more tired. She has trouble climbing stairways at school, and becomes lightheaded when she stands up. Within the past month, she has noticed numbness in her fingers. Her mother feels that she appears pale and tired, compared with 1 year ago. In private discussion, the patient concedes that she stopped taking her vitamin and mineral treatments, both pills and injections, between 2 and 3 years ago, because it was too difficult to remember to take them, the shots were uncomfortable, and because she has been eating well and does not feel that she needs the extra medication anymore. You suspect a nutritional anemia to explain this patient's symptoms.

Question 8-1

Which of the following statements is most accurate regarding the clinical approach to this patient?
A) Iron deficiency anemia may be excluded if the patient's red cells are normocytic.
B) Folate deficiency can be distinguished from vitamin B_{12} deficiency on blood smear by the presence of hypersegmented neutrophils.
C) The presence of paresthesia raises suspicion for vitamin B_{12} deficiency.
D) Folate deficiency can be distinguished from vitamin B_{12} deficiency on the CBC by the presence of macrocytosis.
E) A therapeutic trial of oral iron, folic acid, and B-complex vitamins will likely correct this patient's symptoms.

Discussion 8-1

The correct answer is "C." This patient, who has short gut syndrome and has been lost to follow up for several years, likely has multiple vitamin and mineral deficiencies. She has symptoms suggestive of progressive anemia, including fatigue, activity intolerance, and orthostatic symptoms; three likely nutritional deficiencies that could be occurring are iron, vitamin B_{12}, and folate deficiency. The additional symptom of paresthesia presented in the vignette is not a symptom of anemia; however, vitamin B_{12} deficiency, particularly if unaddressed and longstanding, is associated with neurologic changes that are often permanent (making option "E" incorrect). Vitamin B_{12} is absorbed in the terminal ileum, therefore; surgical removal or inflammation can result in vitamin B_{12} deficiency. Diagnosis is best made by checking levels of each of the above-listed nutrients individually and providing therapeutic doses as appropriate. However, initial evidence may be obtained from the CBC and manual smear evaluation. Because this patient likely has multiple anemia-associated deficiencies, it will be difficult to rule in or out a specific deficiency based on the mean corpuscular volume (MCV); this patient may appear normocytic in the face of a microcytosis-associated iron deficiency and concomitant macrocytosis-associated folate or B_{12} deficiency, or both (making option "A" incorrect). Folate and B_{12} deficiencies are both associated with macrocytosis, and cannot be distinguished based on blood counts and red cell indices (option "D"). Both conditions are also associated with the presence of hypersegmented neutrophils (six or more lobes per nucleus), as shown in Figure 4–4 (option "B"). Other, nonnutritional causes of macrocytic anemia in children are fairly rare. Relative macrocytosis may be seen in spherocytosis syndromes, hypothyroidism, myelodysplastic diseases, trisomy 21, and in any condition that causes significant reticulocytosis, as reticulocytes have increased MCV with respect to mature erythrocytes. Also note that red cells with increased levels of fetal hemoglobin have an increased MCV; therefore, neonates will exhibit an "elevated"—but normal for age—MCV at birth (ie, 106 ± 10 fL in term neonates), which over 3 to 4 months trends down to the "normal" levels expected of children and adults (ie, 88 ± 8 fL).

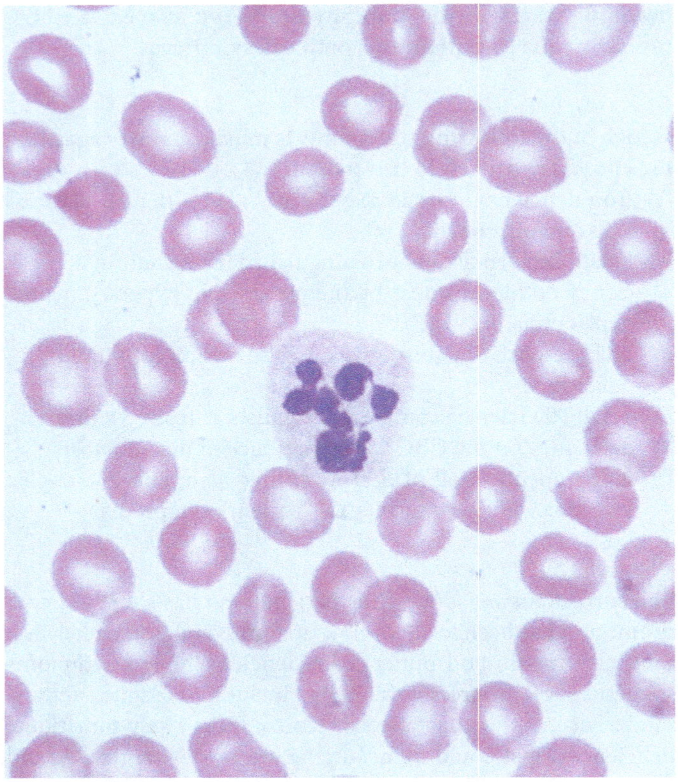

FIGURE 4–4. Hypersegmented neutrophil. This finding accompanies megaloblastic anemia secondary to folate or vitamin B_{12} deficiency. Macrocytosis of red blood cells is also noted. (Reproduced with permission from Laposata M, ed. *Laboratory Medicine: The Diagnosis of Disease in the Clinical Laboratory*, 2nd ed. New York, NY: McGraw-Hill Education, Inc; 2014, Figure 10-13.)

> ▶ **CASE 9**

An 11-month-old boy is brought to your clinic because his parents are concerned that he has become pale. He has had regular health supervision, has no medical problems, and takes no medications. His diet is varied and appropriate for age. He is up-to-date on recommended vaccinations. All developmental milestones have been met appropriately to date. Physical exam reveals a pale, tired-appearing boy who is otherwise awake and interactive. Lab work reveals anemia with hemoglobin 7.3 g/dL and replete iron stores as measured by serum iron and ferritin.

Question 9-1

Which of the following additional exam or laboratory findings would make you concerned that this child is at increased risk of malignancy during his first three decades of life?

A) Reticulocytopenia.
B) Triphalangeal thumbs.
C) Tall stature (height > 95th percentile).
D) Neutropenia.
E) Intoeing with ambulation.

Discussion 9-1

The correct answer is "B." This previously healthy toddler presents with non–iron deficiency anemia, and while the differential diagnosis remains broad, two conditions that can appear similarly are transient erythroblastopenia of childhood (TEC) and Diamond-Blackfan anemia (DBA). Both conditions are forms of pure red cell aplasia found in children. While the clinical findings of TEC and DBA substantially overlap, DBA is often diagnosed in infancy, while TEC is typically diagnosed around 2 years of age. The prognosis and approach to management of these conditions are very different. TEC is thought to be, in part, an immune-mediated postinfectious process; some authors have posited a relationship to viral infection, while others have been unable to find an association with specific viruses. The precise mechanism of TEC is therefore still obscure. TEC is an acquired condition that is self-limited, and the reticulocytopenia/anemia should improve with observation over the ensuing weeks to months. Transfusion is typically only recommended for children with severe, symptomatic anemia (ie, hemoglobin < 5 g/dL) and persistent reticulocytopenia. On the other hand, DBA is a congenital pure red cell aplasia linked to deficient ribosomal protein production, most commonly due to mutations in the *RPS19* or *RPSA24* genes. Syndromic features are present in nearly 50% of patients with DBA and can include upper extremity physical anomalies involving the thumbs, cardiac and genitourinary anomalies, and facial anomalies. DBA is a cancer predisposition syndrome, and patients with DBA have a nearly 50% chance of developing a hematologic or solid malignancy by age 30. Management of DBA depends on severity; supportive care includes chronic transfusion therapy, and many respond to corticosteroid therapy. Cure is affected by hematopoietic stem cell transplantation, although this may not be recommended in patients who do not have a matched related stem cell donor. Table 4–2 offers a clinical comparison of TEC and DBA.

⧖ QUICK QUIZ

What is NOT a cause of pure red cell aplasia in pediatric patients?

A) Systemic lupus erythematosus.
B) Parvovirus.
C) Isoniazid.
D) Malnutrition.
E) Hypothyroidism.

Discussion

The correct answer is "E." In addition to TEC and DBA, other items in the differential for pure red cell aplasia include collagen vascular disease, viral bone marrow suppression (eg, with parvovirus B19, usually in the setting of a patient with a chronic hemolytic syndrome such as hereditary spherocytosis), severe renal disease, medications, and nutritional deficiencies.

TABLE 4–2 COMPARISON OF TRANSIENT ERYTHROBLASTOPENIA OF CHILDHOOD (TEC) AND DIAMOND-BLACKFAN ANEMIA (DBA)

Finding	TEC	DBA
Age at diagnosis	Mean: 26 months	Mean: 11 months
	Median: 23 months	Median: 3 months
Infection history	Antecedent viral illness	None
Macrocytosis	Rare at diagnosis, likely during recovery	Frequent
Reticulocyte count	Low at diagnosis, elevated during recovery	Low
Fetal hemoglobin	Rarely elevated	Frequently elevated
Nonhematologic findings	None	Up to 25% of cases:
		Low birthweight
		Growth retardation
		Microcephaly
		Cleft palate
		Hypoplastic, bifid, or triphalangeal thumbs
		Cardiac abnormalities
		Genitourinary abnormalities
Increased malignancy risk	None	Acute myeloid leukemia
		Myelodysplastic syndrome
		Osteosarcoma, other sarcomas
		Hodgkin lymphoma
		Hepatocellular carcinoma
Initial management	Observation	Corticosteroids

Data from Handin RI, Lux SE, Stossel TP, eds. *Blood: Principles and Practice of Hematology*. Philadelphia, PA: Lippincott, Williams and Wilkins; 2003.

► CASE 10

An 8-year-old girl presents to the emergency department because of lumps on the right side and back of her head. Her parents first noticed them several weeks ago and thought they were "zits" because they were soft and painless. Now, the lumps have grown and are still soft and painless. The patient has previously been healthy, although the parents report that she has been getting up five to eight times each night to void, and is drinking more than usual for the past 2 to 3 weeks. Vital signs are within normal limits. Physical exam is remarkable for soft, nontender nodules over the right temporal bone and right occipital scalp. You also notice a rash on the right pinna, which is scaly and erythematous, and which the patient reports has been there for months; it is occasionally pruritic. A skeletal X-ray series is performed, and reveals a 1.5 × 1.5 cm round, lytic lesion in the right temporal bone and another 2.5 × 3 cm similar lesion in the right occipital bone, the latter of which is shown in Figure 4–5.

Question 10-1

Which of the following is the most likely diagnosis for this patient?
A) Ewing sarcoma.
B) Osteosarcoma.
C) Non-Hodgkin lymphoma.
D) Trauma with contusion of the skull.
E) Langerhans cell histiocytosis.

Discussion 10-1

The correct answer is "E." Langerhans cell histiocytosis (LCH) is a proliferative disorder of dendritic cells. While it is not a clonal disease, and therefore not considered a malignancy, it can involve multiple organs and cause significant and destructive systemic disease. The average age of presentation is young, approximately 2.5 years, but LCH can present at any age. LCH may present with solitary or multiple bony or soft tissue tumors that may or may not be painful; in more ill-appearing children one should suspect additional organ

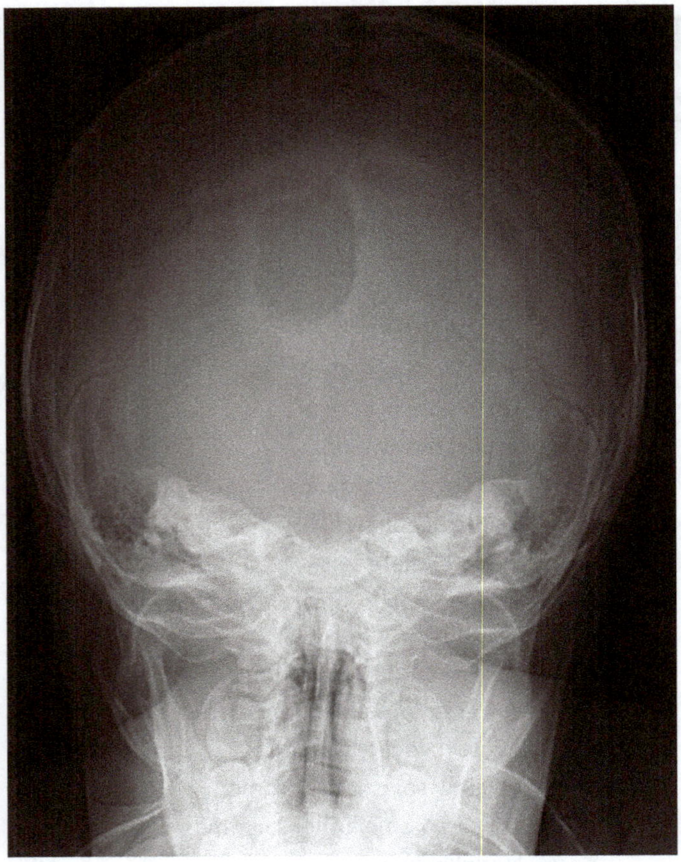

FIGURE 4–5. Skull finding in Langerhans cell histiocytosis (LCH). This plain film exhibits a large lytic lesion in the right occipital bone. There is minimal sclerosis and no periosteal reaction. This appearance is consistent with skull lesions common in LCH. (Used with permission from Adam D. Wolfe, MD, PhD.)

involvement. (See Table 4–3 for a summary of organs that may be involved.) Diagnosis is suspected based on clinical imaging findings, and may be confirmed by biopsy. LCH classically will stain immunohistochemically positive for CD1a and S100. Involvement of specific bones of the skull (ie, mastoid, orbital, sphenoid, and temporal bones) carries additional risk of intracranial progression. This may involve the neurohypophysis (posterior pituitary gland) and cause central diabetes insipidus, as was seen in the vignette, and merits MRI of the pituitary for evaluation, as well as endocrinology consultation. Patients who have LCH involvement of the liver, spleen, and bone marrow are at highest risk of treatment failure. Frontline therapy for LCH includes chemotherapeutic agents and corticosteroids, typically given over 1 year. Cure rates for even high-risk patients are greater than 80%, although significant rates of recurrence (25–40%) dictate retreatment with salvage chemotherapy for many patients before the disease resolves. None of the other option choices given would be expected to cause a lytic lesion of the skull that lacks surrounding sclerotic changes or periosteal reaction.

▶ CASE 11

You are rounding in the newborn nursery, and have been asked to perform circumcision on a 48-hour-old baby boy. He was born by spontaneous vaginal delivery at 39-4/7 weeks' gestation after an uncomplicated pregnancy and has been doing well. His mother has no medical problems and is on no medications. On screening family history, the infant's mother reports that she has never had any bleeding problems. She does note that the infant's maternal grandfather became significantly disabled due to joint problems in his 40s, and that her brother, the infant's uncle, has "some kind of bleeding problem" and has to take medication several times per week to treat his disease. The paternal family history is negative.

Question 11-1

Which of the following factor deficiencies is most likely to affect this baby?
A) Factor V.
B) Factor VII.
C) Factor VIII.
D) Factor XII.
E) von Willebrand factor

Discussion 11-1

The correct answer is "C." The family history described by the mother is most suggestive of a bleeding disorder that follows an X-linked recessive inheritance pattern, of which factor VIII deficiency—hemophilia A—is the most common. Factor VIII deficiency affects an estimated 1 in 5000 male births, and approximately two thirds of cases are inherited; the remainder are due to spontaneous mutation. Factor IX deficiency—hemophilia B, also X-linked—affects approximately 1 in 30,000 male births. Severity of hemophilias is based on the level of factor activity: severe hemophilia results from less than 1% factor activity, moderate hemophilia occurs with 1% to 5% activity, and mild hemophilia is defined as greater than 5% factor activity. Bleeding associated with hemophilias includes joint and muscle bleeding, unusual bruising and hematomas, mucosal bleeding, retroperitoneal bleeding, and postoperative bleeding. Patients with severe and often moderate hemophilia require prophylactic dosing of recombinant factor replacement products throughout their lives to prevent joint bleeding and the development of disabling chronic hemophilic arthropathy. Patients with mild and some moderate hemophilias may not require scheduled prophylactic dosing, and may be treated episodically in the setting of injury, surgery, or dental procedures. In the neonatal period, the greatest bleeding risks in hemophilia are associated with circumcision, heel sticks, and intracranial hemorrhage. Postvaccination intramuscular bleeding is also likely during the infant period. Von Willebrand disease (vWD, option "E") is among the most common bleeding disorders, and vWD and the hemophilias together account for at least 90% of bleeding disorder

TABLE 4–3 COMMON ORGAN INVOLVEMENT IN LANGERHANS CELL HISTIOCYTOSIS

Organ system	Symptoms and Findings	Evaluation	Complications and Outcomes
Bone	Skull is most frequent, then femur, ribs, humerus, vertebrae; may cause pain with associated adjacent soft tissue extension; vertebral lesions may cause spinal compression	Plain film, computed tomography scan	Pathologic fracture, calvarial weakness
Gingiva/mandible	"Floating" teeth	Plain film, computed tomography scan	Can lead to tooth loss
Skin	Scaly, erythematous plaque; associated pruritus	None or biopsy	May resolve spontaneously; new rash may present as sign of relapse
Lymphatic tissues	Lymphadenopathy	Computed tomography scan, biopsy	
Lung	Often asymptomatic, may have cough or dyspnea	Computed tomography scan	Previously considered a "risk organ," but no specific association with treatment failure
Pituitary	Polydipsia, polyuria; rarely other pituitary hormone deficiencies	Magnetic resonance imaging brain + pituitary; serum electrolytes, urine / plasma osmolality, urinalysis, water deprivation test	Likely permanent diabetes insipidus, increases risk for neurodegenerative syndrome in later life
Spleen	Abdominal distension, easy bruising or bleeding, fatigue	Computed tomography scan	"Risk organ" = increased chance of recurrence
Bone marrow	Easy bruising or bleeding; fatigue; fevers and infections	Complete blood count, bone marrow aspirate and biopsy	"Risk organ" = increased chance of recurrence
Liver	Abdominal distension, jaundice, icterus, pruritus	Computed tomography scan	"Risk organ" = increased chance of recurrence; risk of sclerosing cholangitis

Data from Allen CE, Kelly KM, Bollard CM. Pediatric lymphomas and histiocytic disorders of childhood. *Pediatr Clin North Am.* 2015;62(1):139–165; and Demellawy DE, Young JL, Nanassy J, et al. Langerhans cell histiocytosis: A comprehensive review. *Pathology.* 2015;47(4):294–301.

diagnoses. Most vWD is inherited in an autosomal dominant fashion. Von Willebrand factor functions as a carrier for factor VIII and is crucial for recruiting platelets to sites of injury and collagen exposure; therefore, bleeding history in patients with vWD often resembles platelet-type bleeding. Symptoms may include mucocutaneous symptoms such as easy bruising, epistaxis, gingival bleeding, and menorrhagia. It is common to encounter young women with mild vWD, who are not diagnosed until after menarche. Factor V and VII deficiencies (options "A" and "B") are inherited in an autosomal recessive pattern and are considerably rarer than the hemophilias and vWD. Factor XII deficiency (option "D") is also inherited in an autosomal recessive pattern, but this condition is not associated with clinical bleeding symptoms; it causes prolongation of the activated partial thromboplastin time but, because of its lack of clinical symptomatology, does not require any therapy.

Helpful Tip

In hemophilia, the activated partial thromboplastin time (aPTT) may be prolonged but the prothrombin time (PT) is normal. If the aPTT is prolonged, a mixing study should be performed. Correction of the aPTT indicates a factor deficiency. Failure to correct indicates the presence of an inhibitor.

▶ **CASE 12**

A 3-year-old girl with hemoglobin SS (ie, sickle cell anemia) presents to the emergency department with fever, wheezing, and chest pain. She has a history of mild asthma, controlled with as-needed use of albuterol metered dose inhaler, but the medication did not correct her symptoms today. Vital signs include temperature 39°C (102.2°F), heart rate 136 beats per minute, respiratory rate 38 breaths per minute. SpO$_2$ on room air is 92%. On physical exam, the patient is awake and alert, but appears anxious and distressed. She coughs frequently. Chest auscultation reveals fine crackles on the right and scattered expiratory wheeze. Cardiac exam reveals a grade II/VI systolic ejection murmur. Chest X-ray identifies a right middle lobe infiltrate. CBC reveals white blood cells 19.3 × 10^3/mm^3 with 80% neutrophils, hemoglobin 6.8 g/dL, and platelets 602 × 10^3/mm^3. You diagnose the patient with acute chest syndrome (ACS).

Question 12-1

In addition to sending a blood culture and type and screen to the lab, which of the following correctly describes your next steps in caring for this patient?

A) Administer supplemental oxygen only if SpO$_2$ drops below 88%.
B) Initiate total exchange transfusion with appropriately cross-matched packed red blood cells (pRBCs).
C) Avoid opioid pain medications to prevent respiratory depression.
D) Begin therapy with a parenteral third-generation cephalosporin and oral macrolide.
E) Keep total IV fluid rate to 0.75 times maintenance to avoid circulatory overload.

Discussion 12-1

The correct answer is "D." ACS is a complication of sickle cell disease that is thought to occur in nearly 13% of patients with hemoglobin SS disease, and in fewer than 10% of patients with other sickle cell syndromes. The syndrome is characterized by acute onset of fever, cough, and chest pain, and has clinical findings of hypoxemia and new infiltrate on chest X-ray. This syndrome's findings overlap completely with acute bacterial and viral pneumonia, and in fact this is likely one of the underlying etiologies of ACS in children with sickle cell disease. Other contributing etiologies are microvascular occlusion by sickled cells in the pulmonary vascular bed, asthma exacerbation, and atelectasis. As the presence of inflammation and airway narrowing can cause local vasoconstriction in pulmonary capillaries, infection and asthma exacerbation may quickly cause local sickling due to relative tissue hypoxia and narrowed vasculature. Therefore, ACS is thought to be multifactorial in most presentations. Untreated ACS may rapidly progress to respiratory failure and death, and for this reason patients diagnosed with ACS merit inpatient admission and management. The management of ACS is aimed at addressing all of the above etiologies simultaneously. As with any patient who has sickle cell disease and fever, blood culture and parenteral antibiotic therapy are warranted. Treatment in children is directed toward pathogens associated with both typical and atypical pneumonias, and therefore ceftriaxone and azithromycin or comparable regimen is recommended. Patients whose hemoglobin is low (institution dependent, but typically < 8 g/dL) benefit from simple blood transfusion to reduce sickled cells and increase oxygen-carrying capacity; most exchange transfusion programs will not perform exchange on patients with low hemoglobin (making option "B" incorrect). Because patients with ACS-associated chest pain may exhibit tachypnea with shallow breathing, supplemental oxygen is often initiated, regardless of oximetry readings (option "A"), and adequate pain management is crucial to allow comfortable, deeper breathing (option "C"). Pain management with sickle cell disease is best accomplished with a combination nonsteroidal anti-inflammatory drug (NSAID), such as ibuprofen, naproxen, or ketorolac, and an opioid. Opioid doses should be titrated for effect, and with close monitoring to avoid oversedation. Initial hydration to improve flow through occluded vasculature is recommended at 1.0 to 1.5 times maintenance (making option "E" incorrect). Other aspects of management of ACS include aggressive therapy for asthma in patients with this diagnosis, and incentive spirometry and early ambulation as tolerated for atelectasis.

⧖ QUICK QUIZ

Which is a complication of sickle cell disease?
A) Acute vasoocclusive crisis.
B) Sepsis.
C) Stroke.
D) Priapism.
E) All of the above.

Discussion

The correct answer is "E."

> **Helpful Tip**
> Fever in a patient with sickle cell disease is a life-threatening emergency. Sickle cell disease causes functional asplenia with increased risk for overwhelming bacterial infections, including sepsis.

▶ CASE 13

A 12-month-old baby girl comes to your clinic for a health supervision visit. She has been healthy, meeting developmental milestones appropriately, and parents have no concerns today. You note on history that the baby suffered a viral-sounding upper respiratory infection with fever 2 to 3 weeks ago, with symptoms lasting 4 days that have now resolved. The patient has continued to track at the 47th percentile for weight and 61st percentile for height. Based on current guidelines for anemia screening, you order a CBC and discover the following: white blood cells 4.3 × 10^3/mm^3, hemoglobin 12.2 g/dL, platelets 244 × 10^3/mm^3. The WBC differential, which you did not order but was nevertheless performed, reveals an absolute neutrophil count of 130/mm^3 and absolute lymphocyte count of 3850/mm^3.

Question 13-1

Which of the following is the next best step in management of this patient's neutropenia?

A) Provide anticipatory guidance regarding the typically benign nature of the condition; observe with close follow up.

B) Admit the patient to receive intravenous antimicrobial therapy.

C) Request bone marrow aspiration and biopsy.

D) Administer a course of granulocyte colony-stimulating factor (G-CSF).

E) Prescribe a course of oral cephalosporin.

Discussion 13-1

The correct answer is "A." This patient's age, well appearance, and isolated neutropenia following a viral illness are most consistent with benign neutropenia of childhood. This condition is fairly commonly discovered incidentally when a blood count is ordered for a different reason. Benign neutropenia of childhood is a transient condition, thought to be due to an autoimmune reaction following the inciting infection. In some patients, antineutrophil antibody testing will reveal the causative antibody; this test is not offered in many centers and lacks sensitivity, and therefore is not routinely utilized in diagnosis. Over several weeks to months following diagnosis, patients are expected to return to normal neutrophil counts. In a well-appearing child with this diagnosis, observation alone is an appropriate approach. In general, benign neutropenia of childhood, regardless of neutrophil count, is not associated with severe infections. Nevertheless, prompt evaluation of fever is recommended in children with an absolute neutrophil count (ANC) of less than 500/mm³. Normal ANC in term newborns in their first week of life is greater than 3000/mm³, and then decreases to greater than 1100/mm³ during the next 2 years. After the age of 2, normal ANC in children and adolescents is greater than 1500/mm³. Table 4–4 defines different categories of neutropenia and their associated infectious risks. In addition to benign neutropenia of childhood, other possible acquired causes of neutropenia include viral suppression (eg, with Epstein-Barr virus infection), medication induced (eg, antiepileptics, beta-lactam antibiotics, chemotherapeutic agents), and other autoimmune diseases (eg, Crohn disease, systemic lupus erythematosus). Options "B" through "E" represent approaches that might be appropriate in some children with neutropenia but would not be required as a frontline approach in a well-appearing child with incidentally diagnosed neutropenia. If a patient with benign neutropenia should become severely ill, administration of G-CSF (option "D") to hasten neutrophil recovery is appropriate.

▶ CASE 14

A 17-month-old boy presents to your clinic because his parents are concerned about his mobility. He is a previously healthy baby, who met all developmental milestones on

TABLE 4–4 DEFINITIONS OF NEUTROPENIA AND COMPLICATIONS

Severity	Absolute Neutrophil Count (per mm³)	Risks
Normal	> 1500 (> 1100 if younger than age 2 years)	None
Mild	1000–1500	None; merits evaluation for cause of abnormal count (history often sufficient)
Moderate	500–1000	Minimal, risk if other immune functions are impaired
Severe	200–500	Increased risk of infection from commensal organisms (eg, gram-positive skin flora, gram-negative enterics)
Profound (ie, agranulocytosis)	< 200	Significant risk of infection by commensals, opportunistic pathogens such as *Pneumocystis jiroveci*

Data from Newburger PE, Dale DC. Evaluation and management of patients with isolated neutropenia. *Semin Hematol.* 2013;50(3):198–206.

time as of his last visit with you at 12 months of age. Mother reports today that the patient has seemed clumsier over the past 1 to 2 months and is not walking as much as he used to. She is unsure of whether he is in pain. He has vomited 4 to 5 mornings this week. Vital signs are within normal limits, and the patient is continuing to track on his previous percentiles for height and weight. Physical exam reveals a boy who is awake, alert, and interactive. He has horizontal nystagmus on neurologic exam. While sitting upright on the exam table, he leans over to the right and nearly falls off the table before you catch and right his posture. He is unwilling to bear weight on his legs for gait testing today. He has no rash, bruising, petechiae, lymphadenopathy, or organomegaly, and the remainder of your exam is unremarkable.

Question 14-1

Which of the following diagnoses is the most likely, given the historical and exam findings?
A) Craniopharyngioma.
B) Acute lymphoblastic leukemia.
C) Neuroblastoma.
D) Germ cell tumor.
E) Medulloblastoma.

Discussion 14-1

The correct answer is "E." This patient presents with signs and symptoms compatible with increased intracranial pressure (ICP), including ataxia, nystagmus, and vomiting, often observed in patients with a tumor that obstructs cerebrospinal fluid outflow from the third or fourth ventricle. Midline posterior fossa tumors, such as medulloblastoma, can present with these findings. Medulloblastoma, a primitive neuroectodermal tumor of the posterior fossa, is the most common malignant brain tumor of childhood, often diagnosed due to symptoms of increased ICP. The next step in evaluation and management when increased ICP is suspected is often urgent CT scan of the head. If a mass is noted, (MR) imaging is recommended to further delineate the mass. If increased ICP is identified, patients will often undergo placement of an externalized ventricular drain or a ventricular shunt to relieve the pressure. Because medulloblastoma may be metastatic to the spine at diagnosis, MR spine and diagnostic lumbar puncture are required to establish staging. A key element of prognosis for medulloblastoma—and most brain tumors in children—is the extent of primary surgical resection. Gross total resection is associated with better outcomes than partial resection, although the extent of resection may be limited by involvement of the brainstem. Following resection, patients with medulloblastoma are treated with multimodal chemotherapy and radiation therapy (XRT) to involved sites. However, in a patient as young as in the vignette, efforts are made to delay or eliminate the use of XRT due to the severe central nervous system toxicity associated with it. Alternatives to XRT in young children include intensification of chemotherapy, and high-dose chemotherapy with autologous stem cell rescue. Craniopharyngioma (option "A") is a tumor of pharyngeal cell rests (remnants of Rathke pouch) in a primarily suprasellar location near the pituitary gland, which most commonly occurs in immediately prepubertal children and is rare in children as young as the patient in the vignette. It may cause cerebral spinal fluid (CSF) obstruction and increased ICP, and is also associated with vision changes, behavioral abnormalities, and pubertal delay. Treatment is surgical, with or without XRT, and lifelong endocrine deficiencies (e.g. panhypopituitarism) occur subsequent to removal or damage of pituitary tissue. Primary germ cell tumors (option "D") may arise intracranially, most often in the pineal gland or suprasellar region. Symptoms depend on location of the tumor, but primarily include deficiencies of anterior pituitary hormones, diabetes insipidus, and visual disturbances. Acute lymphoblastic leukemia (option "B"), which may involve the central nervous system, does not readily form solid tumors and is unlikely to cause the posterior fossa symptoms described for the patient in the vignette. Neuroblastoma

(option "C") is a small round blue cell tumor derived from neuroepithelial cells of the neural crests during embryonic development. Neuroblastoma rarely penetrates the dura, making it unlikely to have caused the patient's symptoms.

⧗ QUICK QUIZ

Which of the following does not have a small round blue cell appearance by histology?
A) Neuroblastoma.
B) Medulloblastoma.
C) Ewing sarcoma.
D) Osteosarcoma.
E) Neuroendocrine tumors.

Discussion

The correct answer is "D." Neuroblastoma, medulloblastoma, other primitive neuroendocrine tumors, and Ewing sarcoma are so-called small round blue cell tumors because of histologic appearance. These tumors are also known as embryonal tumors, given their origin in early ontogeny; they have substantial migratory and growth potential, making them typically clinically aggressive.

▶ CASE 15

A previously healthy 4-year-old boy presents to your acute care clinic with bilateral leg weakness. He had episodes over the past 3 weeks consisting of pain, weakness, and numbness in his thighs, legs, and feet, which resolved after 1 to 2 hours, and therefore was not brought to medical attention. There is no history of trauma. Today, he has been experiencing another, more severe, episode over the past 4 hours: he woke up unable to stand or walk. He has not voided today. The patient is sitting in a wheelchair, in no apparent pain, alert and answering questions appropriately. Vital signs are within normal limits. On exam, the patient has normal muscle tone, bulk, and strength in all upper extremity muscle groups; the lower extremities exhibit increased tone and 2/5 strength in all muscle groups. Deep tendon reflexes are 2+ in the biceps and 4+ in the patellae. Sensation is diminished in the lower extremities bilaterally. The patient is unwilling to attempt gait testing. Capillary refill in fingers and toes is 2 to 3 seconds, and radial and dorsalis pedis pulses are 2+ bilaterally. You send the patient by ambulance to the emergency department.

Question 15-1

Which of the following are most likely to be part of the immediate management of this patient?
A) Magnetic resonance imaging (MRI) of the spine, consults to neurosurgery and radiation oncology.
B) MRI of the spine, consults to oncology and radiation oncology.

C) MRI of the spine, consults to oncology and neurosurgery, initiation of corticosteroids.

D) Computed tomography (CT) of the spine, consults to oncology and neurosurgery.

E) CT of the spine, consults to oncology and radiation oncology, initiation of corticosteroids.

Discussion 15-1

The correct answer is "C." Spinal cord compression is an onco-logic emergency, and can be seen with solid malignancies such as neuroblastic tumors and soft tissue sarcomas, hematologic malignancies such as extramedullary acute myeloid or lympho-blastic leukemias and lymphomas, and with vascular tumors such as vertebral hemangiomas. Prompt diagnosis and therapy are required to preserve neurologic function. Based on the type of tumor, the approach to initial therapy may vary. One tumor that is known to present with cord compression, neu-roblastoma, is amenable to chemotherapeutic, neurosurgical, and radiotherapeutic interventions, as are many spinal tumors. However, while radiation therapy may successfully treat the tumor, it is often not the initial treatment of choice in pediat-ric patients with tumors in the spine due to long-term adverse effects on growth and function. Emergent imaging with MRI, which can illustrate the source of the tumor as well as extent of epidural and soft tissue disease, is preferred, and will assist in the preliminary differential diagnosis and in establishing whether neurosurgical or chemotherapeutic intervention will be favored. For tumors that are chemotherapy-responsive, such as neuroblastoma, chemotherapy is often preferred over lami-nectomy and resection, again to minimize long-term effects on spinal growth. Corticosteroids are often initiated prior to che-motherapy to reduce peritumoral edema. Neurosurgical inter-vention may be reserved for cases of lack of response to medical therapy within the first 1 to 2 days.

▶ CASE 16

You are seeing an 8-year-old boy in your clinic to estab-lish care following a recent hospital admission. His family recently emigrated from Saudi Arabia, and you are con-ducting today's visit through an Arabic language phone interpreter. The patient was admitted for 2 days last week during a febrile influenza-like illness, because of extreme fatigue and because his eyes became "more yellow than usual." The parents report that the patient has otherwise been healthy. You review the hospital records, which show that the patient was admitted with fever, fatigue, dys-pnea, icterus, jaundice, and anemia with a hemoglobin of 6 g/dL and red blood cells with dark purple inclusions with supravital staining on blood smear. He received 1 unit of ABO-matched, packed red blood cells, tolerated this well, and his symptoms resolved within 48 hours. This had never happened to the patient before, although the par-ents inform you that the patient's 10-year-old brother and his maternal uncle have had jaundice and occasional blood

transfusions in the past, and that the patient's mother, father, and 5-year-old sister do not have these problems. On today's exam, the patient appears normal apart from subtle icterus.

Question 16-1

Which of the following tests is most likely to reveal this patient's diagnosis?

A) Bone marrow aspirate and biopsy.

B) Direct antiglobulin (Coombs) test.

C) Erythrocyte osmotic fragility test.

D) Glucose-6-phosphate dehydrogenase (G6PD) enzyme activity.

E) Hemoglobin electrophoresis.

Discussion 16-1

The correct answer is "D." This patient exhibits evidence of baseline hemolysis, has suffered symptomatic hemolytic ane-mia in the setting of an acute febrile illness, and has a fam-ily history suggestive of an X-linked disorder. Of the choices, these findings best fit with G6PD deficiency. G6PD deficiency is the most common red cell enzymopathy, and carrier sta-tus is most prevalent in families from malaria-endemic areas of the world, including Africa, the Middle East, southern and southeastern Asia, and South America. G6PD is an enzyme critical for function of the pentose phosphate pathway, which restores important reducing substances such as NADPH and glutathione, in red blood cells. Because G6PD-deficient indi-viduals cannot effectively utilize this pathway, their red cells are at risk of oxidant-induced damage and lysis at times of oxidative stress. Oxidative damage can cause precipitation of denatured hemoglobin, seen as Heinz bodies on staining with methyl violet, as with the patient in the vignette. Stress may come from acute infectious or inflammatory insults, such as occurred in the vignette, or due to medications and dietary causes. The most commonly discussed dietary cause is from fava beans, which are often used in Mediterranean and Middle Eastern cooking. Medications to avoid include sulfonamide antibiotics, dapsone, nitrofurantoin, and quinine-containing antimalarials, as well as naphthalene (mothballs). As an aside, for the family in this vignette, providing information on this disease and a list of medications and foods to avoid in their native language may be challenging, but will be crucial to helping them avoid complications for the affected boys. Some individuals with G6PD deficiency will have more severe phe-notypes than others, with some children experiencing hemo-lytic episodes in the newborn or infant periods. Severity is suggested by G6PD enzyme activity assay: patients with less than 10% activity have more severe disease, while those with 10% to 60% activity have more moderate disease. In general, families of east Asian and Mediterranean descent appear to exhibit more severe phenotypes. Regarding the G6PD activ-ity assay, it is recommended that the test be performed after a patient's hemolytic episode has resolved. In most patients, maximal residual enzyme activity is retained in younger red cells (ie, reticulocytes) which comprise the bulk of available cells at the time of a hemolytic event. Therefore, testing during an event increases the chance of a falsely elevated enzyme activity result. Of the other answer choices, hereditary spherocytosis (assayed in option "C") could have a similar clinical presentation, but this condition is usually inherited in an autosomal dominant fashion. One would expect a patient with acute leukemia or bone marrow failure (assayed in option "A") to have additional blood count abnormalities, and a less acute symptomatology to indicate malignancy. Autoimmune hemolytic anemia (assayed in option "B") would not be expected to exhibit an X-linked inheritance pattern, and is not associated with Heinz bodies. Hemoglobinopathies such as sickle cell disease or thalassemia major (assayed in option "E") could cause anemia with hemolysis and jaundice in an episodic fashion, but would be expected to have additional chronic symptoms and would not be expected to exhibit X-linked inheritance.

▶ CASE 17

A 5-day-old baby boy is scheduled for an establishing well-newborn visit in your clinic. All you know about the baby is that he was born at home and has not yet seen a physician or medical provider. The mother called on day of life 2 to make the patient's appointment with you and reported that he was born without complications at 38-6/7 weeks' gestation and was doing well. The clinic receives a call from the baby's mother on the day of the appointment, in which she tells you that she is concerned that the baby is not waking from his nap this morning, is breathing shallowly, and over the past 10 minutes began shaking his right arm and leg. You advise the mother to call 9-1-1.

Question 17-1

When you call ahead to the emergency department to inform them of this patient, which of the following will you recommend be performed first?

A) Magnetic resonance imaging (MRI) of the head with IV contrast.
B) Computed tomography (CT) scan of the brain without IV contrast.
C) Coagulopathy screening with platelet count, prothrombin time (PT), and activated partial thromboplastin time (aPTT).
D) Intravenous administration of vitamin K.
E) Transfusion with fresh frozen plasma.

Discussion 17-1

The correct answer is "E." This term neonate presents with symptoms suggestive of intracranial hemorrhage (ICH), and since he presumably did not receive prophylactic vitamin K at birth and appeared well initially, is likely experiencing the classic form of vitamin K deficiency bleeding (VKDB). Very likely, all of the actions represented in the answer choices above will be taken, as imaging (options "A" and "B") and lab work (option "C") will be used in planning further management, but the most immediate task is to administer a therapy most likely to ameliorate the bleeding. This will most rapidly be accomplished by replenishing

the vitamin K–dependent clotting factors, which are present in physiologic quantities in fresh frozen plasma (FFP). Administering vitamin K is also recommended (option "D"), but will not yield an immediate change in the patient's bleeding diathesis. The symptoms and signs of ICH vary depending on the location of bleeding and the age of the patient. Presenting symptoms of ICH in neonates include seizures, focal weakness, feeding problems, and apneas or other respiratory events. These symptoms are similar to those of neonates who experience ischemic stroke, although arterial ischemic stroke and cerebrospinal venous thrombosis tend to present in neonates less than 72 to 96 hours of age. VKDB risk can be classified into three timeframes. Very early VKDB occurs within the first day after birth, and is associated with maternal medication use that interferes with vitamin K–dependent factor production (eg, warfarin). Classic VKDB presents within the first week of life, as with the patient in the vignette, and is often associated with mucocutaneous bleeding symptoms. Late VKDB can occur after 1 week of life, up to several weeks after birth. The latter two categories of VKDB are often associated with breastfed infants, due to the paucity of vitamin K in breast milk. Prophylactic administration of intramuscular vitamin K, which is recommended for all newborns, has been shown to significantly decrease the incidence of classic and late VKDB. Oral vitamin K is also available, although a single neonatal dose does not appear to reduce the risk of late VKDB. Depending on the normative ranges used in the laboratory, be aware that neonates, and particularly preterm neonates, will have coagulation screening tests that fall out of the "normal" ranges. This is largely due to relatively poor synthetic liver function seen in newborns. Both PT and aPTT prolongation are common in the first few days of life, due to low vitamin K–dependent factors in the former test and due to low propagation (ie, intrinsic) pathway factor levels in the latter case. Exceptions to this include factor VIII and von Willebrand factor levels, as these factors are not liver dependent and may, in fact, be elevated at birth.

> **Helpful Tip**
> Factor VIII and von Willebrand factor are synthesized in the vascular endothelium rather than the liver like all other coagulation factors.

▶ CASE 18

You are following a previously healthy 17-year-old adolescent girl for acute hepatitis. She was admitted to your service with suspected viral hepatitis last week, in the setting of acute diarrhea, nausea, pruritus, jaundice, hepatomegaly, and transaminitis. Since diagnosis, her transaminases, serum bilirubin, and serum chemistries have been checked daily and are stable. This morning, she is reporting increasing fatigue and shortness of breath. Apart from the jaundice and hepatomegaly, you find no other abnormalities on today's exam. You obtain a CBC, which reveals white blood cell count of $2.4 \times 10^3/mm^3$ with 18% neutrophils and 78% lymphocytes, hemoglobin 7.2 g/dL, and platelets of $64 \times 10^3/mm^3$. Erythrocyte sedimentation rate is 100 mm/h (reference range 0–20). Results of hepatitis A, B, and C serologies are negative.

Question 18-1
Which of the following diagnoses best explains this patient's blood count findings today?
A) Acquired aplastic anemia.
B) Acute lymphoblastic leukemia.
C) Chronic myelogenous leukemia.
D) Hepatocellular carcinoma.
E) Epstein-Barr virus infection.

Discussion 18-1
The correct answer is "A." This patient presents with acute seronegative hepatitis with subsequent pancytopenia, consistent with a working diagnosis of autoimmune aplastic anemia. Antecedent autoimmune hepatitis is a frequently encountered historical finding in patients with acquired aplastic anemia. Confirmatory testing with bone marrow aspirate and biopsy is required. Acute lymphoblastic leukemia (option "B") could present with these blood count findings and is certainly in the differential diagnosis, but it would be unexpected to see this acute drop in blood counts shortly after onset of hepatitis with

this diagnosis. The bone marrow assessment in this patient will also be used to rule out leukemia prior to therapy. Chronic myelogenous leukemia (option "C") can exhibit organomegaly, due to widespread extramedullary hematopoiesis, but is associated with marked splenomegaly, a significantly elevated white blood cell count, and many differently maturing cell forms seen on the white cell differential. Hepatocellular carcinoma (option "D") is a possible consequence of chronic hepatitis B or C infection, but should not be associated directly with acute pancytopenia. Epstein-Barr virus (EBV; option "E") can cause viral hepatitis and can be associated with bone marrow suppression, and EBV serologies probably would be tested in this patient; however, the absence of lymphadenopathy and relatively acute onset of pancytopenia should reduce suspicion for this diagnosis. Severe aplastic anemia (SAA) is diagnosed by hypocellularity (< 25%) on bone marrow aspirate. Management of SAA depends on the etiology. Acquired SAA may be caused by medications, such as certain antiepileptic drugs; in these cases discontinuation of the causative medication should be therapeutic. In a patient found to have SAA without a clear etiology, bone marrow failure syndromes are typically evaluated before an autoimmune cause is assumed. Selected bone marrow failure syndromes that are evaluated during a workup of newly diagnosed SAA are reviewed in Table 4–5. Management

TABLE 4–5 SELECTED BONE MARROW FAILURE SYNDROMES CONSIDERED IN THE DIFFERENTIAL DIAGNOSIS OF SEVERE APLASTIC ANEMIA

Condition	Etiology	Inheritance	Common Clinical Findings	Confirmatory Testing
Fanconi anemia	Mutations in multiple FA core complex genes	Variable: AR, XLR (*FANCB* mutation)	Short stature, radial and thumb abnormalities	Chromosomal breakage with diepoxybutane or mitomycin C
Dyskeratosis congenita	Mutations in multiple telomere maintenance enzyme complex genes	Variable: AR, AD, XLR	Dystrophic nails, skin thickening, leukoplakia	Telomere length analysis
Shwachman-Diamond syndrome	Mutation in Shwachman-Bodian-Diamond gene	AR	Pancreatic insufficiency, skeletal abnormalities, neutropenia	Pancreatic enzymes, fecal elastase, SBDS gene testing
Diamond-Blackfan anemia	Ribosome protein (*RPS*) genes	AD	Short stature, microcephaly, thumb abnormalities, cardiac abnormalities, urogenital abnormalities	Erythrocyte adenosine deaminase evaluation
Paroxysmal nocturnal hemoglobinuria	Mutation in *PIGA* gene, codes for a GPI linkage protein	Acquired	Hemoglobinuria, thrombosis, hemolysis, new pancytopenia	Flow cytometry for CD55 and CD59, which are GPI-dependent complement inhibitors

Abbreviations: AD, autosomal dominant; AR, autosomal recessive; GPI, glycophosphatidylinositol; XLR, X-linked recessive.
Reproduced with permission from Chirnomas SD, Kupfer GM: The inherited bone marrow failure syndromes, *Pediatr Clin North Am* 2013 Dec;60(6):1291–1310.

of most bone marrow failure syndromes involves hematopoietic stem cell transplant. For the patient in the vignette, if she is confirmed to have acquired SAA, supportive care with transfusions and prompt attention to infectious symptoms will be the initial management. If an antigen-matched full sibling is available, she would be a candidate for hematopoietic stem cell transplant. For patients without a matched sibling stem cell donor, current standard of care is immune suppressive therapy with antithymocyte globulin, corticosteroids, and cyclosporine A; approximately 70% of patients respond to this intervention within 2 to 3 months.

► **CASE 19**

You are following a 13-year-old adolescent girl with iron deficiency anemia (IDA), which you diagnosed 1 week ago and attributed to menorrhagia. Her bleeding has been lasting 7 days per cycle, requiring seven to eight pads per day, for 2 years. At last week's visit, she was complaining of fatigue, pallor, and exercise intolerance. Initial bloodwork revealed hemoglobin 7.9 g/dL, mean corpuscular volume (MCV) 63 fL, red cell distribution width (RDW) 15%, reticulocyte count 1.3% (reference range 0.2–1.5%), and serum ferritin 4 ng/mL (reference range 11 – 300). The patient was started on a combined oral contraceptive at that time, and began treatment with ferrous sulfate 325 mg tablets (65 mg elemental iron per tablet), 1 tablet by mouth twice daily. She weighs 40 kg. Today, the patient reports that she has had no menstrual bleeding in the past week, but that her other symptoms are largely unchanged from the last visit. She reports compliance with all doses of medication. Lab work today reveals hemoglobin 8.1 g/dL, MCV 69 fL, RDW 19%, reticulocyte count 5.2%, and serum ferritin 10 ng/mL.

Question 19-1

Which of the following would you recommend to the patient?
A) Increase iron dose to 2 tablets twice daily.
B) Continue current iron therapy and follow up in 1 month.
C) Refer to hematology for intravenous iron sucrose infusion.
D) Discontinue iron therapy and follow up in 1 month.
E) Perform hemoglobin electrophoresis.

Discussion 19-1

The correct answer is "B." This patient has findings suggestive of IDA in the setting of excessive menstrual losses and is showing an appropriate response to iron therapy. Patients with IDA will exhibit microcytic anemia, and often elevated RDW reflective of anisocytosis due to irregular red cell production in the iron-deficient bone marrow. Therapy is recommended with oral elemental iron (elemental iron is the bioavailable form; one must distinguish this from total iron often reported on over-the-counter tablet preparations), 3 to 6 mg/kg/day in one or two divided doses. Despite this wide dosing range, there are no consistent data to suggest that 6 mg/kg/day is more effective than 3 mg/kg/day (option "A"), and the patient is responding to

the current approximately 3 mg/kg/day she is taking. The initial response to therapeutic iron will be seen as reticulocytosis. Note that this patient's initial reticulocyte count was within the reference range, but was inappropriately low for her degree of anemia. One week following initiation of therapy, this number increased appropriately. Consequently, and since reticulocytes are larger than mature erythrocytes, the MCV and RDW have increased as well. These findings are reassuring that the patient is complying with medication and experiencing a physiologic response to it. While very rare individuals are refractory to oral iron due to a defect in absorption, a patient who is tolerating and responding to oral iron therapy would not be a candidate for IV iron infusion (option "C"). A measurable rise in hemoglobin may take several weeks to occur, and restoration of normal counts may take 2 to 3 months. Similarly, as the liver iron stores were presumably depleted initially, this patient's iron stores are far from restored, and the ferritin would not be expected to normalize for up to several weeks. Standard iron replenishment therapy is expected to require approximately 3 months before the patient can resume a maintenance or dietary dose (making option "D" incorrect). Patients with thalassemia trait also present with mild-to-moderate anemia and microcytosis and can be mistaken for having IDA. Particularly in young patients, the two conditions can coexist. It is important to follow markers of iron stores, and replenish iron as needed, before contemplating a diagnosis of thalassemia trait. Children who are iron replete, yet remain anemic and microcytic, may be clinically diagnosed with thalassemia trait; the family history may also assist in this diagnosis. Genetic testing is rarely used to confirm this diagnosis, although hemoglobin electrophoresis (option "E") can assist in the diagnosis of beta-thalassemia minor. In this condition, the level of hemoglobin A_2 (consisting of $\alpha_2\delta_2$ globins) is often found to be elevated. However, this finding is obscured in iron-deficient patients, which is why correction of iron deficiency is essential before pursuing the thalassemia trait diagnosis. Patients with alpha-thalassemia minor (2 gene α globin deletion) or minima (1 gene α globin deletion) will not exhibit changes on standard hemoglobin electrophoresis.

► **CASE 20**

A 3-year-old boy is brought to urgent care clinic for fever, pain, and fatigue. He was previously healthy until 3 to 4 weeks ago, when he started seeming more tired to his parents. He developed fevers 6 days ago, with oral temperatures up to 39.1°C (102.4°F), which have been occurring daily and are responsive to acetaminophen. His parents also feel that he has seemed paler to them, and he has bruising on his legs. Vital signs include temperature 38.1°C (100.6°F), heart rate 136 beats per minute, and respirations 24 breaths per minute. On exam, the patient is awake, alert, but tired-appearing. He falls asleep during the exam, awakens easily but wants to be held by his mother and is unwilling to participate in gait testing. He has conjunctival pallor; bilateral cervical lymphadenopathy; grade II/VI systolic ejection murmur; nontender splenomegaly with the tip palpable 4 cm below the left costal margin; bruising on the lower extremities, hips, back, and neck; and scattered petechiae on flexural surfaces. Respiratory effort and lung exam are normal. CBC reveals white blood cells of $36 \times 10^3/mm^3$, hemoglobin 6.1 g/dL, and platelets $9 \times 10^3/mm^3$. The automated white blood cell differential reported 90% lymphocytes, but the lab technician called to say that a manual pathology review is underway because the cells appear atypical.

Question 20-1

Which of the following will be the most crucial to obtain as you are arranging to admit this patient to the hospital?
A) Epstein-Barr virus (EBV) serologic panel.
B) Computed tomography (CT) of the chest with intravenous contrast.
C) Prothrombin time (PT) and activated partial thromboplastin time (aPTT).
D) Serum electrolytes and uric acid.
E) Child abuse consult.

Discussion 20-1

The correct answer is "D." This patient presents with findings concerning for acute leukemia, most likely acute lymphoblastic leukemia (ALL). In many cases, the blood smear will reveal presence of leukemic blasts as shown in Figure 4–6, which speeds diagnosis, although the absence of circulating blasts does not exclude ALL. It is also not possible to diagnose the subtype

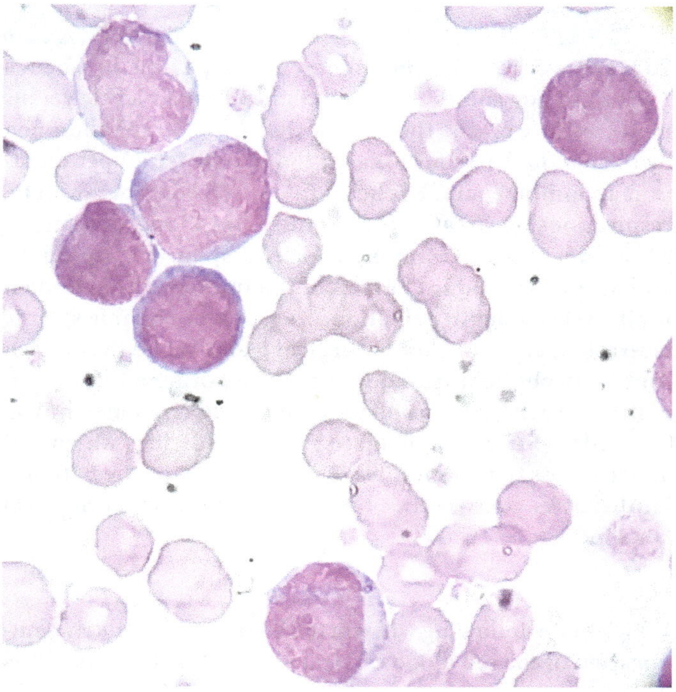

FIGURE 4–6. Leukemic blasts. The abundant white blood cells shown are from the blood smear of a patient with B-lymphoblastic leukemia. They are abnormal in their large, irregular, heterochromatic nuclei, as well as the presence of scant blue cytoplasm lacking granules. (Used with permission from Adam D. Wolfe, MD, PhD.)

of acute leukemia based on the morphologic appearance of the blasts; flow cytometric analysis and molecular genetic evaluations are required. He has symptomatic anemia and thrombocytopenia, as well as fever, and will require hospital admission for diagnostic procedures and blood product transfusions, followed by chemotherapy if the diagnosis is confirmed. Despite the elevated white blood cell count, patients with newly diagnosed ALL are assumed to be functionally neutropenic and the presence of fever in this patient will warrant blood culture and empiric antimicrobial therapy. One potentially threatening complication at this time is tumor lysis syndrome (TLS). TLS is brought about by a sudden lysis of a substantial quantity of leukemic cells simultaneously, creating a massive serum increase in intracellular constituents that can be life-threatening. A chest X-ray is often obtained to rule out the presence of a mediastinal mass, which is most frequently encountered with T-lymphoblastic leukemia and some lymphomas; however, a CT scan is generally not required urgently (option "B"), and presence of a mediastinal mass can cause respiratory obstruction if the patient is placed supine for the scan. Some patients with subtypes of newly diagnosed acute myeloid leukemia are at elevated risk of coagulopathy and disseminated intravascular coagulation, and screening with PT and aPTT is appropriate (option "C"), but this is not the most urgent concern for the patient in the vignette. Because of the patient's systemic symptoms, lymphadenopathy, and organomegaly, suspicion for EBV infection is appropriate (option "A"). However, the degree of leukocytosis and refusal to bear weight on his legs makes this patient's diagnosis more likely to be malignancy. Some of the findings, including the ill appearance, bruising, and refusal to bear weight, may be consistent with nonaccidental trauma (option "E"), but this would not be expected to lead to the blood count findings, organomegaly, or lymphadenopathy.

⌛ QUICK QUIZ

Which is NOT a laboratory finding of acute tumor lysis syndrome?
A) Hypokalemia.
B) Hyperphosphatemia.
C) Hypocalcemia.
D) Hyperuricemia.
E) Elevated serum creatinine.

Discussion

The correct answer is "A." Findings of tumor lysis syndrome (TLS) can include hyperkalemia, hyperphosphatemia, hyperuricemia, and hypocalcemia (secondary to precipitation of calcium phosphate). For these reasons, any patient with a suspected diagnosis of a hematologic malignancy should be screened for these changes, and treated immediately for any abnormal findings. Cardiac instability can be brought about by hyperkalemia, neurologic findings may result from hypocalcemia, and acute renal failure may be seen in patients who precipitate urate or calcium phosphate crystals in the renal tubular system.

The greatest risk of TLS is during the initiation of induction chemotherapy, but TLS can also occur spontaneously before treatment. Patients with TLS should be started on approximately twice-maintenance fluid infusion without potassium. This patient would receive a medication to reduce uric acid: allopurinol is used in patients without hyperuricemia, while rasburicase (recombinant urate oxidase) is administered to patients with established hyperuricemia.

▶ CASE 21

A term baby boy is found on day of life 1 to have petechiae in his antecubital and popliteal fossae, and around the base of the neck. A CBC reveals a platelet count of $13 \times 10^3/mm^3$, and the platelets appear small in size on blood smear evaluation. Family history reveals that the patient has two brothers, ages 6 and 2 years; the older brother has eczema, frequent nose bleeds, bruises easily, and has been admitted to the hospital several times with bacterial pneumonia, while the other brother is healthy. The patient's mother has no chronic illness; her older brother died as a teenager from prolonged bleeding following a motorcycle accident.

Question 21-1

Which of the following additional findings would you anticipate in this patient?

A) Absence of radii on upper extremity X-rays.
B) Marked decrease in megakaryocytes on bone marrow aspirate.
C) Mutation in *WAS* gene on genetic testing.
D) Mutation in *RUNX1* gene on genetic testing.
E) Hyperpigmentation and microcephaly on physical exam.

Discussion 21-1

The correct answer is "C." This patient presents with congenital microthrombocytopenia and an X-linked inheritance pattern with family history of atopic disease and immunodeficiency, all consistent with Wiskott-Aldrich syndrome (WAS). WAS is caused by a defective WAS protein, which participates in cytoskeletal connections that are essential for platelet and leukocyte function. The classic diagnostic triad for WAS is thrombocytopenia, immunodeficiency, and eczema. The platelets in WAS are small in size. Neonates with WAS are at increased risk of significant hemorrhage and merit support with platelet transfusion. Because of the substantial risk of life-threatening bleeding or infection, long-term management includes hematopoietic stem cell transplant (HSCT) if a suitable donor is available. None of the conditions referenced in the other answer choices are inherited in an X-linked fashion, but they are associated with neonatal thrombocytopenia. Absence of radii in a thrombocytopenic neonate (option "A") is associated with the aptly named thrombocytopenia and absent radii (TAR) syndrome. This autosomal recessive condition has an unclear molecular mechanism, but it is associated with a decrease or absence in megakaryocytes in the bone marrow (option "B"). Management of individuals with

TAR syndrome is generally supportive; patients who avoid severe hemorrhage during the infant period will typically see resolution of the thrombocytopenia during the second year. Another condition associated with congenital thrombocytopenia and skeletal abnormalities is Fanconi anemia (FA). This is an inherited bone marrow failure and cancer predisposition syndrome with associated radial and thumb abnormalities, pigmentation abnormalities, genitourinary malformations, microcephaly, and short stature (option "E"). FA is most often inherited in an autosomal recessive pattern, and conveys increased risk of developing myelodysplasia, leukemia, head and neck tumors, and liver tumors. Patients with FA exhibit chromosome instability diagnosed by exposure to diepoxybutane; management typically includes referral for HSCT. Mutations in *RUNX1/AML* gene (option "D") are associated with congenital and familial thrombocytopenias and predisposition to myelodysplasia and acute myeloid leukemias; this condition is quite rare and is curable by HSCT. In neonatal alloimmune thrombocytopenia, the fetus/neonate inherits a platelet antigen from the father that the mother lacks. Maternal IgG antibodies to this antigen cross the placenta causing alloimmune hemolysis. In autoimmune thrombocytopenia occurring in mothers with autoimmune diseases such as lupus or immune thrombocytopenia (ITP), maternal antibodies react with both the mother and the fetus/neonate's platelets. Additional causes of neonatal thrombocytopenia include drug induced, thrombosis, hypersplenism, disseminated intravascular coagulation, and preeclampsia.

▶ CASE 22

You are working in the emergency department when a 7-year-old boy comes in by ambulance after a bicycle versus motor vehicle crash. The patient was struck in the abdomen by the handle bars and suffered immediate left upper quadrant abdominal pain. His heart rate is 166 beats per minute, respirations 36 breaths per minute, and blood pressure is 82/44 mm Hg. On exam, he is pale, diaphoretic, dyspneic, and deeply bruised in the area of the trauma. The abdomen is diffusely tender to palpation. You suspect possible splenic laceration, and consult the surgical team. While they are en route, you obtain intravenous access and order a CBC, coagulation screening labs, and blood type and cross match. You also order O-negative blood to give immediately, which will arrive in less than 5 minutes. During this time, the patient's mother asks you whether the blood transfusion will harm her son.

Question 22-1

Which of the following will you tell her is the most likely complication of the red blood cell transfusion for this patient?

A) Fever.
B) HIV infection.
C) Transfusion-related acute lung injury (TRALI).
D) Gram-positive bacterial infection.
E) Acute hemolytic event.

Discussion 22-1

The correct answer is "A." Clearly, the patient in the vignette is experiencing a severe internal hemorrhage and will require probable massive transfusion, with the benefits far outweighing the risks. However, it is not uncommon for parents to have questions and concerns relating to the safety of blood product transfusion. The overall incidence of fever associated with blood transfusion is approximately 1 per 100 units transfused, making it one of the most common adverse effects. Premedication or as-needed therapy with acetaminophen can prevent or treat this reaction; typically it is self-limited following transfusion. Infectious complications of blood transfusion, which used to be more frequent, are now quite rare. The estimated incidence of bacterial infection, primarily due to gram-positive skin flora, with red cell transfusions (option "D") is between 0.2 and 7.4 per million units. Platelet transfusions are associated with higher rates of gram-positive infection, up to 1 per 2000 units transfused if the platelets were stored at room temperature prior to administration. Viral infections are also potentially transmitted. Cytomegalovirus (CMV) may be transmitted from seropositive donors to seronegative recipients, although products that have been leukoreduced and screened are considered CMV-safe and should be appropriate for most indications. Individually tested, CMV-negative blood products are also available for use, largely with immunocompromised recipients. HIV (option "B") and hepatitis C virus transmission from blood products approaches 1 per 1 to 2 million units, making this quite a rare concern. Hepatitis B virus transmission is slightly more common, at between 1 in 200,000 to 500,000 units. TRALI (option "C") is a rare complication of blood transfusion, associated with transference of antineutrophil antibodies or neutrophil-activating metabolites to the recipient. This leads to neutrophil activation and trapping in pulmonary microvasculature and development of acute respiratory distress syndrome that can be life-threatening. The rate of TRALI in pediatrics is uncertain, but it likely occurs in fewer than 1 in 10,000 units. The reaction is self-limited, and with aggressive hemodynamic and respiratory supportive care, often resolves within several days. Acute hemolytic events (option "E") are also rare; they result typically from administration of an ABO-mismatched unit. Symptoms include fever, chills, hypotension, flank pain, oliguria, and cola-colored urine. Supportive care is aimed at keeping the renal system hydrated until the reaction abates. Incidence of acute hemolytic reactions is estimated at 1 in 75,000 units. A delayed hemolytic reaction may occur in up to 1 per 1500 transfusions, more often due to minor blood group antigen mismatch, up to 10 days after the transfusion. The hemolysis is generally less pronounced, and symptoms less dramatic, than seen in the acute reactions.

▶ CASE 23

A 2-month-old girl comes to the urgent care clinic for evaluation of fever. Her mother reports that the baby has been completely healthy since birth, is growing and developing normally, but developed temperature up to 38.6°C (101.5°F) last night and has been febrile through today. The baby did not want to nurse much this morning. She has had three wet diapers over the past 8 hours and normal stools daily. Vital signs reveal temperature 38.5°C (101.3°F), pulse 124 beats per minute, and respirations 22 breaths per minute. Physical exam reveals a baby who is alert and cries throughout the exam. The anterior fontanelle is open, soft, and flat, not sunken. Mucous membranes are moist. The left tympanic membrane exhibits circumferential erythema, dull light reflex with bulging, and purulent material behind the drum. Heart, lung, and neurologic exams are normal. Because of the fever, a CBC is obtained, which reveals white blood cell count $12.5 \times 10^3/\text{mm}^3$ with a normal white cell differential, hemoglobin 9.2 g/dL, and platelets $360 \times 10^3/\text{mm}^3$. The mean corpuscular volume (MCV) is 88 fL.

Question 23-1

Which of the following is the next best step in management of this patient?
A) Intravenous ceftriaxone.
B) Hemoglobin electrophoresis.
C) Transfusion with packed red blood cells.
D) Bone marrow aspiration and biopsy.
E) Oral amoxicillin.

Discussion 23-1

The correct answer is "E." This patient has been inadvertently identified as "anemic" during her physiologic red cell nadir of infancy, while being evaluated for left acute otitis media. Although practice may vary regarding "obligatory" lab work for 2-month-old infants with fever, most practice guidelines do not suggest this when the patient has an etiology for fever identified on exam. Shortly after birth, infant erythropoiesis decreases due to an abundance of oxygen. As hemoglobin concentrations drift lower, infant erythropoietin production is stimulated and drives new erythropoiesis. The period of decreased hemoglobin concentration is referred to as the physiologic nadir and is not a pathologic process. Nadir occurs between 6 and 12 weeks of life, although the timing can vary and nadir tends to be earlier, more pronounced, and more prolonged in preterm infants. Hemoglobin levels in term infants can drop to 9 to 11 g/dL; as this is a normal finding for age, this patient does not require transfusion support (option "C"). Having only acute symptoms associated with her ear infection, this patient is a candidate for outpatient management, and should not require parenteral antibiotics (option "A") as frontline therapy. Since she has otherwise normal blood counts, evaluation of bone marrow (option "D") is not warranted. Hemoglobin electrophoresis (option "B") might be helpful for diagnosing beta-thalassemia trait in an iron replete child with persistent microcytic anemia, or if hemoglobinopathy is suspected, but the vignette does not provide any data to suggest these diagnoses.

> **Helpful Tip**
> Remember hemoglobin and MCV vary by age in infants and children. Consult pediatric reference tables when interpreting values. Both are highest in the neonatal period, then decrease to adult values in adolescence.

▶ CASE 24

A 4-year-old boy with sickle cell anemia (hemoglobin SS disease) presents to the emergency department with acute onset of fever, fatigue, and pallor that began this morning. He has previously been admitted to the hospital, once for an acute vaso-occlusive event with lower extremity pain, requiring intravenous opioid medications for 48 hours, but has otherwise been well at home. Medications include daily oral penicillin, folic acid, and hydroxyurea. The hydroxyurea dose was recently increased at a clinic visit with the hematologist 2 weeks ago. Vital signs currently include temperature 38.7°C (101.6°F), heart rate 170 beats per minute, and respirations 34 breaths per minute. In general, the patient appears very tired, pale, and dyspneic. A grade III/VI systolic ejection murmur is heard over the left sternal border but is audible throughout the chest. The spleen is palpable to 7 cm below the left costal margin. You are considering the diagnosis of a splenic sequestration event versus an aplastic crisis.

Question 24-1

Which of the following subsequent findings would make you more suspicious for splenic sequestration?

A) Reticulocyte count of 0.2%.
B) Hemoglobin 3 g/dL below the patient's baseline.
C) Platelet count of $55 \times 10^3/mm^3$.
D) Absolute neutrophil count of $940/mm^3$.
E) Left lower lobe infiltrate on chest X-ray.

Discussion 24-1

The correct answer is "C." This patient with sickle cell disease presents with a febrile illness and symptoms suggestive of an acute drop in hemoglobin. In children with hemoglobin SS and an intact spleen (ie, those younger than 5 to 6 years of age), the most dangerous complication with this presentation is a splenic sequestration event. During sequestration, a large proportion of the patient's red blood cells become trapped in the spleen, which can subsequently expand to fill much of the abdomen. Patients with severe sequestration can drop acutely to hemoglobin levels at a fraction of their baseline, putting them at risk for cardiac compromise or hypoxic-ischemic events. Because of entrapment of blood in the spleen, platelets also become trapped in the splenic sinusoids, leading to thrombocytopenia. Patients will also typically exhibit a reticulocytosis in an effort to replace the entrapped red cells. As a life-threatening event, prompt attention to sequestration is critical. Parents of young children are educated to palpate the patient's spleen at home in the setting of severe illness or anemia symptoms, and to seek medical attention immediately if the spleen becomes palpable. If sequestration is suspected and severe anemia confirmed, the event may be reversed by aggressive fluid resuscitation. This often will allow release of the entrapped red cells and restoration of safer hemoglobin concentrations. Transfusion with packed red cells may also be necessary. In this patient's case, management of his fever along with obtaining blood cultures and treating with empiric parenteral antimicrobial therapy is also warranted. Another complication of sickle cell disease in children is an aplastic crisis, associated with parvovirus B19 infection and transient suppression of bone marrow erythropoiesis. The patient in the vignette might be experiencing red cell aplasia, although the acuity and severity of symptoms are not typical. Although parvovirus B19 can cause transient suppression of erythropoiesis in children without sickle cell disease, children with normal red cell lifespan recover their red cell production before becoming symptomatically anemic. Children with conditions causing reduced red cell life span, including those with sickle cell anemia, hereditary spherocytosis, or G6PD deficiency, are at increased risk of exhibiting symptomatic anemia before their marrow recovers from the infection. Because it is a condition of marrow suppression, patients with aplastic crisis exhibit reticulocytopenia (option "A"). Both aplastic crisis and splenic sequestration can exhibit a significant drop in hemoglobin from the patient's baseline (option "B"), although the anemia from sequestration can be more severe and more acute. A patient with sickle cell disease who presents with fever and a new infiltrate on chest X-ray (option "E") might be suspected of having acute chest syndrome, but infiltrate on imaging is not a finding associated with splenic sequestration or aplastic crisis. Moderate neutropenia (option "D") is also not associated with splenic sequestration. It is more probable that the patient's recent dose increase of hydroxyurea would be responsible for this finding.

▶ CASE 25

A previously healthy 8-year-old girl suffered severe inhalational lung injury during a house fire 10 days ago, and has been in the intensive care unit on an extracorporeal membrane oxygenation (ECMO) circuit for 8 days, stably anticoagulated per protocol with unfractionated heparin (UFH). She has been afebrile. This morning, the patient exhibits right lower extremity soft tissue edema; Doppler ultrasound imaging reveals an occlusive deep venous thrombus in the right femoral vein. Lab work reveals white blood cell count of $8.2 \times 10^3/mm^3$ with a normal differential, hemoglobin 10.4 g/dL, and platelets $34 \times 10^3/mm^3$.

Question 25-1

Which of the following is the next best step in the evaluation and management of this patient?

A) Transfuse 10 mL/kg platelets.
B) Replace heparin with a different anticoagulant in the ECMO circuit.

C) Send testing for factor V Leiden (FVL) mutation.
D) Send testing for heparin-induced thrombocytopenia (HIT) antibody.
E) Increase the heparin dose.

Discussion 25-1

The correct answer is "B." This patient likely has HIT, an immune response to heparins that occurs in approximately 0.3% to 0.6% of critically ill patients receiving UFH and low-molecular-weight heparins (LMWH; eg, dalteparin, enoxaparin). HIT suspicion is based on the so-called "4 Ts," described in Table 4–6. When the likelihood of HIT is high, the immediate next step is to eliminate all heparins. Although diagnostic testing for HIT antibody is appropriate (option "D"), it is not recommended to obtain this result before cessation of heparin. This patient, who likely has HIT associated with UFH in the ECMO circuit, will be increasingly challenging to manage. She will require anticoagulation with a nonheparin agent: for example, the direct thrombin inhibitor argatroban is considered an appropriate anticoagulant in children with HIT. Once a patient has been diagnosed with HIT, she should not receive UFH or LMWH in the future. The HIT antibody is directed against platelet factor 4. While it ultimately causes rapid clearance of platelets, the antibody usually has a platelet-activating effect. Therefore, it is important to note that the most common presenting finding of HIT is thrombosis, rather than bleeding, despite the coexistence of thrombocytopenia. Due to the risk of further clotting with HIT, platelet transfusion (option "A") is not recommended unless the patient is experiencing an emergent bleeding event due to the thrombocytopenia. This patient may have an underlying inherited thrombophilic condition, such as FVL, that increases her lifetime risk of deep venous thrombosis (option "C"), but it would be less likely that a patient with FVL on an anticoagulated ECMO circuit would develop a new DVT with thrombocytopenia; HIT is a more likely etiology, and genetic testing would not be the next step in management for this patient. Likewise, increasing the heparin (option "E") in this clinical situation would not be appropriate given the development of new thrombus and thrombocytopenia while on an appropriately heparinized circuit.

> **Helpful Tip**
> Thrombosis is the most common presenting sign of heparin-induced thrombocytopenia (HIT) as the HIT antibody activates platelets.

▶ CASE 26

You are rounding on a term newborn girl in the nursery, who was born yesterday at 40-3/7 weeks' gestation by normal spontaneous vaginal delivery to a healthy, primiparous mother following an uncomplicated delivery. The baby appears healthy, is feeding well, and has voided and passed meconium since birth. The patient's mother is concerned that several members of her family have had cancers at young ages and wants to get your opinion about the risks of future cancers for her new baby. You consider the possibility of an inherited cancer predisposition syndrome.

Question 26-1

Regarding these syndromes, which of the following molecular changes is correctly matched to an associated malignancy?
A) Trisomy 21—osteosarcoma.
B) *Neurofibromin-1 (NF1)* mutation—vestibular schwannoma.
C) *p53* deletion—basal cell carcinoma.
D) *TSC* mutation—optic pathway glioma.
E) Abnormal 11p15 imprinting—Wilms tumor.

TABLE 4–6 4-T SCORING SYSTEM FOR SUSPICION OF HEPARIN-INDUCED THROMBOCYTOPENIA (HIT)

Clinical Finding	Score (range 0–2 for each criterion)		
	0	**1**	**2**
Thrombocytopenia (with respect to prior to heparin initiation)	< 30% drop in platelets, or nadir < 10 × 10³/mm³	30–50% drop in platelets, or nadir 10–19 × 10³/mm³	< 50% drop in platelets, and nadir ≥ 20 × 10³/mm³
Timing of thrombocytopenia or thrombosis (assuming heparin-naïve patient)	Within 4 days	Uncertain timing, likely within 5–10 days; or after 10 days	During days 5–10
Thrombosis	None	Suspected thrombosis or progression/recurrence of preexisting thrombus	New thrombosis
Other cause of thrombocytopenia?	Definite other cause identified	Possible other cause identified	No other cause identified

Scoring: 0–3, low probability of HIT; 4–5, intermediate probability of HIT; 6–8, high probability of HIT.

Reproduced with permission from Warkentin TE: Heparin-induced thrombocytopenia in critically ill patients, *Semin Thromb Hemost* 2015 Feb;41(1):49–60.

Discussion 26-1

The correct answer is "E." A comprehensive understanding of cancer predisposition syndromes goes beyond the general pediatrics board content specifications; however, it is helpful to understand how to link abnormal physical exam findings and family history to future cancer risk. This will aid the pediatrician in identifying next diagnostic steps, and in making appropriate referrals. Abnormal imprinting at 11p15 is associated with Beckwith-Wiedemann syndrome (BWS), which is associated with hemihypertrophy, macroglossia, omphalocele, neonatal hypoglycemia, and increased risk of Wilms tumor and hepatoblastoma. Screening with abdominal ultrasound is recommended every 3 to 6 months until age 8 years. Hepatoblastoma may also be screened by serum alpha-fetoprotein levels obtained every 3 months until age 4 years. There is often no family history in individuals with BWS. Trisomy 21, or Down syndrome (option "A"), is most commonly associated with increased risk of hematologic malignancy. This includes increased risk of developing acute lymphoblastic leukemia, and increased risk of acute myeloid leukemia, frequently of the megakaryoblastic subtype. Children with trisomy 21 are exquisitely chemosensitive, and have more severe adverse effects from chemotherapy than children without this difference. Therefore, leukemia treatment protocols often have different therapeutic dosing and supportive care recommendations for children with trisomy 21.

Mutation of *NF1*, the causative genetic change in neurofibromatosis type 1 (option "B"), is associated with formation of neurofibromas, optic pathway gliomas, other low-grade gliomas, and peripheral nerve sheath tumors. Vestibular schwannomas are associated with neurofibromatosis type 2, which is a rarer condition caused by mutations in the *merlin* gene.

The Li-Fraumeni cancer predisposition syndrome is associated with mutations in tumor suppressor gene *p53* (option "C"). This syndrome includes unusual tumors of many types that arise in young individuals within a pedigree. Common tumors associated with Li-Fraumeni syndrome include those that start with "B"—blood (ie, leukemias), brain, bone (eg, osteosarcoma), and breast. Many other cancers have been associated with this condition, although skin cancers are not among them. Mutations in *TSC* complex genes (option "D") are associated with tuberous sclerosis, a condition with presenting symptoms that include seizures, intellectual disability, and facial angiofibromas. Tumors associated with tuberous sclerosus are often benign and include cardiac rhabdomyomas, subependymal giant cell astrocytomas, and renal angiomyolipomas.

▶ CASE 27

An 8-year-old boy presents to the emergency department with spreading bruising on his legs and buttocks. The symptoms started 1 week ago, with isolated, painful bruises on the legs, which increased and expanded until becoming nearly confluent across the entire lower extremities. Two days ago, the bruising also began to include the penis and scrotum. Today, the patient has been unwilling to walk because of pain.

On exam, the patient is in significant pain and cries out when the palpable purpura on the buttocks, genitalia, and lower extremities are touched. The tissue has alternating areas of violaceous purpura and blue-black bullous changes. Lower extremity pulses are faint and thready. Skin on the trunk, abdomen, chest, back, upper extremities, head, and neck is unaffected. When an antecubital peripheral intravenous line is placed, there is substantial and continuous oozing around the site. Lab work reveals white blood cells $15.8 \times 10^3/\text{mm}^3$ with 80% neutrophils and 15% lymphocytes, hemoglobin 9.1 g/dL, platelets $33 \times 10^3/\text{mm}^3$, prothrombin time (PT) 22 s (reference range 12–15 s), activated partial thromboplastin time (aPTT) 74 s (reference range 24–36 s).

Question 27-1

In addition to pain management, blood culture, and antimicrobial therapy, which of the following is the next best intervention?
A) Platelet transfusion.
B) Fresh frozen plasma (FFP) transfusion.
C) Unfractionated heparin (UFH) loading dose and maintenance infusion.
D) Intravenous immunoglobulin (IVIG) infusion.
E) Induction chemotherapy.

Discussion 27-1

The correct answer is "B." This unfortunate patient presents with purpura fulminans and associated disseminated intravascular coagulation (DIC), a life- and limb-threatening condition. Thrombi form in the microvasculature causing ischemic/necrotic damage to the skin and tissue. The most appropriate intervention is to identify and treat the underlying cause, and to attempt to restore the balance of pro- and anticoagulant factors in the patient's blood as soon as possible. Of the choices given, FFP is the best therapy to initiate. Neonates with homozygous protein C deficiency present with neonatal purpura fulminans, an often fatal condition. In older children, the condition is due to sepsis or antithrombotic factor dysfunction. For example, this patient's presentation could be consistent with meningococcemia, a known inciting event of DIC with or without associated purpura fulminans. Patients who are started on the oral vitamin K antagonist warfarin are at risk of warfarin-induced skin necrosis, which is a form of purpura fulminans caused by microthrombi in the skin following warfarin's depletion of proteins C and S. Some patients develop an autoantibody to protein S, causing a clinical presentation similar to that described in the vignette. For reasons that are not clear, the purpura in this clinical entity preferentially affect the lower body segment. There is no clear consensus in the critical care or hematology literature to support the use of anticoagulation in pediatric purpura fulminans (making option "C" less desirable). Because the patient has consumed his procoagulant factors and platelets in microvascular thromboses, the bleeding risk is elevated; heparin would further increase the risk of hemorrhage. Should the patient develop a severe hemorrhage, platelet transfusion (option "A") might be considered, but as the platelets are currently being consumed in thrombi that are injuring his skin, platelet transfusion would generally be avoided until the coagulopathy is better controlled. Another clinical entity that can exhibit lower body segment purpura is Henoch-Schönlein purpura (HSP). This is a vasculitis mediated by IgA, with the clinical triad of abdominal pain, arthritis, and lower segment palpable purpura. Patients with HSP generally do not become as ill as the patient in the vignette, and since HSP is not a consumptive coagulopathy, the platelet count would be expected to be normal or elevated in this condition.

The patient's presentation has some overlapping features with acute myeloid leukemia (AML). The promyelocytic form of this condition may present with multiple cytopenias and DIC, due to a tissue factor-like substance released by the blasts. However, this patient's differential did not report any blasts, and the purpura fulminans would be unexpected for AML. This patient might undergo bone marrow assessment during his evaluation, but chemotherapy (option "E") would not be started empirically as the next step.

▶ CASE 28

A 2-day-old neonate is ready for hospital discharge with his mother, and you are conducting his discharge physical exam. The pregnancy and delivery were uncomplicated, and the mother was on no medications and had no infections. Delivery was at 37-1/7 weeks' gestation, by normal spontaneous vaginal delivery, Apgar scores were 9 and 9 at 1 and 5 minutes. On your evaluation today, the baby has normal vital signs, nondysmorphic features, normal extremities, and a normal heart and lung exam. During the eye screening, you note leukocoria on the left, and a normal red reflex on the right. There is no family history of eye problems, including cataracts or tumors, or cancers of any kind.

Question 28-1

Which of the following is most likely to be identified on subsequent evaluation?
A) Increased alpha-fetoprotein for age.
B) Germline *p53* mutation.
C) Increased urinary catecholamines.
D) Germline *Rb* mutation.
E) Germline *NF1* mutation.

Discussion 28-1

The correct answer is "D." Of the options presented, this patient most likely has congenital retinoblastoma (RB). While RB is not the sole cause, or most common cause, of loss of red reflex in a newborn, it is in the differential diagnosis for this patient. RB may occur broadly in two categories: hereditary and sporadic. While the nomenclature may be misleading, hereditary RB is defined based on the presence of a germline mutation in the *Rb* gene, even in the absence of a family history. Patients with a single germline mutation are at high risk of acquiring a second, somatic mutation during embryonic retinal development (the so-called "second hit"), which leads to development of RB early, often diagnosed within the first year of life. Because of the presence of

the initial germline mutation, patients with hereditary RB are at high risk of development of tumors in both eyes, even though these may not both present concurrently. RB is the most common malignant tumor affecting the eye in children and carries a substantial risk of intracranial extension if not promptly identified and treated. Treatment is based on extent of disease, and whether both eyes are affected. In unilateral RB with smaller tumors, local treatment such as laser or cryotherapy may be appropriate, while larger tumors may require enucleation. Chemotherapy may be administered via intravitreous, intra-arteriolar, or intravenous routes, depending again on tumor size and extent of invasion. Children with hereditary RB are also at higher risk of developing intracranial involvement, which most often involves the pineal gland (so-called "trilateral" RB). Therefore, for the patient in the vignette, ophthalmologic evaluation under anesthesia and MRI of the brain will be appropriate next steps for evaluating extent of disease. *Rb* codes for the tumor suppressor protein RB. Patients with germline mutations are at increased risk during their lifetimes of multiple malignancies associated with loss of this protein if a second, somatic mutation occurs in other tissues. The nonocular malignancy most often associated with hereditary RB is osteosarcoma. Sporadic RB is thought to be due to acquisition of two somatic mutations later during development, and for this reason often presents later, around or after 2 years of age. These patients are at low risk of bilateral and trilateral RB (bilateral eyes and brain), although the initial evaluation and therapeutic options are the same as described above. Other tumors found within the neonatal period include hepatoblastoma, teratoma, and neuroblastoma. In the former two conditions, serum tumor markers alpha-fetoprotein (option "A") and beta-human chorionic gonadotropin may be elevated, while in neuroblastoma urine catecholamines vanillylmandelic acid (VMA) and homovanillic acid (HVA) may be elevated (option "C"). None of these is specifically associated with newborn leukocoria. As stated earlier, *p53* mutation (option "B") is associated with the Li-Fraumeni syndrome (LFS), another hereditary cancer predisposition syndrome due to loss of a tumor suppressor gene. Neurofibromatosis type 1, characterized by mutation of the *NF1* gene (option "E"), is associated with development of café-au-lait macules, neurofibromas, and optic gliomas.

> **Helpful Tip**
> Leukocoria ("white pupil") is concerning and requires urgent referral to an ophthalmologist. Etiologies include cataracts and retinoblastoma. Checking the red reflex is important especially in infants.

▶ CASE 29

A 19-month-old girl presents to the emergency department with bruising on her chest. Parents report that she was running in the backyard with her older brother, fell forward, and struck her chest on a rock approximately 2 hours ago. She has been complaining of pain at the site of injury, and parents note a large bruise developing at that site. They gave the patient a dose of ibuprofen for pain 2 hours ago. On your physical exam, the patient is alert, interactive, and appropriate. A large, firm, tender hematoma with surrounding contused tissue is noted across the sternum and midchest in an oval shape, approximately 15 cm across and 5 cm high. There are multiple old bruises, in varying states of healing, on the extremities and buttocks. The medical student who is seeing this patient with you asks whether this patient's injury might have been due to nonaccidental trauma (NAT).

Question 29-1

Which of the following most accurately describes the hematologic evaluation of a patient with suspected NAT?

A) If the history, physical exam, and skeletal evaluation are consistent with accidental trauma, a bleeding disorder laboratory screening evaluation is recommended.

B) CBC, prothrombin time (PT), activated partial thromboplastin time (aPTT), and platelet function analyzer (PFA-100) evaluation are recommended as screening tests.

C) The recommended bleeding disorder screening tests can vary depending on the presenting injuries that yielded the NAT suspicion.

D) Consultation with pediatric hematology is recommended during evaluation of all suspected cases of NAT.

E) Presence of petechiae at pressure sites, such as at edges of clothing, should increase suspicion for NAT.

Discussion 29-1

The correct answer is "C." This patient presents with hematoma and contusion suggestive of a blunt force injury to the chest, which may have been due to the mechanism described, or may have occurred in the context of NAT or physical child abuse. Multiple old bruises are present, mostly in typically innocent sites (eg, the extremities), but also at a more unusual site, the buttocks. Distinguishing innocent from suspicious bruising in a toddler can be very challenging. In the case of unusual bruising, distinguishing NAT from a bleeding disorder may also be difficult, and the two entities are not mutually exclusive. Recently, the American Academy of Pediatrics issued clear, evidence-based guidelines to assist in hematologic screening of patients with suspected NAT. The guidelines allow the pediatrician to defer bleeding disorder screening in cases of NAT that were clearly witnessed or clearly established through the history and other objective data (making option "A" incorrect). These guidelines suggest a different coagulopathy workup for patients with bruising versus those with intracranial hemorrhage (ICH; making option "C" correct). The initial workup in both cases includes CBC with platelet count, PT, aPTT, and factor VIII and IX levels. For patients with bruising, screening for von Willebrand disease (vWD) with von Willebrand factor level and activity is added. For patients with ICH, in lieu of vWD screening, it is recommended to evaluate for disseminated intravascular coagulation with fibrinogen level and D-dimer. PFA-100 evaluation (option "B"), because it is difficult to interpret in children, subject to multiple physiologic confounders, and lacks sensitivity for mild disorders, is not recommended in this initial screening process.

Referral to hematology (option "D") is only suggested in cases in which an abnormal screen is identified, or when additional testing is desired. On physical exam, the presence of petechiae (subcutaneous bleeds smaller than 3 mm, usually smaller than 1 mm) at sites of pressure or on flexural surfaces is more suggestive of a quantitative or qualitative platelet problem than NAT (making option "E" incorrect).

▶ CASE 30

A 15-year-old young man with no past medical history presents to the urgent care clinic for evaluation of right leg pain. He notes that he has had a dull, aching pain, ranging from 3 to 6 out of 10 on the pain scale, over the past 5 to 6 months. Over time, this pain seems to be increasing in intensity, and during the past week he has been waking from sleep with pain of severity 6 to 8 out of 10. The patient is an active high school football player, and while the pain persists during this activity, it does not seem to worsen. The pain improves temporarily with ibuprofen. Review of systems is otherwise negative. On physical exam, the patient is ambulatory, with an antalgic gait that favors the right leg. There is a minimally tender, palpable hard tissue mass along the lateral right tibia, which is ovoid and approximately 3 × 5 cm. X-ray series of the right thigh, knee, and leg is ordered.

Question 30-1

Which of the following statements is most accurate regarding possible bone tumors this patient may have?

A) Tumor appearance on radiographic imaging will accurately distinguish osteosarcoma from Ewing sarcoma.

B) Presence of nodules on computed tomography (CT) of the chest favors osteosarcoma over osteoid osteoma.

C) Both osteosarcoma and Ewing sarcoma metastasize to bone marrow.

D) Primary tumors of osteoid osteoma tend to be larger than those of osteosarcoma.

E) The prognoses of osteosarcoma, Ewing sarcoma, and osteoid osteoma are similar, although the therapeutic approach differs for each.

Discussion 30-1

The correct answer is "B." Osteosarcoma (OS) is a malignant tumor of bone-forming cells, arising preferentially in long bones, which most often metastasizes to the lungs. OS is fairly uncommon in younger children, with a peak incidence during adolescence. The prognosis of multifocal or metastatic OS is considerably poorer than that of solitary OS, making accurate staging with CT chest and bone scan essential. OS is a chemotherapy-sensitive tumor, but it is not sensitive to radiation therapy (XRT). Therefore, frontline therapy includes multimodal chemotherapy, followed by resection of all sites of tumor, and additional chemotherapy. The extent of tumor necrosis (greater or less than 90%) at resection, which indicates the relative chemosensitivity of the tumor, has significant prognostic value. Osteoid osteoma, in contrast, is a benign tumor found in long bones, most often seen in the femur or tibia. It does not metastasize (making option "E" incorrect). It tends to be associated with dull, constant pain that is not associated with activity and may be more severe at night in children. This tumor tends to be small, often less than 1.5 cm (making option "D" incorrect). On plain film, there is a characteristic, lucent nidus with sclerotic rim; the surrounding inflammation is responsible for the pain, and explains the efficacy of nonsteroidal anti-inflammatory drugs (NSAIDs) in managing it. Osteoid osteoma may resolve over several years, particularly if treated with chronic NSAIDs, although surgical resection or radiofrequency ablation is often used for definitive therapy and to alleviate pain. Ewing sarcoma is an embryonal small round blue cell tumor, which commonly arises from bone but may be associated with soft tissues. Unlike OS, Ewing sarcoma has affinity for either flat or long bones. Metastasis is most commonly to lungs and bone marrow (option "C"). Management of Ewing sarcoma includes neoadjuvant chemotherapy, surgical resection, XRT of primary tumor, or a combination of these and subsequent chemotherapy. On plain film, shown in Figure 4–7, malignant bone tumors

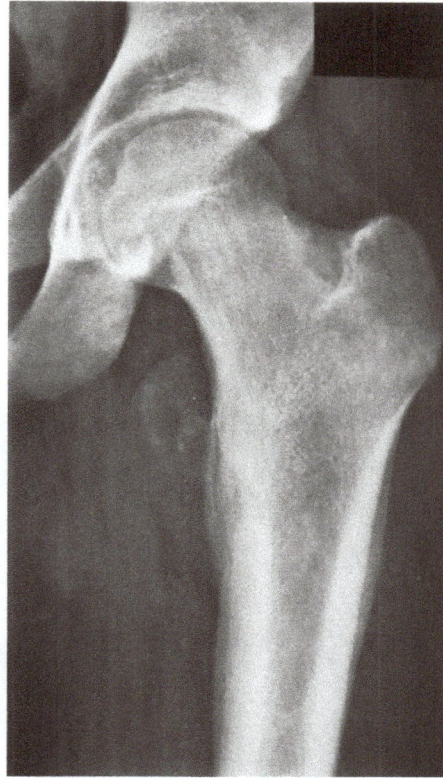

FIGURE 4–8. X-rays of Ewing sarcoma may show an onion-skin appearance due to multiple thin layers of woven bone deposited over the rapidly growing tumor site. (Reproduced with permission from Kantarjian HM, Wolff RA, & Koller CA, eds. *The MD Anderson Manual of Medical Oncology*, 2nd ed. New York, NY: McGraw-Hill Education, Inc; 2011, Figure 40-7 Part B.)

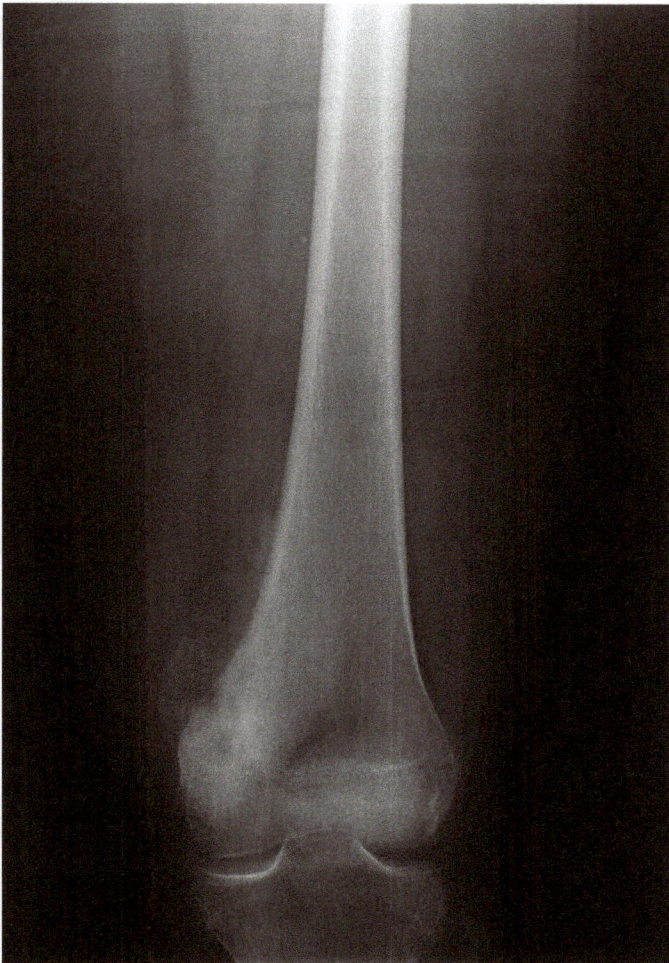

FIGURE 4–7. Osteosarcoma. This plain film of the distal femur exhibits sclerotic changes of the distal metaphysis and diaphysis, and an adjacent soft tissue mass containing calcifications. The lifting of periosteum by tumor expansion often produces a triangular shape, known as a Codman triangle. (Used with permission from Adam D. Wolfe, MD, PhD.)

often exhibit periosteal reaction, poorly defined margins, a moth-eaten lytic pattern, adjacent soft tissue involvement, and larger size when compared with benign tumors. A characteristic onion-skin appearance may be seen with rapidly growing tumors such as Ewing sarcoma, resulting from multiple thin layers of woven bone deposition over the site of tumor expansion. (See Figure 4–8.) When new bony spicules are laid down perpendicular to the tumor growth, they may yield the "sunburst" pattern on X-rays. (See Figure 4–9.) Location of tumor can also yield important information: for example, OS tends to involve the long bone metaphysis, while Ewing sarcoma is more often seen arising in the diaphysis. However, no radiographic criteria offer adequate specificity to distinguish these two tumors on X-rays alone (making option "A" incorrect).

Helpful Tip
With Ewing sarcoma or osteosarcoma, a sunburst pattern (both) or onion-skin appearance (Ewing) may be seen on X-ray, though, X-ray alone cannot differentiate between the two.

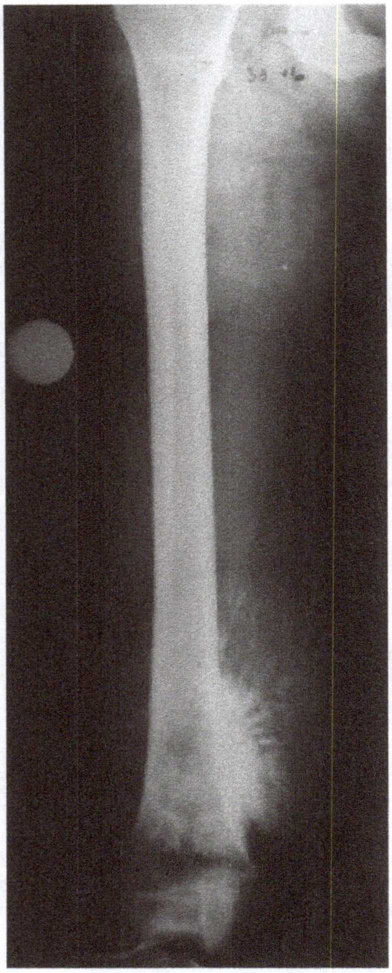

FIGURE 4–9. X-ray of an osteosarcoma showing the characteristic sunburst pattern resulting from the formation of new bony spicules perpendicular to the tumor growth. (Reproduced with permission from Kantarjian HM, Wolff RA, & Koller CA, eds. *The MD Anderson Manual of Medical Oncology*, 2nd ed. New York, NY: McGraw-Hill Education, Inc; 2011, Figure 40-7 Part A.)

> **Helpful Tip**
> Bone awakening in the middle of the night is a red flag sign for malignancy.

▶ CASE 31

A 10-month old girl is admitted to the pediatric intensive care unit with severe respiratory distress. She presented last night with progressive cough, fever, and dyspnea and has been treated with intravenous antibiotics and aggressive fluid resuscitation. She appears no better today, with persistent fever, tachypnea, cough, and fine crackles throughout the chest. There is no palpable lymphadenopathy. Review of the medical history reveals that this patient has been closely followed by her pediatrician for failure to thrive, and is below the first percentile for weight.

She has had ongoing problems with diarrhea and recurrent oral and anogenital thrush. Vaccination history is unavailable. Blood counts on admission included a white blood cell count of $17 \times 10^3/mm^3$ (differential: 95% neutrophils, < 1% lymphocytes, 4% monocytes, 1% eosinophils), hemoglobin 10.5 g/dL, and platelets $585 \times 10^3/mm^3$. Flow cytometry indicated an absence of T and B lymphocytes. Bronchoalveolar lavage performed this morning revealed the presence of *Pneumocystis jiroveci*.

Question 31-1

After management of this acute illness, which of the following long-term interventions is most likely to improve this patient's prognosis?

A) Monthly infusion of intravenous immunoglobulin (IVIG).
B) Highly active antiretroviral therapy.
C) Strict adherence to recommended childhood vaccination schedule.
D) Referral for hematopoietic stem cell transplant.
E) Regular prophylaxis for opportunistic and fungal infections.

Discussion 31-1

The correct answer is "D." This critically ill infant exhibits findings of failure to thrive, chronic diarrhea, recurrent infections with fungal and opportunistic organisms (eg, *Pneumocystis*), lymphopenia, and absence of T and B cells, most consistent with severe combined immunodeficiency (SCID). The absence of reactive lymphoid tissue (lymph nodes, tonsils), also described in the vignette, is noted with this condition. Affected patients often die from infection before their second birthday, and early stem cell transplant offers the only known cure. SCID has multiple subtypes; the T-B- presentation described in the vignette is inherited in an autosomal recessive fashion. T-B+NK- SCID is inherited as an X-linked recessive condition. Within the United States and internationally, newborn screening programs are adopting successful screening programs for SCID, facilitating diagnosis and early transplant before severe infections occur. Lack of antibody production may also be seen in other conditions, such as common variable immunodeficiency. This condition most often presents after adolescence with frequent sinopulmonary infections, decreased IgA, IgG, and IgM levels, but with detectable lymphocytes, and is treated with regular administration of IVIG (option "A"). The presentation of an infant with failure to thrive and frequent infections with opportunistic pathogens is also suspicious for human immunodeficiency virus (HIV) infection (treated by option "B"), but the absence of lymphadenopathy, normal hemoglobin and platelet counts, and absence of B lymphocytes—often elevated with HIV—make this diagnosis less likely. Because this patient has no lymphocytes, she will be unresponsive to vaccinations and should not receive live viral vaccines (making option "C" ineffective). While she will require antimicrobial prophylaxis (option "E") prior to and following her transplant, this patient's overall prognosis is not likely to improve simply with this intervention.

Helpful Tip

Eosinophilia may be present in patients with severe combined immunodeficiency (SCID). The combination of eosinophilia and lymphopenia in the context of a patient with frequent infections should make you consider SCID.

► CASE 32

A 7-year-old boy is seen in the acute care clinic for epistaxis. He has been having nosebleeds from both nostrils, occurring spontaneously, approximately once per week, for several years. The nosebleeds last between 5 and 15 minutes and eventually resolve with pressure. The patient was seen in the emergency department last week for epistaxis lasting longer than 45 minutes, requiring nasal packing to stanch the bleeding. Historically, his mother describes him as bruising easily on his extremities, back, and face. He was circumcised as a neonate and had no unusual bleeding. He has never had bleeding problems associated with vaccinations. He has never appeared to have any joint pain or difficulty walking. There is no family history of individuals with bleeding disorders or bleeding symptoms. The physical exam is entirely normal, apart from several violaceous purpura noted on the lower extremities.

Question 32-1

Which of the following would be appropriate as initial screening tests in evaluation of this patient?

A) Bleeding time (BT), prothrombin time (PT), and activated partial thromboplastin time (aPTT).
B) Platelet count, platelet function assay, factor VIII activity, and factor IX activity.
C) CBC with white cell differential and platelets, factor VIII activity, and factor IX activity.
D) Platelet count, BT, von Willebrand factor (vWF) antigen, and vWF activity.
E) Platelet count, PT, aPTT, vWF antigen, and vWF activity.

Discussion 32-1

The correct answer is "E." While there may be substantial variation in practice in the initial workup for a patient suspected of a bleeding disorder, it is helpful to plan screening based on the most likely etiology of bleeding derived from the history. The patient in the vignette exhibits mucocutaneous bleeding in the form of epistaxis and bruising, common in disorders of primary hemostasis most consistent with platelet-related bleeding or von Willebrand disease (vWD). Confirming an adequate platelet count is crucial in the initial workup. While the prevalence of qualitative platelet function disorders in pediatrics is not precisely known, it is nevertheless rare, and platelet function testing is not currently considered necessary as a first-line screening test (making option "B" incorrect). The most dramatic platelet function defects include Bernard-Soulier

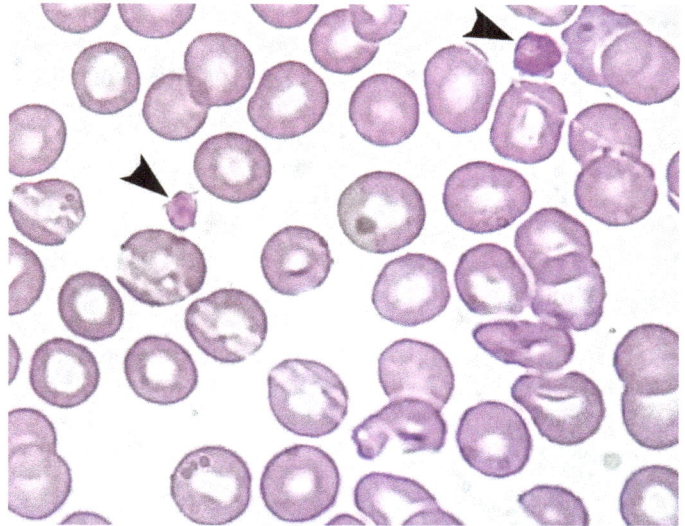

FIGURE 4–10. Macrothrombocytopenia. This blood smear was taken from a patient with Bernard-Soulier syndrome, associated with thrombocytopenia and large platelet size (*arrowheads*). Abnormally large platelets may also be seen in antibody-mediated platelet disorders, such as immune thrombocytopenia (ITP), as well as in myeloproliferative neoplasms. (Used with permission from Adam D. Wolfe, MD, PhD.)

syndrome (BSS; caused by deficient platelet glycoprotein Ib/IX, the vWF receptor) and Glanzmann thrombasthenia (caused by deficient platelet glycoprotein IIb-IIIa, the fibrinogen receptor), and are often diagnosed with severe mucocutaneous bleeding in early childhood. Of note, BSS is one of very few inherited conditions that causes macrothrombocytopenia, or low numbers of large platelets, illustrated in Figure 4–10. The BT, while still available in many centers, has fallen out of favor as a screening test, and is particularly unhelpful in children with suspected bleeding disorders. There is considerable interlaboratory variability, and the BT may be affected by factors independent of bleeding risk, such as age, gender, skin temperature, skin thickness, and hematocrit. The test has largely been supplanted by other laboratory assessments (making options "A" and "D" incorrect). Hemophilia A and B (factor VIII and IX deficiency, respectively) also may cause mucocutaneous bleeding symptoms, although the bleeding with these conditions is most often related to defective secondary hemostasis, such as intramuscular (eg, following vaccination) and intra-articular (ie, joint bleeds and hemophilic arthropathy). The patient in the vignette had no personal or family history to raise suspicion for hemophilia, although screening with PT and aPTT is typically included in initial evaluation to ensure that there are no factor deficiencies within the initiation (ie, extrinsic, measured by PT) or propagation (ie, intrinsic, measured by aPTT) pathways of coagulation (making option "C" less appropriate). The most likely diagnosis for the patient in the vignette is vWD. Most vWD types are inherited in an autosomal recessive manner, making a family history less frequent in affected individuals. Patients with a diagnosis of vWD, or any bleeding disorder, are discouraged from participating in contact sports (such as football, basketball and wrestling) and some limited contact sports (such as baseball, gymnastics and volleyball), based on provider comfort. They require prompt attention to head injury or concussive symptoms, due to the risk of intracranial hemorrhage. Emergency management involves administration of vWF:factor VIII complex, to restore appropriate vWF levels and activity. Type 1 vWD, due to quantitative vWF deficiency, and some subtypes of type 2 vWD, due to qualitative defects in vWF, are responsive to desmopressin (DDAVP). This hormone stimulates immediate mobilization of vWF stores and can cause transient increase in circulating vWF, but is only effective in patients who can produce vWF at baseline. The advantage of DDAVP is that it may be administered intranasally and is therefore easily given at home as a rescue medication. Patients with vWD often undergo DDAVP challenge in the hematology clinic to establish whether they exhibit a response to the medication.

> **Helpful Tip**
> Platelet dysfunction and von Willebrand disease (vWD) cause mucocutaneous bleeding (epistaxis, bruising, gingiva). In addition to mucocutaneous bleeding, factor deficiencies cause bleeding into tissues (joints, muscles).

► CASE 33

You are seeing a 1-month-old baby girl in clinic for a follow-up visit. She has been growing and developing well, and her parents have no concerns today. The baby's initial newborn hemoglobinopathy screen was flagged as abnormal by the state lab, exhibiting a hemoglobin FS pattern suggestive of sickle cell disease. There is no family history of sickle cell disease, and the parents are unaware of any individuals with sickle cell trait. A repeat screen was sent at 2 weeks, with the same result. You are discussing this finding with the family today, and are in the process of referring the patient to pediatric hematology.

Question 33-1

Which of the following statements is most accurate regarding a newborn diagnosed with sickle cell disease?

A) The patient should be protected from sickle cell complications during the first 6 months of life due to the presence of fetal hemoglobin.

B) Penicillin prophylaxis will need to be initiated once the spleen has involuted, usually around 5 to 6 years of age.

C) Starting hydroxyurea by age 12 months should help to protect the child from developing ischemic strokes during childhood.

D) Because of development of functional asplenia, infants with sickle cell disease should receive the 23-valent pneumococcal polysaccharide vaccine instead of the standard 13-valent pneumococcal conjugate vaccine (PCV-13).

E) Parents should be taught to respond promptly to any febrile episodes with acetaminophen, and follow up with their hematologist within 48 hours of fever.

Discussion 33-1

The correct answer is "A." A normal newborn hemoglobinopathy screen exhibits hemoglobins F (HbF, comprised of globin subunits $\alpha_2\gamma_2$) and A (HbA, $\alpha_2\beta_2$). The baby in the vignette exhibits hemoglobins F (fetal) and S (HbS, $\alpha_2\beta^S_2$). Note that the newborn screen reports hemoglobins in descending order of quantity, and HbF will be most abundant in newborns. The patient's inability to produce HbA indicates that she lacks any normal β-globin production. This pattern fits best with either hemoglobin SS disease, or hemoglobin S-β⁰ thalassemia, a heterozygous condition with a similar phenotype. The distinction between these diagnoses should not affect the initial counseling and management of the patient. Under physiologic stress, HbS polymerizes within red blood cells, causing a shape change to the classic sickle cell shape illustrated in Figure 4–11. Stressors include hypoxemia, dehydration, and infection. These abnormally shaped cells may then aggregate and occlude microvasculature, causing tissue hypoxia and endothelial inflammation and damage. The presence of HbF in excess of 30% is protective against this phenomenon, as HbF incorporates into HbS polymers and terminates their extension. Therefore, infants with sickle cell disease do not usually exhibit complications until at least the latter half of the infant period, or after HbF levels drop below 30%. Children with sickle cell disease are at risk of multiple complications. The greatest early risk comes from infection. Patients with sickle cell disease are considered functionally asplenic, regardless of the presence of a spleen; this can be confirmed by the appearance of Howell-Jolly bodies visible on the blood smear, shown in Figure 4–11. These patients are at elevated risk of sepsis due to encapsulated organisms. For this reason, penicillin prophylaxis is typically initiated by 2 months of age and continued

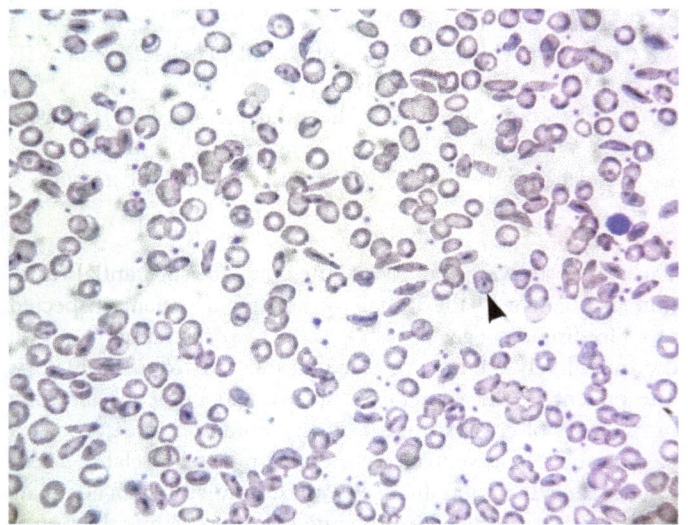

FIGURE 4–11. Sickle cell anemia. This blood smear exhibits many cells with characteristic sickle shape. Multiple cells also exhibit Howell-Jolly bodies, basophilic inclusions of red cells representative of remnant DNA (eg, *arrowhead*). The presence of circulating cells with Howell-Jolly bodies, which are normally cleared by the spleen, indicates functional asplenia. (Used with permission from Adam D. Wolfe, MD, PhD.)

until splenic involution, around 5 to 6 years of age (making option "B" incorrect). Patients with sickle cell disease should receive all recommended childhood vaccinations, including pneumococcal vaccination with PCV-13. They also should additionally receive the 23-valent vaccine between ages 2 and 5 (option "E"). The risk of bacterial sepsis in these patients remains high, and patients with sickle cell disease who develop fever (≥ 38°C [100.4°F]) must be seen immediately for blood culture and empiric parenteral antibiotic therapy (making option "D" incorrect). Sickle cell disease also can cause vaso-occlusive episodes, which can lead to pain, respiratory complications, renal disease, and stroke, depending on the location. Hydroxyurea stimulates increased production of HbF, and has been demonstrated in large clinical trials to provide effective prophylaxis against vaso-occlusion, painful episodes, and acute chest syndrome. Unfortunately, hydroxyurea was not shown to be effective prophylaxis against stroke in sickle cell disease (making option "C" incorrect). Patients with sickle cell disease should undergo screening of middle cerebral artery flow velocities by transcranial Doppler ultrasound, performed annually between ages 2 and 16, and those found to be at risk of stroke are referred for chronic transfusion therapy to reduce stroke risk.

▶ CASE 34

A 12-year-old adolescent girl presents to the acute care clinic due to fatigue. She underwent menarche 4 months ago, and has had fairly heavy flow lasting 5 to 7 days every 4 weeks since then. Her mother describes her as always being pale and easily tired, and she has always been at the low end of the weight and height curves for her age. The fatigue has become more severe over these past 4 months. The patient has never had a blood test before. Her mother reports that she was diagnosed with anemia during pregnancy, and required a blood transfusion after childbirth; no other family members have known anemia or bleeding problems. The patient overall appears well, is alert and answering questions. The patient is afebrile. Exam reveals faint scleral icterus, conjunctival and gingival pallor, tachycardia and a grade I/VI systolic ejection murmur over the left sternal border. There is no lymphadenopathy, organomegaly, or bruising. A CBC reveals white blood cell count of $5.4 \times 10^3/$mm^3, hemoglobin 7.8 g/dL, and platelets $500 \times 10^3/$mm^3. Red cell indices include mean corpuscular volume (MCV) 54 fL and red cell distribution width 15%.

Question 34-1

Which of the following is the most likely diagnosis for this patient?

A) von Willebrand disease.
B) Beta-thalassemia minor.
C) Beta-thalassemia intermedia.
D) Beta-thalassemia major.
E) Alpha-thalassemia minor.

Discussion 34-1

The correct answer is "C." This patient presents with a history of acute-on-chronic fatigue, and symptoms suggestive of a chronic mild anemia with hemolysis (eg, pallor, scleral icterus, fatigue, growth delays). Her symptoms worsened after menarche, suggesting that she was unable to compensate for menstrual blood losses. Her laboratory evaluation reveals a significant microcytosis. The best choice from the answers given, of a microcytic anemia that is chronic but may not be diagnosed until late childhood or adolescence, is beta-thalassemia intermedia. Thalassemia is a collection of syndromes of varying severity, which all result from an imbalance in production of α and β globins in maturing cells of the erythrocyte lineage. The imbalance leads to formation of homotetramers of the overabundant globin subunit, and these hemoglobins are often ineffective or unstable, leading to reduced red cell lifespan and resilience. In the case of beta-thalassemia syndromes, one (minor) or both (intermedia, major) β globin genes is defective. Beta-thalassemia minor is not considered a disease, as adequate β globin production is sustained by the normal copy of the gene, and patients will exhibit a lifelong, mild microcytic anemia that does not cause symptoms and should not require transfusion (making option "B" incorrect). Beta-thalassemia major results from the absence of functional β globin, leaving patients dependent on fetal hemoglobin; these patients become symptomatically anemic usually during the first 1 to 2 years of life and require lifelong blood product support (making option "D" incorrect). Patients with beta-thalassemia intermedia typically inherit one null β globin gene, and one gene with a mutation that decreases production of β globin. They therefore have more severe anemia than patients with thalassemia minor, but less than if they had thalassemia major. These patients may not be diagnosed until later childhood, or in the case of this patient, after menarche. Alpha-thalassemia syndromes are caused by inheritance of mutations in one or more of the four α globin genes. Alpha-thalassemia minima, resulting from a single gene deletion, is asymptomatic and has no reliable associated laboratory abnormalities. Alpha-thalassemia minor, resulting from two gene deletions, resembles beta-thalassemia minor clinically, with lifelong mild microcytic anemia that tends not to cause symptoms (making option "E" incorrect). Hemoglobin H disease results from three deleted α globin genes and is associated with more severe anemia, particularly during acute illnesses, and the presence of hemoglobin H (β$_4$ globin tetramer) on electrophoresis. Alpha-thalassemia major, deletion of all α globin genes, results in inability to produce any hemoglobin F or A, and is not compatible with life unless it is diagnosed in utero and intrauterine blood transfusions are administered. A patient such as the one in the vignette, who presents with anemia after menarche, may also be suspected of having a bleeding disorder; von Willebrand disease (vWD) is the most common of these. In this case, one would expect the patient to have a normocytic anemia, consistent with acute blood loss. If the blood loss were chronic, microcytosis with iron deficiency might be seen with menorrhagia associated with vWD, but the history of lifelong fatigue, pallor, growth issues, and icterus would not be expected (making option "A" incorrect).

► CASE 35

A 4-year-old boy is being evaluated in the urgent care clinic for fever and cough. His mother reports that he has been having frequent febrile illnesses since he was around 6 months of age, with symptoms of ear infections, sinus infections, and at least three diagnosed pneumonias. He "always" seems ill, without any periods of being asymptomatic. Mom has been told on two previous occasions that the patient had abnormally low white blood cell counts. The patient was adopted at birth, and the biologic family history is unknown. On exam, the patient is tired and appears small for age. The oropharynx reveals multiple mucosal ulcerations. Tender cervical nodes are palpable in the anterior and posterior groups bilaterally. Lung exam reveals fine crackles in the upper lobes bilaterally. A CBC includes white blood cells $9.7 \times 10^3/mm^3$ with 2% neutrophils and 91% lymphocytes, hemoglobin 12.3 g/dL with normal red cell indices, and platelet count $266 \times 10^3/mm^3$. Chest X-ray reveals consolidation in the right and left upper lobes, consistent with multifocal pneumonia.

Question 35-1

Which of the following evaluations is most likely to yield an etiology for this patient's infectious history?
A) Bone marrow aspirate and biopsy.
B) Vitamin B_{12} and folate levels.
C) Antineutrophil antibody testing.
D) CBC with differential three times weekly for 6 weeks.
E) Epstein-Barr virus (EBV) serologic panel.

Discussion 35-1

The correct answer is "A." The patient exhibits findings of chronic neutropenia starting in infancy, with multiple febrile sinopulmonary infections, previous low white cell counts, mucositis, and profound neutropenia (absolute neutrophil count = $10,100 \times 0.02$ = $194/mm^3$). The differential diagnosis of infant and childhood neutropenia is broad, and includes nutritional, medication-associated, immune-mediated, and inherited causes. For this patient, severe congenital neutropenia and cyclic neutropenia are strong considerations. In the former case, diagnosis is suggested by maturation arrest at the promyelocyte stage of neutrophil development in the bone marrow. In cyclic neutropenia, neutrophils nadir with a periodicity of approximately 21 days, yielding a history of febrile illnesses and other neutropenic symptoms that coincide with the neutropenia. Other cytopenias may also occur on the same schedule. Diagnosis is made by establishing neutrophil periodicity by obtaining CBC with differential 3 times per week for at least two cycles (ie, 6 weeks; option "D"). The patient's history does not indicate a periodic symptomatic pattern, making this diagnosis less likely. Although the patient in the vignette may have a nutritional deficiency, as vitamin B_{12} and folate deficiencies are associated with acquired childhood neutropenia (option "B"), the absence of abnormalities noted in the red blood cells (eg, anemia, macrocytosis) reduces suspicion for this etiology. Antineutrophil antibodies (option "C") are associated with either

congenital neutropenia due to transplacental transfer of maternal antibody, or an autoantibody produced after a childhood infection. In the former case, severe infections are likely during the first few months of life, but the neutropenia should typically resolve by 6 months of age as maternal antibody wanes. In the latter case, neutropenia may persist for up to several years but typically is not associated with frequent or severe infections. Viral infections, such as EBV, can be associated with prolonged systemic illness and various acquired cytopenias including neutropenia (option "E") that can last for several months. However, this patient's history of frequent sinopulmonary infections with neutropenia lasting at least 3 years makes convalescent or prolonged EBV infection less likely. Patients with neutrophil counts of less than $500/mm^3$ are at greatest risk of bacteremia, and should receive prompt attention to fevers, with blood cultures obtained and empiric treatment with parenteral antibiotics. The patient in the vignette would benefit from intervention with granulocyte colony-stimulating factor (GCSF). This has been shown to increase neutrophil counts in patients with inherited and acquired neutropenias, and to diminish frequency, duration, and severity of infections. In some cases, patients with refractory neutropenia and recurrent life-threatening infections may be considered candidates for hematopoietic stem cell transplantation.

► CASE 36

A previously healthy, 15-year-old adolescent boy presents to the emergency department with cough and dyspnea. He has been noticing progressive difficulty catching his breath for several weeks now and has been unable to sleep on his back for the past week because of the sensation of pressure in his chest. He has not had fever or acute upper respiratory symptoms. Vital signs on presentation include temperature 37.5°C (99.5°F), heart rate 110 beats per minute, and respiratory rate 28 breaths per minute. The patient is awake, alert, and answering questions appropriately. You suspect that this patient has a mediastinal mass.

Question 36-1

Which of the following findings on your initial evaluation is most likely to warrant treatment before a biopsy can be performed?
A) White blood cell count $60 \times 10^3/mm^3$ with 64% blasts.
B) Spleen tip palpable 8 cm below the left costal margin.
C) Edema in the face and neck.
D) Palpable cervical, supraclavicular, axillary, and inguinal lymphadenopathy.
E) Serum alpha-fetoprotein (AFP) 3600 ng/dL (reference range < 10 ng/dL).

Discussion 36-1

The correct answer is "C." This patient presents with indolent progression of dyspnea and orthopnea consistent with a mediastinal mass. A chest X-ray will be helpful in confirming this suspicion. Causes of mediastinal masses in children include malignancy, infection, and venous thrombosis. Mass effect within the mediastinum can lead to the superior vena cava (SVC) syndrome. Symptoms relate to obstruction of venous drainage through the SVC and include those in the vignette; there can also be associated dysphagia and hoarseness. Physical exam findings in patients with SVC syndrome may include edema of the head, neck, and upper extremities with or without cyanosis, wheezing, and stridor. In the latter case, tracheal compression should be suspected. SVC syndrome is an emergency that may require intubation to secure the airway. Patients may decompensate if sedated or placed supine for a prolonged period (eg, for advanced imaging or diagnostic procedures). Patients with progressive symptoms, which can lead to central neurologic findings of headache, confusion, lethargy, and visual disturbance, may require therapy before the cause of the SVC syndrome is identified. Emergency management may include radiation therapy, chemotherapy, or anti-inflammatory medication such as corticosteroids. The differential diagnosis of mediastinal mass in pediatric oncology includes leukemia, lymphoma, neuroblastoma, germ cell tumor, and sarcoma. The hematologic malignancies are suggested by findings including leukocytosis and circulating blasts (option "A"), splenomegaly (option "B"), and lymphadenopathy (option "D"). Elevated tumor markers including AFP (option "E") and beta-human chorionic gonadotropin would raise suspicion for germ cell tumor. If neuroblastoma is favored, urine catecholamines vanillylmandelic acid (VMA) and homovanillic acid (HVA) may be obtained. However, none of these suspicious findings on initial evaluation constitutes an immediate life-threatening state that would merit treatment prior to obtaining a tissue diagnosis.

QUICK QUIZ

Which is NOT an oncologic emergency?
A) Tumor lysis syndrome.
B) Spinal cord compression.
C) Hyperleukocytosis.
D) Typhlitis.
E) All of the above.

Discussion

The correct answer is "E." Hyperleukocytosis causes hyperviscosity and leukostasis affecting the lungs, gastrointestinal tract, and central nervous system. In typhlitis or neutropenic enterocolitis, the bowel wall becomes inflamed in the setting of prolonged neutropenia and may perforate. Additional emergencies include SVC syndrome, increased intracranial pressure, and stroke.

► CASE 37

A 16-year-old adolescent boy has recently completed 39 months of chemotherapy for T-cell acute lymphoblastic leukemia (ALL). He has been in remission since the first month of induction therapy and currently feels well.

His mother notes that the family was advised that be lifelong follow up will be required, due to increased risk of complications from chemotherapy.

Question 37-1

Which of the following is a risk that is likely to decrease over the first year following completion of chemotherapy?
A) Infertility due to alkylating agents.
B) Development of cardiomyopathy secondary to anthracycline exposure.
C) Leukemia secondary to alkylating agents.
D) Immune system dysfunction secondary to myelosuppressive agents.
E) Leukemic relapse in the central nervous system (CNS) and testes.

Discussion 37-1

The correct answer is "D." Treatment with chemotherapy carries numerous short-term and long-term risks. Each class of agents is associated with specific toxicities that must be acknowledged with families during informed consent discussions surrounding cancer therapy. It is crucial to understand that many of the risks associated with chemotherapeutic agents persist indefinitely and require lifelong follow up with a specialist or primary care physician knowledgeable about cancer survivorship. Of the choices presented, the risk most likely to decrease shortly after completion of therapy is immune dysfunction. Some immune suppression is seen with chemotherapy that directly suppresses leukocyte production, which is a potential effect of nearly all chemotherapeutic drugs with the exception of vinca alkaloids (inhibitors of cell division). Other immune suppressive effects are due to the alteration of lymphocyte maturation induced by chemotherapy. Restoration of normal white cell function is usually assumed by approximately 6 months after cessation of chemotherapy. Alkylating agents such as cyclophosphamide are well known to be associated with future infertility, particularly when these agents are administered to adolescents (option "A"). The exact incidence of infertility associated with chemotherapy is unknown, but the risk for this is lifelong. Prior to initiation of chemotherapy, patients are expected to receive counseling regarding this risk, and efforts at fertility preservation should be offered. Anthracycline antibiotics (eg, doxorubicin and daunorubicin) are known to preferentially enter cardiomyocytes and cause oxidative damage. Evidence of anthracycline-associated cardiomyopathy can be identified years, or decades, after exposure (option "C"). Survivorship follow up includes echocardiography performed every 1 to 5 years, depending on cumulative drug exposure, as recommended by the Children's Oncology Group. An ironic and difficult-to-face complication of chemotherapy is the increased risk of secondary malignancy, most often associated with alkylating agents and topoisomerase inhibitors (eg, etoposide). The most frequently encountered malignancies are hematologic, including myelodysplastic syndrome and acute myeloid leukemia, although secondary solid tumors may also be seen. Radiation therapy also increases the risk of developing hematopoietic and solid malignancies. This risk persists lifelong. The other cancer-related risk to survivors following chemotherapy is relapse (option "E"). Close follow up for disease recurrence is therefore essential for any patient who has completed treatment for childhood malignancy. Leukemic relapse, which is most fearsome if it occurs shortly after completion of therapy but may occur many years later, may occur in the bone marrow, CNS, and testes. The possibility of testicular relapse is the reason that boys with leukemia receive maintenance therapy for approximately 12 months longer than girls (ie, approximately 27 months total duration for girls, 39 months for boys).

> ## ▶ CASE 38

A 2-year-old boy is admitted to the nephrology service on Tuesday for acute onset of hematuria, oliguria, and hypertension. On Monday, the patient was picked up by his mother from his father's home (they share custody of the patient). Mom was informed that the patient had fevers of 37.8 to 38.3°C (100.1–101°F) throughout the weekend, for which he received antipyretics that provided relief. By Tuesday morning, the day of admission, the mother noticed a cola-colored tint to the urine, and overall decreased wet diapers that made her concerned. The working diagnosis is postinfectious glomerulonephritis. Blood work on admission revealed white blood cell count $7.4 \times 10^3/mm^3$ with a normal differential, hemoglobin 11.1 g/dL, platelets $194 \times 10^3/mm^3$, creatinine 2.8 mg/dL, and blood urea nitrogen (BUN) 70 mg/dL. No abnormal red cell forms were noted on manual smear evaluation. The patient is scheduled for renal biopsy on Thursday morning. A preprocedure platelet function assay (PFA) is performed for screening purposes on Tuesday, revealing a closure time of greater than 300 seconds (reference range 60–180 s) in the initial screen.

Question 38-1

Which of the following is the most appropriate next step for this patient?
A) Proceed with biopsy as planned, transfuse 1 unit of platelets prior to procedure.
B) Repeat the PFA on Wednesday.
C) Perform plasmapheresis for suspected hemolytic uremic syndrome (HUS).
D) Perform bone marrow aspiration and biopsy.
E) Obtain testing for von Willebrand factor (vWF) antigen and activity.

Discussion 38-1

The correct answer is "B." This patient has renal disease that merits further evaluation and was incidentally discovered to have a prolonged platelet closure time on PFA. This screen may be performed in the setting of renal disease prior to a surgical procedure, as elevated BUN is a known cause of acquired qualitative platelet dysfunction. However, most patients with BUN of less than 100 mg/dL are unlikely to exhibit clinically significant platelet dysfunction. The most likely etiology for the patient's abnormal PFA is drug-induced platelet dysfunction, given the

history of recent antipyretic use, likely ibuprofen. Nonsteroidal anti-inflammatory drugs that inhibit cyclooxygenase-1 enzyme interfere with platelet production of thromboxane A_2 (TXA_2) from arachidonic acid, and the diminished TXA_2 reduces the ability of platelets to activate. This effect caused by ibuprofen is reversible upon withdrawal of the drug, and the alteration of platelet function will largely resolve within less than 72 hours of the most recent dose. In the vignette case, before major changes in the patient's treatment plan are contemplated, it would appropriate to repeat the PFA and observe for improvement. If the patient were to have confirmed non–medication-related platelet dysfunction, transfusion with healthy platelets (option "A") periprocedurally would reduce the likelihood of bleeding. The likelihood of HUS (option "C") in this case is low, as the hemoglobin and platelet counts are normal, and no schistocytes were observed on the blood smear. Further, prior to plasmapheresis for HUS, therapy with eculizumab (monoclonal antibody that inhibits terminal complement pathway activation) might be attempted. As no abnormalities were noted on blood count, bone marrow assessment (option "D") is not warranted. While von Willebrand disease (option "E") often also causes prolongation of the PFA, no other data were provided in the case description to suggest a bleeding disorder, and an acquired platelet problem is more likely.

> ## ▶ CASE 39

During rounds on a 22-hour-old term newborn boy in the nursery one morning, you notice jaundice to the lower abdomen that was not reported at birth. The chart indicates that the mother is G_2P_1 with one spontaneous abortion prior to this pregnancy, took no medications during pregnancy, and received no prenatal care. She reports a history of requiring several blood transfusions following trauma in a motor vehicle accident 3 years ago. Her blood type is O, Rh negative. The baby's father has chronic anemia with mild jaundice, and required several blood transfusions as a child. The baby's vital signs are all normal. The physical exam is unremarkable apart from the jaundice. CBC on the baby reveals hemoglobin 12.8 g/dL, mean corpuscular volume (MCV) 105 fL, and all other values are normal. Total bilirubin is 8.4 mg/dL. The baby is blood type A, Rh negative.

Question 39-1

Which of the following etiologies best explains this baby's jaundice?
A) ABO incompatibility.
B) G6PD deficiency.
C) Rh incompatibility.
D) Beta-thalassemia major.
E) Folate deficiency.

Discussion 39-1

The correct answer is "A." This patient presents within 24 hours of life with hyperbilirubinemia and asymptomatic, mild anemia for age, suggestive of a mild hemolytic condition. The mother has a history of a previous pregnancy and previous blood transfusion in an emergency setting, and may have become sensitized to blood group antigens from these exposures. Infants with A blood group born to mothers with O blood group and history of exposure to A antigen from previous pregnancy or transfusion are at highest risk of alloimmune hemolysis, called hemolytic disease of the fetus and newborn (HDFN). It is important to note that unexposed individuals make IgM type antibodies against mismatched major blood group antigens (ie, this mother likely has circulating anti-A and anti-B IgM), but these do not cross the placenta. Prior exposure to the mismatched blood group, however, stimulates IgG production, and these antibodies are able to cross the placenta and lead to HDFN in subsequent pregnancies. Rh incompatibility (option "C") yields an anti-D IgG, which also causes HDFN, often with greater severity than ABO mismatch, but the mother and infant in this case are both Rh-negative.

Most cases of ABO mismatch–associated HDFN do not cause problematic anemia, and hyperbilirubinemia, when present, may be treated with observation or phototherapy alone. However, some affected infants, mainly those with Rh-associated HDFN, exhibit severe symptoms with significant anemia and a greater degree of hyperbilirubinemia necessitating exchange transfusion. This condition may be diagnosed on prenatal ultrasound with evidence of hydrops, subcutaneous edema, and third space effusions in the abdominal, pericardial, and pleural spaces. G6PD deficiency (assayed by option "B") may be the diagnosis for this patient's father, based on his history provided, and this can be associated with neonatal hemolysis. However, G6PD is inherited in an X-linked recessive fashion, and the patient would not have inherited it from his paternal genome. Beta-thalassemia major (option "D") is associated with chronic hemolysis and jaundice, but since newborns have relatively little β globin production, relying mainly on γ globin present in fetal hemoglobin, they are not expected to exhibit substantial symptoms for several months. Folate deficiency (option "E") causes a nonhemolytic macrocytic anemia. Note that this patient's MCV is within the normal range for newborns, which is higher than older children due to the predominance of fetal hemoglobin. Further, newborns generally have adequate folate stores to last at least several months after birth.

BIBLIOGRAPHY

Albisetti M, Monagle P. Bleeding disorders. In: de Alarcón PE, Werner EJ, Christensen RD, eds. *Neonatal Hematology: Pathogenesis, Diagnosis, and Management of Hematologic Problems*. New York, NY: Cambridge University Press; 2013:286–301.

Allen CE, Kelly KM, Bollard CM. Pediatric lymphomas and histiocytic disorders of childhood. *Pediatr Clin North Am*. 2015;62(1):139–165.

Alter BP, D'Andrea AD. Inherited bone marrow failure syndromes. In: Handin RI, Lux SE, Stossel TP, eds. *Blood: Principles and Practice of Hematology*. Philadelphia, PA: Lippincott, Williams and Wilkins; 2003:209–272.

Anderst JD, Carpenter SL, Abshire TC; Section on Hematology/Oncology and Committee on Child Abuse and Neglect of the American Academy of Pediatrics. Evaluation for bleeding disorders in suspected child abuse. *Pediatrics*. 2013;131(4):e1314–1322.

Armenian SH, Robison LL. Childhood cancer survivorship: An update on evolving paradigms for understanding pathogenesis and screening for therapy-related late effects. *Curr Opin Pediatr*. 2013;25(1):16–22.

Baker RD, Greer FR; Committee on Nutrition, American Academy of Pediatrics. Diagnosis and prevention of iron deficiency and iron-deficiency anemia in infants and young children (0–3 years of age). *Pediatrics*. 2010;126(5):1040–1050.

Boscainos PJ, Cousins GR, Kulshreshtha R, et al. Osteoid osteoma. *Orthopedics*. 2013;36(10):792–800.

Branchford BR, Monahan PE, Di Paola J. New developments in the treatment of pediatric hemophilia and bleeding disorders. *Curr Opin Pediatr*. 2013;25(1):23–30.

Cairo MS, Coiffier B, Reiter A, Younes A; TLS Expert Panel. Recommendations for the evaluation of risk and prophylaxis of tumour lysis syndrome (TLS) in adults and children with malignant diseases: An expert TLS panel consensus. *Br J Haematol*. 2010;149(4):578–586.

Cappellini MD, Fiorelli G. Glucose-6-phosphate dehydrogenase deficiency. *Lancet*. 2008;371(9606):64–74.

Chalmers E, Cooper P, Forman K, et al. Purpura fulminans: recognition, diagnosis and management. *Arch Dis Child*. 2011;96(11):1066–1071.

Chirnomas SD, Kupfer GM. The inherited bone marrow failure syndromes. *Pediatr Clin North Am*. 2013;60(6):1291–1310.

Christensen RD. Reference ranges in neonatal hematology. In: de Alarcón PE, Werner EJ, Christensen RD, eds. *Neonatal Hematology: Pathogenesis, Diagnosis, and Management of Hematologic Problems*. New York, NY: Cambridge University Press; 2013:385–408.

Committee on Sports Medicine and Fitness. Medical conditions affecting sports participation. *Pediatrics*. 2001;107(5):1205–1209.

Da Costa L, Galimand J, Fenneteau O, Mohandas N. Hereditary spherocytosis, elliptocytosis, and other red cell membrane disorders. *Blood Rev*. 2013;27(4):167–178.

de Alarcón PE, Fernández KS. Congenital thrombocytopenias and thrombocytopathies. In: de Alarcón PE, Werner EJ, Christensen RD, eds. *Neonatal Hematology: Pathogenesis, Diagnosis, and Management of Hematologic Problems*. New York, NY: Cambridge University Press; 2013:172–207.

De Bernardi B, Balwierz W, Bejent J, et al. Epidural compression in neuroblastoma: Diagnostic and therapeutic aspects. *Cancer Lett*. 2005;228(1–2):283–99.

Demellawy DE, Young JL, Nanassy J, Chernetsova E, Nasr A. Langerhans cell histiocytosis: A comprehensive review. *Pathology*. 2015;47(4):294–301.

Dimaras H, Kimani K, Dimba EAO, et al. Retinoblastoma. *Lancet*. 2012;379(9824):1436–1446.

Fisher MJ, Rheingold SR. Oncologic emergencies. In: Pizzo PA, Poplack DG, eds. *Principles and Practice of Pediatric*

Oncology. Philadelphia, PA: Lippincott Williams and Wilkins; 2011:1125–1151.

Fleisher T. Primary immune deficiencies: Windows into the immune system. *Pediatr Rev.* 2006;27(10):363–372.

Friedman AD. Wilms tumor. *Pediatr Rev.* 2013;34(7):328–330.

Gajjar AJ, Robinson GW. Medulloblastoma-translating discoveries from the bench to the bedside. *Nat Rev Clin Oncol.* 2014;11(12):714–722.

Harrison P, Mackie I, Mumford A, Briggs C, et al; British Committee for Standards in Haematology. Guidelines for the laboratory investigation of heritable disorders of platelet function. *Br J Haematol.* 2011;155(1):30–44.

Islam MS, Anoop P. Current concepts in the management of stroke in children with sickle cell disease. *Childs Nerv Syst.* 2011;27(7):1037–1043.

Kett JC. Anemia in infancy. *Pediatr Rev.* 2012;33(4):186–187.

Matthews DC. Inherited disorders of platelet function. *Pediatr Clin North Am.* 2013;60(6):1475–1488.

Miller ST. How I treat acute chest syndrome in children with sickle cell disease. *Blood.* 2011;117(20):5297–5305.

Mughal TI, Ejaz AA, Foringer JR, Coiffier B. An integrated clinical approach for the identification, prevention, and treatment of tumor lysis syndrome. *Cancer Treat Rev.* 2010;36(2):164–176.

Neunert C, Lim W, Crowther M, et al; American Society of Hematology. The American Society of Hematology 2011 evidence-based practice guideline for immune thrombocytopenia. *Blood.* 2011;117(16):4190–4207.

Newburger PE, Dale DC. Evaluation and management of patients with isolated neutropenia. *Semin Hematol.* 2013;50(3):198–206.

Parker RI. Transfusion in critically ill children: Indications, risks, and challenges. *Crit Care Med.* 2014;42(3):675–690.

Powers JM, McCavit TL, Buchanan GR. Management of iron deficiency anemia: A survey of pediatric hematology/oncology specialists. *Pediatr Blood Cancer.* 2015;62(5):842–846.

Price VE, Ledingham DL, Krumpel A, Chan AK. Diagnosis and management of neonatal purpura fulminans. *Semin Fetal Neonatal Med.* 2011;16(6):318–322.

Reverdiau-Moalic P, Delahousse B, Body G, et al. Evolution of blood coagulation activators and inhibitors in the healthy human fetus. *Blood.* 1996;88:900–906.

Rund D, Rachmilewitz E. Beta-thalassemia. *N Engl J Med.* 2005;353(11):1135–1146.

Scheinberg P, Young NS. How I treat acquired aplastic anemia. *Blood.* 2012;120(6):1185–1196.

Shields CL, Shields JA. Retinoblastoma management: Advances in enucleation, intravenous chemoreduction, and intra-arterial chemotherapy. *Curr Opin Ophthalmol.* 2010;21(3):203–212.

Teplick A, Kowalski M, Biegel JA, Nichols KE. Educational paper: Screening in cancer predisposition syndromes: guidelines for the general pediatrician. *Eur J Pediatr.* 2011;170(3):285–294.

Thornburg CD, Files BA, Luo Z, et al.; BABY HUG Investigators, Impact of hydroxyurea on clinical events in the BABY HUG trial. *Blood.* 2012;120(22):4304–4310; quiz 4448.

Vagace JM, Bajo R, Gervasini G. Diagnostic and therapeutic challenges of primary autoimmune haemolytic anaemia in children. *Arch Dis Child.* 2014;99(7):668–673.

van der Spek J, Groenwold RH, van der Burg M, van Montfrans JM. TREC based newborn screening for severe combined immunodeficiency disease: A systematic review. *J Clin Immunol.* 2015;35(4):416–430.

Vlychou M, Athanasou NA. Radiological and pathological diagnosis of paediatric bone tumours and tumour-like lesions. *Pathology.* 2008;40(2):196–216.

Warkentin TE. Heparin-induced thrombocytopenia in critically ill patients. *Semin Thromb Hemost.* 2015;41(1):49–60.

Webb J, Kwiatkowski JL. Stroke in patients with sickle cell disease. *Expert Rev Hematol.* 2013;6(3):301–316.

Yu AL, Gilman AL, Ozkaynak MF, et al; Children's Oncology Group. Anti-GD2 antibody with GM-CSF, interleukin-2, and isotretinoin for neuroblastoma. *N Engl J Med.* 2010;363(14):1324–1334.

Cardiology

5

Benton Ng

▶ CASE 1

A 3-year-old boy comes for his yearly well-child check. His mother's only concern is that he is a picky eater. He has been tracking on his growth curve for both height and weight, and is developmentally appropriate. On exam, he has a grade II/VI systolic murmur that you have not previously heard.

Question 1-1

What is the next best step in evaluation?
A) Additional physical exam maneuvers.
B) Electrocardiogram (ECG).
C) Echocardiogram.
D) Chest X-ray.
E) Both B and D.

Discussion 1-1

The correct answer is "A." Innocent murmurs are common in children and most often present in the toddler years. These murmurs are never louder than grade III/VI and rarely radiate. They are louder when the child is supine and softer when standing, but usually do not completely disappear with standing. These murmurs also come and go, and are more prominent during times of increased cardiac output, such as during a febrile illness.

Question 1-2

What is the closest estimate for the percentage of children who have an innocent murmur?
A) 15%.
B) 30%.
C) 50%.
D) 65%.
E) 80%.

Discussion 1-2

The correct answer is "E." The majority of children have an innocent murmur at some time. Some studies report that 85% of children have an innocent murmur. This is in contrast to the incidence of congenital heart disease, which is commonly reported to be around 1%.

Question 1-3

Which of the following is NOT a characteristic of an innocent murmur?
A) Systolic murmur.
B) Diastolic murmur.
C) Continuous murmur.
D) Palpable thrill.
E) Both A and D.
F) Both B and D.
G) Options B, C, and D.

Discussion 1-3

The correct answer is "F." An innocent murmur does not produce a palpable thrill (grade IV or higher). Solely diastolic murmurs are never innocent. The majority of innocent murmurs are systolic murmurs. The venous hum is the one innocent murmur that is a continuous murmur.

> **Helpful Tip**
> In addition to being the only continuous murmur, the venous hum is also the one innocent murmur that is louder while sitting than supine, contrary to other innocent murmurs. It is most easily heard on the low anterior part of the neck, just lateral to the sternocleidomastoid. Turning the patient's head toward the side of the murmur can diminish or eliminate the murmur.

▶ CASE 2

A 16-year-old adolescent boy comes to you for his preparticipation physical. He has not been seen by you in 3 years. There is a family history of coronary artery disease, including his grandfather, who suffered a myocardial infarction at the age of 55. His mother has both hypertension and hyperlipidemia. His weight is at the 95th percentile, his height is at the 75th percentile, his body mass index (BMI) is at the 93rd percentile, heart rate is 63 beats per minute (bpm), and blood pressure is 142/88 mm Hg. His physical exam is otherwise normal.

Question 2-1
What is his diagnosis?
A) Normal blood pressure.
B) Prehypertension.
C) Stage I hypertension.
D) Stage II hypertension.
E) None of the above.

Discussion 2-1
The correct answer is "E." Hypertensive children are more likely to become hypertensive adults. Blood pressure percentiles depend on the child's age, sex, and height. Prehypertension or high normal blood pressure is defined as a blood pressure in the 90th to less than 95th percentile. Stage I hypertension is a blood pressure in the 95th to 99th percentile plus 5 mm Hg. Stage II hypertension is any blood pressure greater than the 99th percentile plus 5 mm Hg. In this case, the patient's blood pressure falls between the 95th and 99th percentiles. But in order for the diagnosis of stage I hypertension to be made, this should be measured on at least three separate occasions. He does not need to be restricted from activities.

Question 2-2
He returns for three more follow ups and his blood pressure measurements are repeatedly in the 90th to less than 95th percentile. What is the most appropriate next step?
A) Therapeutic lifestyle changes.
B) Urinalysis.
C) Echocardiogram.
D) CBC.
E) Electrolytes, glucose, blood urea nitrogen (BUN), creatinine.

Discussion 2-2
The correct answer is "A." Therapeutic lifestyle changes are appropriate for patients who have prehypertension. Counseling should be done with the aim of gradual weight loss. Moderate exercise of 30 to 40 minutes per day, 3 to 5 days per week, is recommended. The goal should be to expend at least 200 kcal/day. Dietary changes are also recommended to decrease intake of salt, sugar, and fat, with 25% to 35% of total calories from fat, 50% to 60% of calories from carbohydrates, and 15% of calories from protein. In general, total caloric intake should be adjusted to prevent further weight gain and help achieve a healthy weight.

Over the next 2 years, his blood pressure measurements are consistently in the 95th to 99th percentile.

Question 2-3
What is the most appropriate next diagnostic step?
A) Serum electrolytes, glucose, BUN, and creatinine.
B) Urinalysis.
C) Echocardiogram.
D) CBC.
E) Renal ultrasound.
F) All of the above.

Discussion 2-3
The correct answer is "F." Workup is recommended in patients with stage I hypertension for further evaluation of the etiology of hypertension and for signs of end-organ damage. This consists of a CBC, electrolytes, renal function, urinalysis, renal ultrasound, echocardiogram, and fasting lipids. The majority of hypertension in adolescents is essential, with the majority of essential hypertension being related to obesity. In the cases of secondary hypertension, the most common etiology is renal. An echocardiogram is done as a screening test to evaluate for left ventricular hypertrophy. This can be an indication for initiating antihypertensive treatment.

▶ CASE 3

A 13-year-old adolescent girl follows up with you after being seen in the emergency department the previous afternoon for chest pain. She began having the pain while running in track practice the day before. She localizes the pain to the middle of the chest and denies radiation. She also denies any palpitations or presyncopal feelings. She does note feeling short of breath. The pain lasted 5 to 10 minutes and resolved when she stopped running.

Question 3-1
What further finding would be most reassuring for a noncardiac cause of chest pain?
A) Pleuritic chest pain.
B) Pain with palpation of her chest wall on exam.
C) Systolic murmur on exam.
D) Normal ECG.
E) History of Kawasaki disease.

Discussion 3-1
The correct answer is "B." Chest pain in children is noncardiac in origin over 98% of the time. Musculoskeletal, gastrointestinal, and pulmonary etiologies are common. Pain with palpation over the costochondral junction on physical exam is consistent with costochondritis. This pain is often self-limited and may be helped by nonsteroidal anti-inflammatory drugs (NSAIDs). Classically, this is characterized by a sharp pain, although description of chest pain can often be unreliable in the pediatric setting. Pleuritic chest pain is often reassuring as well, although this may be the presenting symptom of pericarditis. In the case of pericarditis, the pain is worse with deep breathing but is relieved by leaning forward. The pain is also usually referred to the scapular ridge. There are also classic ECG changes seen with pericarditis (diffuse ST-segment elevation for acute pericarditis). A harsh systolic murmur, especially heard with a systolic click, would be consistent with aortic stenosis. With more

severe stenosis, this could lead to decreased oxygen delivery in the face of increased demand during exercise, resulting in exertional chest pain. Although an abnormal ECG would help with the diagnosis of pericarditis, myocarditis, and anomalous left coronary artery from the pulmonary artery (ALCAPA), a normal ECG does not completely rule out the possibility of a cardiac etiology of the chest pain. For example, other types of anomalous coronaries, such as an anomalous left coronary from the right coronary cusp, have a normal resting ECG. A history of Kawasaki's disease increases a patient's risk for having coronary artery involvement. If patients have never had coronary artery involvement as part of their Kawasaki disease, then this is less likely to be related. But patients who have coronary artery aneurysms as a result of Kawasaki disease are at increased risk for thrombosis or stenosis of their coronary arteries.

Question 3-2

What is the order of ECG findings you would expect to see over the first 1 to 2 months after diagnosis of acute pericarditis?

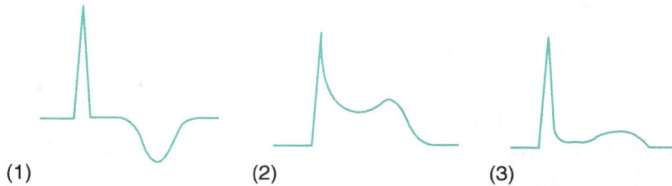

(1) (2) (3)

A) 1,2,3.
B) 2,1,3.
C) 2,3,1.
D) 1,3,2.
E) 3,2,1.

Discussion 3-2

The correct answer is "C." ECG findings seen over time with acute pericarditis have three stages before normalization. Initially there is subepicardial myocardial damage that results in diffuse ST-segment elevation. This is most prominent in leads representing the left ventricle. Within 2 to 3 days, the ST segments return to normal. Two to 4 weeks later, the T waves become inverted. This may persist for up to 1 to 2 months before complete normalization.

> **Helpful Tip**
> An echocardiogram can be useful when pericarditis is suspected to rule out a large pericardial effusion or tamponade physiology, which would require pericardiocentesis.

Question 3-3

All of the following are risk factors for acute pericarditis EXCEPT:

A) Recent cardiac surgery.
B) Recent respiratory infection.
C) Renal failure.
D) Liver failure.
E) Malignancy.
F) Autoimmune disease.

Discussion 3-3

The correct answer is "D." Up to 90% of cases of acute pericarditis are infectious or idiopathic in etiology. Causative viruses include coxsackie B, echovirus, adenovirus, influenza A and B, enterovirus, mumps, Epstein-Barr virus (EBV), and many others. Coxsackievirus is the most classic cause of acute pericarditis in children. Pneumococcus and tuberculosis are the most common bacterial causes. Aspirin or NSAIDs are first-line treatments and are effective. In other cases of acute pericarditis, treatment of the underlying cause is necessary.

▶ CASE 4

A 13-year-old girl who experienced an episode of syncope is being seen for follow up. She participates in band and had an episode during practice. She recalls feeling hot and as if her vision was starting to black out. The next thing she remembers is waking up on the floor. She is unsure of how much time passed. She felt a bit dazed when she woke up, but recovered.

Question 4-1

Which of the following are most likely to be abnormal?

A) ECG.
B) Echocardiogram.
C) Electroencephalogram (EEG).
D) Resting heart rate.
E) Blood pressure.
F) None of the above.

Discussion 4-1

The correct answer is "F." The girl's symptoms are most consistent with neurally mediated syncope (vasovagal syncope). Workup of these patients is often unremarkable. In contrast, cardiac syncope classically has an abrupt onset without presyncopal symptoms (tunnel vision, dizziness, lightheadedness). This patient's history is classic for neurally mediated syncope, which occurs when someone has been standing for a prolonged period of time, such as during band practice or at church. One theory is that prolonged standing results in exaggerated venous pooling and temporary decreased cerebral perfusion leading to syncope. Neurally mediated syncope also occurs after strong emotional or situational triggers.

Question 4-2

Which finding is the most likely to be abnormal for a cardiac cause of syncope?

A) Physical exam.
B) Echocardiogram.
C) Family history.
D) Resting heart rate.
E) Blood pressure.

Discussion 4-2

The correct answer is "C." Often the most suspicious piece of information for a cardiac cause of syncope when working up a patient is family history. An ECG is often part of the initial workup, but a normal ECG does not completely rule out a cardiac cause. Cardiac causes for syncope include hypertrophic cardiomyopathy, long QT syndrome, anomalous coronary arteries, arrhythmogenic right ventricular cardiomyopathy (ARVC), Brugada syndrome, and catecholaminergic polymorphic ventricular tachycardia (CPVT). Whereas the ECG is abnormal in long QT syndrome, Brugada syndrome, and many cases of hypertrophic cardiomyopathy, it can also be normal in some cases of hypertrophic cardiomyopathy, ARVC, CPVT, and with abnormal coronary arteries. The echocardiogram is abnormal with anomalous origins of the coronary arteries, if they are well visualized on the study. Hypertrophic cardiomyopathy should also demonstrate an abnormal echocardiogram, but it can be normal in genotype-positive patients, especially if obtained early in life before development of significant hypertrophy. Echocardiographic criteria exist for the diagnosis of ARVC but these are insufficient to make the diagnosis alone. The echocardiogram is normal in cases of long QT syndrome, Brugada syndrome, and CPVT. Family history of sudden death is not positive in the index case, but if present is often the most concerning part of the history that triggers further workup and referral.

Question 4-3

Which of the following is the most common cause of sudden cardiac death in the young?
A) Long QT syndrome.
B) Hypertrophic cardiomyopathy.
C) Anomalous coronary arteries.
D) Mitral valve prolapse.
E) Commotio cordis.

Discussion 4-3

The correct answer is "B." Hypertrophic cardiomyopathy is by far the most likely cause of sudden death in young athletes (up to 40% of cardiovascular causes). Hypertrophic cardiomyopathy is an autosomal dominantly inherited disease present in 1 in 500 people. There is a great deal of phenotypic heterogeneity, so an identified mutation does not correlate with any specific risk factors for sudden death. A murmur may or may not be present at rest. Having the patient perform the Valsalva maneuver (bear down) will decrease the intensity of most systolic murmurs. In contrast, a murmur caused by obstruction secondary to hypertrophic cardiomyopathy will increase in intensity with the Valsalva.

▶ CASE 5

A 2-month-old previously healthy boy presents to your clinic for a well-child visit. His parents have no major concerns. He is afebrile, his heart rate is 168 bpm, and his respiratory rate is 68 breaths per minute. He has gained 7 g/day since you saw him last at 1 month. On exam, he has a grade II/VI systolic ejection murmur and his liver is palpated 3 cm below the costal margin. You obtain a chest X-ray. The heart looks like a snowman. He does not appear cyanotic, but you ask the nurse to check his oxygen saturation (Spo$_2$).

Question 5-1

What is the most likely Spo$_2$ you will obtain?
A) 100%.
B) 89%.
C) 72%.
D) 65%.
E) 40%.

Discussion 5-1

The correct answer is "B." The child you see is showing clinical signs of volume overload heart failure. He has had poor weight gain and is mildly tachycardic as well as tachypneic. He also has hepatomegaly on exam as well as cardiomegaly by chest X-ray. No significant pulmonary edema is noted on the chest X-ray. Two months of age is common timing for a left-to-right shunt to appear clinically. After birth, pulmonary vascular resistance drops significantly compared to that in utero, and it continues to decrease for the first 6 weeks of life before reaching normal levels. As the pulmonary vascular resistance decreases, there is an increase in the amount of left-to-right shunting, leading to symptoms of volume overload heart failure, which are very rarely present at birth. The most common congenital heart disease to present in this way is a ventricular septal defect (VSD). A hemodynamically significant VSD would cause many of the findings that were noted in this infant. Normal oxygen saturations would be expected with a VSD; but the murmur would be a holosystolic murmur rather than an ejection-type murmur. While there would be cardiomegaly on chest X-ray, you would not expect to see a "snowman sign." Total anomalous pulmonary venous return (TAPVR) can also be relatively asymptomatic in the neonatal period, especially if the pulmonary venous return is unobstructed. Once the pulmonary vascular resistance has dropped, these children develop similar symptoms of heart failure. The murmur in this anatomy results from a pulmonary outflow murmur related to increased volume of blood. This would present as an ejection-type murmur. A "snowman sign" on chest X-ray is classic for supracardiac TAPVR with the pulmonary veins returning to the innominate vein. These children do not appear clinically cyanotic, but when their oxygen saturation is checked, it is lower than normal given the right-to-left shunt across the atrial septum. They are not usually significantly hypoxic (SpO$_2$ < 80%) unless there is some obstruction to pulmonary venous return. There are multiple types of TAPVR. Supracardiac TAPVR occurs when the anomalous pulmonary veins drain above the heart. (See Figure 5–1.) Commonly, all the veins come together into a confluence posterior to the left atrium. This confluence then drains superiorly through a vertical vein into the innominate vein. The oxygenated blood then enters

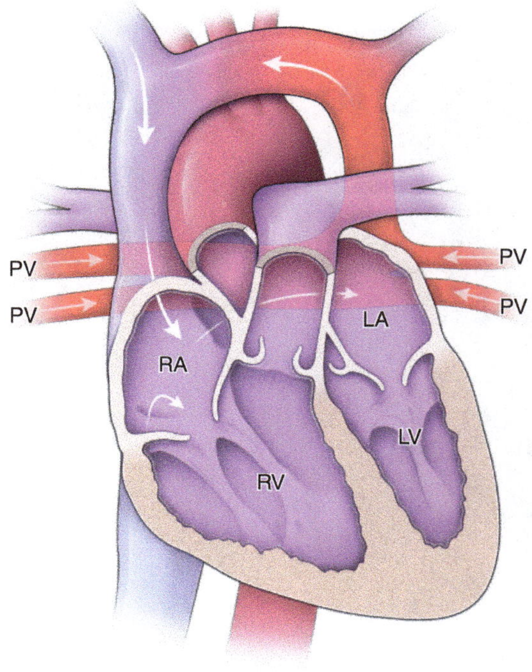

FIGURE 5–1. Supracardiac total anomalous pulmonary venous return (TAPVR). The anomalous pulmonary veins drain above the heart into the innominate vein. The oxygenated blood enters the heart through the superior vena cava. LA, left atrium; LV, left ventricle; PV, pulmonary vein; RA, right atrium; RV, right ventricle. (Used with permission from Benton Ng, MD.)

the heart through the superior vena cava (SVC) into the right atrium. Intracardiac TAPVR occurs when the anomalous veins drain into a confluence that enters the heart through the coronary sinus. This then empties the oxygenated blood into the right atrium. Infracardiac TAPVR occurs when the veins come together into a confluence posterior to the left atrium. Rather than draining superiorly through a vertical vein, the confluence drains through a vein inferiorly, through the diaphragm, and empties into the hepatic vasculature. The oxygenated blood returns to the heart through the inferior vena cava (IVC) into the right atrium. There can also be a mixture of these three types of pulmonary venous return. The severity of presentation of TAPVR is related to any obstruction to pulmonary venous return that can occur at the individual veins, confluence, vertical veins, or atrial septum. Infracardiac TAPVR almost always has some degree of obstruction and requires prompt surgical repair. Patients with severe obstruction present with significant hypoxia and a white-out chest X-ray secondary to pulmonary edema.

⧖ QUICK QUIZ

A patent ductus arteriosus (PDA) is necessary for TAPVR.
A) True.
B) False.

Discussion

The correct answer is "B." A PDA is not required for TAPVR and may worsen the degree of pulmonary edema and subsequent oxygen desaturations as measured by pulse oximetry. There is already significant pulmonary overcirculation with this anatomy and maintenance of the PDA with prostaglandins may worsen the degree of pulmonary overcirculation. In cases of severe hypoxia from obstruction, a PDA will only worsen the pulmonary edema and would not be expected to improve oxygenation.

> 🧑‍🏫 **Helpful Tip**
> Muscular ventricular septal defects (VSDs) are more likely to spontaneously close compared with perimembranous VSDs.

Question 5-2

Suppose the 2-month-old has a holosystolic murmur, cardiomegaly on chest X-ray, and normal SpO$_2$. What condition is she at risk for developing if her congenital heart defect is not repaired?
A) Pulmonary hypertension.
B) Aortic insufficiency.
C) Aortic stenosis.
D) Endocarditis.
E) All of the above.

Discussion 5-2

The correct answer is "E." She has a VSD. Pulmonary hypertension can occur from a longstanding left-to-right shunt. Permanent pulmonary vascular disease is unlikely to occur in the first year of life and with smaller VSDs. With unrepaired VSDs, prolapse of an aortic valve cusp into the VSD can lead to aortic insufficiency. The insufficiency is usually not audible on exam. In the United States, this condition is most frequently seen with perimembranous VSDs. In Asians, it is more likely to occur with subpulmonary VSDs (also known as outlet, supracristal, or conotruncal hypoplasia VSDs). The development of aortic insufficiency with subpulmonary VSDs is much more common than with perimembranous VSDs. Prolapse of the aortic valve cusp can obstruct some of the flow across the VSD, which decreases the amount of left-to-right shunt. VSDs are also associated with subaortic obstruction, which is usually a discrete fibrous or fibromuscular ridge below the aortic valve. Endocarditis is rare, but is seen more often in unrepaired VSDs than in repaired defects.

⧖ QUICK QUIZ

Which of the following is least likely to lead to pulmonary hypertension?
A) Ventricular septal defect (VSD).
B) Atrial septal defect (ASD).
C) Atrioventricular septal defect (AVSD).
D) Patent ductus arteriosus (PDA).
E) Dextro-transposition of the great arteries (DTGA).

Discussion

The correct answer is "B." As stated above, a longstanding VSD with a large left-to-right shunt can lead to pulmonary hypertension secondary to medial hypertrophy and intimal hyperplasia. It is unusual for an unrepaired ASD to lead to pulmonary hypertension even decades later. AVSD or atrioventricular (AV) canal can result in a large left-to-right shunt (usually if there is a large VSD component), which can then lead to pulmonary hypertension if unrepaired. A majority of patients with an AV canal also have trisomy 21 (Down syndrome), which itself is a risk factor for pulmonary hypertension. In the case of a VSD and PDA, the large pressure differential between the left ventricle (LV) and right ventricle (RV) (ie, VSD physiology) and aorta and pulmonary artery (ie, PDA physiology) can lead to large left-to-right shunts and future pulmonary hypertension. Pulmonary hypertension is also seen with increased frequency and with accelerated development in patients with DTGA. Cardiac defects that cause pulmonary overcirculation (ie, left-to-right shunts) may cause pulmonary hypertension.

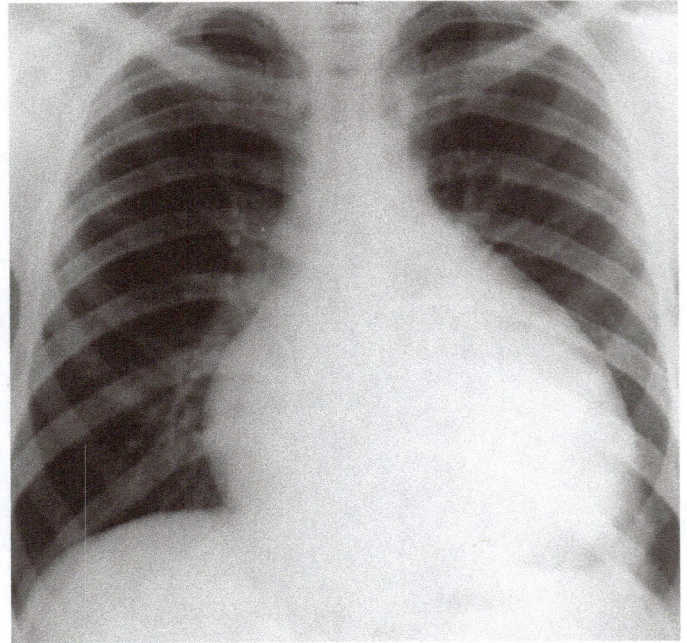

FIGURE 5–2. This chest X-ray shows cardiomegaly with clear lung fields and normal pulmonary vasculature. (Reproduced with permission from Fuster V, Walsh RA, Harrington RA, eds. *Hurst's The Heart*. 13th ed. New York, NY: McGraw-Hill Education; 2011, Fig. 17-20A.)

> **Helpful Tip**
> A holosystolic murmur is heard with VSDs and mitral or tricuspid regurgitation.

▶ CASE 6

A 15-year-old girl is seen for an acute care visit for complaints of a cough. She has had a nonproductive cough for the last 2 weeks. She denies any rhinorrhea, sneezing, or recent sick contacts. She is afebrile. Her heart rate is 122 bpm, her respiratory rate is 38 breaths per minute. On exam, she has a grade III/VI holosystolic murmur. Her chest X-ray shows cardiomegaly with clear lung fields. (See Figure 5–2.)

Question 6-1

Which of the following is the most likely diagnosis?
A) Vascular ring.
B) Ventricular septal defect (VSD).
C) Dilated cardiomyopathy.
D) Pneumonia.
E) Foreign body aspiration.

Discussion 6-1

The correct answer is "C." Although tachycardia, tachypnea, a holosystolic murmur, and cardiomegaly can be consistent with a VSD, this presentation is unlikely to be seen in a 15-year-old. Primary cardiomyopathies are the most likely cause of heart failure in people with structurally normal hearts. Given that the patient is 15 years old, it is unlikely that she has unrecognized significant congenital heart disease, especially if she has been cared for in developed nations. Dilated cardiomyopathy is due to a genetic mutation in sarcomeric, cytoskeletal, or cell membrane proteins. This leads to systolic heart failure and dilation of the ventricles. The murmur heard on exam is due to mitral regurgitation that results from the ventricular dilation and poor function.

▶ CASE 7

A different 15-year-old girl is seen for an acute care visit for complaints of a cough and fatigue. She had a cold with fever, rhinorrhea, congestion, and cough 2 weeks ago, but most of her respiratory symptoms have resolved. She is afebrile. Her heart rate is 122 bpm, and respiratory rate is 38 breaths per minute. On exam, she has a grade III/VI holosystolic murmur. Her chest X-ray shows an enlarged heart with clear lungs fields. (See Figure 5–2.)

Question 7-1

What is the most likely cause of her antecedent respiratory infection?
A) Cytomegalovirus (CMV).
B) Enterovirus.
C) Parvovirus B19.
D) Hepatitis C.
E) Human immunodeficiency virus (HIV).

Discussion 7-1

The correct answer is "B." The most common cause of myocarditis classically is coxsackievirus B (a type of enterovirus), but recent studies have identified adenovirus in a large number of patients. CMV, parvovirus B19, hepatitis C, and HIV are also linked with myocarditis, but at lower frequencies. Biopsy is considered the gold standard for diagnosis of myocarditis, but yields clinical information in only 10% to 20% of cases. A significantly greater number of samples is required for accurate diagnosis than is clinically feasible. Serum biomarkers, such as troponin I and inflammatory markers, are frequently drawn but also have low predictive value. Patients with mildly decreased ventricular function typically improve within weeks to months. Of the group that present with more severe dysfunction, 50% develop chronic dysfunction, 25% progress to death or need for transplantation, and 25% have spontaneous improvement.

► CASE 8

A 2-week-old infant girl is seen in the ED for poor feeding. The mother had an uncomplicated pregnancy and delivery, but the infant has not been interested in eating for the last day. She has also vomited after the few feedings she has taken. It has been over 12 hours since her last wet diaper. She is alert, but not vigorous. She is afebrile, her heart rate is 192 bpm, and respirations are 76 breaths per minute. On exam, she is tachycardic without a murmur. Her liver is 2 cm below the costal margin. Capillary refill in her toes is delayed.

Question 8-1

What is the most likely cause of her symptoms?
A) Systolic dysfunction.
B) Diastolic dysfunction.
C) Volume overload.
D) Hypoxia.
E) Both A and B.

Discussion 8-1

The correct answer is "A." The timing and presentation is consistent with ductal-dependent systemic blood flow, such as a severe coarctation of the aorta or hypoplastic left heart syndrome (HLHS). (See Figure 5–3.) Although the patent ductus arteriosus (PDA) commonly closes within the first day of life, some ducts may remain partially open. The vast majority close within the first 10 days of life. With a severe coarctation or HLHS, once the PDA closes, the patient has insufficient systemic blood flow and presents with signs of shock and poor perfusion. This is an example of ductal-dependent systemic blood flow. While the PDA is open, there should be a predominantly right-to-left shunt from the pulmonary artery to the aorta. This results in lower oxygen saturations in the legs compared with the arms (in cases with prograde flow in the ascending aorta). Severe obstruction causes systolic dysfunction. Diastolic dysfunction is frequently present as well, but the systolic dysfunction and inability to overcome the degree of stenosis are what lead to the problems. It is uncommon for a volume overload lesion, such as a VSD, to present with poor perfusion and shock. Severe hypoxia can eventually lead to insufficient oxygen delivery and resulting acidosis and poor perfusion, but this is not as common.

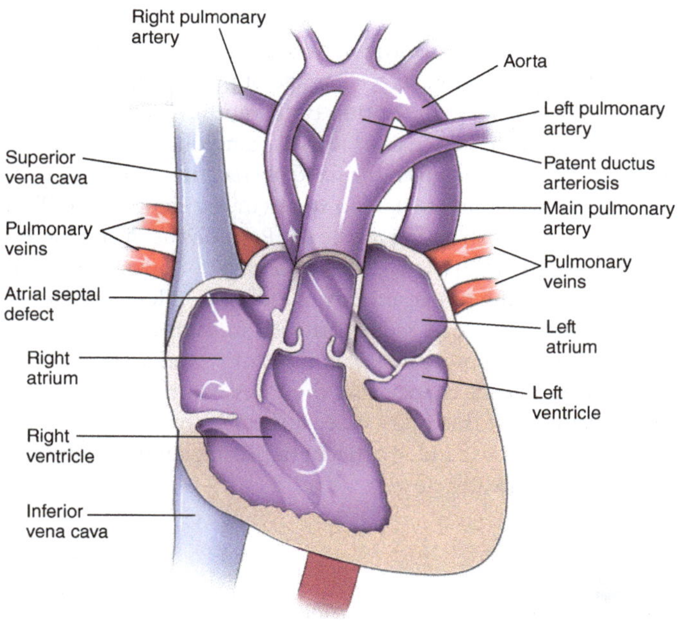

FIGURE 5–3. Hypoplastic left heart syndrome (HLHS). The left ventricle, ascending aorta, and aortic arch are hypoplastic. Infants are dependent on a right-to-left shunting patent ductus arterious for systemic blood flow. LA, left atrium; LV, left ventricle; RA, right atrium; RV, right ventricle. (Used with permission from Benton Ng, MD.)

> **Helpful Tip**
> Ductal-dependent lesions are most likely to present very close to birth and usually within the first 1 to 2 weeks after birth. Volume overload and left-to-right shunt lesions are most likely to present around 2 months of age. This is related to the natural decrease in pulmonary vascular resistance that occurs after birth.

> **Helpful Tip**
> If heart failure is suspected in a child, further evaluation would consist of a pediatric cardiology consult and likely an echocardiogram. Acute management relies on diuretics in all types of heart failure. Milrinone is also used in severe cases for its afterload reduction and chronotropic effects. Heart failure secondary to overcirculation can usually be managed with oral medications in an outpatient setting.

You obtain a blood pressure reading in her right arm, which is 108/72 mm Hg.

Question 8-2

Which medication is your first choice for treatment?
A) Esmolol.
B) Prostaglandin.
C) Milrinone.
D) Dopamine.
E) Indomethacin.

Discussion 8-2

The correct answer is "B." The signs of poor perfusion and upper extremity hypertension, as well as age of presentation, are consistent with a severe coarctation of the aorta. Using a medication to treat the hypertension, such as esmolol, risks decreasing lower body perfusion given the fixed obstruction. The first medication should be prostaglandin to attempt to reopen the PDA and relieve the obstruction. Once the PDA has been completely opened and is unrestrictive, there should no longer be a gradient between the upper and lower extremity blood pressures. At this point, afterload reduction with milrinone can be used if necessary to promote systemic flow. At 2 weeks of age, there is also a significant chance that the PDA will not reopen with prostaglandins. If this is the case, surgery is the only treatment option. Why choose indomethacin (a prostaglandin inhibitor)? The ductus is already closed.

> **Helpful Tip**
> Premature infants with clinically significant PDA require closure with medical treatment using indomethacin or ibuprofen (prostaglandin inhibitors) or surgical ligation.

Question 8-3

Coarctation of the aorta is associated with an increased risk for which of the following?
A) Endocarditis.
B) Intracranial aneurysm.
C) Gastroschisis.
D) Tracheoesophageal fistula.
E) Club foot.

Discussion 8-3

The correct answer is "B." Studies have shown that anywhere from 10% to 50% of patients with coarctation of the aorta have intracranial aneurysms. This may be related to a diagnosis of hypertension. There is currently no recommendation for screening patients with coarctation of the aorta for intracranial aneurysms.

▶ CASE 9

A 14-year-old boy comes to see you for a preparticipation physical. He has normal height and weight. His heart rate is 62 bpm, respirations 18 breaths per minute, and blood pressure 114/68 mm Hg. On exam, he has no murmur, but you notice a click. You refer the patient to the cardiology service, and he is diagnosed with a bicuspid aortic valve without stenosis or insufficiency.

Question 9-1

The patient is at increased risk for all of the following EXCEPT:
A) Aortic stenosis.
B) Aortic insufficiency.

C) Need for lifetime spontaneous bacterial endocarditis (SBE) prophylaxis.
D) Dilated aorta.
E) Presence of bicuspid aortic valve (BAV) in a first-degree relative.

Discussion 9-1

The correct answer is "C." A BAV is commonly asymptomatic in childhood. Over time, the valve can become calcified, stenotic, or insufficient. There is also a risk of aortic dilation unrelated to any stenosis. Recent studies show that cellular abnormalities lead to aortic dilation independent of stenosis and flow dynamics. The aortic dilation increases the risk of aortic dissection. There is a 9% prevalence of BAV in first-degree relatives of patients with BAV, so screening echocardiograms are recommended in first-degree relatives. In the past, the risk of endocarditis with BAV was estimated to be between 10% and 30%. More recent estimates place the risk between 0.3% and 2% per year. With the change to the bacterial endocarditis prophylaxis guidelines, prophylaxis is no longer recommended in patients with straightforward BAV.

In addition to the stated findings of this patient's echocardiogram, described above, it is noted that he has a normal-sized ascending aorta and aortic root.

Question 9-2

He should be allowed to participate in full activity until which of the following occurs?
A) Moderate aortic stenosis or moderate insufficiency.
B) Severe aortic stenosis/aortic insufficiency and dilated aortic root (> 4 cm).
C) Severe aortic stenosis/aortic insufficiency or dilated aortic root (> 4 cm).
D) All of the above.
E) None of the above.

Discussion 9-2

The correct answer is "C." No restrictions are recommended for patients who have an aortic root/ascending aorta size of less than 4 cm.

▶ CASE 10

A boy is born to a 25-year-old G_1P_0 (now P_1) mother by spontaneous vaginal delivery at 39 weeks' gestation. He requires minimal resuscitation. The neonate's Apgar scores are 8 and 8 at 1 and 5 minutes, respectively. He is then moved to the newborn nursery with his mother. The next day, on evaluation, you notice down-slanting palpebral fissures, low-set ears, a webbed neck, and a grade II/VI systolic ejection murmur. You check pulse oximetry, which reads 75%. As the echocardiogram is started, you are told that the child appears to have severe pulmonic stenosis.

Question 10-1

What additional finding is least likely to be present?

A) Large PDA with left-to-right shunt (aorta to pulmonary artery).

B) Right ventricular hypertrophy.

C) Patent foramen ovale with right-to-left shunt (right atrium to left atrium).

D) Moderate-sized PDA with right-to-left shunt (pulmonary artery to aorta).

E) Left ventricular hypertrophy.

Discussion 10-1

The correct answer is "D." The infant in this case has Noonan syndrome, which is associated with pulmonary stenosis. As his PDA has begun to close, he has developed significant hypoxia. An infant with right ventricular hypertrophy is likely to be present with the severe stenosis. The shunting across the patent foramen ovale (PFO) is also likely to be right to left instead of the normal left to right, secondary to the pulmonary outflow tract obstruction. Although the PDA is likely not large given the low oxygen saturations, the direction of shunting is expected to be left to right. You would not expect to have right-to-left shunting across the PDA in the setting of pulmonic stenosis. Initial treatment in this infant would be to start prostaglandins to reopen the PDA to allow for more pulmonary blood flow. An early intervention, either balloon valvuloplasty or surgical valvuloplasty, is required.

> **Helpful Tip**
> The pulmonary valve in Noonan syndrome can be thick and dysplastic, which decreases the chance of successful transcatheter ballooning. It is also associated with hypertrophic cardiomyopathy.

> **Helpful Tip**
> Pulmonary valve stenosis not due to a dysplastic pulmonary valve can often be ballooned by transcatheter intervention successfully. In general, milder to moderate degrees of pulmonary stenosis rarely progress to severe stenosis and may even have a decrease in the gradient over time.

► CASE 11

You see a 9-year-old boy in clinic for complaints of leg pain. He has been experiencing pain for the last week and his parents report that they think his knees and ankles have looked swollen at times. On review of symptoms, they note that he had a sore throat last month that resolved. They deny any rhinorrhea, congestion, or fever. On exam today, his left knee is swollen and tender. The remainder of his musculoskeletal exam is normal.

Question 11-1

Which of the following additional findings would help you make a diagnosis?

A) Fever.

B) Elevated erythrocyte sedimentation rate (ESR).

C) Elevated white blood cell count (WBC).

D) Subcutaneous nodules.

E) Aspiration of synovial fluid.

Discussion 11-1

The correct answer is "D." The patient has a history of sore throat without rhinorrhea or congestion, which is suspicious for previous strep pharyngitis. On exam, he has evidence of monoarticular arthritis with swelling and pain of his knee, which raises concern for rheumatic fever. The Jones criteria are used to diagnose acute rheumatic fever. (See Table 5–1.) Diagnosis is made by fulfilling two major, or one major and two minor, criteria. The major criteria include arthritis, carditis, subcutaneous nodules, erythema marginatum, and chorea. The presence of chorea alone is sufficient to make the diagnosis. Minor criteria include fever, arthralgia, elevated ESR or C-reactive protein (CRP), and prolonged PR interval on ECG. There should also be supporting evidence of a previous strep infection with a positive throat culture or elevated or rising strep antibody titer. Arthritis is the most common symptom and is classically described as a migratory polyarthritis responsive to NSAIDs. Large joints, such as the knees, ankles, elbows, and wrists, are most frequently involved. Carditis clinically is associated with a murmur and is the next most common manifestation. The mitral and aortic valves are the dominant valves involved and of most clinical importance. Moderate to severe regurgitation can lead to heart failure. Pericarditis can also be present but is almost always associated with mitral or aortic valve disease. Isolated pericarditis is unlikely to be secondary to rheumatic fever. Subcutaneous nodules are uncommon and tend to occur over extensor surfaces. Erythema marginatum is also uncommon and is described as a pink macule or papule with serpiginous borders and central clearing. The

TABLE 5–1 JONES CRITERIA FOR ACUTE RHEUMATIC FEVER	
Major Criteria	**Minor Criteria**
Polyarthritis	Fever
Carditis	Arthralgias
Subcutaneous nodules	Elevated inflammatory markers (ESR/CRP)
Erythema marginatum	Prolonged PR interval
Chorea	

CRP, C-reactive protein; ESR, erythrocyte sedimentation rate.

Supportive evidence of a group A streptococcal infection is also required (positive throat culture or rapid strep or elevated streptococcal antibody titer).

Primary episode of rheumatic fever diagnosed by 2 major or 1 major and 2 minor criteria plus evidence of previous streptococcal infection.

rash is evanescent and may change quickly. A hot bath or shower can accentuate the rash. Both erythema marginatum and nodules are associated with the presence of carditis. Sydenham chorea consists of involuntary, purposeless movements and emotional lability. The onset of chorea is usually delayed compared with arthritis and carditis. Chorea may occur 1 to 6 months after the initial infection in contrast to arthritis, which manifests between 10 days and 5 weeks postinfection.

Question 11-2

All of the following are recommendations for treatment of mild to moderate acute rheumatic carditis EXCEPT:

A) High-dose aspirin.
B) Steroids.
C) Activity restrictions.
D) Primary antibiotic prophylaxis.
E) Secondary antibiotic prophylaxis.
F) Intravenous immunoglobulin (IVIG).

Discussion 11-2

The correct answer is "F." High-dose aspirin (80–100 mg/kg/day) is recommended for mild to moderate carditis. Anti-inflammatory agents are considered standard of care as some patients improve with resolution of inflammation. There is no evidence that steroids (2 mg/kg/day for 2 weeks with a taper) are superior to aspirin, but they are recommended in moderate to severe cases of carditis. If steroids are used, aspirin is initiated with the steroid taper. Activity restrictions of some kind are recommended for 4 to 6 weeks, with some experts recommending bed rest. Primary antibiotic prophylaxis, most commonly with penicillin, is used for treatment of acute streptococcal infection. Secondary antibiotic prophylaxis is required in rheumatic carditis, with the duration depending on the severity. The highest risk period for recurrence of rheumatic fever is the first 1 to 2 years following an episode. Patients who have carditis in their initial episode of rheumatic fever are likely to have carditis as part of recurrent episodes. Recurrent rheumatic fever can lead to more severe valve dysfunction and chronic rheumatic heart disease. IVIG is not recommended for rheumatic carditis.

▶ CASE 12

A 3-year-old girl is admitted for evaluation of persistent fever. She has had a daily fever for the last 7 days of at least 38.8°C (102°F). Her mother describes her as generally more irritable over this time. She developed a diffuse maculopapular rash yesterday. On exam, you find her quite irritable and uncooperative with the exam. She is febrile to 39.5°C (103.2°F). She has bilateral conjunctivitis, dry, peeling lips, swollen hands, and a diffuse maculopapular rash.

Question 12-1

She is expected to have all of the following laboratory abnormalities EXCEPT:

A) Anemia.
B) Thrombocytopenia.
C) Hypoalbuminemia.
D) Elevated CRP.
E) Elevated gamma glutamyl transpeptidase.

Discussion 12-1

The correct answer is "B." Clinically, the young girl can be diagnosed with Kawasaki disease with her course of fevers, rash, conjunctival injection, extremity changes, and peeling lips. Additional clinical findings include erythema of the soles and palms, strawberry tongue, and cervical lymphadenopathy. The rash can take on various forms, including an urticarial exanthem, scarlatiniform, erythema multiforme–like, or micropustular rash. Within 2 to 3 weeks after onset of fever, desquamation of the fingers and toes begins in the periungual region. The conjunctival injection spares the limbus. There should be no exudate or pain associated with the conjunctivitis. The cervical lymphadenopathy is usually unilateral in the anterior cervical triangle.

She subsequently receives IVIG and an echocardiogram to evaluate for coronary aneurysms. No aneurysms were seen on this study. She becomes afebrile after receiving IVIG with down-trending inflammatory markers and is discharged home.

Question 12-2

What treatment and follow up are needed?

A) High-dose aspirin (80–100 mg/kg/day).
B) Follow-up echocardiogram.
C) Warfarin.
D) Steroids.
E) Cardiac catheterization.

Discussion 12-2

The correct answer is "B." High-dose aspirin is needed only for the acute illness until the patient has been afebrile for 48 hours. Warfarin is not indicated without giant aneurysms. Steroids can be considered for failed convalescence with IVIG. A cardiac catheterization is also not indicated, especially soon after acute illness. A follow-up echocardiogram is needed, even without aneurysms seen on the initial study. Coronary involvement in Kawasaki disease follows multiple stages. The first stage occurs between 0 and 9 days and consists of acute endarteritis of the coronary arteries with pericarditis, valvulitis, and myocarditis. From days 12 to 25, aneurysm and thrombus formation occur, with intimal proliferation. From days 28 to 31, coronary granulation and marked intimal thickening can occur. From day 40 out to 4 years, there can be scarring, stenosis, and calcification of the coronary arteries. More than 50% of aneurysms resolve in 1 to 2 years. Low-dose aspirin is recommended for at least 6 to 8 weeks, or until the inflammatory markers and coronary arteries are normal. (See Table 5–2.)

▶ CASE 13

A 17-year-old adolescent boy with a history of tetralogy of Fallot previously palliated as an infant undergoes pulmonary valve replacement with a bioprosthetic valve. His

TABLE 5–2 LONG-TERM MANAGEMENT OF KAWASAKI DISEASE—AMERICAN HEART ASSOCIATION GUIDELINES

Risk	Drugs	Restrictions	Follow up	Invasive tests
No aneurysms ever	None beyond 6–8 weeks	None beyond 6–8 weeks	Normal cardiovascular counseling every 5 years	None
Transient ectasia disappearing in 6–8 weeks	None beyond 6–8 weeks	None beyond 6–8 weeks	Normal cardiovascular counseling every 5 years	None
1 small to medium aneurysm	Low-dose aspirin until regression of aneurysm	None beyond 6–8 weeks for patients younger than 11 years; further evaluation recommended for patients older than 11 years to guide restrictions	Annual cardiology follow up with echo and ECG; stress test/ perfusion scan every 2 years	Angiography if abnormal perfusion scan or stress test
≥ 1 large or giant aneurysm	Long-term antiplatelet and warfarin or low-molecular-weight heparin	Avoid contact sports	Every-6-month follow up with echo and ECG; stress test/ perfusion scan yearly	Angiography 6–12 months after acute illness or if other tests are abnormal
Coronary artery obstruction	Long-term low-dose aspirin and warfarin or low-molecular-weight heparin	Avoid contact sports	Every-6-month follow up with echo and ECG; stress test/ perfusion scan yearly	Angiography 6–12 months after acute illness or if other tests are abnormal

ECG, electrocardiogram; echo, echocardiogram.

initial postoperative period is uncomplicated, but he develops fevers on postoperative day 7 with temperatures up to 39°C (102.2°F). Laboratory tests and blood cultures are drawn and he is started on broad-spectrum antibiotics. Both his white blood cell count and inflammatory markers are elevated. Two days later, viridans group streptococci are identified on his initial blood culture. Subsequent daily blood cultures are also preliminarily positive.

Question 13-1

Which of the following would NOT fulfill the diagnosis of definite infective endocarditis?
A) Increasing intensity of systolic murmur as compared with immediate postoperative period.
B) Evidence of an oscillating mass on the prosthetic valve by echocardiogram.
C) Glomerulonephritis.
D) Conjunctival hemorrhage.
E) Rheumatoid factor.

Discussion 13-1

The correct answer is "A." The Duke criteria provide a diagnostic strategy for making the diagnosis of infective endocarditis due to the variability in presentation. The criteria combine clinical, microbiologic, and echocardiography findings to stratify patients into "definite," "possible," and "rejected" cases. (See Table 5–3.) The patient currently fulfills one major criterion: blood culture positive for infective endocarditis. Bacteremia secondary to infective endocarditis should be continuous. Therefore it is not required that cultures be drawn only when the patient is febrile. The timing for obtaining blood culture is not strict, but three cultures drawn over the first 24 hours is felt to be sufficient. Viridans group streptococci (alpha-hemolytic streptococci) and *Staphylococcus aureus* are the two most common etiologies of infective endocarditis. He also fulfills two minor criteria with fever and his congenital heart disease and prosthetic valve. Although an increasing intensity of a murmur may be a result of increasing obstruction secondary to a large vegetation, this is insufficient to meet criteria. Evidence of an oscillating mass by echocardiogram is a major criteria. The remainder of the findings would be minor criteria.

Question 13-2

Which of the following is not an immunologic phenomenon of infective endocarditis?
A) Osler nodes.
B) Glomerulonephritis.
C) Janeway lesions.
D) Roth spots.
E) Rheumatoid factor.

TABLE 5–3 MODIFIED DUKE CRITERIA FOR INFECTIVE ENDOCARDITIS

Definite infective endocarditis

1. Pathologic criteria
   - Microorganism demonstrated by culture or histology in a vegetation
   - Pathologic lesions: vegetation or abscess confirmed by histologic examination.
2. Clinical criteria
   - 2 major or
   - 1 major and 3 minor or
   - 5 minor

Possible infective endocarditis

1. Presence of 1 major and 1 minor criterion or
2. Presence of 3 minor criteria

Rejected infective endocarditis

1. Alternative diagnosis found
2. Resolution of infective endocarditis symptoms with antibiotics for ≤ 4 days
3. No pathologic evidence of infective endocarditis at surgery/autopsy with antibiotic therapy for ≤ 4 days
4. Does not meet criteria for possible infective endocarditis

Criteria

Major criteria

1. Blood culture positive
   a. Typical organisms consistent with infective endocarditis from 2 separate blood cultures
      - Viridans streptococci, *Streptococcus bovis*, HACEK group, *Staphylococcus aureus*
      - Community-acquired enterococci in absence of primary focus
   b. Microorganisms consistent with infective endocarditis from persistently positive blood cultures; at least 2 positive cultures drawn > 12 hour apart
   c. All of 3 or majority of ≥ 4 separate cultures with first and last samples drawn ≥ 1 hour apart
   d. Single positive culture for *Coxiella burnetii*
2. Evidence of endocardial involvement
   a. Echocardiogram positive for infective endocarditis
      - Oscillating intracardiac mass on valve or supporting structures, in the path of regurgitant jets, or on implanted material in the absence of alternative explanation
      - Abscess
      - New partial dehiscence of prosthetic valve
   b. New valvular regurgitation (increase or change in preexisting murmur is not sufficient)

Minor criteria

1. Predisposition, at-risk heart condition, or intravenous drug use
2. Fever (temperature > 38°C [100.4°F])
3. Vascular phenomena: major arterial emboli, septic pulmonary infarcts, mycotic aneurysm, intracranial hemorrhage, conjunctival hemorrhages, and Janeway lesion
4. Immunologic phenomena: glomerulonephritis, Osler nodes, Roth spots, rheumatoid factor
5. Microbiologic evidence: positive blood culture, but does not meet major criteria

HACEK, *Haemophilus* species, *Actinobacillus actinomycetemcomitans*, *Cardiobacterium hominis*, *Eikenella corrodens*, and *Kingella* species.

Discussion 13-2

The correct answer is "C." Janeway lesions are due to vascular phenomena. The other findings are immunologic phenomena. Other vascular findings include major arterial emboli, septic pulmonary infarcts, mycotic aneurysms, intracranial hemorrhage, and conjunctival hemorrhage.

Question 13-3

Which of the following is NOT considered a cardiac condition associated with the highest risk for adverse outcome from endocarditis?

A) Previous episode of infective endocarditis.
B) Bicuspid aortic valve with moderate stenosis and moderate insufficiency.
C) Status 4 months postoperative from patch closure of a perimembranous VSD.
D) Unrepaired tetralogy of Fallot.
E) Mechanical aortic valve.

Discussion 13-3

The correct answer is "B." Cardiac conditions considered to be associated with the highest risk for which SBE prophylaxis with dental procedures should be considered include:

- Prosthetic valve or prosthetic material used for valve repair
- Previous infective endocarditis
- Congenital heart disease
- Unrepaired cyanotic heart disease, including shunts and conduits
- Completely repaired defects with prosthetic material during the first 6 months after procedure
- Repaired defects with residual defects at or near the site of prosthetic patch or device, which may inhibit endothelialization
- Heart transplant with valvulopathy

Question 13-4

Which of the following etiologies of infective endocarditis (native valve) requires the shortest course of treatment?
A) Penicillin-susceptible viridans group streptococci.
B) Penicillin-resistant viridans group streptococci.
C) Oxacillin-susceptible staphylococci.
D) Oxacillin-resistant staphylococci.
E) Length of therapy is the same for all bacterial etiologies.

Discussion 13-4

The correct answer is "A." Endocarditis due to staphylococci (oxacillin susceptible or resistant) requires 6 weeks of intravenous (IV) antibiotics. Cases caused by penicillin-susceptible viridans streptococci require 4 weeks of IV antibiotics. If medical therapy is unable to clear the vegetation, surgery may be needed.

▶ CASE 14

A 5-month-old immunized boy is brought to your clinic by his parents, who are concerned about increased sleepiness and poor feeding. They deny any symptoms of cough, rhinorrhea, or congestion. They report that he had previously been feeding every 2 to 3 hours but now must be woken up each time to feed. He is also taking less with each feed. On exam, he is alert and afebrile. His heart rate is 280 bpm and respiratory rate is 70 breaths per minute. His cardiac exam is significant for tachycardia. His abdomen is soft, with the liver palpable 3 cm below the costal margin. His capillary refill time is 2 to 3 seconds.

Question 14-1

What is the next best treatment?
A) Obtain an ECG.
B) Administer intramuscular (IM) ceftriaxone.
C) Place an IV and administer adenosine.
D) Urinalysis and urine culture.
E) Cardioversion.

Discussion 14-1

The correct answer is "A." This infant has signs of compensated heart failure secondary to arrhythmia. Infection should always be considered in a child with decreased activity, but this 5-month old is afebrile and without signs of localizing infection. In addition, the physical exam finding of hepatomegaly would be less consistent with infection but is a sign of heart failure. While he is quite tachycardic, with a heart rate of 280 bpm, he is hemodynamically stable. Therefore, there is time to obtain an ECG for diagnosis of his arrhythmia. The ECG will show a heart rate greater than 220 bpm, absence of P waves, and no R-R variability. Synchronized cardioversion is reserved for those patients who are hemodynamically unstable. The infant may require an IV and adenosine to break the arrhythmia, but other vagal maneuvers, such as ice to the face, should be attempted first.

You obtain an ECG, shown in Figure 5–4.

Question 14-2

Which of the following is most true?
A) He will require lifelong medication.
B) His heart function is likely to recover.
C) He is at high risk for sudden death.
D) He will have a normal baseline ECG.
E) He will require SBE prophylaxis.

Discussion 14-2

The correct answer is "B." The ECG shows supraventricular tachycardia (SVT). The most common causes of SVT in pediatrics are atrioventricular reentrant tachycardia (AVRT), atrioventricular nodal reentrant tachycardia (AVNRT), and atrial flutter. (See Figure 5–5.) His heart failure is secondary to prolonged tachycardia, or an arrhythmia-mediated cardiomyopathy. Once he is converted out of the abnormal rhythm, his heart function is likely to recover. Given the infant's age at presentation, he is most likely to have AVRT and there is a 50% chance that this will spontaneously resolve as the accessory pathway may become nonconductive tissue. SVT rarely causes sudden death and is well tolerated in children for prolonged periods. In the case of AVRT, there is a small increased risk for sudden death if there is antegrade conduction across the accessory pathway. This may allow for atrial fibrillation to be conducted quickly to the ventricle and result

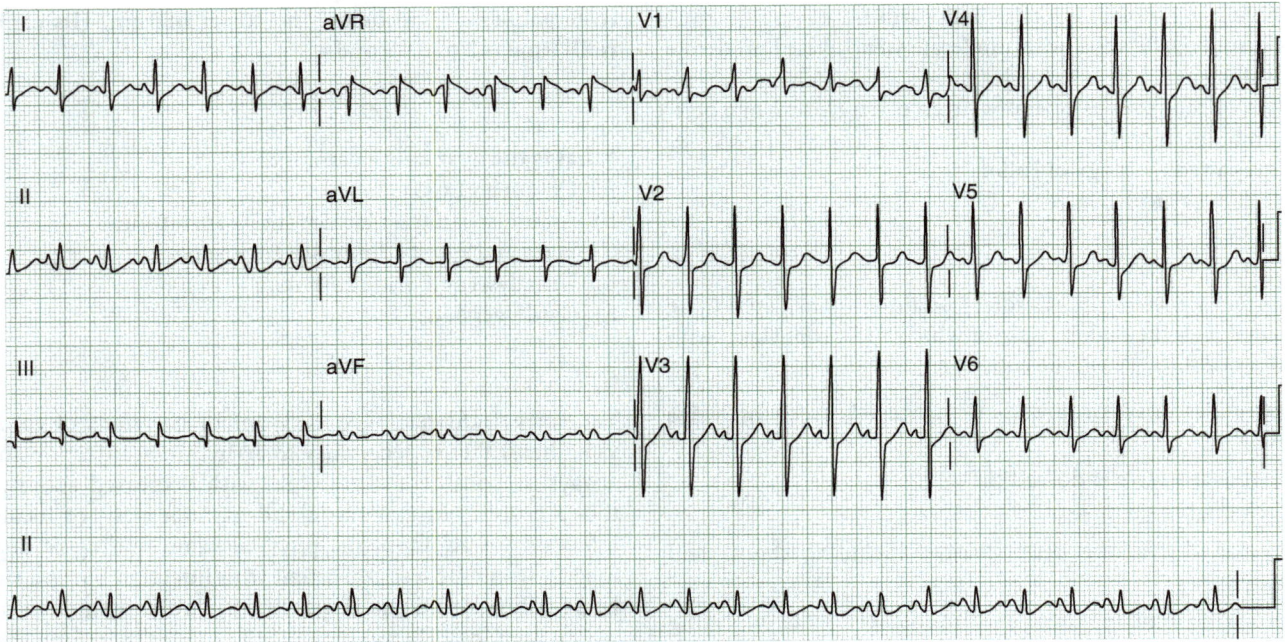

FIGURE 5–4. Supraventricular tachycardia (SVT). ECG showing heart rate greater than 220 bpm, narrow QRS, and no R-R variability. (Reproduced with permission from Klamen DL, Hingle ST, eds. *Resident Readiness: Internal Medicine.* New York, NY: McGraw-Hill Education; 2014, Fig. 11-1.)

in ventricular fibrillation, which is a life-threatening arrhythmia. With AVRT, preexcitation (delta wave) can be seen on a baseline ECG. (See Figure 5–6.) The delta wave occurs due to initial antegrade conduction through the accessory pathway. In AVNRT, the reentrant pathway occurs essentially in the AV node. It is not possible to differentiate AVRT from AVNRT by ECG. In contrast to AVRT, AVNRT is unlikely to resolve spontaneously. AVNRT is a more common presentation in teenagers than infants. Adenosine terminates the SVT caused by both AVRT and AVNRT by blocking conduction through the AV node, which stops the reentrant cycle. In atrial flutter, the reentrant loops are located in the atrium and do not involve the AV node. In these cases, the atrial rate may be as high as 400 to 500 bpm and is conducted to the ventricle in a 2:1 fashion through the AV node, resulting in a ventricular rate of 200 to 250 bpm. In this case, adenosine will block the AV node, but the reentrant loops in the atrium continue. This will result in a ventricular pause, but flutter waves will become apparent on ECG. Once the adenosine wears off, the SVT will resume.

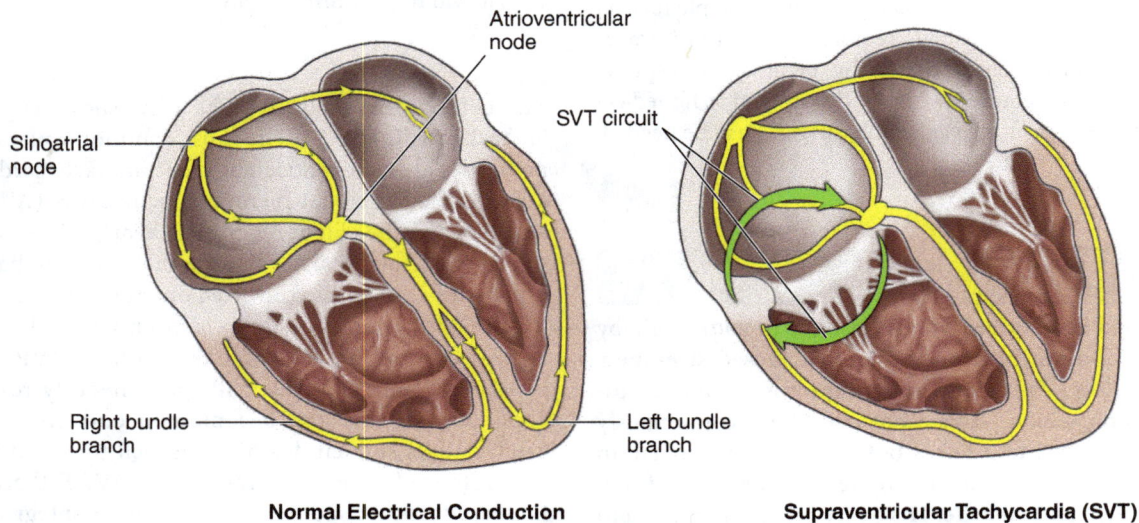

FIGURE 5–5. Supraventricular tachycardia. AV, node; atrioventricular node; AVNRT, atrioventricular nodal reentrant tachycardia; AVRT, atrioventricular reentrant tachycardia; SA node, sinoatrial node. (Used with permission from Benton Ng, MD.)

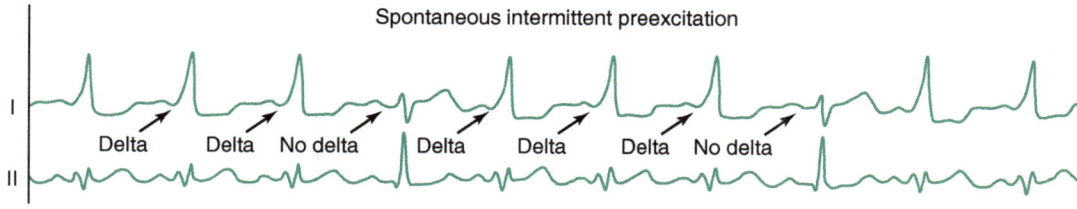

FIGURE 5–6. Delta wave in Wolff-Parkinson-White (WPW) syndrome. This ECG shows findings consistent with WPW syndrome: short PR interval (< 0.2 seconds), delta waves, and widened QRS complexes. Preexcitation (delta wave) results from antegrade conduction via the accessory pathway. (Reproduced with permission from Hay WW, Levin MJ, Deterding RR, Abzug MJ, eds. *Current Diagnosis and Treatment Pediatrics.* 22nd ed. New York, NY: McGraw-Hill Education; 2014, Fig. 20-7.)

Question 14-3
Which of the following rhythms requires defibrillation?

A)

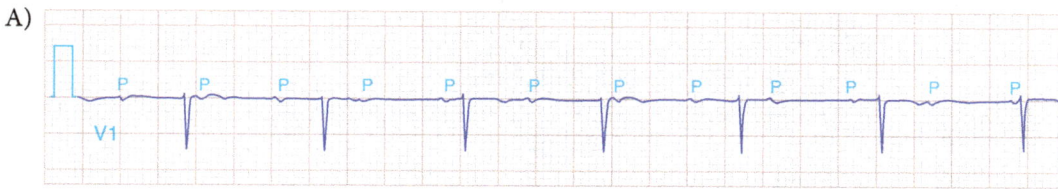

A

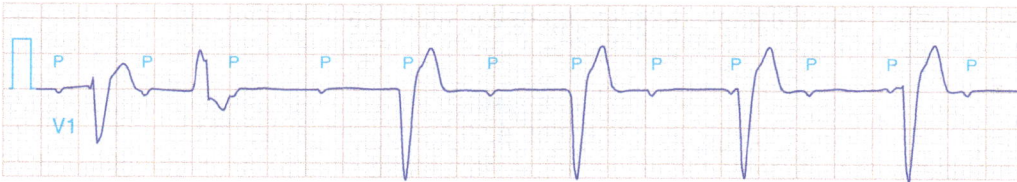

B

(Reproduced with permission from Kasper DL, Fauci AS, Hauser SL, et al: *Harrison's Principles of Internal Medicine,* 19th ed. McGraw-Hill Education, Inc., 2015. Fig 275-4.)

B)

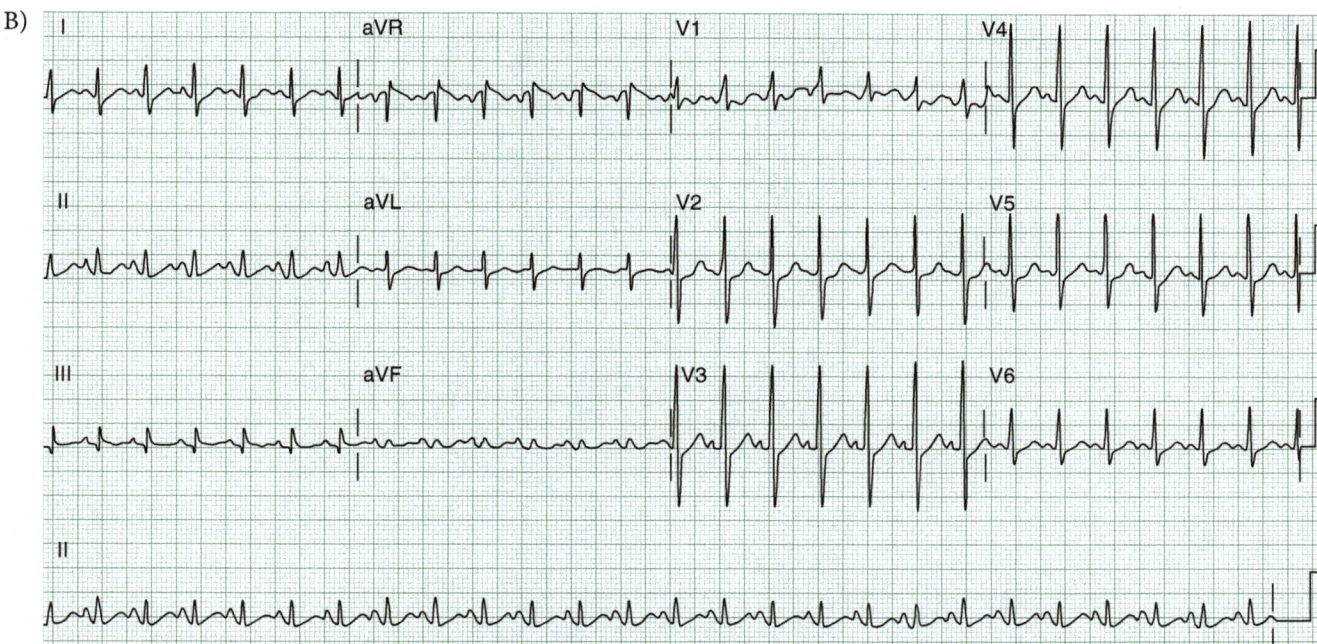

(Reproduced with permission from Klamen DL, Hingle ST, eds. *Resident Readiness: Internal Medicine.* New York, NY: McGraw-Hill Education; 2014, Fig 11-1.)

C)

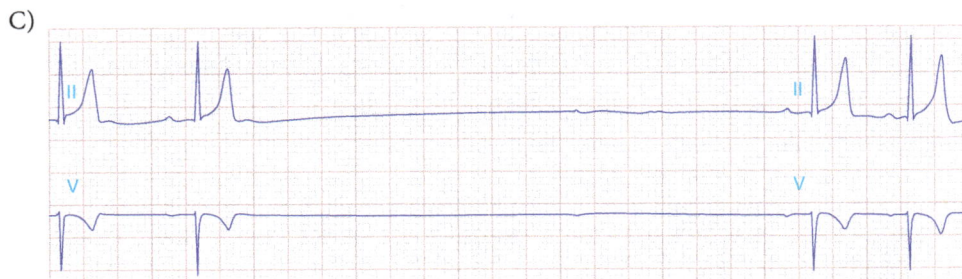

(Reproduced with permission From Longo DL, Fauci AS, Kasper DL, et al, eds. *Harrison's Principles of Internal Medicine.* 19th ed. New York, NY: McGraw-Hill Education; 2015, Fig 274-3.)

D)

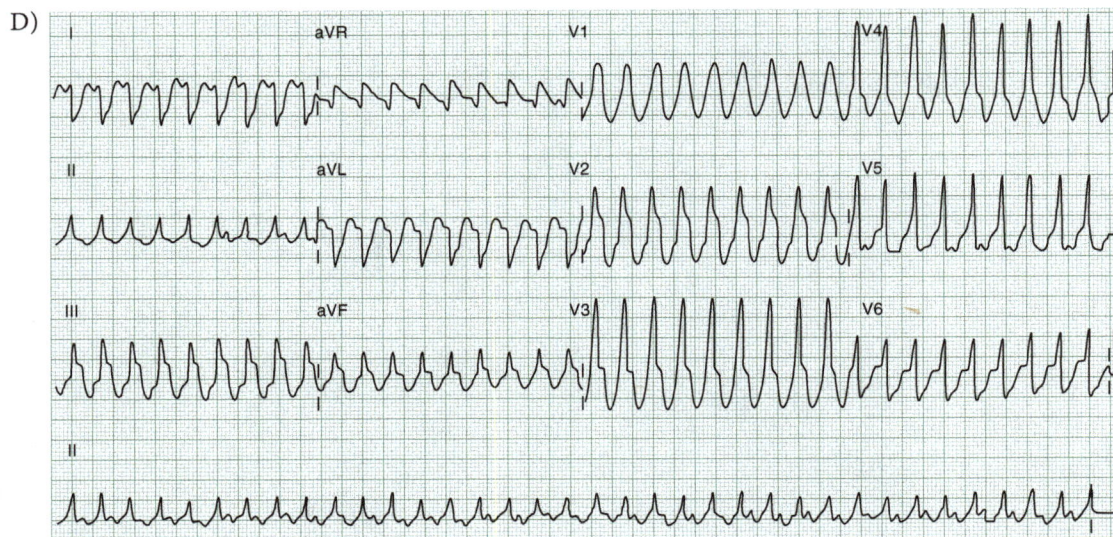

(Reproduced with permission from Klamen DL, Hingle, ST (Eds). *Resident Readiness: Internal Medicine.* McGraw-Hill Education, Inc., 2014. Fig 13-1.)

E)

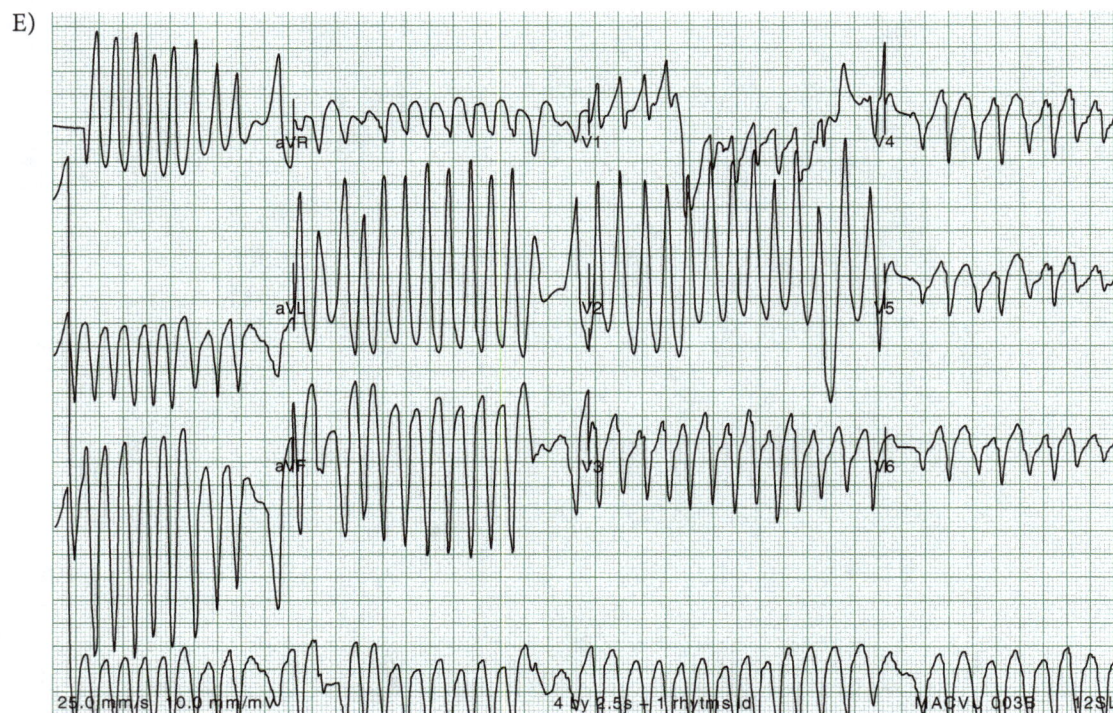

(Reproduced with permission from Klamen DL, Hingle ST, eds. *Resident Readiness: Internal Medicine.* New York, NY: McGraw-Hill Education; 2014, Fig. 14-1.)

Discussion 14-3

The correct answer is "E." Option "A" is an example of third-degree heart block. Symptoms are related to the rate of the underlying junctional or ventricular rhythm. Option "B" is an example of SVT with a heart rate of greater than 220 bpm. SVT is often treated with vagal maneuvers or adenosine. Electricity is only indicated for hemodynamic instability or SVT refractory to medication. In those cases, synchronized cardioversion instead of defibrillation is required. Option "C" is an example of a long pause (> 6 seconds) or asystole. Defibrillation is not indicated for asystole. Epinephrine and chest compressions are recommended by pediatric advanced life support (PALS). Option "D" is an example of a wide-complex tachycardia (180 to 220 bpm), which may represent ventricular tachycardia or SVT with aberrancy. In either case, synchronized cardioversion would be appropriate if needed, not defibrillation. Option "E" is an example of ventricular fibrillation. Defibrillation would be appropriate in this case as part of the PALS algorithm.

> **Helpful Tip**
> Sinus tachycardia is slower than SVT, and P waves are present on the ECG. It has many causes, including fever, dehydration, stress, anemia, and hyperthyroidism.

▶ CASE 15

A 16-year-old adolescent girl presents with complaints of palpitations for the last week. She has had some mild lightheadedness but is not restricted by her symptoms. She denies any episodes of syncope. Her exam is normal except for some irregularity in her heart rate. Upon further questioning, she informs you that she had been camping in Wisconsin last month. You obtain an ECG. (See Figure 5–7.) Eventually, laboratory tests of *Borrelia burgdorferi* infection are positive.

Question 15-1

Which of the following is true?
A) She requires a pacemaker.
B) She requires a myocardial biopsy.
C) Her carditis will resolve with or without antibiotics.
D) Her carditis will require intravenous (IV) antibiotics for resolution.
E) Her carditis will require oral (PO) antibiotics for resolution.

Discussion 15-1

The correct answer is "C." Lyme carditis may be the only presenting symptom of Lyme disease. Carditis occurs in up to 10% of untreated adults. This may manifest as varying degrees of atrioventricular (AV) block, myocarditis, left ventricle (LV) dysfunction, or pericarditis. Rarely, temporary pacing is required for high-degree heart block with symptomatic bradycardia. The carditis may resolve spontaneously, but standard of care is for treatment with antibiotics with the goal of shortening duration. IV antibiotics (ceftriaxone) are recommended for severe cardiac disease, whereas PO antibiotics (amoxicillin or doxycycline) are used for mild to moderate disease.

⧖ QUICK QUIZ

Which of the following is false regarding AV heart block?
A) First-degree AV block is defined as a PR interval greater than 0.2 seconds.
B) There are three types of second-degree AV block.
C) In third-degree AV block, the escape rate is slower than the atrial rate.
D) Mobitz Type I second degree AV block is known as Wenckebach phenomenon.
E) In third-degree AV block, the AV node doesn't conduct any impulses from the atria to the ventricle.

Discussion

The correct answer is "B." The electrical impulse from the atria is delayed or not conducted to the ventricle in AV block. In first-degree AV block, the PR interval is prolonged (> 0.2 seconds). In second-degree AV block, P waves are not always followed by a QRS complex (dropped beats). In Mobitz type I (Wenckebach phenomenon), there is progressive prolongation of the PR interval until one QRS is dropped. In Mobitz type II, a QRS is dropped at random without change in the PR interval. Finally, in third-degree AV block, atria and ventricle depolarizations are independent of each other, and the QRS rate is slower than the P rate.

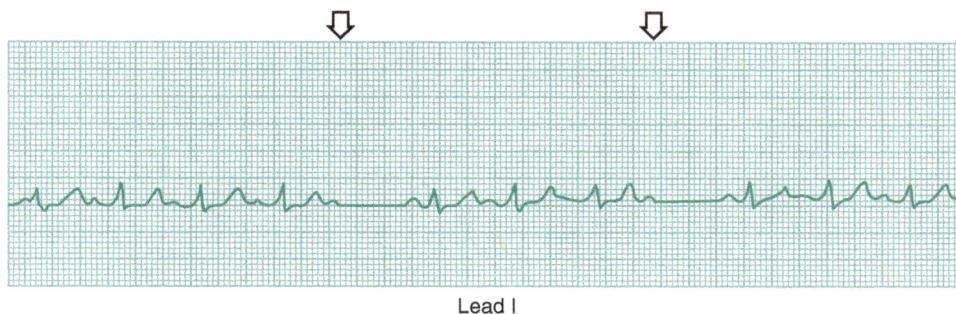

Lead I

FIGURE 5–7. ECG with Mobitz type 1 second-degree atrioventricular (AV) block (Wenckebach). The PR interval gets progressively longer until a P wave is not conducted. (Reproduced with permission from Hay WW, Levin MJ, Deterding RR, Abzug MJ, eds. *Current Diagnosis and Treatment Pediatrics*. 22nd ed. New York, NY: McGraw-Hill Education; 2014, Fig. 20-10.)

▶ CASE 16

You are seeing a 16-year-old adolescent girl for palpitations. She reports that she has sporadic palpitations that are not associated with activity. She feels lightheaded when standing but has not experienced syncope. She is otherwise generally healthy. Her only medication is diphenhydramine as needed for allergies. Her vital signs and physical exam findings are normal. On ECG, her QTc interval is 0.49 seconds.

Question 16-1

All of the following can contribute to the ECG finding EXCEPT:

A) Genetics.
B) Medication.
C) Stroke.
D) Myocardial ischemia.
E) Female sex.

Discussion 16-1

The correct answer is "E." The ECG shows a prolonged QTc interval (rate-corrected QT interval). (See Figure 5–8.) This is calculated most frequently in lead II by measuring the QT interval and dividing by the square root of the previous R-R interval. The exact value that constitutes a prolonged QTc is not straightforward as the value varies based on age and gender. In general, a value greater than 0.46 seconds is prolonged and values between 0.45 and 0.46 seconds are borderline. Congenital long QT syndrome can be secondary to multiple genetic mutations of potassium or sodium channels.

Jervell-Lange-Nielsen and Romano-Ward are two syndromes associated with long QT. Jervell-Lange-Nielsen is inherited in an autosomal recessive fashion and is associated with congenital deafness. Romano-Ward syndrome is inherited in an autosomal dominant fashion. Numerous medications are known to prolong the QT interval, including diphenhydramine. These medications should be avoided in patients with known congenital long QT syndrome due to the risk of further prolonging the QT interval and torsades de pointes. Both stroke and myocardial ischemia are associated with prolonged QT. Female sex is a risk factor for drug induced torsades de pointes but does not contribute to the prolonged QT interval itself.

▶ CASE 17

A 21-year-old man followed for congenital heart block had a transvenous pacemaker inserted at 16 years of age. His only medication is lisinopril for hypertension. He now presents with progressive facial swelling. He also complains of some headache. On exam, his face and neck are noticeably swollen. His cardiac exam is normal.

Question 17-1

What is the next best step?

A) Stop lisinopril.
B) Start furosemide.
C) ECG.
D) Chest x-ray.
E) Echocardiogram.

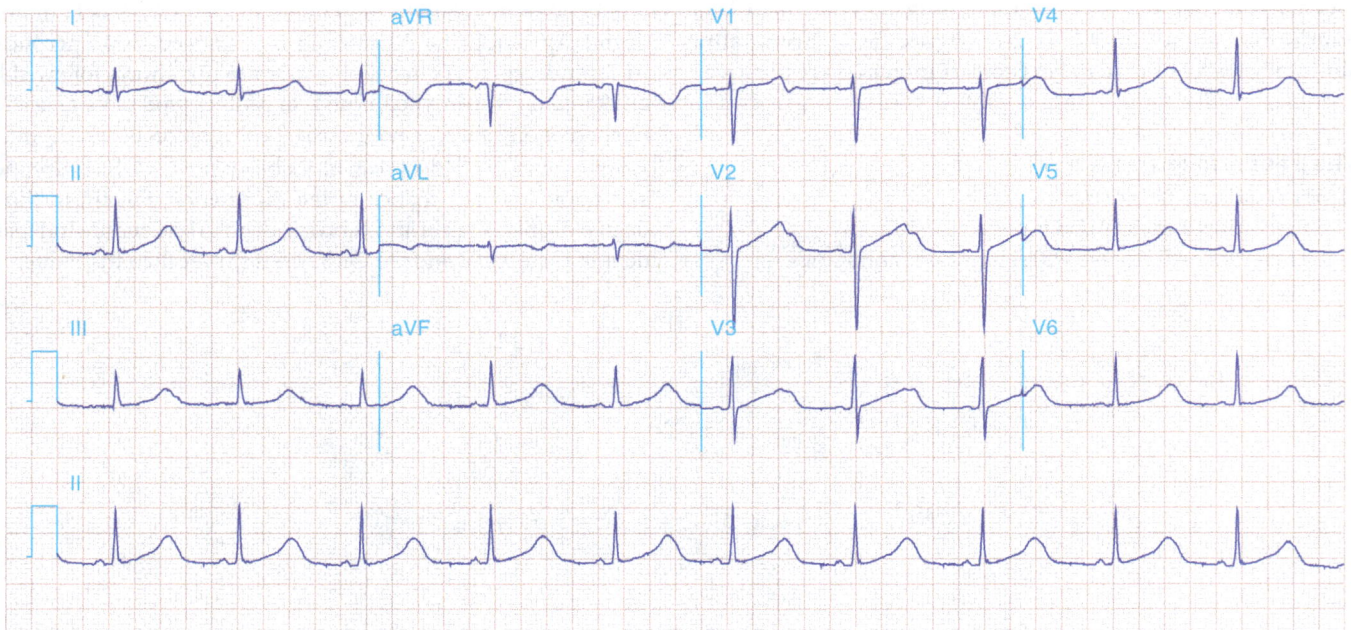

FIGURE 5–8. Long QT syndrome. The QTc (0.6 seconds) is prolonged on this ECG from a patient with hereditary long-QT syndrome. (Reproduced with permission from Kasper DL, Fauci AS, Hauser SL et al: *Harrison's Principles of Internal Medicine*, 19th McGraw-Hill Education, Inc., 2015. Fig 278e-23.)

Discussion 17-1

The correct answer is "E." The patient presents with symptoms that are concerning for superior vena cava (SVC) syndrome, especially given his risk factors of an intravascular device. SVC syndrome is rare with transvenous pacemakers (causes internal thrombosis of SVC) and more commonly associated with mediastinal masses (external compression of SVC). SVC syndrome is characterized by venous distension of the neck, facial and upper extremity edema, mental changes, cyanosis, papilledema, and even coma. Change in posture may exacerbate the symptoms. Facial swelling is the most common symptom. Angiotensin-converting enzyme (ACE) inhibitors can cause angioedema, but the presence of a pacemaker increases suspicion for other causes of facial swelling. An echocardiogram may be able to show the course of the pacemaker leads entering the heart through the SVC. Treatment options include thrombolysis, pacemaker removal, stenting, or surgery.

> **Helpful Tip**
> Superior vena cava (SVC) syndrome results from extrinsic compression or intrinsic obstruction of the SVC. Symptoms include head, neck, and upper extremity edema and dilated neck veins.

▶ CASE 18

You are seeing an 8-year-old girl for the first time in your practice for a well-child visit. She is otherwise healthy with an unremarkable past medical history. Her vital signs are within normal limits but her height plots at less than the fifth percentile. She also has a low posterior hairline and a webbed neck.

Question 18-1

All of the following are associated with her syndrome EXCEPT:
A) Bicuspid aortic valve.
B) Dilated aorta.
C) Coarctation of the aorta.
D) Pulmonary stenosis.
E) Partial anomalous pulmonary venous return.

Discussion 18-1

The correct answer is "D." All of the other lesions are associated with Turner syndrome. The incidence of aortic dissection is eight to nine times that of the general population. Girls with Turner syndrome should continue to be screened for aortic dilation. A magnetic resonance imaging (MRI) scan is recommended once the patient can tolerate the exam without sedation if there are no indications for an earlier MRI because echocardiography is limited in its ability to image the entire aorta. In the absence of other risk factors or dilation, screening with imaging is recommended every 5 to 10 years.

▶ CASE 19

A 2-month-old infant with known tetralogy of Fallot is seen in the emergency department for cough. He is afebrile with a respiratory rate of 30 breaths per minute, heart rate of 120 bpm, and an initial oxygen saturation rate of 82%. He becomes increasingly uncooperative with your examination. Upon initial auscultation of his heart, you hear a grade III/VI harsh systolic ejection murmur. As you listen closely for a variable click associated with pulmonary stenosis, you notice that his once-prominent murmur has significantly decreased in intensity.

Question 19-1

Which of the following is most likely to happen next?
A) Increasing oxygen saturations due to closure of the VSD.
B) Decreasing oxygen saturations due to increasing obstruction.
C) Mottling from decreased systemic perfusion.
D) Development of extremity edema from volume overload heart failure.
E) Pulmonary edema from pulmonary overcirculation.

Discussion 19-1

The correct answer is "B." Tetralogy of Fallot includes a ventricular septal defect (VSD), overriding aorta, variations of pulmonary stenosis, and right ventricular hypertrophy. (See Figure 5–9.) There is a great amount of variability in the severity of tetralogy of Fallot, which is related to the degree of right ventricular outflow tract obstruction. In the mildest forms (pink variant), there is relatively little obstruction; these patients present and have symptoms similar to a VSD. In the most severe forms, there can be severe obstruction due to muscle below the

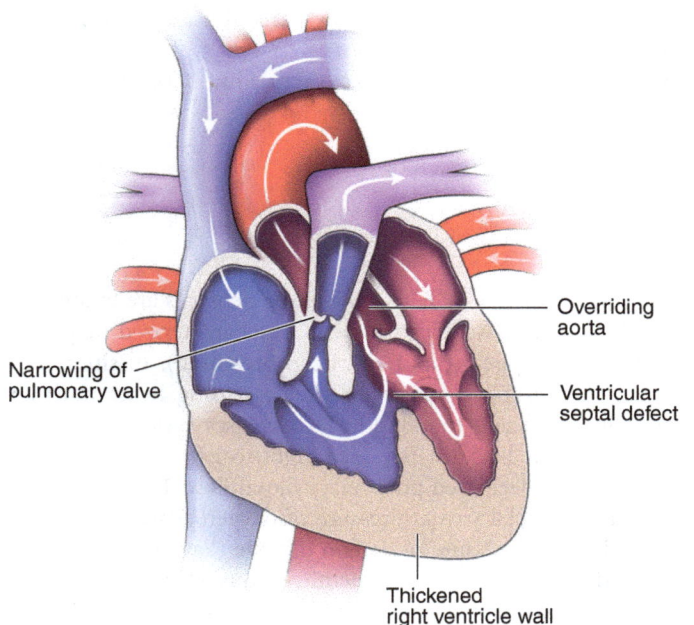

FIGURE 5–9. Teratology of Fallot includes right ventricular hypertrophy, pulmonary outflow tract obstruction, ventricular septal defect, and an overriding aorta. (Used with permission from Benton Ng, MD.)

pulmonary valve with hypoplasia of the pulmonary valve, main pulmonary artery, and branch pulmonary arteries. The degree of hypoxia is related to the degree of pulmonary obstruction. The obstruction related to muscle in the right ventricular outflow tract is dynamic.

Question 19-2

The murmur heard in tetralogy of Fallot is caused by which lesion?
A) Ventricular septal defect (VSD).
B) Overriding aorta.
C) Pulmonary stenosis.
D) Right ventricular hypertrophy.
E) Atrial septal defect (ASD).

Discussion 19-2

The correct answer is "C." A murmur is a result of turbulent blood flow. In tetralogy of Fallot, the VSD is large and unrestrictive. Therefore, there is mainly laminar flow across this defect and no murmur. Instead the murmur is related to pulmonary stenosis. The lesions listed in the other option choices will not cause a murmur. The variables that affect the intensity of a murmur are the size of the orifice through which blood travels, the volume of blood that crosses the orifice, and the pressure gradient across the orifice. Decrease volume of blood flow will decrease the intensity of the murmur if other factors are held constant. Because the right ventricular outflow tract obstruction in tetralogy of Fallot is dynamic, there is a risk for transient severe right ventricular outflow tract obstruction, also known as a Tet spell. In these cases, the first thing to change will be the absence of a previous murmur. This represents complete occlusion of the right ventricular outflow tract. This will be quickly followed by severe cyanosis.

Question 19-3

Which of the following is considered treatment for a Tet spell?
A) Extracorporeal membrane oxygenation (ECMO).
B) Oxygen.
C) Morphine.
D) Phenylephrine.
E) All of the above.

Discussion 19-3

The correct answer is "E." All the answer choices are treatments for Tet spells. These hypoxic spells are characterized by paroxysms of hyperpnea (rapid and deep breathing), fussiness and crying, increasing cyanosis, and a decreasing heart murmur intensity. An event that suddenly decreases systemic vascular resistance can lead to increased right-to-left shunting across the VSD and decreased pulmonary blood flow. This results in a decreased arterial partial pressure of oxygen (PaO_2), increased arterial partial pressure of carbon dioxide ($PaCO_2$), and hyperpnea. This causes increased systemic venous return, which in the setting of fixed right ventricular outflow tract obstruction due to the Tet spell causes increased right-to-left shunt and worsening hypoxia. Treatment includes multiple maneuvers. Holding the infant in a manner that brings the knees to the chest aims to

calm the infant as well as increasing systemic vascular resistance and decreasing systemic venous return. Morphine can be used to decrease respiratory effort to terminate the hyperpnea to break the cycle. Oxygen may increase saturation slightly. Phenylephrine is a vasoconstrictor and will increase the systemic vascular resistance. This is done with the goal of decreasing the amount of right-to-left shunting across the VSD to improve oxygen saturation. In addition, bicarbonate can be given to correct acidosis, as acidosis leads to increased respiratory drive. Ketamine both sedates the patient and increases the systemic vascular resistance. If none of the maneuvers or medications are successful in terminating the Tet spell, venovenous ECMO can be used to stabilize the patient and provide oxygenation.

> **Helpful Tip**
>
> In a Tet spell, the infant becomes upset; pulmonary resistance goes up, increasing pulmonary outflow tract obstruction, right-to-left shunting across the VSD, and subsequent cyanosis. On exam, the murmur is decreased. For an older child, have them squat or pull their knees to the chest.

▶ CASE 20

A boy born after 38-3/7 weeks' gestation by spontaneous vaginal delivery cries immediately with good respiratory effort. His heart rate is strong, at 160 bpm. No murmurs are heard on exam. You notice that he is cyanotic and administer supplemental oxygen through a face mask. No change in color is noted. As the infant is otherwise stable, he is transferred to the neonatal intensive care unit (NICU). He is trialed off oxygen, resulting in an oxygen saturation of 72%. He is placed back on supplemental oxygen by nasal cannula, with an increase in saturation to 78%.

Question 20-1

Which of the following is the most likely possible diagnosis?
A) VSD.
B) D-transposition of the great arteries.
C) Cor triatriatum sinister.
D) Cor triatriatum dexter.
E) Scimitar syndrome.

Discussion 20-1

The correct answer is "B." A VSD will not cause such significant cyanosis. Immediately after birth, a VSD will not cause symptoms and a murmur is unlikely to be present. This is due to relatively elevated pulmonary pressures, which are normal in the immediate newborn period. This prevents significant shunting across the VSD. Cor triatriatum sinister and cor triatriatum dexter result from subdivision or partitioning of the left or right atrium respectively by a membrane. In cor triatriatum sinister, this can present as pulmonary venous obstruction in severe forms and be asymptomatic in mild forms. Both are quite rare. Scimitar syndrome includes partial anomalous pulmonary

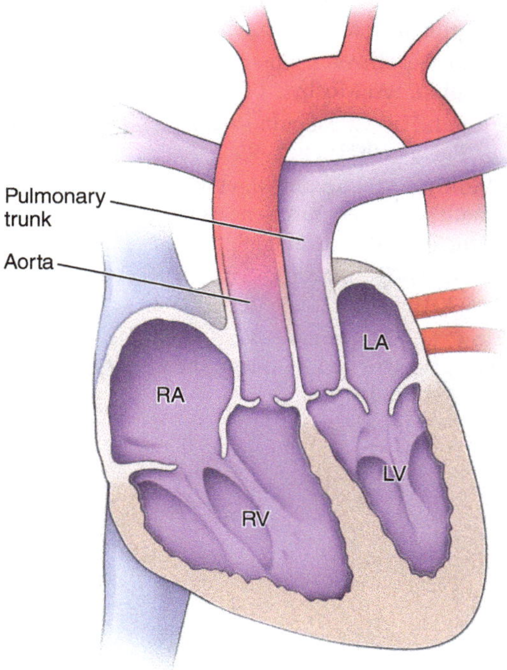

FIGURE 5–10. D-transposition of the great arteries (DTGA). The aorta arises from the right ventricle and the pulmonary artery arises from the left ventricle. (Used with permission from Benton Ng, MD.)

venous return from the right lung, often with right lung hypoplasia, and dextroposition of the heart. Administration of oxygen that does not significantly increase the oxygen saturations is suspicious for a cyanotic heart disease. Of the options listed, D-transposition of the great arteries (DTGA) is the only cyanotic congenital heart defect. DTGA results when the aorta arises from the right ventricle and the pulmonary artery arises from the left ventricle. (See Figure 5–10.) There may or may not be a VSD. This results in two parallel circulations. Life is dependent on mixing of the blood, either through the patent ductus arteriosus, atrial septal defect (ASD), or VSD. Mixing through an ASD is often the most effective shunt as significant bidirectional shunt can occur, to allow both deoxygenated blood to flow to the lungs and oxygenated blood to flow to the body. If the existing ASD is restrictive, a balloon atrial septostomy (Rashkind procedure) can be performed in the cardiac catheterization lab to improve mixing of blood.

> **Helpful Tip**
> While the chest X-ray for DTGA commonly is unremarkable, the classic description is the "egg on a string," with a narrow mediastinum due to the anterior posterior positioning of the great vessels. DTGA is now treated surgically with the arterial switch procedure, which involves transecting both the aorta and pulmonary artery to create an LV-to-aorta and RV-to-pulmonary artery connection. This is often done within the first 10 days of life.

> **Helpful Tip**
> When evaluating a newborn with cyanosis that is not responsive to oxygen, consider the 5 Ts mnemonic in their differential: (1) **T**runcus arteriosus (one vessel), (2) D**T**GA (switching of the two arteries), (3) **T**ricuspid atresia, (4) **T**etralogy of Fallot, and (5) **T**otal anomalous pulmonary venous return (TAPVR; 5 letters in the acronym). Other complex heart diseases can also cause significant desaturations in newborns, including pulmonary atresia, severe Ebstein anomaly, and hypoplastic left heart syndrome.

BIBLIOGRAPHY

Allen HD, Driscoll DJ, Shaddy RE, Feltes TF. *Moss & Adams' Heart Disease in Infants, Children, and Adolescents: Including the Fetus and Young Adult.* 7th ed. Philadelphia, PA: Lippincott Williams and Wilkins; 2008.

Bondy CA; Turner Syndrome Consensus Study Group. Care of girls and women with Turner syndrome: A guideline of the Turner syndrome study group. *J Clin Endocrinol Metab.* 2007;92:10–25.

Chalard F, Ferey S, Teinturier C, Kalifa G. Aortic dilatation in Turner syndrome: The role of MRI in early recognition. *Pediatr Radiol.* 2005;35:323–326.

Cheng S. Superior vena cava syndrome: A contemporary review of a historic disease. *Cardiol Rev.* 2009;17(1):16–23.

Corone P, Doyon F, Gaudeau S, et al. Natural history of ventricular septal defect. A study involving 790 cases. *Circulation.* 1977;55(6):908–915.

Curtis SL, Bradley M, Wilde P, et al. Results of screening for intracranial aneurysms in patients with coarctation of the aorta. *AJNR Am J Neuroradiol.* 2012;33(6):1182–1186.

Gielen H, Daniels O, van Lier H. Natural history of congenital pulmonary valvar stenosis: An echo and Doppler cardiographic study. *Cardiol Young.* 1999;9(2):129–135.

Krause PJ, Bockenstedt LK. Cardiology patient pages. Lyme disease and the heart. *Circulation.* 2013;127(7):e451–455.

Lanzarini L, Larizza D, Prete G, et al. Aortic dimensions in Turner's syndrome: Two-dimensional echocardiography versus magnetic resonance imaging. *J Cardiovasc Med (Hagerstown).* 2007;8:428–437.

Lanzarini L, Larizza D, Prete G, et al. Prospective evaluation of aortic dimensions in Turner syndrome: A 2-dimensional echocardiographic study. *J Am Soc Echocardiogr.* 2007;20:307–313.

Lin AE, Silberbach M. Focus on the heart and aorta in Turner syndrome. *J Pediatr.* 2007;150:572–574.

Little WC, Freeman GL. Pericardial disease. *Circulation.* 2006;113(12):1622–1632.

Lurbe E, Cifkova R, Cruichkshank JK, et al. Management of high blood pressure in children and adolescents: Recommendations of the European Society of Hypertension. *J Hypertens.* 2009;27(9):1719–1742.

Magnani JW, Dec GW. Myocarditis: current trends in diagnosis and treatment. *Circulation.* 2006:113(6):876–890.

Maron BJ, Maron MS. Hypertrophic cardiomyopathy. *Lancet.* 2013;381(9862):242–255.

Matura LA, Ho VB, Rosing DR, Bondy CA. Aortic dilatation and dissection in Turner syndrome. *Circulation.* 2007;116:1663–1670.

Newburger JW, Takahashi M, Gerber MA, et al. Diagnosis, treatment, and long-term management of Kawasaki disease: A statement for health professionals from the Committee on Rheumatic Fever, Endocarditis and Kawasaki Disease, council on Cardiovascular Disease in the Young, American Heart Association. *Circulation.* 2004;110(17):2747–2771.

Ostberg JE, Brookes JAS, McCarthy C, et al. A comparison of echocardiography and magnetic resonance imaging in cardiovascular screening of adults with Turner syndrome. *J Clin Endocrinol Metab.* 2004;89:5966–5971.

Park MK, *Pediatric Cardiology for Practitioners.* 4th ed. Philadelphia, PA: Mosby; 2002.

Park, MK, Guntheroth WG. *How to Read Pediatric ECGs.* Philadelphia, PA: Mosby; 2006.

Reddy SR, Singh HR. Chest pain in children and adolescents. *Pediatr Rev.* 2010;31(1):e1–9.

Ruge H, Wildhirt SM, Poerner M, et al. Severe superior vena cava syndrome after transvenous pacemaker implantation. *Ann Thorac Surg.* 2006;82(6):e41–42.

Siu SC, Silversides CK. Bicuspid aortic valve disease. *J Am Coll Cardiol.* 2010;55(25):2789–2800.

Tinker J, Howitt G, Markman P, Wade EG. The natural history of isolated pulmonary stenosis. *Br Heart J.* 1965;27:151–160.

Cognition, Language, and Learning Disabilities 6

Amy L. Conrad, Todd Kopelman, and Tammy L. Wilgenbusch

> **Helpful Tip**
> An intellectual disability is characterized by onset during early development and includes both intellectual and adaptive functioning deficits across conceptual, social, and practical domains.

► CASE 1

A 30-month-old social and healthy boy presents at his pediatrician's office with his mother, who has concerns about his development. He has a limited vocabulary of about 30 words and does not yet combine words. His parents say that at times he points to items that he wants and follows simple directions that his parents give him. His parents have not noticed any difficulties with his motor development.

Question 1-1

What would be the most appropriate recommendation for his mother?
A) Closely monitor his development for the next 6 months.
B) Recommend a speech and language evaluation.
C) Recommend a full evaluation of his intellectual and developmental skills.
D) Recommend a physical therapy evaluation.
E) All of the above.

Discussion 1-1

The correct answer is "B." At this time, there is evidence of a potential expressive language disorder and this should be further assessed. In general, boys have a higher incidence of language disorders and it is important to begin intervention services as early as possible, so a simple "watch and wait" approach would not be appropriate. In addition, at this time there is no evidence of a global intellectual disability. Children with mild or moderate intellectual disabilities will likely have delays in language; and while their overall sequence of development will be similar to that of other children, it will be at a much slower rate. His mother reports that he follows directions (receptive language) and has adequate motor development so at this time a full intellectual and developmental assessment is not warranted. If his development in other areas of functioning does not continue to keep pace with his peers, then a more extensive evaluation may be warranted at a later time. Other things to consider with expressive language delay include hearing impairment, autism spectrum disorders, and selective mutism (form of anxiety). A hearing screen is reasonable in this case, as well.

> **Helpful Tip**
> The *diagnosis* of an intellectual disability still requires performance on an intelligence quotient (IQ) test to be about 2 or more standard deviations below the norm (usually < 70). The *severity* of an intellectual disability is based on adaptive functioning and level of supports needed (this is a change from the previous method of using IQ cutoffs to define mild, moderate, severe, and profound disability).

The child is now 36 months old. His speech and language evaluation resulted in a diagnosis of an expressive and receptive language disorder. However, his mother reports that his fine motor coordination and gross motor skills are not developing at the same rate as his peers. Family history is significant for a maternal cousin and uncle with mild intellectual disability.

Question 1-2

Which of the following would be appropriate next steps for evaluating his intellectual and developmental functioning?
A) Obtaining a detailed pregnancy, birth, and family history.
B) Referral for formal genetic testing.
C) Referral to a psychologist for intellectual assessment.
D) Both A and B.
E) Options A, B, and C.

Discussion 1-2

The correct answer is "E." A thorough evaluation of a suspected intellectual disability should include a detailed pregnancy, birth, and medical history to determine if there are any possible risk factors. (See Table 6–1.) A detailed family history helps determine if there may be a familial pattern suggesting a genetic or chromosomal link. Formal genetic testing or other laboratory testing provides further information about possible genetic or medical causes. Physical exam and evaluation of growth factors or unusual features of the face or limbs can also be helpful. Formal intellectual testing determines if the child meets criteria for the diagnosis of intellectual disability. Let's hope you did not choose watchful waiting after the first evaluation.

⧖ QUICK QUIZ

What is the best test to investigate the cause of intellectual disability in a child?
A) Brain magnetic resonance imaging (MRI).
B) Urine organic acids.
C) Chromosomal studies.
D) Lead level.
E) Testing should be individualized to the particular case.

Discussion

The best answer is "E." In an era of medical overuse of diagnostic testing, it is always good to individualize testing to the particular case. The list of possible diagnostic tests for developmental delay and intellectual disability is long. Many of these should be used at the discretion of a specialist unless you have suspicion for a specific disorder or syndrome. Possible diagnostic tests include:

- Comparative genomic hybridization microarray
- Fluorescent in situ hybridization (FISH) testing
- Chromosomal and DNA analysis
- Metabolic testing
- Analysis of amino acids in blood, urine, or cerebrospinal fluid
- Analysis of urine organic acids
- Blood levels of lactate, pyruvate, very-long-chain fatty acids, free and total carnitine, and acyl carnitines
- Blood lead level
- Assays of specific enzymes in cultured skin fibroblasts
- Head imaging
- Methylation testing
- Cerebrospinal fluid analysis
- Electroencephalogram

Following evaluation, he has been diagnosed with intellectual disability, linked to a polygenetic family syndrome.

Question 1-3

Given this diagnosis, his care will now include collaboration with all of the following professionals EXCEPT:

TABLE 6–1 PARTIAL LISTING OF ETIOLOGIC FACTORS ASSOCIATED WITH INTELLECTUAL DISABILITY

	Prenatal	Perinatal / Postnatal
Chromosomal causes and genetic syndromes	Down syndrome	
	Fragile X syndrome	
	Williams syndrome	
	Neurofibromatosis	
	Myotonic dystrophy	
	Polygenic familial syndromes	
	Chromosomal microdeletion, translocations, or trisomy	
Metabolic causes	Tay-Sachs disease	
	Hurler syndrome	
	Phenylketonuria	
Medical conditions	Mitochondrial disorders	Premature birth
	Primary microcephaly	Birth injury
		Hypoxia/anoxia
		Fetal malnutrition–placental insufficiency
		Seizures
		Cranial trauma/traumatic brain injury
Infectious causes	Toxoplasmosis	Meningoencephalitis
	Hepatitis B	Encephalitis
	Syphilis	Encephalopathy of various causes
	Herpes zoster	
	Rubella	
	Cytomegalovirus	
	Herpes simplex II	
Teratogenic causes	Exposure to mercury	Maternal drug/alcohol use
		Exposure to lead and radiation
Psychosocial causes	Advanced parental age	Psychosocial deprivation
		Lack of access to prenatal care
		Child abuse resulting in brain injury
		Neglect resulting in malnutrition

A) Primary medical provider.
B) School personnel.
C) Therapists, including speech, language, occupational and physical
D) Legal/financial services.
E) None of the above (all may be included in care).

Discussion 1-3

The correct answer is "E." Families need much support to help care for children with intellectual disability. The level of support will likely vary based on the severity of the diagnosis and comorbid medical conditions. Families will need information and support to ensure appropriate education for their children, manage potential financial issues, and deal with special needs in regards to transportation, as well as respite care for those caring for the child.

⧗ QUICK QUIZ

What percentage of people diagnosed with an intellectual disability fall into the mild severity range?
A) 15%.
B) 30%.
C) 50%.
D) 60%.
E) 85%.

Discussion

The correct answer is "E." The majority of people diagnosed with an intellectual disability (85%) fall into the mild severity range. With support, academic success can often be achieved through and sometimes beyond elementary school. Independent living can also be achieved with supports (extended time, reminders, extra or modified instruction). About 10% of people diagnosed with an intellectual disability fall into the moderate severity range. While basic communication skills are adequate to function, they often have difficulty with more complex concepts and nuances of social interaction. Academic skills are usually at a basic, elementary school level. Self-care is often sufficient (eg, ability to bathe, dress, and feed self), but daily living requires consistent moderate support (eg, group home living, simple/repetitive jobs with close supervision).

▶ CASE 2

An 18-month-old girl presents to your clinic for a well-child appointment. Her parents express several concerns about their daughter's development. She has not yet started to talk, often does not respond when her parents say her name, makes limited eye contact with family members, does not point at objects around her or gesture, rarely smiles or shows happiness, shows no interest in toys, and has recently started to repetitively bang objects. She has passed her vision screening and you do not identify any medical concerns.

Question 2-1

What is an appropriate next step to address these concerns?
A) Complete an autism screening instrument and refer for more specialized evaluation if warranted.
B) Provide developmental guidance and encourage her parents to closely monitor her until her 24-month well-child appointment.
C) Encourage her parents to enroll her in a daycare facility so that additional stimulation will result in improvements in her language and overall development.
D) Complete a broad-based developmental screening to evaluate for other developmental concerns.
E) All of the above are equally valid options.

Discussion 2-1

The correct answer is "A." She is exhibiting several characteristic red flags of an autism spectrum disorder (ASD), so completion of an autism-specific screening is warranted. (See Table 6–2.) Several autism-screening instruments are available. The most commonly used screening instrument with toddlers is the Modified Checklist for Autism in Toddlers–Revised (M-CHAT-R). Option "B" is not recommended as core symptoms of autism can often be identified by the age of 18 to 24 months even though a

TABLE 6–2 EARLY AUTISM RED FLAGS	
Domain	**Symptoms**
Communication	Limited babbling
	Rarely looks at face of speaker
	Fails to respond to name
	Rarely follows a point to reference an object
	Limited pointing to request or share interest
	Limited use of gestures
	Lack of basic imaginative play (pretending to talk on phone, pretending to feed doll)
Responsiveness and regulation	Poor eye contact
	Failure to orient to caregiver
	Reduced positive affect (infrequent social smile)
	Limited showing of things to others
	Limited imitation (waving, clapping)
	Lower activity level
	Irritable, difficult to soothe
	Sleep difficulties
	Feeding difficulties
	Unusual sensory behaviors (repetitive spinning, rotating, tapping)
	Visual examination (holding object close to eyes)

diagnosis of ASD is often not conferred until a child is at least 4 years old. Most parents of a child diagnosed with ASD initially become concerned about his or her development by age 2 and a trained clinician can typically make a stable diagnosis of ASD by age 3. Participation in an intensive early intervention program that uses evidence-based practices has been demonstrated to result in improved performance for many young children with autism compared to participation in a general daycare program (option "C"). Although it will be important for a specialist to rule out other developmental disorders such as a specific language impairment or global developmental delay that may account for her presentation, this patient is exhibiting multiple hallmark features of autism and so a broad developmental screen is not indicated. Compared to an autism-specific screening instrument, a general developmental screening tool is not a good predictor of autism because it assesses different developmental domains.

> **Helpful Tip**
> The American Academy of Pediatrics (AAP) recommends routine screening for an autism spectrum disorder with an autism-specific instrument at 18 and 24 months. The M-CHAT-R is currently the most commonly used screener for this age group and is available in multiple languages. Referral for more specialized assessment is recommended if a child fails an autism-specific screener.

Using the *Diagnostic and Statistical Manual of Mental Disorders, Fifth Edition* (*DSM-5*), you diagnosis the child with autism spectrum disorder. You continue to read in the manual so you can use the correct term in the child's electronic medical record.

Question 2-2

Which is an acceptable term to use?
A) Asperger syndrome.
B) Autism spectrum disorder.
C) Autistic disorder.
D) Pervasive developmental disorder not otherwise classified.
E) None of the above.

Discussion 2-2

The correct answer is "B." Diagnostic criteria for autism were significantly revised in the fifth edition of the *Diagnostic and Statistical Manual of Mental Disorders* (*DSM-5*). Critical changes include replacement of the umbrella term *pervasive developmental disorders* with autism spectrum disorder, and removal of the diagnoses autistic disorder, Asperger syndrome, and pervasive developmental disorder not otherwise specified. A single diagnosis, autism spectrum disorder (ASD), is used to describe a persistent pattern of deficits in the area of social communication combined with the presence of restricted, repetitive, and rigid patterns of interest and behavior. ASD is a heterogeneous disorder with significant variability in presentation. Along with documenting the presence of an ASD, clinicians and researchers

using *DSM-5* guidelines should also specify whether there is an accompanying intellectual disability, language impairment, medical, genetic, environmental, mental, or behavioral disorder. The level of symptom severity in the areas of social communication and restricted and repetitive behaviors should also be indicated.

> **Helpful Tip**
> Early identification of autism spectrum disorder (ASD) is important because early intervention services have been associated with improved child outcomes and with lower reported levels of parent stress.

Question 2-3

ASD can often be distinguished from specific language impairment (SLI) based upon:
A) More difficulty with understanding nonliteral language.
B) Speech delays that emerge during the second year of life.
C) More difficulty with language production.
D) More difficulty with language comprehension.
E) Significant social difficulties and presence of restricted and repetitive behavior patterns.

Discussion 2-3

The correct answer is "E." The core deficits of autism (difficulties in social communication and the presence of restricted and repetitive interests and behaviors) overlap with other disorders, including language impairment, intellectual disability, hearing impairment, and mental health disorders. Differential diagnosis can be challenging and it is important that clinicians possess expertise in the areas of child development, speech and language, and common medical and psychiatric comorbidities.

Communication disorders can be separated into two broad categories of speech and language. Speech disorders consist of difficulties with articulation, including sound production, atypical speech patterns, and voice modulation. Language disorders are characterized by difficulties with language learning, and one or more domains of language (syntax, phonology, morphology, pragmatics, semantics) may be impacted. SLI, also referred to as a language delay, developmental language disorder, and dysphasia, is characterized by difficulties in the areas of language comprehension and expression. Symptoms of SLI typically emerge in preschool or in early elementary school. In contrast to ASD, with a prevalence rate of about 1.3%, SLI has a prevalence of approximately 7%. The features of SLI, by definition, are limited to language. Broader impairments in cognition, social-emotional development, or the presence of restricted and repetitive behaviors may indicate the presence of ASD or another disorder.

⏳ QUICK QUIZ

Current prevalence data indicate that 1 out of every ____ school-aged children in the United States has an autism spectrum disorder (ASD) and that males are ___ more likely to have ASD than females.

A) 150; 2×.
B) 150; 5×.
C) 68; 2×.
D) 68; 5×.
E) 50; 8×.

Discussion

The correct answer is "D." Findings from a surveillance summary report published by the Centers for Disease Control and Prevention in 2014 indicate that approximately 1 in 68 school-aged children has an autism spectrum disorder. This number represents a 30% increase from the previous prevalence estimate of 1 in 88 children. ASD has consistently been identified more commonly in males.

> **Helpful Tip**
> Approximately 70% of individuals with ASD have a comorbid mental health diagnosis, with about 40% of individuals having two or more comorbid diagnoses. The most common mental health diagnoses that co-occur with ASD are attention deficit hyperactivity disorder (ADHD), anxiety disorders (ie, specific phobias, social anxiety, obsessive compulsive disorder), Tourette syndrome, and depression.

▶ CASE 3

A mother brings her 7-year-old boy with trisomy 21 and moderate intellectual disability (ID) to the clinic because she is concerned that he may also have an ASD. She reports that he rarely initiates social interactions with adults or other children, has delayed speech, does not engage in imaginative play, flaps his hands, has an unusually high pain tolerance, and becomes agitated when there are changes to familiar routines.

Question 3-1

What percentage of individuals with ASD have co-occurring ID?

A) 1% to 20%.
B) 21% to 40%.
C) 41% to 59%.
D) 60% to 79%.
E) 80% to 99%.

Discussion 3-1

The correct answer is "D." Substantial overlap exists between the symptoms of ASD and ID and approximately 60% to 70% of individuals with ASD also have a comorbid ID. Of note, reported rates of ID in the ASD population have varied considerably across studies, likely due to differences in methodology and inclusion criteria for ID and ASD. Adaptive functioning (necessary to live independently and interact socially) is often lower than cognitive

performance for people with comorbid ASD and ID. Individuals with ASD and ID may be at greater risk of engaging in challenging behaviors such as aggression and self-injury, and having more psychiatric complications such as anxiety, schizophrenia, and ADHD, compared with those who have ID alone. Particularly for children who are very young or who present with significant intellectual impairment (severe to profound ID), it can be difficult to determine whether social difficulties, communication delays, and repetitive and rigid behaviors are due solely to the cognitive impairment or are better accounted for by the additional presence of ASD. Identification of comorbid ID in a child with ASD is important because different interventions are indicated to address learning and adaptive needs. From an outcome perspective, the presence of ID and language impairments in individuals with ASD is often predictive of response to treatment, as children with stronger cognitive abilities generally make greater progress.

You decide to test his hearing as he has speech delay.

Question 3-2

The area of greatest symptom overlap between ASD and hearing impairment is:

A) The presence of repetitive motor behaviors (stereotypies).
B) Better nonverbal than verbal communication skills.
C) Communication impairments.
D) Reduced frequency of social interaction.
E) Recurrent ear infections.

Discussion 3-2

The correct answer is "C." While there can be substantial symptom overlap between ASD and hearing impairment in the area of communication difficulties, children with ASD are more likely to experience social difficulties and display a pattern of restricted interests and repetitive behaviors. Children with profound hearing loss can also have ASD, and this subgroup tends to be diagnosed with autism much later compared with non–hearing impaired children due to diagnostic overshadowing. An autism-specific instrument, the BISCUIT, has been demonstrated to be sensitive in discriminating children with ASD from children with hearing impairment. Ten points if you knew that BISCUIT was an acronym for Baby and Infant Screen for Children with autism Traits. Recurrent ear infections are a cause of hearing loss but not ASD.

The previous patient you diagnosed was a toddler but this child is older. You pull out your smartphone to find an age-appropriate autism screening tool.

Question 3-3

All of the following are common autism screeners EXCEPT:

A) Social Communication Questionnaire (SCQ).
B) Social Responsiveness Scale (SRS).
C) Denver Developmental Screening Test II (DDST-II).
D) Modified Checklist for Autism in Toddlers–Revised (M-CHAT-R).
E) Screening Tool for Autism in Toddlers and Young Children (STAT).

Discussion 3-3

The correct answer is "C." The DDSD-II is a commonly used screening measure of general developmental progress but does not include items sensitive to ASD symptoms. The M-CHAT-R is a commonly used autism screener for toddlers (aged 16 to 30 months). You should know that one already. The SCQ and SRS are both screeners for children aged 4 years and older. The STAT is a second-level screener that includes semistructured direct observation of a young child's social responsiveness and communication. It is appropriate for children between the ages of 24 and 36 months.

⧗ QUICK QUIZ

Which is NOT a potential factor associated with an increased risk for autism?
A) Measles, mumps, rubella (MMR) vaccine.
B) Advanced paternal age.
C) A sibling with autism.
D) Toxin exposure.
E) Genetic mutation.

Discussion

The correct answer is "A." Evidence does not exist to support a link between either MMR vaccines or exposure to thimerosal as a preservative in vaccines and autism. In 1998, a silly man named Andrew Wakefield published an article in a journal you may have heard of, *The Lancet*. His conclusion linking the MMR vaccine to autism caused a national panic. Despite finding his data to be bogus, this myth persists. Autism is a complex, heterogeneous neurodevelopmental disorder with a multifactorial etiologic pathway. ASD is highly heritable and multiple genes have been implicated that increase susceptibility to the disorder. Clinicians can now identify the genetic basis of ASD in up to 20% of cases. Concordance rates for ASD in monozygotic twins have been estimated at 60% to 70%, and the likelihood that the younger sibling of a child with ASD will also have the disorder (10% to 20%) is significantly higher than the overall likelihood in the general population. In at least 30% of cases, autism is the result of de novo genetic mutations. Certain environmental events can also play a role in influencing the likelihood that an individual will acquire ASD. Currently, information on the relationship among different environmental factors, timing of exposure, and presence of susceptibility genes is limited. Inconsistent findings have been reported regarding the link between parental age and autism, with some studies identifying advanced paternal and maternal age as risk factors. Other environmental factors that may increase the likelihood of ASD include maternal infection to rubella during pregnancy, and toxins such as pesticides and air pollution.

▶ CASE 4

A 3-year-old boy was recently diagnosed with ASD. He presents with delays in the areas of learning, communication, fine motor skills, and social interactions. He is engaging in aggression and self-injurious behavior and is experiencing sleep difficulties. His parents request guidance regarding appropriate intervention services.

Question 4-1

What do you recommend?
A) Speech and language therapy.
B) Occupational therapy.
C) Applied behavior analysis.
D) Educational interventions.
E) All of the above.

Discussion 4-1

The correct answer is "E." Similar to this child, children with ASD often present with multiple areas of concern and treatment must be tailored to individual need. There is no "one size fits all" approach that is effective in working with all children with ASD. It is common for children with ASD to receive intervention through a combination of school programming and private, community-based services. Although a cure for autism does not exist, evidence-based interventions have been identified that, in many cases, can lead to improvements in overall functioning. Applied behavioral analysis (ABA) is an intervention that focuses on changing behaviors by understanding the relationship between behavior and the environment. It has been shown to improve cognitive functioning, social skills, communication, and play skills, though not all children demonstrate equal success. Early intensive ABA programming, typically defined as 25 to 40 hours per week of evidence-based services prior to age 4 years and parental involvement can be instrumental in targeting core difficulties associated with ASD. Medical care is an important treatment component, and referral to subspecialists may be indicated based on specific concerns. Several genetic and neurodevelopmental syndromes are associated with ASD at a much higher rate than in the general pediatric population. There include Angelman, CHARGE (coloboma, heart defect, choanal atresia, retarded growth and development, genital abnormality, and ear abnormality), Cornelia DeLange, Klinefelter, and Sotos syndromes; fragile X; trisomy 21; neurofibromatosis; and tuberous sclerosis. Children with ASD are more likely than the general pediatric population to experience difficulties with feeding, sleep, gastrointestinal disorders (including constipation), seizures, and psychiatric conditions. Several alternative treatments for ASD exist. Many lack scientific support and, in some cases, they may be costly and result in physical harm.

▶ CASE 5

A child's mother brings him in for his annual well-child check. She is concerned because instead of using words to communicate his wants or needs, he is pointing and grunting. Further discussion with the mother and review of his medical record indicates that he is the youngest of three children with highly involved parents who read to him frequently and provide him with daily opportunities for verbal interaction. He has had a high number of ear infections, without tympanostomy tubes.

Question 5-1

This is developmentally appropriate behavior, unless the child is older than age:
A) 4 months.
B) 9 months.
C) 16 months.
D) 24 months.
E) 36 months.

Discussion 5-1

The correct answer is "C". Pointing and grunting in place of using words to communicate his developmentally appropriate until roughly 11 months of age. Continued use of this mode of communication is a red flag if still present after 14 months of age. (See Tables 6–3 and 6–4.)

> **Helpful Tip**
> It is important to understand the distinction between language and speech. Language is our symbolic system through which humans communicate with each other and can be accomplished in various ways (eg, verbally, using sign language, through writing). Speech refers to specific oral and verbal output of language and includes specific sounds, articulation, fluency, and voice quality.

Given that he is currently 24 months old, there is concern that he may have a language delay.

Question 5-2

An appropriate evaluation to determine the presence and extent of his delay would include:
A) Screening of language production.
B) Referral to a speech/language pathologist for a full evaluation of expressive and receptive skills.
C) Hearing evaluation with possible tympanostomy tubes placement and screening of language production.
D) Hearing evaluation with possible tympanostomy tubes placement and referral to a speech/language pathologist for a full evaluation of expressive and receptive skills.
E) Only a hearing evaluation and tympanostomy tubes placement if hearing is low. Further evaluation can be done later if there is continued delay.

Discussion 5-2

The correct answer is "D". A key here is the recurrent ear infections, which is a risk factor for conductive hearing loss. If you cannot hear, it makes sense that you may have speech issues. Appropriate language development requires responsive exposure (positive interactions with adults who demonstrate language sounds and usage), ability to adequately hear and process

TABLE 6–3 RECEPTIVE LANGUAGE DEVELOPMENT: AVERAGE AGE OF ACQUISITION AND AGE INDICATING SIGNIFICANT DELAY OR RED FLAG

Receptive Language Milestones	Average Age of Acquisition	Significant Delays and Red Flags
Alerts or quiets to sound	Birth to 1 mo	2 mo
Turns to the source of sound	Birth to 1 mo, then again 3–5 mo	6 mo
Responds to own name	6–8 mo	10 mo
Follows verbal routines/games ("*Wave by-bye*")	8–10 mo	12 mo
Understands simple questions ("*Where's mommy?*")	9–11 mo	15 mo
Stops when told "No"	9–10 mo	15 mo
Understands at least 3 different words	10–13 mo	15 mo
Points to 3 different body parts	12–16 mo	18 mo
Follow simple commands ("*Show me the ball*" or "*Get your shoes*")	12 mo	18 mo
Follows 2-part commands ("*Get your shoes and give them to Dad*")	24 mo	30 mo
Answers simple questions ("*Who is that?*" or "*What are you doing?*")	24–30 mo	36 mo

Reproduced with permission from Carey WB, Crocker AC, Elias ER, et al: *Developmental-Behavioral Pediatrics*, 4th edition. Philadelphia, PA: Elsevier;2009.

the sounds, and ability to accurately reproduce speech sounds. Disruption of any of these factors may result in language delay. Psychosocial neglect or abuse can result in impoverished verbal input. High rates of otitis media and resulting hearing loss or impaired auditory processing can disrupt exposure to language sounds. Further, abnormalities in the oral cavity (eg, with oral clefts), oral motor dysfunction, or neural injury can impair speech production. Children with cerebral palsy may have speech delay from impaired oral motor function rather than intellectual disability. These are all possible etiologies for delays in language development, and evaluation of environment,

TABLE 6–4 EXPRESSIVE LANGUAGE DEVELOPMENT: AVERAGE AGE OF ACQUISITION AND AGE INDICATING SIGNIFICANT DELAY OR RED FLAG

Expressive Language Milestones	Average Age of Acquisition	Significant Delays and Red Flags
Cooing	2–3 mo	6 mo
Babbling	6–8 mo	10 mo
Nonverbal purposeful messages (requests with a reach; shows objects)	9–10 mo	12 mo
Pointing	10–11 mo	14 mo
Says 3 different spontaneous words	12–15 mo	16 mo
Vocabulary at least 25–50 words	18–22 mo	24 mo
Production of 2-word phrases ("*Mommy sock*"; "*No water*")	18–22 mo	24 mo
Simple sentences ("*I want juice*"; "*Where's my ball?*")	24–30 mo	36 mo
Intelligibility to unfamiliar adult at > 50%	30–36 mo	42 mo
Able to tell about a past event with parent asking questions (personal narrative)	24–30 mo	36 mo
Able to tell or retell a familiar story	36–48 mo	54 mo
Fully intelligible to an unfamiliar adult (despite some immature sounds, such as consonant clusters or /r/ and /l/)	48–54 mo	60 mo
Fully mature speech sounds	Up to 72 mo	> 72 mo

Reproduced with permission from Carey WB, Crocker AC, Elias ER, et al: *Developmental-Behavioral Pediatrics*, 4th edition. Phladelphia, PA: Elsevier;2009.

medical conditions, auditory processing, and speech production should be conducted. This child is 24 months old, and his delay is substantial enough that simply testing hearing and waiting to see if things resolve with tubes (and improved hearing) or conducting a simple language screening would miss out on crucial time for intervention and might further hinder his language development. Assessing his hearing and obtaining a full evaluation will provide greater information to plan the most appropriate intervention for this child.

Question 5-3

What would be an appropriate initial management strategy for a 24-month-old child with a speech or language disorder?

A) Monitor for 6 to 9 months.
B) Teach family members to create an optimal language learning environment and how to stimulate language development.
C) Refer to a speech/language pathologist for articulation therapy.
D) Refer to a speech/language pathologist for therapy to improve vocabulary, varying sentence structure, or lengthening conversations.
E) Options B, C, and D.

Discussion 5-3

The correct answer is "E." Assuming normal hearing, appropriate management of a speech or language disorder is multifaceted and includes optimizing the child's environment to stimulate language as well as addressing specific areas of deficit. In regard to language, this could include direct teaching and exposure to vocabulary, rules of grammar, and conversational exchanges in clinic and other environments (classroom, daycare setting, playground). Therapy may also focus on articulation and sound production and teach appropriate tongue placement, mouth and lip movement, and nasal resonance to improve intelligibility. In general (or at least for the Boards), if a child's development is delayed, waiting is not the right path to choose.

► CASE 6

A sixth-grade girl is doing poorly in all academic areas. Teachers say she understands information when it is read to her or presented verbally. She was referred for testing and was found to have difficulties with memory, but her verbal comprehension and visual-spatial reasoning were age appropriate. Her math skills were found to be on grade level, but her word decoding and reading fluency were at a second-grade level. She was diagnosed with dyslexia by the psychologist and found to be eligible for special education services.

Question 6-1

Which of the following may be associated with a specific learning disability (SLD), as opposed to an intellectual disability?

A) Academic struggles.
B) Significantly low cognitive skills across all areas.
C) Memory deficit.
D) Deficits in daily living skills.
E) Both A and C.

Discussion 6-1

The correct answer is "E." An intellectual disability is defined by significantly below-average global functioning (across all domains) and deficits in adaptive functioning. However, SLDs are characterized by a *relative* deficit in specific domains and normal or higher functioning in other domains. Adaptive functioning is typically age-appropriate. Areas often impacted by an SLD include reading, writing, math, language, and motor skills. Disabilities may be noted early in elementary school, while some children may not be identified until later elementary or middle school.

> **Helpful Tip**
> Children with a specific learning disability are able to comprehend and learn material at their grade level, but their disability may lead to low performance in different academic subjects (a child with a reading disability may perform poorly on math word problems). Appropriate treatment will include accommodations so that they are not penalized for their disability in these different subjects (having math word problems read aloud to the student and allowing them to dictate their answers).

After her diagnosis of dyslexia, she received specialized reading instruction as well as specific classroom accommodations.

Question 6-2

Which of the following could be expected of her by her junior and senior years in high school?

A) Her reading accuracy and fluency will not improve much and she will require intensive accommodations and assistive technologies.
B) Her reading accuracy will likely improve, but her fluency will remain very slow and she will require intensive accommodations and assistive technologies.
C) Her reading accuracy will likely improve, but her fluency will remain slightly slower and she may continue to benefit from some accommodations or assistive technologies.
D) Her reading fluency will likely improve, but her reading accuracy will remain low and some accommodations and assistive technologies will continue to be useful.
E) Her reading skills will all be within normal limits and accommodations and assistive technologies will no longer be required to keep up with her class.

Discussion 6-2

The correct answer is "C." Dyslexia is a synonym for specific reading disability characterized by difficulties with spelling, word recognition, and decoding abilities (recognizing letters in a word, connecting each letter to a sound, blending the sounds to determine the word, assigning a meaning to the word). Fluency disorder is a collective term for stuttering and difficulties speaking smoothly. Children with dyslexia who are identified and provided appropriate reading instruction early often show improvement in reading accuracy, but continue to be slightly slower than same-aged peers. They often do not have an issue with "easy" material, but may struggle with highly complex, technical material or with new terms (eg, when starting a biology or chemistry course). As with specific learning disabilities in general, if appropriate remediation (specialized instruction) is provided some improvement is expected over time. However, these specialized skills will likely continue to be areas of weakness for the child and he or she may continue to benefit from accommodations depending on the severity of the disability.

> **Helpful Tip**
> Specific learning disability can vary in severity. Children with extreme disabilities have deficits in more than one domain or skill whereas those with mild disabilities may have only one affected domain or skill that is minimally low. As the severity and number of deficits increase, the amount of remediation and accommodations also increase. Long-term struggles and high accommodations need will persist in these cases.

> **Helpful Tip**
> Parents may make red flag statements that could indicate the need to screen for a specific learning disability. They may mention struggles in school, low grades, increased frustration with homework, or failure to succeed despite continued instruction. Ask about specific skills and processes in order to determine if referral for further testing is warranted. Ask specifically about performance in classes (reading, math, writing) and the difficulty in each skill area (avoids homework, requires excessive amounts of time, gets overly frustrated).

▶ CASE 7

A second-grade boy has had an unstable living environment and moved frequently with his mother, which has resulted in switching schools frequently and missing a great deal of his kindergarten and first-grade years. Academically he is behind in reading and his mother is concerned that he has a learning disability.

Question 7-1

Which of the following factors contribute to underachievement in children?

A) Familial environment, inconsistent education, mental health and behavioral issues, low motivation.
B) Dominant handedness, familial environment, inconsistent education, mental health and behavioral issues.
C) Familial environment, gender, mental health and behavioral issues, low motivation.
D) Inconsistent education, mental health and behavioral issues, low motivation, and age.
E) Dominant handedness, gender, familial environment, inconsistent education, low motivation.

Discussion 7-1

The correct answer is "A." Many factors beyond cognitive functioning can impact a child's academic achievement. (See Figure 6–1.) Disruption in the family/home environment, interference of systematic education (through minimal attendance or moving from school to school), other medical or mental diagnoses (chronic illness, depression, or anxiety), and even individual temperament can have a negative impact on academic achievement. Factors of age, gender, and handedness have shown no significant impact on achievement. (If handedness mattered, would ambidexterity be a good or bad thing? Trying to provide a chance for a mental break.)

Question 7-2

What will your next steps be in the child's care?

A) Immediately refer him for a full learning disability evaluation with a local psychologist.
B) Follow up with some more specific questions about his environment growing up and his past experiences. Develop a plan based on your findings for the next step in care, which could include further evaluation by a specialist, discussing interventions with the school, or psychological counseling.
C) Follow up with more specific questions about his environment growing up and his past experiences. Based on the level of disruption, contact the Department of Human Services (DHS) for suspected neglect.
D) Suggest that his mother discuss his lack of progress with his teacher and see what the school can do.
E) Tell his mother that he is still fairly young and he will likely grow out of it, but she should monitor his improvement over the next year.

Discussion 7-2

The correct answer is "B." That answer should seem obvious. With the exception of an emergency, more history is always a good option. Given the extent of disruption to both his home life and educational progress, these factors should be considered first before referring for a full evaluation of a learning disability. However, just talking to the school or "waiting to see" may not be enough and could delay appropriate interventions. Helpful information would include details on what stress may be present at the home, if moves have involved disruptions to friendships or cultural norms, at what time points he was out of school or switched schools, and how he is currently functioning (ie, his mood and behavior). This information will help guide appropriate referrals and next steps. Although his environment has been disrupted to a high degree, this does not constitute neglect. Educational neglect is the failure to enroll a child in school or provide appropriate homeschooling or specialized education. His mother has continually enrolled him in school and is appropriately seeking assistance when she noted a problem. It may be helpful to ask why the family keeps moving to identify a modifiable factor so they stay in one place.

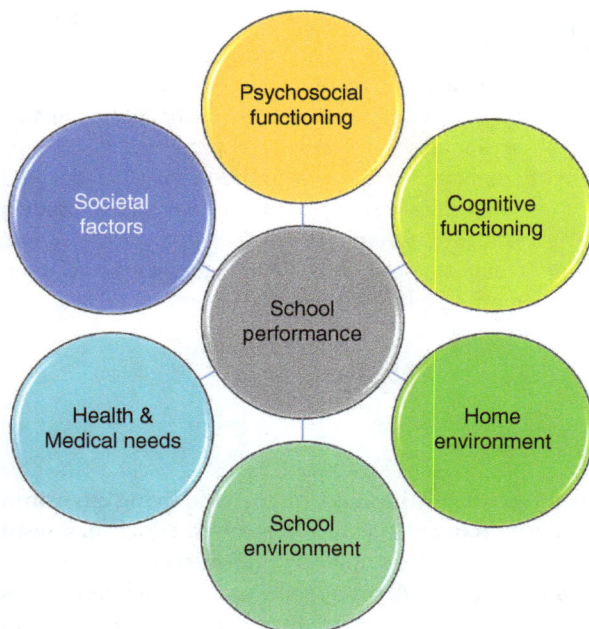

FIGURE 6–1. Etiologies of school-related difficulties.

► CASE 8

Parents of a 2-year-old boy bring him to an appointment because they are concerned about his language and behavior skills. They report that he produces few sounds and does not respond when they talk to him. They are wondering if he is being oppositional because he does not want to listen when they tell him not to do something. In clinic you notice that when he was playing on the floor with his truck he did not respond when you called his name or when there was a loud noise in the hallway outside the exam room. You begin to question if he might have some hearing loss and make a referral to an audiologist and speech/language pathologist.

Question 8-1

Which of the following has NOT been clearly implicated as a factor that can impact developmental outcomes of children who have hearing impairment?

A) Etiology of the hearing loss.
B) Family environment.

C) Early parental bonding.
D) Degree of hearing loss.
E) Timing and appropriateness of interventions.

Discussion 8-1

The correct answer is "C." No one factor will impact developmental outcomes of children with hearing impairment, and factors will affect all children differently. However, currently research does not indicate that early parental bonding has a notable impact on developmental and behavioral outcome in this population. The degree of hearing loss is important because early amplification tools may help children with milder hearing loss. The cause of the hearing loss is very important because sometimes it may lead to additional neurologic dysfunction or other system involvement, such as vision or other medical difficulties. The age at which the hearing loss occurs is a factor. Children who are deaf prelingually are at significant disadvantage in regard to language development compared with those who have been exposed to language during the critical early years. Family climate is a factor that could impact development. In families with prior experience to hearing impairment, parents and families may know sign language and be able to foster communication skills early on. As with most disabilities, early diagnosis and intervention is crucial.

> **Helpful Tip**
> Delayed speech and language development may be the first signs of a hearing impairment. There is a higher prevalence of educationally significant associated disabilities, such as learning disorders, vision problems, and cerebral palsy, in school-aged children who have hearing impairment.

Question 8-2

Which of the following statements about the developmental outcomes of children with hearing impairment is supported by research?
A) Children with hearing impairment develop compensatory skills, such as more efficient visual processing abilities.
B) The primary impact of hearing impairment is that children are unable to hear sounds; however, their ability to develop spoken language is not affected.
C) Hearing impairment limits intelligence.
D) Children with hearing impairment are more socially mature than typically developing peers.
E) Both A and D are supported by research.

Discussion 8-2

The correct answer is "A." Research has shown that children with hearing impairment develop compensatory skills, and often these have to do with visual processing. Language and speech skills tend to be significantly affected in children with hearing impairment, likely because they are not able to appropriately hear sounds in order for appropriate speech production. However, there is no specific indication that hearing impairment itself limits an individual's intelligence. The child's overall ability may be difficult to assess because of the nature of standardized assessments, but this does not mean that he or she has an intellectual disability as a result of the hearing loss. Socially, research suggests that children with hearing impairment are actually less socially mature, not more mature. This may be related to language difficulties, parental overprotectiveness, and decreased opportunities for social interactions.

> **Helpful Tip**
> Children with visual impairment are at risk for sensory deprivation given the noncontinuous nature of auditory and tactile cues. Intensive hands-on training paired with verbalizations is critical in the development of children with visual impairment.

Question 8-3

Which of the following would NOT be considered part of a pediatrician's role in treating a child with a hearing or visual impairment?
A) Etiologic workup and referral to additional medical specialists.
B) Ongoing and routine medical care.
C) Thorough developmental and cognitive testing and evaluation.
D) Anticipatory guidance of developmental, school-based, community-based, and transition needs and assistance to parents in finding resources for these needs.
E) Of course, pediatricians are all-knowing and can fulfill all of the above roles.

Discussion 8-3

The correct answer is "C." As a pediatrician, you will be the medical home for children with sensory impairment. Your job will likely entail education and support of parents, routine medical care, and referral and assistance with finding resources for the child's care. However, while pediatricians may screen for developmental skills, they do not have the time or (often) the specialized training to conduct thorough testing of developmental and cognitive skills and often refer children to a psychologist, occupational/physical/speech therapist, vision teacher, or local schools to complete such evaluations. (Someone mentioned time. Is it time for intermission? If you have procrastinated in studying, buckle down and keep reading.)

> **Helpful Tip**
> Adaptive and motor skill performance is usually impacted more by visual impairment than by communication skills.

QUICK QUIZ

Which of the following is NOT typically seen in children with visual impairment?
A) Stereotyped behavior.
B) Development of smooth grading of movement.
C) Difficulties in sensory integration.
D) Difficulties with proximal stability of the head.
E) None of the above.

Discussion

The correct answer is "B." Motor milestones are often impacted by children with blindness or visual impairment. Some specific motor skills that are often delayed include sensory integration (using sensory input from the environment and body); optic righting (reflex using vision to restore posture and head position); proximal stability of the head, neck, scapula, trunk, and pelvis; lateral and diagonal weight shift; and rotational, protective, and balance reactions. Children with visual impairment often have difficulty with grading of their movements. Movements may be jerky, and all or none rather than graded (coordinated). While developmental milestones may be impacted, it is not uncommon for children with visual impairment to engage in stereotyped behavior such as rocking, eye pressing, or finger flicking. It is theorized that this is the child's attempt to gain additional sensory input given the noncontinuous nature of auditory and tactile cues.

> **Helpful Tip**
> The age at which visual impairment occurs is crucial in the impact on development because so much of how we learn and interact with the world as a child is through sight. Even a brief time of having visual input can benefit development.

▶ CASE 9

A 9-year-old girl whom you have seen for her well-child appointments returns for ongoing problems with reading. Her mother reports that she continues to struggle in reading, despite enrollment for 2 years in the school's Title 1 reading program and tutoring over the summer. The child is becoming increasingly frustrated at school and it is starting to affect her self-esteem. You have decided that she would benefit from an evaluation for a possible SLD.

Question 9-1

Which of the following would *not* be an appropriate professional to refer a child to for achievement and intellectual assessment?
A) A psychometrician.
B) A psychologist.
C) A psychiatrist.
D) A specialized school professional.
E) All of the above would be appropriate professional referrals.

Discussion 9-1

The correct answer is "A." The diagnostic evaluation of achievement and intelligence testing must be conducted by a trained and credentialed professional in assessment and interpretation. This may be a psychologist, psychiatrist, or school professional. While psychometricians may administer tests, it is the credentialed professional that interprets the results and provides diagnosis and recommendations. The diagnostic evaluation often includes a structured interview/history, review of past school or testing records, and standardized assessments of achievement, intellectual, and neuropsychological functioning.

The girl has been evaluated by a psychologist and you are reviewing the report. She has been diagnosed with dyslexia and a memory deficit. However, when you look at the scores provided, you notice that her Full Scale IQ is 105. Knowing that this is within the average range of functioning, you are confused as to how there is a diagnosed disability.

Question 9-2

Which of the following describes your response?
A) The psychologist is obviously a fraud and you will need to refer the family for further testing by a more qualified professional.
B) You leave it alone; the psychologist is trained and credentialed and must know what he or she is talking about.
C) You look more closely at the other scores and notice a large discrepancy between the girl's performance on different tests, with above-average verbal and nonverbal scores but significantly below-average memory scores. This explains it.
D) You look more closely at the other scores and notice a large discrepancy between her performance on different tests, with significantly below-average verbal and nonverbal scores but above-average memory scores. This explains it.
E) None of the above.

Discussion 9-2

The correct answer is "C." It is very dangerous to limit interpretation of an intellectual assessment to the Full-Scale Intelligence Quotient (FSIQ). Although the most common intellectual assessments do have some differences, each typically is made up of different domains (verbal, nonverbal, reasoning, memory, processing speed) that are combined to create the FSIQ. Often for children with SLD, there can be significant discrepancies between those domains. When there are discrepancies, interpretation should be at the domain level.

QUICK QUIZ

What is the average standardized score for cognitive testing?
A) 5.
B) 10.
C) 25.

D) 50.

E) 100.

Discussion

The correct answer is "E." Sorry; a score of 100 does not equal 100%. Many different scales can be used in cognitive, psychological, and achievement testing and it is important to understand what the average range entails. Here are some of the most common you might come across:

- Standardized scores: Average score is 100, with 86 to 114 often being considered the average range.
- Scaled scores: Average is 10, with 8 to 12 often being considered the average range.
- T-scores: Average is 50, with 41 to 59 often being considered the average range.

▶ CASE 10

A father comes to your office because his son has been diagnosed with attention ADHD by a psychologist. The psychologist found that the son's intelligence was below average on testing. While looking at the report you notice that the psychologist commented on the fact that the boy was constantly out of his seat, looking out the window, and missed a lot of easy questions but got more difficult ones correct. You spend time discussing with the father how this likely affected the boy's scores, and emphasize that the psychologist did not diagnose him with below-average intelligence.

Question 10-1

In which of the following testing situations is a factor present that needs to be considered as it may have an influence on the child's performance?

A) During testing, the child was often out of his seat and would answer questions before the examiner finished the directions.

B) The child had a fever that morning and was complaining of a runny nose, but she received ibuprofen before testing and is no longer febrile.

C) During his evaluation, the adolescent mentioned that he was up really late the night before watching fireworks and did not get a lot of sleep.

D) A teenager had his phone on during testing and got a text in the middle of the evaluation that his girlfriend was breaking up with him.

E) All of the above.

Discussion 10-1

The correct answer is "E." It is important to realize that every testing situation is different and there are always factors that need to be taken into consideration when interpreting results. Some things to be aware of include the child's behavior (eg, attention, compliance, fatigue, anxiety, illness), the environment or room in which the testing is taking place

in (eg, adequate lighting, a quiet room free of distractors), the child's past experience with testing, the examiner's experience and effectiveness at working with the child, and the rapport that is established between the child and the examiner. The results will not necessarily be invalid because there was a factor that negatively affected testing, but these things need to be taken into consideration, both by the examiner and by you as a pediatrician, in determining how accurate the assessment was.

▶ CASE 11

Your 10-year-old patient was recently seen for standardized intellectual and achievement tests. His reported intellectual scores included Full-Scale Intelligence Quotient (FSIQ) 113, Verbal Index 105, Visual-Spatial Index 120, Fluid Reasoning Index 125, Working Memory Index 110, and Processing Speed Index 115. The reported achievement scores included Word Reading 88, Reading Fluency 86, Reading Comprehension 90, Math Problem Solving 115, and Written Expression 100.

Question 11-1

Which of the following is the most important factor to pay attention to related to his diagnosis?

A) Determine if the value of the FSIQ falls above the below-average range, which indicates no disability.

B) Determine if the value of the FSIQ falls below the average range, which indicates a disability.

C) Determine if any individual achievement scores are below average, which indicates a disability.

D) Determine if any individual achievement scores are significantly lower (difference of more than 1 standard deviation, or 15 Index points) than FSIQ, which indicates a disability.

E) When significant differences between intellectual domain scores (difference of more than 15 Index points) are present, do not rely on the FSIQ alone and evaluate significant differences between intellectual domains and academic achievement.

Discussion 11-1

The correct answer is "E." To start, remember that 100 is an average score, with a range of 86 to 114 on standard scoring. Intellectual and achievement tests cover a wide range of domains or skill sets. (See Table 6–5.) Variance between these domains (relative strengths and weaknesses for the child) is expected. This means that basing a diagnosis on just one composite score (FSIQ) would mask the variability across domains. Therefore, diagnosis based only on FSIQ (options "A" and "B") is not appropriate. Option "C" would be correct for those using the strict criterion cutoff model of special learning disabilities (SLD). However, this model misses disabilities in children with higher intellectual performance. For this child, his overall intellectual functioning is in the high-average to average range. His academic achievement scores are all above 85, but his reading scores are over 20 Index points lower than his overall intellectual functioning.

TABLE 6–5 COMPONENTS OF INTELLECTUAL, ACADEMIC ACHIEVEMENT, AND ADAPTIVE BEHAVIORAL ASSESSMENTS

Intellectual Assessment	Academic Achievement Assessment	Adaptive Behavioral Assessment
Intellectual Battery (Wechsler, Kaufman, Stanford-Binet)	*Reading Achievement*	*Conceptual*
Verbal comprehension	Phonological awareness	Communication
Visual-spatial	Rapid naming	Functional academics
Fluid reasoning	Reading accuracy/decoding	Self-direction
Working memory	Reading fluency	*Socialization*
Processing speed	Reading comprehension	Play and leisure
Select Neuropsychological Tests	Spelling	Interpersonal skills
Receptive and expressive language	*Math Achievement*	*Practical Skills*
Visual-spatial/motor integration	Computation	Community use
Working memory	Problem solving	Self-care
Processing speed	*Written Expression*	Health and safety
Fine motor coordination	Penmanship	Home living
	Grammar	*Motor Skills* (for young children)
	Fluency	

Reading is a relative weakness for him and this meets criteria for a diagnosis of a reading disorder based on the discrepancy model of SLD. It appears that option "D" should then be correct. However, there are large discrepancies (20 Index points) between his verbal and fluid reasoning indices within his total score (FSIQ), making interpretation using only FSIQ as the criterion line invalid. For this child, the entire pattern of strengths and weaknesses between his intellectual and achievement scores must be compared. He has disabilities in his verbal index of his total intellectual score (FSIQ) and reading in achievement scores.

> ▶ **CASE 12**

A 10-year-old boy is in the winter term of the fourth grade. As his pediatrician, you are aware that reading has been a struggle for him since he started school. He has participated in the Title 1 reading program for the past 3 years, with little improvement. His father has been talking to the school and they are going to move forward with evaluating him for possible special education services. His father is worried and uncertain about what will happen and asks you to discuss what you know about what the school will be doing as they evaluate his son.

Question 12-1

Which of the following is an appropriate method the child's school may use to determine the specialized education services he may or may not qualify for?
A) The school will require his father to hire a tutor outside of school to assist with his reading.
B) The school will refer the child to a specialist, who will evaluate his intellectual abilities and academic achievement to determine if he meets criteria for a reading disability and place him in a specialized reading class if he does.
C) The school has been monitoring his progress through both general classroom instruction and supplemental instruction (Title 1). Because he has failed to respond to these interventions, the school will place him in a specialized reading class for more intense instruction.
D) Either A or B may be appropriate.
E) Either B or C may be appropriate.

Discussion 12-1

The correct answer is "E." The need for special classroom placement is not measured consistently across the nation, or even within states or school districts. The qualification for placement is governed by the Individuals with Disabilities Act (IDEA), and there are three different methods that may be used. A specific learning disability (SLD) may be identified through testing (option "B"); either by (1) a discrepancy between the child's ability and achievement, or (2) evaluation of strengths and weaknesses. In 2004, IDEA was modified and included a third method of identification of children in need of specialized classroom placement. Children who failed to respond to "scientifically research-based" intervention also qualified (option "C"). This approach is referred to as Response to Intervention (RTI) and is employed within the school system, without outside evaluation of intellectual or academic functioning. Instead, students' progress is monitored through three tiers of instruction. Tier 1 is core classroom instruction. Students who struggle with this general instruction are taken to tier 2, where they are provided supplemental instruction for a brief period of time (perhaps 30 minutes per day). Students who continue to struggle after the implementation of tier 2 are taken to tier 3, which involves intense specialized instruction outside the general classroom.

> **Helpful Tip**
> Public law mandates braille instruction services for children with visual impairment who are deemed to need it.

► CASE 13

You are contacted by a local school. They have questions about a 5-year-old girl who is deaf and is about to start school. You explain that according to the Health Insurance Portability and Accountability Act (HIPAA), discussion of the child's protected health information is not permitted without the permission of the minor's legal guardian. You call the mother to discuss school options for her deaf child.

Question 13-1

What might be an appropriate school placement for her?
A) A specialized braille school because there are no special schools for children who are deaf in the area.
B) A specialized school for children who are deaf.
C) The public school where she has an individualized education plan (IEP) and an interpreter.
D) A private school where she is in regular classes without an interpreter.
E) Both B and C would be appropriate placements.

Discussion 13-1

The correct answer is "E." Many educational options are available for children who are deaf or have another sensory impairment, and the appropriate placement will depend on many factors. Such factors include the child's individual skills, the resources and qualifications of the staff at the potential settings, the goals of parents and educators, and the philosophy of the potential setting. Parents will need to decide what placement (specialized school, public school, private school, or homeschooling) is best for their child based on the individual needs of the child and family. As a pediatrician, you will be an important person in starting this conversation and helping parents understand and review their options. Regardless of the setting, children with sensory impairment need a team approach to education. Teams include parents, general and special education teachers, and specialists such as physical therapists, occupational therapists, and speech therapists. For children with a visual impairment, the educational team often contains a vision teacher, orientation and mobility specialist, early interventionist or special education teacher, and general teacher. Children who are deaf will likely have a sign language interpreter.

Helpful Tip

The individualized education program is mandated by law to help children with disabilities succeed in school. An individualized education plan (IEP) is created for the child based on his or her needs. If a child does not qualify for an individualized education program, he or she may be enrolled in a 504 plan. (See Table 6–6.) For non–school-age children, an individual family service plan (IFSP) specifies and provides early intervention services for children from birth to 3 years of age.

TABLE 6–6 COMPARISON OF A 504 PLAN AND AN INDIVIDUALIZED EDUCATION PLAN (IEP)

504 Plan	IEP
US Rehabilitation Act of 1973	Individuals with Disabilities Education Act (2004)
Modified education program	Modified education program
General classroom setting	May include special education setting
Monitored by classroom teacher	Monitored by additional support staff
Parental approval/involvement optional	Parental approval/involvement required
No documentation of growth	Documentation of measurable growth required
Can be applied in college	Cannot be applied in college

► CASE 14

A 12-year-old boy was recently diagnosed with a math disorder by a local psychologist. His mother is upset because his private school refuses to provide him services he qualifies for based on the Individuals with Disabilities Education Act (IDEA).

Question 14-1

What steps can you recommend to his mother to make sure he receives appropriate instruction?
A) The rights of children with disabilities are not the same within private schools. His mother will need to move to a public school to obtain resources provided through either a 504 plan or an IEP.
B) The rights of children with disabilities are not the same within private schools. However, individual schools may be willing to provide recommended accommodations or instruction outside of a 504 Plan or an IEP. His mother should discuss possibilities with the school.
C) The rights of children with disabilities are not the same within private schools. However, he may be able to enroll part-time in a nearby public school to obtain needed specialized instruction. His mother should discuss possibilities with the school.
D) The rights of children with disabilities are the same within private schools, and IDEA should apply to this child. His mother can request a hearing to challenge the eligibility decision.
E) Options A, B, and C may be appropriate.

Discussion 14-1

The correct answer is "E." The rights of children with disabilities are *not* the same within private schools. Services such as classroom accommodations and specialized instruction are

Balancing remediation and accommodations

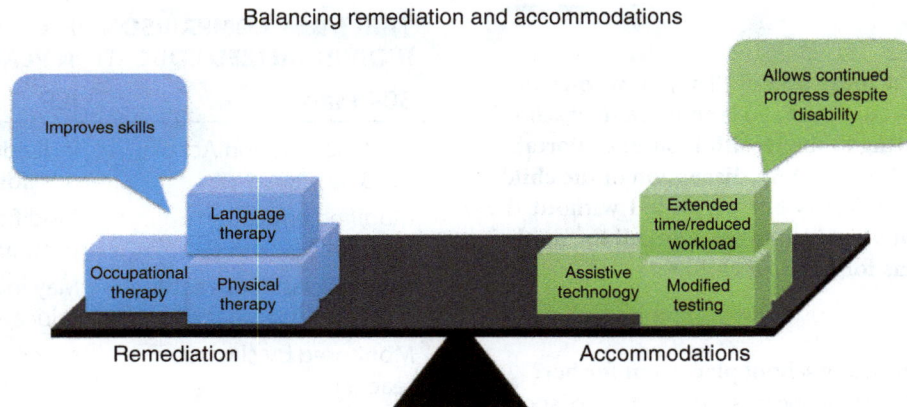

FIGURE 6–2. Balancing remediation and accommodations.

provided at the discretion of the school. Some private schools are willing to provide these services, and his mother should consult with the school to see what options are possible. If the school refuses to provide any services, another option would be to dual enroll him in a local public school, where he would qualify for services. The final option would be to enroll him full-time in a public school (or homeschool). Note that for parents who disagree with IEP determination within the *public* school setting, it is possible to request a hearing and challenge eligibility decisions.

> **Helpful Tip**
>
> The purpose of *remediation* (specialized instruction, language therapy, physical therapy, or occupational therapy) is to help improve the student's skills in areas where there are deficits. If the student's skills do not reach proficient levels, accommodations become important. *Accommodations* allow students to work around their deficit so they can continue to progress in other areas of instruction. Examples would include having math problems read aloud to a child with dyslexia or allowing a child with a written expressive disorder to dictate answers on a test. (See Figure 6–2.)

► CASE 15

A sixth grader at a middle school has dyslexia, but she has well developed cognitive skills in all areas. She does well academically as long as she has help with her reading requirements. She has most classes in the general education setting and has an IEP with accommodations. For many children with an IEP at this middle school, the special education teachers spend time in the regular education classrooms to help children with the curriculum and assist with implementation of accommodations.

Question 15-1

Is this an appropriate setting for her?
A) Yes; since she is able to comprehend and learn grade-level material she does not necessarily need pull-out services, and having accommodations and someone available if she is struggling may be sufficient for her.
B) Yes; it would not be appropriate to pull any child out of the regular classroom so all instruction should be done there.
C) No; any student with an IEP should receive pull-out services.
D) It does not matter; she should not have an IEP since she only has dyslexia.
E) No; obviously the school does not know what it is doing and her parents should consider transferring to another school.

Discussion 15-1

The correct answer is "A." Extra services can be delivered in many ways in the school setting and, as with anything, determining the best place for a student requires consideration of many things. With regard to this child, it is appropriate for her to have an IEP, and given her good cognitive skills and the fact that she is able to learn material with accommodations, there is no indication that she would need to be pulled out of the classroom. There are varying levels of support that schools can provide and it is important to provide the most inclusive education while meeting the student's educational goals. Some children with learning disabilities do not need any pull-out services if they have accommodations in the classroom. Other students may need to be pulled out of the classroom if they require specialized instruction. They might receive a half hour of instruction in one area, or receive all core curriculum in the pull-out classroom. It is important to consider the student's ability to understand and comprehend classroom material, the number and severity of learning disabilities, and the social development of the student.

CASE 16

A 16-year-old sophomore in high school has a significant medical history of difficult-to-control seizures. He has special education services at school, which includes assistance within the general education classroom. He is enrolled in regular sophomore-level courses. His parents feel that school is very difficult for him, even with the special education services. He recently came home in tears and told his parents that he had cheated on a Spanish test in order to get a good grade because he was not able to learn the material. His parents are concerned that he is not learning skills that will help him function independently after high school. He was referred for neuropsychological testing to determine his specific learning difficulties. Testing found that his FSIQ was 65 (with no significant variability between skills) and all of his academic skills were at an elementary level. His adaptive functioning was also low. He was diagnosed with intellectual disability, and recommendations were made for changes in his academic curriculum to focus on functional skills that were more at his level.

Question 16-1

Is this an appropriate setting for him?
A) Yes; he can learn basic skills to function independently after high school his education should focus on core curriculum subject matter.
B) Yes; his accommodations already include pulling him out of the classroom.
C) No; he should be homeschooled since his self-esteem is being negatively affected in public school.
D) It does not matter; his schooling should focus on socialization opportunities.
E) No; his educational goals should focus on acquiring adaptive skills to prepare him to live independently.

Discussion 16-1

The correct answer is "E." You knew the answer would be "no," which narrowed it down to two options, so you had a 50-50 chance of getting the question right. In contrast to the prior case involving the sixth-grade girl with dyslexia, this child does not have ability to comprehend classroom material and will need specialized, pull-out instruction so he can learn skills at his level that would allow him to function best. In his current curriculum, he was not learning and practicing skills that would help him be the most independent. He was very aware that he did not understand classroom material and was upset by this, and by the fact that he had cheated to help himself get a good grade because he did not understand the material. The constant exposure to the realization that he did not know the material was negatively affecting his self-esteem. His difficulties are more global and therefore he will need more support. The educational goals of these two children are likely very different. The high school boy's parents want him to be able to live independently and have a job, and his education should focus on this because

he will need more instruction to learn these basic skills. However, the sixth-grade girl wants to go to college and is able to comprehend classroom material, so she would benefit from taking classes that will help prepare her for college.

> **Helpful Tip**
> The main goal of *early intervention* (provided in preschool or early elementary school) is to provide remediation at the earliest point possible. Earlier intervention allows more time to work on deficient skills, leading to better outcomes, and in the setting of reading disabilities accommodations may not be needed later in school.

CASE 17

Your patient is in her first semester of junior high school. She was diagnosed with ADHD when she was 9 years old and is followed by you for her stimulant medication. The medication does help her focus, but she struggles with skills of organization and memory. Maria has an active 504 plan and in the sixth grade, her teachers followed recommendations to increase communication with her parents regarding assignments and her progress. She was able to achieve A's and B's. However, in the junior high, students are expected to organize and remember their assignments independently. Despite encouragement from her parents and effort on her part, she consistently forgets and misplaces weekly assignments. She is at risk of failing two of her classes. Her parents think that her medication dose should be increased to address these issues.

Question 17-1

What do you suggest?
A) Temporarily increase her dose and instruct her parents to monitor her progress closely. If things at school do not improve you will return her to the original dosage and suggest her parents consult with the school.
B) Suggest that her parents discuss her need for classroom accommodations with the school. With her 504 plan still active, she is eligible to receive these services.
C) Suggest that her parents discuss possible special education placement, such as a homeroom or study hall where a teacher can monitor her progress.
D) Increase her medication dose and suggest that her parents also discuss possible classroom accommodations with the school.
E) None of the above.

Discussion 17-1

The correct answer is "B." Environmental or behavioral interventions should always be closely evaluated before making decisions about stimulant medication dosage. The child's classroom environment has drastically changed, imposing strong requirements on areas in which she has known weaknesses (ie, organization and memory). It is doubtful that changes to her medication will improve her performance. The transition to junior high can be especially difficult for students with ADHD. While their peers may be able to take on responsibility for organization of their assignments, this is often a skill children with ADHD are not yet ready for. They still require accommodations that provide organizational assistance. Specialized instruction placement can be very helpful for children who need it. However, if the same achievement levels can be reached within the general classroom with some accommodations, then this would be the optimum placement. Given the success of the accommodations in the sixth grade, it would be beneficial to reimplement accommodations before putting her in a specialized classroom.

► CASE 18

A third-grade boy with average intelligence is sensitive and seems concerned about what his peers think of him. However, he gets along well with peers in his class and has several close friends in his grade. He has recently received a diagnosis of dyslexia and has begun special education services. His parents are wondering if they should retain him in third grade next year to allow him to catch up with his peers so that he would not have to have special education.

Question 18-1

Which of the following would be an appropriate response to the parents?

A) Suggest they retain him because even though he has a learning disability, the repeated exposure would be good and he can just make new friends.

B) Suggest they not retain him because he is so sensitive it may be bad for his self-esteem.

C) Discuss in more detail their reasoning for wanting to retain him.

D) Ask if either of them were retained and how they liked it.

E) Discuss with them the factors that should be considered, their goals for his education, and reason they feel retention would be good.

Discussion 18-1

The correct answer is "E". The decision to retain a child is not an easy one and should take into consideration many different factors. Without a thorough discussion with parents about their goals, reasons for wanting to retain the child, and other relevant factors, a pediatrician should not make a specific suggestion as to whether to retain the child. One factor to consider is the child's intellectual, developmental, and academic skills. If the child has a delay and it is felt that, given the extra year, his skills would reach grade level it may be appropriate to consider retention. However, if the child's ability to learn and reason is the same as that of his same-age peers but he has a specific

learning disorder; it is unlikely that an extra year in a grade will help him catch up. It is also important to take social and emotional factors into consideration. If the child is particularly shy or sensitive, holding him back may negatively affect his socialization or self-esteem. The grade at which a child is retained also plays a factor. Holding back children in kindergarten, when development is progressing rapidly, has different implications than holding them back in fifth grade, when they have established solid friendships and development and skills are growing more slowly.

► CASE 19

A 6-year-old boy has been displaying a pattern of challenging behaviors at home and school. His mother reports that he frequently argues and disobeys rules, refuses to complete homework or do his chores, and is constantly fighting with his younger sibling and classmates. His teacher expressed concern about his academic performance and challenging behavior at a recent parent–teacher conference.

Question 19-1

Which of the following is an appropriate response to these concerns?

A) Refer him for a specialized evaluation to address learning, attention, and behavioral concerns.

B) Refer him to a local play therapist.

C) Encourage careful monitoring of his progress over the next year.

D) Discuss pharmacologic options with his mother.

E) Encourage increased participation in community-based activities to give him an appropriate "outlet" for his energy.

Discussion 19-1

The correct answer is "A." Based on the available information, he is experiencing significant behavioral difficulties in two settings (home and school) and is displaying several symptoms of oppositional defiant disorder (ODD); however, learning and attentional concerns may also be contributing to his difficulties. Disruptive behaviors can take the form of frequent and intense tantrums, refusal to follow rules, argumentativeness, lying and stealing, and aggression. It is important to distinguish developmentally appropriate oppositional behaviors from the more severe and pervasive behaviors that characterize a diagnosis of ODD. An interdisciplinary mental health evaluation can help with diagnostic clarification and with identifying appropriate interventions. Although options "B" and "D" may be appropriate components of a treatment plan, it is important to first conduct a thorough assessment. Option "C" is not recommended because he is experiencing functional impairment, and challenging behaviors do not typically decrease without intervention. Option "E" is not recommended because it is not an evidence-supported intervention for challenging behaviors.

He is seen by a pediatric psychologist, child psychiatrist, educational consultant, and social worker for a comprehensive assessment.

Question 19-2

What types of assessment measures would you anticipate being administered at the evaluation?

A) Achievement and cognitive testing to rule out possible learning disabilities.

B) Structured clinical parent interview to gather information about his developmental and family histories, and to clarify the presence of coexisting disorders.

C) Physical examination and medical interview to rule out a possible medical cause.

D) Standardized parent and teacher behavior rating scales.

E) All of the above.

Discussion 19-2

The correct answer is "E." History and physical exam are always the first steps, so having these listed as separate choices told you that option "E" had to be correct. The assessment should be multimethod, including the use of parent and child interviews, standardized teacher and parent rating scales, evaluation of comorbid psychiatric disorders, and a review of the patient's social, medical, and family histories.

At the conclusion of the evaluation, he is diagnosed with ODD.

Question 19-3

Which of the following are appropriate frontline treatments for management of this diagnosis?

A) Behavioral parent training.

B) Classroom-based behavioral interventions.

C) Cognitive behavioral therapy.

D) Pharmacologic intervention.

E) Options A, B, and C.

Discussion 19-3

The correct answer is "E." Behavioral interventions targeting oppositional behaviors have a strong evidence base. Cognitive behavioral treatments, such as problem-solving skills training, have also been demonstrated to result in significant decrease in problem behaviors and increases in appropriate social behaviors. In comparison to the strong evidence base for use with ADHD, psychostimulant medications have more limited research support in the treatment of ODD and, in most cases, behavioral interventions should be considered before medication.

▶ CASE 20

An 8-year-old girl was recently diagnosed with a significant reading disability and ADHD. Her parents express concern that she is becoming increasingly withdrawn and anxious, and appears to be experiencing social difficulties with classmates.

Question 20-1

What types of approaches should be considered to address these concerns?

A) Systematic phonics instruction and vocabulary development.

B) A reinforcement-based program focused on increasing on-task behavior.

C) Individual counseling to address anxiety and increase her self-concept.

D) Peer buddy program to increase opportunities for positive peer interactions

E) All of the above.

Discussion 20-1

The correct answer is "E." As a group, children with learning disabilities are at higher risk for anxiety, depression, social difficulties, learned helplessness, and low academic and social self-concept (impression of self) compared with students who do not have a learning disability. It is important to keep in mind that, while students with a learning disability are more likely to struggle and require individualized intervention, many students with a learning disability do not experience these difficulties. The cause for the association between learning disabilities and higher likelihood of anxiety, depression, and low self-concept does not appear to be straightforward. Students' difficulties may result from repeated failure to master academic concepts and an emerging awareness (and embarrassment) over poor performance relative to classmates. Treatments targeting academic performance, attention difficulties, and symptoms of anxiety, depression, and low self-concept have been shown to be effective. For younger students with learning disabilities, academic interventions have resulted in improvements in self-concept. Treatments that focus on improving social skills, interpersonal problem solving, and self-control have been shown to increase self-concept for older students with learning disabilities.

BIBLIOGRAPHY

AAIDD Ad Hoc Committee on Terminology and Classification. *Intellectual Disability: Definition, Classification, and Systems of Supports.* 11th ed. Washington, DC: American Association on Intellectual and Developmental Disabilities; 2010.

American Academy of Pediatrics. Policy statement: Ethical and policy issues in genetic testing and screening of children. *Pediatrics.* 2013;131:620–622. Available online at http://pediatrics.aappublications.org/content/131/3/620. Accessed October 10, 2015.

American Psychiatric Association. *Diagnostic and Statistical Manual of Mental Disorders.* 5th ed. Washington, DC: APA; 2013.

Autism and Developmental Disabilities Monitoring Network Surveillance Year 2010 Principal Investigators; Centers for Disease Control and Prevention. Prevalence of autism spectrum disorders—Autism and Developmental Disabilities Monitoring Network, 14 sites, United States, 2010. *MMWR Surveill Summ.* 2014;63:SS-2.

Bradley R, Danielson L, Hallahan DP. *Identification of Learning Disabilities: Research to Practice.* Mahwah, NJ: Lawrence Erlbaum Associates; 2002.

Center for Disease Control. Prevalence of Autism Spectrum Disorders Among Children Aged 8 Years – Autism and Developmental Disabilities Monitoring Network. *MMWR Surveill Summ*. 2014;63(2).

Carey WB, Crocker AC, Coleman WL, et al. *Developmental-Behavioral Pediatrics*. 4th ed. Philadelphia, PA: Elsevier-Health Sciences Division; 2009.

Christopherson ER, VanScoyoc SM. Diagnosis and management of disruptive behavior disorder. In Christopherson ER, VanScoyoc SM, eds. *Treatments that Work with Children: Empirically Supported Strategies for Managing Childhood Problems*. 2nd ed. Washington, DC: American Psychological Association; 2013:9–34.

Demouy J, Plaza M, Xavier J, et al. Differential language markers of pathology in autism, pervasive developmental disorder not otherwise specified and specific language impairment. *Res Autism Spectrum Disord*. 2011;5:1402–1412.

Dykens EM, Lenze M. Intellectual disabilities and autism spectrum disorder: A cautionary note. In Amaral DG, Dawson G, Geschwind DH, eds. *Autism Spectrum Disorders*. Oxford, England: Oxford University Press; 2011:315–329.

Fletcher-Janzen E, Reynolds CR, eds. *Neuropsychological Perspectives on Learning Disabilities in the Era of RTI: Recommendations for Diagnosis and Intervention*. Hoboken, NJ: John Wiley; 2008.

Harpin V, Mazzone L, Raynaud JP, et al. Long-term outcomes of ADHD: A systematic review of self-esteem and social function. *J Attention Disord*. 2013; May 22. [Epub ahead of print]

Learning Disabilities Association of America. Doctor-to-Doctor: Information on learning disabilities for pediatricians and other physicians. http://ldaamerica.org/doctor-to-doctor-information-on-learning-disabilities-for-pediatricians-and-other=physicians/. Accessed January 22, 2015.

Lecavalier L, Snow AV, Norris M. Autism spectrum disorders and intellectual disability. In Matson JL, Sturmey P, eds. *International Handbook of Autism and Pervasive Developmental Disorders*. New York, NY: Springer Science; 2011;37–51.

Mather N, Wendling BJ. *Essentials of Dyslexia Assessment and Intervention*. Hoboken, NJ: John Wiley; 2012.

Matson JL, Neal D. Differentiating communication disorders and autism in children. *Res Autism Spectrum Disord*. 2010;4:626–632.

Matson JL, Shoemaker M. Intellectual disability and its relationship to autism spectrum disorders. *Res Dev Disabil*. 2009;30:1107–1114.

Nelson JM, Harwood H. Learning disability and anxiety: A meta-analysis. *J Learning Disabil*. 2011;44:3–17.

Shaywitz S. *Overcoming Dyslexia: A New and Complete Science-based Program for Reading Problems at Any Level*. New York, NY: Vintage Books; 2003.

Tomblin JB, McGregor K, Bean A. Specific language impairment. In Amaral DG, Dawson G, Geschwind DH, eds. *Autism Spectrum Disorders*. Oxford, England: Oxford University Press; 2011:315–329.

Worley JA, Matson JL, Kozlowski AM. The effects of hearing impairment on symptoms of autism in toddlers. *Devel Neurorehabil*. 2011;14:171–176.

Collagen Vascular and Other Multisystem Disorders

7

Sandy Hong

► CASE 1

A 14-year-old adolescent girl presents with a history of low-grade fevers for 1 week, a rash on her face, painful swelling of her knee, and calf swelling. She reports chest pain when she takes a deep breath. On exam she has oral ulcers on the hard palate and butterfly-shaped redness on her cheeks and the bridge of her nose. Her knee is swollen, warm, and painful to move. The cardiac exam is normal. (See Figure 7–1.)

Question 1-1
What is the diagnosis?
A) Acute rheumatic fever.
B) Influenza.
C) Systemic lupus erythematosus.
D) Fibromyalgia.
E) Endocarditis.

Discussion 1-1
The correct answer is "C." Painless oral ulcers and her malar "butterfly" rash shout that this is systemic lupus erythematosus (SLE). SLE is a chronic autoimmune disease that affects multiple organ systems. It is more common in females and African Americans. It can occur in any age group but is uncommon in young children. The severity varies and intermittent flares are common.

Question 1-2
What is NOT a diagnostic criterion for SLE from the American College of Rheumatology (ACR)?
A) Photosensitivity.
B) Arthritis.
C) Proteinuria.
E) Pericardial effusion.
D) Thrombocytosis.

Discussion 1-2
The correct answer is "D." SLE is associated with thrombocytopenia not thrombocytosis. SLE is a clinical diagnosis with antibodies to nuclear antigens present. According to the ACR, 4 of 11 criteria should be present. (See Table 7–1.) Constitutional symptoms, fever, fatigue, and myalgia, are common. For the 14-year-old patient, her criteria for lupus are malar rash, arthritis, renal disease (clue was the calf swelling and edema), oral ulcers, and serositis (pleuritic chest pain). Renal involvement makes this unlikely to be rheumatic fever.

> **Helpful Tip**
> Early laboratory abnormalities in SLE include cytopenias such as leukopenia or thrombocytopenia (think petechiae) and abnormal urinalysis indicative of renal disease. So if you are thinking lupus, *do* obtain a complete blood count (CBC) and urinalysis! An antinuclear antibody (ANA) test is usually positive but is only one of the ACR criteria. (See Table 7–2.)

She is being treated with steroids and cyclophosphamide and is in remission. Four months later she presents with constant right knee pain that occurs during the day and night. It is not relieved with movement. The knee exam is normal.

Question 1-3
What is the cause of her pain?
A) Arthritis from an SLE flare.
B) Growing pains.
C) Avascular necrosis.
D) Bursitis.
E) Torn ligament.

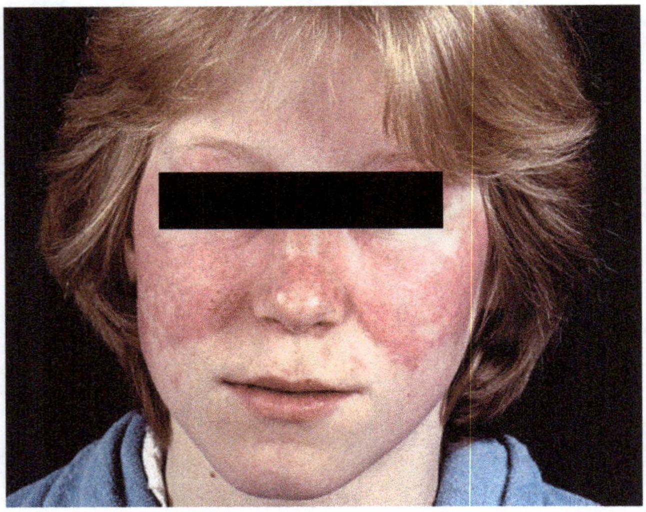

FIGURE 7–1. Malar rash of systemic lupus erythematosus. Classic butterfly rash of systemic lupus erythematosus covering both cheeks and the bridge of the nose. The nasolabial folds are spared. (Reproduced with permission from Wolff K, Johnson RA, and Saavedra AP, eds. *Fitzpatrick's Color Atlas and Synopsis of Clinical Dermatology*. 7th ed. New York, NY: McGraw-Hill Education; 2013, Fig. 14-33.)

TABLE 7–1   REVISED CRITERIA FOR CLASSIFICATION OF SYSTEMIC LUPUS ERYTHEMATOSUS FROM THE AMERICAN COLLEGE OF RHEUMATOLOGY (ACR)

Malar rash
Discoid rash
Photosensitivity
Oral ulcers
Arthritis
Serositis
   Pleuritis (pleuritic pain, rub, effusion)
   Pericarditis (documented by ECG, rub, effusion)
Renal disorder
   Casts (red cell or other)
   Proteinuria
Neurologic disorder
   Seizures
   Psychosis
Hematologic disorder
   Leukopenia
   Lymphopenia
   Thrombocytopenia
   Hemolytic anemia
Immunologic disorder
   Anti-DNA antibody
   Anti-Smith antibody
   False-positive rapid plasma reagin (RPR) for syphilis
Positive antinuclear antibody (ANA)

Adapted with permission from Tan EM, Cohen AS, Fries JF et al: The 1982 revised criteria for the classification of systemic lupus erythematosus, *Arthritis Rheum*. 1982 Nov;25(11):1271–1277.

TABLE 7–2   COMMON LABORATORY FINDINGS IN SYSTEMIC LUPUS ERYTHEMATOSUS (SLE)

Leukopenia
Lymphopenia
Thrombocytopenia
Anemia: hemolytic or chronic disease
Elevated erythrocyte sedimentation rate (ESR)
Elevated C-reactive protein (CRP)
Antinuclear antibody (ANA)
Anti–double-stranded DNA antibody (dsDNA)
Anti-Smith antibody
Antiphospholipid antibody
Decreased C3, C4 (complement levels)
Urinalysis: hematuria, proteinuria, casts, pyuria

Discussion 1-3

The correct answer is "C." The treatment of SLE depends on the severity. Mild cases can be treated with nonsteroidal anti-inflammatory drugs (NSAIDs) and antimalarial drugs. Severe cases require steroids or immunosuppressive therapies such as cyclophosphamide, or both. Avascular necrosis (osteonecrosis) can occur at any time during treatment with steroids and for 2 to 3 years after treatment with high-dose steroids is completed. The pathogenesis is unknown. Pain is the most common presenting symptom. Magnetic resonance imaging (MRI) without contrast is the diagnostic test of choice as plain films can be normal early in the disease, but always obtain plain films first. Other adverse effects of steroids include osteoporosis, cataract, diabetes mellitus, adrenal suppression, immunosuppression, poor growth, Cushing syndrome, and obesity. The patient is likely *not* growing on steroids. Growing pains are usually bilateral, localized to the calves, and present primarily at night. She lacks classic inflammatory symptoms (swelling, warmth) for arthritis. The physical exam would be abnormal for bursitis (swelling, tenderness) and a torn ligament.

> **Helpful Tip**
> Inflammatory joint symptoms of arthritis include:
> - Swelling or effusion, or both
> - Warmth
> - Pain
> - Limitation of movement
> - Morning stiffness or stiffness after sitting (gelling phenomenon)
> - Mild relief of stiffness with movement

> **Helpful Tip**
> Arthritis from rheumatologic conditions involves inflammation of the joint. Synovitis is inflammation of the synovium (joint lining). Both cause joint swelling, effusion, warmth, pain, and loss of motion.

> **Helpful Tip**
> Avoidance of sunlight is important in SLE as it may trigger rashes in those with photosensitivity.

QUICK QUIZ

Which is NOT a feature of acute rheumatic fever (ARF)?
A) Polyarthritis.
B) Erythema marginatum.
C) Carditis.
D) Chorea.
E) Malar rash.

Discussion

The correct answer is "E." ARF is a sequela of untreated group A streptococcal pharyngitis. Diagnosis is based on the modified Jones criteria, requiring evidence of infection and two major or one major and two minor manifestations. (See Table 7–3.) However, chorea alone makes the diagnosis. (See Figure 7–2.) The arthritis is migratory and very responsive to NSAIDs. If not reconsider the diagnosis. In carditis, a murmur is usually present from involvement of the valves.

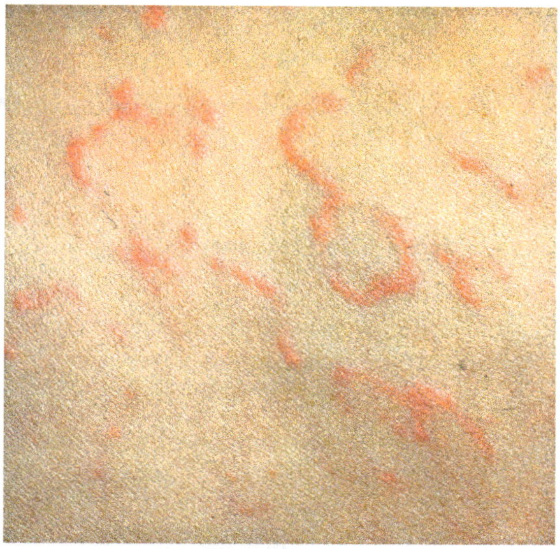

FIGURE 7–2. Erythema marginatum is one of the major criteria in the Jones criteria for diagnosing acute rheumatic fever. It is described as pink rings located on the trunk and extremities. The face is spared. The lesions expand and move from one location to another. (Reproduced with permission from Goldsmith LA, Katz SI, Gilchrest BA, et al, eds. *Fitzpatrick's Dermatology in General Medicine.* 8th ed. New York, NY: McGraw-Hill Education; 2012, Fig. 160-5.)

▶ CASE 2

An 8-year-old girl presents with bilateral ankle pain, a purpuric/petechial rash on her legs, and swelling of her feet. She has no fever. She reports having had rhinorrhea a week ago. Laboratory tests show a normal CBC, and Lyme and ASO titers are negative. She has mild hematuria and no proteinuria.

TABLE 7–3 JONES CRITERIA FOR DIAGNOSIS OF ACUTE RHEUMATIC FEVER

Major manifestations (PECCS mnemonic)

Polyarthritis

Erythema marginatum

Chorea

Carditis

Subcutaneous nodules

Minor manifestations

Fever

Arthralgias

Elevated CRP or ESR

Prolonged PR interval (PR > 0.2 seconds)

Evidence of group A streptococcal infection

Positive throat culture or rapid antigen tests

Elevated antibody titer (ASO, DNase B)

CRP, C-reactive protein; ESR, erythrocyte sedimentation rate.

Question 2-1

What is the diagnosis?
A) Post-streptococcal arthritis.
B) Lyme disease.
C) Systemic lupus erythematosus.
D) Henoch-Schönlein purpura.
E) Immune thrombocytopenia.

Discussion 2-1

The correct answer is "D." Henoch-Schönlein purpura (HSP), or IgA vasculitis, causes a characteristic rash (nonthrombocytopenic palpable purpura); arthritis or arthralgias, or both; colicky abdominal pain; and renal disease. The history of a recent upper respiratory tract infection is classic for HSP. For the diagnosis to be HSP, the platelet count and coagulation studies must be normal. (See Table 7–4 and Figure 7–3.) Patients with lupus usually present with an abnormal CBC, indicating leukopenia, thrombocytopenia, anemia, or a combination of these. The patient's Lyme titer is negative, and Lyme arthritis tends to be in the knees. This is unlikely streptococcal disease as the patient's ASO titer is negative, she has no history of pharyngitis, and it would not explain the rash. Her platelet count is normal, ruling out immune thrombocytopenia.

Question 2-2

What treatment do you recommend for HSP?
A) NSAIDs.
B) Prednisone.
C) IVIG.
D) Morphine.
E) Nothing.

TABLE 7–4 MANIFESTATIONS OF HENOCH-SCHÖNLEIN PURPURA

Rash	Dark-red and purple lesions on the lower extremities and buttocks (classic)
	Symmetric
Edema/Swelling	Hands and feet
	Scrotum
	Around the eyes
Gastrointestinal	Colicky abdominal pain
	Vomiting
	Intussusception
	Hematemesis, hematochezia, melena
	Perforation, ischemia
Renal	Hematuria
	Proteinuria
	Nephritis
	Nephrotic syndrome
	Hypertension
	End-stage kidney disease
Neurologic	Headaches
	Seizures
	Ataxia
Constitutional	Fever
	Malaise
Musculoskeletal	Arthralgia
	Arthritis

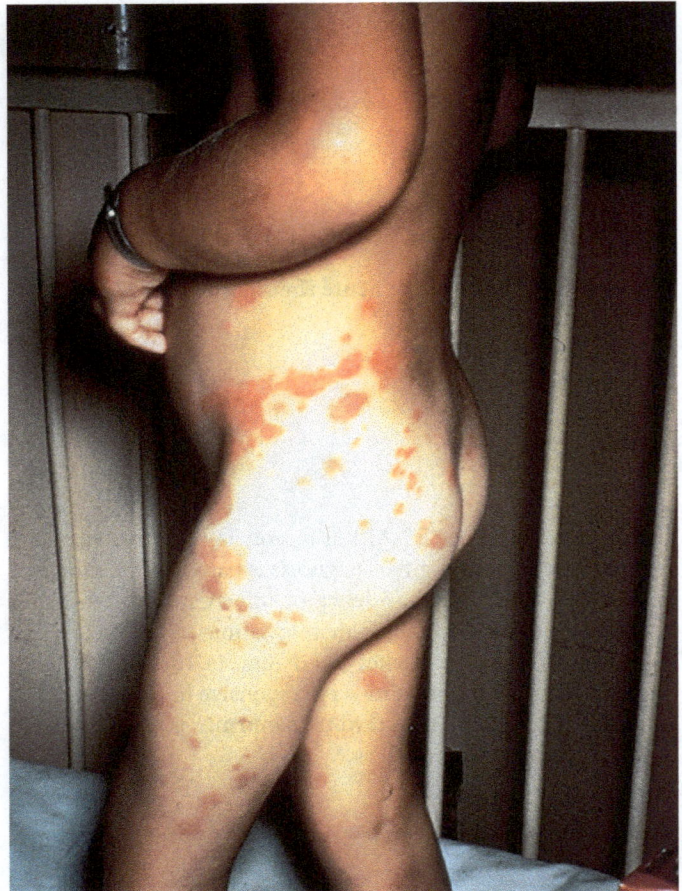

FIGURE 7–3. Henoch-Schönlein purpura (HSP). Symmetric palpable purpura on the lower extremities and buttocks of a child with HSP. (Reproduced with permission from Knoop KJ, Stack LB, Storrow AB, et al: *The Atlas of Emergency Medicine*, 3ed. McGraw-Hill Education, Inc., 2010. Fig 15-23. Photo contributor: Ralph A. Gruppo, MD.)

Discussion 2-2

The correct answer is "A." NSAIDs are given for relief of joint and abdominal pain. Avoid NSAIDs if the patient has significant kidney disease or active gastrointestinal bleeding. Save corticosteroids (prednisone) for patients with severe abdominal pain or inability to walk due to arthritis; otherwise try to avoid prescribing them.

> **Helpful Tip**
> All patients with HSP should have follow-up urinalysis and blood pressure checks monthly for 6 months. Renal involvement may develop up to 6 months after presentation.

> **Helpful Tip**
> In atypical cases, abdominal pain or arthritis will be the presenting sign of HSP. The diagnosis becomes clear when the rash develops. If in doubt, you can obtain a biopsy the skin or kidney to look for IgA deposits.

QUICK QUIZ

What is the most characteristic renal finding in patients with HSP?

A) Macroscopic hematuria
B) Microscopic hematuria
C) Proteinuria
D) Hypertension
E) Elevated serum creatinine

Discussion

The correct answer is "B." Renal involvement occurs in 20% to 50% of children with HSP but less than 5% go on to develop end-stage renal disease. Any of the findings listed may occur, but microscopic hematuria is most common. Signs and symptoms of renal disease usually develop 2 to 6 weeks after presentation. Nephrotic range proteinuria, elevated serum creatinine, and hypertension are signs that progressive kidney disease will develop.

► CASE 3

A 5-year-old boy presents with 7 days of fever to 39.4°C (103°F) daily. He is irritable and has a morbilliform rash, conjunctivitis, swelling of his feet, and large adenopathy of the neck. Laboratory tests show leukocytosis, anemia, elevated alanine aminotransferase (ALT), and pyuria.

Question 3-1

What is the diagnosis?
A) Measles.
B) Stevens-Johnson syndrome.
C) Kawasaki disease.
D) Scarlet fever.
E) Adenovirus infection.

Discussion 3-1

The correct answer is "C." Kawasaki disease is a vasculitis affecting children typically between 6 months and 6 years of age. Symptoms self-resolve after 2 weeks. However, without treatment up to 25% of patients will develop coronary artery aneurysms. Table 7–5 shows characteristic laboratory abnormalities. The differential diagnosis includes viral infections (adenovirus, measles), Stevens-Johnson syndrome, and scarlet fever.

⧗ QUICK QUIZ

Which is NOT a diagnostic criterion of Kawasaki disease?
A) Exudative conjunctivitis.
B) Lymphadenopathy.
C) Strawberry tongue.
D) Feet swelling.
E) Urticarial rash.

TABLE 7–5 LABORATORY ABNORMALITIES IN ACUTE KAWASAKI DISEASE

Neutrophilic leukocytosis

Elevated C-reactive protein

Elevate erythrocyte sedimentation rate

Anemia for age

Thrombocytosis after the first week (can exceed 1 million/mm³)

Thrombocytopenia from disseminated intravascular coagulation (DIC)—*rare*

Hyponatremia

Hypoalbuminemia

Elevated serum gamma glutamyl transpeptidase (GGT)

Elevate serum liver transaminases

Sterile pyuria

Cerebral spinal fluid pleocytosis

Leukocytosis in synovial fluid

Discussion

The correct answer is "A." The diagnosis of Kawasaki disease requires fever for 5 or more days plus four or more of the following five clinical characteristics:

- Conjunctivitis: bilateral, nonexudative, bulbar with limbus sparing (key)
- Oropharyngeal changes: cracked lips, pharyngeal erythema, strawberry tongue
- Cervical lymphadenopathy: unilateral, typically painless
- Extremity changes: swelling of the hands or feet, erythema of the palms or soles
- Rash: erythematous, polymorphic

Pharyngitis with exudates or ulcers, purulent conjunctivitis, and bullous or vesicular rash are not seen in Kawasaki disease. Check the perineum for the rash as it is more prominent there and may desquamate early. Weeks after the fever, peeling under the nail beds of the fingers and toes may occur. Abdominal complaints (pain, diarrhea, and vomiting) are common. (See Figures 7–4 through 7–6.)

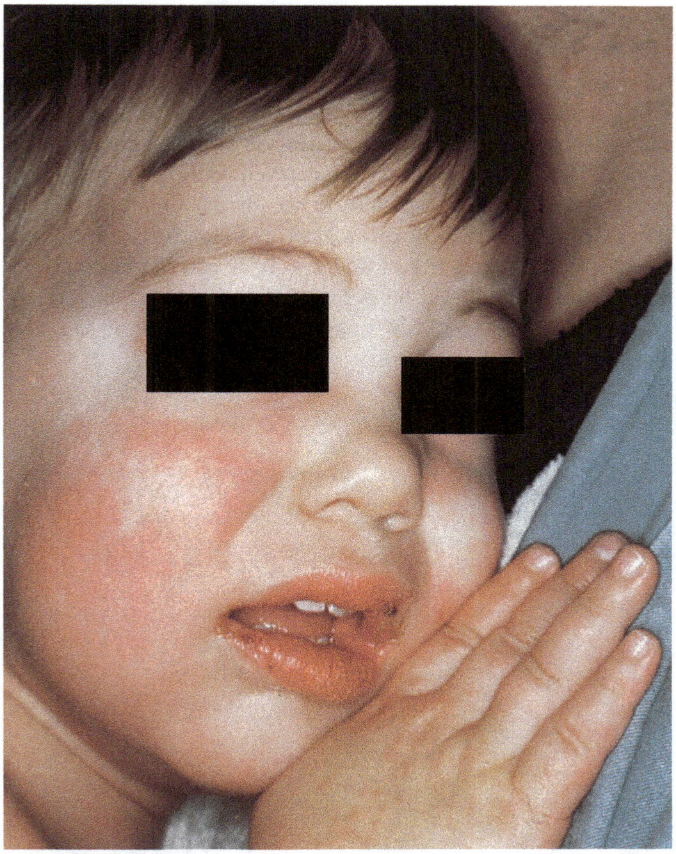

FIGURE 7–4. Kawasaki disease. A young boy with prolonged fever and (1) red, cracked lips; (2) red, edematous hands; (3) nonexudative conjunctivitis; and (4) morbilliform rash. He has four of five diagnostic criteria consistent with Kawasaki disease. (Reproduced with permission from Wolff K, Johnson RA, Saavedra AP, eds. *Fitzpatrick's Color Atlas and Synopsis of Clinical Dermatology*. 7th ed. New York, NY: McGraw-Hill Education; 2013, Fig. 14-66.)

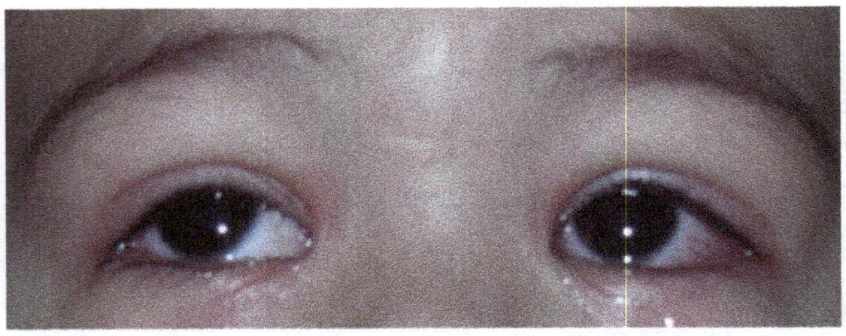

FIGURE 7–5. In Kawasaki disease, the conjunctiva is injected and the limbus is spared, and without exudate. (Reproduced with permission from Goldsmith LA, Katz SI, Gilchrest BA, et al, eds. *Fitzpatrick's Dermatology in General Medicine*. 8th ed. New York, NY: McGraw-Hill Education; 2012, Fig. 167-5.)

Question 3-2

What tests do you order now?

A) Abdominal ultrasound.
B) Echocardiogram.
C) Rapid streptococcal antigen test of the oropharynx.
D) Blood culture.
E) Urinalysis.

Discussion 3-2

The correct answer is "B." You already established that he has Kawasaki disease so additional laboratory testing to support or look for an alternative diagnosis is not needed. A baseline echocardiogram should be performed as soon as the diagnosis is suspected. Treatment should not be delayed waiting for the test or its results. Aneurysms typically do not form before day 10 of the illness, so the initial echocardiogram is frequently normal. For uncomplicated cases (heart and coronary arteries normal), an echocardiogram should be performed at diagnosis, at 2 weeks and at 6 to 8 weeks after the onset of Kawasaki disease to evaluate for coronary artery aneurysms.

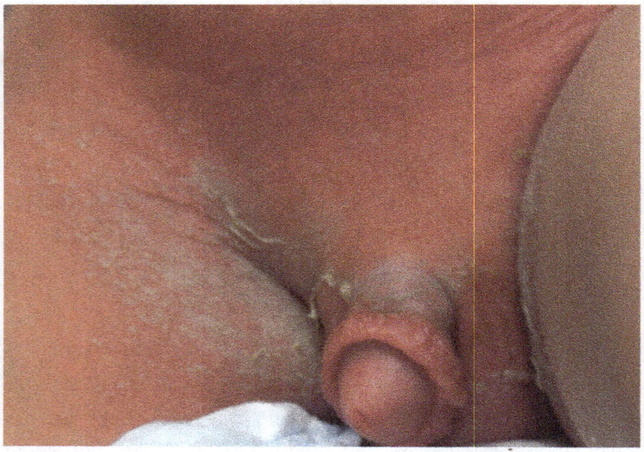

FIGURE 7–6. Desquamation and erythema of the perineum in a boy with Kawasaki disease. The rash frequently starts in the perineum. (Reproduced with permission from Goldsmith LA, Katz SI, Gilchrest BA, et al, eds. *Fitzpatrick's Dermatology in General Medicine*. 8th ed. New York, NY: McGraw-Hill Education; 2012, Fig. 167-3.)

Helpful Tip
Hydrops of the gallbladder (distention not due to stones) can be seen at presentation in patients with Kawasaki disease.

Question 3-3

When is the ideal time to treat this patient with IVIG (intravenous immunoglobulin)?

A) By day 12 of fever.
B) By day 5 of fever.
C) By day 10 of fever.
D) Never.
E) After systemic steroids fail to resolve the fever.

Discussion 3-3

The correct answer is "C." Once the diagnosis is made, acute Kawasaki disease is treated with a single dose of IVIG and high-dose aspirin. Treatment is indicated until 10 days after the onset of fever (earlier is better). The reason IVIG is effective is unknown. About 15% of patients fail to respond (defined as fever that persists or returns ≥ 36 hours after completion of the initial IVIG infusion). A second dose of IVIG is usually given. Other options include steroids and infliximab but these are usually reserved for third-line therapy. Patients should be afebrile for at least 48 hours after completion of their IVIG infusion before discharge. Once the patient has been afebrile for 48 hours (some sources recommend waiting 2 weeks), aspirin can be decreased to a low dose for thrombosis prevention. Low-dose aspirin is continued for 6 to 8 weeks. It can be stopped if the echocardiogram at that time is normal. If aneurysms are present, aspirin is continued indefinitely. Measles and varicella vaccines should be delayed for 11 months after administration of IVIG. When lose-dose aspirin is being taken, use of ibuprofen should be avoided. The child should receive a seasonal influenza vaccine because of the risk of Reye syndrome.

Helpful Tip
Treating a patient with Kawasaki disease before day 10 of fever decreases the risk of coronary disease. Treatment before day 5 is sometimes associated with increased resistance and need for retreatment.

Helpful Tip
Urethritis causes the sterile pyuria seen in Kawasaki disease. Urine collected by catheter or suprapubic aspirate will be normal. Order a bag or clean-catch specimen.

Helpful Tip
A child with fever lasting for 5 days or longer and two or three clinical criteria should be evaluated for incomplete Kawasaki disease. A diagnostic algorithm for this condition was created in 2004 by the American Heart Association.

Helpful Tip

IVIG can cause hemolytic anemia. This has been described in children treated for Kawasaki disease.

▶ CASE 4

A 9-year-old girl presents with fever, rash, and bilateral joint swelling of the wrists and knees. Once per day, she has a fever associated with a rash. Her temperature is 39°C (102.2°F). On exam, she appears ill and uncomfortable. She has tachycardia, tachypnea, hepatosplenomegaly, and warm, painful swelling of multiple joints. A rub is present on cardiac exam. Salmon-colored macules are present on her back and abdomen.

Question 4-1

What is the diagnosis?
A) Parvovirus B19 infection.
B) Lyme disease.
C) Systemic-onset juvenile idiopathic arthritis.
D) Leukemia.
E) None of the above.

Discussion 4-1

The correct answer is "C." Juvenile idiopathic arthritis (JIA) is a group of chronic diseases causing arthritis of unknown etiology affecting children and adolescents younger than 16 years of age. Arthritis must be present in the same joint for more than 6 weeks to diagnosis JIA. Disorders described by the term *JIA* are grouped into seven categories. (See Table 7–6 and Figure 7–7.) In Lyme disease, the rash is annular, red, and expands to classically form a bull's eye (erythema migrans). Lyme arthritis differs from JIA in that joints have large effusions and minimal pain. Malignancy (especially leukemia) mimics JIA. Typically only one joint is involved and pain is severe. Bone pain and pain during the night are red flags for malignancy. Fever is not intermittent and arthritis is transient in parvovirus B19 infections. In this patient, the fever, rash, and arthritis should point you toward the diagnosis of systemic-onset JIA (sJIA). Infection and malignancy are always included in the differential diagnosis for sJIA.

Helpful Tip

Early in the course of JIA, symptoms of joint pain, swelling, and stiffness are present in the morning and after inactivity (gel phenomenon) and improve with activity. Children may refuse to walk for several hours in the morning.

Question 4-2

Which physical exam finding is NOT associated with sJIA?
A) Hepatomegaly.
B) Lymphadenopathy.
C) Arthritis.
D) Stomatitis.
E) Pericardial rub.

TABLE 7–6 INTERNATIONAL LEAGUE OF ASSOCIATIONS FOR RHEUMATOLOGY (ILAR) CLASSIFICATION CRITERIA FOR JUVENILE IDIOPATHIC ARTHRITIS (JIA)

Systemic JIA	Abrupt onset
	Fever, rash, and arthritis
	Serositis
	Organomegaly
	Lymphadenopathy
	Onset: any age
	Girls and boys equally affected
Oligoarticular JIA	≤ 4 joints involved
	Onset: 1–2 years of age
	Girls > boys
	ANA positive
	Persistent: no change in number joints
	Extended: over time increases to 4 or more joints involved
Polyarticular JIA (RF negative)	≥ 5 joints involved
	Onset: 1–2 years of age
	Girls > boys
Polyarticular JIA (RF positive)	≥ 5 joints involved
	Onset: adolescence
	Girls > boys
Psoriatic arthritis	Arthritis and psoriasis
	Dactylitis
	Nail pitting or onycholysis
	Psoriasis in a first-degree relative
Enthesitis-related arthritis	Arthritis and enthesitis
Inflammation of the tendon, ligament, or fascia attachment site to bone	Onset of arthritis in a boy aged 6 years or older
	HLA-B27 positive
	Sacroiliitis or sacroiliac joint tenderness
	Uveitis
	Family history of ankylosing spondylitis, enthesitis-related arthritis, sacroiliitis with inflammatory bowel disease, Reiter syndrome, or acute anterior uveitis in a first-degree relative

RF, rheumatoid factor.

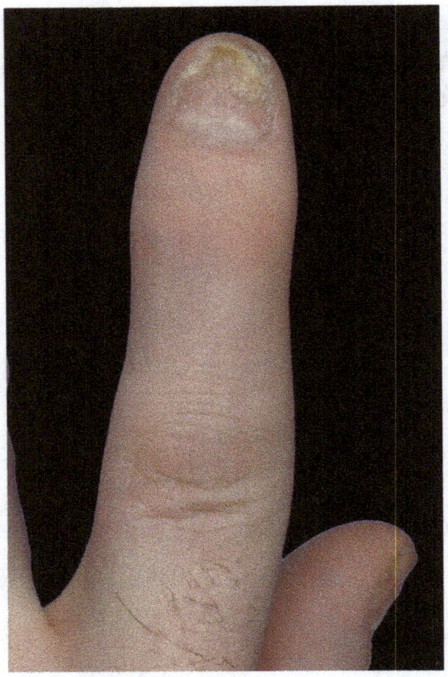

FIGURE 7–7. Psoriatic arthritis. Sausage-like thickening over the interphalangeal joints and psoriasis of the nail. (Reproduced with permission from Wolff K, Johnson RA, Saavedra AP, eds. *Fitzpatrick's Color Atlas and Synopsis of Clinical Dermatology.* 7th ed. New York, NY: McGraw-Hill Education; 2013, Fig. 3-15.)

Discussion 4-2

The correct answer is "D." Systemic-onset JIA (formerly Still disease) classically causes once-daily (quotidian) spiking fever accompanied by an evanescent (fades when afebrile) salmon pink–colored macular rash. Fever is typically intermittent, and children may look well between fevers. Arthritis most commonly involves the wrists, knees, and ankles. Hepatomegaly, splenomegaly, and lymphadenopathy are common. Serositis, pericarditis, or pleuritis may be present with pericardial or pleural effusions. Stomatitis is a feature of Kawasaki disease, not sJIA.

Question 4-3

What is NOT a current medication used in the treatment of JIA?
A) Methotrexate.
B) Sulfasalazine.
C) NSAIDs.
D) Steroids.
E) IVIG.

Discussion 4-3

The correct answer is "E." Medication treatment options include NSAIDs, disease-modifying antirheumatic drugs (DMARDs, including methotrexate), biologic response modifiers (eg, tumor necrosis factor-alpha inhibitors, anakinra), and steroids. Children with JIA should be under the management of a rheumatologist.

She presents to the emergency department with a 3-day history of fever, bruising, headache, and lethargy. On exam,

she appears ill, with hepatomegaly and extensive bruising over her arms and legs, and is somnolent. Her laboratory testing reveals the following results (normal values in parentheses):

White blood cell count 3000/mm³ (5000–15,500/mm³)
Hemoglobin 8 mg/dL (11.5–15 g/dL)
Platelet count 81,000/mm³ (150,000–400,000/mm³)
Alanine aminotransferase (ALT) 75 units/L (10–25 units/L)
Aspartate aminotransferase (AST) 70 units/L (10–30 units/L)
Ferritin 4000 ng/mL (7–140 ng/mL)
Fibrinogen 90 mg/dL (200–400 mg/dL)
Triglycerides 250 mg/dL (< 150 mg/dL)
INR 2.5
ESR 20 mm/h (0–15 mm/h)

Question 4-4

How do you interpret her laboratory results?
A) She has macrophage activation syndrome.
B) Her results are normal.
C) She has a flare of her sJIA.
D) She has leukemia not sJIA.
E) She has hemolytic uremic syndrome.

Discussion 4-4

The correct answer is "A." Macrophage activation syndrome (MAS) is a life-threatening complication of sJIA. It is similar to hemophagocytic lymphohistiocytosis with uncontrolled macrophage and T-cell proliferation. Bone marrow aspirate shows phagocytosis of bone marrow cells by macrophages. Clinical symptoms overlap with other disorders. Distinguishing clinical characteristics are bleeding and central nervous system dysfunction. In sJIA, the white blood cell count, platelet count, and ESR are elevated not decreased as in MAS. Other clues pointing to MAS include the low fibrinogen, highly elevated ferritin, and elevated triglyceride levels. Hemolytic uremic syndrome causes thrombocytopenia and anemia but not leukopenia or a coagulopathy (prolonged INR). Leukemia would not cause elevated triglycerides or, typically, a coagulopathy.

> **Helpful Tip**
> All rheumatologic diseases can present with joint swelling. Systemic lupus erythematosus, dermatomyositis, arthritis, and vasculitis are just a few examples. Joint swelling does not equal juvenile arthritis.

> **Helpful Tip**
> Patients with JIA require serial eye exams to monitor for uveitis. A positive ANA increases the risk for developing uveitis.

▶ CASE 5

A 6-year-old girl is at the clinic because of joint pain with fatigue. She denies morning stiffness. She has no diarrhea, but on review of symptoms you note abdominal pain intermittently. The following laboratory tests are obtained: CBC, ESR, rheumatoid factor (negative), and ANA (negative). Her physical exam findings are normal. She has no synovitis suggestive of inflammatory arthritis.

Question 5-1

What is included in your differential diagnosis of arthralgia?
A) Guaiac stool to look for inflammatory bowel disease.
B) Celiac disease.
C) Joint hypermobility.
D) Hypothyroidism.

Discussion 5-1

The correct answer is "B." She has no elevation in ESR or diarrhea consistent with inflammatory bowel disease. Her joints are normal and not hypermobile. She has no findings of coarse hair and normal reported growth. The abdominal pain makes celiac disease as a cause of arthralgias more likely.

▶ CASE 6

A 3-year-old girl with a new baby sister presents with recent refusal to walk. She is crawling now and refuses to stand by herself, wanting to be carried. She has a previous history of eczema. On exam, she has a rash over the knuckles, elbows, and knees; gum hyperemia; and nail beds that show periungual erythema and swelling. Her laboratory testing shows the following results (normal values in parentheses):

ALT 200 units/L (10–25 units/L)
AST 350 units/L (10–30 units/L)
Creatine kinase (CK) 600 units/L (20–200 units/L)
Lactate dehydrogenase (LDH) 400 units/L (110–295 units/L)
ESR 27 mm/h (0–15 mm/h)
Urinalysis normal
CBC normal

Question 6-1

What is the diagnosis?
A) Malignancy.
B) Discitis.
C) Psoriasis.
D) Juvenile dermatomyositis.
E) Stress of a new sibling.

Discussion 6-1

The correct answer is "D." Juvenile dermatomyositis (JDM) is an autoimmune vasculopathy that causes proximal muscle weakness and distinct rashes. Young children can present with loss of

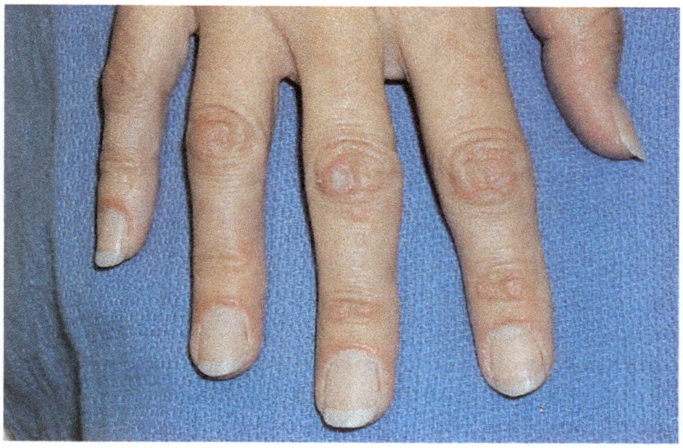

FIGURE 7–8. Dermatomyositis often involves the hands as erythematous flat-topped papules over the knuckles (Gottron sign). Periungual telangiectases are also evident. (Reproduced with permission from Kasper DL, Fauci AS, Hauser SL et al: *Harrison's Principles of Internal Medicine*, 19th ed. McGraw-Hill Education, Inc., 2015. Figure 76e-64.)

milestones as the marker of weakness. Swallowing and breathing may be affected. The rashes of JDM are very characteristic and may be mistaken for eczema. (See Figure 7–8.) They are (1) heliotrope rash—violet discoloration of the upper eyelids; (2) Gottron papules—pink, thickened, scaly plaques classically over the proximal interphalangeal joints and distal interphalangeal joints; and (3) photosensitivity—shawl sign (a pattern of erythema that develops over the chest and neck when exposed to sunlight). Diagnosis of JDM requires rash plus three of the following criteria: muscle weakness, elevated muscle enzymes, abnormal electromyogram (EMG), abnormal muscle biopsy, or MRI evidence of myositis.

> **Helpful Tip**
> The weakness of JDM is symmetric and proximal, causing difficulty climbing stairs and raising the arms above the head. On exam, patients have difficulty lifting their head, doing a sit up, and standing up from the floor (positive Gower sign).

▶ CASE 7

A 9-year-old left-handed boy presents with fourth finger swelling of 2 months' duration, morning stiffness, and rash. He can no longer straighten the end of his finger. He says the skin on his arm has become thick and darker in color compared with the rest of his skin. On exam, he has a lesion with faint erythema and a blue border on his left biceps. The skin over his forearm, wrist, dorsum of hand, and fourth finger is hyperpigmented with scarring and atrophy. He has swelling of his left four metacarpophalangeal joint, and a flexion contracture of his proximal interphalangeal joint (PIP).

Question 7-1

What is the diagnosis?

A) JIA.
B) Linear scleroderma.
C) Methicillin-resistant *Staphylococcus aureus* infection.
D) Systemic lupus erythematosus.
E) None of the above.

Discussion 7-1

The correct answer is "B." Juvenile scleroderma causes skin fibrosis and may be localized to the skin (morphea) or affect other organs (systemic sclerosis). Localized scleroderma is usually self-limited and has many different subtypes. In localized scleroderma, an area of "waxy" swelling with a blue or red border develops into an indurated hypopigmented or hyperpigmented skin lesion with atrophy. In systemic sclerosis, extracutaneous involvement includes pulmonary and cardiac fibrosis, Raynaud phenomenon, renal artery hypertension, and gastrointestinal dysmotility. Heart failure from cardiopulmonary fibrosis is the most common cause of death. The patient has linear scleroderma, a type of localized scleroderma. Lesions can extend through the subcutaneous tissues and muscle to the bone. Lesions crossing joints cause contractures and limb-length discrepancies. Arthritis may be present in some children. (See Figure 7–9.)

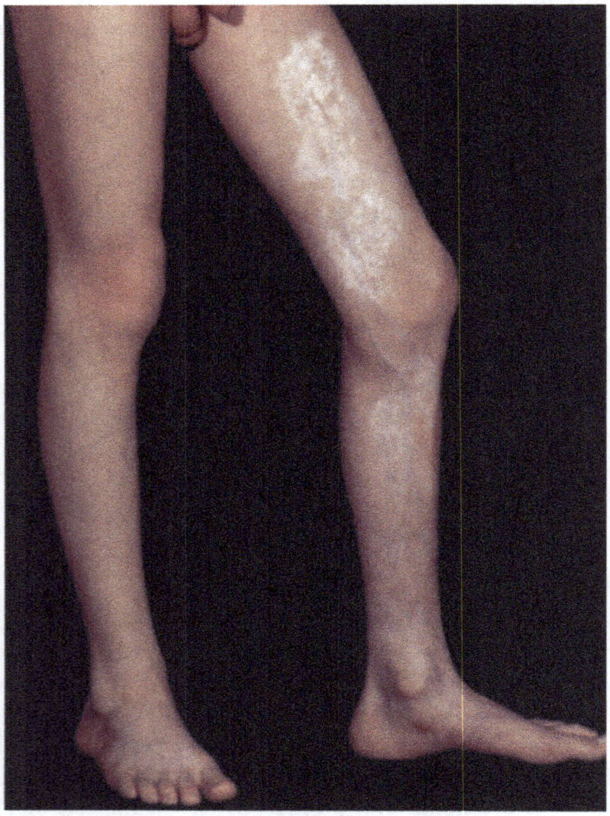

FIGURE 7–9. This boy has linear scleroderma, a form of localized scleroderma (morphea) that causes skin fibrosis. Linear lesions can extend to the bone, causing contractures of joints. He has an indurated, waxy, hypopigmented lesion extending from his thigh to his foot. (Reproduced with permission from Wolff K, Johnson RA, Saavedra AP, eds. *Fitzpatrick's Color Atlas and Synopsis of Clinical Dermatology.* 7th ed. New York, NY: McGraw-Hill Education; 2013, Fig. 14-51.)

⧖ QUICK QUIZ

What is NOT a clinical feature of sarcoidosis?

A) Hilar lymphadenopathy.
B) Pulmonary fibrosis.
C) Uveitis.
D) Erythema nodosum.
E) Seizures.

Discussion

The correct answer is "E." Sarcoid is rare in children and results in the formation of noncaseating (no necrosis) granulomas in multiple organs. Presentation varies by age. Older children have lung and lymph node involvement (hilar or mediastinal lymphadenopathy, or both, and pulmonary infiltrates). Rash, uveitis, and arthritis occur in children younger than 4 years of age. Definitive diagnosis is made by biopsy.

▶ CASE 8

A 15-year-old male wrestler presents with a 4-month history of hip and buttock pain. He has trouble sleeping due to the pain. In the mornings, his low back is stiff but improves after he starts to move. On exam, he has pain upon palpation of the sacroiliac joint, decreased ability to bend forward, and thickening in the left ankle with mild warmth. His hips are normal.

Question 8-1

Which of the following laboratory results is NOT expected with his diagnosis?

A) Positive HLA-B27.
B) Normal ESR.
C) Normal CBC.
D) Positive ANA.
E) Negative rheumatoid factor.

Discussion 8-1

The correct answer is "D." He has juvenile ankylosing spondylitis (JAS) a type of spondyloarthropathy involving the spine and sacroiliac joints, causing pain and limited motion of the lumbar spine and sacroiliitis detectable on MRI. Ninety percent of patients with JAS who have sacroiliac disease are HLA-B27 positive. The juvenile spondyloarthropathies are a group of disorders that cause enthesitis and arthritis. They are considered a subset of JIA (enthesitis-related arthritis; see Table 7–6). Key clinical clues are:

- Boy older than 6 years
- HLA-B27 positive
- Arthritis of the lower extremities
- Enthesitis of the Achilles tendon and plantar fascia
- Back and sacroiliac joint pain and stiffness
- Usually ANA and rheumatoid factor negative

► CASE 9

A 10-year-old boy was diagnosed with erythema infectiosum (fifth disease) 2 weeks ago after developing fever and the classic "slapped cheek" rash. Now he presents with a 1-week history of joint pain when writing and playing the flute. He reports morning stiffness. On exam he has arthritis of the ankle and knee. You decide to treat him with NSAIDs and reevaluate as symptoms have been present for only 1 week. At follow up 6 weeks later, he is symptom free.

Question 9-1

What is the diagnosis?
A) Postinfectious/reactive arthritis.
B) Acute rheumatic fever.
C) Septic arthritis.
D) Oligoarticular juvenile idiopathic arthritis.
E) Polyarticular juvenile idiopathic arthritis.

Discussion 9-1

The correct answer is "A." Reactive and postinfectious arthritis develop 1 to 4 weeks after a viral or bacterial infection. Most cases are preceded by gastroenteritis. Classically, reactive arthritis (formerly known as Reiter syndrome) developed after an enteric or genitourinary tract infection. The classic triad of arthritis, urethritis, and conjunctivitis is uncommon in children. Many are positive for HLA-B27. Arthritis typically involves the large joints of the legs, responds to NSAIDs, and resolves within weeks to months. Common pathogens in reactive arthritis include *Salmonella, Shigella, Yersinia, Campylobacter, Giardia intestinalis,* and *Chlamydia trachomatis.* Common pathogens in postinfectious arthritis include parvovirus B19, rubella, varicella-zoster, herpes simplex, cytomegalovirus, Ebstein-Barr virus, hepatitis B, adenovirus, enteroviruses, group A streptococcus, and mycoplasma. Differentiating between poststreptococcal reactive arthritis (PSRA) and acute rheumatic fever (ARF) is challenging. Some clinicians consider PSRA to be incomplete ARF and treat with penicillin prophylaxis. Unlike the arthritis of ARF, PSRA does not migrate and is less responsive to NSAIDs.

► CASE 10

A 17-year-old adolescent girl presents with fatigue and widespread joint pain that is getting progressively worse. For the last year, her hands, knees, back, and ankles have ached constantly. The pain is worse with activities. She can no longer participate in gym class and is constantly tired. On exam, she can hyperextend both elbows, lay her palms flat on the floor when standing without bending her knees, touch both thumbs to her forearms, and extend both pinky fingers to 90 degrees. Her Beighton score is 7/9.

Question 10-1

What is NOT a recommended treatment for her condition?
A) Reassurance.
B) NSAIDs.
C) Physical therapy.
D) Narcotics.
E) All of the above are recommended for treatment of her condition.

Discussion 10-1

The correct answer is "D." Her symptoms and a Beighton score of 6 or higher is consistent with benign joint hypermobility syndrome (BJHS). Physical therapy builds muscle strength to stabilize joints. NSAIDs may be useful to treat pain. Symptoms improve with age and are not associated with long-term complications. People with BJHS are double jointed and have musculoskeletal pain. The syndrome tends to run in families. Girls and younger children are most often affected as hypermobility decreases with age. BJHS is diagnosed clinically using the Beighton score. (See Table 7–7.) It is important to rule out other conditions associated with hypermobile joints, such as Marfan syndrome and Ehlers-Danlos syndrome.

TABLE 7–7 BEIGHTON SCORING SYSTEM FOR DIAGNOSING BENIGN JOINT HYPERMOBILITY SYNDROME

> 10 degrees of hyperextension of the knees	1 point for each side
> 10 degrees of hyperextension of the elbows	1 point for each side
Passive flexion of the thumb to forearm	1 point for each side
Passive extension of the fifth finger > 90 degrees	1 point for each side
Touch the floor with both palms with knees straight	

Score ≥ 6 indicates hypermobility.

⧖ QUICK QUIZ

Which of the following statements about classic Ehlers-Danlos syndrome (EDS) is NOT true?

A) It is caused by mutation in the genes (*COL5A1, COL5A2*) encoding type V collagen.
B) Patients can have associated cardiac defects.
C) It is an autosomal recessive condition.
D) Patients are prone to easy bruising.
E) Diagnosis is based on clinical exam and family history.

Discussion

The correct answer is "C." EDS is an autosomal dominant condition, not autosomal recessive. Classic EDS is an inherited connective tissue disorder known for hyperelastic skin (stretches easily and snaps back), poor wound healing with stretched scars, and joint hypermobility. The skin is smooth, velvety, and fragile. Those affected bruise easily and are prone to joint dislocation. Mitral valve prolapse and aortic root dilation are uncommon. Hernias and rectal prolapse may occur. It is one of six different types of EDS. (See Table 7–8 and Figure 7–10.)

⧖ QUICK QUIZ

Which is NOT a clinical feature of Marfan syndrome?

A) Aortic root dilation.
B) Ectopia lentis.
C) Scoliosis.
D) Pectus deformities (excavatum or carinatum).
E) Hyperopia.

A

B

FIGURE 7–10. Ehlers-Danlos syndrome is an inherited connective tissue disorder characterized by hyperextensible skin, poor wound healing, and joint hypermobility. (A) The skin stretches when pulled then snaps back when released. (B) Joint hypermobility is measured using a scoring system. One criterion is the ability to passively flex the thumb to the forearm, as shown here. (Reproduced with permission from Fuster V, Walsh RA, Harrington RA, eds. *Hurst's The Heart*. 13th ed. New York, NY: McGraw-Hill Education; 2011, Fig. 14-8A,B.)

TABLE 7–8 DIAGNOSTIC CRITERIA FOR CLASSIC EHLERS-DANLOS SYNDROME

Major criteria 3 required	Hyperextensible skin
	Wide, atropic scars
	Joint hypermobility (Beighton score ≥ 6; see Table 7–7)
Minor criteria 1 required	Smooth, velvety skin
	Molluscoid pseudotumors
	Subcutaneous spheroids
	Joint complications (dislocations, sprains, pes planus)
	Muscle hypotonia, gross motor delay
	Easy bruising
	Hernias, rectal prolapse, cervical insufficiency
	Family history

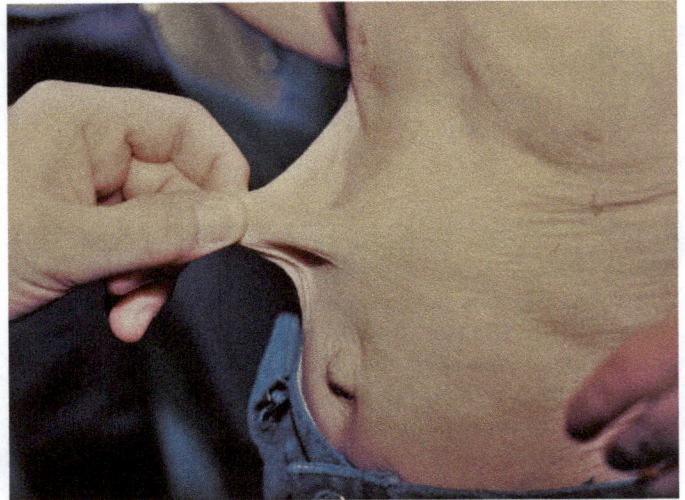

Discussion

The correct answer is "E." Myopia, not hyperopia, is associated with Marfan syndrome. Marfan syndrome is an autosomal dominant connective tissue disorder caused by a mutation in the *FBN1* gene. It is important to recognize the condition to monitor for its cardiac complications. Patients are tall, thin, and have long extremities (arm span > height), pectus deformities, ligamentous laxity, flat feet (pes planus), and arachnodactyly (long, thin fingers and toes). The face is long and narrow with deep-set eyes, high-arched palate,

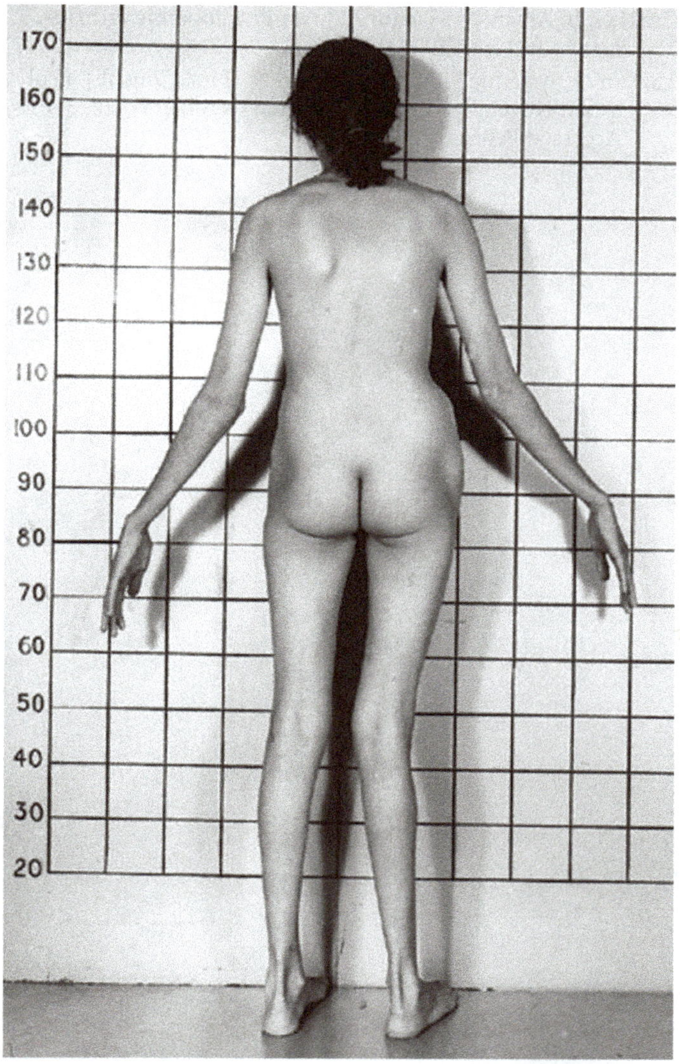

FIGURE 7–11. This teenage girl has Marfan syndrome. She has long limbs and fingers, scoliosis, and genu valgum (knock knees). (Reproduced with permission from Valle D, Beaudet AL, Vogelstein B et al: *The Online Metabolic and Molecular Bases of Inherited Disease*, 8ed. McGraw-Hill Education, Inc; 2014. Fig 206-2.)

dental crowding, and a small chin. (See Figure 7–11.) Marfan syndrome is associated with aortic dilation, mitral or tricuspid valve prolapse (or both), and an increased risk for aortic dissection. Spontaneous pneumothorax may occur as well.

► CASE 11

A 13-year-old adolescent boy who plays basketball presents with complaints of knee pain with running. He does not have stiffness and his knees do not swell. His symptoms seem to occur after activities. Physical exam is normal, with a negative lateral patellar compression exam, no crepitus or snapping of the knees, and no tibial pain to palpation.

Question 11-1
What is the diagnosis?
A) Functional joint pain.
B) Plica syndrome.
C) Chondromalacia patella.
D) Osgood-Schlatter disease.

Discussion 11-1
The correct answer is "A." This is not plica syndrome as the patient has no joint snapping on exam. It is not chondromalacia patella as there is no pain to lateral compression of the patella. This is not Osgood-Schlatter disease as he does not have tibial pain to palpation. Sometimes there is not a good anatomic or pathologic correlate to joint pain, and we call it "functional joint pain." No treatment is necessary, but people commonly use NSAIDs to treat the discomfort.

BIBLIOGRAPHY

Berard R, Whittemore B, Scuccimarri R. Hemolytic anemia following intravenous immunoglobulin therapy in patients treated for Kawasaki disease: A report of 4 cases. *Pediatr Rheumatol.* 2012;10(1):10.

Burke RJ, Chang C. Diagnostic criteria of acute rheumatic fever. *Autoimmun Rev.* 2014;13(4–5):503–507.

Cassidy JT, Laxer RM, Petty RE, Lindsley CB. *Textbook of Pediatric Rheumatology.* 6th ed. Philadelphia, PA: Saunders; 2011.

Dietz HC. Marfan syndrome. (Published April 18, 2001 [Updated June 12, 2014]). In Pagon RA, Adam MP, Ardinger HH, et al, eds. *GeneReviews* [Internet]. Seattle, WA: University of Washington; 1993–2015. http://www.ncbi.nlm.nih.gov/books/NBK1335/. Accessed February 19, 2015.

Gurion R, Lehman TJ, Moorthy LN. Systemic arthritis in children: A review of clinical presentation and treatment. *Int J Inflamm.* 2012;2012:271569.

Kliegman RM, Stanton BF, St. Geme JW, et al. *Nelson Textbook of Pedaitrics.* 19th ed. Philadelphia, PA: Saunders, 2011.

Lanzkron S. Henoch-Schönlein purpura. [First Consult]. (Published October 3, 2012 [Updated October 2, 2012]). Accessed February 23, 2015.

Malfait F, Wenstrup R, DePaepe A. Ehlers-Danlos syndrome, classic type. (May 29, 2007 [Updated August 18, 2011]). In Pagon RA, Adam MP, Ardinger HH, et al, eds. *GeneReviews* [Internet]. Seattle, WA: University of Washington; 1993–2015. Available from http://www.ncbi.nlm.nih.gov/books/NBK1244/. Accessed Feburary 20, 2015.

Newburger JW, Takahashi M, Gerber MA, et al. Diagnosis, treatment, and long-term management of Kawasaki disease: A statement for health professionals from the Committee on Rheumatic Fever, Endocarditis and Kawasaki Disease, Council on Cardiovascular Disease in the Young, American Heart Association. *Circulation.* 2004;110(17):2747–2771.

Petty RE, Southwood TR, Manners P, et al; International League of Associations for Rheumatology. International League of Associations for Rheumatology classification of juvenile idiopathic arthritis: Second revision, Edmonton, 2001. *J Rheumatol*. 2004;31(2):390–392.

Prakken B, Albani S, Martini A. Juvenile idiopathic arthritis. *Lancet*. 2011;377(9783):2138–2149.

Yazdany J. Systemic lupus erythematous. [First Consult]. (Published November 1, 2013 [Updated October 31, 2013]). Accessed February 23, 2015.

Critical Care

Ashley Loomis and Niyati Patel

8

▶ CASE 1

A 4-month-old infant arrives in the emergency department with a 2-day history of fever, decreasing interest in oral (PO) intake, and little to no urine output today. Mother notes that the patient is more lethargic today. Upon examination you note a well-nourished infant who arouses and moans to your exam but quickly falls back asleep in his mother's arms. Vital signs are heart rate (HR): 170 beats per minute (bpm), respiratory rate (RR): 60 breaths per minute, blood pressure (BP): 80/60 mm Hg, temperature (T): 38°C (100.4°F). Multiple attempts to obtain intravenous (IV) access are unsuccessful.

Question 1-1

What is the most appropriate next therapy?

A) Administer PO acetaminophen for fever.
B) Administer isotonic PO fluids.
C) Obtain intraosseous (IO) access and administer a 20-mL/kg isotonic fluid bolus via IO.
D) Administer PO broad-spectrum antibiotic therapy.
E) Obtain an ultrasound of his abdomen.

Discussion 1-1

The correct answer is "C." This patient is in compensated shock. Recognize that blood pressure is often the last vital sign to decline in pediatric shock. (See Figure 8–1.) Shock is a syndrome characterized by inadequate oxygen delivery to meet metabolic demands, often resulting in acidosis, organ dysfunction, and death if not treated adequately and efficiently. Recall that when treating shock, one should obtain IV/IO access and give fluids within the first 5 minutes of the patient's arrival.

▶ CASE 2

While examining your patients prior to rounds in the pediatric intensive care unit (PICU), you note that a 3-year-old with otherwise normal vital signs for age has a capillary refill of 3 seconds.

Question 2-1

Which of the following is most accurate?

A) Capillary refill is unaffected by the use of vasopressors.
B) Environmental temperature can affect capillary refill.
C) Capillary refill greater than 3 seconds is always indicative of abnormal perfusion.
D) Inter-observer reliability does not affect measurement of capillary refill.
E) I have never heard of capillary refill.

Discussion 2-1

The correct answer is "B." Although capillary refill is a common clinical test used in pediatrics, the inter-observer variability makes it a very insensitive tool. Studies have demonstrated a tremendous amount of inconsistency in how this test is performed, thus making the interpretation of the results quite difficult. It is known that certain vasopressors—specifically those that are pure vasoconstrictors (eg, Neo-Synephrine)—can affect capillary refill time. Additionally, environmental temperature can affect capillary refill time in an otherwise perfectly healthy individual. Therefore, while traditionally a capillary refill of greater than 3 seconds is considered abnormal, it may not always indicate abnormal perfusion. If you read the preceding explanations, option "E" is no longer applicable.

▶ CASE 3

You are admitting a 23-month-old girl to the pediatric PICU secondary to new-onset gait abnormality and recent early morning headaches associated with vomiting. As you perform your initial examination, you note that she is arousable, but irritable, and her respiratory rate is 60 bpm, which is a new finding according to the emergency medical services (EMS) team that transported her to your institution.

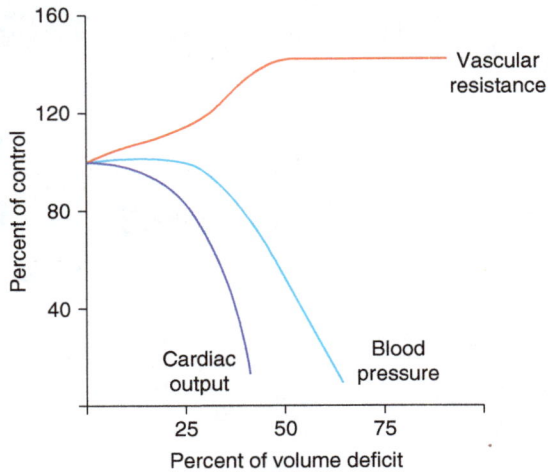

FIGURE 8–1. Hemodynamics in pediatric shock. In compensated shock, a child may continue to maintain a normal blood pressure for age with adequate perfusion to the brain and heart provided by increased cardiac output—as a result of tachycardia, and increased systemic vascular resistance. Although blood pressure remains normal, other organs may be hypoperfused and if left untreated, the patient could progress to decompensated shock.

Question 3-1

What is the most likely explanation for this new-onset tachypnea?

A) Impending coma from elevated intracranial pressure (ICP).
B) Respiratory viral illness.
C) Foreign body aspiration secondary to impaired gag reflex.
D) Anxiety secondary to increased personnel and PICU setting.
E) Dehydration secondary to a history of emesis.

Discussion 3-1

The correct answer is "A." This patient's constellation of symptoms, including gait abnormality, headaches, and vomiting, should prompt the reader to think of a mass-occupying lesion. Understanding of the Monro-Kellie doctrine (Figure 8–2) leads

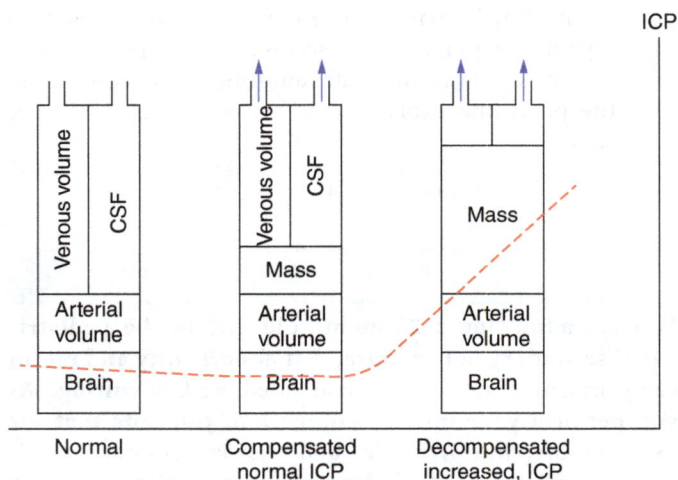

FIGURE 8–2. The Monro-Kellie doctrine states that the cranial vault is a closed, rigid box with a fixed volume. An increase in the volume of any of its components—brain, blood, or cerebrospinal fluid—will result in increased pressure on the vault and displacement of one of the other components.

us to the conclusion that this child, in compensating for the lesion-induced increased intracranial pressure, is limiting blood flow to the brain by hyperventilating and causing vasoconstriction of the cerebral vasculature.

▶ CASE 4

A 3-year-old boy is in the operating room being prepared for a tonsillectomy and adenoidectomy after a sleep study demonstrated significant sleep apnea. Shortly after the surgery has begun the anesthesiologist notes an end-tidal CO_2 of 90 mmHg, HR 175 bpm, and T 40°C (104°F).

Question 4-1

All of the following are associated with increased risk for development of these clinical changes EXCEPT:

A) Family history of malignant hyperthermia.
B) Exposure to volatile anesthetic agents.
C) Treatment with succinylcholine.
D) Dantrolene therapy.
E) History of muscular dystrophy.

Discussion 4-1

The correct answer is "D." The boy in this case is demonstrating clinical signs consistent with malignant hyperthermia (MH). MH has an autosomal dominant inheritance pattern with variable penetrance; thus, a family history of MH is a known risk factor. MH typically occurs after a trigger, most commonly by volatile anesthetic agents or succinylcholine. Clinical signs consistent with MH include rapid increase in end-tidal CO_2, tachycardia, hyperthermia, hyperkalemia, myoglobinuria, muscle rigidity, and, if not treated adequately, disseminated intravascular coagulopathy, cardiac failure, and renal failure. Patients with existing muscular dystrophy are at higher risk for development of this syndrome. Dantrolene therapy, which is used to treat MH, inhibits release of ionized calcium by the sarcoplasmic reticulum, thus interfering with muscle contraction. The use of dantrolene does not increase the risk of developing MH.

▶ CASE 5

A 5-year-old previously healthy boy is seen in the emergency department with complaints of decreased activity tolerance and breathlessness for the past 2 days. He has not been febrile today; however, he recently recovered from what his mother thought was the flu. His vital signs are HR 140 bpm, RR 40, BP 70/50 mm Hg, and T 37.5°C (99.5°F). The emergency department physician obtains IV access, sends off laboratory studies and a blood culture, administers a total of 40 mL/kg of isotonic fluid, and administers broad-spectrum IV antibiotics. The patient is now noted to be more tachycardic, with increased work of breathing, and pulses that are difficult to palpate.

Question 5-1

What is the most likely cause of this child's decompensation?
A) Septic shock.
B) Viral bronchiolitis.
C) Bacterial pneumonia.
D) Systemic inflammatory response syndrome (SIRS).
E) Congestive heart failure.

Question 5-2

Which of the following statements regarding this child's diagnosis is most accurate?
A) A 12-lead ECG will confirm the diagnosis.
B) An elevated C-reactive protein will confirm the diagnosis.
C) A stat 2-dimensional echocardiogram will confirm the diagnosis.
D) The patient is in fluid refractory distributive shock.
E) The patient is in primary respiratory failure.

- -

You decide to admit this patient to the PICU.

Question 5-3

Which of the following is the best initial choice of therapy?
A) Continue to administer another 20-mL/kg bolus followed by a vasopressor if hemodynamics do not improve.
B) Initiate bronchodilator therapy and systemic steroids.
C) Initiate epinephrine and milrinone infusions with conservative fluid replacement (5–10 mL/kg) as needed.
D) Initiate vasopressin infusion alone.
E) Administer supplemental oxygen.

- -

After transfer to the PICU, prior to initiating therapy the child develops jugular venous distention, muffled heart sounds, palpable liver edge, worsening tachycardia, and BP of 60/50 mm Hg.

Question 5-4

What is the best next step in management?
A) Augment preload and prepare for emergent pericardiocentesis with echocardiogram guidance.
B) Aggressive diuretic therapy.
C) Initiate a milrinone infusion to improve ventricular filling.
D) Initiate an epinephrine infusion to help improve cardiac output.
E) Perform endotracheal intubation.

Discussion 5-1 through 5-4

The correct answers are "E," "C," "C," and "A." When approaching a patient in shock, remember to continually reassess after each therapy. Although fluid resuscitation is the appropriate initial management for any patient in shock, the reassessment helps to determine what type of shock the patient is experiencing. After fluid resuscitation, the presence of rales, hepatomegaly, worsening tachycardia, and worsening perfusion are all signs consistent with cardiogenic shock. In patients with septic shock or systemic inflammatory response syndrome (SIRS), one would not expect a worsening clinical status following aggressive fluid resuscitation. In a patient with viral bronchiolitis or bacterial pneumonia, work of breathing may continue to progress with fluid resuscitation; however, worsening perfusion would not be expected. Once

the diagnosis of cardiogenic shock is suspected, a 2-dimensional echocardiogram is needed to confirm the diagnosis. This will help determine if the patient is suffering from impaired systolic or diastolic function (eg, myocarditis), or tamponade physiology (eg, pericardial effusion). With impaired systolic function epinephrine can augment contractility. Recall that epinephrine does increase myocardial oxygen demand and has the potential to lead to myocardial ischemia and infarction. If impaired diastolic function is present, milrinone can help relaxation and filling. Recall that milrinone will also lead to vasodilation and must be used cautiously in the hypotensive patient. The triad of tachycardia, jugular venous distention, and narrowed pulse pressure is tamponade physiology until proven otherwise. The definitive diagnosis is clinically made, and the therapy of choice is echocardiogram-guided pericardiocentesis if a pericardial effusion is to blame. Aggressive diuresis in the setting of tamponade physiology could result in significantly diminished systemic venous return and cardiac arrest.

▶ CASE 6

A 13-year-old girl with a past medical history significant for school avoidance is brought to your office by her mother. The girl states that she is "fine," but Mom states that she has not seemed like herself for the past 4 days. Mom reports that her daughter has been sleeping much more than usual, her appetite is much less than normal, and she has had occasional emesis. Mom also notes that the girl has intermittently been "talking nonsense." Physical exam reveals the following: oral T 38°C (100.4°F), HR 85 bpm, RR 18, BP 100/65 mm Hg, and oxygen saturation (SpO_2) of 100% on room air. Your patient looks down at the floor and will not engage with you. Her heart and lung sounds are normal. When you palpate her abdomen, she yelps when you feel her right upper quadrant and bats your hand away. With repeat palpation of that area, you note guarding without rebound and a firm liver edge 1 cm below the right costal margin. Bowel sounds are present and the remainder of her abdomen is nontender. On neurologic exam, cranial nerves II through XII are intact. Reflexes are brisk throughout, and strength is 5/5 in all extremities. When you ask her to touch her nose and then your finger, she touches her right eye and then misses your finger completely. At the end of your exam, she is mumbling unintelligibly and then lies down on the exam table.

Question 6-1

Your next best step is:
A) Reassure her mother that this is normal early teenage behavior.
B) Schedule an appointment for her next month with your child psychiatry colleague.
C) Obtain a chest X-ray and clean catch urinalysis.
D) Order a CBC with white blood cell count differential, electrolytes, BUN, creatinine, glucose, calcium, magnesium, phosphorus, AST, ALT, GGT, alkaline phosphatase, total and direct bilirubin, PTT, INR, and fibrinogen.
E) Schedule her for an abdominal ultrasound next week.

Discussion 6-1

The correct answer is "D." This girl's history of somnolence, anorexia, emesis, and mental status changes indicate that an immediate diagnostic workup is required. Abdominal pain, hepatomegaly, brisk reflexes, and spatiotemporal disorientation are signs consistent with hepatic dysfunction necessitating laboratory evaluation. These subtle signs are the most common presentation of fulminant hepatic failure in children. Jaundice may be present or absent depending on the etiology of the liver disease. "Classic" findings of liver failure in adults, such as a history of drug or alcohol use, ascites, spider angiomata, palmar erythema, and asterixis, occur very late in the course of pediatric patients following progression to chronic liver disease or are absent altogether. In infants, irritability, failure to thrive, a high-pitched cry, and a change in sleep rhythm may be the only symptoms noted.

The girl's laboratory results return and demonstrate normal blood count and differential, electrolytes, BUN, creatinine, calcium, magnesium, and phosphorus. Her glucose is low at 70. Her AST and ALT are significantly elevated at 3523 and 4278, respectively. GGT and alkaline phosphatase are normal. Total bilirubin is slightly elevated at 3.2, with a direct fraction of 0.2. PTT is normal, INR is prolonged at 2.6, and fibrinogen is normal. Upon further questioning when discussing these abnormalities with the girl and her mother, she admits that she ingested a bottle of pills in a suicide attempt 4 days ago.

Question 6-2

Which of the following substances could account for her current clinical condition?

A) Acetaminophen.
B) Aspirin.
C) Diphenhydramine.
D) Prenatal vitamins.
E) None of the above.

Discussion 6-2

The correct answer is "A." Acetaminophen ingestion is the most common etiology of acute hepatic failure in children and adolescents in the United States. If caught early and treated with intensive medical therapy, survival and recovery are good. However, some patients have severe damage by the time the ingestion is discovered or progressively deteriorate and ultimately need liver transplantation. Since it has been 4 days since this girl's suicide attempt, it is too late for *N*-acetylcysteine treatment, and she should be transferred to a hospital with a PICU and solid organ transplant capability.

> ► **CASE 7**

A 3-year-old boy with no significant past medical history is admitted to the PICU in respiratory distress secondary to a presumed viral bronchiolitis. Viral studies have been sent but are still pending. Upon arrival to the PICU he is placed on continuous positive airway pressure (CPAP); however, despite this intervention he continues to have subcostal and supraclavicular retractions, grunting, and nasal flaring. His nurse is concerned that he seems more lethargic and recently began "head bobbing." As the PICU team prepares to intubate and mechanically ventilate the child, the attending physician asks you what size endotracheal tube you would like for this child.

Question 7-1

Assuming this child has a normal airway the best answer is:

A) 2.0 uncuffed tube.
B) 2.0 cuffed tube.
C) 3.0 uncuffed tube.
D) 3.0 cuffed tube.
E) 4.5 cuffed tube.

Discussion 7-1

The correct answer is "E." The traditional formula used to determine the internal diameter of the endotracheal tube is age based: (age + 16)/4. For the patient in this vignette, (3 + 16)/4 = 4.75. Thus, the best choice of the endotracheal tube sizes listed above is the 4.5 cuffed tube. The length-based Braslow tape recommendations are also an acceptable guide to help determine appropriate size. Cuffed tubes in a hospital setting are generally regarded as safe outside of the neonatal age group. Additionally, patients with some disease processes (eg, poor lung compliance, elevated airway resistance, large glottic leak) may have improved mechanical ventilation with a cuffed tube.

The pediatric resident gives the patient ketamine, midazolam, and rocuronium as induction medications. He then places the endotracheal tube and attaches a carbon dioxide (CO_2) detector to the end of the tube. After several bagged breaths the color on the detector turns yellow. Upon auscultation, the resident notes that breath sounds are asymmetric, with right greater than left.

Question 7-2

The most likely reason for this is?

A) Esophageal intubation.
B) Tracheal intubation.
C) Right mainstem intubation.
D) Left mainstem intubation.
E) Resident inexperience; get the attending.

Discussion 7-2

The correct answer is "C." The persistent color change on the CO_2 detector indicates that the endotracheal tube is not in the esophagus. With appropriate tracheal intubation, one would expect to see color change on the CO_2 detector in addition to hearing bilateral air entry over both lung fields. The presence of louder breath sounds over the right lung field than the left is pathognomonic for a right mainstem intubation. The right main bronchus branches off at a less acute angle from the trachea than the left, making it the more likely bronchus to be intubated if the endotracheal tube is advanced too far.

The respiratory therapist adjusts the endotracheal tube to the appropriate position as confirmed by chest X-ray. Before leaving the room, the bedside nurse calls your attention to the patient's rising heart rate and declining blood pressure. His saturations remain at 98% and you continue to hear symmetric breath sounds.

Question 7-3

What is the next best step in management?
A) Naloxone bolus to treat narcotic side effects.
B) 20 mL/kg isotonic fluid bolus for impaired venous return from elevated intrathoracic pressures.
C) Needle decompression of a tension pneumothorax.
D) Dopamine infusion for septic shock.
E) Bolus stress-dose steroids for adrenal suppression.

Discussion 7-3

The correct answer is "B." Upon intubation of a patient, be aware of the changes that occur when going from negative pressure ventilation to positive pressure ventilation. The overall pressure in the intrathoracic cage increases with lung expansion and can directly impair systemic venous return, especially in a patient such as this one, who has likely had a fair amount of insensible water losses with tachypnea and increased work of breathing. The patient did not receive any narcotics prior to intubation, so naloxone will do nothing to reverse his hypotension. The patient continues to have adequate SpO_2 and symmetric breath sounds, making a tension pneumothorax very unlikely. Although the patient may have a SIRS response to his virus, the first-line treatment would not be a pressor but fluid, making option "D" incorrect. Lastly, while some drugs (eg, etomidate, chronic steroid therapy) can cause adrenal suppression, there would be no reason to assume this in a previously healthy child.

▶ CASE 8

A mother brings her 5-year-old daughter to your clinic with significantly increased work of breathing for several days. When you ask the nurse to obtain a pulse oximetry reading she calls you to the bedside urgently as the child is difficult to arouse.

Question 8-1

What are the first steps you should take to manage this patient?
A) Transfer to the emergency department immediately.
B) Give 2.5 mg of nebulized albuterol.
C) Assess airway and breathing and check for pulses.

D) Finish your well check; the child is just getting some much-needed rest.
E) None of the above.

Discussion 8-1

The correct answer is "C." Always remember the initial assessment when approaching a difficult-to-arouse child. Your initial evaluation should include assessment of the patency of the airway, effectiveness of breathing, and adequate circulation as evidenced by the presence of a pulse. Think of your **ABCs**—**A**irway, **B**reathing, and **C**irculation. Remember to palpate pulses centrally—brachial in infants, carotid or femoral in older children. Although this child may need to be transferred to the emergency department, it is not appropriate to move her in this state with no further intervention.

You note this child has a patent airway, continues to have some shallow, gasping breaths, and has a carotid pulse of 84 bpm.

Question 8-2

What is the next best step in management?
A) Call 9-1-1 and activate the emergency response system.
B) Deliver breaths using an appropriately sized bag-valve-mask (BMV).
C) Begin chest compressions.
D) Perform a blind finger sweep of the airway.
E) Both A and B are correct.

Discussion 8-2

The correct answer is "E." Recall that pediatric arrests are primarily respiratory in origin as opposed to their adult counterparts. Adequate breaths and oxygenation in an acutely decompensating child may be all that is needed to stabilize him or her. At this time someone should be assigned the task of activating the emergency response system, so they will be on their way while the team continues to work on the child. After providing good breaths and oxygenation be sure to reassess ABCs.

After delivering several adequate breaths by BVM, you reassess the patient. She continues to be unresponsive, has ongoing gasping breaths, and her carotid pulse is now 40 bpm and thready.

Question 8-3

What is your next step?
A) Continue BVM ventilation at a rate of 10 to 12 breaths per minute and await emergency medical services.
B) Start chest compressions at a rate of 60 bpm to a depth of one quarter the anterior-posterior diameter of the chest.
C) Start chest compressions at a rate of 80 bpm to a depth of more than one third the anterior-posterior diameter of the chest.
D) Start chest compressions at a rate of 100 bpm to a depth of more than one third the anterior-posterior diameter of the chest.
E) Continue BVM ventilation and find the office automated external defibrillator (AED).

Discussion 8-3

The correct answer is "D." Symptomatic bradycardia (HR < 60 bpm in a child or < 100 bpm in a neonate) or pulselessness requires immediate initiation of chest compressions. Chest compressions must be hard—depth greater than one third the anterior-posterior diameter of the chest with full recoil—and fast—100 bpm.

> **Helpful Tip**
>
> Hum the 70s tune "Stayin' Alive" and compress to the beat to get the right rate. The ratio of compressions to ventilation if an advanced airway is not present is 30:2 for single rescuer and 15:2 for two rescuers. Once cycle of cardiopulmonary resuscitation (CPR) equals 15 or 30 compressions (whichever is applicable) and 2 breaths. Assessments are done every 5 cycles (about 2 minutes). The ultimate goal is to limit interruptions of chest compressions. If an advanced airway is present the rescuer should aim for a goal of 8 to 10 breaths per minute.

While you and the nurse continue CPR your colleague brings the office AED and attaches the pad. After 5 full cycles of CPR you pause to assess the rhythm and see the rhythm below. A weak pulse is present.

Question 8-4

What is the best course of action?

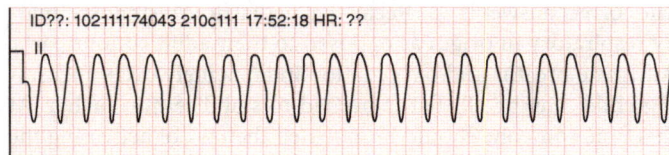

ID??: 102111174043 210c111 17:52:18 HR: ??

A) Clear everyone from the patient and deliver a synchronized shock of 0.5 J/kg of body weight then immediately resume chest compressions.
B) Clear everyone from the patient and deliver a nonsynchronized shock of 2 J/kg of body weight then wait to analyze the rhythm.
C) Obtain peripheral intravenous access (PIV) and deliver adenosine 0.1 mg/kg.
D) Place a bag of ice to the child's face.
E) Resume chest compressions; this is not a shockable rhythm.

Discussion 8-4

The correct answer is "A." The rhythm shown above is ventricular tachycardia. This can be distinguished from supraventricular tachycardia (SVT) due to a wide QRS complex. Options "C" and "D" are appropriate therapies to try if the patient had SVT. Ventricular tachycardia is a shockable rhythm, and the algorithm for therapy is first a synchronized shock at 0.5 to 1 J/kg followed by immediate chest compressions, upon reassessment of the rhythm if the patient continues to have a nonperfusing ventricular tachycardia *with* a pulse increase to 2 J/kg synchronized cardioversion.

QUICK QUIZ

Which is true regarding ventricular tachycardia?
A) Nonsynchronized shocks should be delivered for pulseless ventricular tachycardia.
B) Shocks should never be synchronized for ventricular tachycardia.
C) AEDs can only be used in children older than 5 years of age.
D) 4 J/kg should always be used per shock.
E) You should have paid more attention during your pediatric advanced life support (PALS) training.

Discussion

The correct answers are "A and E." In the setting of ventricular tachycardia, always check for a pulse first to guide what to do!

- Pulse + poor perfusion = perform cardioversion
  - Synchronized shocks, start at 0.5 to 1 J/kg, and escalate to 2 J/kg.
- Pulseless = perform defibrillation
  - Nonsynchronized shocks, start at 2 J/kg, and escalate to 4 J/kg.

AEDs can be used for defibrillation but not synchronized cardioversion. AEDs can be used for infants and children if a manual machine is not available.

▶ CASE 9

A 17-year-old previously healthy adolescent boy presents to the emergency department with a 1-day history of headache, fever, myalgias, and decreased activity. He has not had urine output for the last 12 hours. Upon physical exam, temperature is 39°C (102.2°F), HR 125 bpm, RR 30, BP 75/45 mm Hg, and SpO$_2$ is 94% on room air. He is unable to answer simple questions. His skin is warm to the touch, pulses are bounding throughout, and capillary refill time is instantaneous. Multiple small petechiae are noted on his chest and abdomen.

Question 9-1

Which of the following signs is/are NOT consistent with a diagnosis of sepsis?
A) Fever > 38°C (100.4°F).
B) Tachycardia.
C) Capillary refill time > 5 seconds.
D) Capillary refill time < 2 seconds.
E) All of the above are consistent with a diagnosis of sepsis.

Discussion 9-1

The correct answer is "E." Children in septic shock may present with signs of either "warm shock," as manifested by the teenager with bounding pulses and flash capillary refill in the vignette, or "cold shock," exemplified by diminished pulses and prolonged capillary refill time. International consensus definitions for pediatric sepsis are shown in Table 8–1. The petechiae

TABLE 8-1 DEFINITIONS OF PEDIATRIC SEPSIS

Infection	Suspected or proven infection caused by any pathogen or a clinical syndrome associated with a high probability of infection
Systemic inflammatory response syndrome (SIRS)	Requires 2/4 of the following criteria, 1 of which must be abnormal temperature or abnormal leukocyte count: 1. Core temperature > 38.5°C (101.3°F) or < 36°C (96.8°F) 2. Tachycardia (may be bradycardia if < 1 year of age) 3. Respiratory rate > 2 standard deviations above normal for age or acute need for mechanical ventilation not related to neuromuscular disease or general anesthesia 4. Leukocyte count elevated or depressed for age (not secondary to chemotherapy) or > 10% immature neutrophils
Sepsis	SIRS in the presence of or as a result of suspected or proven infection
Severe sepsis	Sepsis + one of the following: 1. Cardiovascular organ dysfunction 2. Acute respiratory distress syndrome (ARDS) 3. Two or more other organ dysfunctions

Septic shock	Sepsis + one of the following despite receipt of > 40 mL/kg isotonic fluid in 1 hour:
	 1. Persistent hypotension
	 2. Need for vasoactive drug to maintain normal blood pressure
	 3. Two of the following:
	    a. Unexplained metabolic acidosis
	    b. Increased lactate
	    c. Oliguria
	    d. Capillary refill time > 5 seconds
	    e. Core to peripheral temperature gap > 3°C

indicate thrombocytopenia from disseminated intervascular coagulation (DIC). Finding petechiae below the nipple line is never a good sign. Ingrain this case in your head! Don't miss septic shock.

> **Helpful Tip**
> For sepsis, an infection must be proven or suspected. The infection does not have to be bacterial!

Question 9-2

Within the first 5 minutes of the previous patient's arrival, which of the following actions should be taken?
A) Begin high-flow oxygen.
B) Establish IV access.
C) Obtain a chest X-ray.
D) Start dopamine at 5 mcg/kg/min.
E) Both A and B.

Discussion 9-2

The correct answer is "E." When managing a critically ill child, the ABCs should always be followed. This patient is maintaining his airway and breathing spontaneously but needs supplemental oxygen to improve his oxygen delivery. In order to improve his circulatory status, vascular access must be obtained immediately. The initial step in shock resuscitation, fluid bolus administration, may then begin.

Question 9-3

Despite multiple attempts by nursing staff in the first 5 minutes, peripheral IV access cannot be obtained. The next best step is:
A) Have another nurse attempt to place an IV.
B) Place an intraosseous (IO) needle.
C) Call the anesthesia service for a peripheral IV start.
D) Call the surgical service for central line placement.
E) Request transfer of the patient to the PICU.

Discussion 9-3

The correct answer is "B." It is crucial that vascular access is obtained in the first 5 minutes of caring for a patient with shock of any type. An IO needle should be placed in a long bone (tibia, sternum, humerus) either manually or using an assistive device. It is appropriately anchored in the intraosseous membrane when it feels stable to touch and flushes easily without extravasation into the tissue. It may then be used to draw blood and infuse fluids or medications, including those that require central access.

Intraosseous access is successfully obtained and the nurse asks what type of fluid you would like to give through it.

Question 9-4

Your response is:
A) D_5NS at 100 mL/h.
B) D_5NS 20 mL/kg over 15 min.
C) NS 20 mL/kg over 5 min.
D) NS 20 mL/kg over 1 h.
E) D_5NS + 20 mEq/L KCl at 50 mL/h.

Discussion 9-4

The correct answer is "C." The established initial step in resuscitation from shock of any type is fluid boluses of isotonic solution. Normal saline (NS) or lactated Ringer (LR) may be used, although NS is the safer choice in patients with poor urine output since LR contains potassium. Volume of 20 mL/kg is given as fast as possible. Up to 60 mL/kg should be given in the first 15 minutes, watching for rales or hepatomegaly, which are signs of cardiac failure. Colloid solution infusion should be considered following the initial 60 mL/kg. Patients with septic shock may require up to 200 mL/kg of fluid resuscitation within the first hour to ensure adequate intravascular volume repletion.

Considering his history and physical exam findings, you suspect that this patient has septic shock caused by *Neisseria meningitidis*.

Question 9-5

The next best step in his evaluation should be:
A) Obtain a computed tomography (CT) scan of the head looking for cerebral edema.
B) Obtain CBC, electrolytes, coagulation studies, venous blood gas, and lactate.
C) Send a blood culture to the lab looking for gram-negative diplococci.
D) No further diagnostic evaluation is needed before antibiotic therapy is begun.
E) Perform a lumbar puncture to collect cerebrospinal fluid (CSF).

Discussion 9-5

The correct answer is "D." All of the other responses could be appropriate items in his diagnostic evaluation, but the most important next step in treating his septic shock is broad-spectrum antibiotic therapy. A third-generation cephalosporin such as ceftriaxone is appropriate treatment. Vancomycin may be added based on risk factors. Antibiotic administration should not be delayed to wait for diagnostic tests or studies. Protect yourself and others from infection by following droplet precautions and giving postexposure antibiotic prophylaxis when indicated.

Following oxygen administration, IO placement, NS 60 mL/kg, and antibiotics, the patient's heart rate has decreased to 115 bpm, SpO$_2$ has improved to 100%, and respiratory rate is in the mid 20s. His BP remains low at 80/50 mm Hg, pulses are still bounding, and capillary refill time is less than 2 seconds.

Question 9-6

The next best step in his management is:
A) Norepinephrine 0.05 mcg/kg/min via IO.
B) Epinephrine 0.05 mcg/kg/min via IO.
C) Repeat NS 20 mL/kg bolus.
D) Central line placement.
E) Activated protein C.

Discussion 9-6

The correct answer is "A." If shock persists despite 60 mL/kg of crystalloid fluid resuscitation, an inotrope should be added. Central line placement is not required as IO access may be used to infuse drugs centrally. This patient demonstrates signs

consistent with warm shock (hypotension, bounding pulses, flash capillary refill from inappropriate vasodilation), and norepinephrine is the drug of choice to treat that entity due to its alpha-adrenergic vasoconstrictor effects. Dopamine could be an appropriate first-line inotropic agent to start in warm shock as well, since it may run safely through a peripheral IV line. Activated protein C was evaluated to see if its benefit to septic adults extends to children, but the trial was closed due to an increased risk of intracranial hemorrhage and poor risk-to-benefit ratio.

► CASE 10

You are paged to the emergency department stat to assist with a patient who is en route. He is a 4-year-old previously healthy boy who suffered a drowning in his babysitter's backyard swimming pool. It is estimated that he was submerged approximately 15 minutes, and the babysitter started rescue breathing and CPR after pulling him out of the water. He was intubated when EMS arrived and CPR is continuing in the ambulance. Upon his arrival to the emergency department, his rectal temperature is 30°C (86°F), pulses are palpable with ongoing compressions, and SpO$_2$ is 90% with bagging occurring through the endotracheal tube (ETT) at a rate of 20 breaths per minute. His pupils are fixed and dilated, he does not respond to verbal stimulation, and he extends his extremities to painful stimuli. His Glasgow Coma Scale (GCS) score is 4. EMS reports that he received two code doses of epinephrine during the 7-minute drive to the hospital through the IO needle they placed at the scene.

Question 10-1

Your management of this patient should include all of the following EXCEPT:
A) Passive and active rewarming measures.
B) Continued CPR, epinephrine doses through the IO needle, and defibrillation if necessary until return of spontaneous circulation or core temperature of 32–34°C (89.6–93.2°F).
C) Ensuring appropriate ventilation and oxygenation via bagging through the ETT or ventilator support.
D) Discontinuation of support as resuscitation is futile.
E) Immediate treatment of seizures or hypoglycemia.

Discussion 10-1

The correct answer is "D." Since this patient's core temperature is hypothermic, aggressive resuscitation efforts should continue regardless of whether the drowning occurred in warm or cold water. Hypothermia can have profound effects on cardiac rhythm and contractility, which may improve rapidly once the body reaches a more normal temperature. Both passive (removal of wet clothes, warm blankets, increasing environmental temperature) and active (warmed IV fluids, external radiant heat, ventilation with heated gas) rewarming should be instituted in this child. Resuscitation should continue following PALS guidelines until return of spontaneous circulation or successful rewarming. Resuscitative efforts should cease if the child has a core temperature of 32–34°C (89.6–93.2°F) and still has not had return of spontaneous circulation. Maintaining appropriate ventilation and oxygenation and immediate treatment of conditions that worsen cerebral injury (seizures, hypoglycemia, hyperthermia) are paramount in the management of this critically ill child.

....

The boy has return of spontaneous circulation 20 minutes into his resuscitation. His core temperature has warmed to 34°C, his HR is 120 bpm, blood pressure is 80/40 mm Hg on an epinephrine continuous infusion, and oxygen saturations are 94% with 60% oxygen delivered through the ventilator. He is not breathing over the set ventilator rate of 25 bpm, his neurologic exam has not changed, and he has not received any sedative or analgesia medication since he was in the ambulance. Right before he is moved to the PICU, his parents ask you about his chances for survival.

Question 10-2

The best prognostic indicator of his future outcome is:
A) His submersion time of 15 minutes.
B) His age and sex.
C) Spontaneous, purposeful movements within the next 24 hours.
D) Absence of measured O_2 saturation (SpO_2) < 90%.
E) Adequate blood pressure on ≤ 1 vasopressor medication.

Discussion 10-2

The correct answer is "C." Significant improvement on serial neurologic exams in the first 24 to 48 hours following injury is the best predictor of prognosis following cerebral anoxia. Submersion times of less than 5 minutes usually result in survival and submersion times of greater than 25 minutes usually result in death, but outcomes vary widely following submersion times of 5 to 25 minutes. Although boys drown more frequently, there is no difference in outcome between the sexes. The incidence of drowning spikes in both the toddler and teenage years but age is not a prognostic factor for outcome. Neither level of hypoxia nor need for vasopressor support indicates future outcome.

....

During the boy's first 24 hours in the PICU, he remains hemodynamically stable on an epinephrine continuous infusion. His oxygenation and ventilation remain acceptable with moderate ventilator support. His core temperature has varied between 35°C and 36°C (95°F and 96.8°F). His pupils remain fixed and dilated, he does not respond to voice, and he extends his extremities to pain. He has not received any sedation, analgesia, or muscle-relaxing drugs. Approximately 36 hours following his drowning event, he suddenly has a spontaneous rise in BP to 130/80 mm Hg with concurrent drop in HR to 65 bpm.

Question 10-3

These changes in vital signs are most likely due to:
A) Worsening cerebral edema.
B) Pneumothorax.
C) Kink in his Foley catheter causing bladder distention.
D) Improvement in his neurologic status.
E) None of the above.

Discussion 10-3

The correct answer is "A." Brain cells respond to anoxic injury by swelling, leading to cerebral edema. This can then worsen the extent of the injury by increasing the amount of ischemic injury. This process occurs over the first 24 to 72 hours following the initial event. Hypertension, bradycardia, and irregular respirations (which this patient cannot demonstrate as his respiratory pattern is set by the ventilator) form the Cushing triad, which is the classic presentation of increased intracranial pressure and impending brainstem herniation. There is no evidence that therapies to reduce intracranial pressure improve outcomes for drowning victims.

....

Over the next 24 hours, the boy's condition worsens. He remains hemodynamically stable and normothermic but he is no longer having any response to painful stimuli. His family relays to you that the PICU physicians have stated the need to perform brain death testing.

Question 10-4

All of the following are criteria for brain death EXCEPT:
A) Flaccid tone and unresponsiveness to deep painful stimuli.
B) Pupils midposition or fully dilated with absence of light reflexes.
C) Absence of corneal, cough, and gag reflexes.
D) Presence of oculovestibular reflexes.
E) Absence of spontaneous respiratory effort while on mechanical ventilation.

Discussion 10-4

The correct answer is "D." The exam is consistent with brain death when oculovestibular reflexes are absent. This brainstem reflex is tested by elevating the head to 30 degrees and then irrigating each auditory canal with 10 to 50 mL of ice water, one ear at a time, waiting several minutes in between. Movement of the eyes in any direction means that the reflex is present. Further required elements of brain death testing are noted in Table 8–2. Each individual institution has its own specific policy on what exactly the process steps are to declare a patient brain dead.

....

The boy's initial brain death exam, including an apnea test, is consistent with brain death. His parents do not want to wait a full 12 hours to perform the second exam as they would like him to be an organ donor. They ask if there is any way the time between exams can be shortened.

TABLE 8–2 REQUIREMENTS FOR ESTABLISHING BRAIN DEATH

Irreversible and known cause of coma	Traumatic brain injury, anoxic brain injury, identifiable metabolic disorder, other
Correction of factors that may interfere with testing	Core temperature > 35°C (95°F), SBP or MAP in acceptable range for age, no drug effects (sedative, analgesic, neuromuscular blocker) or metabolic intoxication
Physical exam	1. Flaccid tone and unresponsive to deep painful stimuli 2. Pupils are midposition or fully dilated and without response to light 3. Corneal, cough, and gag responses are absent 4. Oculovestibular reflexes are absent 5. Spontaneous respiratory effort while on mechanical ventilation is absent
Apnea test	1. Patient remains hemodynamically stable and is not hypoxic during testing 2. No respiratory effort is observed despite final $PaCO_2 > 60$ mm Hg or ≥ 20 mm Hg above baseline
Waiting period between 2 exams performed by separate qualified attending physicians	≥ 24 hours in patients who are term newborns to 30 days old; ≥ 12 hours in patients 31 days to 18 years old

MAP, mean arterial pressure; $PaCO_2$, partial pressure of carbon dioxide in arterial blood; SBP, systolic blood pressure.

Question 10-5

Appropriate confirmatory testing that may shorten the interval between brain death exams is:

A) Electroencephalographic documentation of electrocerebral silence.
B) Radionuclide cerebral blood flow determinations that document the absence of cerebral blood flow.
C) Computed tomography of the head demonstrating brainstem herniation.
D) All of the above.
E) Both A and B.

Discussion 10-5

The correct answer is "E." An electroencephalogram (EEG) demonstrating electrocerebral silence and cerebral blood flow

(CBF) studies documenting the absence of cerebral blood flow are both confirmatory tests for brain death declaration. Only one of them need be performed. These may be used when complete brain death testing is not possible due to the underlying condition of the patient, for example hypoxia or hypotension during apnea testing. They may also function as a confirmatory test when family members request a shorter time frame between exams. In this case, the second clinical exam should still be performed immediately following the EEG or CBF study and all must demonstrate no cerebral activity. Cerebral imaging is not a part of brain death declaration.

▶ **CASE 11**

A previously healthy 15-year-old boy is brought to the emergency department after being thrown from his snowmobile. He was wearing a helmet; opens his eyes to command; is oriented to person, place, and time; localizes to painful stimuli; and is in mild respiratory distress. His vital signs are HR 115 bpm, RR 22, T 37.5°C (99.5°F), SpO_2 94% on 100% FiO_2 via nonrebreathing facemask.

Question 11-1

What is his Glasgow Coma Scale (GCS) score?

A) 8.
B) 10.
C) 12.
D) 13.
E) 15.

Discussion 11-1

The correct answer is "D." Remember, the GCS is based on three components: eye opening, verbal response, and motor response. (See Table 8–3.) The patient in this vignette loses 1 point for eye opening and 1 point for motor response, giving him a GCS score of 13. Strongly consider intubation for any patient with a GCS of 8 or less, or with a rapidly declining GCS score. A modified GCS is available for preverbal infants and children.

> **Helpful Tip**
> To remember the Glasgow Coma Scale, think:
> 4 eyes—4 points for eye opening
> Jackson 5—5 points for verbal
> V6 engine—6 points for motor

> **Helpful Tip**
> Traumatic brain injuries can cause abnormal posturing of the body spontaneously or in response to stimuli. In decorticate posturing, the upper body is flexed. In decerebrate posturing, the upper body is extended. In both, the lower body is extended and internally rotated. Both are grave signs. (See Figure 8–3.)

TABLE 8-3 GLASGOW COMA SCALE

Behavior	Response	Response (preverbal children)	Score
Eye opening	Spontaneously	Spontaneous	4
	To command/speech	To sound	3
	To pain	To pain	2
	No response	No response	1
Verbal response	Oriented to person, place, and time	Vocalizations, smile, interacts	5
	Confused, but answers questions	Cries, irritable	4
	Inappropriate words	Cries to pain	3
	Incomprehensible sounds	Moans to pain	2
	No response	No response	1
Motor response	Obeys commands	Spontaneous movement	6
	Localizes to pain	Withdraws from touch	5
	Withdraws from pain	Withdraws from pain	4
	Abnormal flexion (decorticate)	Abnormal flexion (decorticate)	3
	Abnormal extension (decerebrate)	Abnormal extension (decerebrate)	2
	No response	No response	1
Total			15

Upon close examination you note that the patient's right chest wall seems to move inward upon inspiration and outward upon exhalation.

Question 11-2

What is the most appropriate course of action?
A) Emergent intubation and mechanical ventilation.
B) Strapping and splinting to stabilize the chest.

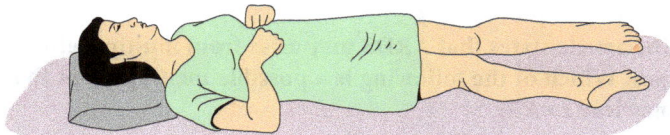

Decorticate or flexor posturing

Decerebrate or extensor posturing

FIGURE 8-3. Abnormal posturing is seen with severe traumatic brain injuries. Decorticate posturing: flexion and adduction of the arms with extension and internal rotation of the legs. Decerebrate posturing: extension and internal rotation of the arms and legs. Decerebrate posturing scores lower on the GCS. (Reproduced with permission from Hall JB, Schmidt GA, Kress JP, eds. *Principles and Critical Care*. 4 ed. New York, NY: McGraw-Hill Education; 2015. Fig. 86-15.)

C) Surgical consult and analgesia with a patient-controlled analgesic (PCA) pump.
D) Initiating continuous positive airway pressure.
E) Both C and D are correct.

Discussion 11-2

The correct answer is "D." The patient in this vignette is suffering from flail chest secondary to a blunt force from a motor vehicle accident. Flail chest typically occurs when there are several anterior and posterior fractures to multiple ribs, creating an unstable or "free" area of the chest wall that no longer contributes to lung expansion. This is clinically evidenced by the characteristic paradoxical movement of the flail area of chest—inward upon inhalation and outward upon exhalation. Although it is tempting to splint or strap the chest to stabilize it, this may actually inhibit chest wall movement and adequate inspiration and pulmonary toilet. While some cases of flail chest are severe enough to require mechanical ventilation, a patient in mild distress with a reasonable GCS should not require such invasive measures. Some cases may require surgical intervention, though the mainstay for flail chest therapy is analgesia and support with noninvasive positive pressure ventilation.

As you continue your evaluation you note the patient is taking shallow breaths, complaining of chest pain, and upon auscultation the right breath sounds are diminished as compared with the left. HR is now 130 bpm, BP 125/80 mm Hg, RR 30, T 38°C (100.4°F), and arterial blood gases demonstrate 7.35/52/75/20 with a hemoglobin concentration of 8.4 g/dL.

Question 11-3

What is the most appropriate next step?

A) Increase the dose of the PCA to improve analgesia.

B) Obtain stat an upright chest X-ray and stop your surgical colleagues before they leave the emergency department for their next consult.

C) Perform stat needle decompression of the right pleural space.

D) Administer broad-spectrum IV antibiotics.

E) None of the above.

Discussion 11-3

The correct answer is "B." This patient has clinical and laboratory signs consistent with a hemothorax: short shallow breaths, chest pain, tachypnea, and a low hemoglobin concentration. Hemothorax typically occurs in the setting of blunt force trauma. Diagnosis of a hemothorax can be confirmed by an upright chest X-ray. While the differential diagnoses includes pneumothorax, unless the patient is acutely demonstrating tension pneumothorax physiology with resultant hemodynamic compromise it is beneficial to obtain a chest X-ray prior to emergently decompressing the pleural space, as a hemothorax would likely not resolve with simple needle decompression. The primary mode of treatment for a hemothorax is a tube thoracostomy with the potential for thoracotomy if bleeding is significant or persistent. Transfusion of blood products may be necessary to correct coagulopathies and maintain adequate intravascular volume and oxygen delivery.

▶ CASE 12

At 4:30 PM on a Friday afternoon, your nurse hears a phone message from the worried father of one of your long-term patients. He states that his child was transferred to the PICU earlier that day and the physicians there have mentioned it was due to "ARDS." He says that he has never heard of this before and asks you to call him to answer his questions about it. You recall that his previously healthy 2-year-old daughter was admitted to the hospital 2 nights ago by one of your partners with a 3-day history of oral temperature 40°C (104°F), cough, and increased work of breathing. The girl was hypoxic and was placed on oxygen via nasal cannula and started on antibiotics for community-acquired pneumonia. Before returning the father's call, you refresh your memory on acute respiratory distress syndrome.

Question 12-1

The review article that you read defines the consensus criteria for ARDS as all of the following EXCEPT:

A) Acute onset (< 7 days) of hypoxia from an identifiable insult.

B) Frontal X-ray with diffuse infiltrates in one lung.

C) Severe hypoxemia as identified by $PaO_2/FiO_2 < 200$.

D) Absence of left atrial hypertension.

E) All of the above are consensus criteria for ARDS.

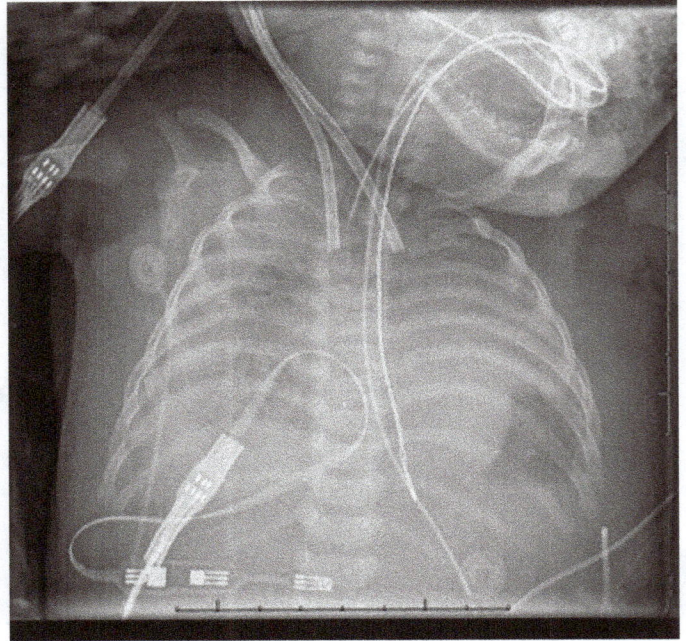

FIGURE 8–4. This radiograph demonstrates typical findings in acute respiratory distress syndrome, including bilateral diffuse alveolar opacities, with obscurement of the pulmonary vascular markings, and asymmetric consolidation.

Discussion 12-1

The correct answer is "B." The definition of acute respiratory distress syndrome (ARDS) requires diffuse bilateral infiltrates. (See Figure 8–4.) ARDS is a disorder marked by profound hypoxia and severely decreased lung compliance. An initial insult activates the inflammatory and coagulation cascades, which increases the usual pulmonary endothelial and epithelial permeability. This results in alveoli filling with protein-rich edema fluid. This leads to difficulty in oxygen transfer, inactivation of surfactant, and worsened ventilation-perfusion mismatch.

Question 12-2

The article states that ARDS may arise from multiple etiologies. Which of the following is a possible inciting event that may lead to ARDS?

A) Pneumonia (bacterial, viral, or fungal).

B) Sepsis.

C) Aspiration.

D) Multiple trauma.

E) All of the above are possible inciting events that may lead to ARDS.

Discussion 12-2

The correct response is "E". These are the most common causes of ARDS. Other entities that may injure the lung and result in ARDS include drowning, embolism, smoke inhalation, acute pancreatitis, blood product transfusions, drug overdose, and cardiac bypass. ARDS can be classified as primary or secondary etiologies. With primary etiologies (eg, pneumonia, lung contusion), the lung injury classic to ARDS is secondary to direct insult to the lung parenchyma. In secondary etiologies (eg, pancreatitis, sepsis), the injury is secondary to a systemic inflammatory response. The distinction between primary and secondary ARDS can have implications on treatment and outcome.

After your quick review, you return the father's call. He relays that his daughter was intubated upon her arrival to the PICU and is still requiring a high amount of oxygen despite several changes to her ventilator made by the pediatric intensivist. Dad is very scared and his first question to you is, "Can my daughter die from ARDS?"

Question 12-3

You reply:

A) No, ARDS is not lethal.
B) Yes, ARDS can be fatal.
C) Complications such as sepsis and multiorgan system failure increase the risk for death.
D) Only children with chronic medical conditions die from ARDS.
E) Both B and C.

Discussion 12-3

The correct answer is "E." Significant mortality occurs from ARDS despite advances in therapeutic options. Complications increase this risk for death. Both previously healthy children and those with chronic medical conditions are at risk to die from ARDS.

Dad then asks, "What methods will the doctors use to increase her chance of survival?"

Question 12-4

You answer:

A) List her for lung transplant immediately.
B) Use lung protective strategies such as low tidal volume ventilation, positive end-expiratory pressure (PEEP), and permissive hypercapnia.
C) Start her on the medicine that treats ARDS.
D) Perform radiation therapy directed at her lungs.
E) None of the above.

Discussion 12-4

The correct answer is "B." These strategies prevent ventilator-induced lung injury due to barotrauma, atelectrauma, and volutrauma. Lung transplant and radiation therapy are not used as therapeutic measures in ARDS. Unfortunately, there is no medicine that treats ARDS. All of the methods used to minimize damage and improve survival are supportive.

BIBLIOGRAPHY

Brierley J, Carcillo J, Choong K, et al. Clinical practice parameters for hemodynamic support of pediatric and neonatal septic shock: 2007 update from the American College of Critical Care Medicine. *Crit Care Med.* 2007;37(2):666–688.

Chameides L, Samson R, Schexnayder S, Hazinski MF. *Pediatric Advanced Life Support Provider Manual.* Dallas, TX: American Heart Association; 2011.

Cornfield DN. Acute respiratory distress syndrome in children: Physiology and management. *Curr Opin Pediatr.* 2013;25(3):338–343.

D'Agostino D, Diaz S, Sanchez MC, Boldrini G. Management and prognosis of acute liver failure in children. *Curr Gastoenterol Rep.* 2012;14:262–269.

Goldstein B, Giroir B, Randolph A. International pediatric sepsis consensus conference: Definitions for sepsis and organ dysfunction in pediatrics. *Pediatr Crit Care Med.* 2005;6(1):2–8.

Holmes JF, Palchak MJ, MacFarlane T, Kuppermann N. Performance of the Pediatric Glasgow Coma Scale in children with blunt head trauma. *Acad Emerg Med.* 2005;12(9):814–819.

Kliegman RM, Stanton BF, Schor NF, et al, eds. *Nelson Textbook of Pediatrics.* 19th ed. Philadelphia, PA: Elsevier/Saunders; 2011.

Lobos AT, Menon K. A multidisciplinary survey on capillary refill time: Inconsistent performance and interpretation of a common clinical test. *Pediatr Crit Care Med.* 2008;9(4):386–391.

McKiernan CA, Lieberman SA. Circulatory shock in children: An overview. *Pediatr Rev.* 2005;26:451–460.

Mews C, Sinatra F. Chronic liver disease in children. *Pediatr Rev.* 1993;14:436–443.

Meyer RJ, Theodorou AA, Berg RA. Childhood drowning. *Pediatr Rev.* 2006;27:163–169.

Nakagawa TA, Ashwal S, Mathur M, Mysore M. Clinical report—Guidelines for the determination of brain death in infants and children: An update of the 1987 task force recommendations. *Pediatrics.* 2011;128:e720–e740.

Nichols DG. *Rogers' Textbook of Pediatric Intensive Care.* Philadelphia, PA: Lippincott Williams and Wilkins; 2008.

Schwaitzberg SD, Bergman KS, Harris BH. A pediatric trauma model of continuous hemorrhage. *J Pediatr Surg.* 1988;23(7):605–609.

Yager P, Noviski N. Shock. *Pediatr Rev.* 2010;31:311–319.

Ear, Nose, and Throat Disorders

9

Derek Zhorne

C) Topical glucocorticoid therapy.
D) Systemic antimicrobial therapy.
E) Systemic glucocorticoid therapy.

▶ CASE 1

A 6-year-old boy presents to your office with worsening right ear pain and itching for several days. His mother has always been concerned about a skin tag in front of his ear and is concerned that it may be infected. Physical exam reveals an isolated right preauricular skin tag with no surrounding erythema; however, he has definite pain with manipulation of his tragus and you see a thick, purulent discharge in the edematous and erythematous external auditory canal.

Question 1-1

Which of the following prophylactic treatments is NOT recommended for his condition?
A) Wearing ear plugs while swimming.
B) Using acidifying ear drops before and after swimming.
C) Removing cerumen from the ear on a daily basis.
D) Drying the ear canal with a hair dryer.
E) Avoiding trauma to the external auditory canal.

Discussion 1-1

The correct answer is "C." Otitis externa, also called *swimmer's ear*, is cellulitis of the external auditory canal. It is often exacerbated by heat, humidity, moisture in the ear, and localized trauma to the ear canal skin. Cerumen provides a protective barrier to the underlying skin of the external ear canal and should not be removed. The old adage "Don't put anything smaller than your elbow in your ear" helps to avoid otitis externa. How does this pertain to a pediatrician's favorite pastime of ear curettage? Prophylactic measures to prevent otitis externa consist of avoiding ear moisture (by wearing ear plugs or using a hair dryer after swimming), using acidifying ear drops to inhibit bacterial and fungal growth and avoiding trauma to the ear canal.

Question 1-2

All of the following therapeutic options may be indicated in the treatment of otitis externa EXCEPT:
A) Oral pain medication.
B) Topical antimicrobial therapy.
C) Topical glucocorticoid therapy.
D) Systemic antimicrobial therapy.
E) Systemic glucocorticoid therapy.

Discussion 1-2

The correct answer is "E." There is currently no indication for the use of systemic glucocorticoids in the treatment of otitis externa. Pain is a significant complaint in otitis externa and responds best to oral pain medications. The use of topical antimicrobials targeted to the common bacterial pathogens of *Staphylococcus aureus* and *Pseudomonas aeruginosa* can be achieved with fluoroquinolone, polymyxin B and neomycin, or aminoglycoside ear drops for 7 to 10 days. Avoid the use of aminoglycoside ear drops if the tympanic membrane is perforated or cannot be visualized as they can be ototoxic. Topical glucocorticoids are often added to antimicrobial suspensions and may help to decrease pain and relieve itching. If the patient is immunocompromised or there is evidence of periauricular cellulitis, then oral antimicrobial therapy is indicated.

> **Helpful Tip**
> Preauricular sinuses, pits, and skin tags are common and frequently noted on routine physical exam. Either inherited in an incomplete autosomal dominant pattern or arising spontaneously, they usually cause no symptoms. However, everyone with a preauricular sinus, pit, or skin tag should have a formal hearing test. Remember that both the external ear structures and the kidneys form during the same period of embryogenesis. Infants with isolated preauricular sinuses, pits, or skin tags do not routinely need a renal ultrasound unless there are other malformations or dysmorphic features, a family history of deafness, or a maternal history of gestational diabetes.

► CASE 2

A 5-year-old girl presents to the emergency department with a chief complaint of left-sided ear pain. Her parents report that the family was at the movie theater when the girl cried "Ouch!" and then told them that her older brother had put something in her ear. The older brother is not saying anything as he calmly eats his popcorn.

Question 2-1

Which of the following is NOT a clinical finding associated with an acute foreign body in the external ear canal?
A) Cellulitis.
B) Ear pruritus.
C) Bleeding.
D) Tinnitus.
E) Ear pain.

Discussion 2-1

The correct answer is "A." Acute foreign bodies in the ear canal are often asymptomatic and identified because of a witnessed event or based on a verbal report by the affected child. Clinical findings may include ear pain, pruritus, bleeding, tinnitus, or even conductive hearing loss. If left unattended, a foreign body may lead to a secondary infection. Remember that organic matter should not be irrigated as it will absorb liquid and swell, causing increased pain and making it more difficult to remove. Batteries (especially button batteries) require immediate removal as they can generate an electric current and cause a severe burn with liquefaction necrosis within 4 hours. (This leaves a person wondering if a battery really could fit in an ear. To be clear, this is not a challenge.)

⧖ QUICK QUIZ

Trauma can result in an ear hematoma (pooled collection of blood) which presents as a boggy purple swelling of the pinna. The normal folds of the ear will be difficult to visualize due to swelling. This is in contrast to an ear bruise, which does not change the shape of the ear.

All of the following are potential complications of an ear hematoma EXCEPT:
A) Infection
B) Conductive hearing loss
C) Cartilage necrosis
D) Development of "cauliflower ear"
E) Reaccumulation of the hematoma

Discussion

The correct answer is "B." Auricular trauma can result in the formation of a hematoma between the perichondrium and the cartilage of the pinna. If untreated, pressure necrosis of the underlying cartilage may occur with subsequent infection, cosmetic deformity, or both. The "cauliflower ear" deformity seen among wrestlers is the result of new and often asymmetric cartilage formation after a hematoma. To prevent these sequelae, patients should be referred to an otolaryngologist for drainage and application of a carefully molded pressure dressing. Drainage should occur within 7 days of the inciting injury.

► CASE 3

An 8-month-old girl is brought to the clinic for evaluation of a fever. She has been healthy and this is her first illness. She has no known drug allergies. Her mother reports that several members of the family "had a cold" last week and the patient had several days of coughing and rhinorrhea that seemed to improve. Physical exam reveals an ill-appearing infant with a temperature of 39.2°C (102.5°F) and a right tympanic membrane (TM) that is erythematous and bulging with white fluid present behind the TM. You perform pneumatic otoscopy and do not appreciate any movement of the TM. (See Figure 9–1.) You explain to the mother that the child has a right-sided acute otitis media (AOM).

Question 3-1

Acute otitis media is commonly caused by any of the following organisms EXCEPT:
A) *Streptococcus pneumoniae*.
B) *Staphylococcus aureus*.
C) Nontypeable *Haemophilus influenzae*.
D) *Moraxella catarrhalis*.
E) *Streptococcus pyogenes*.

Discussion 3-1

The correct answer is "B." The most commonly identified bacterial organisms to cause AOM include *S. pneumoniae* (35–40%), nontypeable *H. influenzae* (30–35%), *M. catarrhalis* (15–18%), and *S. pyogenes* (4%). Remember that AOM occurs most frequently as a consequence of a viral upper respiratory tract infection (URI), which leads to eustachian tube inflammation and dysfunction with subsequent negative middle ear pressure and movement of secretions containing the pathogenic bacteria from the nasopharynx into the middle ear.

Question 3-2

Which of the following is the most appropriate initial treatment for this patient?
A) Clindamycin.
B) Cefuroxime.
C) Cefdinir.

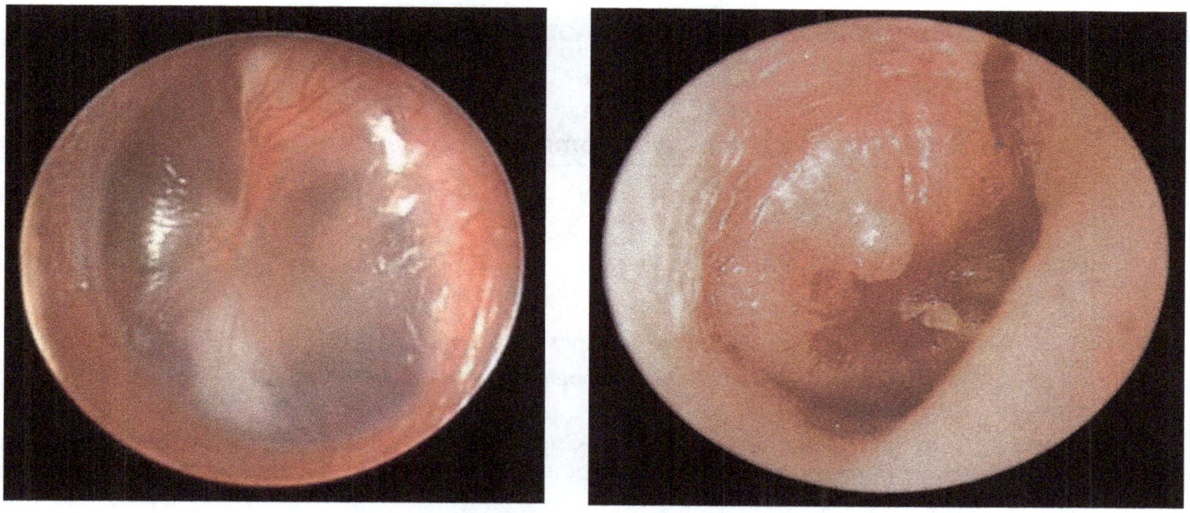

FIGURE 9–1. Acute otitis media. (A) A normal tympanic membrane is shown with a shiny light reflex. (B) The tympanic membrane is inflamed (red), bulging, and has a purulent effusion consistent with acute otitis media. The light reflex is gone. (Used with permission from Dr. Shelagh Cofer, Department of Otolaryngology, Mayo Clinic.)

D) Amoxicillin and clavulanic acid (Augmentin).
E) Amoxicillin.

Discussion 3-2

The correct answer is "E." According to the 2013 American Academy of Pediatrics (AAP) Clinical Practice Guideline for the diagnosis and management of AOM in children, first-line therapy for AOM is high-dose amoxicillin (80–90 mg/kg of body weight/day divided twice daily). *S. pneumoniae* often is resistant to lower dose amoxicillin. This resistance mechanism is via alteration of penicillin-binding proteins (not beta-lactamase production) and can usually be overcome by increasing the dose of amoxicillin. If the patient (1) has been treated with amoxicillin in the past 30 days, (2) has a history of recurrent AOM unresponsive to amoxicillin (3) has concurrent purulent conjunctivitis, or (4) has shown no improvement after 48 hours of amoxicillin therapy, then clinicians should prescribe an antibiotic with additional beta-lactamase coverage (option "D"). Concurrent conjunctivitis suggests *H. influenzae* infection. *H. influenzae* often is resistant to penicillin via beta-lactamase production. Addition of the beta-lactamase inhibitor clavulanate usually is able to overcome this resistance mechanism. If the patient has a penicillin allergy, then alternative agents include cefdinir, cefuroxime, or cefpodoxime. If the patient is unable to take oral medications or compliance is a concern, then you may consider ceftriaxone 50 mg/kg given intramuscularly once daily for 3 days. Remember that AOM is painful and all patients should receive oral pain medication as well. Children younger than 2 years of age should be treated for 10 days, children older than 2 years should be treated for 7 days, and children older than 6 years should be treated for 5 days. See Table 9–1 for recommendations on the initial management of AOM.

Helpful Tip

AOM is the most common condition for which children in the United States are prescribed antibiotics. It is imperative that clinicians follow strict diagnostic criteria to make an accurate diagnosis and avoid prescribing unnecessary antibiotics. See Figure 9–2 for normal TM landmarks. The diagnosis of AOM can be made in children who present with moderate to severe bulging of the TM *or* new onset of otorrhea not due to acute otitis externa *and* the presence of a middle ear effusion proven by pneumatic otoscopy or tympanometry. In a nonverbal child, the diagnosis of AOM can be made with mild bulging of the tympanic membrane *and* recent (< 48 hours) onset of ear pain (manifest as holding, tugging, or rubbing of the ear) *or* intense erythema of the tympanic membrane *and* evidence of a middle ear effusion.

Helpful Tip

Risk factors for AOM include daycare attendance, which increases the likelihood of recurrent viral URIs, bottle-propping in the crib, smoke exposure, eustachian tube dysfunction, and impaired host immune defenses (especially consider immunoglobulin A [IgA] deficiency).

Question 3-3

Which of the following is NOT a potential complication of AOM?
A) Bezold abscess.
B) Tympanosclerosis.
C) Tympanic membrane perforation.
D) Facial nerve paralysis.
E) Mastoiditis.

TABLE 9–1 RECOMMENDATIONS FOR THE INITIAL MANAGEMENT OF ACUTE OTITIS MEDIA (AOM)

Age	Otorrhea with AOM[a]	Unilateral or Bilateral AOM[a] with Severe Symptoms[b]	Bilateral AOM[a] without Otorrhea	Unilateral AOM[a] without Otorrhea
6 mo–2 y	Antibiotic therapy	Antibiotic therapy	Antibiotic therapy	Antibiotic therapy or additional observation
≥ 2 y	Antibiotic therapy	Antibiotic therapy	Antibiotic therapy or additional observation[c]	Antibiotic therapy or additional observation[c]

[a]Applies only to children with well-documented AOM and a high certainty of diagnosis.

[b]A toxic-appearing child, persistent otalgia for more than 48 hours, temperature greater than 39°C (102.2°F) in the past 48 hours, or if there is uncertain access to follow-up after the visit.

[c]This plan of initial management provides an opportunity for shared decision making with the child's family for those categories appropriate for initial observation. If observation is offered, a mechanism must be in place to ensure follow-up and begin antibitoics if the child worsens or fails to improve within 48–72 hours of AOM onset.

Reproduced with permission from Friedman NR, Scholes MA, Yoon PJ. Ear, nose, and throat. In: Hay WW, Levin MJ, Deterding RR, Abzug MJ, eds. *Current Diagnosis & Treatment: Pediatrics.* 22nd ed. New York, NY: McGraw-Hill; 2013.

Discussion 3-3

The correct answer is "A." A Bezold abscess is a laterocervical abscess between the digastric and sternocleidomastoid muscles and may be seen as a complication of mastoiditis. Tympanosclerosis is an acquired disorder of calcification and scarring of the TM and middle ear structures from inflammation and may result in conductive hearing loss if the ossicles are involved. Patients with AOM and subsequent TM perforation often have rapid relief of pain and subsequent otorrhea. These perforations usually heal spontaneously within several weeks, although patients should receive topical antimicrobial ear drops for 10 to 14 days and be referred to an otolaryngologist for a follow-up exam and hearing evaluation. The facial nerve travels through the middle ear as it courses through the temporal bone and may be exposed to inflammation during an episode of AOM with resulting facial nerve paralysis. It is a rare complication that requires both systemic antibiotics and referral to an otolaryngologist for prompt myringotomy and tube placement. Mastoiditis is covered in detail later. Other potential complications of AOM include development of retraction pockets, cholesteatoma, chronic suppurative otitis media, intracranial infections (meningitis, epidural abscess, brain abscess), and lateral or cavernous sinus thrombosis.

Helpful Tip

Children with three or more distinct and well-documented episodes of AOM within 6 months or four or more episodes within 12 months should be referred to an otolaryngologist for tympanostomy tube placement.

You appropriately treated your patient with 10 days of high-dose amoxicillin for her right AOM and are now seeing her back for her 9 month well-child check. She is doing well and her mother has no complaints. Her physical exam at this time reveals the presence of clear fluid behind the TM without any bulging,

Right tympanic membrane

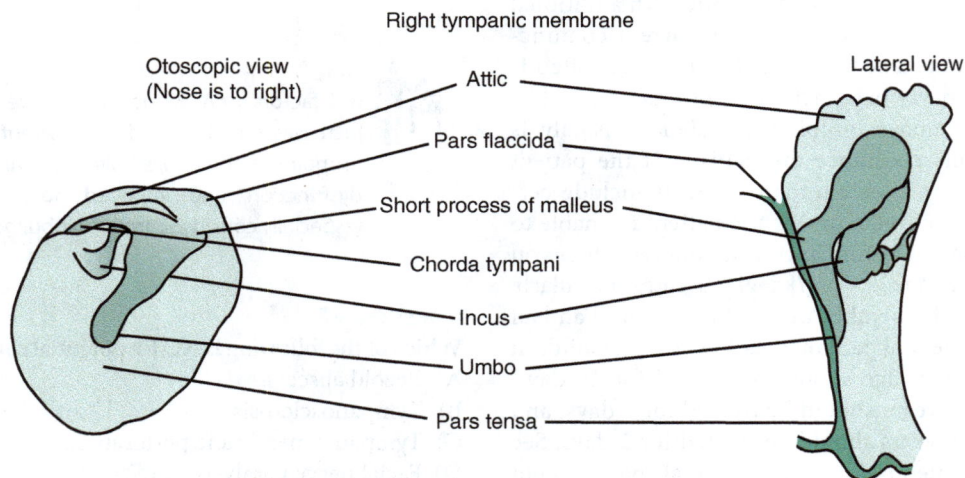

Otoscopic view (Nose is to right)

Lateral view

- Attic
- Pars flaccida
- Short process of malleus
- Chorda tympani
- Incus
- Umbo
- Pars tensa

FIGURE 9–2. Tympanic membrane landmarks. (Reproduced with permission from Hay WW, Levin MJ, Deterding RR, Abzug MJ, eds. *Current Diagnosis and Treatment Pediatrics.* 22nd ed. McGraw-Hill Education; 2014, Fig. 18-1.)

erythema, or otorrhea. You explain to the mother that the patient now has evidence of otitis media with effusion (OME).

Question 3-4

All of the following statements regarding OME are correct EXCEPT:

A) Most episodes will resolve spontaneously within 3 months.
B) OME is often associated with allergic rhinitis, adenoidal hypertrophy, and eustachian tube abnormalities.
C) Referral for tympanostomy tube placement is indicated for hearing loss > 20 decibels (dB).
D) The initial treatment option is "watchful waiting" for 3 months.
E) 5% to 10% of episodes will last 1 year or longer.

Discussion 3-4

The correct answer is "C." OME is defined as the presence of fluid in the middle ear space without associated signs or symptoms of inflammation. It may occur spontaneously due to poor eustachian tube function or as the result of an inflammatory process following AOM. Most episodes resolve spontaneously within 3 months, although 30% to 40% of children have recurrent OME and 5% to 10% of episodes last 1 year or longer. OME is often associated with allergic rhinitis, adenoidal hypertrophy, and eustachian tube abnormalities. As most cases resolve, it is recommended to pursue "watchful waiting" for 3 months if the patient is not at risk for hearing problems. Children at risk for speech or language delays are likely further affected by hearing problems from OME and should be evaluated sooner. This includes children with craniofacial anomalies (eg, Down syndrome, cleft palate, Robin sequence, or CHARGE association [coloboma, heart disease, atresia of the choanae, retarded growth and development, genitourinary anomalies, and ear defects with associated deafness]), permanent hearing loss, autism spectrum disorders, severe visual impairments, or syndromes that adversely affect cognitive and linguistic development. A hearing test should be obtained in any child with OME that persists for 3 months or longer, or at any time that language delay, learning problems, or a significant hearing loss is suspected. If the patient has hearing loss of 40 dB or greater, then referral for tympanostomy tube placement is indicated because persistent hearing loss of this magnitude has been shown to impact speech, language, and academic performance. If the patient has hearing loss of 21 to 39 dB, then he or she should have formal language testing and may benefit from strategies to optimize the learning and listening environment. If the patient has hearing loss of less than 20 dB, then a repeat hearing test should be performed in 3 to 6 months if the OME persists.

> **Helpful Tip**
>
> Children with OME lasting 3 months or longer and who have had a normal hearing test should be reexamined at 3- to 6-month intervals until the effusion is no longer present or they have developed symptoms warranting referral to an otolaryngologist. Pressure equalization (PE) tubes are indicated for hearing loss of greater than 40 dB or structural abnormalities of the eardrum or middle ear. See Table 9–2 for potential complications associated with OME.

TABLE 9–2 POTENTIAL COMPLICATIONS OF OTITIS MEDIA WITH EFFUSION

Potential Physical, Behavioral, Developmental Complications

Mild intermittent ear pain, fullness, or "popping"

Secondary manifestation of ear pain in infants such as ear rubbing, sleep disturbances

Failure of infants to respond appropriately to voices or environmental sounds (eg, not turning toward the sound source)

Hearing loss suggested by lack of attentiveness, failure to respond to normal conversational level speech, need for excessively high sound levels when using audio equipment or watching TV

Recurrent episodes of AOM with persistent OME between episodes

Problems with school performance

Balance problems, unexplained clumsiness, or delayed gross motor development

Delayed speech or language

AOM, acute otitis media; OME, otitis media with effusion.

Data from Rosenfeld RM, Culpepper L, Doyle KJ, et al: Clinical practice guideline: Otitis media with effusion, *Otolaryngol Head Neck Surg.* 2004 May;130(5 Suppl):S95-118.

You are now seeing your patient for her 2-year-old well-child check. She had five episodes of AOM in a 12-month-period and subsequently had tympanostomy tubes placed at 19 months of life. Mom reports that the patient has had persistent white discharge from her left ear for several weeks and wonders if it is related to her tubes or a sign of another ear infection.

Question 3-5

Which of the following is the most likely pathogen to cause chronic suppurative otitis media (CSOM)?

A) *Pseudomonas aeruginosa.*
B) *Klebsiella* species.
C) Anaerobic bacteria.
D) Fungi.
E) *Escherichia coli.*

Discussion 3-5

The correct answer is "A." CSOM is the most common cause of hearing impairment in the developing world and one of the most common childhood infectious diseases worldwide. The World Health Organization (WHO) defines CSOM as "otorrhea through a perforated tympanic membrane present for at least 2 weeks." It is often the sequelae of AOM. The most commonly isolated organisms in decreasing order of frequency are *P. aeruginosa* (18–67%), *Staphylococcus aureus* (14–33%), and gram-negative organisms such as *Proteus* species, *Klebsiella* species, and *Escherichia* species (4–43%). Both anaerobic bacteria such as *Bacteroides* and *Fusobacterium* species as well as fungi such as *Candida* and *Aspergillus* have also been reported. There is no standard of therapy and recommended regimens vary widely. In developing countries, antiseptic ear drops (eg, aluminum acetate, boric acid, iodine powder, or povidone-iodine) are commonly used due to low cost and ease of availability. Most clinicians in the United States use a combination of topical fluoroquinolone ear drops for 14 days with the initiation of the so-called "aural toilet," which includes dry mopping, ear wicking, or gentle suctioning to keep the ear canal consistently dry and free of debris.

> **Helpful Tip**
>
> Otorrhea simply means drainage from the ear and results from either problems with the external ear canal or middle ear disease with a TM perforation. See Table 9–3 for causes of purulent otorrhea. Bloody otorrhea is less common and typically is seen with trauma to the external canal from a foreign body or overly aggressive cleaning of the ear canals, neoplasm, longitudinal temporal bone fracture causing TM and external canal laceration, or in the setting of traumatic cerebrospinal fluid otorrhea associated with a basilar skull fracture.

> **Helpful Tip**
>
> A cholesteatoma is a squamous epithelium–lined sac that may fill with desquamated keratin and behave in a locally destructive manner. Usually caused by prolonged eustachian tube dysfunction with subsequent chronic negative middle ear pressure that draws in the upper flaccid portion of the tympanic membrane, a cholesteatoma can erode into bone and penetrate into the mastoid bone or disrupt the ossicular chain. Early cholesteatomas start with slowly progressive hearing loss, but patients may also have ear pain, headache, or a sensation of "ear fullness." On physical exam, you may see a retraction pocket or apparent TM perforation that exudes keratin debris or granulation tissue. Treatment is surgical marsupialization of the sac or its complete removal. See Figure 9–3 for an example of a cholesteatoma. For those scratching their heads, the top part of the TM is sucked in making a little pouch. The pouch fills with sloughed squamous epithelial cells. The filled pouch accumulates in the middle ear and mastoid, destroying structures as it grows. It has to go, so call a surgeon.

Question 3-6

Which of the following is an indication for tympanostomy tube insertion?

A) Two episodes of AOM within 6 months.

B) Three episodes of AOM within 12 months.

C) Persistent TM perforations.

TABLE 9–3 **CAUSES OF PURULENT OTORRHEA**
Acute otitis media with perforated tympanic membrane
Infectious complications of acute otitis media (ie, acute mastoiditis, intracranial infection)
Otitis externa
Chronic suppurative otitis media
Cholesteatoma
Tympanostomy tube drainage

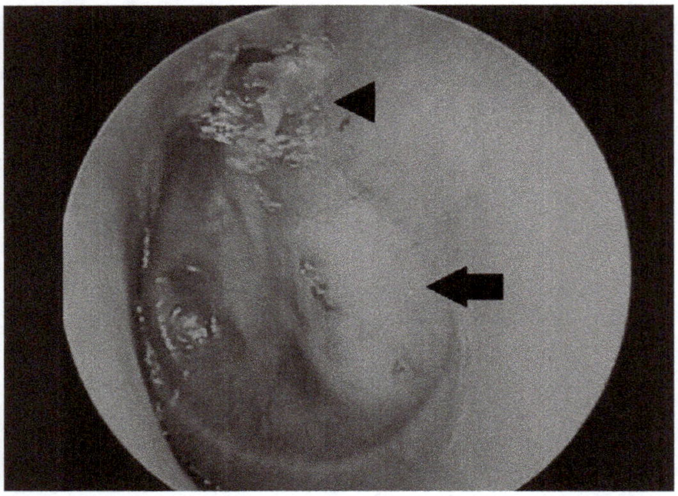

FIGURE 9–3. Cholesteatomas result from invagination of the pars flaccida (see Figure 9–2) part of the tympanic membrane, with accumulation of keratin debris and sloughed squamous epithelial cells. Cholesteatomas are locally erosive and require surgical excision. The arrowhead points to retraction and the arrow to the cholesteatoma sac behind the tympanic membrane. (Reproduced with permission from Lalwani AK, ed. *Current Diagnosis & Treatment in Otolaryngology: Head and Neck Surgery*. 3rd ed. McGraw-Hill Education; 2011, Fig. 50-2.)

D) Conductive hearing loss > 40 dB associated with a middle ear effusion.

E) Tympanosclerosis.

Discussion 3-6

The correct answer is "D." This was a test to see if you had been reading the helpful tips, which are helpful for this question. Indications for tympanostomy tube insertion include (1) recurrent episodes of AOM (defined as three or more distinct and well-documented episodes of AOM within 6 months or four or more episodes within 12 months), (2) conductive hearing loss greater than 40 dB associated with a middle ear effusion, or (3) prevention of acquired cholesteatoma due to a retraction pocket of the TM. Options "A" and "B" are both incorrect because the patient must have had three or more episodes of AOM within 6 months or four or more episodes within 12 months. Options "C" and "E" are incorrect because they are potential complications of tympanostomy tube insertions and not indications for placement. Other potential complications include myringosclerosis, tympanosclerosis, tympanostomy tube otorrhea, and focal atrophy of the tympanic membrane, which increases the risk of developing retractions pockets and cholesteatomas.

> **Helpful Tip**
>
> Quick Diagnosis: Benign paroxysmal positional vertigo (BPPV) manifests as paroxysmal vertigo and nystagmus that only occurs with certain head positioning. It is diagnosed using the Dix-Hallpike maneuver, in which the patient is moved from the sitting position to recumbency with the head tilted 30 to 40 degrees over the end of the examination table and 30 to 45 degrees to one side. The dysfunctional ear is the one that is downward when symptoms are elicited.

▶ CASE 4

You are seeing a 20-month-old boy in your office with a chief complaint of "fever and ear swelling." On physical exam, you see an irritable child and notice that his right auricle appears displaced inferiorly and outward. He has swelling, erythema, and extreme tenderness over his right mastoid area. His tympanic membrane is bulging with loss of the normal landmarks.

Question 4-1

What is the most appropriate next step in the management of this patient's condition?
A) Discharge home with a prescription for high-dose oral amoxicillin.
B) Admit to the hospital and start intravenous clindamycin.
C) Order a plain X-ray of the skull.
D) Admit to the hospital and start intravenous ampicillin.
E) Order a computed tomography (CT) scan of the head and temporal bones.

Discussion 4-1

The correct answer is "E." This patient has acute mastoiditis which is a bacterial infection of the mastoid bone and air cells. It arises from middle ear space infection that spreads by means of boney erosion or through the emissary vein of the mastoid and can occur at any age although greater than 60% of cases are in children younger than 2 years of age. There is usually a preceding history of AOM, and patients present with fever, headache, and ear pain as well as postauricular swelling, redness, and tenderness. On physical exam, the mastoid process is swollen, erythematous, and tender while the auricle is displaced both anteriorly and inferiorly and the ipsilateral tympanic membrane shows signs of AOM. In children 2 years of age or younger, the auricle appears to be pushed "down and out." Mastoiditis is a clinical diagnosis, although you should obtain a CT scan of the head and temporal bones to evaluate for a subperiosteal or intracranial abscess.

The CT scan shows clouding of the middle ear and mastoid air cells with loss of definition of the bony septae that define the mastoid air cells. There is no apparent subperiosteal

abscess or intracranial involvement. You have consulted the otolaryngology service, who will see the patient later today.

Question 4-2

What is the most appropriate next step in the management of this patient's condition?
A) Discharge home after being seen by the otolaryngologist with a prescription for high-dose oral amoxicillin.
B) Admit to the hospital for mastoidectomy.
C) Order a plain X-ray of the skull.
D) Admit to the hospital and start intravenous (IV) broad-spectrum antibiotics.
E) Consult the pediatric surgery department.

Discussion 4-2

The correct answer is "D." The most common bacterial cause of mastoiditis is *Streptococcus pneumoniae*, although *Staphylococcus aureus* (including methicillin-resistant strains), *Streptococcus pyogenes,* and gram-negative bacilli such as *Pseudomonas aeruginosa* and nontypeable *Haemophilus influenza* have all been implicated. Accordingly, the next most appropriate step is to start broad-spectrum IV antibiotics to cover likely pathogens, including methicillin-resistant *S. aureus* (MRSA). Surgical drainage with mastoidectomy is indicated for a subperiosteal or intracranial abscess or a patient who does not improve after 24 to 48 hours of IV antibiotics. A tympanocentesis or myringotomy with or without tympanostomy tube placement, with the middle ear fluid sent for Gram stain and culture, can help guide antimicrobial therapy. A typical course of therapy for uncomplicated mastoiditis is 7 to 10 days of IV antibiotics and then transitioning to oral therapy for a total 4-week course of treatment.

> **Helpful Tip**
>
> There are many possible causes of ear pain—or otalgia, if you want to use medical terminology. (See Table 9–4.)

TABLE 9–4 CAUSES OF EAR PAIN

Location	Etiologies
Auricle	Trauma, hematoma, eczema, impetigo, insect bites, herpes zoster
Meatus	External otitis media, eczema, hard cerumen, foreign body, herpes zoster, trigeminal neuralgia (CN V3)
Middle ear	AOM, mastoiditis, cholesteatoma, malignancy
Referred pain through cranial nerves V, IX, X, and the second and third cervical nerves	Unerupted lower molar, dental caries, TMJ dysfunction, tonsillitis, carcinoma or sarcoma of the pharynx, cervical lymphadenitis, thyroiditis, trigeminal neuralgia

AOM, acute otitis media; TMJ, temporomandibular joint.

▶ CASE 5

You are working in the emergency department and see a 3-week-old infant girl for "trouble breathing." The parents report that the infant has had apparent trouble breathing since birth, with frequent clear right-sided nasal discharge. Review of the birth records show that the patient was born at 40 weeks' gestation by uncomplicated vaginal delivery and had a normal newborn nursery stay. The infant is breastfeeding and the mother feels that she frequently stops feeding to "catch her breath."

Question 5-1

Given this presentation, your clinical suspicion is for:
A) Meningitis.
B) Viral upper respiratory infection.
C) Choanal atresia.
D) *Chlamydia trachomatis* infection.
E) Heart failure.

Discussion 5-1

The correct answer is "C." This patient may have choanal atresia (blocked posterior nasal opening), which is the most common congenital anomaly of the nose and occurs in approximately 1 in 7000 live births. It is typically unilateral and is twice as common in females. Remember that neonates are obligate nasal breathers and anything that creates nasal obstruction (such as choanal atresia) may present as respiratory distress. Option "A" is incorrect because the clinical picture does not fit meningitis. Option "B" is incorrect because you would not expect unilateral discharge with a viral URI. Option "D" is incorrect because you would most commonly see conjunctivitis or pneumonia as a result of neonatal *C. trachomatis* infection. Although you should think of possible heart failure whenever a young child is having difficulty with feedings, the case description is clearly focusing on an upper airway issue; thus option "E" is incorrect.

> **Helpful Tip**
> Unilateral choanal atresia occurs more frequently on the right side and usually presents later in life with unilateral nasal obstruction or discharge. Bilateral choanal atresia presents at birth with respiratory distress and may have "cyclical cyanosis" wherein the cyanosis improves with crying and worsens with feeding. Suspect the diagnosis if you are unable to pass a 6-French catheter through the nose to a depth of about 3 to 4 cm. Confirm the diagnosis with an axial CT scan with intranasal contrast that will show a narrowing of the posterior nasal cavity at the level of the pterygoid plate.

> **Helpful Tip**
> Remember, approximately 50% of patients with bilateral choanal atresia have CHARGE association. Other syndromes that may include choanal atresia include Treacher-Collins, Kallmann, and VACTERL/VATER association (**V**ertebral anomalies, **A**nal atresia, **C**ardiac defects, **TE**F [tracheoesophageal fistula] and/or esophageal atresia, **R**enal anomalies, and **R**adial or **L**imb defects).

⏳ QUICK QUIZ

All of the following are potential therapies for epistaxis (nose bleeding) EXCEPT:
A) Firm pressure on the soft part of the nose below the nasal bones for 5 to 10 minutes.
B) Application of topical vasoconstrictor such as oxymetazoline or phenylephrine.
C) Intranasal packing.
D) Vigorous nose blowing to clean out the nasal passages.
E) Chemical cautery with topical silver nitrate.

Discussion

The correct answer is "D." Epistaxis is conservatively treated by application of firm pressure to the soft part of the nose below the nasal bones for 5 to 10 minutes while sitting up and leaning forward to avoid swallowing the blood. If the bleeding persists, then a one-time application of a topical vasoconstrictor or chemical cautery with silver nitrate may be used. For persistent bleeding, you should obtain an otolaryngology consult as the patient may require anterior or posterior intranasal packing or more advanced surgical interventions. Option "D" is incorrect as it will likely contribute to further bleeding. The evaluation of a patient with epistaxis should include a directed history to evaluate for prior or recurrent episodes of epistaxis, history of nasal trauma, prior head and neck procedures, family history of bleeding disorders, as well as the use of nonsteroidal anti-inflammatory drugs (NSAIDs), warfarin, heparin, aspirin, cocaine, or alcohol. Most cases of epistaxis arise from the anterior portion of the nasal septum at Kiesselbach plexus. Less common posterior bleeding may arise from branches of the anterior ethmoid or sphenopalatine artery and require an urgent otolaryngology consult for posterior packing and admission with pulse oximetry monitoring. After resolution of the acute bleeding, patients with epistaxis often benefit from increased nasal moisture with a daily application of water-based ointment such as petroleum jelly (eg, Vaseline) into the nose or with twice-daily nasal saline irrigation and humidifier use.

⏳ QUICK QUIZ

In a patient with an episode of epistaxis, a hematology workup is warranted for any of the following EXCEPT:
A) Frequent nose picking.
B) Family history of a bleeding disorder.
C) Medical history of easy bleeding such as with circumcision or dental extraction.
D) Spontaneous bleeding at any site.
E) Onset before age 2 years.

Discussion

The correct answer is "A." See Table 9–5 for the differential diagnosis of epistaxis, and remember that digital trauma (nose picking) is a common cause of epistaxis in children. Children love to

TABLE 9–5 DIFFERENTIAL DIAGNOSIS OF EPISTAXIS

Trauma (nose picking, blunt trauma)	Neoplasms (nasopharyngeal carcinoma, rhabdomyosarcoma, lymphoma, juvenile nasopharyngeal angiofibroma)
Medications (especially nasal sprays)	Bleeding disorders (hemophilia, thrombocytopenia, von Willebrand disease, hereditary hemorrhagic telangiectasia)
Nasal polyps	Sinusitis

Helpful Tip

Nasal foreign bodies often present with unilateral foul-smelling rhinorrhea, nasal obstruction, epistaxis, or even halitosis (bad breath). Treatment options include a trial of vigorous nose blowing or the application of a nasal decongestant (eg, oxymetazoline spray) and then removal with alligator forceps. Refer to an otolaryngologist if the object is unlikely to be removed on the first attempt or appears wedged in place. Remember that disk-type batteries are very dangerous nasal foreign bodies as they can generate an electrical current and cause necrosis of mucosa and cartilage in less than 4 hours! (The real question is, why do children put things in their nose and ears?)

pick their noses but are not likely to admit to it. Although epistaxis is caused by a bleeding disorder in less than 5% of cases, a hematology workup would be indicated for all of the other situations listed above.

► CASE 6

You are working in the emergency department and see a 17-year-old adolescent boy who was involved in a physical altercation at school. He was hit in the face with a baseball bat (don't ask!) and is complaining of severe nose pain and difficulty breathing through his nose. On physical exam, you notice a boggy, widened nasal septum that is very tender to palpation and appreciate a whistling noise with each inspiration. You inform the patient that he has a hematoma of the nasal septum and needs immediate referral to an otolaryngologist.

Question 6-1

All of the following are potential complications of an untreated nasal septal hematoma EXCEPT:
A) Odontogenic infection.
B) Development of a "saddle-nose deformity."
C) Nasal abscess formation.
D) Cavernous sinus thrombosis.
E) Meningitis.

Discussion 6-1

The correct answer is "A." Early referral of a nasal septal hematoma to an otolaryngologist for evaluation of the hematoma and packing of the nose with antibiotic prophylaxis is important. If unattended, the septal cartilage may undergo fibrosis, necrosis, and then perforate within 3 to 4 days. The subsequent loss of structural support results in the characteristic "saddle-nose deformity." The other complications listed above as options "C," "D," and "E" are due to secondary infection with subsequent spread through the cavernous sinus. It is always good to know the worst-case scenario. Do not miss out on the opportunity to encourage the teenage boy to use his words when angry.

► CASE 7

You are seeing a 15-year-old adolescent boy with a past medical history of allergic rhinitis who has a chief complaint of "a persistent cold." A review of the chart shows that he was seen 2 weeks ago with similar complaints of daytime cough and rhinorrhea. He reports feeling worse now, with new fevers up to 39.0°C (102.3°F) as well as fatigue and headache. Physical exam is notable for clear rhinorrhea and tenderness to palpation of his face. His posterior oropharynx is clear without any erythema or exudates.

Question 7-1

Which of the following is the most appropriate next step in the management of this patient?
A) Order a plain film X-ray of his skull.
B) Order a CT scan of his head.
C) Offer supportive care therapies with nasal saline rinses and pain medication.
D) Prescribe a 5-day course of amoxicillin and clavulanic acid.
E) Prescribe a 14-day course of amoxicillin.

Discussion 7-1

The correct answer is "E." Acute bacterial sinusitis is a common complication following viral upper respiratory tract infections and is more common in patients with allergic inflammation. Many of the presenting symptoms of sinusitis are very similar to those of a viral respiratory infection, such as daytime cough, nasal discharge, fever, and fatigue. However, it is the persistence (or worsening) of these symptoms without improvement that is suggestive of sinusitis. Adolescent patients may have associated facial pain and tenderness on exam. First-line therapy is amoxicillin with or without clavulanic acid as the most commonly identified pathogens are *Streptococcus pneumoniae* (~30% cases), *Haemophilus influenza* (30% cases), *Moraxella catarrhalis* (~10% cases), and respiratory anaerobes in the presence of acute maxillary sinusitis associated with odontogenic infections. Options "A" and "B" will not help distinguish between acute bacterial sinusitis and a viral respiratory infection as both produce nonspecific signs of sinus inflammation. However, a

CT scan of the head or magnetic resonance imaging (MRI) of the brain and orbits should be obtained if there is clinical concern for orbital or central nervous system involvement. Option "C" describes appropriate supportive therapies for patients with sinusitis, but the mainstay of treatment for acute bacterial sinusitis is antimicrobial therapy. Although length of therapy is somewhat controversial, most experts recommend treating for 10 to 28 days or until the patient has been asymptomatic for at least 7 days.

Question 7-2

According to the AAP, all of the following statements are true in the diagnosis of acute bacterial sinusitis EXCEPT:
A) Persistent illness lasting more than 10 days without improvement.
B) Worsening course after initial improvement.
C) Clear rhinorrhea that subsequently turns yellow-green.
D) Severe onset of symptoms with fever and purulent nasal discharge for at least 3 consecutive days.
E) Symptoms may consist of nasal discharge or daytime cough.

Discussion 7-2

The correct answer is "C." Although it is a commonly held belief that clear rhinorrhea comes from viral colds and purulent (ie, yellow-green) nasal discharge comes from bacterial infections, this is incorrect. The other statements are all correct. According to the AAP, the diagnosis of acute bacterial sinusitis is made when a child with an acute URI presents in one of the following ways:

- Persistent illness (nasal discharge of any quality or daytime cough or both) lasting more than 10 days without improvement or a worsening course (worsening or new onset of nasal discharge, daytime cough, or fever after initial improvement)
- Severe onset (concurrent fever defined as temperature of 39°C (102.2°F) or higher and purulent nasal discharge for at least 3 consecutive days

Question 7-3

All of the following are potential complications of acute bacterial sinusitis EXCEPT:
A) Orbital cellulitis.
B) Orbital subperiosteal abscess.
C) Cavernous sinus thrombosis.
D) Nasal abscess formation.
E) Brain abscess.

Discussion 7-3

The correct answer is "D." The most common complication of acute bacterial sinusitis is orbital involvement (ie, orbital cellulitis [option "A"]) in young children with ethmoid sinusitis. Other potential complications include orbital subperiosteal abscess formation (option "B"), cavernous sinus thrombosis (option "C"), and brain abscess (option "E") resulting from intracranial extension of infection. The most common complication of frontal sinusitis is Pott puffy tumor, or osteomyelitis of the frontal bone.

⏳ QUICK QUIZ

Which of the following sinus cavities are present at birth?
A) Maxillary and ethmoid.
B) Maxillary and frontal.
C) Maxillary and sphenoid.
D) Ethmoid and frontal.
E) Ethmoid and sphenoid.

Discussion

The correct answer is "A." The maxillary and ethmoid sinuses are present at the time of birth. The frontal and sphenoid sinuses begin to develop at ages 1 to 2 years but do not appear radiographically until ages 5 to 8 years.

Question 7-4

All of the following are known associations or risk factors for chronic sinusitis EXCEPT:
A) Recurrent viral upper respiratory infections.
B) Allergic rhinitis.
C) Ciliary dyskinesia.
D) Cystic fibrosis.
E) Young children in daycare.

Discussion 7-4

The correct answer is "E." Although at risk of contracting (and spreading!) many opportunistic infections, young children in daycare do not appear to be at risk for having chronic sinusitis, which is defined as an inflammatory disorder of the paranasal sinuses and linings of the nasal passage that lasts 12 weeks or longer. Risk factors include recurrent viral upper respiratory infections, asthma, allergic rhinitis, cigarette smoking, ciliary dyskinesia, cystic fibrosis, and immunodeficiency (especially hypogammaglobulinemia).

> **Helpful Tip**
> Remember to order a CT scan and consult an otolaryngologist if there is concern for sinus trauma.

▶ CASE 8

You are seeing a 12-year-old adolescent girl with no significant past medical history in your office for the chief complaint of "sore throat." Her mother states that the patient has had 5 days of low-grade fevers, malaise, and a sore throat. This morning she appeared more ill, with temperature of 39.4°C (103°F), a severe sore throat, and neck pain, and she does not want to open her mouth. Physical exam is notable for unilateral left-sided tonsillar swelling, uvular deviation to the right, and trismus.

Question 8-1

Based on this history and physical exam, the most likely diagnosis is:
A) Viral upper respiratory infection.
B) Sinusitis.
C) Peritonsillar abscess.
D) Strep throat.
E) Mononucleosis.

Discussion 8-1

The correct answer is "C." Classic physical exam findings for a peritonsillar abscess include severe sore throat, unilateral tonsillar swelling, trismus, and deviation of the uvula away from the affected side. Patients may also present with fever, drooling, odynophagia, and a muffled or "hot potato" voice. Hot potato voice is a buzz word for this infection. It is usually seen in older children and adolescents after an antecedent infection such as tonsillitis (option "E"), strep throat (option "D") or a viral URI (option "A"). The physical exam is not consistent with sinusitis (option "B").

Question 8-2

Which of the following is the most appropriate next step in the management of this patient?
A) Order a CBC and blood culture.
B) Order a lateral X-ray of the neck.
C) Start therapy with oral corticosteroids.
D) Start therapy with oral cephalexin.
E) Arrange for an incision and drainage procedure.

Discussion 8-2

The correct answer is "E." A peritonsillar abscess should be drained with either needle aspiration or a formal incision and drainage procedure. The fluid should be sent for Gram stain and routine culture of aerobic and anaerobic organisms. Option "A" is incorrect because lab tests are not needed to make the diagnosis or start therapy. Option "B" is incorrect as a lateral X-ray of the neck may be indicated for evaluation of a retropharyngeal abscess but will not help make the diagnosis of a peritonsillar abscess. Option "C" is incorrect as there is little data to support the use of corticosteroids in the treatment of pediatric peritonsillar abscesses. Option "D" is incorrect because, although starting antibiotics is important and cephalexin will cover two of the common organisms (*Streptococcus pyogenes* and *Staphylococcus aureus*), it will not cover respiratory anaerobes.

Question 8-3

All of the following are potentially appropriate antibiotics for treatment of a peritonsillar abscess EXCEPT:
A) Oral metronidazole.
B) IV ampicillin-sulbactam.
C) Oral clindamycin.
D) IV clindamycin.
E) IV ampicillin-sulbactam and vancomycin.

Discussion 8-3

The correct answer is "A." The most common pathogens in a peritonsillar abscess include group A streptococcus (*Streptococcus pyogenes*), *Staphylococcus aureus,* and respiratory anaerobes.

Metronidazole (option "A") will only provide anaerobic coverage and thus is not appropriate therapy. The other options all provide appropriate therapy. Option "E" would be the ideal combination in an area with a high prevalence of methicillin-resistant *S. aureus* (MRSA) because the ampicillin-sulbactam would provide coverage for group A streptococcus, respiratory anaerobes, and methicillin-sensitive *S. aureus* (MSSA), while vancomycin provides optimal coverage for MRSA. Remember that the bioavailability of oral and IV clindamycin is essentially equivalent, so either is appropriate as long as the patient is not vomiting and is able to keep down the oral medication. Antibiotics should be continued for a total 14-day course of therapy, and the patient may transition to oral antibiotics once clinically improved.

> ### ► CASE 9

You are seeing an 8-year-old boy in your office with a chief complaint of "sore throat." His mother reports that the older sibling was diagnosed with strep throat earlier in the week and she "wants to make sure that is not what is going on here." Further history reveals the patient has had 2 days of fever higher than 39.4°C (103°F) and a sore throat without any rhinorrhea or cough. Physical exam is notable for erythematous tonsils with exudates, palatal petechiae, and tender cervical lymphadenopathy.

Question 9-1

Which of the following is the next most appropriate step in the care of this patient?
A) Order a CBC and blood culture.
B) Obtain a rapid group A strep antigen test.
C) Order Epstein-Barr virus serologies.
D) Order a urinalysis.
E) Start therapy with oral clindamycin.

Discussion 9-1

The correct answer is "B." This patient most likely has group A streptococcus (GAS) pharyngitis or "strep throat." The most appropriate step is to confirm the diagnosis as untreated GAS pharyngitis can lead to acute rheumatic fever, cervical adenitis, peritonsillar abscess/cellulitis, otitis media, or sepsis. The diagnosis of GAS can be made with a rapid antigen test as it has a specificity of 95% or greater and a sensitivity of approximately 80%. Thus, if the rapid antigen test is positive, you should treat for strep throat. However, a negative rapid antigen test requires confirmation by performing a throat culture. CBC and blood cultures (option "A") are not helpful in the diagnosis of strep throat. Epstein-Barr virus serologies (option "C") may help diagnosis mononucleosis, which can have a similar presentation of fever, pharyngitis, and tender cervical lymphadenopathy but may also include fatigue, malaise, periorbital edema, and mild hepatomegaly or splenomegaly. Checking a urinalysis (option "D") would be appropriate if you are concerned about post-streptococcal glomerulonephritis, which typically occurs 1 to 3 weeks following an episode of GAS pharyngitis and does not fit with the timing of this patient's illness. Oral clindamycin (option "E") is not the first-line therapy for GAS pharyngitis.

Question 9-2

Which of the following is an appropriate treatment regimen for GAS pharyngitis?
A) Trimethoprim-sulfamethoxazole.
B) Amoxicillin.
C) Ceftriaxone.
D) Ciprofloxacin.
E) Doxycycline.

Discussion 9-2

The correct answer is "B." GAS pharyngitis is treated with either oral penicillin or amoxicillin for 10 days or a single intramuscular injection of penicillin G benzathine if there are concerns for adherence or the patient is vomiting. For penicillin-allergic patients, alternative treatments include cephalexin, azithromycin, or clindamycin. A third-generation cephalosporin such as ceftriaxone (option "C") is not indicated for GAS pharyngitis, which can be treated with a more narrow-spectrum cephalosporin such as cephalexin. GAS pharyngitis should not be treated with tetracyclines (option "E"), trimethoprim-sulfamethoxazole (option "A"), or fluoroquinolones (option "D").

▶ CASE 10

A 4-year-old girl presents to the emergency department with a chief complaint of "fever." Her mother reports that she was previously healthy but seemed to have a common cold last week. She has now had 3 days of fever, difficulty and pain with swallowing, as well as apparent neck pain. Physical exam is notable for cervical lymphadenopathy, neck tenderness, and a refusal to perform cervical neck extension or lateral rotation. Her posterior pharyngeal wall is erythematous and appears to be bulging.

Question 10-1

Based on this history and physical exam, the most likely diagnosis is:
A) Viral upper respiratory infection.
B) Diphtheria.
C) Retropharyngeal abscess.
D) Strep throat.
E) Mononucleosis.

Discussion 10-1

The correct answer is "C." This patient has a retropharyngeal abscess. Younger children often present with a preceding history of viral URI symptoms while an older patient usually has a history of pharyngeal trauma such having had an endoscopy procedure, dental procedure, intubation, or penetrating injury such as a pencil to the back of the throat (think falling asleep at school while chewing on a pencil!). The most common symptoms include fever, neck pain, neck swelling, sore throat, and odynophagia, although children may also have a muffled voice or drooling. The exam is notable for neck tenderness, limitation of cervical movements (especially neck extension), torticollis, and cervical lymphadenopathy. Know that in reality a toddler is not going to be overly cooperative. So be suspicious.

Question 10-2

All of the following are common pathogens in a retropharyngeal abscess EXCEPT:
A) *Streptococcus pyogenes* (group A streptococcus).
B) *Staphylococcus aureus*.
C) *Fusobacterium* species.
D) *Prevotella* species.
E) *Streptococcus pneumoniae*.

Discussion 10-2

The correct answer is "E." Although a common cause of both community-acquired pneumonia and acute otitis media in children, *S. pneumoniae* is not a common pathogen in retropharyngeal abscesses. Most of these infections tend to be polymicrobial with a combination of group A streptococcus, *Staphylococcus aureus* (MSSA and MRSA) and respiratory anaerobes such as *Fusobacterium*, *Prevotella*, *Bacteroides*, and *Peptostreptococcus*.

Question 10-3

Which of the following is the most appropriate antimicrobial therapy for a retropharyngeal abscess?
A) Ampicillin-sulbactam.
B) Cephalexin.

C) Ceftriaxone.
D) Vancomycin.
E) Metronidazole.

Discussion 10-3

The correct answer is "A." As mentioned earlier, empiric therapy for a retropharyngeal abscess should include coverage of group A streptococcus, *Staphylococcus aureus*, and respiratory anaerobes, all of which can be achieved with ampicillin-sulbactam monotherapy. If there is significant concern for MRSA, then consider adding vancomycin (option "D"). Another option would be to use clindamycin monotherapy. Cephalexin (option "B"), ceftriaxone (option "C"), and vancomycin (option "D") are incorrect because they do not provide anaerobic coverage. Metronidazole (option "E") does not provide coverage for group A streptococcus or *S. aureus*.[25]

> **Helpful Tip**
> Although the diagnosis of a retropharyngeal abscess can be made on clinical grounds alone, imaging may be helpful to plan a surgical approach if necessary. A screening lateral neck X-ray will show widened prevertebral soft tissues that exceed the anterior-posterior dimension of the adjacent vertebral body. For a lateral neck X-ray, the child must sit still with her head up and neither extended nor flexed as either will distort the retropharyngeal space. An ultrasound or CT scan of the neck can identify the size of the abscess and identify important surrounding structures. Immediate surgical drainage is indicated if the patient has airway compromise or a fluctuant abscess. Not all patients require surgical intervention. Intravenous antibiotics should be continued until the patient is afebrile and clinically improved; he or she can then be switched to oral clindamycin or amoxicillin-clavulanic acid for a total 14 days of therapy.

> **Helpful Tip**
> Also known as a lateral pharyngeal abscess, a parapharyngeal abscess is similar to a retropharyngeal abscess. Neck motion is not typically impaired but a prominent bulge of the lateral pharyngeal wall may be seen. It is treated with IV antibiotics with or without surgical drainage.

> **Helpful Tip**
> The two most common indications for tonsillectomy and adenoidectomy are recurrent throat infections (pharyngitis) and sleep-disordered breathing. Table 9–6 summarizes information about indications, complications, and contraindications of common "T&A." Pain control is important to prevent dehydration. (If it hurts with swallowing, why would a child want to drink? Good luck rationalizing with a toddler.)

TABLE 9–6 TONSILLECTOMY AND ADENOIDECTOMY

Indications for Tonsillectomy
- Most common indications:
  (1) Recurrent throat infections (pharyngitis)
     - 7 episodes in past year *and*
     - 1 or more of the following: fever, cervical adenopathy, tonsillar exudate, or positive test for group A streptococcus
  (2) Sleep-disordered breathing
     - Concurrent tonsillar hypertrophy *and*
     - Associated comorbidities (poor growth, poor school performance, enuresis, behavioral problems) *or*
     - Abnormal polysomnography
- Other indications include need to exclude a tumor and treatment of PFAPA syndrome (periodic fever with aphthous stomatitis, pharyngitis and adenitis).

Indications for Adenoidectomy
- Indications relate to adenoidal hypertrophy causing nasal obstruction with subsequent symptoms and include:
  - Severe nasal obstruction
  - Refractory chronic sinusitis
  - Recurrent acute otitis media
  - Chronic otitis media with effusion
  - Repeat tympanostomy tube placement
- Consideration can also be given to patients with dental malocclusion from persistent mouth breathing, hyponasal speech and "adenoid facies" (long and narrow face, narrow maxilla, steep mandible and an overbite)

Complications of a Tonsillectomy and Adenoidectomy
- Bleeding is most common complication (rate of 0.1–8.1%)
- Other operative complications include trauma to teeth or soft palate, laryngospasm, and aspiration
- Postoperative complications include nausea, vomiting, pain, dehydration, postobstructive pulmonary edema, nasopharyngeal stenosis, or velopharyngeal insufficiency (weak pharyngeal muscles) with hypernasal speech.
- Mortality rate is reported to approximate that of general anesthesia alone

Contraindications to Tonsillectomy and Adenoidectomy
- Contraindications include cleft palate or submucous cleft palate due to risk of velopharyngeal insufficiency with resultant hypernasal speech, bleeding disorder, or acute tonsillitis
- Taking out angry infected tonsils is generally avoided but may be required for tonsillitis or peritonsillar abscess unresponsive to medical therapy (called a "quinsy" tonsillectomy)

> **Helpful Tip**
> Velopharyngeal insufficiency (specifically the sphincter) results in improper closing of the soft palate muscle in the mouth during speech. Air escapes out the nose rather than the mouth when talking, making it hard to pronounce certain consonant sounds.

▶ CASE 11

You are attending in the newborn nursery and the lactation consultant has concerns that a full-term, 2-day old male infant is not feeding well due to a short lingual frenulum. On exam, you notice that the infant is unable to protrude the tongue past the alveolar ridge and his weight is down 8% from birthweight. The mother has experience breastfeeding her other two children and feels that the infant does not latch on well during feeding.

Question 11-1

Which of the following is the most appropriate next step in the management of this infant?

A) Order a CBC with white blood cell count differential, C-reactive protein, and blood culture.
B) Start empiric IV ampicillin and gentamicin for presumed early-onset sepsis.
C) Start intravenous fluids for dehydration.
D) Arrange for a frenulectomy.
E) Instruct the mother to increase the frequency of feeding attempts to every 2 hours.

Discussion 11-1

The correct answer is "D." This infant has a tongue-tie (ankyloglossia), which results from a short lingual frenulum and subsequent difficulty with protrusion and elevation of the tongue. Tongue-tie may result in neonatal feeding difficulties or dental and speech problems later in childhood. If the infant is having difficulty with breastfeeding and the tongue cannot protrude past the alveolar ridge, a frenulectomy should be performed by a trained provider in the newborn period. A quick clip is all this infant needs.

▶ CASE 12

An 8-month-old boy is brought to the emergency department for evaluation of a skin rash. He has been healthy and this is his first illness. He has no known drug allergies. His mother reports that he developed a red raised rash on his cheeks and around his mouth earlier today. The rash does not appear to bother the infant. He is afebrile and otherwise acting normally while eating a popsicle in the room.

Question 12-1

Given this presentation, your clinical suspicion is for:

A) Facial cellulitis.
B) Hives.
C) Cold panniculitis.
D) Eczema.
E) Pressure erythema.

Discussion 12-1

The correct answer is "C." Cold panniculitis is sometimes called "popsicle panniculitis" as it commonly occurs in association with eating frozen treats. The absence of systemic symptoms such as fever combined with a history of cold exposure (ie, eating popsicles) are very suggestive of cold panniculitis. It represents acute cold injury to the subcutaneous fat and the development of erythematous indurated nodules or plaques on the exposed skin. Lesions usually appear 24 to 72 hours after exposure to cold and gradually return to normal in 2 weeks to 3 months, although postinflammatory hyperpigmentation may remain.

⧗ QUICK QUIZ

Infectious causes of pediatric parotitis (inflammation of the parotid glands) include all of the following EXCEPT:

A) Mumps
B) Epstein-Barr virus
C) Parainfluenza virus
D) *Staphylococcus aureus*
E) *Clostridium difficile*

Discussion

The correct answer is "E." *C. difficile* may cause diarrhea, bloody diarrhea, pseudomembranous colitis, or fulminant colitis but does not cause parotitis. (Having a bacteria that lives in fecal matter in your salivary gland doesn't sound appetizing.) As a result of mumps immunization, parotitis is now uncommonly seen in children. Bacterial parotitis typically presents in infants younger than 2 months of age (especially premature infants in the neonatal intensive care unit [NICU]) and occasionally in children older than 10 years of age as acute-onset of fever, unilateral swelling, and tenderness of the parotid gland with overlying erythema. The most common pathogen is *Staphylococcus aureus*, although streptococci (including group B streptococcus in neonates), gram-negative bacilli, and anaerobic bacteria can all be involved. Management should include obtaining a culture of purulent fluid expressed from the Stenson duct and antibiotic therapy (eg, clindamycin) to cover both *S. aureus* and anaerobes. Viral parotidis is usually seen in children aged 3 to 10 years secondary to mumps or a multitude of other viruses (eg, Epstein-Barr virus, cytomegalovirus, enteroviruses, parainfluenza viruses, influenza viruses, human immunodeficiency virus [HIV], herpes simplex viruses, coxsackievirus and lymphocytic choriomeningitis virus). Viral parotitis typically presents with several days of fever, malaise, and headache followed by parotid gland swelling that eventually becomes bilateral, with one side more affected than the other. Management includes pain control, adequate hydration, sialogogues (eg, lemon drops or sour candy to facilitate ductal secretions), heat packs, and gland massage as well as good oral hygiene.

> **Helpful Tip**
> The parotid gland extends from in front of the ear, to the jawline, to behind the ear. On exam, the angle of the mandible is not palpable when the gland is enlarged.

> **Helpful Tip**
> A ranula is a sublingual salivary gland retention cyst that occurs on the floor of the mouth and appears as a thin-walled, bluish cyst. Refer the patient to an otolaryngologist for surgical management.

⌛ QUICK QUIZ

You have been asked to lecture the third-year medical students on infectious and benign lesions of the oral cavity. In preparation for your talk, you review the important clinical findings to differentiate among these entities.

Which is NOT a cause of a benign oral lesion?
A) Fibroma.
B) Mucocele.
C) Geographic tongue.
D) Aphthous ulcer.
E) Fissured tongue.

Discussion

The correct answer is "D." See Table 9–7 for the differential diagnosis of oral lesions in childhood.

▶ CASE 13

You attend the delivery of an infant girl who was noted to have a cleft lip on prenatal ultrasound. On your initial exam, she is found to have a complete unilateral cleft lip and palate. (See Figure 9–4.) The family has lots of questions regarding this diagnosis.

Question 13-1

All of the following are true regarding cleft lip and palates EXCEPT:
A) Cleft lip occurs most often on the left side.
B) Right-sided clefts are more commonly associated with syndromes.
C) There is no association between a bifid uvula and a cleft palate.
D) Cleft lip is more common in males and cleft palate in females.
E) Almost all children with cleft lip and palate require myringotomy and tympanostomy tube placement due to eustachian tube dysfunction.

Discussion 13-1

The correct answer is "C." A bifid uvula is present in approximately 3% of children but there is an association with submucous cleft palate. A submucous cleft palate is diagnosed by the classic triad of a bifid uvula, central thinning of the soft palate, and a palpable notch in the posterior border of the hard palate. It is important to identify this abnormality because affected children have a 40% risk of developing persistent middle ear effusions and are at risk for velopharyngeal incompetence resulting in hypernasal speech.

> **Helpful Tip**
> Cleft lips are classified as complete or incomplete and unilateral or bilateral. A complete cleft lip implies a separation of the lip that extends through the nasal sill (floor of nasal opening) and the alveolus into the palate. An incomplete cleft lip may present as a cleft of variable width with an intact bridge of skin below the nasal sill.

> **Helpful Tip**
> Although many congenital syndromes include clefting as a manifestation of a genetic abnormality, these syndromes make up less than 20% of all clefts. Most cases (cleft lip or palate, or both) are sporadic but can run in families. Conditions commonly associated with a cleft palate include the following:
>
> - Velocardiofacial (Shprintzen) syndrome—an autosomal dominant disorder caused by deletion in chromosome 22q11; it likely represents a phenotypic variant of DiGeorge syndrome
> - Van der Woude syndrome—an autosomal dominant disorder with a high degree of penetrance that is characterized by lower lip sinus tracts or pits
> - Stickler syndrome or hereditary arthroophthalmopathy—an autosomal dominant condition characterized by a flat face, severe nearsightedness (myopia) and hypermobile joints
> - Treacher-Collins syndrome or mandibulofacial dysostosis—an autosomal dominant disorder characterized by underdeveloped facial bones (small cheek bones, jaw and chin), downslanting eyes, cleft zygomatic bone, dental malocclusion (overbite), eye (eyelid coloboma, missing eyelashes) abnormalities, and abnormal ears
> - Pierre Robin sequence—results from abnormal formation of the mandible and may occur in isolation or as a feature of a genetic syndrome

TABLE 9–7 DIFFERENTIAL DIAGNOSIS OF ORAL LESIONS IN CHILDHOOD

Diagnosis	Cause	Clinical Appearance	Treatment
Hand-foot-mouth disease	Enteroviruses, group A and B coxsackie viruses	Fever, oral vesicles on the buccal mucosa and tongue and small, tender cutaneous lesions on the hands, feet, buttocks and genitalia	Supportive with pain medications and fluid hydration
Herpangina	Coxsackie A viruses	Fever and odynophagia due to painful posterior pharyngeal ulcers; mainly occur in summer and early fall	Supportive with pain medications and fluid hydration Topical therapy with 1:1 mixture of Maalox and Benadryl may be helpful[a]
Acute herpetic gingivostomatitis	Primary HSV-1 infection in childhood	Multiple small 1–3 mm ulcers on inner lips, buccal mucosa, gingiva, tongue, and anterior tonsillar pillars; associated fever and tender cervical lymphadenopathy	Treatment is symptomatic Oral acyclovir therapy can decrease symptom duration if started in the first 3–4 days of illness
Aphthous ulcer "canker sore"	Unknown	Painful small, shallow, round to oval ulcers with a grayish base; occur on nonkeratinized mucosal surfaces, so lesions on the lips and perioral lesions exclude this diagnosis; no associated fever or cervical lymphadenopathy	Topical corticosteroid (triamcinolone dental paste) may help Avoid salty or acidic food Pain control with acetaminophen or ibuprofen
Benign lesions of oral cavity	1. *Fibroma*—smooth, pale pink protuberances with a sessile or pedunculated base that occur on any mucosal surface secondary to connective tissue hyperplasia from chronic irritation 2. *Traumatic ulcer*—most common oral ulcer in children; caused by mechanical, chemical or thermal injury with the appearance depending on the inflicted trauma 3. *Geographic tongue* (benign migratory glossitis)—chronic, recurring disorder characterized by red-pink, slightly depressed lesions with irregularly elevated white or yellow borders; more common in girls 4. *Fissured tongue* (lingua plicata)—developmental anomaly with a prominent central figure on the tongue from which smaller fissures radiate laterally; common finding in Down syndrome 5. *Hemangioma*—red or bluish-red, slightly raised lesions that can occur in any soft tissue location but more commonly on the lip, dorsum of tongue, gingiva and buccal mucosa 6. *Lymphangiomas*—benign tumors of the lymphatic vessels that may be pink to reddish-blue, soft and compressible; most commonly seen on the tongue, lips, and buccal mucosa 7. *Mucocele*—painless swelling on the lower lip buccal mucosa, usually < 1 cm diameter and translucent or bluish in color		

HSV, herpes simplex virus.

[a] Maalox = aluminum hydroxide and magnesium hydroxide; Benadryl = diphenhydramine.

⏳ **QUICK QUIZ**

The clinical features of Pierre Robin sequence are micrognathia, glossoptosis (posteriorly displaced tongue), and cleft palate, with the tongue tending to prolapse backward and cause airway obstruction that can be life-threatening.

All of the following are appropriate initial interventions for a patient with Pierre Robin sequence EXCEPT:

A) Tracheostomy.
B) Glossopexy or tongue-lip plication surgery.
C) Insertion of nasopharyngeal airway.
D) Mandibular distraction surgery.
E) Placing the patient in the prone position.

Discussion

The correct answer is "A." In most cases, the respiratory obstruction associated with Pierre Robin sequence is seen in the immediate neonatal period and will improve over time as the mandible grows to accommodate the tongue. Conservative measures include placing the infant in the prone positioning to allow the tongue to "fall forward" and alleviate the obstruction, placing a nasogastric feeding tube, or inserting an oral or

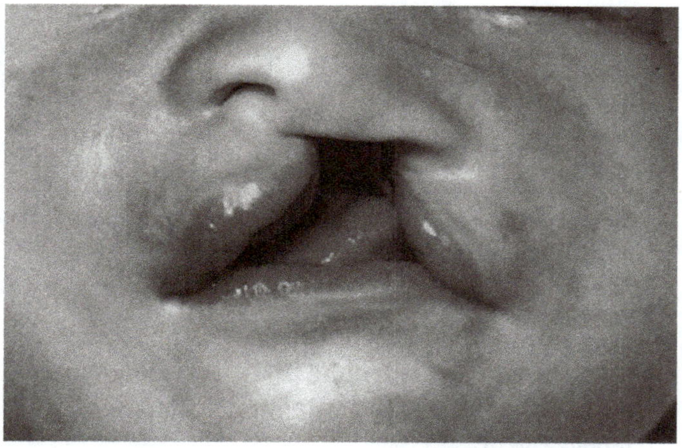

FIGURE 9–4. This infant has a complete unilateral cleft lip that extends into the nasal sill. (Reproduced with permission from Lalwani AK, ed. *Current Diagnosis & Treatment in Otolaryngology: Head and Neck Surgery*. 3rd ed. McGraw-Hill Education; 2011, Fig 20-4.)

nasopharyngeal airway as a temporizing measure. However, if these measures fail then surgical intervention is warranted. The goal of surgery is to avoid a tracheostomy (option "A"). Glossopexy or tongue-lip plication surgery is a procedure in which the tongue is essentially sutured in place anteriorly to the lip. More recently, mandibular distraction surgery has been used to elongate the mandibular ramus and bring the tongue forward with the mandible.

> **Helpful Tip**
> Primary teeth begin to erupt at around 7 months of age (range: 3–16 months). The first teeth seen are the mandibular central incisors followed by the maxillary central incisors.

> **Helpful Tip**
> The prognosis for viability worsens rapidly the longer a tooth is outside the mouth. Ideally, an avulsed permanent tooth should be reimplanted into its socket as soon as possible after a gentle rinsing with clean water, and the patient should seek emergency dental care. The best storage and transport media in order of preference is Hank's balanced salt solution (found in the commercially available "Save-A-Tooth" kit), milk, saline, saliva, or water.

> **Helpful Tip**
> The loss of a primary tooth may either accelerate or delay eruption of the underlying permanent tooth. A generalized delay in tooth eruption may be associated with medical conditions such as hypothyroidism, hypopituitarism, cleidocranial dysplasia, trisomy 21, or rickets.

> ▶ **CASE 14**

You are attending on the general pediatric service and have a 4-year-old male patient who was admitted with fever and unilateral neck swelling. Exam reveals a 3 × 4 cm area of right-sided cervical swelling that has central fluctuance. It is tender to palpation and the overlying skin is erythematous. The patient was previously healthy and has no known animal exposures. He does not appear to have poor dentition.

Question 14-1

Acute unilateral cervical lymphadenitis is commonly caused by all of the following EXCEPT:
A) *Streptococcus pyogenes* (GAS).
B) *Staphylococcus aureus*.
C) Atypical mycobacteria.
D) *Bartonella henselae*.
E) Human immunodeficiency virus.

Discussion 14-1

The correct answer is "E." This patient has acute, unilateral cervical lymphadenitis, which is most often caused by either *Streptococcus pyogenes* (GAS) or *Staphylococcus aureus*. Atypical mycobacteria are usually a more indolent presentation with a characteristic violaceous appearance overlying matted lymph nodes. *Bartonella henselae* causes cat-scratch disease and should be considered if there is a history of cat exposure (especially kittens). In a young infant, you should consider group B streptococcus (GBS) cellulitis-adenitis, which can be a manifestation of late-onset GBS infection. Tularemia caused by *Francisella tularensis* after contact with an infected animal such as a rabbit or pet hamster may present as the ulceroglandular syndrome, which is characterized by a papular lesion in the drainage field of the inflamed lymph node. Older children with a history of dental disease may have acute unilateral cervical lymphadenitis due to anaerobic bacteria. The clinical history is very important in a child with cervical lymphadenitis as a detailed exposure history may help elicit possible infectious associations such as brucellosis from ingesting unpasteurized animal milk or goat exposure, atypical mycobacterium from ingesting unpasteurized milk, tularemia from a rabbit or pet hamster exposure, bubonic plague from prairie dog exposure, cat scratch disease from kitten exposure, or tuberculosis from travel to an endemic area.

Question 14-2

What is the most appropriate next step in the care of this patient?
A) Order a CBC with white blood cell count differential and blood culture.
B) Arrange for an incision and drainage procedure.
C) Order a tuberculin skin test (PPD).
D) Start antibiotic therapy with oral azithromycin.
E) Order a rapid strep test and throat culture.

Discussion 14-2

The correct answer is "B." This patient's exam is notable for an area of central fluctuance, which indicates a drainable fluid collection. Although it is appropriate to start antibiotics effective against both *Streptococcus pyogenes* and *Staphylococcus aureus*, the most important first step is to drain the fluid collection. In a young infant with possible GBS cellulitis-adenitis, it would be important to send blood for culture as such children are often bacteremic. If you suspect either tuberculosis or atypical mycobacteria as a possible etiology, then administering a tuberculin skin test (PPD) would be appropriate.

> **Helpful Tip**
>
> It is useful to separate chronic cervical lymphadenopathy into unilateral or bilateral categories, as the unilateral form is usually caused by cat-scratch disease or atypical mycobacteria, whereas the bilateral form is more commonly caused by viral infections such as Epstein-Barr virus (EBV) or cytomegalovirus (CMV). Remember to consider the possibility of leukemia, lymphoma, or other malignancies or immunodeficiencies if a patient presents with chronic cervical lymphadenopathy.

► CASE 15

A mother brings her 10-year-old daughter in for evaluation of a "neck mass." She reports that the child has a history of recurrent midline neck swelling for the past several years. The patient was healthy until last week when she developed a low-grade fever, rhinorrhea, and coughing. Mom then noticed a prominent midline neck swelling that appears erythematous and tender to palpation. You observe that the swelling moves upward when the patient sticks out her tongue during your exam.

Question 15-1

Which of the following is the most likely diagnosis?

A) Lymphoma.
B) Infected brachial cleft cyst.
C) Cystic hygroma.
D) Reactive viral lymphadenopathy.
E) Infected thyroglossal duct cyst.

Discussion 15-1

The correct answer is "E." The differential diagnosis for a pediatric neck mass is extensive and most easily understood by grouping into broad categories of infectious or inflammatory neck masses, congenital neck masses and neoplastic neck masses. (See Table 9–8.) A thyroglossal duct cyst is an epithelium-lined cyst resulting from the persistence of any segment of the thyroglossal duct along its migration from the foramen cecum of the tongue to the pyramidal lobe of the thyroid. It is the most common midline neck mass in children. Remember that, during formation, the thyroid migrates down from the base of the tongue to its location in the neck. Thyroglossal duct cysts are typically found near the level of the hyoid bone in the midline of the neck. Clinically, they most often appear as a painless, fluctuant midline neck mass that moves upward with a

TABLE 9–8 DIFFERENTIAL DIAGNOSIS OF PEDIATRIC NECK MASSES

Infectious or Inflammatory Neck Masses	Congenital Neck Masses	Neoplastic Neck Masses
Reactive viral lymphadenopathy (adenovirus, rhinovirus, enterovirus, EBV, etc)	Thyroglossal duct cysts	Lymphoma
Bacterial lymphadenitis (*Staphylococcus aureus*, group A streptococci [GAS], tularemia, brucellosis, etc)	Branchial cleft cysts	Rhabdomyosarcoma
Mycobacterium tuberculosis	Dermoid cysts	Neuroblastoma
Atypical mycobacterium	Teratomas	Metastatic adenopathy
Cat-scratch disease (*Bartonella henselae*)	Lymphangioma (cystic hygroma)	Thyroid cancer
Toxoplasmosis	Thymic cysts	
Histoplasmosis	Laryngoceles	
Actinomycosis	Lymphatic malformations	
HIV-associated lymphadenopathy	Hemangioma	
Sarcoidosis	Fibromatosis colli	
Kawasaki disease		

Adapted with permission from Tintinalli JE, Stapczynski J, Ma O, et al. eds. *Tintinalli's Emergency Medicine: A comprehensive study guide*, 8th ed. New York, NY: McGraw-Hill; 2015.

protruding tongue or during swallowing. It is important to evaluate thyroid function because thyroglossal duct cysts may contain ectopic thyroid tissue with associated hypothyroidism. By comparison, branchial cleft cysts are round, smooth, mobile lateral neck masses found along the anterior border of the sternocleidomastoid muscle. Most of these arise from incomplete obliteration of the second branchial cleft. Patients may have a history of recurrent swelling or infection in the same lateral neck area. Both thyroglossal duct cysts and branchial cleft cysts are often asymptomatic until they become infected in the setting of an upper respiratory tract infection. Acutely infected cysts require antibiotics to cover typical skin flora and anaerobes. Definitive treatment is elective surgical excision. A cystic hygroma or lymphangioma is a painless lymphatic malformation commonly located above the clavicle.

► CASE 16

You are seeing a 15-year-old adolescent girl with a chief complaint of "neck swelling." She reports noticing a small bump in the midline of her neck for the past several weeks that seems to have gotten significantly larger in the past several days. Physical exam is notable for bilateral anterior cervical lymphadenopathy and a nontender, 2 cm right-sided thyroid nodule. You notice that her voice sounds rather hoarse. Given the history and physical exam, you are concerned that she may have thyroid cancer.

Question 16-1

All of the following are clinical features that may be associated with thyroid carcinoma EXCEPT:

A) History of external radiation to the head or neck, or both.
B) History of exposure to nuclear fallout.
C) Bradycardia.
D) Dysphagia.
E) Vocal cord paralysis.

Discussion 16-1

The correct answer is "C." The most common presentation of a patient with thyroid cancer is the presence of a solitary thyroid nodule or mass. Although approximately 2% of children have palpable thyroid nodules, most of these are benign adenomas or cystic lesions. Patients with thyroid cancer may have a history of external radiation to the head and neck, exposure to nuclear fallout, a history of rapid growth of the thyroid nodule, a firm or fixed neck mass, hoarseness, dysphagia, or cervical lymphadenopathy. Thyroid cancer is divided into four main types: papillary, follicular, medullary, and anaplastic. In children, the vast majority of masses are differentiated thyroid cancer, which includes both papillary and follicular thyroid carcinomas. Medullary thyroid carcinoma (MTC) is notable due to the production of calcitonin from the parafollicular or C cells of the thyroid gland, and it may be associated with multiple endocrine neoplasia type 2A (MEN 2A) or MEN 2B. Diagnosis of thyroid carcinoma is made by fine needle aspiration biopsy.

⧗ QUICK QUIZ

You are the attending in the newborn nursery and have been asked to give a lecture to the medical students and nursing staff regarding universal hearing screening.

All of the following regarding hearing tests are true statements EXCEPT:

A) The AAP recommends that all infants have a hearing screen performed by 1 month of age.
B) A behavioral audiogram is the gold standard for hearing testing.
C) Mild hearing loss is present when the quietest sounds that a person can hear with his or her better ear is between 20 and 40 dB

D) A child should be referred for formal hearing testing if the caregiver has a concern regarding hearing, speech, language, or developmental delay at any age
E) A failed otoacoustic emission test (OAE) indicates an abnormality in the auditory nerve or brainstem.

Discussion

The correct answer is "E." An OAE does not assess the neuronal transmission of sound from the eighth cranial nerve to the brainstem as does an auditory brainstem response (ABR). OAE detects conductive hearing loss and ABR detects conductive and sensorineural hearing loss. The remaining statements are all true. Universal hearing screening is recommended because some degree of hearing loss is present in 1 to 6 per 1000 newborn infants, and congenital or acquired hearing loss in children has been shown to adversely affect speech development, language development, academic achievement, and social-emotional development. According to the "Year 2007 Position Statement: Principle and Guidelines for Early Hearing Detection and Intervention Programs" endorsed by the AAP, the hearing of all infants should be screened at no later than 1 month of age. Those who do not pass screening should have a comprehensive audiologic evaluation at no later than 3 months of age. Additionally, the AAP recommends hearing screening for all children at ages 4, 5, 6, 8, and 10 years. Any child with a risk factor for hearing loss, regardless of the newborn hearing screen result, should be referred for an audiologic assessment at least once by 24 to 30 months of age. (See Table 9–9.)

TABLE 9–9 RISK FACTORS ASSOCIATED WITH HEARING LOSS IN CHILDHOOD

Caregiver concern regarding hearing, speech, language, or developmental delay

Family history of hearing impairment

NICU stay of > 5 days or any of the following: ECMO, assisted ventilation, exposure to ototoxic medications, hyperbilirubinemia requiring exchange transfusion

Confirmed neonatal infections associated with hearing loss such as CMV, herpes, rubella, syphilis, or toxoplasmosis

Anatomic malformations of the head and neck

A syndrome that is associated with hearing loss such as neurofibromatosis, osteogenesis imperfecta, Usher, Waardenburg, Alport, Pendred, Jervell, or Lange-Nielson

Neurodegenerative disorders such as Hunter syndrome

Sensory motor neuropathies such as Friedreich ataxia and Charcot-Marie-Tooth syndrome

Confirmed incidence of infectious disease associated with hearing loss, such as bacterial or viral (especially herpes virus and varicella) meningitis

Chemotherapy

Recurrent or persistent otitis media for at least 3 months

History of significant head trauma (especially involving the basilar skull or temporal bone)

CMV, cytomegalovirus; ECMO, extracorporeal membrane oxygenation; NICU, neonatal intensive care unit.

Helpful Tip

Mild hearing loss is present when the quietest sounds that a person can hear with his or her better ear is between 20 and 40 dB. These individuals have some difficulty keeping up with conversations, especially in noisy surroundings. Moderate hearing loss is in the 41 to 70 dB range, and affected people have difficulty keeping up with conversations without a hearing aid. Severe hearing loss is in the 71 to 95 dB range, and affected people benefit from hearing aids but often rely on lip reading and may use sign language.

Helpful Tip

A variety of objective tests have been developed for hearing screening. The choice of which to use depends on the child's age, degree of cooperation, and available resources.

- *Tympanometry* measures relative changes in tympanic membrane movement as air pressure changes in the external auditory canal. It provides the best objective middle ear assessment and is useful in the evaluation of suspected hearing loss.
- *Evoked otoacoustic emissions (OAEs)* are acoustic signals generated within outer hair cells of the cochlea that travel in a "reverse direction" through the middle ear space and tympanic membrane out to the ear canal. These signals are generated in response to an auditory stimulus and may be detected with a very sensitive microphone-and-probe system placed in the external ear canal. The benefits of an OAE test are that you can obtain ear-specific results, it can be performed quickly at any age, it does not depend on whether the child is asleep or awake, and it provides a simple "pass/fail" report. However, an OAE test does not assess the neuronal transmission of sound from the eighth cranial nerve to the brainstem and thus will not identify nerve abnormalities (sensorineural hearing loss). A "failed" OAE test only implies that a hearing loss of greater than 30 to 40 dB may exist or that the middle ear is abnormal. A physical obstruction of the ear canal (eg, vernix in a newborn) will also give a false "failed" result.
- An *automated brainstem response (ABR)* test involves placing surface electrodes on the child's head and recording neural activity generated in the cochlea, auditory nerve, and brainstem in response to acoustic stimuli presented through earphones or ear inserts. The benefit of an ABR is the assessment of the eighth cranial nerve and brainstem auditory pathway in addition to the peripheral auditory system that is evaluated by an OAE. The main disadvantages of an ABR are the increased time required to perform the test (about 15 minutes) and the need for the child to remain quiet and not move. Consequently, infants may require sedation. A "failed" ABR test implies a hearing loss of greater than 40 dB.

Helpful Tips

It is important to remember that OAEs or ABRs are only testing the integrity of the auditory pathway and are not true tests of hearing. Hearing cannot be definitively considered normal until a child is mature enough to participate in a behavioral audiogram, which is the gold standard for hearing evaluation. Everyone remembers the behavioral audiograms in school when you were given earphones and asked to raise a hand when a sound was heard.

⧗ QUICK QUIZ

At the end of your lecture regarding universal hearing tests, a medical student remains confused regarding the difference between conductive hearing loss and sensorineural hearing loss (SNHL).

All of the following are true statements regarding hearing loss EXCEPT:

A) The most common congenital infection associated with sensorineural hearing loss is toxoplasmosis.
B) Conductive hearing loss results from a mechanical problem in the outer or middle ear and involves the pinna, external auditory canal, tympanic membrane, or ossicles.
C) Sensorineural hearing loss results from inner ear problems involving the cochlea, eighth cranial nerve, internal auditory canal, or the brain.
D) The most common childhood disorder associated with conductive hearing loss is otitis media.
E) In general, patients need to have severe to profound bilateral SNHL and little or no benefit from hearing aid use after 6 months before being considered for a cochlear implant.

Discussion

The correct answer is "A." Congenital CMV is the most common infection associated with SNHL. SNHL results from an inner ear or nerve problem and may be caused by congenital anomalies, infection (bacterial meningitis, CMV, toxoplasmosis, rubella, or syphilis), exposure to ototoxic medications, or due to genetic inheritance. SNHL is more prevalent among premature infants with low birth weights, likely due to other factors including administration of ototoxic drugs and perinatal complications, including hyperbilirubinemia. Medications known to be associated with permanent SNHL include aminoglycosides, macrolides, vancomycin, tetracycline, aspirin, NSAIDs, high-dose loop diuretics, and chemotherapy agents such as cisplatin, 5-fluorouracil, and bleomycin. In comparison, conductive hearing loss results from a mechanical problem in the outer or middle ear and may be caused by congenital anomalies, infection (such as otitis externa or otitis media), penetrating trauma, tympanic membrane perforation, otosclerosis, cholesteatoma, or malignant tumors such as squamous cell carcinoma.

► CASE 17

You are seeing a 12-year-old boy whose chief complaint is that "my nose is constantly dripping." The patient and his mother report that he has had persistent rhinorrhea and sneezing for the past 2 months. It is not associated with changes in the temperature or exposure to tobacco smoke but is definitely worse when he is asked to mow the lawn outside. On physical exam his nasal turbinates are swollen and erythematous bilaterally and there is a cobblestone appearance to the posterior pharyngeal wall. You diagnose him with allergic rhinitis and begin to discuss treatment options.

Question 17-1

Which of the following is the first-line medication therapy for allergic rhinitis?
A) Oral antihistamines.
B) Leukotriene antagonists.
C) Intranasal antihistamines.
D) Intranasal corticosteroids.
E) Nasal saline rinses.

Discussion 17-1

The correct answer is "D." The differential diagnosis of chronic rhinitis includes allergic or nonallergic rhinitis. Allergic rhinitis affects up to 40% of children in the United States and represents an IgE-mediated inflammatory response to allergen exposure. Symptoms include nasal congestion, rhinorrhea, sneezing, and an itchy nose, throat, or eyes. Physical exam may reveal swollen and erythematous nasal turbinates. The most important treatment modality is the use of intranasal corticosteroids, which has been shown to improve symptoms and help prevent progression to more severe disease. Other treatment options include oral and intranasal antihistamines as well as leukotriene antagonists. Nasal saline rinses have been shown to be helpful by washing away the allergens. Nonallergic rhinitis presents with similar symptoms, but does not seem to involve an immunologic reaction. Triggers may include environmental temperature changes or air pollution. Rhinitis medicamentosa is "rebound" nasal congestion that may occur after the discontinuation of chronic nasal decongestant spray use. Look for the allergic salute—a horizontal crease across the nose from rubbing the tip of the nose.

On close exam, you notice a pale grapelike mass in his right nostril. He does not remember being previously told about it. He has no history of chronic cough, greasy stools, or recurrent nosebleeds.

Question 17-2

What is NOT a cause of his intranasal mass?
A) Cystic fibrosis.
B) Chronic allergic rhinitis.
C) Aspirin-sensitive asthma.
D) Viral rhinitis.
E) Chronic bacterial sinusitis.

Discussion 17-2

The correct answer is "D." Nasal polyps frequently present as smooth, pale, spherical mucosal masses that protrude from the middle meatus. A classic description is a "gray or pale appearing grapelike mass." They develop after recurrent episodes of mucosal edema such as may be seen in longstanding allergic rhinitis, aspirin-sensitive asthma, chronic infectious sinusitis, or cystic fibrosis. Not all polyps are benign, and they may represent malignancy such as glioma, lymphoma, neuroblastoma, juvenile nasopharyngeal angiofibroma, or rhabdomyosarcoma. Children with polyps and symptoms of allergic rhinitis should be evaluated for allergies, as they will likely benefit from using a topical nasal corticosteroid or receiving a course of oral corticosteroids. Any child with multiple benign nasal polyps should be evaluated for cystic fibrosis—the most common cause of polyps in children. Polyps and recurrent infections should trigger an immunologic workup. Surgical removal is an option if medical management has failed or the polyps are very large in size. However, it is not uncommon for nasal polyps to recur after surgical removal. The use of intranasal corticosteroids after polyp removal may help prevent this recurrence.

> **Helpful Tip**
> The most common cause of nasal polyps in children is cystic fibrosis. Typical respiratory and digestive symptoms might be absent. Sweat the patient!

⧗ QUICK QUIZ

Instead let us say the 12-year-old presented for evaluation of rhinorrhea during the winter. He has cough and congestion. He still claims "my nose is constantly dripping." With more questioning, he admits that his symptoms improve for a day or two before fully returning. He is in school and has younger siblings. On exam, he has erythematous nasal mucous with clear drainage. His throat is mildly erythematous. You diagnosis him with the common cold and recommend supportive care.

Which of the following statements about acute viral rhinitis is false?
A) It is the most common pediatric infectious disease.
B) Recurrent episodes only occur in children with an immunodeficiency.
C) Healthy children may have over 10 illnesses per year.
D) Multiple different viruses are to blame.
E) A single episode typically last 7 to 10 days.

Discussion

The correct answer is "B." A viral upper respiratory tract infection is the most common pediatric infectious disease. Children younger than 5 years of age often have 6 to 12 illnesses per year with each episode lasting up to 10 days. No wonder parents always feel that their young children are "always sick!" Rhinoviruses are the most commonly isolated agents (30–40% of cases), with other identified viruses including adenoviruses, coronaviruses, enteroviruses, influenza, parainfluenza, and respiratory syncytial virus. The typical clinical course consists of clear or mucoid rhinorrhea, nasal congestion, and a sore throat that lasts 7 to 10 days. Fever may be present and is more commonly seen in younger children. Recurrent bacterial sinopulmonary infections would be a red flag for an immunodeficiency.

► CASE 18

You are seeing a 4-year-old, former 26-week-premature boy in your office for his well-child check. A review of his chart shows that he was intubated in the neonatal intensive care unit (NICU) for 2 weeks but subsequently discharged home without supplemental oxygen, has a history of gastroesophageal reflux for which he takes omeprazole, and was diagnosed with mild global developmental delay. His mother reports that he is doing well but that "he sounds hoarse" all the time. She reports that he frequently clears his throat and seems to have a new chronic cough that developed over the past week. He had a low-grade fever several days ago, and his younger sister has been ill recently.

Question 18-1

All of the following are potential causes of his new symptoms, EXCEPT:

A) Acute viral laryngitis.
B) Subglottic stenosis.
C) Gastroesophageal reflux.
D) Vocal fold granuloma.
E) Vocal fold nodule.

Discussion 18-1

The correct answer is "E." Vocal fold nodules are a common cause of chronic hoarseness in school-aged children and develop from repeated traumatic abuse of the vocal folds, such as from screaming or shouting. This patient is young to have developed vocal fold nodules and there is no supporting information provided to make you worry that he is "abusing his voice." The remaining choices are all potential causes of hoarseness in this particular patient.

Although hoarseness in children is most often secondary to acute viral laryngitis or benign lesions of the vocal cords, the differential diagnosis is quite broad. Acute viral laryngitis may persist for up to a week after other symptoms of an upper respiratory tract infection have resolved. Gastroesophageal reflux with associated laryngopharyngeal reflux may cause chronic inflammation of the vocal folds. Subglottic stenosis and vocal fold granulomas usually occur secondary to traumatic or prolonged intubation. Vocal cord paralysis is a common cause of stridor in neonates or infants who have undergone a surgical intervention that may be associated with damage to the recurrent laryngeal nerve (such as certain congenital heart disease surgeries). Papillomas secondary to human papillomavirus (HPV) types 6 and 11 typically become symptomatic in children by causing progressive hoarseness and stridor over weeks

to months. Congenital anomalies that may cause hoarseness include laryngeal webs, laryngeal clefts, or hemangiomas. Any patient with hoarseness that has persisted beyond 2 weeks should be evaluated by an otolaryngologist and undergo laryngoscopy.

BIBLIOGRAPHY

American Academy of Pediatrics. Group A streptococcal infections. In: Pickering LK, ed. *Red Book: 2012 Report of the Committee on Infectious Diseases*. 29th ed. Elk Grove Village, IL: American Academy of Pediatrics; 2012.

American Academy of Pediatrics, Joint Committee on Infant Hearing. Year 2007 position statement: Principles and guidelines for early hearing detection and intervention programs. *Pediatrics*. 2007;120(4):898–921.

Baugh RF, Archer SM, Mitchell RB, et al; American Academy of Otolaryngology–Head and Neck Surgery Foundation. Clinical practice guideline: Tonsillectomy in children. *Otolaryngol Head Neck Surg*. 2011;144(1 suppl):S1–S30.

Brown JC, Osincup DP. Pediatric procedures: Nasal and otic foreign bodies. In: Tintinalli JE, Stapczynski J, Ma O, et al, eds. *Tintinalli's Emergency Medicine: A Comprehensive Study Guide*. 7th ed. New York, NY: McGraw-Hill; 2011.

Brown KD, Banuchi V, Selesnick SH. Diseases of the external ear. In: Lalwani AK, ed. *Current Diagnosis & Treatment in Otolaryngology: Head & Neck Surgery*. 3rd ed. New York, NY: McGraw-Hill; 2012.

Burrow TA, Saal HM, de Alarcon A, et al. Characterization of congenital anomalies in individuals with choanal atresia. *Arch Otolaryngol Head Neck Surg*. 2009;135(6):543.

Busaidy N, Habra M, Vassilopoulou-Sellin R. Endocrine malignancies. In: Kantarjian HM, Wolff RA, Koller CA. eds. *The MD Anderson Manual of Medical Oncology*. 2nd ed. New York, NY: McGraw-Hill; 2011.

Friedman NR, Scholes MA, Yoon PJ. Ear, nose, and throat. In: Hay WW, Levin MJ, Deterding RR, Abzug MJ, eds. *Current Diagnosis & Treatment: Pediatrics*. 22nd ed. New York, NY: McGraw-Hill; 2013.

Goldstein NA, Hammerschlag MR. Peritonsillar, retropharyngeal and parapharyngeal abscesses. In: Feigin RD, Cherry JD, Demmler-Harrison GJ, Kaplan SL, eds. *Textbook of Pediatric Infectious Diseases*. 6th ed. Philadelphia, PA: Saunders; 2009:177–185.

Harlor AD, Jr, Bower C; Committee on Practice and Ambulatory Medicine, Section on Otolaryngology–Head and Neck Surgery. Hearing assessment in infants and children: Recommendations beyond neonatal screening. *Pediatrics*. 2009;124:1252–1263.

Hoffman WY. Cleft lip and palate. In: Lalwani AK, ed. *Current Diagnosis & Treatment in Otolaryngology: Head & Neck Surgery*. 3rd ed. New York, NY: McGraw-Hill; 2012.

Joint Committee on Infant Hearing, American Academy of Audiology, American Academy of Pediatrics, American Speech-Language-Hearing Association, Directors of Speech and Hearing Programs in State Health and Welfare Agencies. Year 2000 position statement: Principles and guidelines for early hearing detection and intervention programs. *Pediatrics*. 2000;106(4):798–817.

Kentab OY, Qureshi N. Neck masses in children. In: Tintinalli JE, Stapczynski J, Ma O, et al, eds. *Tintinalli's Emergency Medicine: A Comprehensive Study Guide*. 7th ed. New York, NY: McGraw-Hill; 2011.

Klein U. Oral medicine and dentistry. In: Hay WW, Levin MJ, Deterding RR, Abzug MJ, eds. *Current Diagnosis & Treatment: Pediatrics*. 22nd ed. New York, NY: McGraw-Hill; 2013.

LeBlond RF, Brown DD, Suneja M, Szot JF. The head and neck. In: LeBlond RF, Brown DD, Suneja M, Szot JF, eds. *DeGowin's Diagnostic Examination*. 10th ed. New York, NY: McGraw-Hill; 2014.

Lichten SR. Retropharyngeal abscess. In: Gerschel J, Rauch D. eds. *Caring for the Hospitalized Child: A Handbook of Inpatient Pediatrics*. Elk Grove Village, IL: American Academy of Pediatrics; 2013.

Lieberthal AS, Carroll AE, Chonmaitree T, et al. The diagnosis and management of acute otitis media. *Pediatrics*. 2013;131:e964–e999.

Lustig LR, Schindler JS. Ear, nose, and throat disorders. In: Papadakis MA, McPhee SJ, Rabow MW, eds. *Current Medical Diagnosis & Treatment 2015*. New York, NY: McGraw-Hill; 2014.

Lye C, Nead JA, Chase L. Parotitis. In: Gerschel J, Rauch D, eds. *Caring for the Hospitalized Child: A Handbook of Inpatient Pediatrics*. Elk Grove Village, IL: American Academy of Pediatrics; 2013.

Macfadyen CA, Acuin JM, Gamble CL. Systemic antibiotics versus topical treatments for chronically discharging ears with underlying eardrum perforations. *Cochrane Database of Syst Rev*. 2006(1):CD005608. doi: 10.1002/14651858.CD005608.

McArdle AJ, Shroff R. Question 3: Is ultrasonography required to rule out congenital anomalies of the kidneys and urinary tract in babies with isolated preauricular tags or sinuses? *Arch Dis Child*. 2013;98:84–87.

Mittiga MR, Gonzalez del Rey JA, Ruddy RM. Pediatric conditions. In: Knoop KJ, Stack LB, Storrow AB, Thurman R, eds. *The Atlas of Emergency Medicine*. 3rd ed. New York, NY: McGraw-Hill; 2010.

Rosenfeld RM, Schwartz SR, Cannon CR, et al. Clinical practice guideline: Acute otitis externa. *Otolaryngol Head Neck Surg*. 2014;150(1 suppl):S1–S24.

Rosenfeld RM, Culpepper L, Yawn, B, Mahoney MC; AAP, AAFP, AAO-HNS Subcommittee on Otitis Media with Effusion. Clinical practice guideline: Otitis media with effusion. *Otolaryngol Head Neck Surg*. 2004;130:S95.

Rubin MA, Ford LC, Gonzales R. Pharyngitis, sinusitis, otitis and other upper respiratory tract infections. In: Longo DL, Fauci AS, Kasper DL, et al, eds. *Harrison's Principles of Internal Medicine*. 18th ed. New York, NY: McGraw-Hill; 2012.

Shah RN, Cannon TY, Shores CG. Infections and disorders of the neck and upper airway. In: Tintinalli JE, Stapczynski J, Ma O, et al, eds. *Tintinalli's Emergency Medicine: A Comprehensive Study Guide, 7th ed*. New York, NY: McGraw-Hill; 2011.

Spiegel JH, Numa W. Nasal trauma. In: Lalwani AK, ed. *Current Diagnosis & Treatment in Otolaryngology: Head & Neck Surgery*. 3rd ed. New York, NY: McGraw-Hill; 2012.

Summers SM, Bey T. Epistaxis, nasal fractures, and rhinosinusitis. In: Tintinalli JE, Stapczynski J, Ma O, et al, eds. *Tintinalli's Emergency Medicine: A Comprehensive Study Guide*. 7th ed. New York, NY: McGraw-Hill; 2011.

Suurna MV. Congenital nasal anomalies. In: Lalwani AK, ed. *Current Diagnosis & Treatment in Otolaryngology: Head & Neck Surgery*. 3rd ed. New York, NY: McGraw-Hill; 2012.

Usatine RP, Smith MA, Chumley HS, Mayeaux EJ. Otitis media: Acute otitis and otitis media with effusion. In: Usatine RP, Smith MA, Chumley HS, Mayeaux EJ, eds. *The Color Atlas of Family Medicine*. 2nd ed. New York, NY: McGraw-Hill; 2013.

Verhoeff M, Van Der Veen EL, Rovers MM, et al. Chronic suppurative otitis media: A review. *Int J Pediatr Otorhinolaryngol*. 2006;70(1):1–12.

Wald ER, Applegate KE, Bordley C, et al. Clinical practice guideline: Diagnosis and management of acute bacterial sinusitis in children aged 1 to 18 years. *Pediatrics*. 2013;132:e262–280.

Wang RY, Earl DL, Ruder RO, Graham JM. Syndromic ear anomalies and renal ultrasounds. *Pediatrics*. 2001;108(2):e32–e38.

Weinberger PM, Terris DJ. Otolaryngology–Head and neck surgery. In: Doherty GM, ed. *Current Diagnosis & Treatment: Surgery*. 13th ed. New York, NY: McGraw-Hill; 2010.

Zhorne D, Nead JA, Chase L. Retropharyngeal abscess. In: Gerschel J, Rauch D, eds. *Caring for the Hospitalized Child: A Handbook of Inpatient Pediatrics*. Elk Grove Village, IL: American Academy of Pediatrics; 2013.

Emergency Care

10

Sarah L. Miller

▶ CASE 1

You are seeing a 10 day-old male infant in clinic for a weight check. He was delivered at term by uncomplicated vaginal delivery. A rectal temperature obtained in triage measured 38.1°C (100.7°F). The child's mother states that he has been taking less with each feeding today. His siblings have had cough, congestion, and fever over the past week. On exam the infant is sleeping but easily arouses. His fontanelle is neither bulging nor sunken. He does have some clear rhinorrhea. Mucous membranes are moist. Lungs are clear with normal work of breathing, and abdomen is benign. Extremities are warm and well-perfused. He is not jaundiced.

Question 1-1

The most appropriate management of this patient includes:

A) Continue to monitor at home as he likely has a cold like his siblings.
B) Administer ceftriaxone intramuscularly (IM) and discharge to home with plan to follow up in clinic tomorrow for reevaluation.
C) Order a chest X-ray and obtain a catheterized urine sample for urinalysis and culture.
D) Transfer to the emergency department for further evaluation and hospital admission.
E) Prescribe an over-the-counter cold medicine.

Discussion 1-1

The correct answer is "D." The neonate in this scenario has a fever and decreased feeding, which should raise immediate concern for neonatal sepsis, requiring a complete infectious workup (including blood, urine, and cerebrospinal fluid [CSF] culture), hospital admission, and empiric antibiotic treatment. This scenario is frequently referred to as "the rule out." Fever in a neonate is defined as 38°C (100.4°F) or higher. In an infant younger than 28 days of age, fever is a medical emergency and requires an infectious workup, including lumbar puncture, intravenous antibiotics, and admission to the hospital. For infants 29 to 90 days old, fever denotes urgency, but treatment may be stratified by risk. Unless your office is remarkably well-supplied, this workup would most likely be performed in a hospital setting with subsequent admission for observation. If you chose option "E," you will frustrate your office colleagues who practice evidence-based medicine but parents will love you. (See Figure 10–1.)

⧖ QUICK QUIZ

What is the most appropriate method of measuring body temperature in pediatric patients?

A) Rectal.
B) Temporal.
C) Axillary.
D) Tympanic.
E) Forehead.

Discussion

The correct answer is "A." The rectal temperature is the most accurate noninvasive assessment of core body temperature. The American Academy of Pediatrics (AAP) recommends that rectal temperature be obtained for children 0 to 3 years old and oral temperatures for children 4 years and older. However, in toddlers it may be technically difficult to measure a rectal temperature because of patient discomfort and resistance. Taking a rectal temperature on a 3-year-old may fall under cruel and unusual punishment. Tympanic temperature measurements are accurate in children 6 months of age and older if the tympanic membrane is not obstructed by wax. Axillary temperature measurements may be used for screening only and are not appropriate for infants. Mercury thermometers should never be used due to risk of ingestion.

```
                              ┌────────────────────────┐
                              │   Non-toxic-appearing, │
                              │   28–90 days and        │
                              │   "Low-risk" (defined below) │
                              └────────────────────────┘
┌──────────────┐                      │
│  < 28 days   │              ┌───────┴───────────────────────────────────┐
└──────────────┘              │                                           │
       │                      │                                           │
      Yes          No                                                    Yes
       │            │                                                     │
       ▼                                                                  ▼
┌──────────────────┐                                      ┌────────────────────────┐
│ Admit to hospital│                                      │ Outpatient management  │
└──────────────────┘                                      └────────────────────────┘
```

┌─────────────────────────┐   ┌──────────────────────────────────────┐   ┌──────────────────────────────┐
│ Blood culture   │   │   **Option 1**   │   │   **Option 2**   │
│ Urine culture   │   │ Blood culture   │   │ Blood culture   │
│ Lumbar puncture   │   │ Urine culture   │   │ Urine culture   │
│ Parenteral antibiotics │   │ Lumbar puncture (CSF culture)   │   │ Reevaluation within 24 hours │
│ Chest radiograph*   │   │ Ceftriaxone 50 mg/kg IV or IM intravenously │ └──────────────────────────────┘
└─────────────────────────┘   │ Reevaluation within 24 hours   │
                              └──────────────────────────────────────┘

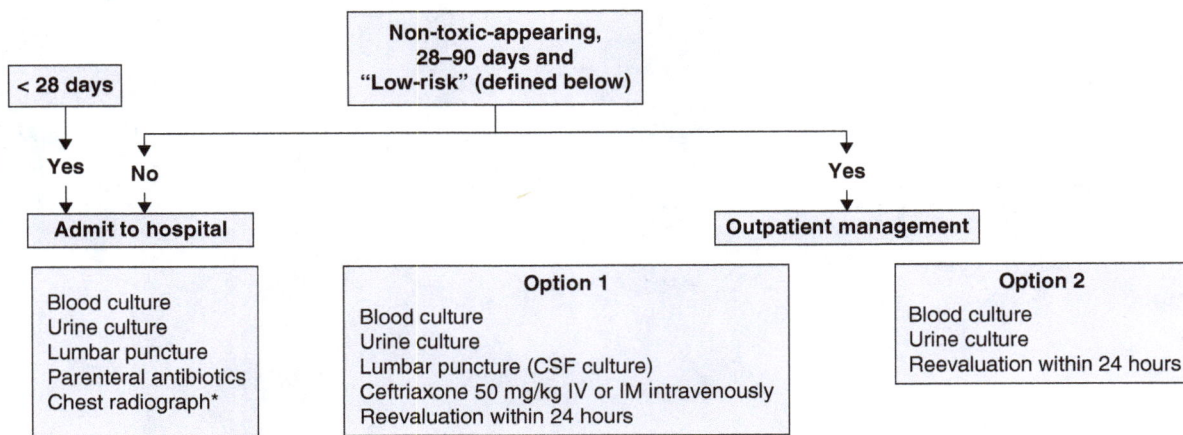

*Chest radiograph if signs of pneumonia: respiratory distress, abnormal breath sounds, tachypnea, pulse oximetry < 95%.

┌───┐
│ **Follow-up of low-risk infants treated as outpatients with positive culture results:**   │
│   │
│ Blood culture positive (pathogen): Admit for sepsis evaluation and parenteral antibiotic therapy pending results │
│ Urine culture positive (pathogen): Persistent fever: Admit for sepsis evaluation and parenteral antibiotic therapy pending results │
│   Outpatient antibiotics if afebrile and well   │
└───┘

┌───┐
│ **Low-risk criteria for febrile infants:**   │
│   │
│ Clinical criteria: │
│   Previously healthy, term infant with uncomplicated nursery stay   │
│   > 28 days old   │
│   Nontoxic clinical appearance   │
│   No focal bacterial infection on examination (except otitis media)   │
│ Laboratory criteria: │
│   WBC count 5–15,000/mm^3, < 1,500 bands/mm^3, or band/neutrophil ratio < 0.2   │
│   Negative gram stain of unspun urine (preferred), or negative urine leukocyte esterase and nitrite, or < 5 WBCs/hpf │
│   When diarrhea present: < 5 WBCs/hpf in stool   │
│   CSF: < 8 WBCs/mm^3 and negative gram stain (option 1 only)   │
└───┘

FIGURE 10–1. Diagnostic evaluation of fever in an infant younger than 90 days of age.

⧖ QUICK QUIZ

How should fever be treated?
A) Acetaminophen.
B) Ibuprofen.
C) Treatment is not required.
D) Cool bath.
E) Both A and B.

Discussion

The correct answer is "C." Fever is a symptom of an underlying infectious or inflammatory process that causes resetting of the hypothalamic thermoregulatory set point followed by the body's response to increase the temperature to match the new set point. Fever, therefore, does not require treatment in and of itself. Parents should be reassured that unless their child appears uncomfortable no medications need to be given. High fever has not been shown to cause brain damage, and the height of fever is not the trigger for febrile seizures. They should avoid excessive bundling when fever is present. Fluids should be encouraged to replace increased insensible losses with fever. Fever should be differentiated from hyperthermia, as hyperthermia can be fatal if left untreated. In hyperthermia, the body temperature increases independently without hypothalamic regulation, exceeding the body's cooling mechanisms. Hyperthermia is due to environmental, metabolic, or pharmacologic factors.

▶ CASE 2

Your next patient is a 10-week-old infant boy brought by his father for fever. He has had a fever of 38.8°C (102°F) since this morning and has not seemed interested in breastfeeding throughout the day. He has had one wet diaper in the past 12 hours. Physical exam reveals a lethargic infant with tachycardia and delayed capillary refill, but no other localizing signs for his fever. He has received his 2-month vaccinations. He is otherwise healthy and was delivered at term. His father states that the patient's mother was diagnosed with influenza yesterday.

Question 2-1

What is the most appropriate management?

A) Continue to monitor at home as he likely has influenza like his mother.
B) Administer ceftriaxone IM and discharge to home with a plan to follow up in clinic tomorrow for reevaluation.
C) Order a chest X-ray and obtain a catheterized urine sample for urinalysis and culture.
D) Transfer to the emergency department for further evaluation and hospital admission.
E) Administer acetaminophen.

Discussion 2-1

The correct answer is "D." The infant in this scenario is an obviously ill-appearing, febrile 70-day-old. Although there is some controversy, infants in this age group who are febrile but well-appearing and otherwise "low risk" (see Figure 10–1) may be managed as outpatients. However, the infant in this scenario is "high risk" and obviously quite ill, with signs of shock. He is at much higher risk of serious bacterial infection (eg, sepsis, meningitis, urinary tract infection). Appropriate disposition of this patient requires rapid transfer to the emergency department for stabilization. Call 9-1-1. This infant needs an ambulance. Workup would include a complete blood count (CBC); cultures of blood, urine, and CSF; antibiotics; fluid resuscitation; and admission.

> **Helpful Tip**
> The most common serious bacterial infection in infants younger than 90 days of age is a urinary tract infection.

▶ CASE 3

An 18-month-old girl is brought to the emergency department with a 2-day history of fever. She has been feeling tired and wants to be held constantly. She is drinking but is not eating. She has no other symptoms or sick contacts. She is a healthy toddler with no past medical history and is up-to-date on her vaccines. On exam, she is ill but not toxic. She is warm to the touch. There is no rash, meningismus, or focal infection on exam.

Question 3-1

The most appropriate management includes:

A) Perform a lumbar puncture.
B) Obtain a blood culture.
C) Prescribe amoxicillin.
D) Obtain a urine specimen for urinalysis and culture.
E) Send her home.

Discussion 3-1

The correct answer is "D." The risk of a serious bacterial infection decreases with age and vaccination. Historically, diagnostic evaluation in a febrile toddler without a source included obtaining blood, urine, and possibly CSF to avoid missing an invasive infection with *Haemophilus influenzae* type B or *Streptococcus pneumoniae*. Now with vaccinations, if the infant (older than 90 days) or child is well appearing the only routine test to consider would be urinalysis and urine culture for (1) all females and uncircumcised males younger than 2 years, (2) all circumcised males younger than 6 months, and (3) all children with genitourinary abnormalities.

▶ CASE 4

A nurse tells you that emergency medical services (EMS) are en route with a 17-year-old adolescent girl who has altered mental status and a measured temperature of more than 41°C (> 106°F). Their estimated arrival time (ETA) is 5 minutes. You have a few minutes to consider your differential diagnosis for this patient.

Question 4-1

What will you be looking for when she arrives?

A) Petechiae.
B) Muscular rigidity.
C) Exophthalmos.
D) Mydriasis.
E) All of the above.

Discussion 4-1

The correct answer is "E." Temperature above 41°C (105.8°F) may be associated with *fever* secondary to bacterial or viral infection or inflammation. It may also be consistent with *hyperthermia* secondary to environmental factors (heat stroke), medications (neuroleptic malignant syndrome, serotonin syndrome, malignant hyperthermia), intoxication (particularly MDMA or anticholinergics), and thyroid storm.

⧗ QUICK QUIZ

Which types of lacerations can be repaired in the office and which should prompt consideration of surgical referral?

A) Simple forehead laceration.
B) Scalp laceration.
C) Lip laceration.
D) Finger laceration with severed ligament.
E) Nonlinear leg laceration.

Discussion

The correct answer is "D." Lacerations are a common presenting complaint in pediatric patients. Most are small, simple lacerations on the head or scalp as a result of falls. Wounds associated with tearing or compression of the skin may create irregular or stellate lacerations, which may be associated with tissue damage and poor healing. Most lacerations can be repaired in the office or emergency department with excellent cosmetic results. Wounds that should prompt further evaluation or referral include

TABLE 10–1 INDICATIONS FOR ADMINISTRATION OF TETANUS VACCINE

Vaccination history unknown or patient has received < 3 doses, all wounds

Patient has received ≥ 3 doses but none in the last 10 years for simple, clean wound

Patient has received ≥ 3 doses but none in the last 5 years for contaminated or complex wound

puncture wounds to the neck, chest, or abdomen; lacerations on the neck; persistent or pulsatile bleeding; tendon or nerve injuries; lacerations with underlying fracture or muscle involvement; large, complicated, or heavily contaminated lacerations; retained foreign bodies; or lacerations on the face with potential for poor cosmetic outcome. Lacerations involving the vermillion border can be sutured without surgical consultation if the pediatrician is experienced and able to achieve a good cosmetic result.

Sutures generally provide the best tensile strength and cosmetic outcome, but are more time consuming and require follow up for removal. For wounds on the scalp or long linear lacerations, staples are appropriate. Skin adhesives are appropriate for small, linear, low-tension wounds without continued bleeding and not located on hands, feet, or joints. Adhesive strips (Steri-Strips) may be used in similar situations as skin adhesive; however, these are more appropriate for additional wound support after removal of sutures or staples. Puncture wounds generally should not be closed owing to the increased risk of infection. Prophylactic antibiotics should be considered for animal or human bites or suspicion for retained foreign body. Puncture wounds through sneakers are at increased risk for infection with *Pseudomonas aeruginosa*. All wounds should be thoroughly irrigated with sterile water, saline, or dilute iodine solution. Tap water is a usable alternative when sterile solutions are not available. Irrigation should be at relatively high pressure (4 to 15 psi) to flush bacteria, debris, and necrotic tissue out of the wound. A minimum volume of 100 mL of irrigation fluid per centimeter of wound is appropriate. Immunizations should be reviewed and tetanus vaccine given if indicated. (See Table 10–1.) Tetanus immune globulin is indicated for complex or contaminated wounds when vaccination history is unknown *or* if patient has received less than 3 doses of tetanus vaccine. Prophylactic antibiotics are not needed for minor wounds.

▶ CASE 5

A 4-year-old is brought to the emergency department after being bitten in the face by a dog with several resultant lacerations to the nose and left cheek.

Question 5-1

Which of the following is true regarding dog bites?
A) Most bites in children are to the hands or forearm.
B) It is more likely that the child was bitten by a stray dog.

C) The wound should be gently irrigated with sterile water to prevent further tissue damage.
D) All victims of dog bites should be treated with antibiotics to prevent infection.
E) None of the above.

Discussion 5-1

The correct answer is "E." Dog bites in children are most common on the face and neck, while in adolescents and adults bites are more often to the extremities. The offending dog is most often one that the victim knows. Antibiotics should be considered for patients with higher risk bites, including bites to the hand or near a prosthetic joint, associated crush injury, those requiring closure, delayed presentation, or a victim with immune compromise.

Question 5-2

Appropriate antibiotic prophylaxis for this child would include all of the following EXCEPT:
A) Cephalexin oral.
B) Amoxicillin/clavulanate oral.
C) Ampicillin/sulbactam intravenous.
D) Clindamycin plus trimethoprim/sulfamethoxazole oral.
E) None of the above.

Discussion 5-2

The correct answer is "A." First-line oral prophylaxis for this child is amoxicillin/clavulanate (Augmentin) orally or ampicillin sulbactam (Unasyn) intravenously (IV). For penicillin-allergic patients options include clindamycin or metronidazole *plus* doxycycline, trimethoprim/sulfamethoxazole, or moxifloxacin. Remember that doxycycline is associated with enamel hypoplasia and tooth discoloration and should not be used in children younger than 8 years of age. Fluoroquinolones should be used with caution owing to risk of tendon rupture. Cephalexin has limited activity against *Pasteurella multocida* and therefore should not be used for bite wound prophylaxis.

The child's parents tell you that the dog that bit their child belongs to their neighbor. They are unsure if its vaccinations are up to date. They are wondering if their child should receive a rabies vaccine.

Question 5-3

What is your response?
A) No, if the bite was provoked.
B) No, if the dog may be observed.
C) Yes, all dog bites require rabies vaccination.
D) Yes, if vaccination status of the dog is unknown.
E) Yes, both the rabies immune globulin and vaccines should be administered.

Discussion 5-3

The correct answer is "B." Signs of rabies in animals include anorexia, difficulty swallowing, ataxia, seizures, and abnormal behavior or vocalizations. If the dog in this scenario does not display any of these symptoms and can be observed for 10 days, no postexposure prophylaxis (PEP) is indicated. Prophylaxis should be considered if the dog is not observable and should be given immediately if the dog is known or suspected to be rabid. Rabies PEP includes rabies immune globulin injected at or proximal to the site of injury at time of presentation and rabies vaccine given on days 0, 3, 7, and 14. For wild animal bites, the animal in question should be assumed to be rabid and PEP should be strongly considered. If the animal in question can be captured and tested, PEP can be discontinued if results are negative. Further evaluation of nonbite exposures and decision to initiate PEP can be made in conjunction with local public health authorities. A listing of state and local resources is available from the Centers for Disease Control and Prevention (CDC; www.cdc.gov/rabies/resources/contacts.html).

CASE 6

You are seeing a 17-year-old adolescent boy with a hand injury. He was brought to the emergency department by his parents after they noticed his hand was becoming increasingly red and swollen. They noticed some "cuts on his knuckles" several days ago when he returned home from a party. When you examine his hand you see several horizontal linear lacerations over his third and fourth dorsal metacarpophalangeal (MCP) joints, with underlying warmth, erythema, and induration. This area is exquisitely tender, and his ability to flex or extend his fingers at the MCP joints is severely limited. There is a small amount of purulent drainage from the area. He initially states he injured his hand after "punching a wall," but when you interview him with his parents out of the room he admits that he had instead punched someone in the face.

Question 6-1

The most appropriate next step in management is:
A) Oral antibiotics and reevaluation in 24 hours.
B) Magnetic resonance imaging (MRI) scan of the hand to evaluate for tendon injury.
C) IV antibiotics and immediate consultation with hand surgeon.
D) IV antibiotics and admission to the pediatric floor for observation.
E) Referral to anger management counseling.

Discussion 6-1

The correct answer is "C." The wounds described are also consistent with a closed fist contacting another person's teeth, or a "fight bite." Patients may withhold this detail of their history, so any injury to the hand with these characteristics should be treated as a fight bite regardless of stated history. Polymicrobial infections are common after this injury, with a spectrum of complications including cellulitis, tenosynovitis, septic joint, and osteomyelitis. Common bacterial isolates include gram-negative bacilli, streptococcal species, *Staphylococcus aureus*, and *Eikenella corrodens*. This patient's presentation is concerning for septic arthritis or tenosynovitis, given his limited range

of motion. Management would include immediate evaluation by a hand surgeon, and admission for IV antibiotics. X-rays may be obtained to evaluate for fracture or retained foreign body (eg, tooth fragments).

> **Helpful Tip**
> Management of other human bite wounds can be more straightforward. All wounds should be thoroughly irrigated. Puncture wounds are generally not closed, and there is some controversy regarding suture closure of larger wounds. Delayed primary closure or loose approximation of wound edges are both proposed management options. Antibiotic prophylaxis is recommended for puncture or other deep bite wounds, those with underlying tendon or bone, or bites to the face.

QUICK QUIZ

Most snake bites in the United States are unprovoked, often due to startling the snake in its natural habitat.
A) True.
B) False.

Discussion

The correct answer is "B." The likelihood of encountering a venomous snake increases as one approaches the equator, therefore these exposures are more common in the southern United States. Poisonous snakes found in the United States include pit vipers (rattlesnakes, cottonmouths, and copperheads) and coral snakes. The majority of deaths attributed to snake bites in the United States are in men who have been intentionally handling or playing with snakes, although innocent victims do exist. Pit viper envenomation is associated with extensive local swelling, which may progress to systemic symptoms including paralysis, rhabdomyolysis, shock, and disseminated intravascular coagulation (DIC). Immediate management includes removing any tight clothing or jewelry in the area. Suctioning of the area in an attempt to remove venom is not recommended. Antivenom should be administered if available. Coral snakes inject venom via repeated bites or "chewing"; therefore, these bites are less likely to result in significant envenomation. Local edema and coagulopathy are not seen with coral snake bites, in contrast to pit viper envenomation. Systemic effects may be delayed for hours and are primarily neurotoxic and myotoxic. Patients should be monitored closely for respiratory depression and rhabdomyolysis. In general, all patients with suspected snake envenomation should be monitored in a facility with intensive care capabilities.

CASE 7

A 12-year-old girl presents with foot pain. She states she was getting ready to head out for a hike with her family in the Arizona desert. She put her foot in her boot and felt a sudden sharp pain on the side of her foot. This occurred about 30 minutes ago. She is feeling well other than some tingling and pain in the area. She did not look into her boot but believes she may have been bitten by a spider. On exam she has a small puncture wound to the lateral aspect of her foot without erythema or swelling. Tapping over this area causes significant increase in her pain and paresthesias.

Question 7-1

Management of this patient's symptoms should include:
A) Cold compress and oral pain medication followed by 4 to 5 hours of observation in the emergency department.
B) Rapid administration of *Loxosceles* antivenom.
C) Admission to the hospital for observation.
D) Irrigation of the wound and discharge to home.
E) Throwing away her boots.

Discussion 7-1

The correct answer is "A." The patient in this scenario has symptoms most consistent with bark scorpion sting, with local reaction only. Scorpions are found primarily in the southwestern United States. She should be treated symptomatically and discharged to home if symptoms have not progressed 4 to 5 hours after envenomation. As her symptoms are mild, antivenom is not indicated. Patients presenting for evaluation of "spider bite" are almost always not, in fact, the victims of arachnid assault. Most of these alleged "spider bites" will be diagnosed as cellulitis or abscess. However, spider bites do occur, and the common species (brown recluse and black widow spiders) are found throughout the United States. *Loxosceles*, or brown recluse, spiders are named for their tendency to build webs in small secluded spaces, such as the back of a closet or dark corner of a garage. They are 8 to 15 millimeters (mm) in length and light to dark brown, with a violin- or fiddle-shaped spot on their dorsal thorax. They are most common in midwestern and southern states. Brown recluse spider bites can cause local skin irritation but are not associated with paresthesias. Effects of bites are generally local skin necrosis, although major complications including DIC, kidney injury, and hemolytic anemia have been reported. Most exposures can be managed with local wound care. Surgical debridement and empiric antibiotic treatment are not recommended. *Latrodectus*, or black widow, spiders are larger (12–16 mm in length) and can be identified by a red or orange "hourglass" on their ventral abdomen. They are not always black, however, with colors ranging from pale brown to gray to black. A black widow spider bite is not associated with significant local reaction or paresthesias. Black widow venom causes very little local reaction, but it does contain a neurotoxin capable of inducing persistent contraction of both smooth and skeletal muscle. Severe abdominal pain, tachycardia, diaphoresis, and muscle spasms are common presenting symptoms. Black widow envenomation is not fatal, and treatment is supportive. Antivenom is available as an adjunct to pain control. More than 40 types of scorpion are found in the United States; however, the Arizona bark scorpion (*Centruroides sculpturatus*) is responsible for most morbidity and mortality associated with scorpion stings. Its primary habitat is in the southwestern

United States. The effects of its venom are primarily neurotoxic, with symptoms ranging from local pain and paresthesias to skeletal muscular hyperactivity to multisystem organ failure. Local pain and paresthesias may be worsened by tapping over the site of the sting. These cases are managed with pain control, and cool compresses. Patients should be monitored for progression of symptoms but if stable 4 to 5 hours after evenomation may be discharged to home. More severely affected patients often present with agitation, writhing, and roving eye movements. These patients with skeletal muscular or cranial nerve involvement can be treated with benzodiazepines and analgesics followed by admission for observation. Antivenom is available for patients with more severe symptoms. (Although many people think that urine is a magical remedy for bites or stings, including those from jellyfish, it's not!)

Suppose the patient had instead been stung by an insect in the order Hymenoptera.

Question 7-2

All of the following are true regarding Hymenoptera stings EXCEPT:
A) The order Hymenoptera includes bees, wasps, and ants.
B) Patients who have systemic reactions to bee stings should be observed for several hours, even if symptoms have completely resolved after treatment.
C) Wasps and bees leave their "stinger" in the skin, which may need to be removed.
D) Systemic reactions from Hymenoptera stings are not possible without prior sensitization.
E) A large local reaction may develop around the sting site.

Discussion 7-2

The correct answer is "D." The order Hymenoptera encompasses a group of stinging insects, including bees, wasps and ants. Envenomation causes immediate pain followed by development of an erythematous wheal at the site of entry. Self-limited local reactions can be treated with cold compresses and oral analgesics or antihistamines as needed. Bee stings may require removal of the "stinger," a modified ovipositor, which is left in the skin. (Kudos if you know what an ovipositor is.) Stings with significant local swelling (eg, in the hand) may benefit from oral corticosteroids. Multiple stings, which usually occur after nest disturbance, can cause significant systemic effects and may be fatal, even in people with no history of anaphylaxis or prior exposure. Think about that the next time you are tempted to kick or knock down a nest. Anaphylactic reactions increase in incidence with increasing age. Presentation of anaphylactic or anaphylactoid reactions may include urticaria, hypotension, bronchospasm, angioedema, vomiting, or diarrhea. Treatment should be rapidly initiated, including epinephrine, steroids, and IV fluids, as well as aggressive airway management and vasoactive medications (pressors) if needed. Patients with systemic reactions should be closely observed for at least 4 to 6 hours after resolution of symptoms because of the risk of biphasic IgE-mediated reaction.

QUICK QUIZ

Treatment of exposure to North American species of jellyfish includes all of the following EXCEPT:
A) Vinegar.
B) Hot water.
C) Sea water.
D) Urine.
E) Use plastic object to remove tentacles.

Discussion

The correct answer is "D." Jellyfish stings are mediated through nematocysts, which are small structures located on the tentacles and near the mouth. Nematocysts are able to attach to the skin and when triggered release venom. Contact or pressure over nematocysts triggers release; thus, it is helpful to inactivate nematocysts prior to removal of tentacles from skin. Vinegar (4–6% acetic acid) has been shown to help prevent nematocyst discharge when applied for 30 minutes. Tentacles can be rinsed off with sea water or scraped off with a credit card. Rinsing with fresh water or urine is not recommended as hypotonic solutions may trigger nematocysts. After removal of nematocysts, soaking in hot water has been shown to deactivate some jellyfish toxins. (Hopefully, some will remember the jellyfish episode from *Friends*.)

► CASE 8

A 6-year-old boy is brought for evaluation of abdominal pain after a bicycle accident. He was wearing a helmet when he struck a curb and fell forward, striking his abdomen on the handlebars.

Question 8-1

He is most likely to have injured which of the following?
A) Stomach.
B) Pancreas.
C) Duodenum.
D) Liver.
E) Kidney.

Discussion 8-1

The correct answer is "D." In blunt abdominal trauma, the liver and spleen are the most commonly injured organs. Hollow organs injuries are less common but may also be life threatening. Duodenal injuries, specifically duodenal hematomas, are associated with blunt trauma from bicycle handlebars but are still less common than solid organ injuries.

► CASE 9

You are evaluating a 13-year-old adolescent girl who was kicked in the abdomen while she was grooming her horse. She is complaining of pain in her upper abdomen and left shoulder. When you examine her you note bruising to her left upper quadrant and significant tenderness to palpation in this area. Her left shoulder exam is completely normal.

Question 9-1

Based on her history and exam, you are suspicious of what type of injury?
A) Splenic injury.
B) Kidney injury.
C) Pancreatic injury.
D) Stomach injury.
E) Ovarian injury.

Discussion 9-1

The correct answer is "A." Acute splenic injury often presents as left upper quadrant abdominal pain that may be referred to left shoulder. Splenic injury should be considered in persistent hypotension or shock after blunt trauma. Negative FAST (Focused Assessment with Sonography in Trauma) does not rule out splenic rupture, as bleeding may be contained within the splenic capsule. Computerized tomography (CT) scan of the abdomen with IV contrast is the preferred diagnostic study to diagnose splenic laceration or rupture. Whenever possible splenic ruptures are managed conservatively given the risk for immunocompromise after splenectomy. Any child with suspected or confirmed splenic rupture requires emergent surgical consult and should be admitted for close observation. Due to the risk of massive hemorrhage and shock, aggressive resuscitation with IV crystalloid fluids is indicated and blood transfusion may also be necessary.

Question 9-2

Which laboratory tests are typically indicated in evaluation of blunt abdominal trauma?
A) CBC.
B) Lipase.
C) Urinalysis.
D) Kidney function.
E) All of the above.

Discussion 9-2

The correct answer is "E." Indicated laboratory tests include CBC (hemoglobin and platelet count), electrolytes, liver panel (elevations of AST and ALT may be seen in liver injury), amylase and lipase, urinalysis (hematuria may be seen in injury to kidney, bladder, or urethra), lactic acid (may be elevated in tissue ischemia/hypoperfusion). Coagulation studies (PT/INR, PTT) are generally not indicated in otherwise healthy children unless there is a history of coagulopathy or in cases of massive hemorrhage.

► CASE 10

An 8-year-old girl is brought to the emergency department from the scene of an accident. Paramedics state that she was riding her bike when she was struck from behind by a car traveling 40 miles per hour (mph). She was not wearing a helmet. On arrival she is agitated and crying.

Question 10-1

Your initial rapid assessment of this patient should include all of the following EXCEPT:

A) Measurement of pulse, blood pressure, respirations, and pulse oximetry.
B) Checking peripheral pulses and capillary refill.
C) Lung auscultation.
D) Removal of clothing to fully expose the patient.
E) Assessing level of responsiveness.
F) Obtaining a detailed history of events surrounding the injury and performing a full head-to-toe exam.

Discussion 10-1

The correct answer is "F." Trauma is responsible for nearly 50% of deaths in children aged 1 to 14 years. Trauma evaluation therefore involves a rapid patient assessment known as the primary survey. This includes identifying and correcting potentially life-threatening abnormalities involving airway, breathing, circulation, and mental status. This is often simplified to ABCDE (**A**irway, **B**reathing, **C**irculation, **D**isability [neurologic exam], **E**xposure). Airway assessment includes identifying airway obstruction or inability to protect the airway, and treatment includes repositioning (with cervical spine immobilization), suctioning, and securing the airway if necessary. This patient's airway appears to be intact as she is awake and crying. Breathing should be assessed using respiratory rate and effort, pulse oximetry, and lung auscultation, with treatments including supplemental oxygen, needle decompression or chest tube for pneumothorax, and bag-valve mask or mechanical ventilation. Circulation assessment includes examining pulse rate, blood pressure, peripheral pulses, and capillary refill. Treatments include securing intravenous access, administration of IV fluids or blood transfusion, hemorrhage

control, or vasoactive mediations (pressors) as needed. Disability includes rating of neurologic status using the Glasgow Coma Scale (see Table 10–2), with treatments aimed at airway protection and maintaining cerebral perfusion. Exposure involves removing all clothing to facilitate full exam for injury while avoiding hypothermia. Further assessment, known as the secondary survey, including detailed head-to-toe exam, obtaining AMPLE history (**A**llergies, **M**edications, **P**ast medical history, **L**ast meal, **E**vents surrounding injury) should proceed after primary survey is completed.

....

When you examine this patient's chest you note abrasions and bruising on the left anterior and lateral chest wall. She is tachypneic and pulse oximetry reads 91% on room air. Her blood pressure is normal although she is tachycardic. You notice crepitus in the subcutaneous tissue in her neck and her trachea is deviated to the right. Her breath sounds are absent on the left.

Question 10-2

Your next step in management is:

A) Immediate chest X-ray.
B) Esophagram to evaluate for esophageal rupture.
C) Immediate CT of the chest with IV contrast to evaluate for pulmonary laceration.
D) Needle decompression of the left chest followed by tube thoracostomy.
E) Administration of supplemental oxygen via nonrebreathing face mask.

Discussion 10-2

The correct answer is "D." Blunt chest trauma is commonly associated with pulmonary contusion, hemothorax/pneumothorax, and rib fractures. Less common injuries include pulmonary or

TABLE 10–2 GLASGOW COMA SCALE (GCS) FOR CHILDREN AND MODIFIED SCALE FOR INFANTS

Behavior	Response	Response (preverbal children)	Score
Eye opening	Spontaneously	Spontaneous	4
	To command/speech	To sound	3
	To pain	To pain	2
	No response	No response	1
Verbal response	Oriented to person, place, and time	Vocalizations, smile, interacts	5
	Confused, but answers questions	Cries, irritable	4
	Inappropriate words	Cries to pain	3
	Incomprehensible sounds	Moans to pain	2
	No response	No response	1
Motor response	Obeys commands	Spontaneous movement	6
	Localizes to pain	Withdraws from touch	5
	Withdraws from pain	Withdraws from pain	4
	Abnormal flexion (decorticate)	Abnormal flexion (decorticate)	3
	Abnormal extension (decerebrate)	Abnormal extension (decerebrate)	2
	No response	No response	1
Total			15

tracheobronchial laceration, myocardial contusion, aortic injury, diaphragmatic rupture, or esophageal rupture. This patient has a tension pneumothorax, as evidenced by unilateral absent breath sounds, subcutaneous emphysema, and tracheal deviation away from the affected side. If untreated, further mediastinal shift can lead to decreased cardiac output, hypotension, and shock, culminating in a pulseless electoral activity (PEA) arrest. Management of a tension pneumothorax requires immediate needle decompression followed by chest tube placement. Physical findings should prompt immediate treatment—do not wait for chest X-ray to confirm the diagnosis. Esophageal rupture is a relatively uncommon complication of blunt chest trauma. Signs and symptoms include chest pain, tachycardia, dyspnea, subcutaneous emphysema, pneumomediastinum, or pneumothorax. Diagnosis is made by esophagram or esophagoscopy. Pulmonary laceration is usually associated with nearby rib fractures; patients may present with respiratory distress, hemoptysis, hemothorax, or pneumothorax. Treatment involves airway management (particularly with hemoptysis), volume resuscitation, tube thoracostomy, and emergent consultation with a pediatric surgeon. (See Figure 10–2.)

Your patient will open her eyes to painful stimuli. She answers questions with inappropriate words. She is moving her arms and legs spontaneously.

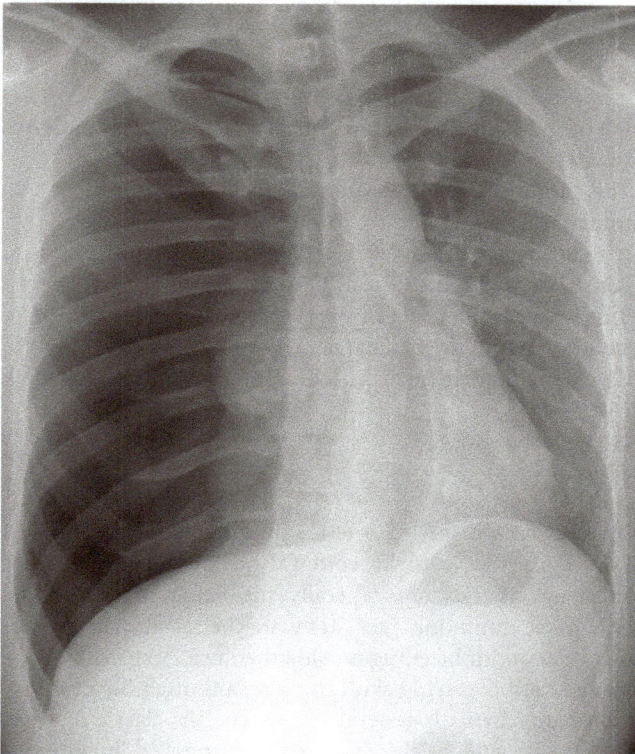

FIGURE 10–2. A tension pneumothorax is present on the right side with no lung markings on the right and shift of the mediastinum to the left. Immediate needle decompression and placement of a chest tube thoracotomy is indicated to prevent cardiopulmonary arrest. (Reproduced with permission from McKean SC, Ross JJ, Dressler DD, Brotman DJ, Ginsberg JS, eds. *Principles and Practice of Hospital Medicine*. New York, NY: McGraw-Hill Education; 2012, Fig. 107-7.)

Question 10-3

What is her GCS score?
A) 20.
B) 2.
C) 11.
D) 0.
E) 16.

Discussion 10-3

The correct answer is "C." The patient's score is 2 (eyes) + 3 (verbal) + 6 (motor) = 11. The minimum and maximum GCS scores are 3 and 15, so the only option was C (see Table 10–2).

You determine this patient's GCS to be 11. The alteration in consciousness leads you to focus your exam to identify signs of serious head injury.

Question 10-4

What is NOT a sign of skull fracture in pediatric patients?
A) Scalp hematoma.
B) A palpable step-off.
C) Post-traumatic clear otorrhea.
D) Bruising behind the ear.
E) Scalp laceration.

Discussion 10-4

The correct answer is "E." Any palpable crepitus or depression on head exam should raise suspicion for skull fracture. Signs of basilar skull fracture include CSF rhinorrhea, CSF otorrhea or bleeding from external auditory canal, hemotympanum, Battle sign (bruising posterior to the ear), and raccoon eyes (periorbital ecchymosis). For suspected depressed, basilar, or open skull fractures, a head CT scan should be performed to look for intracranial injuries. (See Figure 10–3.) A simple linear skull fracture in a patient without concern for nonaccidental trauma

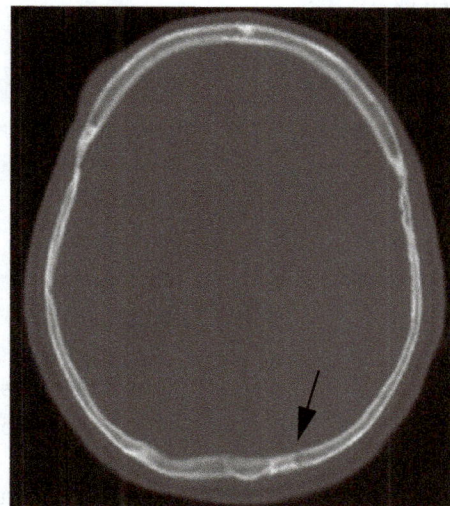

FIGURE 10–3. A left occipital linear skull fracture is visible on head CT scan in bone window view. (Reproduced with permission from Hall JB, Schmidt GA, Kress JP, eds. *Principles of Critical Care*. 4th ed. New York, NY: McGraw-Hill Education; 2015, Fig. 118-2.)

and otherwise normal exam requires no additional workup. Treatment includes reassurance and analgesia.

Question 10-5

All of the following are signs of acute increased intracranial pressure or brain herniation EXCEPT:
A) Altered mental status.
B) Bradycardia.
C) Fixed, nonreactive pupils.
D) Diarrhea.
E) Impaired external ocular abduction.

Discussion 10-5

The correct answer is "D." Symptoms of increased intracranial pressure and brain herniation overlap as increased intracranial pressure may lead to brain herniation. You must act immediately if concerned about herniation (ie, posturing, nonreactive pupil dilation). (See Table 10–3.)

Question 10-6

Which is NOT an indication for head CT scan in trauma patients?
A) Frontal scalp hematoma.
B) Severe headache.
C) Papilledema.
D) Open skull fracture.
E) Known diagnosis of hemophilia.

Discussion 10-6

The correct answer is "A." Prolonged loss of consciousness, worsening or severe headache, penetrating injury, GCS score less than 14, focal neurologic exam, signs of increased intracranial

TABLE 10–3 COMPARISON OF FINDINGS IN INCREASED INTRACRANIAL PRESSURE VERSUS HERNIATION

Acute Increased Intracranial Pressure	Herniation
Altered mental status/ Depressed GCS	Altered mental status/ Depressed GCS
Full fontanel	Obtunded
Irritability	Cushing triad:
Severe headache	• Hypertension
Seizure	• Bradycardia
Papilledema	• Irregular breathing (Cheyne-Stokes)
Neck stiffness	Fixed, dilated pupil(s)— "blown pupil"
Photophobia/phonophobia	Decerebrate posturing
Vomiting	Extraocular movement paralysis

GCS, Glasgow Coma Scale.

pressure or herniation, exam concerning for depressed or basilar skull fracture, delayed or prolonged seizure, bleeding disorder, clinical deterioration during the period of observation, or concern for nonaccidental trauma are all indications for imaging. In the absence of the preceding findings, consider imaging versus observation for high-speed motor vehicle crash, child struck by car, falls (> 5 feet for children younger than 2 years of age or > 3 feet for infants), persistent vomiting, nonfrontal scalp hematoma (in children younger than 2 years), or parental concern for significant behavior change. Head injuries with low-risk mechanisms, GCS score of 15, normal behavior, and exam do not require imaging. A simple frontal scalp hematoma in a well-appearing child with a normal neurologic exam does not require imaging. Kids' heads are heavy and their balance is terrible during the early phase of walking, making them prone to face plants.

You note a large boggy hematoma on this patient's right temporal/parietal scalp. You have ordered a head CT scan to evaluate for skull fracture or intracranial injury. While the CT is being performed on your patient, you are called to see another patient who was just brought to the emergency department by EMS for acute respiratory distress. Twenty minutes later you are called back to the trauma room because your first patient has become unresponsive. As you are securing the patient's airway you receive a call from the radiology department, reporting the patient's head CT results. The radiologist describes a biconvex lens–shaped area of acute hemorrhage overlying the right lateral cerebrum with midline shift.

Question 10-7

Which of the following statements is true about this patient's diagnosis?
A) This finding is almost always associated with injury to underlying brain parenchyma.
B) A majority of patients with this finding report brief loss of consciousness at the time of injury.
C) This injury is the result of shearing forces causing tearing of small vessels in the pia mater.
D) Operative management with craniotomy is necessary in all cases.
E) None of the above.

Discussion 10-7

The correct answer is "E." The CT findings described in this case are consistent with an epidural hematoma (EDH). (See Figure 10–4.) EHDs are generally the result of blunt head trauma, most commonly falls. They are the result of arterial or venous injury with bleeding outside the dura. Sixty to 80% are associated with overlying skull fracture, although direct injury to brain parenchyma is generally not seen. The classic scenario of head injury with brief loss of consciousness → "lucid interval" → rapid deterioration is often seen in Board questions but is much less common in clinical practice. Patients may present instead with headache and persistent nausea. When the diagnosis of EDH is made emergent consultation with a neurosurgeon is mandated owing to the risk of expansion and herniation. The patient in this case would certainly require craniotomy with

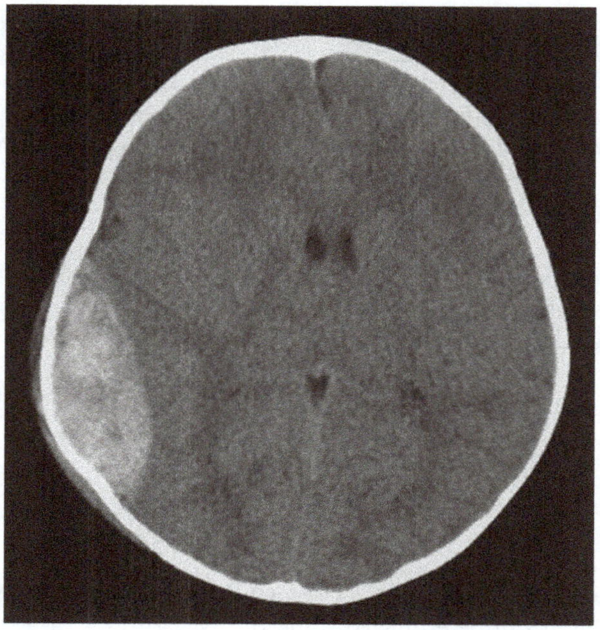

FIGURE 10–4. A biconvex lens–shaped hemorrhage overlying the parietal area, consistent with an acute epidural hematoma. Epidural hematomas are located between the skull and the dura and do not cross suture lines. (Reproduced with permission from Doherty GM, ed. *Current Diagnosis & Treatment: Surgery*. 14th ed. New York, NY: McGraw-Hill Education; 2015, Fig. 36-8.)

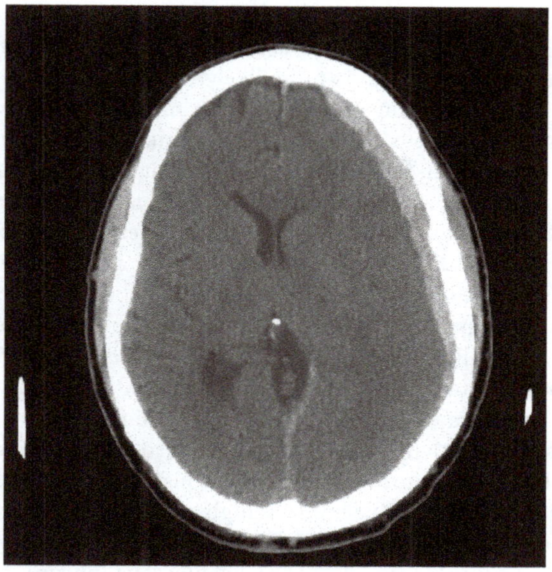

FIGURE 10–5. A subdural hematoma is present over the left frontotemporoparietal area. There is mass effect with mild midline shift. Subdural hematomas are located between the arachnoid and dura and cross suture lines. (Reproduced with permission from Hall JB, Schmidt GA, Kress JP, eds. *Principles of Critical Care*. 4th ed. New York, NY: McGraw-Hill Education; 2015, Fig. 118-4.)

evacuation of the hemorrhage. Small epidural hematomas may not require operative intervention; however, all patients should be admitted to the hospital for close observation.

Imagine instead that the radiologist had reported bilateral crescent-shaped areas of hemorrhage.

Question 10-8

Which of the following is true of this diagnosis?

A) This finding is likely to be associated with injury to underlying brain parenchyma.
B) If found in infants this injury is pathognomic for child abuse.
C) This finding is usually the result of arterial bleeding.
D) Compared to epidural hemorrhages, this finding has a better long-term prognosis for complete recovery.
E) None of the above.

Discussion 10-8

The correct answer is "A." A crescent-shaped area of hemorrhage on CT scan describes a subdural hematoma (SDH). (See Figure 10–5.) This is usually the result of tearing of bridging veins that pierce the dura after falls or direct blows to the head. Associated brain injury is common; however, skull fracture is not. Because of this association with underlying brain injury, SDH is associated with 10% to 20% mortality and long-term neurologic sequelae are more common than in EDH. SDH should raise suspicion for nonaccidental trauma in infants but is not pathognomic. Presenting symptoms include headache, seizure, vomiting, or other signs of increased intracranial

pressure. SDH also mandates emergent neurosurgical consultation; however, small or chronic SDHs often are not managed operatively.

▶ CASE 11

You are seeing a 14-year-old boy who is brought from a local swimming pool with neck pain after diving into the shallow end of the pool. He did not lose consciousness; however, he has complained of persistent neck pain and is refusing to turn his head due to pain. He is also complaining of weakness and tingling in his arms.

Question 11-1

Which of the following statements is true regarding cervical spine injury in children?

A) Cervical spine fracture is most common in children younger than 8 years old.
B) Hypoventilation and apnea are suspicious for high cervical spine injury with cord compromise.
C) Focal neurologic deficit is concerning for brain injury, but not for cervical spine injury.
D) Most cervical spine injuries occur in females.
E) None of the above are true.

Discussion 11-1

The correct answer is "B." Spinal cord injuries are uncommon in children occurring most frequently in teenage males. Cervical spine injuries result from blunt trauma and may involve the bones, ligaments, blood vessels, peripheral nerves, or spinal cord. Cervical spine fracture is rare in children younger than 8 years. This age group is more likely to injure the upper cervical spine. Common mechanisms are motor vehicle crashes, diving, sports-related injuries, and violence. Maintain a high index of suspicion for cervical spine injury in patients with neck pain, torticollis, altered mental status, focal neurologic deficits, or substantial torso injury. Apnea or hypoventilation also can be signs of high cervical spinal cord injury disrupting innervation to the diaphragm. Management of pediatric cervical spine injury involves immobilization of the cervical spine with a cervical collar. Radiologic evaluation includes plain X-rays (anterior posterior, cross-table lateral, and odontoid views) to evaluate for fracture or dislocation/subluxation. CT scan offers increased sensitivity and specificity but also increased risk due to radiation exposure. CT should be considered if clinical suspicion for cervical spine injury is high and plain films are inadequate or if plain films are suspicious for acute injury. MRI is more sensitive for spinal cord or ligamentous injuries. MRI is generally not part of emergent evaluation but is indicated for patients with persistent neurologic abnormalities.

Question 11-2

Which types of injuries discovered as part of your trauma assessment should also raise suspicion for thoracic or lumbar spinal injury?
A) Facial fracture.
B) Duodenal perforation.
C) Femoral fracture.
D) Bladder perforation.
E) None of the above.

Discussion 11-2

The correct answer is "B." Injury to the thoracic or lumbar spine is associated with small bowel or pancreatic injury, pneumothorax or hemothorax, lung contusion, aortic injury, and head injury. Compression fractures are the most prevalent, most often occurring in the lower thoracic or upper lumbar spine. They are associated with lower energy mechanisms (eg, falls and sports) involving axial loading and flexion. They are usually not associated with neurologic deficit. Burst fractures (vertebral body is smashed into fragments) are the result of axial load injury, also occurring most commonly at the thoracolumbar junction. They may be associated with neurologic deficit if significant retropulsion of fragments into the spinal canal occurs. Flexion-distraction injuries (vertebrae are pulled apart) are generally associated with more severe mechanism. They may be osseous, ligamentous, or both.

> **Helpful Tip**
>
> Children with a history of blunt trauma and neurologic findings suggestive of spinal cord injury but with normal X-rays and CT findings are described as having a spinal cord injury without radiographic abnormality (SCIWORA). A spinal cord injury may still be present and the child should have an MRI.

▶ CASE 12

A 3-month-old girl is brought to the emergency department by ambulance for evaluation of hot water burns. The child is sleepy but arousable. There are bright read burn marks from the umbilicus down with sparing of the buttocks and no splash marks above the umbilicus.

Question 12-1

The most accurate method of estimating the total body surface area involved in a burn patient is:
A) The rule of 9s.
B) Palmar surface area.
C) Lund and Browder chart.
D) All of the above are equally accurate.
E) None of the above.

Discussion 12-1

The correct answer is "C." The total body surface area (TBSA) involved can be estimated using the Wallace Rule of 9s (see Table 10–4); however, this is less accurate in young children. The surface area of a patient's palm is approximately 1% TBSA and can be used to approximate small burns. The Lund and Browder chart is a more accurate method of estimation. This chart includes a diagram of the body with the measured area of the burn adjusted for age. (See Figure 10–6.) Only partial-thickness and full-thickness burns are included in the TBSA. Superficial burns are not included. Burns involving greater than 10% TBSA require fluid resuscitation, due to increased insensible losses and systemic inflammatory response. The Parkland formula is typically used to calculate additional fluid requirements. (See Table 10–5.)

Question 12-2

For a 20-kilogram (kg) child with a 20% TBSA burn the volume of intravenous fluid required over the next 24 hours in addition to maintenance intravenous fluids is:
A) 1000 milliliters (mL).
B) 1600 mL.
C) 800 mL.
D) 1500 mL.
E) None of the above.

TABLE 10–4 WALLACE RULE OF 9s.

Body Part	% TBSA
Head	9
Anterior torso	18
Posterior torso	18
Arm	9
Leg	18
Perineum	1

TBSA, total body surface area.

The Lund-Browder burn chart

Burn estimate diagram

Age and area

Initial evaluation*

Signature

_____

Date of burn

_____

Date completed

_____

*To be completed by the admitting resident or LIP admission

☐ N/A, please refer to OPD COMPlan or 1st admission burn diagram

This is a working burn estimate diagram only. It is not as accurate as photography

CODE:
Crosshatch - 2°
Solid - 3°

Area	Birth-1 yr	1-4 yrs	5-9 yrs	10-14 yrs	15 yrs	Adult	2°	3°	Total
Head	19	17	13	11	9	7			
Neck	2	2	2	2	2	2			
Anterior trunk	13	13	13	13	13	13			
Posterior trunk	13	13	13	13	13	13			
Right buttock	2.5	2.5	2.5	2.5	2.5	2.5			
Left buttock	2.5	2.5	2.5	2.5	2.5	2.5			
Genitalia	1	1	1	1	1	1			
Right upper arm	4	4	4	4	4	4			
Left upper arm	4	4	4	4	4	4			
Right lower arm	3	3	3	3	3	3			
Left lower arm	3	3	3	3	3	3			
Right hand	2.5	2.5	2.5	2.5	2.5	2.5			
Left hand	2.5	2.5	2.5	2.5	2.5	2.5			
Right thigh	5.5	6.5	8	8.5	9	9.5			
Left thigh	5.5	6.5	8	8.5	9	9.5			
Right lower leg	5	5	5.5	6	6.5	7			
Left lower leg	5	5	5.5	6	6.5	7			
Right foot	3.5	3.5	3.5	3.5	3.5	3.5			
Left foot	3.5	3.5	3.5	3.5	3.5	3.5			

** Only 2° and 3° burns are included in the total TBSA burn percent total

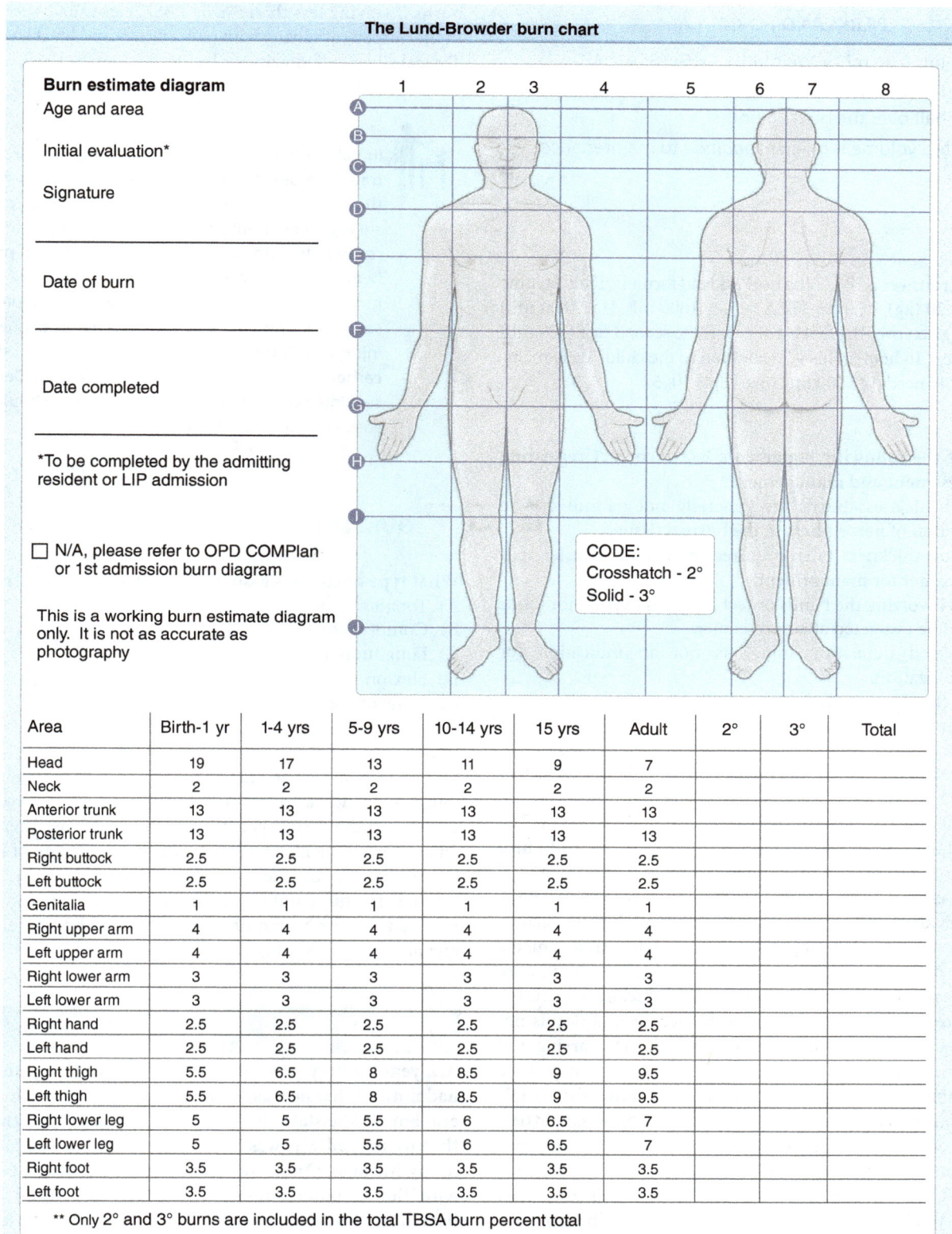

FIGURE 10–6. The Lund-Browder chart provides the best estimate of the burn extent, accounting for changes in body proportions with age. (Reproduced with permission from Goldsmith LA, Katz SI, Gilchrest BA, et al, eds. *Fitzpatrick's Dermatology in General Medicine.* 8th ed. New York, NY: McGraw-Hill Education; 2012, Fig. E95-4.1.)

TABLE 10–5 PARKLAND FORMULA

Fluid volume (in mL) = Weight (kg) × % TBSA × 4

Half of this volume is given over the first 8 hours, the second half over the next 16 hours

Calculated volume is given *in addition* to maintenance fluids

Discussion 12-2

The correct answer is "B." Using the Parkland formula, Fluid volume (in mL) = 20 (kg) × 20 (% TBSA) × 4 = 1600 mL. Half (800 mL) should be given over the first 8 hours and the second half (800 mL) over the next 16 hours. This is in addition to the child's daily maintenance fluid needs of 1500 mL. (See Table 10–5.)

Question 12-3

Which of the following statements is/are correct regarding burn assessment and management?

A) Partial-thickness burns are generally not painful due to disruption of nerve fibers in the burned tissue.

B) Any full-thickness burn requires immediate transfer to a burn center for management.

C) Burns involving the hands or feet or burns over major joints should be evaluated at a burn center.

D) Associated inhalation injury is not an indication for hospitalization.

E) All of the above are true.

Discussion 12-3

The correct answer is "C." Burns involving the hands or feet or burns over major joints should be evaluated at a burn center. Superficial or first-degree burns involve the epidermis only. The affected skin may be red or painful but can be expected to heal fully without scarring. A sunburn is an example of a superficial burn. Superficial burns are *not* used in calculations of TBSA. Partial-thickness (or second-degree) burns involve the dermis. They may involve blistering but the underlying skin remains pink and moist and is still viable. Partial-thickness burns are further classified as superficial or deep. Full-thickness burns (or third degree) involve destruction of the dermis and skin is not able to regenerate. Full thickness burns result in scarring and require skin grafting. Only in full-thickness burns may pain be absent if the nerves are affected. In the period immediately following injury it can be difficult to distinguish between partial-thickness and full-thickness burns, and the extent of injury may evolve over time. Management of burns depends on severity, extent of TBSA affected, and location. Patients with superficial or partial-thickness burns involving less than 5% TBSA or full-thickness burns involving less than 2% TBSA may be managed as outpatients. Those with partial-thickness burns involving 5% to 10% TBSA or full-thickness burns involving 2% to 5% TBSA or suspected inhalational injury should be admitted to the hospital for observation. Any burn encompassing greater than 10% TBSA or any burns to the head, genitalia, hands, or feet or burns involving joints should be referred to a burn center. Superficial burns involving less than 5% of TBSA can usually be managed in the outpatient setting with pain control and local wound care. Topical silver sulfadiazine or bacitracin may be used.

> **Helpful Tip**
> Initial assessment of burn injuries is similar to the trauma assessment outlined earlier, which follows the ABCDEs of initial stabilization and primary survey. Care should be taken during evaluation and resuscitation to minimize fluid losses and prevent hypothermia. Presence of soot around the nares, mouth, or both, or stridor/hoarse voice should raise suspicion for possible airway involvement (inhalation injury) in burns related to fires, as well as possible carbon monoxide or cyanide toxicity. Delay in seeking treatment or immersion patterns should raise suspicion for child abuse.

QUICK QUIZ

What type of stress is associated with a greenstick fracture?

A) Torsion.

B) Compression.

C) Longitudinal.

D) Flexion.

E) None of the above.

Discussion

The correct answer is "C." A greenstick fracture results when longitudinal force causes a bone to bend with disruption of one side of the cortex, generally in the diaphysis. There may be an associated buckle fracture on the opposite side of the bone. Greenstick fractures are often seen in the forearm. They are unstable fractures and require immobilization to promote healing. Reduction may require completion of the fracture to correct angulation. (See Figure 10–7.)

► CASE 13

A 2-year-old boy presents with arm pain. His grandmother had noticed that he was not using his left arm for the last several hours. She states that they were crossing the street when the boy slipped. She was holding his left hand and pulled him up by his arm. On exam the patient is holding his left arm with the shoulder adducted and internally rotated, elbow flexed, and forearm pronated. He is holding his left hand with his right hand to keep it against his abdomen. There is no swelling or ecchymosis of the elbow, forearm, or wrist. You do not elicit any bony tenderness with palpation over the distal humerus, wrist, or hand. He cries and resists when you attempt to supinate his hand. His grandmother is concerned that she may have broken his arm and wants to know if he needs X-rays.

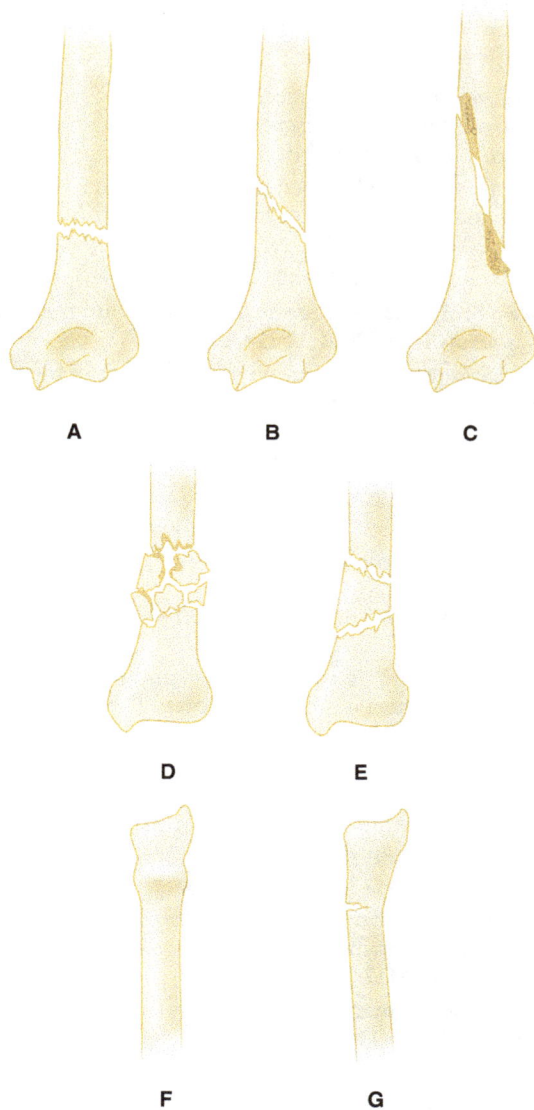

FIGURE 10–7. Fracture patterns in children: (A) Transverse, (B) oblique, (C) spiral, (D) comminuted or fragmented fracture, (E) segmental, (F) torus—buckling/compression of the cortex on one side only, and (G) greenstick—cortex fractures under tension on one side while the other side remains intact. (Reproduced with permission from Tintinalli JE, Stapczynski JS, Ma OJ, et al, eds. *Tintinalli's Emergency Medicine: A Comprehensive Study Guide*. 8th ed. New York, NY: McGraw-Hill Education; 2016, Fig. 267-2.)

Question 13-1

What is your response?

A) X-rays are not needed as clinically he has a fracture of the distal radius.
B) X-rays are needed because he won't supinate his forearm.
C) X-rays are not needed because a fracture won't be evident this early.
D) X-rays are not needed as he has a subluxed radial head.
E) X-rays should always be obtained when a child aged 2 years or younger injures an extremity.

Discussion 13-1

The correct answer is "D." The history and exam described for this patient are typical for "nursemaid's elbow," or subluxation of the radial head under the annular ligament. It is common in children up to 8 years old, with peak incidence around 2 years of age. With a consistent history and exam, as in this case, routine X-rays are not indicated. Always palpate the distal radius and obtain X-rays if you are worried about a fracture of the distal radius. Reduction should be attempted by supination of the forearm followed by flexion of the elbow and shoulder, or by hyperpronation of the forearm. You may feel a pop. After several minutes, and with distraction, the child should begin to use the arm normally again. Owing to apprehension from prior pain, the child may need prompting to move the affected arm. This can be accomplished by immobilizing the unaffected arm while offering an object of interest to the child.

> **Helpful Tip**
> Children commonly sustain fractures rather than dislocations or sprains as their ligaments are stronger than their bones.

► CASE 14

A 17-year-old adolescent boy presents with shoulder pain. He was tackled while playing rugby and fell, landing on his right shoulder. He had immediate pain over the superior aspect of his shoulder. On exam he has tenderness over the distal clavicle and acromioclavicular joint without visible deformity or crepitus. He is able to move his shoulder but complains of pain with abduction.

Question 14-1

You suspect he sustained an injury to:
A) Clavicle.
B) Acromioclavicular joint.
C) Scapula.
D) Both A and B.
E) All of the above.

Discussion 14-1

The correct answer is "D." The clavicle is the most commonly fractured bone in the shoulder region, with 90% of clavicular fractures occurring in the midshaft. Medial or lateral clavicular fractures are less common. The mechanism described in this case would be typical for both clavicular fracture and acromioclavicular (AC) separation. Given the location of tenderness on exam there is concern for lateral clavicular fracture or AC separation. AC separation refers to strain or disruption of the AC ligament, which in severe cases is accompanied by disruption of the coracoclavicular ligament. Physical exam findings include tenderness or deformity over the AC joint. Pain may be exacerbated by adducting the shoulder across the body to compress the AC joint. Plain films (X-rays) may show a widened AC joint space or elevation of the distal clavicle. Stress views obtained with the patient holding 5- to 10-pound weights in the affected arm may help to further delineate the degree of separation but are not part of routine evaluation. AC injuries are graded from I to VI according to degree of ligamentous disruption, with types I to III managed with pain control and brief immobilization in a sling for comfort. Types IV to VI may require surgical correction; however, these injuries are associated high-energy mechanisms resulting in complete disruption of both ligaments with gross deformity of the shoulder. Clavicular fractures are managed similarly, with surgical referral indicated for open fractures, or displacement of fracture causing neurovascular compromise or tenting of the skin.

Question 14-2

Which orthopedic injuries should raise suspicion for injury to vasculature or nerves?

A) Supracondylar humeral fracture.
B) Posteriorly displaced clavicular fracture.
C) Pelvic fracture.
D) Anterior shoulder dislocation.
E) All of the above.

Discussion 14-2

The correct answer is "E." Medial clavicular fractures with displacement posterior to the sternum may have laceration of subclavian vessels or injury to the recurrent laryngeal nerve. Anterior shoulder dislocations may result in injury to the axillary nerve. Fractures of the supracondylar humerus, if displaced, may also injure the median nerve and brachial artery (with medial displacement of the proximal humeral segment) and the radial nerve (with lateral displacement of the proximal fragment). The ulnar nerve is less commonly involved but may be affected with posterior displacement of the proximal humeral fragment. Supracondylar fractures as well as fractures of the tibia or fibula, or both, are at risk for compartment syndrome. Elevation of the muscle compartment pressure impairs blood flow, causing nerve and muscle injury. Remember the 6 Ps: pain (earliest), paresthesia, pallor, poikilothermia, paralysis, and pulselessness (late). Look for horrible pain despite analgesics and pain with passive muscle stretch. Dislocation of the tibia and femur at the knee is associated with injury to the popliteal artery. Careful assessment of pulses, measurement of ankle-brachial index, and duplex ultrasound are mandatory. If all are normal the patient should be admitted for serial vascular exams. If any of the preceding parameters are abnormal emergent consultation with a vascular surgeon, as well as an arteriogram and

CT angiogram, should be obtained. In children, pelvic fractures may cause injury to the pelvic vessels, but this is significantly less common than in adult patients.

BIBLIOGRAPHY

Arora R, Mahajan P. Evaluation of child with fever without source: Review of literature and update. *Pediatr Clin North Am.* 2013;60:1049–1062.

Avarello JT, Cantor RM. Pediatric major trauma: An approach to evaluation and management. *Emerg Med Clin North Am.* 2007;25:803–836.

Avner, JR. Acute fever. *Pediatr Rev.* 2009;30:5–13.

Balhara KS, Stolbach A. Marine envenomations. *Emerg Med Clin North Am.* 2014;32:223–243.

Baraff LJ. Management of fever without source in infants and children. *Ann Emerg Med.* 2000;36:602–614.

Daniels AH, Sobel AD, Eberson CP. Pediatric thoracolumbar spine trauma. *J Am Acad Orthop Surg.* 2013;21:707–716.

DeBoard RH, Rondeau DF, Kang CS, Sabbaj A, McManus JG. Principles of basic wound evaluation and management in the emergency department. *Emerg Med Clin North Am.* 2007;25:23–39.

Friday B, Depenbrock P. Land envenomations. *Curr Sports Med Rep.* 2014;13:120–125.

Jamshidi R, Sato TT. Initial assessment and management of thermal burn injuries in children. *Pediatr Rev.* 2013;34:395–404.

Kennedy SA, Stoll LE, Lauder AS. Human and other mammalian bite injuries of the hand: Evaluation and management. *J Am Acad Orthop Surg.* 2015;23:47–57.

Leonard JC: Cervical spine injury. *Pediatr Clin N Am.* 2013;60:1123-1137.

Leonard JC, Kupperman N, Olsen C, et al. Factors associated with cervical spine injury in children after blunt trauma. *Ann Emerg Med.* 2010;58(2):145–155.

Schunk JE, Schutzman A. Pediatric head injury. *Pediatr Rev.* 2012;33:398–411.

Skolnik AB, Ewald MB. Pediatric scorpion envenomation. *Pediatr Emer Care.* 2013;29:98–106.

Spiro DM, Zonfrillo MR, Meckler GD. Wounds. *Pediatr Rev.* 2010;31:326–334.

Steere M, Sharieff GQ, Stenklyft PH. Fever in children less than 36 months of age—questions and strategies for management in the emergency department. *J Emerg Med.* 2003;25:149–157.

Wing R, Dor MR, McQuilkin PA. Fever in the pediatric patient *Emerg Med Clin North Am.* 2013;31:1073–1096.

Endocrine Disorders

11

Vanessa Curtis

▶ CASE 1

An infant is born at 39 weeks' gestation to a healthy Gravida 1 now Para 1 Caucasian woman. Pregnancy and delivery were uncomplicated. On newborn exam, the neonate is noted to have ambiguous genitalia with a 1.5 cm phallic structure, no palpable testicles, and pigmented labial scrotal folds.

Question 1-1
Which of the following is the most appropriate first step?
A) Confirm that electrolytes are normal and then discharge the infant with outpatient follow-up by endocrinology.
B) Obtain karyotyping and then discharge the infant with outpatient follow-up by endocrinology.
C) Order a pelvic ultrasound; obtain 17-hydroxyprogesterone, luteinizing hormone, and testosterone levels; obtain karyotyping; and arrange for an inpatient endocrine consult.
D) Reassure the family that they can let the child choose its sex when older and advise a gender-neutral name such as Pat.
E) Consult the urology service and arrange for cosmetic genital surgery as soon as possible.

Discussion 1-1
The correct answer is "C." In early fetal development, both XX and XY fetuses are undifferentiated in terms of reproductive structures. In normal sexual differentiation, the bipotential gonad differentiates beginning around 7 weeks' gestational age into a testicle or ovary based on multiple genes. If the gonads become testicles, they secrete müllerian-inhibiting substance, causing the müllerian ducts to regress, and they secrete testosterone, causing the wolffian ducts to persist (which develop into the epididymis, vas deferens, and seminal vesicles). If the gonads become ovaries, the lack of müllerian-inhibiting substance allows the müllerian structures to persist (which become the oviducts, uterus, cervix, and upper vagina), and the lack of testosterone results in wolffian duct regression. The external genitalia respond to testosterone, which is converted peripherally into the more potent dihydrotestosterone, with posterior fusion of the genital folds and growth of the genital tubercle into

a phallic structure. (See Figure 11–1.) In this infant, physical exam alone cannot tell you whether it is an undervirilized male or an overvirilized female; however, the most immediately dangerous diagnosis in the differential is that the infant is a virilized female as a result of congenital adrenal hyperplasia (CAH). In female infants with classic 21-hydroxlyase deficiency CAH, excess adrenal androgen during gestation can cause ambiguous genitalia with clitoral enlargement, a urogenital sinus, and fusion of the labial folds. The internal reproductive organs are normal. In male infants with 21-hydroxlyase deficiency, genitalia are typically normal, though these infants are at risk for salt-wasting crisis. Neonates with CAH are at risk for adrenal crisis because of their inability to make cortisol and aldosterone. (See Figure 11–2.) They may be identified on newborn screen or based on ambiguous genitalia. An infant suspected of CAH should be monitored closely until the diagnosis is evident.

The infant is found to have a markedly elevated 17-hydroxyprogesterone (17-OH-P), 46,XX karyotype, müllerian structures on pelvic ultrasound, and normal luteinizing hormone (LH), testosterone, and estrogen levels, confirming a diagnosis of CAH. The team discusses results with the family and advises that the child was meant to be a female.

Question 1-2
The infant will likely require all of the following medical therapies EXCEPT:
A) Oral hydrocortisone.
B) Oral fludrocortisone.
C) Estrogen.
D) Injectable hydrocortisone for illness or stress.
E) Salt supplementation.

Discussion 1-2
The correct answer is "C." Infants with classic salt-wasting 21-hydroxylase CAH require glucocorticoid supplementation with hydrocortisone, with a goal of replacing the cortisol deficiency and also suppressing the overactive hypothalamic-pituitary axis (HPA) and preventing further androgen excess. Infants also

219

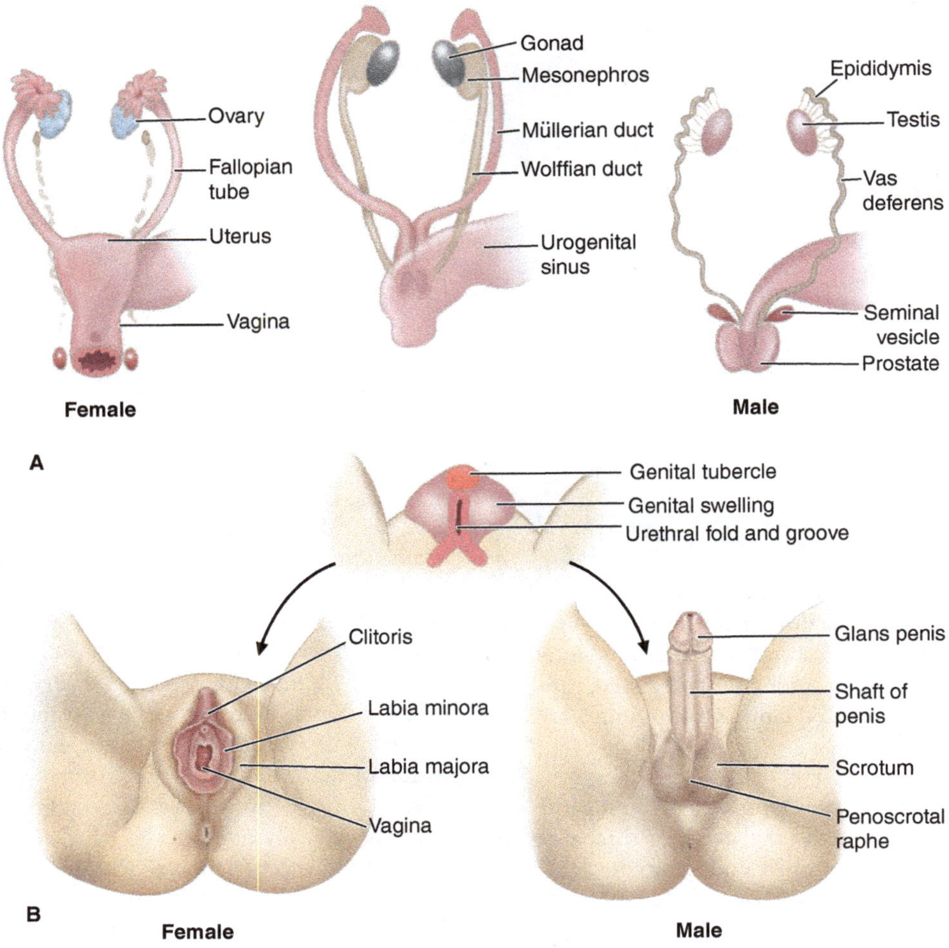

FIGURE 11–1. Sexual Development. Development of the male and female internal and external urogenital tracts. (Reproduced with permission from Braunwald E et al: *Harrison's Principles of Internal Medicine*, 15th ed. New York: McGraw-Hill; 2001.)

require mineralocorticoid supplementation with fludrocortisone to maintain appropriate serum sodium and potassium and blood pressure. Finally, owing to the low salt content in an infant diet, newborns often require a supplemental salt solution until they are eating more table foods. For any patient who is cortisol-dependent, additional therapy is needed when ill. Typically this includes tripling the hydrocortisone dose for high fevers or other significant illness. Patients are also taught to administer intramuscular (IM) hydrocortisone if illness prevents oral intake.

> **Helpful Tip**
> If a child with CAH (or any child who requires cortisol replacement) presents with severe illness and inability to take things by mouth, do not hesitate to administer parenteral hydrocortisone at a dose of 100 mg/m². This works out to:
> - 25 mg hydrocortisone IV/IM for a small child or infant
> - 50 mg hydrocortisone IV/IM for a medium-sized child
> - 100 mg hydrocortisone IV/IM for a large child.
>
> When in doubt, give more.

The family is planning on having more children in the future.

Question 1-3
Which of the following is an accurate statement to help the family as they consider future pregnancies:
A) There is a 1% chance of having another child affected with CAH.
B) Mothers can be treated prenatally with dexamethasone to reduce the virilization of female fetuses with CAH.
C) Fathers can be treated preconception with prednisone to reduce the virilization of female fetuses with CAH.
D) There is a 12.5% chance of having another child affected with CAH.
E) With the rising cost of college these days, discourage another pregnancy.

Discussion 1-3
The correct answer is "B." 21-Hydroxylase deficiency is an autosomal recessive condition (like many enzyme deficiencies—hint, hint), and thus the chance of having another affected

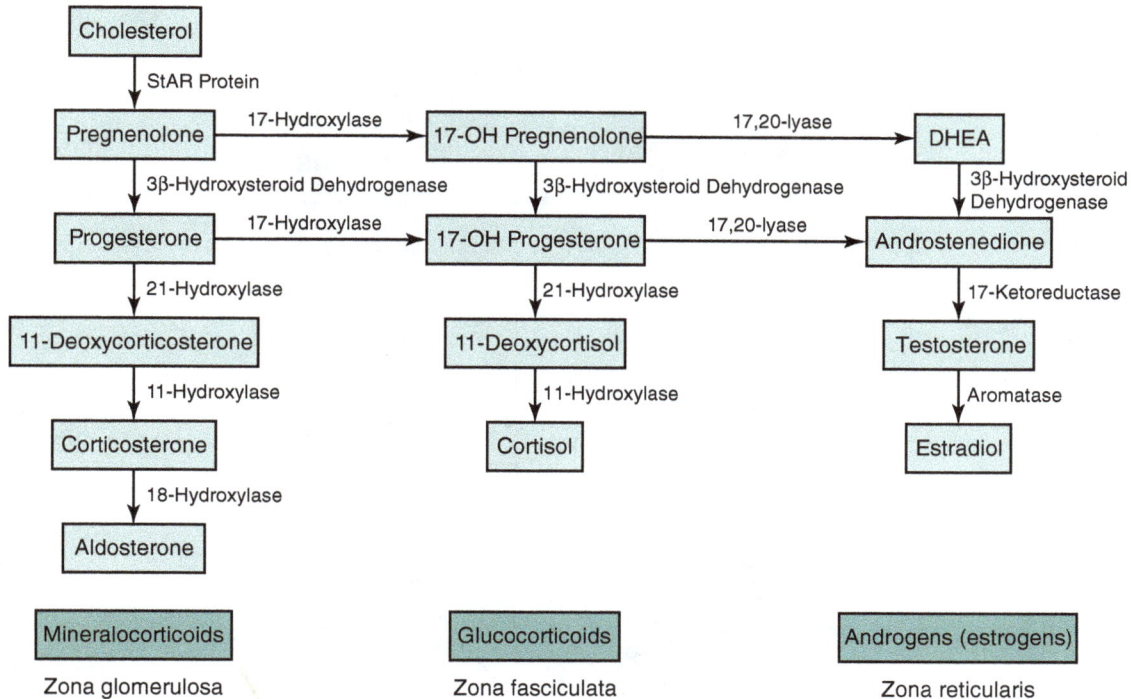

FIGURE 11–2. Steroid Pathway. Synthesis of endogenous steroids: mineralocorticoids, glucocorticoids, and sex steroids. DHEA, Dehydroepiandrosterone. (Reproduced with permission from Hay WW, Levin MJ, Deterding RR, Abzug MJ, eds. *Current Diagnosis and Treatment Pediatrics*. 22th ed. New York, NY: McGraw-Hill Education; 2014, Fig. 34-8.)

child would be 1 in 4 (25%). Mothers can be treated prenatally with dexamethasone, which suppresses fetal pituitary adrenocorticotropic hormone (ACTH), causing less overproduction of adrenal androgen, and theoretically reduces virilization in female fetuses. The treatment must be done very early in the pregnancy (prior to knowing if the fetus is affected by CAH or the fetal sex) and can have adverse effects on both the fetus and mother, and thus is not considered standard of care.

► CASE 2

A 16-year-old adolescent girl presents with primary amenorrhea. She has had excellent growth and is several inches taller than her older sisters. She has Tanner 3 breasts and scant pubic hair. Her clitoris is prominent. Workup reveals a 46,XY karyotype, pubertal LH levels, and markedly elevated testosterone level for a female.

Question 2-1

This presentation is consistent with which of the following syndromes?
A) Klinefelter syndrome.
B) Turner syndrome.
C) Androgen insensitivity syndrome.
D) Trisomy 21.
E) Mayer-Rokitansky-Küster-Hauser syndrome.
F) Curtis-Peterson syndrome.

Discussion 2-1

The correct answer is "C." Disorders of androgen action are a common form of 46,XY disorders of sexual development and occur when the internal genitalia and gonads and testosterone levels are consistent with 46,XY (male) but there is insensitivity at the level of the androgen receptor. These patients have a variable phenotype ranging from a phenotypic woman with no pubarche (complete androgen insensitivity syndrome) to an undervirilized male to a phenotypic man to isolated infertility (partial androgen insensitivity syndrome).

Helpful Tip
(But really a fun fact.) Complete androgen insensitivity syndrome is overrepresented in elite female athletes and fashion models. Think about it.

► CASE 3

A 10-year-old boy presents for his well-child check. His mother raises concern that he has started youth soccer and is doing well but seems so much shorter than his peers. He has no chronic medical conditions and is not taking any medications. Review of his growth charts shows that he was born at term and was average for gestational age (AGA). He has been at the fifth percentile since his first birthday for both height and weight. His growth velocity has been 6 cm/y for the past year.

2 to 20 years: Boys
Stature-for-age and Weight-for-age percentiles

NAME _____Alfred_____

RECORD # _____

Mother's Stature	5' 0"	Father's Stature	5' 5"	
Date	Age	Weight	Stature	BMI*
3/4/05	2 weeks	7 lb 9 oz		

*To Calculate BMI: Weight (kg) ÷ Stature (cm) ÷ Stature (cm) x 10,000
or Weight (lb) ÷ Stature (in) ÷ Stature (in) x 703

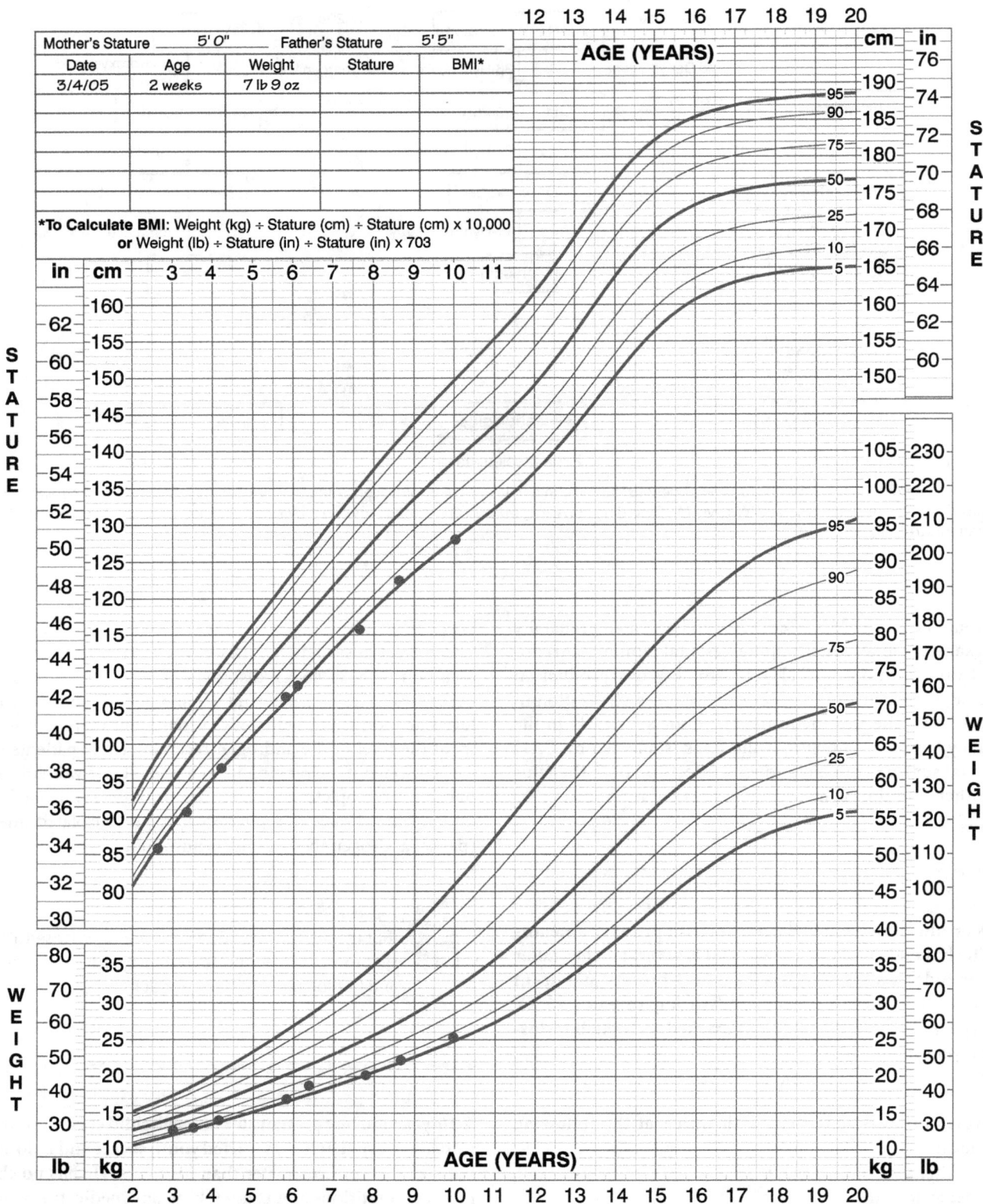

AGE (YEARS)

STATURE

WEIGHT

Published May 30, 2000 (modified 11/21/00).
Reproduced with permission from the National Center for Health Statistics in collaboration
with the National Center for Chronic Disease Prevention and Health Promotion (2000).
http://www.cdc.gov/growthcharts.

CDC
SAFER · HEALTHIER · PEOPLE™

Question 3-1

Which of the following is most likely to reveal his diagnosis?

A) A growth hormone stimulation test.
B) Karyotype.
C) Parents' pubertal timing.
D) Mother's and father's heights.
E) Mother's height and the milkman's height.

Discussion 3-1

The correct answer is "D." In this case, if the parents are short, the child needs no further workup since he has a normal growth rate (5 cm/y) and is otherwise healthy. Parental heights are important pieces of evidence when considering a child with short stature. Short parents have short children. (See following growth curve.) Children with familial short stature are born AGA and should track along an appropriate growth curve at a normal growth *rate*. They typically have a normal

bone age and normal growth hormone secretion. To calculate a midparental height, you must first consider if the child is male or female. If the child is male, add 5 inches (13 cm) to the mother's height and then average with the father's height. If the child is female, subtract 5 inches (13 cm) from the father's height and average with the mother's height.

▶ CASE 4

A 15-year-old adolescent boy presents for his well-child check. His mother raises concern that he seems to be growing poorly, and there is a widening discrepancy between his height and that of his peers. On review of his growth charts you note that, indeed, he was previously at the 15th percentile but since age 13 years his height percentile has gradually declined and is currently at the 3rd percentile. See following growth curve.

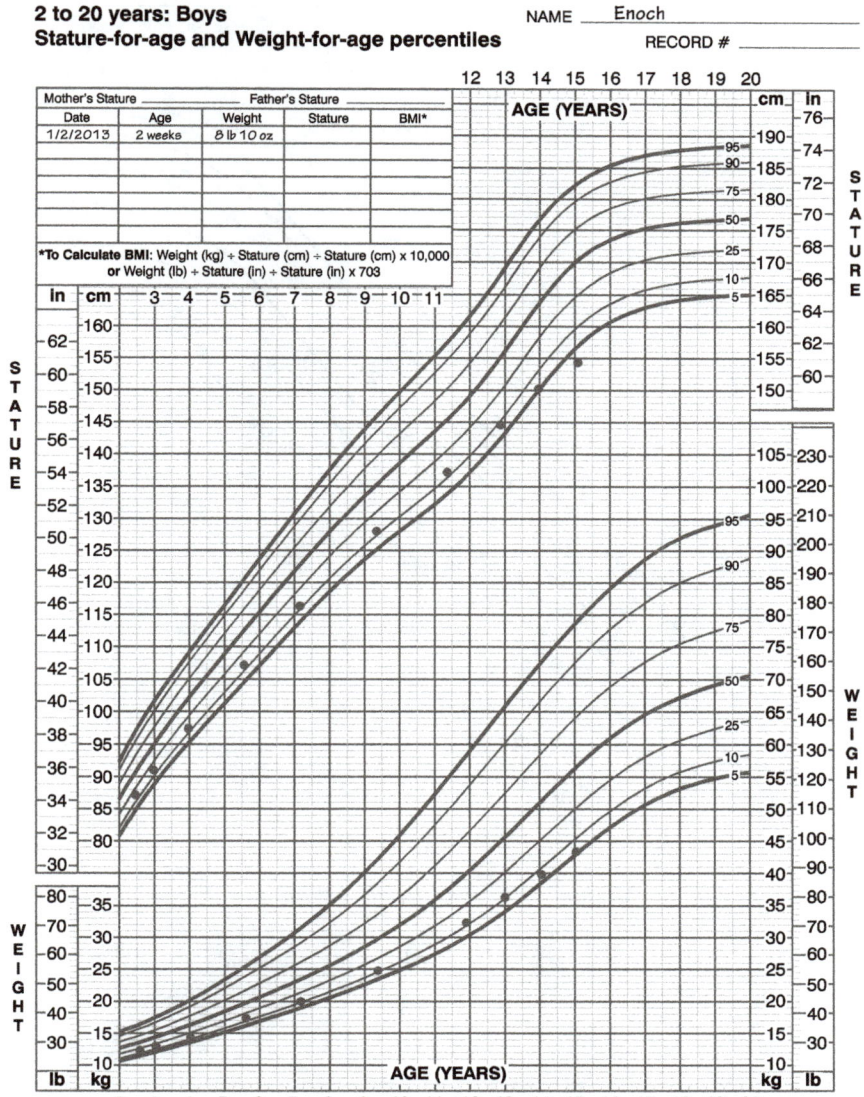

2 to 20 years: Boys
Stature-for-age and Weight-for-age percentiles
NAME Enoch
RECORD #

Published May 30, 2000 (modified 11/21/00).
Reproduced with permission from the National Center for Health Statistics in collaboration
with the National Center for Chronic Disease Prevention and Health Promotion (2000).
http://www.cdc.gov/growthcharts.

Weight has been appropriate for height. He will be a freshman next month and would rather go out for football than cross-country, but his parents are worried that he may be injured because of his small size.

Question 4-1

Which of the following would be a reassuring finding on history and physical exam with regard to his prognosis?

A) Mother and father are both tall.
B) Mother had menarche at age 11 years.
C) Father was shaving by the time he started high school.
D) He has Tanner 3 pubic hair and testicles are 10 mL.
E) He has Tanner 1 pubic hair and testicles are 4 mL.

Discussion 4-1

The correct answer is "E." Constitutional delay of growth and puberty (CDGP) is a common cause of short stature. Known collectively as "late bloomers," children with CDGP are of normal size at birth; however, a downward shift in growth rate during the first 2 years of life results in a childhood height that is lower than expected for genetic potential. The child then remains with a normal growth rate during childhood but has late entry into puberty. During the time when the child is growing at a prepubertal growth rate and friends are starting their pubertal growth spurt, the child experiences an increased height discrepancy between his or her height and that of peers and downward crossing of percentiles. The child eventually does enter puberty, exhibits catch-up growth, and achieves appropriate height for their family. (See Figure 11–3.)

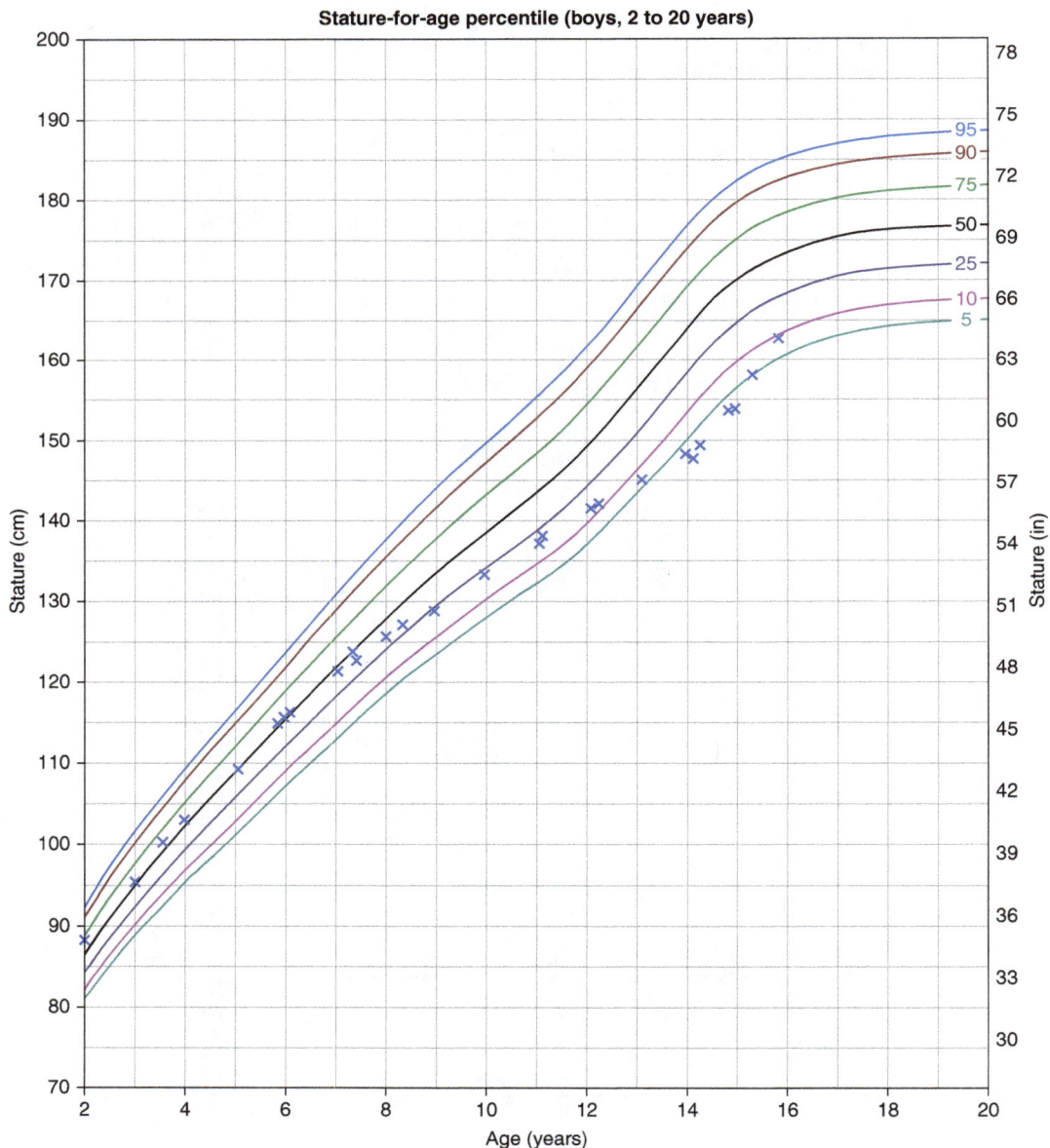

FIGURE 11–3. This boy has constitutional delay of growth and puberty. (Reproduced with permission from Centers for Disease Control and Prevention (CDC).)

In evaluating the adolescent in this case, CDGP would be suspected if there is a family history of late bloomers (eg, mother had late menarche or father was still growing after high school) and the adolescent is prepubertal on physical exam.

....

Based on history and physical exam, a diagnosis of CDGP is suspected. The family is still concerned and hoping for some further testing to confirm this suspicion.

Question 4-2

Appropriate workup may include which of the following?
A) Thyroid-stimulating hormone (TSH) and free thyroxine (T_4).
B) Insulin-like growth factor-1 (IGF-1).
C) Luteinizing hormone (LH), follicle-stimulating hormone (FSH), and testosterone.
D) Bone age X-ray.
E) Watchful waiting.
F) All of the above.

Discussion 4-1

The correct answer is "F." If the history is supportive, watchful waiting may be all that is necessary. Though nonspecific, a delayed bone age would be reassuring; a delayed bone age predicts that growth is expected to continue longer than normal allowing catch-up growth. If the history and physical exam are not supportive of CDGP, you may want to consider screening for thyroid disease (TSH and free T4), growth hormone deficiency (IGF-1) and for other causes of delayed puberty (LH, FSH, testosterone).

▶ CASE 5

A 12-year-old adolescent girl presents for her well-child check. Her family does not have any concerns. She has previously been healthy and is not taking any medications. On review of her growth charts, she is currently at the 5th percentile; however, she was previously growing along the 50th percentile until 2 to 3 years ago. See following growth curve.

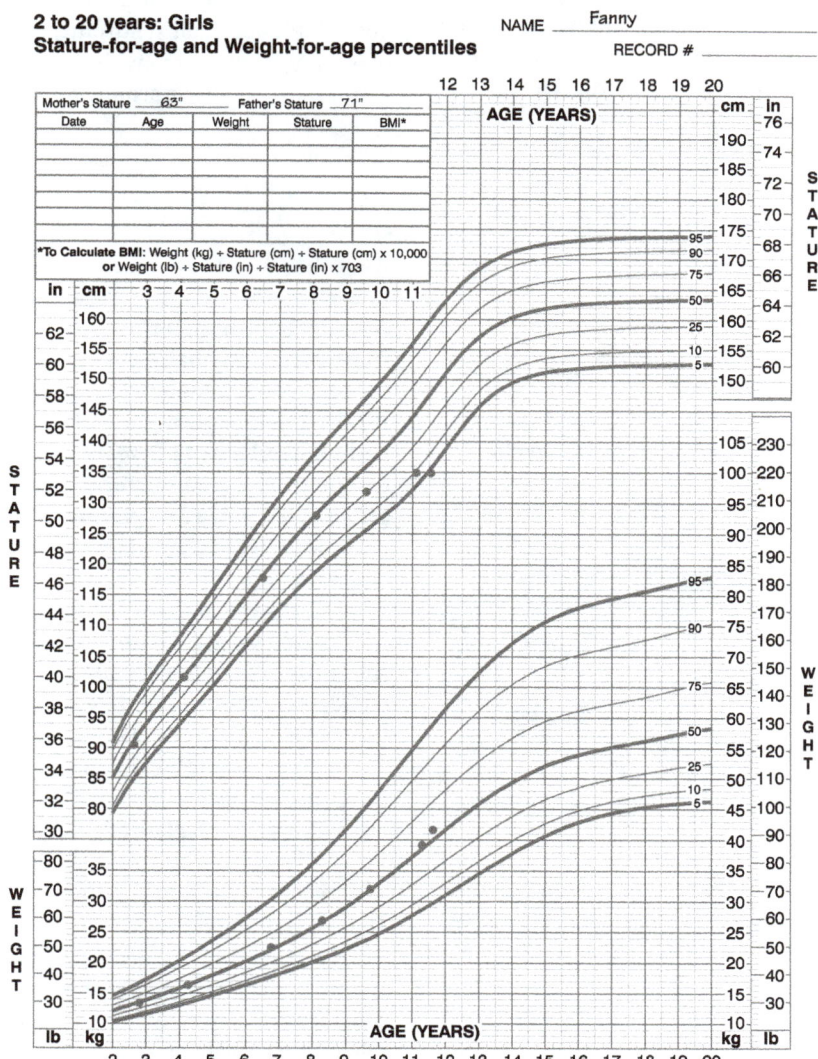

Her weight has continued to track along the 50th percentile. Mother is 5 feet, 3 inches tall and father is 5 feet, 11 inches.

Question 5-1

Appropriate workup may include which of the following?

A) TSH and free T_4.

B) IGF-1.

C) Bone age X-ray.

D) Growth hormone level.

E) Options A, B, and C.

F) No workup is necessary since she is not below the 5th percentile.

Discussion 5-1

The correct answer is "E." This child is not pathologically short (height is at the 5th percentile); however, her slow growth velocity and downward crossing of height percentiles is concerning and must be evaluated. Furthermore, her family is not short (midparental target height is 5 feet, 4.5 inches, which is approximately the 50th percentile), which is another red flag for her. In a child with growth deceleration or growth failure, endocrine causes must be considered such as hypothyroidism, growth hormone (GH) deficiency, and cortisol excess. Appropriate screening lab tests for hypothyroidism include TSH and free T_4. IGF-1 with or without IGF-binding protein 3 (BP3) are appropriate screening tests to assess for GH deficiency. A random GH level would not be helpful. Finally, a bone age is nonspecific but can provide further information about height potential.

> **Helpful Tip**
>
> If IGF-1 and IGF-BP3 are low, this raises concern for growth hormone deficiency (GHD) but is not diagnostic. To diagnose GHD, children must undergo provocative growth hormone testing, which is typically done by a pediatric endocrinologist.

▶ CASE 6

A 6-year-old girl is brought in by her parents to evaluate for tall stature. She recently had her kindergarten winter concert, and her family noted that she was a head taller than her peers and had to stand in the back row (with the naughty boys). She has no significant past medical history and no concerns on review of systems. Her height is at the 97th percentile. Her weight is at the 99th percentile.

Question 6-1

Differential diagnosis includes all of the following EXCEPT:

A) Growth hormone excess.

B) Precocious puberty.

C) Familial tall stature.

D) Overnutrition.

E) Prader-Willi syndrome.

F) Hyperthyroidism.

Discussion 6-1

The correct answer is "E." Tall stature can simply be related to genetics (familial tall stature). Calculate a midparental height to consider whether this is the case. Children with simple familial tall stature should have a growth rate at the upper end of normal, a normal bone age, and no dysmorphic features. If the family is not tall, then it is appropriate to consider pathologic causes of the tall stature. Hormones that promote linear growth include growth hormone, sex steroids, and thyroid hormone. Growth hormone excess is very rare in children but can result in extreme tall stature. Children with precocious puberty experience their pubertal growth spurt early, resulting in a period of tall stature. They ultimately do not end up tall for their family, however, as they will have premature epiphyseal closure (advanced bone age). Excess thyroid hormone also leads to increased linear growth with early epiphyseal closure, resulting in ultimate normal or short stature. Overnutrition or exogenous obesity also drives linear growth, resulting in modest overgrowth in childhood, and is a common cause of tall stature in children. As with precocious puberty and hyperthyroidism, this is associated with increased skeletal maturation resulting in a final height that is *not* tall. Prader-Willi syndrome, as with most endocrine causes of obesity, is associated with short stature. Look for small hands with Prader-Willi syndrome.

▶ CASE 7

A mother makes an urgent visit for her 9-year-old daughter to evaluate breasts that she noticed the other day when they were trying on swimsuits for a family vacation. Mother is frantic that "my baby is developing too early!" She is hopeful that you can determine what is wrong and put a stop to it ASAP. While taking the history, you learn that the mother had menarche at 11.5 years of age. On physical exam of the daughter, you find bilateral breast buds, some long straight pubic hairs, and a few pimples.

Question 7-1

What is the most appropriate course of action?

A) Consult surgery to remove the breast buds.

B) Order lab tests to include LH, FSH, and estradiol.

C) Reassure the mother that this is normal.

D) Order a magnetic resonance imaging (MRI) scan of the brain to determine the cause of central puberty.

E) Order lab tests to include 17-OH-progesterone, dehydroepiandrosterone sulfate (DHEA-S), and androstenedione.

Discussion 7-1

The correct answer is "C." Typical female puberty is first heralded by breast budding and starts at 10 years of age; however, any time after 8 years of age can be normal. It is important to consider the family history, race or ethnicity, and any medical conditions when assessing an individual child. In this case, she is older than 8 years old. Her mother had menarche at 11.5 years, which suggests that she was a slightly early bloomer as well. Furthermore, the girl has early Tanner 2 pubic hair, which is also consistent. We can expect that she will have another 2+ years before menarche, which is often the parent's main concern. Males have a later initiation of puberty, with testicular enlargement starting around 12 years of age. Males should be evaluated for pathologic precocious puberty if they demonstrate any signs of virilization prior to 9 years of age. It is important to become comfortable with the Tanner stages and the normal timing and tempo. (See Figures 11–4 and 11–5.) If the child was younger than 8 years of age, part of the workup would likely include gonadotropins (LH, FSH) and estradiol. If the child was found to have central precocious puberty (elevated LH, FSH), a brain MRI would be indicated. If the child demonstrated signs of androgen (as opposed to estrogen), you would consider checking the adrenal studies mentioned in option "E."

> **Helpful Tip**
> **Rule of 2s**
> - Normal female puberty is 10 years ± *2 years*
> - The time from thelarche to menarche is a little over *2 years*
> - Boys are about *2 years* behind girls

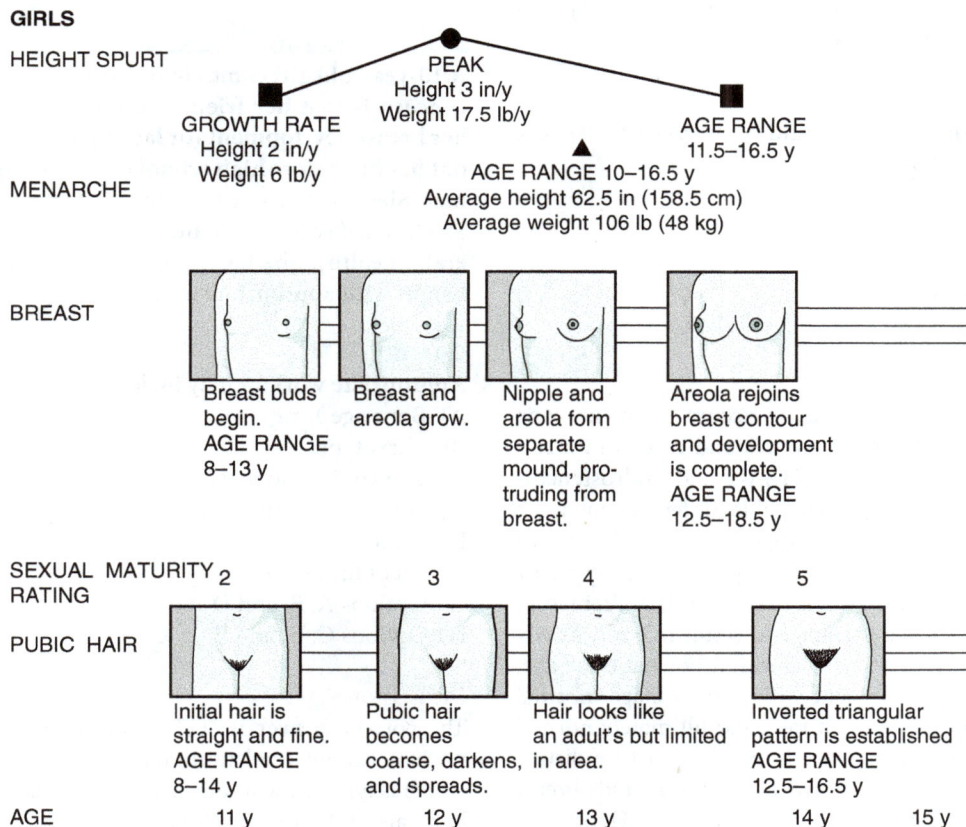

⏳ **QUICK QUIZ**

At what age is puberty (thelarche onset) considered precocious in girls?

A) 7.
B) 9.
C) 11.
D) 13.
E) 15.

Discussion

The correct answer is "A." Onset of puberty before age 8 years in girls and 9 years in boys is considered precocious.

▶ **CASE 8**

An 8-year-old girl is referred by her second-grade teacher for body odor. (We are talking teenage boy hockey locker-room quality!) On history, you learn that she has had gradually progressive pubic hair for the past 2 years. She has had some mild acne, which is controlled with over-the-counter preparations. She denies breast changes or menstrual bleeding. Her mother had menarche at 13 years of age; her father just blushes and

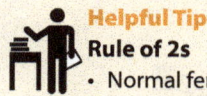

GIRLS

HEIGHT SPURT — PEAK / Height 3 in/y / Weight 17.5 lb/y
GROWTH RATE / Height 2 in/y / Weight 6 lb/y
AGE RANGE / 11.5–16.5 y
AGE RANGE 10–16.5 y / Average height 62.5 in (158.5 cm) / Average weight 106 lb (48 kg)

MENARCHE

BREAST
- Breast buds begin. AGE RANGE 8–13 y
- Breast and areola grow.
- Nipple and areola form separate mound, protruding from breast.
- Areola rejoins breast contour and development is complete. AGE RANGE 12.5–18.5 y

SEXUAL MATURITY RATING   2   3   4   5

PUBIC HAIR
- Initial hair is straight and fine. AGE RANGE 8–14 y
- Pubic hair becomes coarse, darkens, and spreads.
- Hair looks like an adult's but limited in area.
- Inverted triangular pattern is established AGE RANGE 12.5–16.5 y

AGE   11 y   12 y   13 y   14 y   15 y

FIGURE 11–4. The Tanner stages of female breast and pubic hair development. (Reproduced with permission from Hay WW, Levin MJ, Deterding RR, Abzug MJ, eds. *Current Diagnosis and Treatment Pediatrics.* 22th ed. New York, NY: McGraw-Hill Education; 2014, Fig. 4-4.)

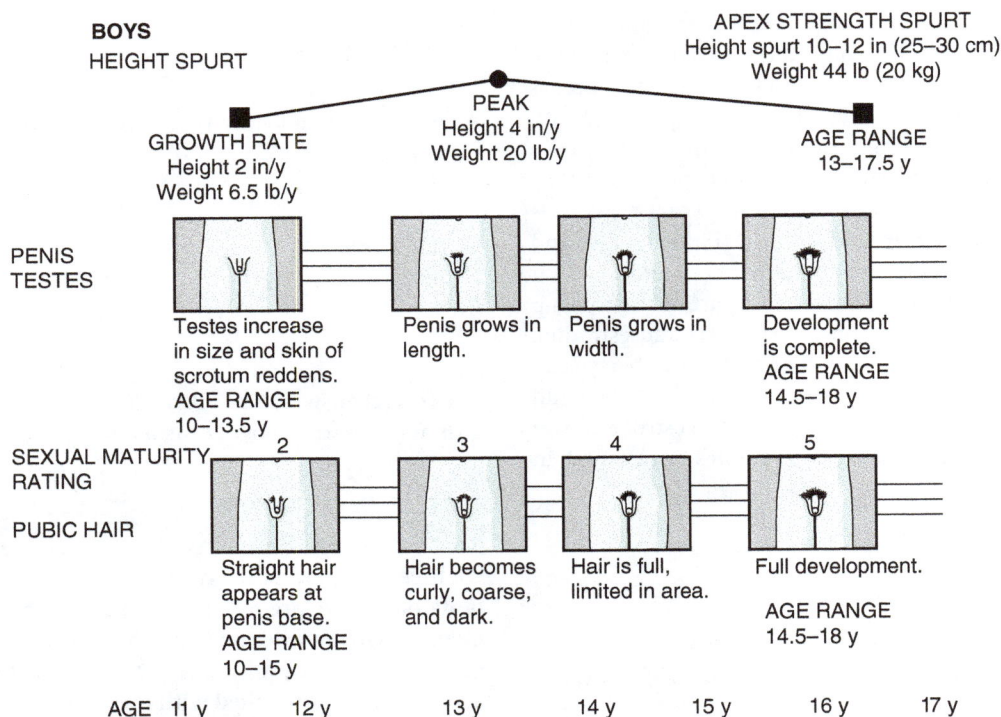

FIGURE 11–5. The Tanner stages of male genital and pubic hair development. (Reproduced with permission from Hay WW, Levin MJ, Deterding RR, Abzug MJ, eds. *Current Diagnosis and Treatment Pediatrics*. 22th ed. New York, NY: McGraw-Hill Education; 2014, Fig 4-3.)

stares at you blankly when you ask about his puberty. On exam, you find Tanner 3 pubic hair.

Question 8-1

Which of the following features would be the most reassuring on your exam and workup?
A) Clitoromegaly.
B) Bone age of 8 years.
C) Bone age of 11 years.
D) Elevated testosterone level.
E) Tanner 4 breasts.

Discussion 8-1

The correct answer is "B." Adrenarche occurs when the zona reticularis of the adrenal cortex matures and results in a rise in adrenal androgens, including DHEA-S and androstenedione. The adrenal androgens are responsible for female pubarche (sexual hair), body odor, and acne. (See Figure 11–2, earlier.) Adrenarche is separate from true central puberty and typically manifests after thelarche; however, it *can* occur first. Premature adrenarche can be a normal variant and result in early, slowly progressive pubarche. It is associated with a normal bone age, adrenal androgen levels consistent with Tanner stage, normal testosterone levels, normal growth rate, and ultimately normal true puberty. "Benign" premature adrenarche must be distinguished from precocious puberty (which would include breast development and advanced bone age), late-onset CAH, or virilizing tumors (both of which would result in virilization/clitoromegaly and advanced bone age).

► CASE 9

A 13-year-old girl comes in for her well-child check. Her only concern is that her friends call her "Flat Stanley" based on her breast development (or lack thereof). She is hoping to fill out her bra before high school cheerleading tryouts this summer. She was born at term with a birth weight of 5 pounds. She has had recurrent acute otitis media but otherwise is generally healthy. She has grown along the third percentile for height with appropriate weight gain.

Question 9-1

Appropriate workup may include which of the following?
A) Bone age X-ray.
B) Karyotype.
C) Growth hormone level.
D) Good family history of heights and pubertal timing.
E) Insulin level.
F) All of the above.
G) Options A, B, and D.
H) Options C, D, and E.

Discussion 9-1

The correct answer is "G." Delayed female puberty can be a normal variant (constitutional delay of growth and puberty) which is typically a familial trait and is associated with a delayed bone age. If there is no family history of delayed puberty or if a girl does not have any signs of breast tissue by 13 years, it is important to consider other causes of delayed puberty. These include hypogonadotropic hypogonadism, which can be functional (due to chronic disease, eating disorders, or high energy expenditure) or pathologic due to a true/permanent gonadotropin-releasing hormone (GnRH) deficiency (ie, Kallmann syndrome). Differential diagnosis of delayed puberty in females also includes hypergonadotropic hypogonadism (ovarian insufficiency), of which the most common cause is Turner syndrome (45,XO karyotype).

> **Helpful Tip**
>
> In addition to delayed puberty, other features of Turner syndrome include short stature (20 cm shorter than midparental height), widely spaced nipples, webbed neck, cubitus valgus, bicuspid aortic valve or aortic coarctation, horseshoe kidney, recurrent otitis media, and high risk of autoimmune disease. (See Figure 11–6.)

⧗ QUICK QUIZ

At what age is puberty (no testicle enlargement) considered delayed in boys?
A) 10.
B) 12.
C) 14.

D) 16.
E) 18.

Discussion

The correct answer is "C." Lack of pubertal changes (in girls, breast buds; in boys, testicular enlargement) by age 12 years in girls and 14 years in boys is considered delayed puberty.

▶ CASE 10

A 14-year-old adolescent girl was seen in her local acute care clinic for an ear infection and was noted to have thyromegaly. She was referred to your clinic for further evaluation. She reports some fatigue and cold intolerance, but admits that it is winter and she has been staying up late texting with her boyfriend. On exam, she has a thyroid that is twice normal size with no discrete nodules. Thyroid function tests show elevated TSH of 25 μIU/mL and mildly low free T_4 of 0.7 ng/dL.

Question 10-1

The most likely cause of her hypothyroidism is:
A) Iodine deficiency.
B) Thyroid cancer.
C) Autoimmune (Hashimoto) thyroiditis.
D) Radiation exposure.
E) Congenital hypothyroidism.

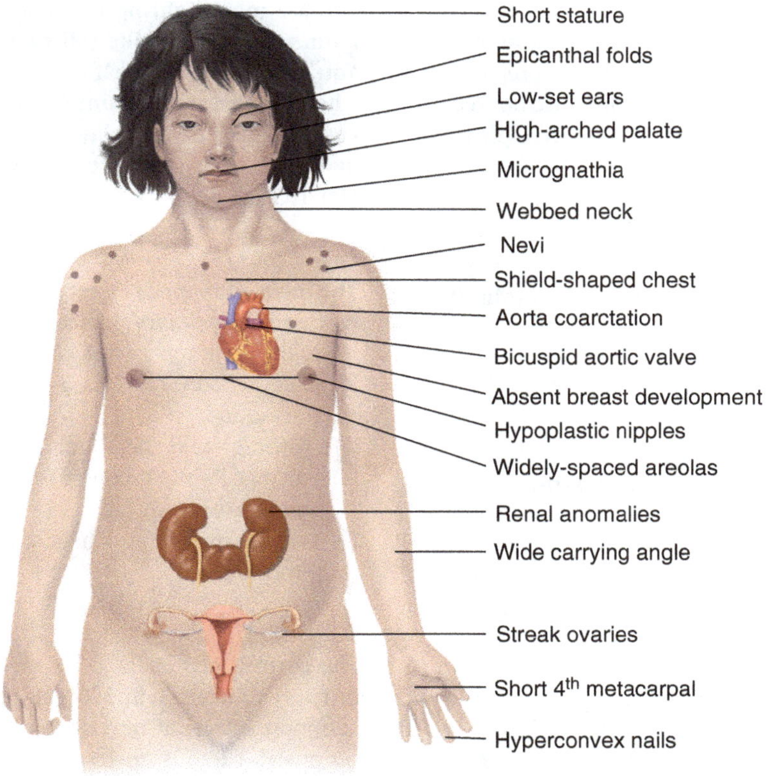

FIGURE 11–6. Features of Turner syndrome (45,XO). (Reproduced with permission from Hoffman BL, Schorge JO, Schaffer JI, et al, eds. *Williams Gynecology*. 2nd ed. New York, NY: McGraw-Hill Education; 2012, Fig. 18-8.)

Discussion 10-1

The correct answer is "C." Acquired hypothyroidism in the United States is most often caused by autoimmune thyroiditis, also known as Hashimoto thyroiditis. Iodine deficiency is the most common cause of hypothyroidism worldwide but is uncommon in North America because of iodine supplementation of salt. Thyroid cancer does not typically affect thyroid function. Children who are treated with radiation for tumors of the head and neck are at higher risk of hypothyroidism; this would be considered based on the history. Congenital hypothyroidism is possible but would typically present before this age. Common symptoms of hypothyroidism in children include fatigue, cold intolerance, constipation, dry skin, and brittle hair. Signs of hypothyroidism include growth deceleration, bradycardia, facial puffiness, and delayed relaxation phase of deep tendon reflexes. There may be a small amount of weight gain (2–4 kg), although this is not typically severe.

Question 10-2

What is the most appropriate treatment for this patient?
A) Synthetic triiodothyronine (T_3).
B) Synthetic T_4.
C) Pork or beef desiccated thyroid.
D) Nothing until her free T_4 decreases further.
E) Synthetic TSH.

Discussion 10-2

The correct answer is "B." Synthetic T_4 (levothyroxine) is the treatment of choice for children with hypothyroidism and is typically started if the TSH is greater than 7 to 10 µIU/mL. With appropriate treatment, children should be expected to resume normal growth and development. Thyroid preparations that contain T_3 alone (liothyronine) or in combination preparations that are made or derived from desiccated glands are not recommended for routine treatment of pediatric hypothyroidism.

⧗ QUICK QUIZ

Which laboratory value is not typical of autoimmune thyroiditis (Hashimoto thyroiditis)?
A) Elevated TSH.
B) Low free T_4.
C) Elevated thyroid peroxidase antibodies.
D) Elevated thyroglobulin antibodies.
E) Elevated thyroid-stimulating immunoglobulins.

Discussion

The correct answer is "E." Thyroid-stimulating immunoglobulins or TSH receptor antibodies are typically seen in Graves disease, which causes hyperthyroidism.

▶ CASE 11

A 15-year-old adolescent boy comes in for his sports physical. He has no concerns whatsoever. He has no significant past medical history and takes no medications. On exam, he is at the 80th percentile for height and weight and is approaching the end of puberty. The only abnormality is thyroid gland asymmetry; he has an approximately 1 × 2 cm firm nodule on the left upper lobe that you can palpate. Lab tests in clinic show a normal TSH.

Question 11-1

What is the most appropriate next step?
A) Reassurance.
B) Obtain a free T_4 level.
C) Order neck/thyroid ultrasound.
D) Follow up in 6 months for repeat thyroid exam.
E) Obtain thyroid peroxidase antibody titer.

Discussion 11-1

The correct answer is "C." Thyroid nodules may be caused by benign conditions, including multinodular goiter, autoimmune (Hashimoto) thyroiditis, simple cysts, or adenomas. However, children presenting with thyroid nodules are more likely to have cancer than adults, and carcinoma needs to be ruled out. It is helpful to start with a TSH level to assess thyroid function. Most children presenting with a thyroid nodule have normal function and will need to then undergo neck/thyroid ultrasound to further characterize the lesion and determine if fine needle aspiration is necessary.

▶ CASE 12

You are moonlighting in the local newborn nursery to earn money for a new bike (all carbon and electronic shifting). You are patting yourself on the back for finding this easy gig when you get a call from the state lab saying that an infant you discharged yesterday has been found to have an abnormal newborn thyroid screen, with a TSH level of greater than 100 µIU/mL.

Question 12-1

The most appropriate next step is:
A) Send the primary pediatrician a note to address the abnormal level at the 2-week check.
B) Call the family and have them take the infant for a thyroid ultrasound.
C) Nothing, since the infant looked fine at discharge.
D) Arrange for the infant go for repeat labs today, and prescribe levothyroxine.
E) Call the family and have the infant go for repeat labs in 2 months.

Discussion 12-1

The correct answer is "D." Congenital hypothyroidism occurs in approximately 1 in 3000 newborns and is one of the most common causes of preventable mental retardation. So take it seriously! There is an inverse relationship between the age at treatment initiation and IQ, making prompt recognition and treatment of utmost importance. The goal is to start supplementation by 2 weeks of age. All states in the United States include congenital hypothyroidism as part of the newborn screen, although exact protocols vary. Serum TSH concentrations rise abruptly at birth due to exposure to cold and then decrease rapidly to about 20 μIU/mL at 24 hours of age. An early collection can cause a false positive on the newborn screen. If a screen is positive, it is important to call the family immediately, confirm the result with a venipuncture TSH and free T_4, and start therapy. The most common cause of congenital hypothyroidism is thyroid dysgenesis (85% of cases); however, patients may also have defects in thyroid hormone metabolism. Thus, thyroid imaging can be helpful to determine etiology but does not dictate treatment and is not routinely done.

> **Helpful Tip**
> The majority of thyroid hormone is bound by thyroid-binding globulin (TBG). Total T_4 assays are affected by TBG amount, although free T_4 assays are not. Hereditary TBG deficiency is an X-linked recessive disorder that results in normal TSH with low total T_4 and has historically caused diagnostic dilemmas. We now have the capability to measure a free T_4, which is normal in this setting of "euthyroid hypothyroxinemia."

▶ CASE 13

A 14-year-old adolescent girl comes to the clinic with her father because of palpitations and exercise intolerance that are interfering with her basketball season. She describes a 2- to 3-month history of the concerns with associated jitteriness and poor sleep. She has had a voracious appetite but has had a stable weight (her friends are jealous that she can eat a whole bag of Flamin' Hot Cheetos every night and maintain her figure). She has not had a menstrual period for the past 2 months despite previously being regular. She gets up once or twice a night to urinate. On exam, the young woman is fidgeting. She is wearing a T-shirt despite the January weather. Her pulse is 120 beats per minute (bpm). Her skin is warm, and she has a tremor. You suspect hyperthyroidism. Her labs show:

TSH <0.01 μIU/mL

Free T4 4.7 ng/dL

Thyroid-stimulating immunoglobulin (TSI) 250%

Thyroid peroxidase (TPO) antibodies negative

Question 13-1

Which of the following is NOT a true statement regarding this girl's condition?

A) Treatment options include medical, surgical, or radioablative therapy.

B) She most likely has Graves disease.

C) It is likely that she has been eating too much iodine-containing seaweed.

D) There is a chance of spontaneous remission.

E) First-line medical therapy is methimazole.

Discussion 13-1

The correct answer is "C." Elevated thyroid hormone with suppressed TSH is consistent with hyperthyroidism. Hyperthyroidism affects many organ systems, and symptoms include palpitations, jitteriness, insomnia, weight loss, polyphagia, polyuria, increased stooling frequency, and heat intolerance. Signs include tachycardia, tremor, brisk reflexes, and weight loss. Hyperthyroidism is most commonly caused by Graves disease due to stimulating autoantibodies but can also be caused by a destructive autoimmune process with passive spilling of thyroid hormone ("hashitoxicosis"). Positive TSI or thyrotropin receptor antibodies (TrAb), markedly enlarged and smooth thyroid gland, exophthalmos (rare in kids), and relative elevation of T_3 greater than T_4 can point to Graves disease. Positive TPO antibodies, mildly enlarged heterogeneous/cobblestone gland, and relative T_4 greater than T_3 can point to hashitoxicosis. Management of hyperthyroidism in pediatric patients includes medical therapy with methimazole or definitive therapy with radioactive iodine ablation or thyroidectomy. Beta-blockers can be used to treat the tachycardia if necessary.

> **Helpful Tip**
> Neonatal Graves disease can occur if there is transplacental passage of maternal stimulatory TSH-receptor antibodies. It occurs in approximately 2% of mothers who have a history of Graves disease, with increased risk in women who have a high antibody titer during their third trimester. Neonatal Graves disease is transient and resolves when maternal antibodies disappear, but it can be life-threatening in the interim. Clinical manifestations include intrauterine growth restriction (IUGR), premature birth, microcephaly, irritability, tachycardia, and poor weight gain. Neonatal Graves disease can be treated with methimazole and beta-blockers.

⏳ QUICK QUIZ

Which sign is NOT associated with a thyroid storm?

A) Normal mental status.

B) Congestive heart failure.

C) Fever of 40°C (104°F).

D) Tachycardia.

E) Death.

Discussion

The correct answer is "A." Thyroid storm is the ultimate manifestation of hyperthyroidism. It can cause life-threatening autonomic and cardiovascular instability (hyperpyrexia, arrhythmias, heart failure, and tachycardia). The skin is sweaty, and the mind is foggy. TSH is low, and free T_4 and T_3 are high. (Nurse, I need a stat beta-blocker please!)

► CASE 14

A 13-year-old girl comes in for follow-up of fatigue. She has also lost weight. She has seen several providers over the past 6 months and has been diagnosed with depression. She returns today because her parents are concerned that she may also have an eating disorder. On exam, you find a thin girl. Her pulse is 115 bpm and blood pressure (BP) 96/60 mm Hg. You astutely note that her skin tone is darker than her family's, and she has clearly hyperpigmented lips and buccal mucosa.

Question 14-1

Which of the following lab results would be consistent with primary adrenal insufficiency?

	ACTH	Cortisol	Sodium	Potassium
A)	Low	Low	Low	High
B)	High	Low	Low	High
C)	High	High	Low	High
D)	High	Low	High	Low
E)	Low	Low	High	Low

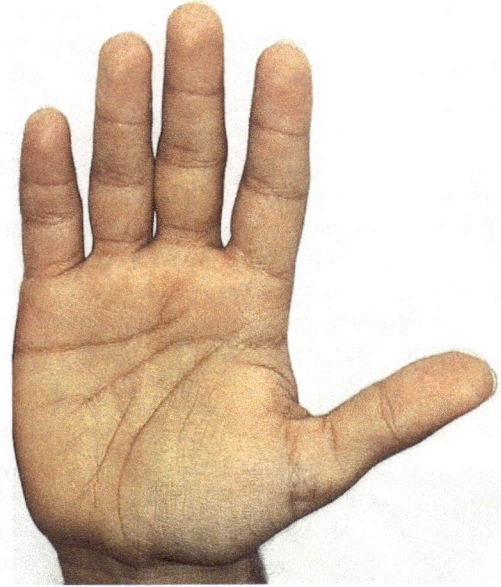

FIGURE 11–7. Hyperpigmentation in Addison disease. (Reproduced with permission from Longo D, Fauci A, Kasper D, Hauser S, Jameson J, Loscalzo J (Eds). *Harrison's Principles of Internal Medicine*, 18th Ed. McGraw-Hill Education, Inc., 2013. Fig 406-15A.)

Discussion 14-1

The correct answer is "B." Acquired primary adrenal insufficiency is most often caused by autoimmune destruction of the adrenal gland (Addison disease). Loss of adrenal gland function results in cortisol and aldosterone deficiency, both of which can be life threatening. Without cortisol, a patient develops hypotension, hypoglycemia, fatigue, weight loss, chronic nausea, and general lassitude. The pituitary gland attempts to compensate by increasing ACTH. Hyperpigmentation of the skin may develop, as well as darkening of the palmar creases, scars, lips, buccal mucosa, and genitals (see Figure 11–7), because ACTH shares a precursor with melanocyte-stimulating hormone (MSH). Without aldosterone, a patient develops hypotension, syncope, hyponatremia, and hyperkalemia. Addison's disease can develop insidiously and present with vague symptoms; it is important to recognize the clinical picture to prevent a life-threatening adrenal crisis. If suspected, initial studies should include ACTH (will be markedly elevated), cortisol (will be low or inappropriately normal for the ACTH level), and electrolytes (will show hyponatremia and hyperkalemia).

> **Helpful Tip**
> Addison disease is associated with the development of other autoimmune diseases, such as type 1 diabetes mellitus, autoimmune thyroid disease, and vitiligo.

Your patient is started on glucocorticoid and mineralocorticoid therapy and now feels like a million bucks! She comes in for follow-up and is a little upset that you ruined her good tan, but is otherwise happy.

Question 14-2

All of the following will be important for her follow-up EXCEPT:
A) She should wear a medical alert bracelet to identify her as steroid-dependent.
B) She should take extra glucocorticoid medication if she is sick.
C) She should never restrict her salt intake.
D) She will need injectable glucocorticoid if she cannot take her oral dose.
E) All of the above.

Discussion 14-2

The correct answer is "E." Patients with primary adrenal insufficiency require glucocorticoid and mineralocorticoid replacement. Glucocorticoid replacement typically consists of hydrocortisone given three times daily for precise dosing, but prednisone or dexamethasone can be used. Patients and families need to be taught to "stress dose" during illness. For febrile illnesses, broken bones, or minor procedures, the patient will need to increase her glucocorticoid dose (typically triple the dose). For severe illnesses in which the patient cannot take an oral glucocorticoid medication or for procedures requiring sedation, an injectable dose of hydrocortisone at 50 to 100 mg/m^2 should be given IV or IM. Patients should be instructed to wear a "steroid-dependent" medical alert bracelet in case of emergency. Mineralocorticoid is replaced with fludrocortisone; the dosage does not change with illness. However, it is adjusted over the long term based on blood pressure, electrolytes, or symptoms of salt craving. Patients with adrenal insufficiency should never be instructed to restrict salt intake.

▶ CASE 15

A 14-year-old boy presents for hypertension that was identified on his sports preparticipation physical exam and has persisted. On review of his growth chart, his height is at the first percentile and has not changed in 2 years. His weight has continued to track along the 40th percentile, leading to an overweight body mass index (BMI). On exam, he has a round face. Skin exam reveals several bruises on his arms and legs, and purplish striae on his abdomen.

Question 15-1

What could explain his hypertension, growth failure, and physical findings?
A) He uses inhaled, intranasal, and topical steroids for his atopic disease and also gets an oral burst of prednisone whenever he has an upper respiratory tract infection.
B) He has been on prednisone at 20 mg daily for his juvenile arthritis for the past 3 years.
C) He has a brain tumor that secretes ACTH.
D) He has an adrenal tumor that secretes cortisol.
E) All of the above.
F) None of the above.

Discussion 15-1

The correct answer is "E." Beware the short and fat child! The combination of growth failure with abnormal fat distribution (moon facies, dorsocervical fat pad ["buffalo hump"],

supraclavicular fat pads, centripedal obesity), hypertension, easy bruising, and violaceous striae should alert you to the possibility of cortisol excess (Cushing syndrome). Patients may also have facial plethora, abnormal glucose tolerance, weakness, and menstrual irregularities or pubertal delay. (See Figure 11–8.) The most common cause of cortisol excess is exogenous and iatrogenic. Oral, injectable, topical, inhaled, and intranasal steroids that are used for many nonendocrine diseases may be implicated, and the history should aim to quantify the glucocorticoid exposure from all sources. Endogenous Cushing syndrome may be caused by excessive secretion of ACTH from the pituitary gland (true Cushing disease) or excessive secretion of cortisol from the adrenal gland as a result of tumor or genetic disease.

You suspect Cushing syndrome. The patient is not on any medications.

Question 15-2

Which of the following is the most appropriate initial test to evaluate for cortisol excess?
A) Morning serum cortisol.
B) Midnight salivary cortisol.
C) Serum ACTH level at noon.
D) Oral glucose tolerance test (OGTT).
E) Spot urinary free cortisol.

Discussion 15-1

The correct answer is "B." The diagnosis of cortisol excess can be difficult and cannot be made on the basis of one test. A random cortisol cannot be used to diagnose cortisol excess. First-line tests include a late-night salivary cortisol level or 24-hour urine collection for free cortisol, or a low-dose dexamethasone suppression test.

▶ CASE 16

An 8-year-old girl presents for her well-child check. Her height today is the same as the height recorded at her 7-year-old check. You initially assume this is an error, but when she also fails her vision screen you start to worry. On a careful review of systems, she admits to nocturia and fatigue. On physical exam, she is short but in no acute distress. Visual field testing on confrontation is suspicious for a bitemporal hemianopsia. You call the ophthalmology service to see if they can get her in today.

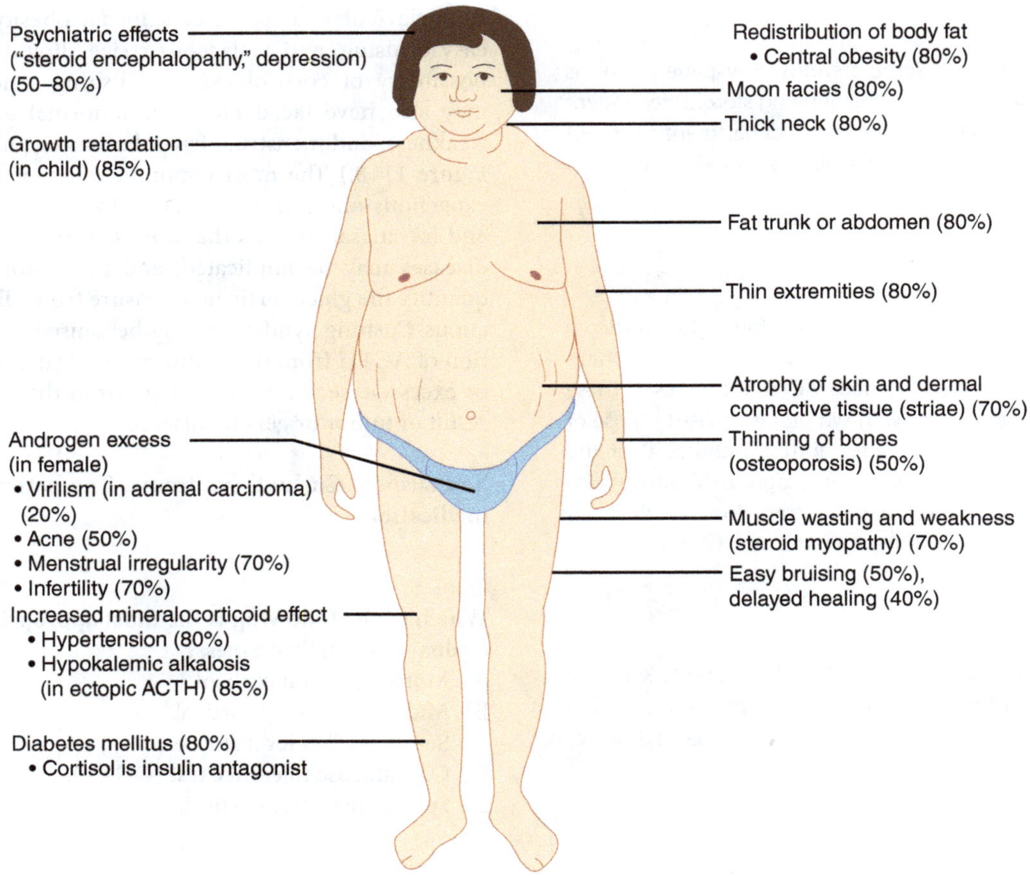

FIGURE 11–8. Common findings from cortisol excess. (Reproduced with permission from Hammer GD, McPhee SJ, eds. *Pathophysiology of Disease: An Introduction to Clinical Medicine.* 7th ed. New York, NY: McGraw-Hill Education; 2014, Fig. 21-11.)

Question 16-1

Which of the following lab tests would be appropriate to order today while you are waiting to hear back from ophthalmology?

A) TSH.

B) Free T₄.

C) Serum sodium and urine osmolality.

D) GH level.

E) Cortisol level.

F) Prolactin.

G) All of the above.

H) Options A, B, and D.

I) Options B, C, E, and F.

J) None of the above

Discussion 16-1

The correct answer is "I." This child has several clinical features that may indicate a central nervous system (CNS) lesion near the pituitary gland (the "master" hormone gland), including signs of optic nerve compression, diabetes insipidus, GH deficiency, and possibly hypothyroidism. In addition to addressing her visual deficits, it will be informative to further evaluate her pituitary function. The anterior pituitary gland secretes

ACTH, GH, LH, FSH, TSH, and prolactin. The posterior pituitary gland secretes antidiuretic hormone (ADH) and oxytocin. (See Figure 11–9.) To screen pituitary function, you need to consider the effect of those pituitary hormones. Appropriate lab tests include free T₄, serum sodium with concurrent urine osmolality, cortisol, and prolactin. A random GH level will not be helpful to assess for GH deficiency, but you could consider IGF-1. A TSH level will not be reliable since you are worried about a central process.

You confirm that she has multiple anterior pituitary deficiencies (low free T₄, low cortisol, low IGF-1), disruption of the pituitary stalk (mildly elevated prolactin), as well as diabetes insipidus (dilute urine with elevated serum sodium).

Question 16-2

What is an important next step to evaluate for causes of her pituitary deficiencies?

A) Brain CT.

B) Brain MRI.

C) GH stimulation test.

D) Head ultrasound.

E) No further workup; just treat the deficiencies.

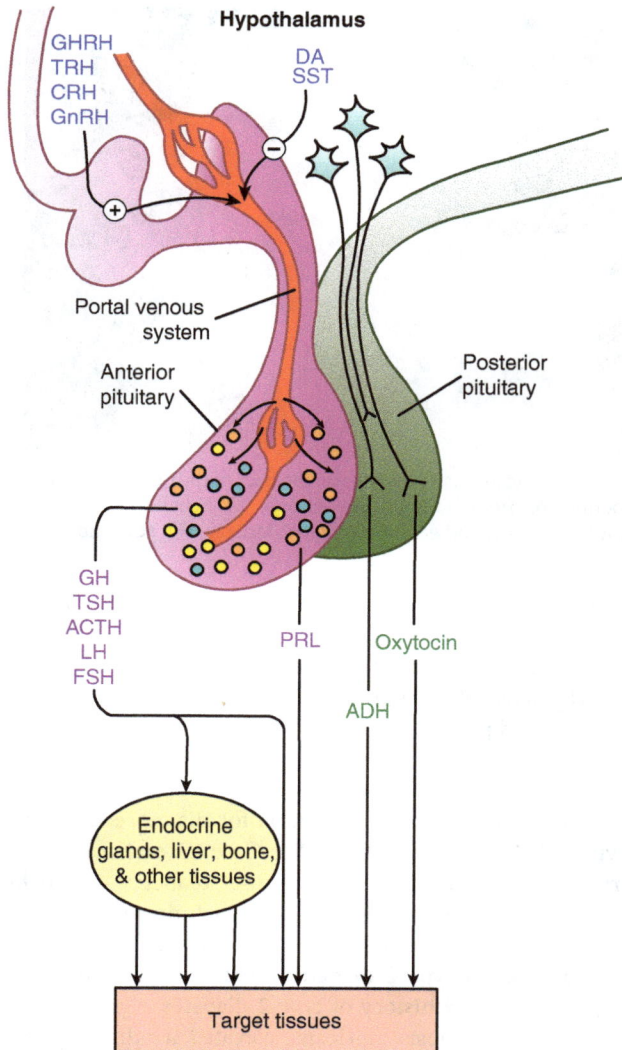

FIGURE 11–9. The pituitary hormones. ACTH, adrenocorticotropin; ADH, antidiuretic hormone (vasopressin); CRH, corticotropin-releasing hormone; DA, Dopamine; FSH, Follicle Stimulating Hormone; GH, growth hormone; GHRH, growth hormone–releasing hormone; GnRH, gonadotropin-releasing hormone; LH, luteinizing hormone; PRL, prolactin; SST, somatostatin; TRH, thyrotropin-releasing hormone; TSH, thyroid-stimulating hormone. (Reproduced with permission from Katzung BG, Trevor AJ, eds. *Basic & Clinical Pharmacology.* 13th ed. New York, NY: McGraw-Hill Education; 2015, Fig. 37-1.)

Discussion 16-2

The correct answer is "B." A child presenting with multiple acquired pituitary deficiencies needs to be urgently evaluated for CNS neoplasm, which could include a pituitary or extrapituitary tumor (eg, craniopharyngioma) or an infiltrative process. This is best done with a brain MRI with and without contrast.

▶ CASE 17

A 7-year-old boy is brought in for nocturnal enuresis. He is very embarrassed since he has been potty-trained for years and now has had 2 weeks of nightly bed-wetting. On further questioning, his mother thinks he had some daytime polyuria

and polydipsia. He has not had a documented weight loss but has failed to gain weight since his last health supervision visit. He has generally been feeling well otherwise, until today when he did not want to eat. On exam, you find a thin, tired-appearing boy. His lips and mucous membranes are dry. He has tachycardia with a normal BP. You suspect he may have diabetes mellitus type 1. Your clinic is on a new cost-saving initiative, so you are only allowed three lab tests.

Question 17-1

What three studies will be most helpful in confirming diagnosis *and* guiding your next steps?
A) Blood glucose, insulin, hemoglobin A_{1c} (Hbg A_{1c}).
B) GAD65 antibodies, islet cell antibodies, islet antigen 2 (IA-2) antibodies.
C) Blood glucose, urinalysis, basic metabolic panel (BMP).
D) Blood glucose, tissue transglutaminase (TTG), TSH.
E) C-peptide, insulin, blood glucose.
F) OGTT (this counts as three, since it is expensive).

Discussion 17-1

The correct answer is "C." Diagnostic criteria for diabetes mellitus include:

- Fasting plasma glucose ≥ 126 mg/dL (7 mmol/L) on more than one occasion; *or*
- Random venous plasma glucose ≥ 200 mg/dL (11.1 mmol/L) in a patient with symptoms (polyuria, polydipsia, polyphagia); *or*
- Hgb A_{1c} ≥ 6.5%; *or*
- 2-hour blood glucose on OGTT ≥ 200 mg/dL (11.1 mmol/L)

In this case, there are symptoms of diabetes mellitus; thus if the blood glucose is greater than 200 mg/dL, you have your diagnosis. The next most important thing is to determine whether the child is ketotic or in diabetic ketoacidosis (DKA), which informs your next step in management. DKA is distinguished by hyperglycemia and anion gap metabolic acidosis due to ketones, and requires more aggressive therapy. If you know whether there are ketones in the urine and the anion gap (based on the BMP), you can determine whether DKA is present. GAD65, islet cell, and IA-2 antibodies can be elevated in type 1 diabetes mellitus but are not part of the diagnostic criteria. TTG and TSH are routinely assessed in new diabetic patients to screen for autoimmune comorbidities. Insulin level would be expected to be low but is not part of the diagnostic criteria.

Your patient did indeed have type 1 diabetes mellitus, and you have treated his DKA.

Question 17-2

What is the most appropriate long-term therapy?
A) Subcutaneous basal insulin given at night.
B) Subcutaneous bolus insulin given with meals.
C) Oral metformin (Glucophage) given twice daily.
D) Subcutaneous basal and bolus insulin.
E) Oral sulfonylurea given with meals.

Discussion 17-2

The correct answer is "D." Standard of care for youth with type 1 diabetes is a basal-bolus insulin regimen. This is typically achieved initially with multiple daily injections, including a long-acting insulin given at bedtime (hs) (glargine or detemir) and a short-acting insulin given at mealtime (lispro or aspart). This can also be achieved with continuous insulin infusion administered using a short-acting insulin via pump.

He returns for a scheduled follow-up. He is feeling great and doing well with his diabetes care regimen.

Question 17-3

Which of the following studies is part of routine screening for patients with type 1 diabetes mellitus?
A) Urine albumin/creatinine ratio.
B) TSH.
C) TTG.
D) Ophthalmology exams.
E) Lipid panel.
F) All of the above.

Discussion 17-3

The correct answer is "F." Routine follow-up for children with type 1 diabetes should be done at least four times a year and include monitoring of height and weight, blood pressure, and thorough physical exam. Lab monitoring includes Hbg A_{1c}, spot urine albumin/creatinine ratio yearly after age 10 years, TSH every 1 to 2 years, celiac disease screening (TTG) every 2 to 3 years or if symptomatic, lipid panel by age 10 years and then at least every 5 years, and a dilated ophthalmologic evaluation for children over 10 years of age and 3 to 5 years after onset of diabetes

▶ CASE 18

A 15-year-old boy comes to the clinic because of concern about increased urination and thirst. His teachers have noticed that he leaves class frequently at school, and he has also been getting up at night to urinate. He is obese but tells you he is pleased to have lost several pounds over the last several weeks. On exam, his height is at the 80th percentile, weight is at the 99th percentile, blood pressure is 130/80 mm Hg, and heart rate is 90 bpm. In general, he is obese but otherwise appears healthy. On exam, you note thickened and darkened skin on his posterior neck and axillae (see Figure 11–10), pink striae on his abdomen, and well-muscled legs and arms. You suspect that he could have type 2 diabetes mellitus but are smart enough to also consider type 1.

Question 18-1

Which of the following features would support a diagnosis of type 2 versus type 1 diabetes mellitus?
A) Recent weight loss.
B) Low C-peptide level.

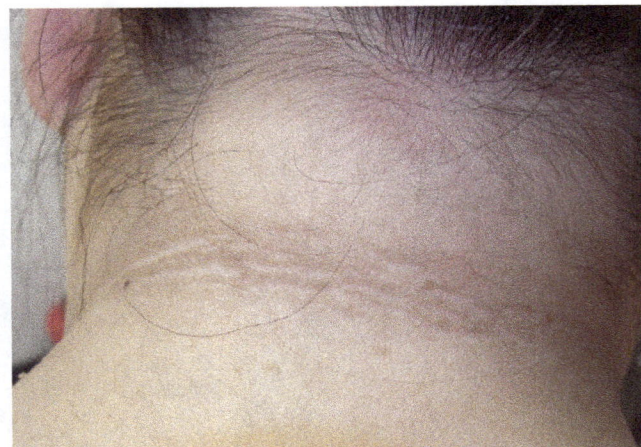

FIGURE 11–10. Acanthosis nigricans on the back of the neck. (Reproduced with permission from Hoffman BL, Schorge JO, Schaffer JI, et al, eds. *Williams Gynecology*. 2nd ed. New York, NY: McGraw-Hill Education; 2012, Fig. 17-6.)

C) Signs of insulin resistance (acanthosis nigricans).
D) Blood glucose of 280 mg/dL.
E) Polyuria and polydipsia.

Discussion 18-1

The correct answer is "C." The criteria for diagnosis of type 1 and type 2 diabetes are identical. (See Case 17, earlier.) In pre-pubertal children, all cases of new-onset diabetes should be considered type 1 unless there is overwhelming evidence to the contrary. In postpubertal children, factors that would support a diagnosis of type 2 diabetes include obesity, insidious onset, positive family history of type 2 diabetes, signs of insulin resistance (acanthosis nigricans, elevated insulin, elevated C-peptide), negative pancreatic antibodies, and high-risk race/ethnicity (ie, non-Hispanic black, Native American, Hispanic, Pacific Islander, and Asian American). If in doubt, it is safer to treat a patient as you would a confirmed case of type 1 diabetes, by administering insulin to prevent DKA.

Question 18-2

You ultimately confirm a diagnosis of type 2 diabetes mellitus. All of the following screening is indicated except?
A) Lipid panel.
B) AST, ALT.
C) TSH.
D) Urine albumin/creatinine ratio.
E) Follow-up elevated blood pressure.

Discussion 18-2

The correct answer is "C." Adolescents with type 2 diabetes mellitus are at risk for comorbidities that include dyslipidemia, nonalcoholic fatty liver disease (NAFLD), hypertension, and microalbuminuria. They must be monitored closely and treated aggressively for these comorbidities. Type 2 diabetes mellitus is often present in a quartet of findings with central adiposity, dyslipidemia (particularly low high-density lipoprotein and elevated triglycerides), and hypertension, which comprise the "metabolic syndrome." Though there are no strict criteria for pediatric metabolic syndrome, it is important to recognize insulin resistance, which underlies the high-risk constellation of features, and address the entire picture. Treatment with lifestyle modification and weight loss are crucial (and difficult), and pharmacologic therapy is added as indicated for each component.

► CASE 19

A 1-week-old term breastfed infant girl presents to the emergency department with a seizure. She has been irritable for the past 3 days. You stabilize her ABCs and then order an initial set of lab tests, which show normal glucose, normal sodium and potassium, low total and ionized calcium, and high phosphorous. A chest X-ray is remarkable for the absence of a thymic shadow.

Question 19-1

What is the most likely additional finding?
A) High parathyroid hormone (PTH).
B) Low PTH.
C) High 1,25-$(OH)_2$ vitamin D.
D) High TSH.
E) High magnesium.

Discussion 19-1

The correct answer is "B." The newborn has DiGeorge syndrome. Neonatal hypocalcemia is common due to the rapid transition necessary at birth when the maternal calcium source is abruptly cut off and the infant must rely on its own intake and PTH system. Neonatal hypocalcemia is divided into early and late, based on timing of presentation. Early hypocalcemia (first 2 to 3 days after birth) is more typically due to circumstances surrounding the birth, such as prematurity, infant of a diabetic mother, asphyxia, and IUGR. Late hypocalcemia is more likely to be caused by hypoparathyroidism, maternal hyperparathyroidism, hypomagnesemia, vitamin D deficiency, or excess phosphate load. (See Figure 11-11.)

Helpful Tip

DiGeorge (velocardiofacial) syndrome is the most common syndrome associated with hypoparathyroidism diagnosed in the neonatal period. Remember CATCH22:

C – Cardiac defects
A – Abnormal facies
T – Thymic hypoplasia
C – Cleft palate
H – Hypocalcemia
22 – 22q11 microdeletion

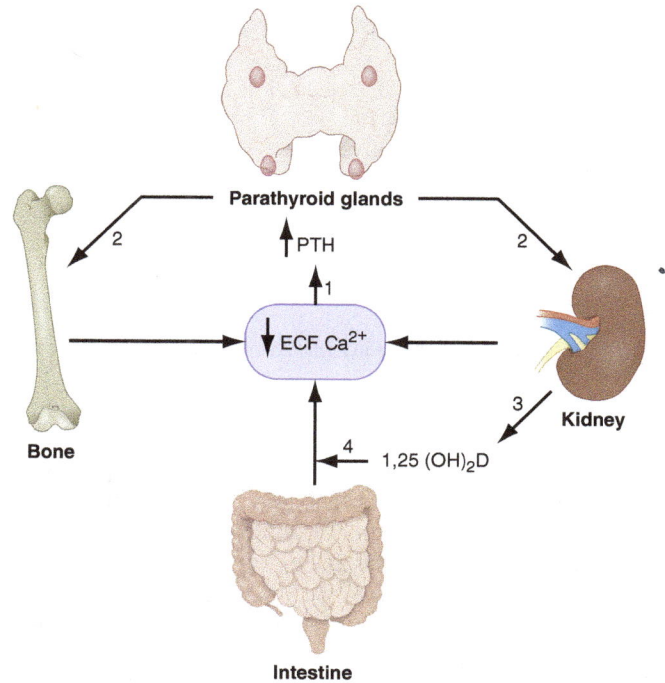

FIGURE 11–11. Calcium homeostasis. ECF Ca²⁺, extracellular ionized calcium; PTH, parathyroid hormone. (Reproduced with permission from Longo D, Fauci A, Kasper D, Hauser S, Jameson J, Loscalzo J, eds. *Harrison's Manual of Medicine*, 18th ed. New York, NY: McGraw-Hill Education; 2013, Fig. 187-1.)

► CASE 20

A 15-year-old adolescent girl was seen in the emergency department for abdominal pain and hematuria that is diagnosed as nephrolithiasis. She has now passed the stone and is in your office for follow-up. On your excellent history, she endorses irritability and fatigue that started insidiously over the past year. She has been struggling to complete her school assignments and is even failing physical education because she complains of weakness.

Question 20-1

The next most appropriate step is:
A) Start a selective serotonin reuptake inhibitor (SSRI) since she has symptoms of depression.
B) Recommend a low-calcium and low-oxalate diet to prevent future stone formation.
C) Check lab values, including calcium, phosphorous, PTH, 25-(OH) vitamin D, and urine calcium.
D) Check lab values, including TSH, cortisol, 1,25-$(OH)_2$ vitamin D.
E) Send for imaging of her parathyroid glands.

Discussion 20-1

The correct answer is "C." Nephrolithiasis combined with symptoms such as fatigue, mood changes, vague weakness, musculoskeletal pains, anorexia/nausea, or polyuria should raise concern for hypercalcemia. (Remember: Bones, Stones, Groans, Psychic

TABLE 11–1 CAUSES OF HYPERCALCEMIA

	Calcium	Phosphorous	PTH	25(OH)D	1,25(OH)$_2$D
Hyperparathyroidism	⇑	⇓	⇑	⇔	⇔
Vitamin D intoxication	⇑	⇑	⇓	⇑	⇔
Immobility	⇑	⇔	⇓	⇔	⇔
• Granulomatous disease	⇑	⇑	⇓	⇔	⇑

PTH, parathyroid hormone; 25(OH)D, 25-hydroxyvitamin D; 1,25(OH)$_2$D, 1,25-dihydroxyvitamin D.

Overtones.) This patient needs a workup before simply treating her symptoms. Differential diagnosis of hypercalcemia includes hyperparathyroidism, vitamin D intoxication, malignancy, immobilization, and granulomatous disease (eg, sarcoidosis, tuberculosis). The first step is to confirm the hypercalcemia and determine if it is PTH-mediated. In hyperparathyroidism, the PTH level is elevated or inappropriately normal for the hypercalcemia, and the phosphorous is low. If you determine that the hypercalcemia is *not* due to excess PTH, consider the other etiologies. (See Table 11–1.)

> **Helpful Tip**
>
> Familial hypocalciuric hypercalcemia is a benign cause of hypercalcemia that typically presents with incidental hypercalcemia in childhood. It is an autosomal dominant condition, and heterozygotes have mild hypercalcemia, hypocalciuria, and normal PTH. It is important to recognize this condition to prevent morbidity from further evaluation and treatment.

▶ CASE 21

A 24-month old boy is brought in by his parents to establish pediatric care. He is short statured. Over the past several months, he has developed progressive leg bowing. On exam, he has frontal bossing, nontender palpable lumps along his costochondral junctions, and wide wrists. His family isn't worried since the patient has an uncle and a brother with a similar features.

Question 21-1
What is the most likely laboratory finding?
A) Elevated 25-(OH) vitamin D.
B) Elevated calcium.
C) Elevated alkaline phosphatase.
D) Elevated phosphorous.
E) Elevated 1,25-(OH)$_2$ vitamin D.

Discussion 21-1
The correct answer is "C." This child has a clinical picture consistent with rickets. Patients with rickets have short stature,

delayed fontanelle closure, frontal bossing, enlarged costochondral junctions (also known as the rachitic rosary), and widening of the wrists with bowing of the distal radius and ulna. When they start walking, they develop bowing of the femur and tibia. (See Figure 11–12.) Normal bone growth requires sufficient calcium and phosphorous levels. Deficiencies in either can result in rickets. In both calcipenic and phosphopenic rickets, the alkaline phosphatase is elevated. Calcipenic rickets is typically acquired and due to nutritional deficiencies, particularly in 25-(OH) vitamin D. Phosphopenic rickets is due to renal

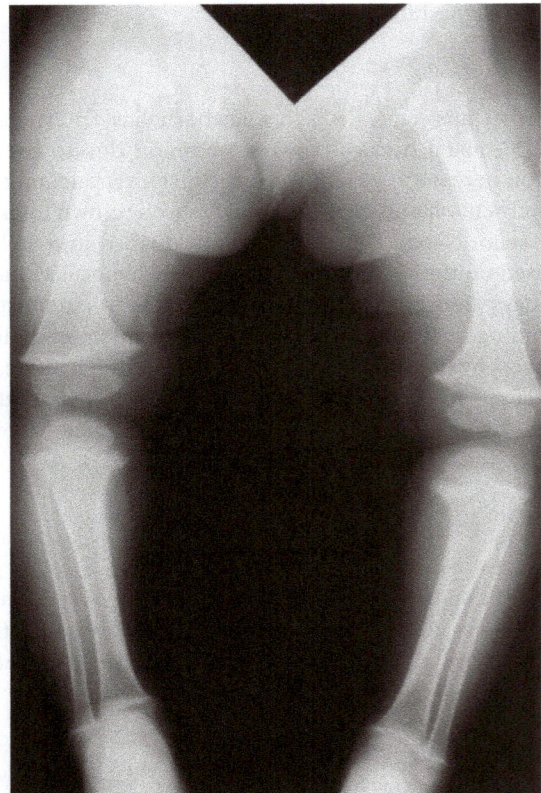

FIGURE 11–12. Bowing of the long bones, metaphyseal widening and irregular physes in hypophosphatemic rickets. (Reproduced with permission from Skinner HB, McMahon PJ, eds. *Current Diagnosis & Treatment in Orthopedics*. 5th ed. New York, NY: McGraw-Hill Education; 2014, Fig. 10-3.)

phosphate wasting. Although it can be due to primary renal disease, it is more often caused by an X-linked inherited disorder. The mainstay of phosphopenic rickets treatment is phosphorous replacement.

BIBLIOGRAPHY

American Academy of Pediatrics, Rose SR: Section on Endocrinology and Committee on Genetics, American Thyroid Association; Brown RS; Public Health Committee, Lawson Wilkins Pediatric Endocrine Society, Foley T, et al. Update of newborn screening and therapy for congenital hypothyroidism. *Pediatrics.* 2006;117(6):2290–2303.

American Diabetes Association. Standards of medical care in diabetes—2011. *Diabetes Care.* 2011;34(suppl 1):S11–61.

Ethics

12

Rebecca Benson and Catherina Pinnaro

► CASE 1

An 11-year-old girl has a serious immunodeficiency, secondary to which she spends a large amount of time in the hospital. Recently, a simple protocol involving venipuncture similar to blood donation was developed to obtain cells from patients with diseases like hers. Researchers believe that studying these cells will give them new information about the immune systems as well as disease-specific information. The girl has already undergone similar procedures without ill effects. Her parents strongly support her participation in the study. Because the study investigator does not want to pressure the girl into agreeing, she asks a bioethics consultant to explain the procedure and solicit the girl's agreement. By the end of the discussion, it is clear that the girl understands the procedure and is not afraid or made anxious by the prospect of undergoing it. However, once she is told that the procedure would not help her and that she can refuse to participate, she quickly states that she would rather spend the 30 minutes playing.

Question 1-1

Are the study coordinators required to obtain the girl's assent for the procedure?

A) No, they do not need to ask her because her parents are the ultimate decision makers for her until she turns 18 years old.

B) No, they only need her assent if her parents are not willing to consent for the procedure.

C) Yes, as the U.S. regulations for research require the assent of children capable of providing it in all cases.

D) Yes, because the procedure will involve collecting a biologic specimen.

Discussion 1-1

The correct answer is "C." The assent requirement in pediatric research refers to obtaining a child's "positive agreement" and assumes that the child's parent(s) have already consented to enroll him or her in a research study. Its purpose is to serve as a nod to the child's developing sense of self. The U.S. regulations require the assent of children *capable* of providing it in all cases but do allow institutional review boards (IRBs) to waive the requirement when the research offers the "'prospect of direct benefit that is important to the health or well-being of the children and is available only in the context of research'" (Emanuel 2008). A patient's reluctance or dissent should also carry considerable weight when the proposed intervention is not essential to his or her welfare or can be deferred without substantial risk, or both. The American Academy of Pediatrics (AAP) has adopted the belief that children become capable of assent at the age of 7 years. This view is linked to the historic Rule of Sevens, which presumes that "children under the age of 7 do not have the capacity necessary to make their own decisions; children 7–14 years of age are presumed not to have this capacity until proven otherwise [and]; children over 14 are presumed to have the capacity to make their own decisions and lead their own lives, unless proven otherwise" (AAP 1995).

► CASE 2

You are seeing a 16-year-old adolescent girl in your pediatric practice. During her last well-child visit, she indicated that she was not sexually active but did have a boyfriend. You counseled her on safe sex practices and encouraged her to contact you if she had any concerns. She comes in today with vaginal discharge and painful urination.

Question 2-1

Do you need to obtain formal informed consent from her legal guardians to test or treat her for sexually transmitted diseases (STDs)?

A) No, because she is a mature minor and may give consent for an elective procedure, as long as it is minor and has a low risk of complications.

B) No, because most states give adolescent patients with decision-making capacity the right to seek confidential health care for certain conditions, such as STDs, pregnancy, and drug or alcohol abuse.

C) Yes, because while care may be provided for an adolescent without consent in emergency situations, it is inappropriate to provide care without consent in nonemergencies.

D) Yes, because she is not an emancipated minor and is dependent on the support of her parents.

Discussion 2-1

The correct answer is "B." Conflicts arise between the rights of adolescents and the rights of their parents to make decisions. Providing medical care to adolescents requires a specific awareness of the minor treatment statutes and common law in each state in which the care is being provided. Although parents have the right and responsibility to nurture and protect their minor child, statutes and court decisions may preempt parental authority when it conflicts with the best interest of the youth and society. In emergencies, medical care may be rendered to a minor without consent from the parent or guardian. Another category of exception to the parental consent rule exists for emancipated minors. Emancipation means the relinquishment by the parent of control and authority over the adolescent, thus terminating the parental duty of support, usually when the child is living apart from the parent and is financially independent. In addition to exceptions for emergency situations and in the case of emancipation, most states have enacted statutes allowing minors to consent to treatment for certain specific medical conditions, often including pregnancy, STDs, contraception, substance abuse, and mental illness. These laws vary from state to state and may or may not contain an age threshold. Some give the physician discretion as to whether to inform the parents about the treatment.

Question 2-2

In the model of shared decision making, which of the following is true?

A) The physician shares information about different treatment options with the patient and family and then tells them what the plan will be based on his or her medical expertise.

B) The physician's goal is not to bias patient and family decision making by giving a recommendation.

C) The physician must follow the treatment plan selected by the patient, regardless of whether it conflicts with his or her conscience.

D) The physician, along with the patient and family, discuss the information together to come to a consensus decision about treatment.

Discussion 2-2

The correct answer is "D." In a shared decision-making model, the goal is to establish a collaborative approach to making medical decisions that takes into account the medical expertise and guidance of the medical provider along with the values and preferences of the patient. This is often contrasted against two other models, the paternalistic approach and the menu option approach. The paternalistic approach assumes the provider knows what the best treatment plan is for the patient but does not take into account the role of the individual patient's experience and goals in determining a plan. In the menu option approach, the provider shares options for treatment but does not learn about patient goals and preferences and use these to make a recommendation and reach a consensus decision with the patient and family. If there is a clearly superior treatment plan, or if the provider has a sense of which treatment plan would best help the patient achieve his or her goals, the provider can certainly make a recommendation. Providers are not required to provide care that is not medically indicated, and if they have a strong moral objection to providing certain care, there is an ethical basis for recusing themselves from a patient's care as long as there are other providers available and willing to assume care.

> **Helpful Tip**
> While the physician provides expertise about the diagnosis, prognosis, and treatment options, the patient is the expert in his or her experience of the illness, goals of care, how values shape the balance of benefits and burdens, and preferences about how much risk he or she is willing to assume to achieve a certain goal.

Question 2-3

Which of the following has been found to be positively correlated with improved accuracy of diagnosis, treatment adherence, and patient functional status?

A) Effective communication of the health care team.

B) Involvement of an ethics consult service.

C) Specialty of the physician involved.

D) Number of years in practice of the primary physician.

E) All of the above.

Discussion 2-3

The correct answer is "A." Communication in health care is the foundation of the therapeutic relationship and it is a skill that taught and improved upon over time. Studies have shown that effective communication is positively correlated with diagnostic accuracy, development of a successful treatment plan, adherence to the agreed-upon treatment plan, and the patient's functional status, as well as other desired outcomes. None of the other answers have been shown to be correlated with all of these areas.

Question 2-4

Which of the following is the correct definition of fidelity?

A) The physician's obligation to protect the patient's privacy.

B) The physician's obligation to the truth.

C) The physician's obligation to be trustworthy.
D) The physician's obligation to put the patient's needs ahead of his or her own.
E) None of the above.

Discussion 2-4

The correct answer is "C." Developing a successful patient-parent-pediatrician relationship requires trust. It is built upon the pediatrician's obligations to uphold confidentiality, veracity, and fidelity. Fidelity, being trustworthy, and altruism (option "D"), putting the patient first, are expectations of the pediatrician when caring for patients and their families. Confidentiality is the physician's obligation to protect a patient's personal health information and not share the information without the patient's permission as per the Health Insurance Portability and Accountability Act (HIPPA) Privacy Rule (option "A"). Confidentiality becomes challenging as a child enters adolescence. It is important that the adolescent, parent(s), and pediatrician be aware of the boundaries surrounding disclosure of information to the parent without the adolescent's permission. A dedication to truth, veracity (option "B"), requires a physician to explore the facts of a case, including verifying the truthfulness of the patient's account.

▶ CASE 3

An expectant mother finds out during the second trimester of her pregnancy that her baby has multiple congenital anomalies, including brain abnormalities, heart defects, and underdeveloped kidneys, leading to oligohydramnios and minimal lung development. She desires to continue the pregnancy but owing to continued severe fetal growth restriction and concern about very poor viability after birth, she is considering comfort care only and does not want resuscitation attempted. You are the pediatrician for this mother's other children, and she asks you to be the pediatrician in attendance at her repeat cesarean delivery.

Question 3-1

Which of the following is true?
A) The infant is an imperiled newborn and must receive full resuscitative efforts according to the "Baby Doe rules" in the 1984 Child Abuse Amendment.
B) Morphine cannot be given as a comfort medicine as it may suppress the infant's respiratory effort, leading to an earlier death.
C) If the infant receives a do not resuscitate (DNR) order after birth, then no treatments, such as oxygen by nasal cannula or mask, should be administered.
D) None of the above.

Discussion 3-1

The correct answer is "D." This infant has a series of congenital anomalies that are not consistent with being able to live a long life, even if resuscitation and other procedures were performed in the neonatal period. The 1984 Child Abuse Amendments were intended to prevent discrimination against infants with disabling disorders, such as trisomy 21, who had a serious illness, such as duodenal atresia, that was amenable to a straightforward surgical treatment with high likelihood of success. The concern was that interventions that could be lifesaving, and that would have been applied to otherwise healthy infants, were being withheld from these infants simply because of their disability. In contrast, exceptions are granted by these regulations for cases in which there is permanent unconsciousness, futile treatment, and virtually futile therapy that imposes excessive burdens of suffering on the infant. In the case described above, if prenatal evaluation remains consistent for multisystem organ dysfunction with little chance of survival, even with maximum resuscitation, this treatment can be said to be quantitatively futile in achieving its desired goals, and overly burdensome to the patient. Choosing a comfort care plan for an infant who is certain to have a limited life does not mean that no treatment or care will be provided. While a DNR order may be placed, that does not mean that medications or oxygen should not be offered if they may provide comfort. Morphine can be given for signs of pain or distressed breathing during the provision of comfort care at end of life. Although there is actually little evidence that appropriately titrated doses of morphine cause respiratory depression or hasten death, the principle of double effect is widely felt to justify the use of morphine for comfort even if there is a foreseeable but unintended effect, such as causing respiratory depression. The principle, doctrine, or rule, of double effect is a way of ethically evaluating an action that intends a good action, but also has a foreseeable, but unintended action that one would normally avoid. The conditions to evaluate the action are as follows: (1) The nature of the intended act must be morally good or neutral; (2) the bad effect must not be the means by which the good effect is achieved; (3) the intention must be the achieving of the good effect, with the bad effect an unintended effect; and (4) the good effect must be at least proportional in importance to the bad effect.

▶ CASE 4

A 4-year-old boy with cerebral palsy and a seizure disorder resulting from complications of prematurity has been admitted for his fourth episode of suspected aspiration pneumonia this year. He has chronic lung disease on bilevel positive airway pressure (BiPAP) at night and is gastrostomy-tube fed. He has currently been intubated for a week and attempts to wean the ventilator have not been successful. His mother feels he has been declining in condition over the past year and has had more discomfort from spasticity and seizures. She asked today to extubate the patient and change to a comfort care plan. The social worker contacts you as you have been a care provider for the patient over the past year. He is concerned that mother's request is based on the fact that his care has become too burdensome for her to manage at home.

Question 4-1

Which of the following would be the best first step in an ethical strategy to address this concern?

A) Recommend that an ethics consult be placed.
B) Ask the social worker to discuss long-term placement options with the mother.
C) Consult otolaryngology for placement of a tracheostomy.
D) Set up a time to talk with the mother about the boy's recent condition and her goals for his care.
E) Develop a comfort care plan and proceed with extubation.

Discussion 4-1

The correct answer is "D." Multiple studies have shown that the parents of children with chronic, complex illness want their physician to provide oversight of the long-term care plan and to treat the parents as the experts in their child's care by factoring in their views and concerns. One way to do this is to periodically review the child's condition and discuss the goals for their care. As a child's condition changes, the goals may shift from an emphasis on prolonging life and treating all reversible illnesses to prioritizing other goals, such as comfort, or remaining at home rather than making frequent trips to the hospital. This also gives the provider the opportunity to affirm the family's efforts and recognize unmet needs. Based on the goals identified in that conversation, a plan can be developed that may incorporate options "B," "C," or "E." It would be premature to recommend an ethics consultation before having had such a discussion, however, if persistent concerns about differences in moral values persist, an ethics consultation could be of value.

The child is eventually extubated, and is able to maintain saturations with spontaneous breathing. A DNR order is placed, as mother does not wish for resuscitation to be attempted due to concerns that it would cause harm and prolong a period of poor quality of life for him. The medical team is able to decrease his number of seizures and improve his spasticity so that he appears more comfortable. The surgeon who placed his gastrostomy tube recommends consideration of a fundoplication or surgical jejunostomy for feedings, to minimize aspiration.

Question 4-2

Which of the following would be the most ethical way to discuss the child's potential code status should he undergo an operation?

A) Inform the mother that she would have to request to change the child's code status to full code for the operation and for 30 days during the perioperative period.
B) Give the mother the option to keep the child's status DNR, but inform her that the anesthesiologist will not be able to keep him as sedated and comfortable during the procedure due to risk of sedation causing hemodynamic instability.
C) Inform the mother that the surgeon, anesthesiologist, and primary attending will discuss the risks and benefits of resuscitation, including specific procedures that they anticipate, with her to decide together how to best help the child.
D) Give mother the option to keep the child's status DNR but inform her that if the anesthesiologist or surgeon who is scheduled to do the procedure objects, he will not be able to have the operation.

Discussion 4-2

The correct answer is "C." The AAP recommends a process of "required reconsideration" that takes into consideration the goals of the patient and family and the specific interventions that could be performed during the procedure should the child's status deteriorate. The primary attending, surgeon, and anesthesiologist should inform the family about the likelihood that the child would require various resuscitative measures to be kept alive during the procedure, their chance of success, the likelihood of reversibility, and the possible outcomes. This should allow the family and medical team determine a plan that will best serve the individual child's needs. A family should not be required to agree to a full code status for a prescribed length of time. If the overall goal for the child is to promote comfort, then the sedation plan for the procedure should not be compromised in a way that would expose the child to discomfort. If a health care professional is unwilling to honor a family's refusal of resuscitation, he or she should withdraw from the case but make a conscientious effort to identify another physician who is willing to honor the DNR request.

▶ CASE 5

An infant was found apneic and pulseless in her crib. Her parents call 9-1-1 and she is resuscitated and transported to the pediatric intensive care unit (PICU). She remains unresponsive but will intermittently breathe over the ventilator. A diagnostic workup is performed to rule out an underlying treatable condition. During this time, she remains intubated and is receiving parental nutrition and hydration. No cause is identified. The infant remains unable to produce voluntary behaviors but does demonstrate sleep-wake cycles. Her parents want a gastrostomy tube for permanent feeding and a tracheostomy for permanent ventilatory support.

Question 5-1

Can the physician decline to perform these procedures?

A) Yes, because the patient is brain dead; thus treatment is medically futile.
B) Yes, because the patient is in a persistent vegetative state; thus treatment is medically futile.
C) No, because it is always a parents' right to determine what is best for the child.
D) No, because while the patient is in a persistent vegetative state, the procedures are not physiologically futile.
E) No, because while the patient is in a coma, the procedures are not physiologically futile.

Discussion 5-1

The correct answer is "D." In this case, the child is not brain dead as she is able to breathe over the ventilator at times and has sleep-wake cycles. She does meet the criteria for persistent vegetative state (PVS) as her brainstem is at least partially intact and she demonstrates sleep-wake cycles. Mechanical ventilation for a patient in PVS is not physiologically futile. Therefore, if the parents believe the child has an acceptable quality of life, a decision to provide mechanical ventilation or nutrition for the child must be respected. When determining futility, physicians must make sure to distinguish physiologic futility from our perception of the patient's quality of life (ie, qualitative futility). Strict physiologic futility means that an intervention would not achieve its intended immediate physiologic effect. The treatment simply would not work. Examples of strict physiologic futility include the use of antibiotics to cure a viral illness or cardiopulmonary resuscitation for a patient who has been pulseless for longer than 1 hour. Qualitative futility weighs the potential benefit of an intervention with the quality of its effects. Providers must recognize that our values and biases play a role in this determination and take into account that patients and families may weigh benefits and burdens differently. This is a situation that would warrant a palliative care consult or an ethics consult to discuss goals of care. If the child did meet brain death criteria, the medical team could not only refuse to perform the gastrostomy tube and tracheostomy, but also could withdraw ventilatory support without the parents' permission. However, there have been cases where parents have sought legal protection to continue life support, and courts have allowed their wishes to continue mechanical ventilation in cases of brain death. (See Table 12–1.)

TABLE 12–1 BRAIN DEATH CRITERIA IN CHILDREN

1. Coexistence of apnea and coma
2. Absence of brainstem function
3. Absence of hypotension for age or hypothermia
4. Flaccid muscle tone/absence of spontaneous movement (except spinal reflexes)
5. Observation and testing according to age
   a. 7 days to 2 months: 2 exams and electroencephalograms (EEGs) separated by 48 hours
   b. 2 months to 1 year: 2 exams and EEGs separated by 24 hours. However, 1 exam is acceptable if concomitant cerebral radionuclide study demonstrates no visualization of the cerebral arteries (ie, cerebral blood flow).
   c. Older than 1 year: If a known irreversible cause exists, an observation of at least 12 hours is recommended. At least 24 hours is recommended if it is difficult to assess the extent and reversibility of brain damage. However, the observation times can be reduced if EEG demonstrates electrocerebral silence *or* cerebral radionuclide study does not visualize cerebral arteries.

Data from Report of Special Task Force. Guidelines for the determination of brain death in children. American Academy of Pediatrics Task Force on Brain Death in Children. *Pediatrics.* 1987 Aug;80(2):298-300.

Helpful Tip

Brain death: Irreversible cessation of all functions of the entire brain, including the brainstem.

Coma: A state of deep, unarousable, sustained (> 1 hour) pathologic unconsciousness with the eyes closed, resulting from dysfunction of the ascending reticular activating system in either the brainstem or both cerebral hemispheres (thus lack of wakefulness and awareness).

Permanent vegetative state: Complete unawareness of self and the environment, with inability to produce purposeful/voluntary behavioral responses accompanied by sleep-wake cycles with either complete or partial preservation of hypothalamic and brainstem autonomic functions. Cranial nerves variably preserved.

Minimally conscious state: Severely altered consciousness in which minimal but definite behavioral evidence of self or environmental awareness is demonstrated

---

The infant undergoes gastrostomy tube and tracheostomy placement and is transferred to a chronic care facility. However, she subsequently develops a significant pneumonia, necessitating readmission to the PICU. She requires increasing ventilator settings and ultimately suffers bilateral pneumothoraxes. Her parents are worried that she is suffering and would like to discontinue all life-sustaining technologies. However, they have seen that she gets agitated at times and are concerned that she will be in pain when mechanical ventilation is discontinued.

Question 5-2

Is it appropriate to offer opioid medications for palliation in a terminally ill patient in whom life-sustaining technologies will be discontinued?

A) No, because it is illegal for a physician to expedite a pediatric patient's death regardless of the circumstances, and opioids have side effects that may do so in addition to alleviating pain.

B) No, because this family cannot choose to withdraw treatment once the treatment has been initiated.

C) Yes, because the medication would be administered with the intent to treat suffering and not to hasten death.

D) None of the above.

Discussion 5-2

The correct answer is "C." Managing pain, dyspnea, or agitation associated with a terminal illness usually requires the use of medications such as opioids that may have undesired respiratory or cardiovascular adverse effects. There is a clinical distinction informing what differentiates palliation from euthanasia. Palliation is defined as symptom-directed therapy aimed at improving quality of life, usually without curative intent. Euthanasia is defined as administration of medications to a patient with the intent of causing death. Palliation and euthanasia have some of the same goals. Both are ultimately spurred by the desire to relieve suffering. In palliation, the primary goal is to treat pain and symptoms, with an understanding that there is some chance that death may happen more quickly. With euthanasia, ending life is the means of ending suffering. In theory, the distinction should be clear. But in clinical practice, it can be harder to differentiate. Whether a physician intends to treat suffering or hasten death when medications are administered can be difficult to discern.

Question 5-3

Is it ever appropriate to withhold hydration or nutrition at the end of life?

A) Yes, because in certain patients who are actively dying it is unlikely that death would come any sooner for lack of nutrition.

B) No, because in some instances if the patient is not actively dying it may hasten death.

C) No, because it will cause the patient more suffering.

D) Both A and B.

Discussion 5-3

The correct answer is "D." Nutrition and hydration are like any other form of medical technology in that they can either be withheld or withdrawn in appropriate circumstances. Withholding feedings is reasonable when the goal is to diminish suffering; examples would be a patient who is actively dying, one who would require a procedure such as tube placement to receive artificial nutrition, or when feeding itself is actually causing suffering. For a patient who is clearly in the last hours or days of life, it is unlikely that death would come any sooner for lack of nutrition. However, in the case of a patient who is not actively dying and who tolerates supplemental nutrition, withholding it becomes more problematic because the sole intent of doing so may be to hasten death. Even though the time frame is different from that of a lethal injection, the end result is still determined by the action, and the only relief of suffering provided is through death itself.

▶ CASE 6

A 6-day-old infant is admitted to the general pediatrics service with fever and undergoes an evaluation for neonatal sepsis. After obtaining the appropriate studies and cultures, she is started on empiric antibiotics. Because the electronic medical record system is down, the resident handwrites the orders and sends them to the pharmacy. The order is misread, and the infant is given 10 times the requested dose of an antibiotic. She appears to have had no immediate adverse effects and is likely to have a full recovery.

Question 6-1

Should the error be disclosed to the parents?

A) No, as the patient has not been acutely harmed by the error, and the parents may lose trust in the physicians caring for their daughter.

B) Yes, but only if harm could arise later based on the antibiotic that was overdosed.

C) Yes, because studies show that parents of pediatric patients almost universally express a desire to receive information about medical errors.

D) Yes, because the principles of professionalism outlined by the American Board of Pediatrics (ABP) include honesty, integrity, reliability, and responsibility.

E) Both C and D.

Discussion 6-1

The correct answer is "E." The ABP's specific guidelines for teaching and evaluating professionalism include honesty and integrity, reliability and responsibility, respect for others, compassion/empathy, self-improvement, self-awareness/knowledge of limits, communication and collaboration, and altruism and advocacy. Honesty and integrity encompass the duty to be intellectually honest and straightforward in interactions with patients and peers in all professional communication. Thus, while it is true that no immediate harm has come upon the patient, it is part of the physician's professional responsibility to convey the error to the parents. While it is important to realize that complications may arise later that will be difficult to explain if the dosing error is not disclosed (ie, acute kidney injury from gentamicin toxicity), the potential for harm is not the primary factor to take into consideration when determining whether or not to disclose an error. Not surprisingly, when asked, adult patients and parents of pediatric patients almost universally express a desire to receive information about medical errors despite its unsettling nature. Further, a solid body of research shows that an overwhelming majority of surveyed physicians believe serious errors should be disclosed to patients and families.

Question 6-2

Should the physician offer an apology?

A) Yes, because it is reflective of your caring and kindness, and in most states cannot be used against you in a malpractice suit.

B) No, because it can be seen as an admission of fault and may ultimately be used against you in court.

C) Yes, but it may be useful to distinguish saying "I am sorry for what happened" from an apology that entails personal or institutional accountability for error.

D) No, because it is inappropriate to attract attention to a mistake that has not yet caused harm.

E) Both A and C.

Discussion 6-2

The correct answer is "E." It may seem like an obvious thing to do, but apologizing in medicine can be difficult given the possibility of future malpractice claims. Apology laws have been implemented in 36 states and are designed to allow professionals to offer words of condolence for adverse medical outcomes without the fear of being sued. In a study conducted by the University of Michigan Health System, faster settlement times and decreased payments by 47% were reported with the advent of its apology and disclosure agreement.

▶ CASE 7

A 17-year-old adolescent boy with cystic fibrosis is a patient in your pediatric practice. You first met him in the newborn nursery and have cared for him since. He is graduating high school in a few months and will be heading out of state for college. He comes in with his parents for a well adolescent physical. During the visit, they present you with a plaque commemorating your service to the community and a picture frame.

Question 7-1

Is it appropriate to accept this gift?

A) Yes, it is appropriate for a pediatrician to accept a modest gift from patients and/or their families.

B) No, it is not appropriate for a pediatrician to accept any gifts from patients and/or their families.

C) No, it is not appropriate for a pediatrician to accept any gifts from patients and/or their families unless it is part of a sanctioned awards benefit.

D) Yes, pediatricians may accept gifts from patients and/or their families, as it can be considered rude to reject them, even if the monetary value makes the physician uncomfortable.

Discussion 7-1

The correct answer is "A." Patients or parents sometimes give pediatricians gifts, especially after providing help for a complex or troubling health-related problem. Under most circumstances, gifts have a far more symbolic than material value. For most pediatricians, accepting modest gifts does not involve serious conflict; in fact, refusal of a gift may constitute a social or cultural affront. As the monetary worth of the gift increases, however, so does the psychological and ethical difficulty in maintaining appropriate boundaries in the professional relationship. When the pediatrician feels uncomfortable with a gift that a family insists on delivering, he or she must voice the concern and suggest acceptable alternatives, such as a charitable donation in the pediatrician's name. Highly valued gifts may indicate that these boundaries have been crossed and caution is urged when the material value of gifts or offered services could seem to influence the pediatrician's professional judgment. Furthermore, the pediatrician must be sensitive to the possibility that the intent of the gift is, in fact, to alter behavior.

Question 7-2

Is it ever acceptable for a pediatrician to treat his or her own children or the children of close family members or friends?

A) No, it represents a conflict of interests as it makes the physician more likely to lack objectivity, function with incomplete information, and have difficulty setting physician-patient boundaries.

B) No, because significant confidentiality issues may arise when caring for minor relatives and the children of close friends.

C) Yes, if limited to minor treatment and decisions, clear emergencies and disasters, or for pediatricians who practice in underserved areas in which there are no other physicians capable of providing pediatric care.

D) All of the above.

Discussion 7-2

The correct answer is "D." Pediatricians should know that caring for one's own children and caring for the minor children of relatives and close friends, particularly outside of the physician–patient relationship, presents significant ethical issues, including issues of confidentiality, and may lead to less-than-optimal medical care. Exceptions exist for treatment of minor conditions or during emergencies and disasters and in underserved areas in which alternatives are unavailable.

⧗ QUICK QUIZ

You have been summoned to provide expert witness testimony in a medical malpractice suit.

Which of the following is true regarding expert witness testimony?

A) A witness is presumed to be qualified if he or she has board certification in the relevant area, even if the witness is not engaged in clinical practice and no longer has a valid license to practice medicine.

B) After accepting the case, the witness should make sure to become an expert in the specialty involved so that he or she can describe the standards of care and acceptable treatment modalities relevant to a particular case.

C) The witness should assume that an identified breach in the standard of care caused the poor outcome for the patient.

D) The witness may be asked to testify about the current clinical state of the patient to assist in determining damage.

E) The witness will not need to help the jury distinguish between an adverse event caused by malpractice (negligent care) and an adverse event that happened for another reason maloccurrence.

Discussion

The correct answer is "D." In order to determine damages, an expert witness may be asked to provide information about the current state of the patient based on his or her review of the records. The AAP Policy Statement, Guidelines for Expert Witness Testimony in Medical Malpractice Litigation, outlines responsible practices that physicians should follow to safeguard their objectivity in preparing and presenting expert witness testimony (Committee on Medical Liability 2002). The policy recommends that physicians demonstrate the following qualifications to be considered to have genuine expertise: hold a current medical license, be certified by the relevant board, and be actively engaged in clinical practice, including knowledge of or experience in performing the skills and practices at issue in the lawsuit. Before accepting the case, the physician should be familiar with the medical standards of care so as not to introduce bias into his or her understanding if trying to become educated on the issues after knowing about the case. The witness should not assume that the breach in the standard of care caused the adverse event, but should provide unbiased and complete testimony in a fair and objective way. The witness may be asked to provide an opinion about whether the breach in care is the most likely cause of the injury. Part of the role of the expert witness is to help the jury distinguish between a bad outcome that occurred although reasonable care was provided and negligence that caused an adverse event.

▶ CASE 8

The mother of a 3-year-old child with trisomy 21 brings him in for a well-child check. You notice bruising on his upper arms, upper legs, and over the torso. He has petechiae on his face and neck. He weighs less today than at his 2-year visit, and he seems very fatigued during the visit.

Question 8-1

Which of the following is true?
A) Children with developmental disabilities are no more likely than the typically developing child to be the victim of maltreatment.
B) Physical discipline such as spanking is a reliable technique to speed the process of toilet training.
C) Intimate partner violence and child maltreatment are closely linked, and living with an adult victim of abuse increases the risk of physical abuse to the child.
D) There is profound disagreement among pediatricians about their role in screening for parental problems and providing anticipatory guidance that can help prevent child abuse.
E) Physical punishment is often indicated for behavior that is unacceptable to the parents, whether it is developmentally normal behavior or not.

Discussion 8-1

The correct answer is "C." In "The Pediatrician's Role in Child Maltreatment Prevention," Flaherty and colleagues report that the majority of pediatricians feel they should be screening for parenting problems and that anticipatory guidance can help prevent child abuse. Child maltreatment is closely linked to adult intimate partner violence. In addition to an increased risk of physical abuse, children with disabilities are affected emotionally, cognitively, and behaviorally. Children with disabilities are approximately three times more likely to be maltreated than those without disabilities. Toilet training is one of the trigger times for child maltreatment, including immersion burns and genital bruising. Physical punishment is not known to speed the process of toilet training but is commonly used by parents who feel that their children should be able to control soiling or enuresis. Physical punishment is not indicated as a means of discipline for behaviors of concern to parents, and parents often misinterpret developmentally normal behavior such as normal negativism and exploratory behavior as unacceptable misbehavior.

▶ CASE 9

A 9-year-old boy who is a patient in your practice was brought here from Ethiopia as an infant by his father. The boy's mother died from AIDS, and he was subsequently found to be HIV positive. He has been stable on antiretroviral therapy since then. His father has not told him that he is positive for HIV, and has been telling him that the antiretroviral tablets are "vitamins." Within the past year, the father stopped refilling his son's antiretroviral prescription, telling the infectious disease specialist that he felt "the medicine was not doing anything" and that "his son did not need it anymore." He refused to bring the boy to clinic to have his blood counts checked. A report was made to child protective services and the boy was placed in foster care so that he could continue receiving the antiretroviral medication.

Question 9-1

Which of the following is true?
A) The AAP recommends that adolescents should know their HIV status and strongly encourages disclosure to school-aged children.
B) Foster parents always have legal authority for medical decision making, so they can choose to tell the child about his HIV status whenever they want and have him decide whether or not he wants to continue treatment.
C) The boy's pediatrician is required to disclose his HIV status to him, regardless of what his father's wishes are.
D) A court order for the boy to continue receiving antiretroviral therapy makes it irrelevant whether he is made aware of his HIV status.
E) Children with chronic health conditions, including HIV, typically have better psychological outcomes when they are not informed about the nature and consequences of their illness.

Discussion 9-1

The correct answer is "A." The AAP recommends that adolescents should know their HIV status so that they can appreciate the consequences of many aspects of their health, including their sexual behavior and participation in treatment decisions. Physicians are encouraged to work with parents to make the disclosure in a way that is mutually acceptable, but they should not accept parental requests not to disclose under all circumstances. If an older child or adolescent asks directly, or if it becomes clear that disclosure of HIV status is important for the child or adolescent to make informed decisions about his or her health, then the physician should disclose. Option "B" is incorrect, as foster parents do not always gain legal authority for medical decision making. This is often retained by the parents or taken on by a guardian appointed by the state. It is also not likely to be appropriate to let a 9-year-old decide whether he wants to continue such a critical therapy unless there are significant burdens to the treatment. The child's pediatrician is not required to disclose his status to him at this age, but may be instrumental in helping his father or appointed guardian to recognize the benefits of sharing this information with the boy, and can help it to happen in a supportive environment at an ideal time. Having a court order for the boy to continue to receive antiretroviral therapy does not change the dynamics at play in providing him with the information about his chronic health condition. Studies have shown that children with chronic diseases had better coping skills and psychological outcomes when informed about what to expect during their illness.

► CASE 10

The parents of a 3-year-old boy with newly diagnosed acute lymphoblastic leukemia tell you that they plan to seek alternative care for their child rather than the recommended chemotherapy. They plan to take him to a practitioner in another state who is not affiliated with a recognized pediatric oncology center.

Question 10-1

If parents cite religious reasons for seeking alternative care, which of the following is true?

A) Parents have as much discretion to choose alternative care based on religious reasons for their child as they would for themselves.

B) Parents are expected to make decisions for their children based on the child's best interests unless it interferes with their religious beliefs.

C) Treatment is most likely to be mandated by the judicial system if the illness is life-threatening, the treatment is highly efficacious, and treatment has low side-effect burden.

D) Unless there is a court order, the physician may not intervene with therapy against parent's wishes even to prevent serious harm from occurring, such as death or severe disability.

E) The physician should report the parents to child protective services before attempting to educate them about the recommended treatment, as this is rarely successful in cases of religious reasons.

Discussion 10-1

The correct answer is "C." Infants and children are unable to make autonomous medical decisions; thus, their parents are expected to do this for them. The arrived-upon choice should reflect the child's best interests. While significant discretion in the interpretation of these interests should be allowed for, parents' choices may be limited when they ultimately pose a danger to the child. Family values are very much a part of a child's best interest; however, there are times when religion and medicine conflict. The courts have consistently ordered lifesaving medical treatment over parental religious objections, making option "B" incorrect. The U.S. Supreme Court famously stated, "Parents may be free to become martyrs themselves. But it does not follow they are free, in identical circumstances, to make martyrs of their children before they have reached the age of full and legal discretion when they can make that choice for themselves" (*Prince v Massachusetts*, 321 US 158, 170 [1944]). Thus, option "A" is incorrect. It would be inappropriate to report the parents to child protective services before attempting to educate them

about the recommended treatment. All parents need to be fully informed before they can consent (or dissent) for a treatment or procedure. Provided it is a non–life-threatening circumstance, if the parents continue to refuse treatment after the risks and benefits have been explained clearly it would be appropriate at that time to report the parents to child protective services and involve the judicial system. Although most circumstances in which parents refuse medical treatment for their children are not urgent and thus there is time to obtain a court order for treatment, sometimes the decision is emergent and comes down to life or death. In *HCA, Inc v Miller*, it was established that where the need for life-sustaining medical treatment is or becomes an emergency while a non–terminally ill child is under a physician's care, a court order is *not* necessary to override parental refusal.

Question 10-2

What if the child in question was an adolescent refusing treatment based on religious beliefs?

A) The adolescent can refuse life-saving treatment if deemed a mature minor by the courts.

B) The adolescent cannot refuse life-saving treatment, regardless of his or her perceived maturity, unless an emancipated minor.

C) The adolescent cannot refuse lifesaving treatment, even if he or she is considered an emancipated minor.

D) The adolescent can refuse treatment if both parent and child are in agreement about treatment refusal.

Discussion 10-2

The correct answer is "B." Some adolescents may possess adequate decision-making capacity to comprehend and evaluate the risks and benefits of medical treatment. The mature minor exception is an ethics-derived concept that reflects the belief widely accepted in pediatrics that, as a child grows and develops, his or her cognitive capacity increases substantially so that he or she may merit being treated as an autonomous decision maker. Interestingly, this exception is not reflected uniformly in the law. Fourteen states permit mature minors to consent to general medical treatment in either all or a restricted range of circumstances, and three states allow minors regardless of their age or maturity to consent to treatment in all or some circumstances. States' requirements for mature minor exceptions vary and comprise a combination of qualities, including age, ability to meet the informed consent standard (ie, capacity), maturity, and having graduated from high school. Patients are legally considered minors until the age of 18 years in most U.S. states, although some states have exceptions for emancipated minors. Emancipation occurs when something in the child's life—marriage, military enlistment, pregnancy—alters the relationship between the child and parents and supersedes the parent–child relationship. In these circumstances, the possibility of coercion should also be considered in the evaluation of whether a capacitated adolescent's dissent is autonomous.

Question 10-3

Would it matter if the parents were Christian Scientists and they were refusing a treatment because consent would violate their religious belief (in contrast with a nonreligious belief such as naturopathy)?

A) No, the standard remains the same whether the parents' reason for refusing an intervention arises from religion, culture, or some other source.

B) No, because parents cannot decline medical treatment that is recommended by a physician.

C) Yes, because the Constitution provides for freedom of religion.

D) Yes, because treatment refusal is considered child neglect unless the treatment is refuted secondary to established religious doctrine.

Discussion 10-3

The correct answer is "A." It is important to recognize that our reasons for interfering with parental decision making are not because the parents have a religious belief but because their decision places a child at substantial risk of serious harm. That standard remains the same whether the parents' reason for refusing an intervention arises from religion, culture, or some other source. The Constitution requires that the government not interfere with religious practice or endorse particular religions. The government also has an interest in protecting children and innocent third parties.

> **Helpful Tip**
>
> Ask yourself these questions to determine whether state interference with parental decision making is justified:
>
> - By refusing treatment, is there significant risk to the child?
> - Is the risk imminent, requiring immediate action to prevent it?
> - Is the intervention that has been refused necessary to prevent the harm?
> - Does the refused intervention have proven efficacy to prevent the harm?
> - Is the refused intervention safe?
> - Is there another option to prevent serious harm?
> - Can the state intervention be generalized to all other similar situations?
> - Would most parents agree that the state intervention was reasonable?

Question 10-4

All of the following should be considered as part of the process to work through an ethical conflict about care based on religious beliefs EXCEPT:

A) If possible, anticipate conflict and take steps to prevent it, such as using a surgical technique that involves minimal blood loss for a patient who is a Jehovah's Witness.

B) Ask for more information about the religious belief system if you are not familiar with it

C) Request help from a hospital chaplain or spiritual services provider, or an ethics consult if available, in situations where there seems to be an impasse.

D) Inform the parents that they may not request advice from a spiritual leader in their faith tradition about health care decisions.

E) Pursue a court order for treatment if the child would likely experience severe harm without receiving treatment.

Discussion 10-4

The correct answer is "D."

▶ CASE 11

You are taking care of a 15-year-old boy who presented with hepatosplenomegaly and abdominal pain, but no other symptoms. He is active in sports, but struggles with academics. In consultation with the genetics service, you send a panel of tests that returns positive for Niemann-Pick disease. When you call the parents and ask them to come in for the results, they come to your office without their son, stating that they did not want to take him out of school. You give them information about the diagnosis and allow them to ask questions, and tell them about referrals to specialists that you plan to make. The parents state that they do not want you to tell their son about his diagnosis as they want to learn more about it themselves before telling him. You recommend that the adolescent refrain from playing contact sports due to his persistent hepatosplenomegaly. Several months later, he comes in for a sports physical. His mother asks to speak to you privately, and tells you that they have decided not to tell him about the specific diagnosis. They want him to enjoy the present, and ask for you to sign his sports physical form so that he can play soccer. You find out that they have not taken their son to see the specialists you referred him to.

Question 11-1

Which of the following is true?

A) The adolescent is a mature minor and so you may tell him his diagnosis and counsel him independently, regardless of his parents' preferences.

B) If you counsel the adolescent's parents about the risks of playing sports with hepatosplenomegaly and they still want you to give him permission to engage in sports, you are obligated to sign the sports physical form.

C) Obtaining a pediatric ethics consult would be appropriate in this situation.

D) Both A and C.

E) All of the above.

Discussion 11-1

The correct answer is "C." The AAP in conjunction with the American College of Medical Genetics and Genomics has written a policy statement on genetic testing and screening of children. The policy specifically indicates that at the time of genetic testing, parents or guardians should be encouraged to inform their child of the test results at an appropriate age. They should also be advised that, under most circumstances, a request by a mature adolescent for test results should be honored. It is unclear whether this pretest counseling occurred in this scenario. Regardless, option "A" is incorrect, because the adolescent has not actually requested the test results, so you are not necessarily obligated to tell him. It is also questionable as to whether he would qualify as a mature minor. States' requirements for mature minor exceptions vary and comprise a combination of qualities, including age, ability to meet the informed consent standard (ie, capacity), maturity, and having graduated from high school. Given this adolescent's underlying condition and noted poor academic performance, depending on his state's interpretation of the mature minor statute, he may not qualify. Option "B" is also inappropriate. Although the adolescent's parents can ultimately accept the risks of his participation in sports, it is the duty of the physician to do no harm to the patient, and the physician is legally obligated to report on medical conditions accurately. An ethics consult would be appropriate in this context for a few reasons. Rather than being simply a mechanism for implementing federal regulations about treatment of disabled infants and children, ethics committees help resolve conflicts about treatment decisions through case consultation, provide a forum for discussion of policies relating to institutional ethics, and educate their health care communities about ethical concepts. They may also be used when problems of communication seem to be impeding patient care. In this case, a lack of effective communication with the parents is impeding patient care. Additionally, the ethics committee should be able to facilitate a discussion about institutional policies (ie, pretest genetic counseling) as well as educate other physicians who may be performing genetic testing about appropriate counseling.

▶ CASE 12

A 5-year-old boy has recently been diagnosed with Duchene muscular dystrophy (DMD). After learning more about the diagnosis, including the fact that female carriers have an increased risk of developing cardiomyopathies, his parents approach their physician, and ask for testing for his 3-year-old brother and 16-year-old sister.

Question 12-1

Which of the following is the best response?

A) Neither of the siblings should be tested at this time. His brother should be tested only if he develops symptoms.

B) His brother should be tested now and his sister should be tested so that she knows if she is a carrier prior to making decisions about reproduction.

C) His brother should be tested now, but testing for his sister should be deferred until she is over 18 years old and can make the decision about testing herself.

D) His brother may be tested now or only if he develops symptoms, and his sister may be tested if she gives assent.

E) His brother should not be tested unless he develops symptoms, but his sister should be tested, whether or not she is willing to give assent.

Discussion 12-1

The correct answer is "D." In a child with symptoms of a genetic condition, the rationale for genetic testing is similar to that of other medical diagnostic evaluations. Parents or guardians should be informed about the risks and benefits of testing, and their permission should be obtained. Ideally and when appropriate, the assent of the child should be obtained. Parents or guardians may authorize predictive genetic testing for asymptomatic children at risk of childhood-onset conditions. Ideally, the assent of the child should be obtained. In this case, the 3-year-old brother is too young to give assent, but testing is still warranted for him as DMD is a childhood-onset condition. Thus, option "E" is incorrect. The AAP and American College of Medical Genetics and Genomics (ACMG) do not support routine carrier testing in minors when such testing does not provide health benefits in childhood. Arguably, this is not routine carrier testing, as the AAP recommends that all carriers should have an ECG and echocardiogram at least every 5 years, starting at age 25 or 30. So, if the boy's sister assented to testing, it would be appropriate to perform the testing now. Additionally, if the 16-year-old sister were a manifesting carrier (ie, had muscle, joint, or cardiac symptoms currently), her parents could request testing now. For pregnant adolescents or for adolescents considering reproduction, genetic testing and screening should be offered as clinically indicated, and the risks and benefits should be explained clearly.

Question 12-2

Which of the following is the best answer about the ethics of genetic screening?

A) Offering newborn screening should not be mandatory so that physicians can decide if it would be in a particular infant's best interest.

B) Parents should not have the right to refuse newborn screening due to the potential harm to the child if a treatable disorder is missed.

C) Potential risks of genetic screening include discovery of misattributed parentage, emotional distress, and distortion of parental expectations.

D) Routine carrier status screening is recommended for conditions even if the status will have no relevancy during childhood.

E) When carrier status is discovered during newborn screening, the results should be withheld until the child reaches the age of majority.

Discussion 12-2

The correct answer is "C." There are risks inherent to genetic screening, and many of them are psychosocial or emotional in nature. Other risks can occur if parents pursue unproven treatments, particularly if they have adverse side effects. The AAP and the ACMG both support the mandatory offering of newborn screening for all children, but feel that parents should have the option of refusing the procedure, and an informed refusal should be respected. Therefore, options "A" and "B" are incorrect. Newborn screening may identify carriers for recessive conditions, such as cystic fibrosis, hemoglobinopathies, and galactosemia. In some cases, this information may have potential medical relevance during childhood or adolescence. As an example, sickle cell trait has been shown to increase the risk of exercise-related splenic infarct and exertional rhabdomyolysis. In any case, the information about carrier status is felt to belong to the child, and the parents are the appropriate surrogates to receive that information, so option "E" is incorrect. In contrast, it is not recommended to pursue screening or testing for carrier status of conditions in which the carrier status has no medical relevance during childhood or adolescence, so option "D" is incorrect.

▶ CASE 13

The parents of a normally developing 10-year-old boy approach you about a referral for growth hormone treatment for their son. The father feels that his own short stature inhibited his ability to participate competitively in sports at the high school and college level. He tells you that he does not want his son to be hindered by his short status. James has been tracking at around the fifth percentile for height for the past 5 years, and has had a normal workup. He is considered to have idiopathic short stature.

Question 13-1

Which of the following is true?

A) If the parents have seen commercials extolling the benefits of growth hormone to improve athletic ability for short children, this indicates that the therapy is generally acceptable to the public and should be supported by the physician.
B) There is concern that unrestricted use of enhancement therapies such as growth hormone would cause social justice conflicts due to inaccessibility of the treatment to low-income and disadvantaged children.
C) There is overwhelming evidence that short stature is a cause of psychological distress that causes limitations for individuals, and that gaining a few inches in height increases quality of life for people treated with growth hormone.
D) As long as the parents have insurance coverage or are willing to pay for the treatment out of pocket, rather than seek reimbursement from public funding, there is no concern about justice related to resource allocation.
E) There is no difference between providing treatments to replace what no longer functions well due to a medical diagnosis and providing treatments to exceed initial limitations and make the body or mind function "better than well."

Discussion 13-1

The correct answer is "B." One of the overarching concerns about enhancement therapies is that due to cost, they are typically inaccessible to low-income families. This creates a social justice concern that those who are already disadvantaged will potentially be subjected to further discrimination. There is also a distributive

justice argument based on the resource allocation issue. Should health care dollars be funneled toward a few inches of height for a select few, or would they be better spent to improve health in areas that are of more widespread concern, such as obesity or malnutrition? Option "A" is incorrect, as the content of direct-to-consumer advertisements should not be accepted as an ethical justification for supporting a particular treatment. Although some studies have suggested population differences in short and tall groups with regard to access to income, academic achievement, self-esteem, and social status, recent studies have not shown a relation between adult height and quality of life (reviewed in the following: American Academy of Pediatrics Committee on Drugs and Committee on Bioethics 1997; Allen and Fost 2004; Gill 2006). The primary goals of medicine are to prevent illness and support healing and recuperation to normal function and ability. Treatments such as performance-enhancing substances that are designed to make the patient "better than well" are considered to be nontherapeutic. There is a difference between providing treatments that are therapeutic in nature and those that are nontherapeutic. Typically, when considering nontherapeutic use, the provider must have an even higher level of concern for the safety profile of the treatment as well as the ethics of utilization.

The 10-year-old has also been having some difficulty with performance in school. He has been evaluated for attention deficit disorder within the past few months and does not meet criteria. He was also assessed for learning disabilities, and nothing of concern was noted. His teacher reports that he is an average student but is not particularly efficient during his study time and is quickly discouraged when he does not understand a new concept easily. The teacher recommends some behavioral modifications to his study time at home, along with some focused attention in the classroom. His mother brings him in to see you and reminds you that she was diagnosed with attention deficit disorder as an adult. She finds that she is able to concentrate better at her job since being started on amphetamines. She asks for a trial of amphetamine treatment for her son, to see if it will help him to do better in school.

Question 13-2

Which of the following would NOT be part of an initial appropriate response?

A) Agree to start a trial of an amphetamine as long as the mother and teacher agree to fill out attention deficit disorder diagnostic rating scales before and during treatment.
B) Support his teacher's approach of study time behavioral modifications and schedule a follow-up to assess how the plan is working.
C) Suggest that he be reassessed for attention deficit disorder again in the future if he does not show improvement with behavioral strategies.
D) Discuss side effects and other risks of amphetamines (such as potential for abuse and addiction) with his mother.
E) Encourage his mother to be accepting of his baseline ability and explain the potential dangers of trying to enhance his cognitive ability with medication.

Discussion 13-2

The correct answer is "A." If the boy has not met criteria for attention deficit disorder, it is not appropriate to initiate treatment with amphetamines at this time despite the request of his mother. It is appropriate to support his teacher's plan of behavioral modification, and to follow up to see how his performance in school is changing. Maintaining a relationship with his mother is important to decrease the likelihood that she will turn elsewhere to try to get him the medication she thinks will help him. Discussing the risks and side effects of the medication she is requesting can help her to be more informed on the topic. Encouraging parents to be accepting of their children's abilities and explaining the potential harms of medical enhancements are ways that pediatricians can provide the best possible care for their patients.

▶ CASE 14

You are the pediatrician assuming care for a family that recently moved into your community. The 5-year-old child has congenital deafness, and the mother is also deaf. Throughout the visit, you and the mother converse using the father as a sign language interpreter. The father and the two other children have no hearing impairments. The father is interested in pursuing cochlear implants for the child, but the mother is adamantly against this. She views them as an "enhancement" and feels it will exclude the child from the deaf community.

Question 14-1

How should you approach this situation?

A) Explain to the mother that it is your responsibility to ensure that the child's best interests are upheld and that it would be ethically inappropriate to deny the child the chance to hear.

B) Present the family with outcome-based data on cochlear implants and allow them to decide whether to pursue cochlear implants for the child.

C) Avoid making any recommendations at this point, as you just met this family and should not interfere in their decision-making process.

D) None of the above.

Discussion 14-1

The correct answer is "B." Cochlear implants were first introduced in 1957, and the technology has continued to advance. In 1990, the Food and Drug Administration (FDA) approved the use of cochlear implants for children over age 2 years. This decision was deplored by the National Association of the Deaf (NAD) for several reasons. First, the NAD saw deafness as a cultural and linguistic minority and felt that it was not appropriate to use scientific tools to modify a child into the majority, even if that might reduce the burdens the child will bear. Additionally, the NAD was worried about outcomes. Early studies showed that many children who received cochlear implants continued to have poor language acquisition and to do poorly in school, likely secondary to later acquisition and fluency in American Sign Language. Later studies showed that outcomes were variable and that while some children who receive implants do well in the hearing world, most continue to require special assistance or use sign language along with spoken language. Thus, option "A" is incorrect. Cochlear implants are not definitively in a child's best interest, as the data show that most children still in fact need assistance after receiving cochlear implants. Also, one must take into account the child's developing sense of identity and culture. The deaf community has its characteristic language, history, and values. The child who is allowed to remain deaf can learn a sign language and ultimately become part of a live cultural and linguistic minority group. The child using a cochlear implant is only nominally within the hearing culture, and may be condemned to be an outsider by the deaf community, which frowns on those who attempt to be "oral." Option "C" is inappropriate as the parents are clearly at discord in terms of treatment for their child, and they depend on physicians to give them objective information to help them make decisions.

BIBLIOGRAPHY

Allen DB, Fost N. hGH for short stature: Ethical issues raised by expanded access. *J Pediatrics*. 2004;144(5):648–652.

American Academy of Pediatrics Committee on Bioethics. Ethics and the care of critically ill infants and children. *Pediatrics*. 1996;98(1):149–152.

American Academy of Pediatrics Committee on Bioethics. Informed consent, parental permission and assent in pediatric practice. *Pediatrics* 1995;95:314–317.

American Academy of Pediatrics Committee on Bioethics. Professionalism in pediatrics: Statement of principles. *Pediatrics*. 2007;120(4):895–897.

American Academy of Pediatrics Committee on Drugs and Committee on Bioethics. Considerations related to the use of recombinant human growth hormone in children. *Pediatrics*. 1997;99(1):122–129.

American Academy of Pediatrics Committee on Pediatric AIDS. Disclosure of illness status to children and adolescents with HIV infection. *Pediatrics*. 1999;103(1):164–166.

American Academy of Pediatrics Section on Cardiovascular and Cardiac Surgery, et al. Cardiovascular health supervision for individuals affected by Duchenne or Becker muscular dystrophy. *Pediatrics*. 2005;116(6):1569–1573.

Benson R, Pinnaro C. Autonomy and autism: Who speaks for the adolescent patient? *AMA J Ethics*. 2015;17(4):305–309.

Bernat JL. Medical futility: Definition, determination, and disputes in critical care. *NCC Neurocrit Care*. 2005;2(2):198–205.

Boothroyd A, Grodin M. Auditory capacity of hearing-impaired children using hearing aids and cochlear implants: Issues of efficacy and assessment. *Scand Audiol Suppl*. 1997;46:17–25

Carter BS, Jones PM. Evidence-based comfort care for neonates towards the end of life. *Semin Fetal Neonatal Med*. 2013;18(2):88–92.

Chan JD, Treece PD, Engelberg RA, et al. Narcotic and benzodiazepine use after withdrawal of life support: Association with time to death? *Chest*. 2004;126(1):286–293.

Coleman DL, Rosoff PM. The legal authority of mature minors to consent to general medical treatment. *Pediatrics*. 2013;131(4):786–793.

Committee on Bioethics. Conflicts between religious or spiritual beliefs and pediatric care: Informed refusal, exemptions, and public funding. *Pediatrics*. 2013;132(5):962–965.

Committee on Bioethics. Policy statement—Pediatrician-family-patient relationships: Managing the boundaries. *Pediatrics*. 2009;124(6):1685–1688.

Committee on Bioethics; Committee on Genetics; American College of Medical Genetics and Genomics; Committee on Social, Ethical, and Legal Issues. Ethical and policy issues in genetic testing and screening of children. *Pediatrics*. 2013;131(3):620–622.

Committee on Medical Liability, American Academy of Pediatrics. Guidelines for expert witness testimony in medical malpractice litigation. *Pediatrics*. 2002;109(5):974–979.

Cornell University Law School Legal Information Institute. Emancipation of minors. http://www.law.cornell.edu/wex/emancipation_of_minors.

Diekema DS. Session 2. Religious, cultural, and philosophical objections to care. *American Academy of Pediatrics Bioethics Resident Curriculum: Case-Based Teaching Guides*, 1995:11–17.

Diekema DS. What is left of futility? The convergence of anencephaly and the Emergency Medical Treatment and Active Labor Act. *Arch Pediatr Adolesc Med*. 1995;149(10):1156–1159.

Eisen MD. Djourno, Eyries, and the first implanted electrical neural stimulator to restore hearing. *Otol Neurotol*. 2003;24(3):500–506

Emanuel EJ. The assent requirement in pediatric research. In: *The Oxford Textbook of Clinical Research Ethics*. Chap 60. Oxford: Oxford UP, 2008.

Fallat ME, Deshpande JK; American Academy of Pediatrics Section on Surgery, Section on Anesthesia and Pain Medicine, and Committee on Bioethics. Do-not-resuscitate orders for pediatric patients who require anesthesia and surgery. *Pediatrics* 2004;114(6):1686–1692.

Flaherty EG, Stirling J Jr; American Academy of Pediatrics; Committee on Child Abuse and Neglect. The pediatrician's role in child maltreatment prevention. *Pediatrics*. 2010;126(4):833–841.

Gathings JT Jr. When rights clash: The conflict between a parent's right to free exercise of religion versus his child's right to life. *Cumberland Law Rev*. 1988–1989;19(3):585–616

Gill DG. "Anything you can do, I can do bigger?": The ethics and equity of growth hormone for small normal children. *Arch Dis Child*. 2006;91(3):270–272.

Guichon J, Mitchell I. Medical emergencies in children of orthodox Jehovah's Witness families: Three recent legal cases, ethical issues and proposals for management. *Paediatr Child Health (Oxford)*. 2006;11(10):655–658

Institutional ethics committees. *Pediatrics*. 2001;107(1):205–209.

Lantos JD. Ethics for the pediatrician: The evolving ethics of cochlear implants in children. *Pediatr Rev*. 2012;33(7):323–326

Lee J. Cochlear implantation, enhancements, transhumanism and posthumanism: Some human questions. *Sci Eng Ethics*. 2015 May 12. [EPub ahead of print]

Levetown M; American Academy of Pediatrics Committee on Bioethics. Communicating with children and families: From everyday interactions to skill in conveying distressing information. *Pediatrics*. 2008;121(5):e1441–e1460.

Matlow AG, Moody L, Laxer R, Stevens P, Goia C, Friedman JN. Disclosure of medical error to parents and paediatric patients: Assessment of parents' attitudes and influencing factors. *Arch Dis Child*. 2009: n. pag. Web.

National Agenda. Moving forward on achieving educational equality for deaf and hard of hearing students. April 2005.

National Association of the Deaf. Cochlear implants in children: A position paper of the National Association of the Deaf. *NAD Broadcaster*. 1991;13(1):1

Saitta N, Hodge SD. Efficacy of a physician's words of empathy: An overview of state apology laws. *J Am Osteopath Assoc*. 2012;112(5):302–306.

Sigman GS, O'Connor C. Exploration for physicians of the mature minor doctrine. *J Pediatr*. 1991;119:520–525.

Trahan J. Constitutional law: Parental denial of a child's medical treatment for religious reasons. *Annu Surv Am Law*. 1989(1):307–341

University of Michigan Health Systems. Full disclosure of medical errors reduces malpractice claims and claim costs for health systems. *Innovations Exchange*. June 23, 2010.

Woods M. Overriding parental decision to withhold treatment. *Virtual Mentor*. 2003;5(8).

Eye Disorders

13

Melanie Schmitt and Judith Sabah

▶ CASE 1

An Asian-American mother brings her 2-month-old daughter to your office for a routine well-child visit. The mother is concerned because her daughter's eyes do not appear to be working together and turn in at times. On exam, the infant gives occasional smiles. Her weight and height have increased appropriately, and she has no apparent neurologic signs.

Question 1-1

What should you tell the mother?

A) The infant needs to be referred to a pediatric ophthalmologist for surgery.
B) Do not worry, as eye coordination does not occur until 4 to 5 months of age.
C) The infant might have an intracranial mass and needs magnetic resonance imaging (MRI).
D) The infant needs to be referred to a pediatric neurologist.
E) None of the above.

Discussion 1-1

The correct answer is "B." The visual system continues to mature after birth, including the vergence system, which allows coordination of vergence movements (ie, when the two eyes move together to track visual stimuli). Infants may exhibit some degree of intermittent esotropia (eye turning in) or exotropia (eye turning out) up to the fifth month of life. It is reasonable to observe the child until this age before obtaining a second opinion from a pediatric ophthalmologist. However, constant strabismus is never normal and should be promptly investigated.

At 6 months of age, the mother brings her daughter back for another routine visit. All is well, except for her eyes. Mom remains concerned that her daughter's eyes continue to turn in. On exam, you agree that both eyes appear to be turned in.

You use your penlight to examine the corneal light reflex. Both reflexes fall in the center of the pupil.

Question 1-2

What is the most likely diagnosis?

A) Pseudostrabismus.
B) Right esotropia.
C) Left exotropia.
D) Alternating esotropia.
E) Alternating exotropia.

Discussion 1-2

The correct answer is "A." Infants with a broad, flat nasal bridge or redundant upper eyelid skin, also known as prominent epicanthal folds, can falsely appear to have in-turned eyes. This pseudostrabismus is more common in infants of Asian and Hispanic descent. The best way to quickly check ocular alignment is by using the corneal light reflex. The infant's eyes are normally aligned if the corneal light reflex falls in the center of each pupil. A child with pseudostrabismus is at higher risk of developing true strabismus as he or she grows older and should be monitored by a pediatric ophthalmologist.

> **Helpful Tip**
>
> Children with a history of retinopathy of prematurity, inherited retinal disorders, or congenital ocular infections (eg, toxoplasmosis) may exhibit pseudostrabismus. These conditions can cause temporal dragging of the fovea, which is the part of the retina in charge of central vision. The ectopically located fovea results in the eyes turning "outward" in order to fixate with the "displaced" fovea. This creates the illusion of exotropia and is termed *pseudoexotropia*. When the cover tests are performed, there is lack of eye movement, contrary to what would be expected with a true exotropia.

► **CASE 2**

A mother with a history of high hyperopia and strabismus asks you if she should have her 8-month-old son evaluated by a pediatric ophthalmologist. The mother has not noticed any eye deviation, which is confirmed on your examination.

Question 2-1

What should your advice be to this mother?
A) Your son's eyes are straight; do not worry, we can observe.
B) Due to your family history of strabismus and high hyperopia, we should refer him to a pediatric ophthalmologist.
C) If your son's eyes have not started deviating by now, he will be fine.
D) We can wait another 2 years before referring your son.
E) None of the above.

Discussion 2-1

The correct answer is "B." Strabismus and high hyperopia (farsightedness) can be familial and with a positive family history, the child should be evaluated. If an obvious deviation is noticed, then immediate referral should be made. In an infant with no obvious strabismus, referral should be made by 1 year of age. Some patients with high hyperopia may not develop strabismus, which is characteristically esotropia, until later in childhood. However, being able to identify these patients early on may prevent the development of possible complications such as amblyopia, or reduced vision. Large-angle deviations should be surgically treated before 24 months of age to allow for the development of binocular motor and sensory function. Nevertheless, the patient should be referred as soon as a deviation is observed. This allows for the early detection and treatment of amblyopia and refractive error. Both glasses and patching therapy can eliminate or decrease an abnormal ocular deviation and may lead to a better surgical outcome if surgery is still necessary.

> **Helpful Tip**
> A child with an abnormal red reflex should be referred urgently to a pediatric ophthalmologist. A white pupillary reflex (leukocoria) with either esotropia or exotropia may represent sensory strabismus, in which deprivation of vision in that eye has led to its drifting. But, keep in mind the differential diagnosis of an abnormal pupillary reflex is extensive. Examples include cataract, retinoblastoma, Coats disease, persistent fetal vasculature, retinal detachment, toxocara, and amblyopia (where the brighter reflex is observed in the amblyopic and deviated eye), to name a few.

Question 2-2

In which of the following situations would urgent neuroimaging be warranted?
A) A 2-year-old girl with a worsening esotropia despite wearing her hyperopic glasses.
B) A 5-month-old boy with a large-angle esotropia.
C) A 4-year-old with a sudden onset of esotropia and limited outward movement of the left eye.
D) A 4-year-old with a history of intermittent esotropia, worsening per mother.
E) A 4-year-old with a new exotropia.

Discussion 2-2

The correct answer is "C." The acute onset of strabismus and limited extraocular motility is concerning for an intracranial process. The sudden onset of esotropia may reflect an acute case of ipsilateral cranial nerve sixth palsy. Hydrocephalus, Arnold-Chiari malformation, intracranial neoplasm, meningitis, cavernous sinus lesions, or trauma are potential causes of a cranial nerve sixth palsy in children. An MRI scan of the brain and orbit with and without contrast should be ordered on an urgent basis. Worsening esotropia in a patient with known history of infantile strabismus, hyperopia, or intermittent esotropia may be an indication for surgery and is not suggestive of an intracranial process.

► **CASE 3**

A mother brings her 8-year-old son for an urgent visit. Her son recently developed "giggly" eyes in conjunction with headaches. On exam, the child is afebrile and you observe eye movements reminding you of a playground seesaw. As one eye rolls in and down, the other eye rises up and out.

Question 3-1

What is the best next step in management?
A) Order an urgent neurology consult.
B) Order an urgent ophthalmology consult.
C) Reassure the mother, because this is likely related to a viral illness and will resolve on its own.
D) Order an urgent MRI scan.
E) Prescribe an antibiotic and follow up in 1 week.

Discussion 3-1

The correct answer is "D." Any acquired nystagmus in a previously well child is concerning for an intracranial process and warrants urgent imaging. Contrast is necessary and special attention should be given to the areas of the suprasellar cistern and posterior fossa. There is one form of acquired nystagmus, called latent nystagmus, which does not require imaging. Patients with latent nystagmus have a history of strabismus, and the nystagmus is observed only when one eye is covered. There are different forms of nystagmus with varying etiologies. Congenital motor nystagmus (CMN), a common cause of infantile nystagmus, is present by 6 months of life and is benign. CMN is not caused by a known ocular or intracranial abnormality; the underlying etiology is idiopathic. Patients usually have good vision, in the 20/40 range, and their nystagmus is dampened by convergence (looking at an object up close), which often leads to esotropia. Because CMN is a benign condition, imaging is not required. Ocular conditions that cause poor vision may be associated with nystagmus due to poor sensory input.

These conditions include congenital cataracts, congenital glaucoma, congenital toxoplasmosis, retinal colobomas, bilateral optic nerve hypoplasia or atrophy, optic nerve colobomas, aniridia (foveal hypoplasia), retinal dystrophies, retinoblastoma, and retinopathy of prematurity. Spasmus nutans is the triad of nystagmus, head nodding, and torticollis, or abnormal neck position. It is an acquired process and usually occurs in the first 2 years of life, resolving by age 3 to 4. Rarely, spasmus nutans has been associated with intracranial lesions. As a result, most clinicians advocate for systematic neuroimaging of these patients. Seesaw nystagmus is associated with a lesion in the rostral midbrain or the suprasellar area, most commonly a craniopharyngioma. Convergence-retraction nystagmus is part of the dorsal midbrain syndrome, defined by paralysis of upward gaze, defective convergence, eyelid retraction, and pupillary-light dissociation. When trying to look up, the eyes jerk irregularly, turn toward the nose, and sink into the socket. This type of nystagmus is associated with aqueductal stenosis or pinealoma. Opsoclonus is very rare and is not a true nystagmus. Rather, it is a bizarre, rapid, and involuntary ocular oscillation. It is usually postinfectious or a paraneoplastic manifestation of occult neuroblastoma. Remember, opsoclonus myoclonus ("dancing eyes, dancing feet") should immediately make you think neuroblastoma. Downbeat nystagmus, when congenital, is usually benign and transient but if acquired, is associated with Arnold-Chiari malformation. Upbeat nystagmus is mild in primary position but worsens in upgaze. It can be seen in patients with multiple sclerosis, cerebellar diseases, or brainstem tumors. Just like downbeat nystagmus, it may be benign when congenital and be transient in normal infants. For those who are not budding ophthalmologists, the take-home point is that acquired nystagmus equals urgent head imaging.

▶ CASE 4

You are seeing a 4-day-old infant for a weight check after discharge from the hospital. The mother had suboptimal prenatal care, and her overall health is not well known. The delivery was uneventful. The newborn's exam is pertinent for low-grade fever and some lethargy leading to poor feeding. In addition, bilateral hyperpurulent discharge, lid swelling, and conjunctival chemosis are present.

Question 4-1

What is the most likely etiologic agent of this case of ophthalmia neonatorum?
A) Herpes simplex virus.
B) Chemical.
C) *Neisseria gonorrhoeae*.
D) *Chlamydia trachomatis*.
E) Adenovirus.

Discussion 4-1

The correct answer is "C." Chemical conjunctivitis causes a mild, self-limited irritation and redness of the conjunctiva, usually within the first 24 hours after instillation of silver nitrate.

In developed countries, silver nitrate has largely been replaced by erythromycin to prevent this potential side effect. Ophthalmia neonatorum caused by *N. gonorrhoeae* has an onset typically in the first 3 to 4 days of life but may be delayed for up to 3 weeks. Affected infants present with conjunctival hyperemia and discharge, which can be severe. Gram stain, showing gram-negative diplococci, and cultures should be obtained. The patient must be admitted for systemic antibiotics and be closely monitored, as rapid corneal deterioration may occur, with ulcer development and subsequent perforation. The patient should be tested for HIV, *Chlamydia trachomatis*, and syphilis. The onset of *C. trachomatis* is usually around 1 week of age but can be earlier in cases of premature rupture of membranes. Palpebral conjunctival scraping is necessary for diagnosis in order to isolate the obligate intracellular organism. Systemic antibiotics are also required due to the risk of pneumonia. Herpes simplex virus is a less common form of ophthalmia neonatorum and typically presents around 2 weeks of age. Adenovirus is not associated with ophthalmia neonatorum.

> **Helpful Tip**
> Infections with *N. gonorrhoeae* or *C. trachomatis* are usually associated with ophthalmia neonatorum. However, if either is the causative agent in a child with conjunctivitis, sexual abuse should be suspected.

▶ CASE 5

A mother brings her 2-year-old daughter to your office to evaluate left eye irritation and redness of several months' duration. On closer examination, you notice multiple umbilicated skin lesions on the left lower lid.

Question 5-1

What is the best next step?
A) Ophthalmology referral for incision and debridement of the central core of each lesion.
B) Artificial tears.
C) Oral acyclovir.
D) Observation.
E) Topical ophthalmic antibiotic.

Discussion 5-1

The correct answer is "A." The patient has the classic lesions of molluscum contagiosum, which is a DNA poxvirus. If lesions are within close proximity of the lid margin, viral particle release onto the conjunctival surface may trigger a chronic follicular conjunctivitis. In this situation, the treatment of choice is complete excision of the lesions. Otherwise, if the patient is asymptomatic, observation is appropriate and resolution often occurs spontaneously. Cryotherapy and cautery are not recommended as they can lead to skin depigmentation and eyelash loss. The peak incidence is between 2 and 4 years of age. Atopic or immunocompromised patients can present with diffuse

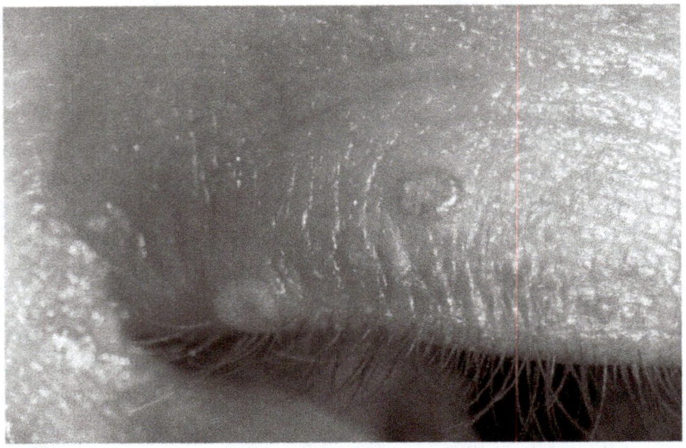

FIGURE 13–1. Molluscum contagiosum is a viral infection of the skin caused by a DNA poxvirus. Look for umbilicated (central depression like an umbilicus) flesh-colored papules. Lesions close to the lash line can cause a chronic follicular conjunctivitis. (Reproduced with permission from Riordan-Eva P, Cunningham ET, eds. *Vaughan & Asbury's General Ophthalmology.* 18th ed. New York, NY: McGraw-Hill Education; 2011, Fig. 5-12.)

lesions present throughout the body. If the patient presents with extensive lesions in the absence of immunosuppressive therapy (eg, transplant history), cancer, or atopy, HIV testing should be strongly considered. (See Figure 13–1.)

Question 5-2

Which of the following forms of conjunctivitis is usually associated with a systemic disease?

A) Parinaud oculoglandular syndrome.
B) Vernal or atopic keratoconjunctivitis.
C) Oculocutaneous conjunctivitis.
D) Blepharoconjunctivitis.
E) All of the above.

Discussion 5-2

The correct answer is "E." Option "A" is also known as "catscratch disease," which can occur after being licked, bitten, or scratched by a cat. It is associated with fever and preauricular or submandibular adenopathy. The treatment is supportive in mild cases or may require the use of azithromycin, doxycycline, or ciprofloxacin in severe cases. Vernal and atopic keratoconjunctivitis are associated with seasonal and perennial allergies, respectively. In addition to topical ophthalmic treatment, a systemic antihistamine and mast cell stabilizer are often need to control symptoms. Vernal keratoconjunctivitis is more prevalent in males, typically presents in the first decade of life, and most often subsides by the late teens. Oculocutaneous conjunctivitis refers to conjunctivitis associated with Stevens-Johnson syndrome/toxic epidermal necrolysis, graft-versus-host disease, or varicella-zoster virus. Blepharoconjunctivitis is a common disorder in all age groups and affects the eyelid margin with or without obvious inflammation. One cause of blepharoconjunctivitis is rosacea, which is more prevalent in adults than children. Rosacea is a systemic disease characterized by overactive sebaceous glands.

> **Helpful Tip**
> Another systemic disease that can be associated with conjunctivitis is infectious mononucleosis ("mono"), which usually occur between 15 and 30 years of age. In addition to fever, widespread lymphadenopathy, and pharyngitis, the patient can present with conjunctivitis and keratitis (inflammation of the cornea). The treatment of the ophthalmic complications is supportive. Lastly, patients with Kawasaki disease can present with bilateral conjunctival injection.

▶ CASE 6

A 3-year-old girl is brought to your clinic by her mother, who is concerned about her daughter's worsening eye redness, tearing, and lid swelling of 1 month's duration. Per parental history, the girl is a constant eye rubber. On exam, in addition to the ocular findings described by the mother, you notice some mild scaly skin inside the elbows and on the upper eyelids. The patient's past medical history is also significant for a nut allergy.

Question 6-1

What is the most likely diagnosis?

A) Ocular rosacea.
B) Viral conjunctivitis.
C) Bacterial conjunctivitis.
D) Molluscum contagiosum.
E) Atopic conjunctivitis.

Discussion 6-1

The correct answer is "E." The patient has several signs pointing to atopic conjunctivitis. She has scaly skin at locations typical for atopic dermatitis (eczema). Her persistent eye rubbing is another indicator and may be secondary chronic papillary conjunctivitis. In addition, she has a history of nut allergy, which is common in atopic patients. The distinction between allergic and infectious conjunctivitis mostly comes from the history. Patients with allergic conjunctivitis often have seasonal symptoms or have other systemic findings consistent with allergies (either annual or perennial). Infectious conjunctivitis is usually acute, self-limited, and associated with mucopurulent or purulent discharge, whereas, allergic conjunctivitis is chronic, recurrent, and associated with clear discharge. It is common for patients with allergic conjunctivitis to have shiners under their eyes. Infectious processes may or may not be associated with fever, otitis media, or upper respiratory infections, which would not be the case in a patient with an allergic conjunctivitis.

Question 6-2

What is most appropriate management of infectious conjunctivitis?

A) Observation.
B) Oral antibiotics.

C) Cool compresses.
D) Topical ophthalmic antibiotics, cool compresses, good hand hygiene, and limit contact with others for 10 days.
E) Good hand hygiene.

Discussion 6-2

The most appropriate answer is "D." It can be very difficult to differentiate between bacterial and viral conjunctivitis as they both can present with mucopurulent discharge, hyperemia, and lid swelling. Both bacterial and viral conjunctivitis are self-limited and resolve without treatment within 2 weeks, typically without complications. However, use of a topical ophthalmic antibiotic, in the case of bacterial conjunctivitis, will decrease symptoms duration to 2 to 4 days (from 7 to 10 days). A culture is rarely obtained unless resolution does not occur after 2 weeks or there is a history of recurrent disease. A bacterial conjunctivitis would most often be associated with otitis media or sinusitis, whereas a viral conjunctivitis is commonly caused by an upper respiratory infection. When the etiology is in doubt, one should prescribe broad-spectrum topical ophthalmic antibiotics in order to treat the causative agent. Cool compresses, good hand hygiene, and limiting contact with others while infectious (around 10 days) is advised in cases of infectious conjunctivitis. Endemic keratoconjunctivitis is a class of conjunctivitis caused by a group of adenoviruses (types 8, 19, and 37) that is highly contagious. It is usually associated with preauricular lymphadenopathy and is particularly infectious (Table 13–1).

> **Helpful Tip**
> Herpetic corneal disease can be diagnosed clinically by conjunctivitis, eye pain, light sensitivity, and fluorescein eye drops. Under cobalt blue light, corneal herpetic dendrites are visible after staining with green fluorescein dye. Oral acyclovir is the treatment of choice in children.

QUICK QUIZ

What is the most common microorganism associated with bacterial conjunctivitis in school-aged children?
A) *Neisseria gonorrhoeae.*
B) *Chlamydia trachomatis.*
C) *Streptococcus pneumoniae.*
D) *Enterococcus* species.
E) *Clostridium perfringens.*

TABLE 13–1 SUMMARY OF THE MAIN TYPES OF CONJUNCTIVITIS

Type of Conjunctivitis	Distinctive Signs	Age of Onset	Treatment
Bacterial[a]	Mucopurulent or purulent discharge. Cat scratch disease is usually also associated with preauricular and submandibular lymphadenopathy.	Any	Topical broad-spectrum antibiotic (trimethoprim/polymyxin) except for *N. gonorrhoeae* or *C. trachomatis*, which are treated systemically with ceftriaxone or doxycycline/azithromycin, respectively. Doxycycline should only be administered in children older than 8 years of age. Cat scratch disease can be observed if mild; more severe cases may be treated with azithromycin, doxycycline, or ciprofloxacin.
Viral	Clear or mucopurulent discharge. If herpetic corneal disease is present the typical dendrite may be observed with cobalt blue light with fluorescein staining.	Any age except for molluscum contagiosum, which peaks at 2 to 4 years of age	Supportive, cool compresses. May have to use topical antibiotic in cases of severe epidemic keratoconjunctivitis associated with corneal epithelial defects. Herpetic disease is treated with oral acyclovir. Molluscum contagiosum should be treated with incision and debridement of the lesion core.
Atopic/vernal	Large conjunctival papillae mostly under the superior tarsus (seen eyelid eversion). Presence of shiners under the eyes. Patients with atopic disease often have scaly skin on the eyelids.	Preponderance in males. Typically occurs in the first decade of life.	Systemic and topical antihistamine and mast cell stabilizer. Recurrent/recalcitrant disease may necessitate the use of topical steroids, which should be done under the supervision of an ophthalmologist to monitor the intraocular pressure.

[a]Special Considerations: If the etiologic agent is *Neisseria gonorrhoeae* or *Chlamydia trachomatis,* it is recommended to check the patient for other sexually transmitted diseases and for sexual abuse, depending on the age.

Discussion

The correct answer is "C." The most common microorganisms associated with bacterial conjunctivitis include *S. pneumoniae*, *Moraxella catarrhalis*, and, to a lesser extent, *Haemophilus influenzae* type B due to widespread immunization. These bacteria mirror the causative agents of sinusitis. In terms of viral conjunctivitis, the most common etiology is adenovirus.

► CASE 7

A mother brings her 4-year-old son to your office due to the acute onset of right eyelid swelling and redness. The swelling started about 2 days ago and is worsening. The patient was wrestling with his brother 3 days prior and scratched the outside corner of his right eye. He is afebrile and denies any pain. On exam, the right upper and lower eyelids are swollen and erythematous. There is a healing scar at the lateral border of his right upper eyelid. Both eyes have intact extraocular movements. His pupils are round and reactive with no relative afferent pupillary defect. The conjunctiva is white and quiet. On vision testing, the patient sees 20/25 out of each eye. Mom reports putting some petroleum jelly (Vaseline) on the scar to try to help it feel better.

Question 7-1

What is the most likely diagnosis?
A) Idiopathic orbital inflammation.
B) Orbital cellulitis.
C) Stevens-Johnson syndrome.
D) Preseptal cellulitis.
E) Atopic conjunctivitis.

Discussion 7-1

The correct answer is "D." The patient shows classic signs of preseptal (sometimes called periorbital) cellulitis. Unlike cases of orbital cellulitis, the patient is typically free of pain with normal eye movements, and shows no evidence of proptosis, inflammation of the globe (ie, no conjunctival chemosis or injection), or pupillary involvement. Children suffering from an orbital cellulitis are usually febrile, lethargic, and systemically unwell. Preseptal cellulitis is located anterior to the septum, which is a dense fibrous sheath that acts as a barrier between the orbit and eyelids. Three main pathways can lead to preseptal cellulitis. Inoculation following trauma or skin infection, direct spread from adjacent sinusitis or dacryocystitis, or bacteremic spread from a distant focus may precipitate cellulitis. Currently, the most common agents causative of preseptal cellulitis include *Streptococcus pneumonia*, other streptococcal species, and *Staphylococcus aureus*. (See Figures 13–2 and 13–3.)

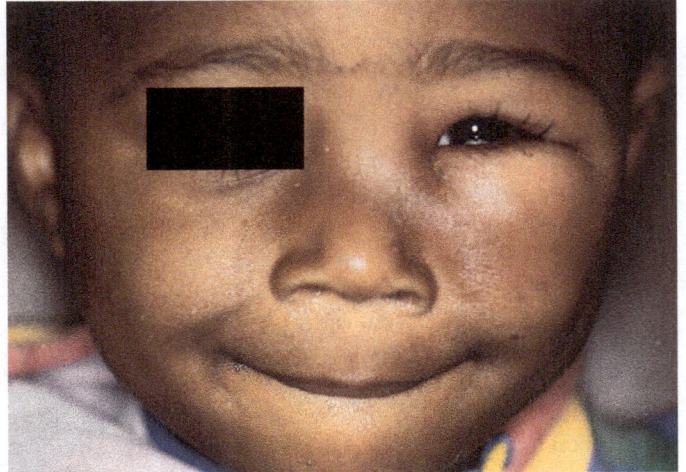

FIGURE 13–2. Preseptal or periorbital cellulitis is an infection of the soft tissues around the eye. The left eye has swollen, erythematous eyelids but the conjunctiva is clear. (Reproduced with permission from Knoop KJ, Stack LB, Storrow AB, Thurman RJ (Eds). *The Atlas of Emergency Medicine*, 3ed. McGraw-Hill Education, Inc., 2010. Photo contributor: Kevin J. Knoop, MD, MS. Fig 14-46.)

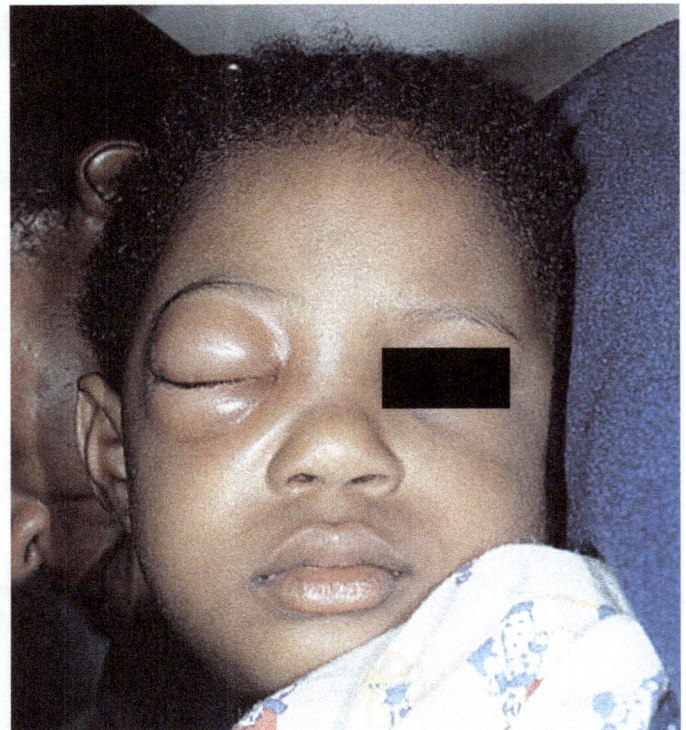

FIGURE 13–3. Orbital cellulitis is an infection of the globe that is typically a complication of ethmoid sinusitis. It must be distinguished from preseptal cellulitis. The right eye is swollen, erythematous, and proptotic. Proptosis is the clue that this is orbital cellulitis. (Reproduced with permission from Shah BR, Lucchesi M. *Atlas of Pediatric Emergency Medicine*. New York, NY: McGraw-Hill; 2006, Fig. 8-14.)

Since the child appears to have mild to moderate preseptal cellulitis, you decide to treat him with oral antibiotics on an outpatient basis. You send him home on amoxicillin and clavulanic acid and tell the mother to bring him back in 2 days. Three days later when they actually return, and the mother reports that the patient would not take the oral medication. His right eyelid is now completely closed secondary to the excessive swelling. He is also febrile now.

Question 7-2

What is the next best course of action?
A) Continue to encourage oral antibiotics and send the patient home.
B) Change oral antibiotics and have them come back in 2 days.
C) Admit the child for computed tomography (CT) of the brain and orbits, cultures, and intravenous antibiotics.
D) Refer the child to an ophthalmologist for drainage of the lid.
E) Admit the child to the hospital for oral antibiotics to ensure compliance.

Discussion 7-2

The correct answer is "C." The patient is noncompliant with treatment, has worsening of symptoms, and is now febrile. He has developed subsequent orbital cellulitis. Imaging will detect the presence of an abscess and determine the extent of the infection (ie, orbital versus preseptal). In a patient with a history of trauma, imaging can also help rule out a foreign body. The culture results may dictate antibiotic coverage especially in cases of resistant microorganisms. In more than 90% of cases, orbital cellulitis occurs secondary to sinusitis, most commonly due to direct extension from the ethmoid sinus. It can also evolve from a complicated preseptal cellulitis, dacryocystitis, or dental infection. Exogenous etiologies include trauma or periorbital or orbital surgery. Orbital cellulitis can also be secondary to intraorbital causes such as endophthalmitis or an endogenous cause such as bacteremia. Orbital cellulitis warrants hospital admission for intravenous antibiotics.

Question 7-3

What is the most common microorganism involved in orbital cellulitis in young children?
A) Gram-negative bacteria.
B) Anaerobic bacteria.
C) Gram-positive cocci.
D) Fungi.
E) Parasites.

Discussion 7-3

The correct answer is "C." The common etiologic agents in orbital cellulitis vary by age. In children younger than 9 years of age, the infection is usually from a single aerobic pathogen, most commonly a gram-positive coccus (*Staphylococcus aureus, Streptococcus pyogenes, Streptococcus pneumoniae,* or *Streptococcus sanguinis*). In children older than 9 years, multiple pathogens can be involved leading to complex infections, involving both aerobic and anaerobic microorganisms. These include *S. aureus, S. pyogenes, S. pneumoniae, M. catarrhalis,* and various anaerobic species. Gram-negative organisms excluding *M. catarrhalis* are mostly found in immunosuppressed patients. Fungal infections are rare but can occur in immunocompromised and diabetic patients. Patients with cystic fibrosis are likely to be infected with *Pseudomonas aeruginosa* or *S. aureus*. Remember *S. aureus* can be either methicillin sensitive or resistant (MSSA or MRSA).

Question 7-4

What is the preferred imaging modality for an orbital infection?
A) MRI.
B) CT scan.
C) Ultrasound.
D) X-ray.
E) Positron emission tomography (PET) scan.

Discussion 7-4

The correct answer is "B." In uncomplicated cases of preseptal cellulitis imaging is generally not needed; these patients may be treated on an outpatient basis with oral antibiotics and close follow-up. If an adequate assessment cannot be performed, for example due to excessive lid swelling, or if the patient is failing oral antibiotics, then imaging is warranted to assess for possible abscess and the extent of involvement (orbital or not). CT is the modality of choice. Although MRI has the advantage of lacking radiation exposure, CT can be obtained quickly and often without sedation. MRI is superior in detecting intracranial complications, such as cavernous sinus thrombosis, and may be obtained secondarily.

Question 7-5

What are the possible complications of orbital cellulitis?
A) Orbital abscess.
B) Subperiosteal abscess.
C) Cavernous sinus thrombosis.
D) Subdural and brain abscess.
E) All of the above.

Discussion 7-5

The correct answer is "E." An abscess should be suspected if there is treatment failure on intravenous antibiotics, worsening proptosis, or globe displacement. Since most orbital cellulitis is secondary to sinusitis, the abscess usually localizes to the subperiosteal space adjacent to the infected sinus. It may also extend through the periosteum into the orbital soft tissues. Not all subperiosteal orbital abscesses necessitate surgical drainage and certain criteria will guide the ophthalmologist and otolaryngologist (ENT) in determining the surgical plan. Orbital infections rarely spread to the cavernous sinus. However, if it occurs, cavernous sinus thrombosis will be characterized by the rapid progression of proptosis, the development of ipsilateral ophthalmoplegia (eye muscle paralysis), and the onset of anesthesia in both the first and second divisions of the trigeminal nerve. Early on cranial nerve VI may be affected with lateral rectus palsy. Rarely, the ophthalmoplegia can spread to the contralateral eye and is virtually diagnostic of cavernous sinus thrombosis. Meningitis and frank brain abscess may also develop. (See Table 13–2.)

> **Helpful Tip**
> Nasal decongestants, such as ephedrine, can help promote intranasal drainage of infected sinuses.

> **Helpful Tip**
> Orbital cellulitis is an emergency that is vision threatening. Distinguishing features from preseptal cellulitis are (1) painful extraocular movements, (2) ophthalmoplegia, (3) vision changes, and (4) proptosis. Both cause eyelid erythema and swelling. If in doubt, order a CT scan.

► CASE 8

A 4-year-old girl presents with a history of a nodule on the right upper lid. It has been present for 2 weeks. The skin over the nodule is mildly erythematous. The child denies any pain. You also notice some scurf on the lashes of both eyes. The girls' mother has a history of rosacea.

Question 8-1

What is the most likely diagnosis?
A) Chalazion.
B) Molluscum contagiosum.
C) Stye.
D) Rhabdomyosarcoma.
E) Capillary hemangioma.

Discussion 8-1

The correct answer is "A." Chalazia are lipogranulomatous inflammations resulting from obstruction of the meibomian

TABLE 13–2 COMPARISON OF CHARACTERISTICS IN PRESEPTAL AND ORBITAL CELLULITIS

	Preseptal Cellulitis	Orbital Cellulitis
Signs and symptoms	Eyelid swelling	Eyelid swelling, fever, proptosis, painful eye movements, chemosis
CT findings	If ordered, sinusitis may be present	Sinusitis, mild soft tissue changes in the orbit
Organisms involved	*Staphylococcus aureus, Streptococcus pneumoniae*	< 9 years old: single organism. *S. aureus, S. pyogenes, S. pneumoniae, S. sanguinis,* and *M. catarrhalis* > 9 years old: multiple aerobic (as above) and anaerobic agents
Etiology	1. Trauma (puncture, laceration, abrasion of eyelid skin) 2. Severe conjunctivitis (atopic, epidemic keratoconjunctivitis), skin infection (impetigo, zoster) 3. URI with sinusitis	1. Extension from periorbital structures (sinuses, face and eyelids, lacrimal sac, teeth) 2. Exogenous causes (trauma, surgery) 3. Endogenous causes (bacteremia with septic embolization) 4. Intraorbital causes (endophthalmitis, dacryoadenitis)
Management	Mild–moderate: outpatient basis, oral antibiotics with close follow-up Severe: admission with IV antibiotics	Admission with IV antibiotics
Complications	Develops into orbital cellulitis	Abscess (subperiosteal, orbit, subdural, brain), cavernous sinus thrombosis, meningitis, death

IV, intravenous; URI, upper respiratory tract infection.

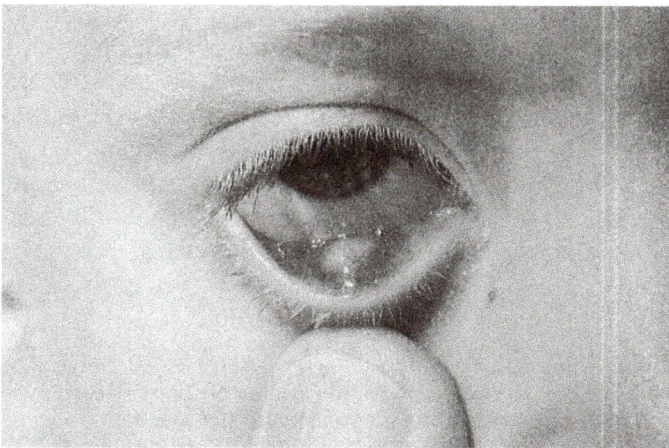

A

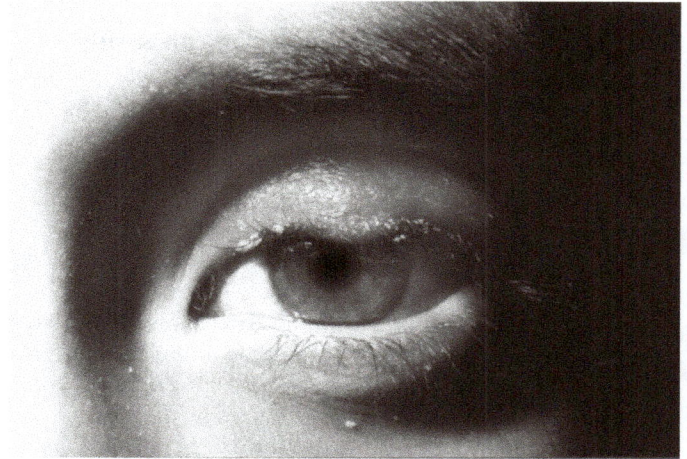

B

FIGURE 13–4. A chalazion develops when a meibomian gland in the eyelid becomes obstructed resulting in the formation of a chronic inflammatory lesion. On the eyelid, a rubbery nodule develops. Unlike a hordeolum (stye), a chalazion is noninfectious, chronic, and nontender. (Reproduced with permission from Hay WW, Levin MJ, Deterding RR, Abzug MJ, eds. *Current Diagnosis and Treatment Pediatrics*. 22nd ed. New York, NY: McGraw-Hill Education; 2014, Fig. 16-11A, B.)

glands, which are modified sebaceous glands. Chalazia are non-infectious in nature. In contrast, a stye (hordeolum) is a painful acute infection often caused by *Staphylococcus aureus.* An external hordeolum involves the glands of Zeis or Molls gland, while an internal hordeolum affects the meibomian glands. The meibomian glands are located in the tarsus, which is more posterior in location. The glands of Zeis are located at the base of eyelash hair follicles and therefore more anterior. Distinguishing clinically between a chalazia and stye can be difficult. Both can be associated with rosacea, which is a disease affecting the sebaceous glands. (See Figures 13–4 and 13–5.)

You advise the girl's mother to proceed with eyelid hygiene procedures, including warm compresses three times a day for 5 to 10 minutes, followed by eyelid scrubs for 1 to 2 minutes. You also recommend a flaxseed oil supplement. You explain that dietary supplementation with omega fatty acids is used

FIGURE 13–5. A hordeolum (stye) is an acute painful infection of the glands of Zeis or Molls gland (external hordeolum) or meibomian glands (internal hordeolum). Unlike a chalazion, a hordeolum is acute, painful, and infectious. The upper lid hordeolum in this picture also has associated blepharitis. (Reproduced with permission from Hay WW, Levin MJ, Deterding RR, Abzug MJ, eds. *Current Diagnosis and Treatment Pediatrics*. 22nd ed. New York, NY: McGraw-Hill Education; 2014, Fig. 16-12.)

to treat meibomian gland dysfunction. A follow-up visit is scheduled in 6 weeks. When the mother brings her daughter back for follow-up, the lesion is larger and there are additional lesions on the lower lid.

Question 8-2
What is the best next step in management?
A) Oral tetracycline.
B) Topical ophthalmic antibiotic–steroid combination.
C) Artificial tears.
D) Oral steroid.
E) Admit the patient for intravenous antibiotics.

Discussion 8-2
The correct answer is "B." Chalazia being an inflammatory process, if conservative management fails, one can try a short course of topical ophthalmic steroid ointment. Usually, the ointment is a mixture of antibiotic and steroid compounds. It can be applied twice a day for 2 weeks, in addition to continuing eyelid hygiene measures. If no improvement occurs, then incision and drainage is usually recommended. As a follow-up question, how would one get a 4-year-old to eat flaxseed oil? That sticker chart would need handsome prizes.

> **Helpful Tip**
> Tetracyclines should not be prescribed for children before their adult teeth are in place to prevent staining. Also, do not prescribe topical steroids without the supervision of an ophthalmologist as their chronic use could lead to increased intraocular pressure, which could cause an optic neuropathy with visual field losses.

Question 8-3

How would you manage a stye (hordeolum) differently?

A) Immediate admission for intravenous antibiotics.
B) Conservative management with warm compresses and eye-lid scrubs.
C) Oral antibiotics.
D) Oral steroids.
E) Proceed directly with incision and drainage.

Discussion 8-3

The correct answer is "B." Although the etiology of a stye is infectious, the initial management is similar to that for a chalazion (ie, conservative management). A course of topical antibiotic ointment may help decrease the size of the lesion and relieve some of the discomfort. Larger lesions or abscesses may require systemic antibiotic or incision and drainage. Rarely, true preseptal cellulitis can arise from a stye.

> **Helpful Tip**
> As in all young children, a lid lesion can be a cause of amblyopia by distorting the globe or partially occluding the visual axis and should not be overlooked.

▶ CASE 9

A 14-month-old girl is brought to your office. Her mother reports tearing from both eyes, which is more noticeable on the left side, since birth. The discharge is usually clear but worsens with upper respiratory infections (URIs), becoming thicker and yellowish-green. During a URI, the lid may also appear mildly swollen and red. The eyes are otherwise white and quiet, and the child is not particularly light sensitive.

Question 9-1

What is the most likely diagnosis?

A) Chronic conjunctivitis.
B) Glaucoma.
C) Congenital nasolacrimal duct (NLD) obstruction.
D) Preseptal cellulitis.
E) Epiblepharon.

Discussion 9-1

The correct answer is "C." All of the listed options are possible causes of epiphora (excessive tearing), except option "D." In this patient, the symptoms are bilateral, worse with an upper respiratory infection, and have been present since birth. Congenital NLD obstruction (dacryostenosis) occurs in about 5% of the full-term newborns and is typically bilateral. The discharge is usually clear or mucoid, except at times of URI when it becomes more mucopurulent. Crusting of the eyelashes is common. With chronic epiphora, the skin around the eye can become

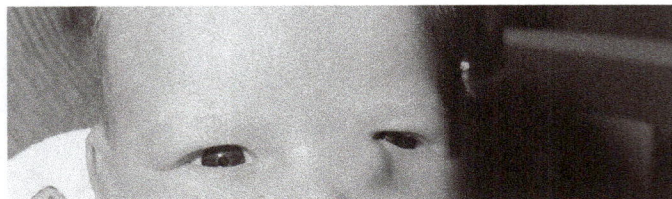

A

B

FIGURE 13–6. Nasolacrimal duct obstruction: (A) a large dacrocystocele from congenital obstruction of the left nasolacrimal duct; (B) the characteristic appearance of a draining dacrocystocele with mattering on both the upper and lower lids. (Reproduced with permission from Hay WW, Levin MJ, Deterding RR, Abzug MJ, eds. *Current Diagnosis and Treatment Pediatrics.* 22nd ed. New York, NY: McGraw-Hill Education; 2014.)

red and excoriated and resemble contact dermatitis. Unlike primary congenital glaucoma, there is a lack of light sensitivity, no blepharospasm, and the conjunctiva is usually white and quiet. If you suspect glaucoma, the infant or child needs to be seen emergently by a pediatric ophthalmologist for treatment. Saving vision is very important. (See Figures 13–6 through 13–8.) Kudos if you knew that an epiblepharon is an extra skinfold along the lower lash margin that may cause in-turning of the eyelashes.

> **Helpful Tip**
> A simple dye disappearance test can be done in clinic by instilling a drop of fluorescein in the affected eye and looking at the tear film with a blue cobalt light. Significant retention after 5 to 10 minutes is suggestive of a nasolacrimal system obstruction. Look for blue drainage from the ipsilateral nostril. Not only will you know that the duct is open but others may think you are a magician.

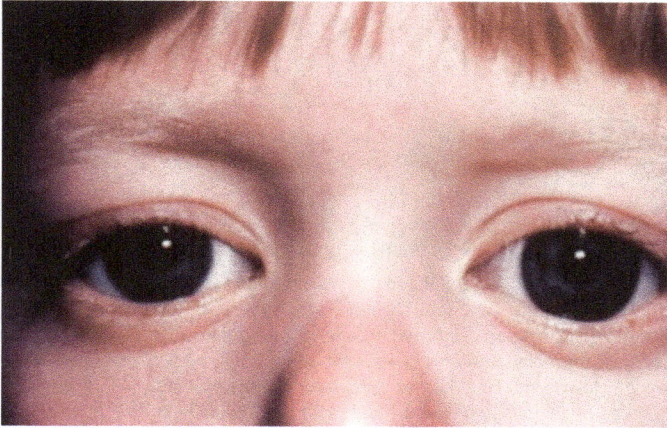

FIGURE 13–7. Primary congenital glaucoma usually presents in the first year of life. Symptoms include tearing, photophobia, and blepharospasm. Look for the following on exam: (1) enlarged, cloudy cornea; (2) injected conjunctiva; (3) tearing; (4) optic nerve cupping; and (5) enlargement of the eye (buphthalmos). If glaucoma is present or suspected, immediately refer the patient to a pediatric ophthalmologist. (Reproduced with permission from Riordan-Eva P, Cunningham ET, eds. *Vaughan & Asbury's General Ophthalmology*. 18th ed. New York, NY: McGraw-Hill Education; 2011, Fig. 11-10.)

FIGURE 13–8. A 3-year-old with primary congenital glaucoma of her left eye. Notice that the eye looks bigger (increased cornea diameter) and has increased tears. (Used with permission from the University of Iowa and EyeRounds.org.)

Helpful Tip
If the child presents with mucopurulent discharge but no other signs of infection suggestive of preseptal cellulitis, especially in the instance of a concomitant URI, a broad-spectrum topical antibiotic such as trimethoprim/polymyxin (Polytrim) can be administered for 4 to 5 days. The chronic use of topical antibiotic is usually not recommended. The dermatitis around the eye can be treated with an ointment combining an antibiotic and steroid, such as sulfacetamide/prednisolone (Blephamide) or neomycin/polymyxin B/dexamethasone (Maxitrol), for a similar duration.

Question 9-2

How should you manage this child?

A) Oral antibiotics.

B) Refer to a pediatric ophthalmologist for surgical management.

C) Crigler massages.

D) Topical ophthalmic antibiotics.

E) Reassurance and observation.

Discussion 9-2

The correct answer is "B." The natural history of congenital NLD obstruction is spontaneous resolution by 12 months of life in up to 80% to 90% of the cases. A short course of topical broad-spectrum antibiotic can be used if a secondary infection is suspected, especially a concomitant URI. Beyond the age of 1 year, most pediatric ophthalmologists will perform NLD probing and irrigation with or without stenting. However, some may advocate further observation until 24 months. If the patient presents during the first year of life, Crigler massages (NLD massages) are recommended. The caretaker is instructed to apply his or her finger in the nasal corner of the eye at the level of the caruncle (fleshy tissue in the inner eye corner) and to apply pressure while sliding the finger downward along the nasal wall 2 to 3 times a day.

Helpful Tip
A raised bluish lesion located just *below and nasal* to the medial canthus (corner of the eye) present at birth is highly suggestive of a *congenital dacryocystocele*. It is caused by trapped fluid (amniotic fluid) inside the nasolacrimal system. A dacryocystocele may be observed during the first week of life and often resolves spontaneously with the help of Crigler massages (nasolacrimal duct [NLD] massages). Past that time period, referral to a pediatric ophthalmologist is recommended for intervention. This would entail probing the NLD system in order to decompress the dacryocystocele. If associated erythema is noted on the overlying skin, an infection or acute dacryocystitis is likely also present. In that case, the newborn should receive systemic antibiotics followed by surgical probing. Any difficulty breathing when feeding or in the presence of a dacryocystocele could be a sign of a concurrent *nasal mucocele* (intranasal extension of the NLD cyst) for which an otolaryngology referral is imperative. A raised lesion *above* the medial canthus is more typical of a nasofrontal *encephalocele*, and neurosurgery should be then consulted. (See Figures 13–9 and 13–10.)

▶ CASE 10

A mother brings her 4-month-old infant for a well-child visit. She has no concerns other than the fact that the infant's left eye does not seem to be as big as the right eye. On exam, you notice a very faint lid crease, eyelid lag on downgaze, barely visible corneal reflex, and poor elevation of the upper lid on the left side. The rest of the exam, including pupils and extraocular movements, is normal.

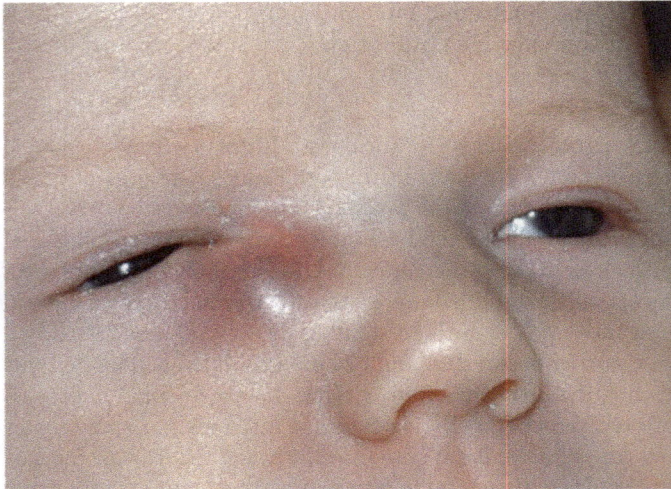

FIGURE 13–9. A dacryocystocele forms when the nasolacrimal duct is obstructed. It appears as a bluish swelling under and nasal to the medial canthus. The mass causes upward slanting of the palpebral fissure. Infants should be referred to a pediatric ophthalmologist as secondary infection may occur. (Used with permission from the University of Iowa and EyeRounds.org.)

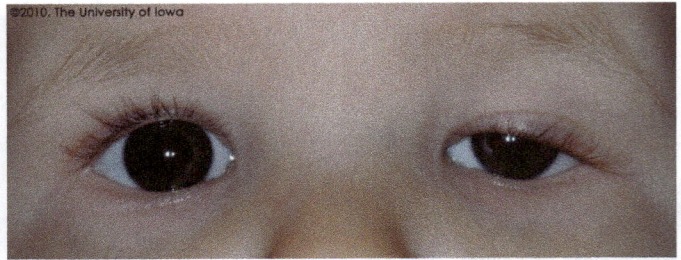

FIGURE 13–10. An encephalocele is a congenital skull defect with herniation of cranial contents through the defect. (Reproduced with permission from Lalwani AK, ed. *Current Diagnosis & Treatment in Otolaryngology: Head and Neck Surgery*. 3rd ed. New York, NY: McGraw-Hill Education; 2011, Fig. 11-5A.)

Question 10-1

This child most likely has:

A) Congenital cranial nerve (CN) III palsy.
B) Congenital ptosis.
C) Congenital Horner syndrome.
D) Acquired aponeurotic ptosis.
E) Marcus Gunn jaw-winking syndrome.

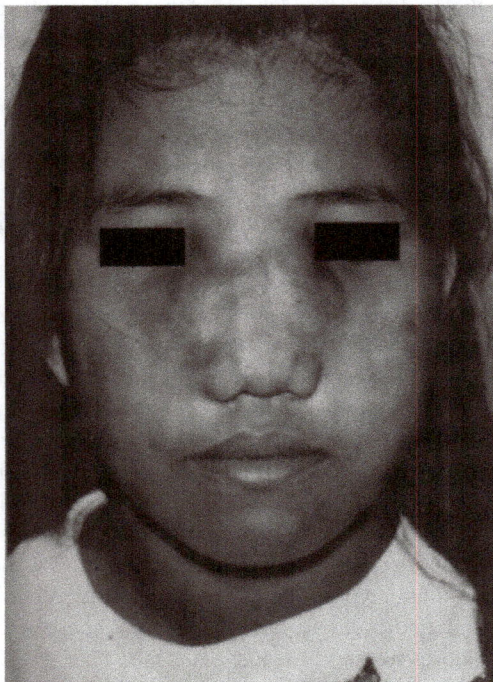

FIGURE 13–11. Congenital ptosis as seen in the left upper eyelid results from poor levator function. The levator muscle is dysgenic, with fatty or fibrotic tissue instead of striated muscle. The dysgenic muscle cannot relax or contract normally, resulting in poor eyelid elevation with upgaze and eyelid lag on downgaze. This patient is at risk for amblyopia as vision is partially blocked by the sagging eyelid. (Used with permission from the University of Iowa and EyeRounds.org.)

Discussion 10-1

The correct answer is "B." Congenital ptosis is secondary to levator muscle dysgenesis (myogenic etiology). The etiology of acquired ptosis is diverse and includes aponeurotic defects, CN III palsy, Horner syndrome, ocular myopathies, myasthenia gravis, and synkinetic neurogenic syndromes such as Marcus Gunn jaw-winking syndrome. The most common cause of acquired ptosis is aponeurotic, with defects at the origin or insertion of the aponeurosis. The distinction between congenital myogenic ptosis (simple congenital ptosis) and acquired aponeurotic ptosis can be made with the clinical observation of a weak or absent lid crease, which would be observed in congenital ptosis. In contrast, in cases of acquired ptosis, the lid crease is higher than normal. The levator function is reduced in congenital ptosis and near normal in acquired aponeurotic ptosis. Lastly, there is eyelid lag in downgaze with congenital myogenic ptosis and eyelid drop (ie, worsening of the ptosis when looking down) in acquired aponeurotic ptosis. (See Figure 13–11.)

> **Helpful Tip**
>
> In a child younger than 7 years of age with severe ptosis, demonstrating a corneal light reflex that is minimally visible or completely obstructed, an emergent referral to a pediatric ophthalmologist is necessary. Severe ptosis may lead to deprivation amblyopia, which could cause permanent vision loss in the ipsilateral eye.

> **Helpful Tip**
>
> Ptosis associated with a miotic pupil is suspicious for *Horner syndrome*. A *third nerve palsy* is associated with ptosis, strabismus (eye pointed down and out), and limited extraocular motility. Mydriasis (dilated pupil) may or may not be present in a third nerve palsy.

► CASE 11

A 6-month-old boy with "big beautiful eyes" is brought to your office by his mother for a routine well-child visit. The mother states that he has experienced excessive tearing since birth. She is convinced that his tear ducts are plugged and, like her previous children, his symptoms will resolve with time. During the exam he appears to be quite bothered by the room light. He becomes even fussier when you attempt to examine his eyes with a penlight. Throughout the examination you also note frequent blinking. The mother wants to know if she should start doing lacrimal massages to help with his symptoms.

Question 11-1

What is the most likely diagnosis in this infant?
A) Nasolacrimal duct obstruction.
B) Conjunctivitis.
C) Congenital glaucoma.
D) Corneal abrasion.
E) Dry eye syndrome.

Discussion 11-1

The correct answer is "C." Primary congenital glaucoma (PCG) has an incidence of approximately 1 in 10,000 to 20,000 live births in Western countries. The classic triad of clinical findings associated with PCG is epiphora, photophobia, and blepharospasm. These signs indicate irritation to the cornea caused by corneal edema resulting from elevated intraocular pressure (IOP). Another consequence of chronically increased IOP in PCG is gross enlargement of the eye (buphthalmos, which means "ox eye"). The most common physical sign in PCG is a cloudy cornea. The classic clinical triad, however, may appear before the onset of any physical findings and therefore is important in the early diagnosis of PCG. The combination of corneal edema and buphthalmos can create the appearance of big, beautiful eyes, leading many patients to be overlooked. PCG is typically bilateral. Males (65%) are more frequently affected than females (35%). (See Figures 13–7 and 13–8, earlier.)

> **Helpful Tip**
>
> Some definitions: *Epiphora* is excessive tearing. Patients may present with increased pooling around the eyes or frank tears rolling down the face. *Photophobia* is hypersensitivity to light. Infants will be observed protesting to light by crying, avoidance (closing eyes), or frequently rubbing the eyes. *Blepharospasm* is involuntary eyelid squeezing or twitching and may be seen as recurrent blinking.

> **Helpful Tip**
>
> If primary congenital glaucoma is suspected, an emergent referral to ophthalmology for immediate intervention is required.

► CASE 12

A 3-month-old infant girl was urgently added to your scheduled clinic appointments. Her mother became concerned when looking at family photos from a few weeks ago. She noticed that the light reflex appeared significantly duller in her daughter's eyes than in the rest of the family. On further inspection, you confirm that the red reflex is diminished bilaterally. In addition, when viewing the patient's eyes with direct ophthalmoscopy you note some cloudiness to her pupils. The mother states that her daughter is otherwise healthy and has received all appropriate vaccinations. The remainder of her examination is normal.

Question 12-1

All the following are associated with the patient's condition EXCEPT:
A) Positive family history.
B) Down syndrome.
C) Galactosemia.
D) Trauma.
E) Intrauterine infection.

Discussion 12-1

The correct answer is "D." The patient's clinical picture is consistent with bilateral congenital cataracts. Congenital cataracts are relatively common, occurring in about 1 in 2000 live births. Although trauma may be associated with a unilateral pediatric cataract, it is not a cause of bilateral congenital cataracts. Other disorders associated with bilateral *congenital* cataracts include congenital TORCH (toxoplasmosis, other [syphilis, varicellazoster, parvovirus B19], rubella, cytomegalovirus, and herpes) infections, maternal drug ingestion, trisomies 13, 18, and 21, Lowe syndrome, Alport syndrome, and aniridia. Inherited cataracts, which are usually transmitted in an autosomal dominant fashion, are the most common cause of bilateral congenital cataracts in the United States. Other family members, therefore, are also often affected but to varying degrees. Steroid use, radiation exposure, hypoparathyroidism, diabetes mellitus, and Fabry disease are potential causes of bilateral *pediatric* cataracts. (See Figure 13–12.)

Question 12-2

What may be a sign or symptom of congenital cataracts?
A) Strabismus.
B) Nystagmus.
C) Leukocoria.
D) Decreased vision.
E) All of the above.

Discussion 12-2

The correct answer is "E." Strabismus, nystagmus, leukocoria, and decreased vision can all be observed with congenital cataracts. Strabismus (ocular misalignment) is more frequently seen with unilateral congenital cataracts. Nystagmus (involuntary,

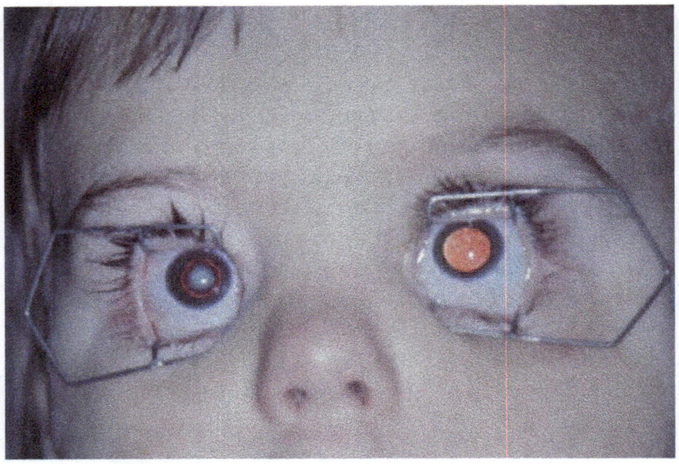

FIGURE 13–12. Congenital cataracts. This child has a cataract of the right eye (pupils are dilated). The red reflex is asymmetric and partially opaque/white (leukocoria) in the affected eye. (Reproduced with permission from Riordan-Eva P, Cunningham ET, eds. *Vaughan & Asbury's General Ophthalmology*. 18th ed. New York, NY: McGraw-Hill Education; 2011, Fig. 8-3.)

rhythmic shaking of the eyes) may occur in bilateral congenital cataracts. The presence of strabismus or nystagmus indicates that the cataracts are significantly affecting visual function. Leukocoria (white pupil) may be present in either bilateral or unilateral cataracts.

> **Helpful Tip**
> Strabismus, nystagmus, leukocoria, and decreased vision are all nonspecific signs and are affiliated with a variety of ocular conditions. The presence of any one of these signs in an infant, however, should prompt an immediate referral to ophthalmology for evaluation and potential treatment.

> **Helpful Tip**
> It is imperative that a patient with a congenital cataract be seen by an ophthalmologist in a timely matter. A delay in treatment may result in significant amblyopia, particularly in the case of a unilateral cataract.

▶ CASE 13

A 10-year-old boy with spina bifida comes to your office because of a worsening headache over the past week. He has a history of congenital hydrocephalus for which a ventriculoperitoneal shunt was placed at the age of 4 months. This morning his headache became unbearable. His visual acuity is tested and is 20/20 in both eyes. You are able to evaluate his optic nerves with direct ophthalmoscopy and notice that the disc margins appear blurred. Additionally, you observe multiple disc hemorrhages.

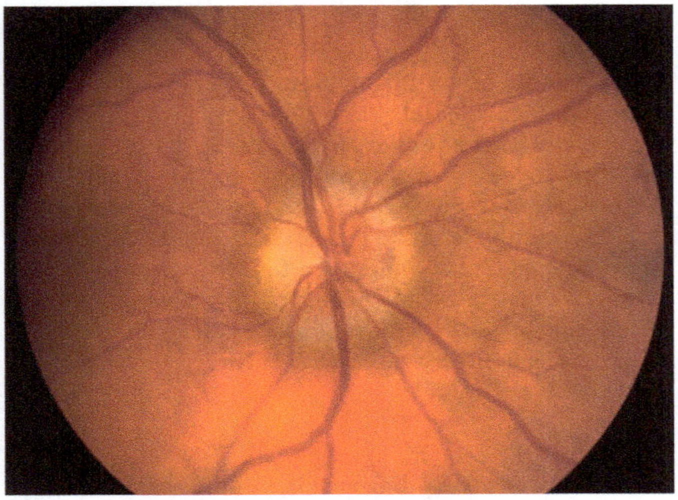

FIGURE 13–13. Papilledema is swelling of the optic disc from increased intracranial pressure. On funduscopic exam the following may be seen: (1) loss of venous pulsations (early), (2) splinter hemorrhages, (3) elevation of the optic disc, (4) blurred disc margins, (5) obliteration of the disc cup, (6) engorged retinal veins, and (7) disc hyperemia. Notice that the optic nerve is elevated with blurred margins and complete loss of the cup. (Used with permission from the University of Iowa and EyeRounds.org.)

Question 13-1
What is NOT a typical finding associated with this condition?
A) Relative afferent pupillary defect.
B) Elevated intracranial pressure.
C) Altered mental status.
D) Double vision.
E) Nausea or vomiting.

Discussion 13-1
The correct answer is "A." The patient's clinical picture is consistent with papilledema, which is defined as optic disc swelling secondary to increased intracranial pressure (ICP). Considering his past medical history, this patient's papilledema is most likely caused by hydrocephalus due to a failed shunt. The patient will thus require emergent referral to a neurosurgeon for potential shunt revision. (See Figure 13–13.) A relative afferent pupillary defect (Marcus-Gunn pupil) is not a typical finding in papilledema because both optic nerves are affected in this condition. Headache, nausea, vomiting, altered mental status, and double vision are all symptoms of increased ICP. Vision may be normal early in the course; however with chronicity asymptomatic vision loss usually ensues.

> **Helpful Tip**
> A relative afferent pupillary defect (RAPD) is seen in conditions that cause unilateral or asymmetric disease of the optic nerve.

Question 13-2
Which condition is associated with papilledema?
A) Dural sinus thrombosis.
B) Idiopathic intracranial hypertension.

C) Intracranial neoplasm.
D) Meningitis.
E) All of the above.

Discussion 13-2

The correct answer is "E." Anything than causes elevated ICP, including dural sinus thrombosis, idiopathic intracranial hypertension, intracranial neoplasm, and meningitis, may result in papilledema. If papilledema is suspected, emergent neuroimaging and evaluation by ophthalmology and neurology is necessary. A lumbar puncture (LP) should not be performed until intracranial herniation or mass is ruled out on imaging. An LP will allow measurement of opening pressure and cerebrospinal fluid analysis.

► CASE 14

A 4-week-old girl was born at 28 weeks' gestation with a birth weight of 1700 g. She required supplemental oxygen for the first two weeks of life. Since this time she has been in good condition, feeding well, and gaining weight appropriately. Her two older siblings at home were both born full-term. Her parents inquire if their daughter will require any additional follow-up compared with their other children.

Question 14-1

At what chronological age should this patient be screened for retinopathy of prematurity (ROP)?
A) This week.
B) 1 week.
C) 2 weeks.
D) 3 weeks.
E) Screening is not necessary.

Discussion 14-1

The correct answer is "A." According to the American Academy of Pediatrics, all infants with a birthweight of 1500 g or less or a gestational age of 30 weeks or less should be screened for ROP. It is recommended that the initial screening examination be performed at 4 weeks' chronological age or 31 weeks' postmenstrual age, which is determined by the later of these two dates.

> **Helpful Tip**
> Screen for retinopathy of prematurity (ROP):
> - At 31 weeks' postmenstrual age if gestational age is 22 to 27 weeks
> - At 4 weeks' chronological age if gestational age is 27 to 30 weeks

Question 14-2

What is an additional reason to consider ROP screening?
A) Twin birth.
B) Family history of ROP.
C) Caesarean delivery.
D) Unstable clinical course.
E) No prenatal care.

Discussion 14-2

The correct answer is "D." Infants who do not fit the criteria previously stated, with a gestational age of more than 30 weeks or birthweight between 1500 and 2000 g, but who have experienced an unstable clinical course and are determined to be at high risk for ROP by their physician, should also be screened for ROP. Twin birth, family history of ROP, caesarean delivery, and lack of prenatal care are not reasons alone to warrant screening.

> **Helpful Tip**
> Additional retinal screening is required after the initial examination if the retina is not fully vascularized in either eye.

► CASE 15

A 3-year-old girl with a history of juvenile idiopathic arthritis (JIA) presents to your office with a red, painful right eye of 2 days' duration. She is being followed regularly by a rheumatologist and documented to have oligoarticular, antinuclear antibody (ANA)–positive JIA, which was diagnosed at age 2. According to the mother, her arthritis has been well controlled on methotrexate. You check her vision and it measures 20/20 in both eyes. Her pupils are equal and reactive with no RAPD; however, she exhibits extreme sensitivity to light during your examination. The conjunctiva of the right eye is very injected, but the left eye appears unaffected. You do not note any discharge in either eye. Her mother denies any recent upper respiratory tract symptoms, sick contacts, or trauma. She was evaluated by an ophthalmologist 6 months ago and had a normal ophthalmic exam at that time.

Question 15-1

What is this patient's most likely diagnosis?
A) Conjunctivitis.
B) Anterior uveitis.
C) Corneal abrasion.
D) Nasolacrimal duct obstruction.
E) Chalazion.

Discussion 15-1

The correct answer is "B." The patient is exhibiting photophobia, conjunctival injection, and eye pain that, along with her diagnosis of JIA, make anterior uveitis the most likely etiology. Risk factors for the development of uveitis in JIA patients include female gender, oligoarticular onset, age at diagnosis 6 years or younger, rheumatoid factor (RF)–negative, and ANA-positive. This patient has all these risk factors and thus is at higher risk for uveitis.

> **Helpful Tip**
> Some definitions: *Anterior uveitis* is inflammation in the front part of the eye. *Oligoarthritis* is arthritis that affects four or fewer joints at the time of disease onset.

Question 15-2

What is a feature that helps distinguish anterior uveitis from conjunctivitis?
A) Redness.
B) Tearing.
C) Pain.
D) Blurry vision.
E) Bilateral.

Discussion 15-2

The correct answer is "C." Redness, tearing, blurry vision, and a bilateral presentation are all features that may be associated with either anterior uveitis or conjunctivitis. Although pain is often a symptom of anterior uveitis, it is not associated with conjunctivitis. It is important to note that the chronic anterior uveitis associated with JIA differs from other forms of uveitis in that it is commonly painless. These children tend to present with grossly white or quiet eyes and only have microscopic evidence of inflammation. This asymptomatic presentation demonstrates the importance of having routine ophthalmic screening examinations in patients with JIA.

▶ CASE 16

A 6-year-old boy presents to your office for his yearly routine examination. He is a very active and bright child. As part of the screening exam, you check his visual acuity, which measures 20/20 and 20/60 in his right and left eye, respectively. His pupils are equal and reactive with no evidence of a RAPD. You perform the cover-uncover and alternate cover tests and do not detect any deviation. His extraocular movements are full and his red reflex appears normal. The remainder of the exam is normal, and he is otherwise healthy with no significant past medical history. His mother recalls her brother being treated for a "lazy eye" at a young age.

Question 16-1

What is the most likely cause of poor vision in this child?
A) Strabismus.
B) Amblyopia.
C) Cataract.
D) Cranial nerve VI palsy.
E) Retinoblastoma.

Discussion 16-1

The correct answer is "B." The patient's history and physical exam are most consistent with amblyopia. The lack of eye movement on cover-uncover and alternate cover tests is not supportive of a diagnosis of strabismus. The presence of a normal red reflex makes both cataract and retinoblastoma unlikely answers. Lastly, the extraocular movements would be limited in a patient with a cranial nerve VI palsy. Amblyopia ("lazy eye"), which has an estimated prevalence of 2% to 4% in the general population, is the most common cause of decreased vision in childhood. For vision to develop, both eyes must see objects clearly and transmit a signal to the brain. If one eye has impaired visual input to the brain, the brain will favor the other eye so that a single clear image

TABLE 13–3 CAUSES OF VISUAL DEPRIVATION AMBLYOPIA

Congenital or traumatic cataract

Corneal opacity

Ptosis

Vitreous hemorrhage

Surgical lid closure

Prolonged eye patching (iatrogenic)

is produced. If the condition goes untreated, the brain will ignore all input from the affected eye, resulting in permanent blindness in the affected eye. Amblyopia often remains undetected until routine vision screening for school or physical exams. Because it is a preventable, treatable, and potentially reversible condition, amblyopia should be detected in a timely manner.

> **Helpful Tip**
> Some definitions: *Amblyopia* is defined as decreased best-corrected visual acuity in the absence of any structural abnormality of the visual pathway or eye. It may be bilateral, but more commonly is unilateral. *Strabismus* ("squint") is due to misalignment of the eyes.

Question 16-2

What is a possible cause of amblyopia?
A) Refractive error.
B) Ptosis.
C) Strabismus.
D) Corneal opacity.
E) All of the above.

Discussion 16-2

The correct answer is "E." Amblyopia may be caused by strabismus, uncorrected refractive error, or visual deprivation. Strabismus is the most common cause of amblyopia. The type of amblyopia present determines which treatment is initiated. For example, in the case of uncorrected refractive error, correction with spectacles is the initial mode of treatment. On the other hand, in order to treat amblyopia related to strabismus various modalities may be required, such as occlusion therapy (eg, eye patch), eye muscle surgery, refractive correction, or a combination of these. Treatment of visual deprivation involves addressing the underlying cause of the disruption. (See Table 13–3.)

▶ CASE 17

A 12-year-old girl is urgently added to your scheduled appointments. On presentation, she is covering her right eye and very reluctant to let you take a look at it. She states that she scratched her eye while applying some of her mother's mascara earlier today. She has experienced pronounced right eye pain ever since the incident. You are able to convince her to let you examine. Her right eye is diffusely injected and tearing profusely. On penlight examination, the cornea appears clear and pupils are equal, round, and reactive with no evidence of a RAPD. You test her visual acuity and she is easily able to read the 20/20 line with both eyes. You next instill fluorescein drops into her right eye, and she complains of burning upon application. With the use of the blue light on the direct ophthalmoscope, you are able to visualize a superficial linear area of corneal staining.

Question 17-1

What does fluorescein staining detect?
A) Corneal abrasion.
B) Intraocular foreign body.
C) Conjunctivitis.
D) Endophthalmitis.
E) Uveitis.

Discussion 17-1

The correct answer is "A." Corneal abrasion is a common childhood injury that is the result of corneal epithelial loss caused by ocular trauma. Fluorescein stains the epithelial defect a bright green when viewed with a cobalt blue light. Patients typically present with tearing, conjunctival injection, pain, and photophobia following the injury. Visual acuity may or may not be affected depending upon the extent of corneal involvement. In young children, injuries often go unwitnessed and the child presents with eyelid edema and conjunctival injection. In this situation, the corneal abrasion may mimic and be mistaken for preseptal cellulitis or conjunctivitis. Infants with corneal abrasions may present with irritability. (See Figure 13–14.)

Question 17-2

What is the most appropriate treatment in this patient?
A) Topical anesthetic.
B) Pressure eye patch.

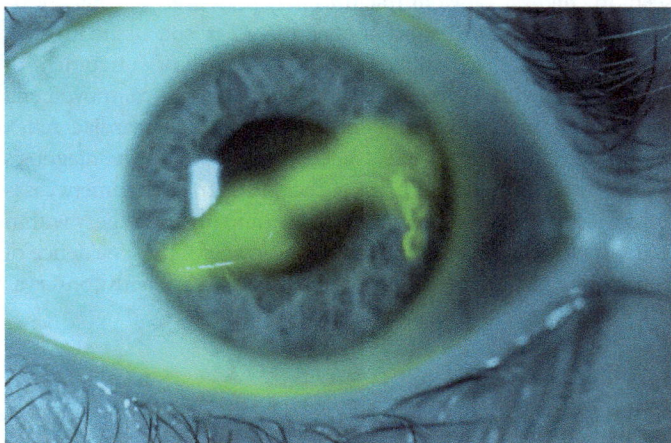

FIGURE 13–14. A corneal abrasion results from traumatic disruption of the corneal epithelium. Fluorescein stains it a bright green when viewed by cobalt blue light. (Reproduced with permission from Knoop KJ, Stack LB, Storrow AB, Thurman RJ (Eds). *The Atlas of Emergency Medicine*, 3ed. McGraw-Hill Education, Inc., 2010. Photo contributor: Lawrence B. Stack, MD. Fig 4-3.)

C) Topical steroid.
D) Ophthalmic antibiotic.
E) Systemic antibiotic.

Discussion 17-2

The correct answer is "D." A short course of broad-spectrum ophthalmic antibiotic drops or ointment should be prescribed to prevent secondary infection. Unless an extensive corneal abrasion is present, the use of a pressure patch to keep eyelids closed is not warranted. Pressure patches may increase the risk of secondary infection (especially if vegetative matter is involved in the injury) and do not speed the healing process. Topical anesthetic provides temporary relief, but its long-term use delays healing, increases the risk of infection, and may cause a secondary ulcer. Therefore, a topical anesthetic should not be prescribed for a corneal abrasion. Topical steroids should also avoided because they similarly increase the risk of infection and delay healing. There is no proven benefit of the use of systemic antibiotics in the treatment of corneal abrasions. Corneal abrasions are generally self-limited and heal within 1 to 2 days of the injury. Follow-up evaluation should be planned for a few days after presentation with the expectation that symptoms will be significantly improved. If clinical improvement is not seen at the follow-up appointment, prompt referral to an ophthalmologist should occur.

⏳ QUICK QUIZ

When ocular trauma occurs as a result of high-velocity injuries, such as car crashes or metal work, one should have a high clinical suspicion of a corneal foreign body.

How would you initially manage a superficial corneal metal foreign body?
A) Removal with a sharp forceps.
B) Observation.
C) Removal with a blunt spatula.
D) Removal with a cotton swab.
E) Forceful irrigation with a saline solution.

Discussion

The correct answer is "E." The most appropriate way to conservatively manage a superficial corneal foreign body is to first vigorously irrigate the eye. This should be performed after instillation of a topical ophthalmic anesthetic for comfort measures. Simply irrigating the eye may act to dislodge the foreign body without causing further damage to the corneal surface. If irrigation fails an attempt may be made with a cotton swab or blunt spatula to carefully remove the object. Care should be taken with this maneuver as being overly aggressive may result in permanent corneal scarring and decreased vision. For this same reason, sharp objects should be avoided. At this point, if the foreign body cannot be removed, evaluation by an ophthalmologist is needed. A rust ring, which can also compromise vision, may occur if a metal foreign body is left in the eye. Furthermore, an exam under sedation or general anesthesia may be necessary in young or uncooperative patients. After the removal of the foreign body, management is similar to that of a corneal abrasion and includes treatment with topical antibiotics.

▶ CASE 18

A 12-year-old boy is brought into your clinic after being elbowed in the left eye by a classmate a few hours before. He exhibits pain and extreme sensitivity to light. His vision is normal in his right eye, but measures only 20/50 in his left eye. His pupils are equal and reactive and no RAPD is present. On penlight exam you are able to see some red layering within the front part of the eye but do not note any staining with fluorescein.

Question 18-1

What is the next important step in workup of this patient?
A) Orbital MRI.
B) Obtain a complete blood count (CBC).
C) Measure intraocular pressure.
D) Coagulopathy workup.
E) Orbital CT.

Discussion 18-1

The correct answer is "C." This patient has a hyphema, which is an accumulation of blood in the anterior chamber of the eye. The most common cause of a hyphema is trauma. Rarely a hyphema may be spontaneous, occurring in association with diseases such as retinoblastoma, juvenile xanthogranuloma, or leukemia. One of the most important initial signs to check in an hyphema patient is intraocular pressure (IOP). IOP can be increased as a result of a hyphema and can result in long-term complications such as corneal blood staining. Elevated IOP can be usually treated with IOP-lowering ophthalmic medications. Another critical part of the hyphema workup is obtaining sickle cell screening in African-American children. Patients with sickle cell disease require very close monitoring as they are at increased risk of complications and may require earlier surgical intervention. Conservative management with a topical steroid and cycloplegic medication is recommended in the treatment of hyphemas. Additionally, a Fox shield over the affected eye, elevating the head of the bed, and bedrest with only bathroom privileges is necessary for at least the first 5 days. In some circumstances a child may be admitted to the hospital for observation. (See Figure 13–15.)

> **Helpful Tip**
> Some definitions: *Hyphema* is the presence of blood within the anterior chamber of the eye. A traumatic hyphema is due to ruptured iris vessels. The *anterior chamber* is the space between the cornea and iris.

The same patient returns to your office 1 month later after being punched in the right eye by the class bully. On exam you note that he is unable to elevate or depress his right eye much

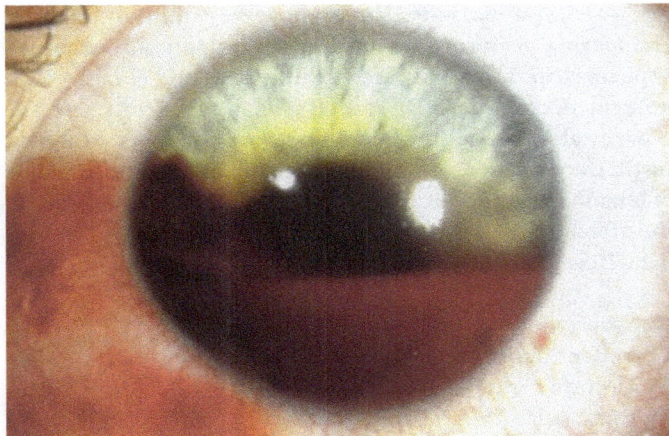

FIGURE 13–15. A hyphema developed after blunt trauma to the eye. Notice the layering of blood in the anterior chamber of the eye. (Reproduced with permission from Riordan-Eva P, Cunningham ET, eds. *Vaughan & Asbury's General Ophthalmology*. 18th ed. New York, NY: McGraw-Hill Education; 2011, Fig. 19-9.)

past midline. He has some mild periorbital edema, but the remainder of the exam is otherwise normal with good vision and no evidence of conjunctival inflammation. Toward the end of your exam he starts complaining of some nausea.

Question 18-2

What are you most suspicious of based on his presentation?
A) Ruptured globe.
B) Hyphema.
C) Corneal abrasion.
D) Blowout fracture.
E) Retinal detachment.

Discussion 18-2

The correct answer is "D." The clinical picture is most consistent with a blowout fracture. With any of the other answers, you would expect to find decreased vision. In the presence of a ruptured globe or corneal abrasion, conjunctival inflammation or hemorrhage should be seen. In children, blowout fractures may present in a "white-eyed" manner with minimal signs of conjunctival or soft tissue involvement. This patient's motility deficit is indicative of entrapment of the inferior rectus within the fracture, limiting vertical movement. Entrapment may produce a life-threatening oculocardiac reflex with bradycardia, heart block, syncope, and nausea. The diagnosis should be confirmed on orbital CT scan. Pediatric entrapment cases are considered an ophthalmic emergency and urgent surgery within 24 hours to relieve the entrapment is warranted. If no evidence of entrapment or motility deficit is found, observation with conservative management of the fracture is appropriate.

> **Helpful Tip**
> Some definitions: *Blowout fracture* is an orbital floor fracture caused by a compressive injury. *"Trapdoor" fracture*, which is the most common cause of strabismus in a blowout fracture, results in the entrapment of the inferior rectus muscle in the floor fracture.

► CASE 19

A 4-month-old girl is brought into your office for a routine check. The infant's mother is concerned because the lesion around her left eye, which appeared as a faint red dot a birth, has grown remarkably. You observe a superficial blanching red lesion on the left upper eyelid with resultant mild ptosis. Her mother also complains that the lesion appears to become more prominent and cause bulging of her eye with excessive crying. She did not notice any worsening with her recent upper respiratory tract infection.

Question 19-1

What is this patient at greatest risk for?
A) Coagulopathy.
B) Amblyopia.
C) Cardiovascular complication.
D) Corneal exposure.
E) Acute lesional hemorrhage.

Discussion 19-1

The correct answer is "B." This is a classic presentation of capillary hemangioma, or infantile periocular hemangioma, which is the most common orbital tumor of childhood. The majority of hemangiomas appear within the first month of life and are clinically insignificant. Most commonly they present as a superficial vascular lesion with a predilection for the upper eyelid or orbit. They less commonly appear as a subcutaneous bluish mass. Caregivers describe a growing red or purple spot. Blanching of the lesion with pressure distinguishes it from a port-wine stain. The natural history involves rapid growth over a 3- to 6-month period of time, followed by stabilization and then regression after the age of 1 year. Amblyopia is a common complication of periocular hemangiomas; as a result ophthalmic evaluation is recommended. Visual deprivation due to mass-induced ptosis is one cause of amblyopia. The subtler finding of astigmatism, which results from corneal distortion, is the most frequent amblyogenic factor. Since most hemangiomas spontaneously regress with excellent cosmesis by 7 years of age, conservative management is recommended in the absence of significant amblyopic risk. If intervention is mandatory, topical or systemic beta-blockers are currently the treatment of choice. (See Figure 13–16.)

Helpful Tip

There are several systemic associations of capillary hemangiomas. *Kasabach-Merritt syndrome* is a rare coagulopathy (thrombocytopenia) with a high mortality rate that results from platelet sequestration in large hemangiomas involving the skin and internal organs throughout the body. *PHACE(S) syndrome* (**P**osterior fossa abnormalities, **H**emangioma, **A**rterial lesions, **C**ardiac abnormalities, **E**ye and **S**ternal abnormalities) is also associated with extensive facial hemangiomas and has potentially life-threatening cardiovascular and neurologic consequences.

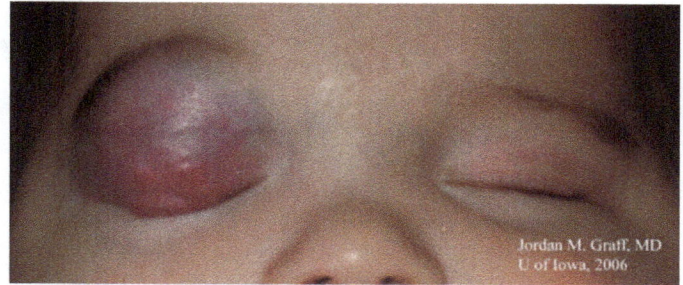

FIGURE 13–16. A periocular hemangioma of the entire right upper eyelid restricts opening of the eye, placing this infant at risk for amblyopia. The lesion has a superficial component (elevated, red area) and a deeper component (smooth, purplish area). This infant requires treatment with a beta-blocker. (Used with permission from the University of Iowa and EyeRounds.org.)

► CASE 20

A 25-month-old boy is brought by his parents for a routine visit. His parents note that he is very healthy and reaching the appropriate developmental milestones. They ask if they should be concerned about his eyes. Over the past month, he has been exhibiting turning in of his eyes. His father states that he had a similar issue as a child, but that it was corrected with eyeglasses. You observe alternating turning in of the infant's eyes during your exam. The turning in appears to be constant. On penlight exam, you note that the light reflex is located near the center of the right cornea, but appears to be displaced outward on the left eye. On the cover-uncover test, you note that the deviated eye moves outward when the deviated eye is uncovered. His ocular motility is full in both eyes.

Question 20-1

What is the most likely diagnosis?
A) Cranial nerve VI palsy.
B) Exophoria.
C) Exotropia.
D) Esophoria.
E) Esotropia.

Discussion 20-1

The correct answer is "E." This is an example of esotropia. "Eso-" indicates that the eye is deviated nasally or inward, whereas "exo-" describes a temporally or outwardly turned eye. "Phoria" describes a latent deviation that is not present under binocular conditions. A phoria is apparent only when binocularity becomes disrupted, such as when one eye is covered. "Tropia," on the other hand, is manifestation of strabismus that is observed under binocular conditions, even when one eye is not covered. A tropia may be constant, as in this case, or intermittent with varying control. Though a cranial nerve VI palsy would result in esotropia, a limitation in the outward movement of the eye would also be present. The Hirschberg test, cover-uncover test, and alternate cover test are important in the evaluation of childhood strabismus.

Helpful Tip

Some definitions: The Hirschberg test, which is performed by shining a light source on the patient's eyes, relies on the corneal light reflex to assess ocular alignment. For accurate assessment, the examiner must be positioned centrally in front of the patient and directly behind the light source. If, for example, the corneal light reflex is displaced outwardly on one eye, then an esotropia is present. Inward displacement of the corneal light reflex is consistent with an exotropia. If the corneal light reflex is centrally located on both corneas, then a tropia is not present (eyes are normally aligned). The cover-uncover test is also used to identify tropias. During this test, the examiner covers one eye at a time for a few seconds and watches for movement of the fellow eye. If the uncovered eye moves in from an outward position, then an exotropia exists. In the case of an esotropia, the uncovered eye moves out from an inward position. A tropia is not present if there is no movement of the uncovered eye. If a tropia is not detected on the cover-uncover test, the alternate cover test, which breaks binocular fusion, can be used to disclose a phoria. The alternate cover test is performed by covering each eye in an alternate fashion. A phoria is present if movement of the uncovered eye is observed.

BIBLIOGRAPHY

Basic and Clinical Science Course. Section 6: Pediatric Ophthalmology and Strabismus. San Francisco, CA: American Academy of Ophthalmology; 2014–2015.

Basic and Clinical Science Course. Section 6: Pediatric Ophthalmology and Strabismus. San Francisco, CA: American Academy of Ophthalmology; 2011–2012.

Basic and Clinical Science Course. Section 7: Orbit, Eyelids, and Lacrimal System. San Francisco, CA: American Academy of Ophthalmology; 2011–2012.

Becker BB. The treatment of congenital dacryocystocele. *Am J Opthhalmol.* 2006;142(5):835–838.

Eustis HS, Mafee MF, Walton C, Mondonca J. MR imaging and CT of orbital infections and complications in acute rhinosinusitis. *Radiol Clin North Am.* 1998;36:1165–1183.

Fierson WM; American Academy of Pediatrics Section on Ophthalmology; American Academy of Ophthalmology; American Association for Pediatric Ophthalmology and Strabismus; American Association of Certified Orthopedists. Screening examination of premature infants for retinopathy of prematurity. *Pediatrics.* 2013;131(1):189–195.

Garcia GH, Harris GJ. Criteria for nonsurgical management of subperiosteal abscess of the orbit: Analyses of outcomes 1988–1998. *Ophthalmology.* 2000;107(8):1454–1458.

Goldberg F, Berne AS, Oski FA. Differentiation of orbital cellulitis from preseptal cellulitis by computed tomography. *Paediatrics.* 1978;62:1000–1005.

Hoyt C, Taylor D. *Pediatric Ophthalmology and Strabismus.* 4th ed. London: Elsevier Saunders; 2013.

Kaiser P, Friedman N, Pineda R. *The Massachusetts Eye and Ear Infirmary Illustrated Manual of Ophthalmology.* 4th ed. London: Elsevier Saunders; 2014.

Mandal A, Netland P. *The Pediatric Glaucomas.* Philadelphia, PA: Elsevier; 2006.

Meyer DR. Congenital ptosis. In: *Focal Points: Clinical Modules for Ophthalmologists.* San Francisco, CA: American Academy of Ophthalmology; 2001, module 2.

Pediatric Eye Disease Investigator Group; Repka MX, Chandler DL, Beck RW, et al. Primary treatment of nasolacrimal duct obstruction with probing in children younger than 4 years. *Opthhalmology.* 2008;115(3):577–584.

Rosenbaum AL, Santiago AP. *Clinical Strabismus Management: Principles and Surgical Techniques.* Philadelphia, PA: Saunders; 1999.

Schanll BM, Christian CJ. Conservative treatment of congenital dacryocystocele. *J Pediatr Ophthalmol Strabismus.* 1996;33(5):219–222.

Sondhi N, Archer SM, Helveston EM. Development of normal ocular alignment. *J. Pediatr Ophthalmol Strabismus.* 1988;25:210.

von Noorden G, Campos E. *Binocular Vision and Ocular Motility. Theory and Management of Strabismus.* 6th ed. St. Louis, MO: Mosby; 2002.

Weiss A, Friendly D, Eglin K, et al. Bacterial periorbital and orbital cellulitis in childhood. *Ophthalmology.* 1983;90:195–203.

Wright K, Strube Y. *Pediatric Ophthalmology and Strabismus.* 3rd ed. New York, NY: Oxford University Press; 2012.

Fetus and Newborn

14

Erin Osterholm and Jessie Marks

▶ CASE 1

A woman comes to the obstetrics clinic for a routine prenatal visit at 32 weeks' gestation. She is healthy and has continued to feel regular fetal movements with no changes or concerns. As her practitioner obtains fetal heart tones by Doppler, a fetal heart rate of 200 beats per minute (bpm) is noted.

Question 1-1

What would be the most appropriate next step to evaluate fetal well-being?

A) At-home kick counts.
B) Contraction stress test.
C) Biophysical profile.
D) Consultation with a pediatric cardiologist for prenatal evaluation.
E) Ultrasound.

Discussion 1-1

The correct answer is "D." Obstetricians utilize a variety of techniques to assess fetal well-being throughout pregnancy. Although kick counts can be useful in minimizing unnecessary interventions in an uncomplicated pregnancy, this is an inappropriate approach for more complex concerns. Nonstress tests (NSTs) monitor fetal heart rate reactivity in response to fetal movement and spontaneous maternal contractions. Contraction stress tests (CSTs) evaluate concerns relating to uteroplacental insufficiency by observing the response of the fetus during induced uterine contractions. CSTs are not preferred due to the high false-positive rate and need to induce contractions. The biophysical profile is designed to estimate the risk of fetal asphyxia within 1 week if no intervention is done; it combines the results of an NST with measurements of amniotic fluid levels and fetal tone, breathing (hiccups count!), and movement. Other methods used to monitor the prenatal health of the fetus include checking fetal heart rate by Doppler and measuring maternal fundal height. Fetal arrhythmias are rare and most resolve prior to delivery, but the potential for significant morbidity and mortality dictates close follow-up and assessment by a pediatric cardiologist during the prenatal period, as some fetuses may require in utero

treatment with maternal or transplacental medications. After birth, an electrocardiogram (ECG), measurement of four-point blood pressures, and possibly an echocardiogram should be performed.

> **Helpful Tip**
> Fetal bradycardia is defined as heart rate less than 100 bpm, most commonly from atrioventricular block. Fetal tachycardia is defined as a heart rate greater than 180 bpm, most commonly due to paroxysmal supraventricular tachycardia. The most common and typically least concerning fetal arrhythmia is an irregular heartbeat. In almost 50% of cases, fetal arrhythmias are associated with congenital heart disease. The presence of maternal SS-A (anti-Ro) or SS-B (anti-La) antibody, associated with autoimmune conditions such as systemic lupus erythematosus and Sjögren syndrome, is also associated with fetal arrhythmias.

The newborn is born healthy at 39 weeks' gestation with resolution of arrhythmia prior to delivery and normal ECG after birth. Later, the mother is concerned about frequent spit-ups. You speak with her about these concerns. The infant is being bottle fed with formula and often has milk running out of his mouth after feeding, especially with burping or when lying flat after a feed. On exam, he appears well. His belly is soft and has good bowel sounds.

Question 1-2

Which of the following is true about spit ups and emesis in newborns?

A) Even small amounts of red or brown blood are always concerning if found in a newborn's spit-up.
B) Bilious emesis is not typically a concerning finding in newborns.
C) It is common for infants to spit up clear, colorless mucus mixed with feedings during the first 24 hours of life.
D) True projectile vomiting can be normal in newborns.
E) Newborns should not spit up.

Discussion 1-2

The correct answer is "C." Previously swallowed amniotic fluid is often regurgitated by itself or with milk in the first 24 hours of life. Small amounts of red or brown blood may be found in the spit-up of normal newborns when it was swallowed during delivery or in breastfed babies whose mothers have cracked and bleeding nipples. Bilious emesis is always an emergency. Potential causes include obstruction, such as malrotation with midgut volvulus, and necrotizing enterocolitis (rare in term infants, but it does occur). True projectile vomiting is never normal and warrants immediate evaluation for gastric obstruction such as pyloric stenosis. Gastroesophageal reflux (spitting up) is very common in infants, improves with age, and is not concerning. Gastroesophageal reflux disease (GERD) indicates complications such as feeding refusal or poor weight gain requiring further evaluation.

> **Helpful Tip**
>
> Acid-blocking medications are associated with increased risk of pneumonia, gastroenteritis, and necrotizing enterocolitis. Do not prescribe these agents for the "happy spitter" with benign gastroesophageal reflux. Instead, have the family invest the money in burp clothes.

Once you have reassured the newborn's mother regarding gastroesophageal reflux, she asks about the newborn metabolic screen that will be done after he is 24 hours old. She wonders if it is necessary and why it is performed.

Question 1-3

Which of the following statements about newborn metabolic screening is true?

A) The diseases included in newborn screening are standardized throughout the country.
B) The importance lies in the availability of significant interventions for each of the diseases screened in this test.
C) Parents are not allowed to opt out of newborn screening for their child for any reason.
D) Newborn screens are not able to be done after an infant is discharged from the birth hospitalization.
E) It is optional for states to perform newborn screening.

Discussion 1-3

The correct answer is "B." States are mandated to perform newborn metabolic screening and hearing screening. All states screen for phenylketonuria (PKU) and hypothyroidism. Although the additional components screened for vary from state to state, the commonality and power of this screening test is that all of the diseases, if found, can have significantly improved long-term health outcomes with the early interventions that are made possible by detecting the disease process at birth. Parents are allowed to opt out of newborn metabolic screening for religious reasons. Screening should be repeated at one of the infant's subsequent outpatient visits if a borderline result or error in testing is identified. Some states routinely do more than one screening

to enhance the likelihood of identifying conditions that require metabolite accumulation for detection.

> **Helpful Tip**
>
> The blood spot specimen for newborn screening should be collected after 24 hours of age. The newborn needs time to build up the abnormal compounds in his or her blood.

While examining the newborn you change his diaper, which is the first urination he has had since birth 20 hours earlier. The medical student with you wonders out loud what is done if an infant does not urinate in the first day of life.

Question 1-4

What should you tell the medical student about the appropriate evaluation and management of an infant who does not urinate in the first 24 hours of life?

A) A complete lack of urination by 24 hours may be a sign of acute kidney injury.
B) Newborns rarely void in the first 24 hours of life.
C) No investigation is warranted until the newborn has reached at least 48 hours of life without urinating.
D) No testing is indicated until 72 hours if prenatal ultrasounds showed normal kidney and bladder structure.
E) Relax, it is only pee.

Discussion 1-4

The correct answer is "A." About 90% of newborns urinate by 24 hours of life, which leaves a relatively large number of newborns (10%) who do not, and most of these do not have pathologic conditions. A complete lack of urination by 24 hours of life may be a sign of congenital renal or urinary tract structural or functional anomalies or acute kidney injury and should be investigated. For a newborn with delayed voiding, check for a prenatal history of oligohydramnios or urinary system abnormalities on ultrasound. Next, make sure the newborn is feeding frequently and that a void was not missed. Examine the abdomen and genitalia closely. If no urination can be documented by 24 hours of life, measure serum electrolytes and blood urea nitrogen (BUN) and creatinine levels, obtain a renal ultrasound, and catheterize the newborn to see if urine is present. Prenatal ultrasounds are good screening tools but are not sufficient to rule out pathologic conditions in a symptomatic infant.

> ► **CASE 2**

You are in the operating room leading a newborn resuscitation team at a scheduled routine repeat cesarean delivery at 40 weeks' gestation. As you instruct the medical student with you on how to set up the equipment while waiting for the delivery, she asks if there is any medical significance to the use of a warmer in the delivery room other than keeping the infant comfortable.

Question 2-1

Of the following, the most appropriate response you could give would be:

A) The main reason for using a warmer is to calm the infant so he or she does not use up extra energy fussing in the first minutes of life.
B) Radiant warmers are useful, without known risk, and require no special considerations for use, especially in premature infants who have a higher likelihood of becoming cold.
C) Because cold stress is rare in newborns even without the use of a warmer, the warmer's main function is to help awaken the infant and ease the transition from the womb into the "outside world."
D) The potential risks of prolonged exposure to radiant warmers must be considered in the care of all infants, but especially the premature.
E) Radiant warmers help heat the operating suite so it is not as cold for the newborn after delivery.

Discussion 2-1

The correct answer is "D." Maintaining an appropriate core temperature in the newborn is critical and is actually the primary objective of most basic care provided during and immediately after resuscitation: drying, use of a warmer, swaddling or skin-to-skin contact, and use of a hat. This is especially important in premature and low birthweight infants. There is a risk of insensible water losses with the use of radiant warmers, which deserves consideration in the postresuscitative care of premature infants due to their propensity for fluid and electrolyte imbalances. Newborns are prone to heat loss because of their high surface area-to-body mass ratio, which is emphasized in any infant of low birthweight. Cold stress in a newborn causes a rapid depletion of essential fat and glycogen stores, putting the infant at risk for developing complications such as hypoglycemia. Hypothermia on admission to the neonatal intensive care unit is a predictor of increased mortality.

> **Helpful Tip**
> The neonatal resuscitation algorithm changes with some regularity. Questions and discussions in this chapter are based on core concepts of infant resuscitation. However, readers should also make themselves familiar with current resuscitation guidelines.

When the infant is delivered, your team appropriately dries and stimulates her. At birth she is apneic, floppy, and blue with a heart rate of 70 bpm. At 1 minute, she remains cyanotic, floppy, and has a heart rate of 70 bpm. She is breathing irregularly at a rate of 15 breaths per minute, and has grimaced a few times during stimulation but is not crying. Your team follows the neonatal resuscitation program (NRP) guidelines appropriately, giving positive-pressure ventilation by bag and mask. By 5 minutes, her heart rate has risen to 90 bpm, her torso has become pink (though her hands and feet remain dusky), she is breathing spontaneously and has flexor tone but is not actively moving. At 10 minutes, the infant is crying, breathing, actively moving, completely pink, and has a heart rate of 120 bpm.

Question 2-2

How would you assign this child's Apgar scores?

A) 4, 7, and 9; a 10-minute score is necessary when the score at birth is below 4.
B) 3 and 6; a 10-minute score is not necessary when the 5-minute score is 6 or higher.
C) 3 and 7; a 10-minute score is not necessary when the 5-minute score is 7 or higher.
D) 3, 6, and 10; a 10-minute score is necessary when the 5-minute score is less than 7.

Discussion 2-2

The correct answer is "D." Apgar scores are assigned at 1 and 5 minutes. If the 5-minute score is less than 7, scoring should be repeated every 5 minutes up to 20 minutes. The Apgar score is used to clinically assess the newborn during the transition to extrauterine life. It is *not* meant to predict neurologic outcomes or development. The components, which are fivefold and tallied on a scale of 0 to 2 for a maximum total score of 10, are as follows: color, heart rate, grimace/reflex irritability, tone, and respiratory effort. One convenient acronym is based on the last name of the scoring method's creator, Virginia Apgar: **A**ppearance, **P**ulse, **G**rimace, **A**ctivity, and **R**espiration. Each receives a score of "0" if not present at all, a "1" if present but below expected level, and a "2" for fully met criteria, as detailed in the Table 14–1.

> **Helpful Tip**
> Peripheral cyanosis (acrocyanosis) is extremely common in newborn infants and may continue through the first 24 to 48 hours of life. It results from vasomotor instability with constriction of the blood vessels in the hands and feet. To ensure central cyanosis is not present, look for a pink tongue (mucous membranes).

⏳ QUICK QUIZ

What percentages of neonates require some form of resuscitation after delivery?

A) 90%.
B) 1%.
C) 10%.
D) 0%.
E) 5%.

Discussion

The correct answer is "C." The majority of neonates will not require resuscitation. Approximately 1% will require extensive resuscitation such as chest compressions. Those not needing resuscitation can usually be identified by the following characteristics: (1) term gestation, (2) crying or breathing, and (3) good muscle tone.

TABLE 14–1 APGAR SCORE

Score	0	1	2
Appearance (color)	Central cyanosis	Acrocyanosis	Completely pink
Pulse	No pulse	Present but < 100 bpm	> 100 bpm
Grimace (reflex irritability)	No response to stimulation	Grimace in response to stimulation	Grimace plus crying or active movement in response to stimulation
Activity (tone)	Flaccid	Flexion with little to no active movement	Active movements
Respiration	No respiratory effort	Slow or irregular breathing	Spontaneous respirations

Helpful Tip
An infant is supposed to be blue immediately after delivery as oxygen saturation is only 60% at delivery. If he or she remains blue, you should take action.

Later that day, the infant is doing well and her parents, who have two other children at home, indicate that they would like an early discharge home from the hospital at 24 hours of life.

Question 2-3
Which of the following would make you uncomfortable sending her home at 24 hours of life?
A) Discharge at around 24 hours of life would occur on a Friday afternoon, and as the family lives in a rural area, they would be unable to attend a follow-up appointment until Monday.
B) The infant's temperature has been stable for the last 12 hours.
C) The infant has only urinated twice and stooled once.
D) The infant has breastfed well twice consecutively.
E) The infant is not jaundiced.

Discussion 2-3
The correct answer is "A." Newborns may stay in the hospital up to 48 hours after a vaginal birth and 96 hours after a cesarean delivery. Discharge before 48 hours of age is considered early. The most recent recommendations for early discharge utilize numerous criteria. Multiple minimum criteria must be met, so leaving early is no easy feat for an infant. Minimum criteria are:

- Term infant
- Vital signs stable for 12 hours before discharge
- Clinically well, with a reassuring exam
- Two successful consecutive feedings
- Voided once
- Passed at least one stool
- Received hepatitis B vaccine
- Newborn screens completed
- No hyperbilirubinemia
- No risk factors for sepsis
- Competent caregivers

- Social concerns addressed
- Follow-up arranged within the next 48 to 72 hours

Both you and the parents feel the infant is doing well according to the discharge criteria outlined above, and follow-up is arranged for tomorrow. As you begin discharge teaching, the parents ask about care of the umbilical cord stump.

Question 2-4
Which of the following would be an appropriate statement for you to make?
A) Daily umbilical cord stump cleansing with alcohol is a universal recommendation.
B) The parents should contact their physician if the cord stump does not fall off within the first week.
C) Umbilical cord infections (omphalitis) are typically rare, even with minimal care.
D) Bleeding is rare when the stump falls off, so even transient spotting at the time of sloughing should be reported immediately to the child's physician.
E) It is fine to pull off the stump if the odor is unpleasant.

Discussion 2-4
The correct answer is "C." Umbilical cord care is minimal, as infection is rare and the stump must essentially rot to fall off, usually within the first 2 weeks of life. Alcohol cleansing has been associated with delayed cord separation without a significant decrease in the infection rate in developed countries, but is an excellent and inexpensive option in low-resource settings or when cutting and clamping of the cord was not done in aseptic fashion. Transient spotting is common as the stump sloughs off, though persistent or recurrent oozing of blood should be evaluated. A cord stump that is still present after 3 weeks of age should be investigated further, as this may represent leukocyte adhesion defect (neutrophil dysfunction) or other pathology.

▶ **CASE 3**

A 16-year-old new mother asks you whether you think her infant girl was born "on time." When you inquire further, she admits she is not sure when she got pregnant and is concerned her newborn might be premature. She is worried because her aunt had a premature infant who had subsequent health issues related to prematurity. She is tearful and would like your best estimate of her newborn infant's gestational age. She had late prenatal care. Based on ultrasound dating in the third trimester, the newborn is term.

Question 3-1

What would you tell this mother?
A) Since the ultrasound occurred in the third trimester, it should be quite accurate.
B) The New Ballard score can stand alone as an accurate measure of the infant's gestational age at birth.
C) Her best recollection of the dates of her last menstrual period is probably the most accurate estimate.
D) Integrating the obstetrician's estimated due date with the infant's New Ballard score gives the best estimate of the infant's gestational age at birth.
E) The fact that the infant is breathing on her own indicates that she is term.

Discussion 3-1

The correct answer is "D." Prenatal ultrasound is most accurate at predicting fetal gestational age when done in the first trimester. The New Ballard score is a useful tool in confirming suspected gestational age, but can under- or overestimate the age of infants born prematurely. Variation between examiners can also occur. Two sets of signs—physical characteristics and neuromuscular maturity—are assessed by physical exam. The sum of the two gives the Ballard score. Note that the raw Ballard score does not equal the gestational age. The score must be placed on a chart to give the corresponding gestational age. (See Figure 14–1.)

⏳ QUICK QUIZ

What gestational age range defines a term infant?
A) 34-0/7 weeks' gestation to 36-6/7 weeks' gestation.
B) 42-1/7 weeks' gestation and older.
C) 38-0/7 weeks' gestation and older.
D) 37-0/7 weeks' gestation to 42-0/7 weeks' gestation.
E) Why are there so many choices?

Discussion

The correct answer is "D." Option "A" defines a late preterm infant. Infants born at or before 33-6/7 week's gestation are premature. Those born after 42 weeks' gestation are postterm. (See Figures 14–2 and 14–3.) Too early or too late is not good; on time is just right!

Question 3-2

Your team estimates this infant's gestational age by New Ballard score and measurements to be 39 weeks' gestation. Assuming this is correct, what would you expect this newborn's calculated mean arterial pressure (MAP) to be?
A) The MAP should be around 30.
B) The MAP should be around 40.

C) The MAP should be around 50.
D) The MAP should be around 60.

Discussion 3-2

The correct answer is "B." A general rule of thumb is that a newborn's MAP should approximately match his or her gestational age. This applies to premature, term, and postterm infants alike.

The mother voices relief when you relay the consensus opinion that her child appears to be a healthy, full-term infant. She then asks about the eye ointment that was applied after you checked the infant's red reflexes. She heard it protects the infant from an eye infection.

Question 3-3

Which sexually transmitted pathogen that causes neonatal conjunctivitis is nearly 100% prevented by the prophylactic erythromycin eye ointment that was applied?
A) *Chlamydia trachomatis*.
B) *Neisseria gonorrhoeae*.
C) *Candida albicans*.
D) *Gardnerella vaginalis*.
E) *Trichomonas vaginalis*.

Discussion 3-3

The correct answer is "B." Application of 0.5% erythromycin ointment is close to 100% effective at preventing neonatal conjunctivitis or ophthalmia neonatorum caused by *N. gonorrhoeae* acquired from the mother at birth. Alternately 1% tetracycline ointment and 1% silver nitrate may be used, but these preparations are not available in the United States. Gonococcal conjunctivitis manifests at 2 to 5 days of age with impressive eye swelling and a large amount of pus. (See Figure 14–4.) Untreated it can cause blindness. Do not miss this one. Erythromycin is not effective against *Chlamydia* conjunctivitis, which presents later (at 1 to 2 weeks of age) and may not be as severe. *Candida* is not sexually transmitted nor a pathogen of neonatal conjunctivitis. *Trichomonas* and *Gardnerella* infection, associated with bacterial vaginosis, increases a woman's risk of preterm labor, premature rupture of membranes, and preterm delivery, as well as miscarriage, endometritis, and chorioamnionitis but is not a known cause of neonatal conjunctivitis.

Question 3-4

Which of the following statements about gestational age at birth is correct?
A) Hematocrit levels are typically higher and have a later nadir in premature infants than term infants.
B) Premature infants generally require less fluid and fewer calories per kilogram of body weight than their term counterparts.
C) Postterm infants are at a higher risk than term infants of suffering neonatal complications such as perinatal asphyxia and persistent pulmonary hypertension.
D) Late preterm infants are no more likely than term infants to have apneic episodes or hypoglycemia during the birth hospitalization.
E) Why is so much emphasis placed on gestational age?

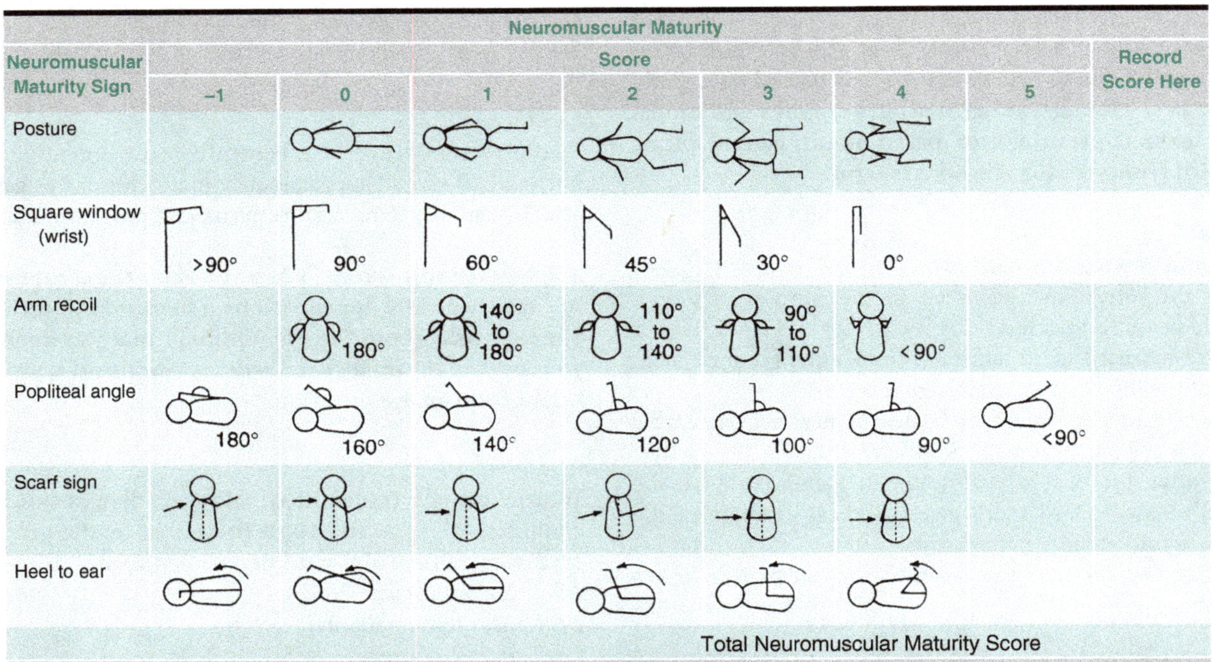

Neuromuscular Maturity								
Neuromuscular Maturity Sign	**Score**							**Record Score Here**
	−1	0	1	2	3	4	5	
Posture								
Square window (wrist)	>90°	90°	60°	45°	30°	0°		
Arm recoil		180°	140° to 180°	110° to 140°	90° to 110°	<90°		
Popliteal angle	180°	160°	140°	120°	100°	90°	<90°	
Scarf sign								
Heel to ear								

Total Neuromuscular Maturity Score

Physical Maturity								
Physical Maturity Sign	**Score**							**Record Score Here**
	−1	0	1	2	3	4	5	
Skin	Sticky, friable, transparent	Gelatinous, red, translucent	Smooth, pink, visible veins	Superficial peeling &/or rash; few veins	Cracking, pale areas; rare veins	Parchment, deep cracking; no vessels	Leathery, cracked, wrinkled	
Lanugo	None	Sparse	Abundant	Thinning	Bald areas	Mostly bald		
Plantar surface	Heel toe 40–50 mm: −1 <40 mm: −2	>50 mm: no crease	Faint red marks	Anterior transverse crease only	Creases anterior 2/3	Creases over entire sole		
Breast	Imperceptible	Barely perceptible	Flat areola; no bud	Stippled areola; 1- to 2-mm bud	Raised areola; 3- to 4-mm bud	Full areola; 5- to 10-mm bud		
Eye/Ear	Lids fused loosely: −1 tightly: −2	Lids open; pinna flat; stays folded	Slightly curved pinna; soft; slow recoil	Well-curved pinna; soft but ready recoil	Formed & firm instant recoil	Thick cartilage; ear stiff		
Genitals (male)	Scrotum flat, smooth	Scrotum empty; faint rugae	Testes in upper canal; rare rugae	Testes descending; few rugae	Testes down; good rugae	Testes pendulous; deep rugae		
Genitals (female)	Clitoris prominent & labia flat	Prominent clitoris & small labia minora	Prominent clitoris & enlarging minora	Majora & minora equally prominent	Majora large; minora small	Majora cover clitoris & minora		

Total Physical Maturity Score

Maturity	Score	−10	−5	0	5	10	15	20	25	30	35	40	45	50
Rating	Weeks	20	22	24	26	28	30	32	34	36	38	40	42	44

FIGURE 14–1. The New Ballard score is a clinical assessment used to estimate the gestational age of newly born infants. An individual score is calculated for neuromuscular maturity and physical maturity. The two numbers are added together to give the maturity score (see bottom of figure), which corresponds to the correct gestational age (rating in weeks under the maturity score). For example, a neuromuscular maturity score of 18 plus a physical maturity score of 17 equals a maturity score of 35, which rates at 38 weeks' gestation. (Reproduced with permission from Ballard JL, Khoury JC, Wedig K, et al: New Ballard Score, expanded to include extremely premature infants, *J Pediatr* 1991 Sep;119(3):417-423.)

Discussion 3-4

The correct answer is "C." Red blood cell production decreases after birth, leading to an eventual physiologic nadir as the prenatally manufactured cells die off. As the newborn's oxygenation status rapidly rises with the onset of breathing and closure of the ductus arteriosus, the body loses the hypoxic push for erythropoiesis. Concurrently erythropoietin production is reduced. This physiologic anemia of infancy occurs at 8 to 12 weeks for a term infant and 3 to 6 weeks for a premature infant. This process combined with lower hematocrits at birth means that premature infants are at risk for anemia of prematurity, a quicker and steeper nadir than

FIGURE 14–2. A postterm infant's weight may be increased or decreased (ie, the placenta can degenerate, causing malnutrition). The skin is cracked, peeling, wrinkly, and loose. Fingernails are long and may have meconium staining. This infant born at 43 weeks' gestation is covered with meconium from delivery. (Reproduced with permission from Cunningham FG, Leveno KJ, Bloom SL, et al, eds. *Williams Obstetrics.* 24th ed. New York, NY: McGraw-Hill Education; 2014, Fig. 43-4.)

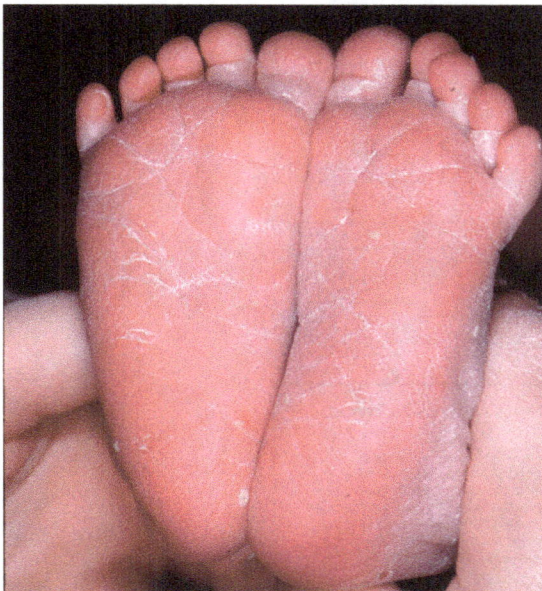

FIGURE 14–3. Postterm infant feet. Dry, multiple creases and scaling feet typical of a postterm infant. Small pustules of transient neonatal pustular melanosis are present. (Reproduced with permission from Goldsmith LA, Katz SI, Gilchrest BA, et al, eds. *Fitzpatrick's Dermatology in General Medicine.* 8th ed. New York, NY: McGraw-Hill Education; 2012, Fig. 107-1.)

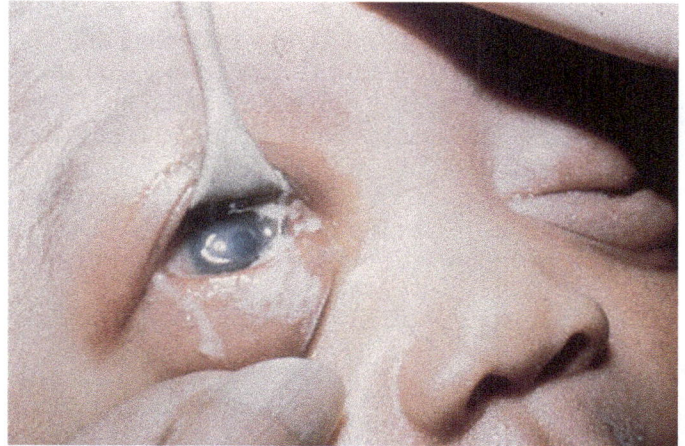

FIGURE 14–4. Ophthalmia neonatorum in a newborn with gonococcal conjunctivitis. This infection can be prevented with administration of 0.5% erythromycin ointment shortly after birth. Untreated, the infection may lead to blindness. (Reproduced with permission from Levinson W, ed. *Review of Medical Microbiology and Immunology.* 13th ed. New York, NY: McGraw-Hill Education; 2014, Fig. 16-3.)

that seen in term infants. Delayed cord clamping in premature infants has been shown to prevent anemia, necrotizing enterocolitis, and intraventricular hemorrhage. Premature infants require more fluid and calories per kilogram of body weight than their term counterparts, not less, due to their high surface area-to-body mass ratio and subsequent propensity for heat and fluid loss. Postterm infants are more likely than term infants to suffer neonatal complications, including birth trauma, perinatal asphyxia, meconium aspiration syndrome, and persistent pulmonary hypertension. Late preterm infants, like their premature friends, are at higher risk of complications during the birth hospitalization (hypoglycemia, temperature dysregulation, feeding difficulties, severe hyperbilirubinemia, respiratory distress, and apnea) and have significantly higher readmission rates compared with term infants.

QUICK QUIZ

Which of the following statements regarding birthweight is incorrect?

A) Large for gestational age (LGA) is defined as greater than 90%.
B) Small for gestational age (SGA) is defined as less than 10%.
C) Low birthweight infants are not always SGA.
D) Gestational age is important for birthweight classification.
E) Studies have shown eating chocolate every day during pregnancy guarantees a LGA infant.

Discussion

The correct answer is "E." Weight, length, and head circumference are measured at birth and plotted on a growth curve according to gestational age to determine the percentile. The percentile classifies the infant as SGA (< 10%), average for gestational age (AGA), or LGA (> 90%). (See Figure 14–5.) Low birthweight (< 2500 g) and macrosomia (> 4000 g) are defined by a specific weight, not the plotted percentile. Thus, an infant can be low birthweight but AGA. When an infant is SGA or LGA, you should ask yourself why and be alert to possible complications (ie, hypoglycemia) to watch for. Chocolate makes people happy, and who doesn't want a happy mother to be.

⧗ **QUICK QUIZ**

Regarding SGA infants, which of the following is FALSE?
A) Maternal substance abuse is a cause of intrauterine growth restriction (IUGR).
B) SGA infants have increased mortality.
C) All SGA infants have IUGR.
D) Symmetric IUGR may be due to chromosome abnormalities.
E) Stop labeling infants; you might make them insecure.

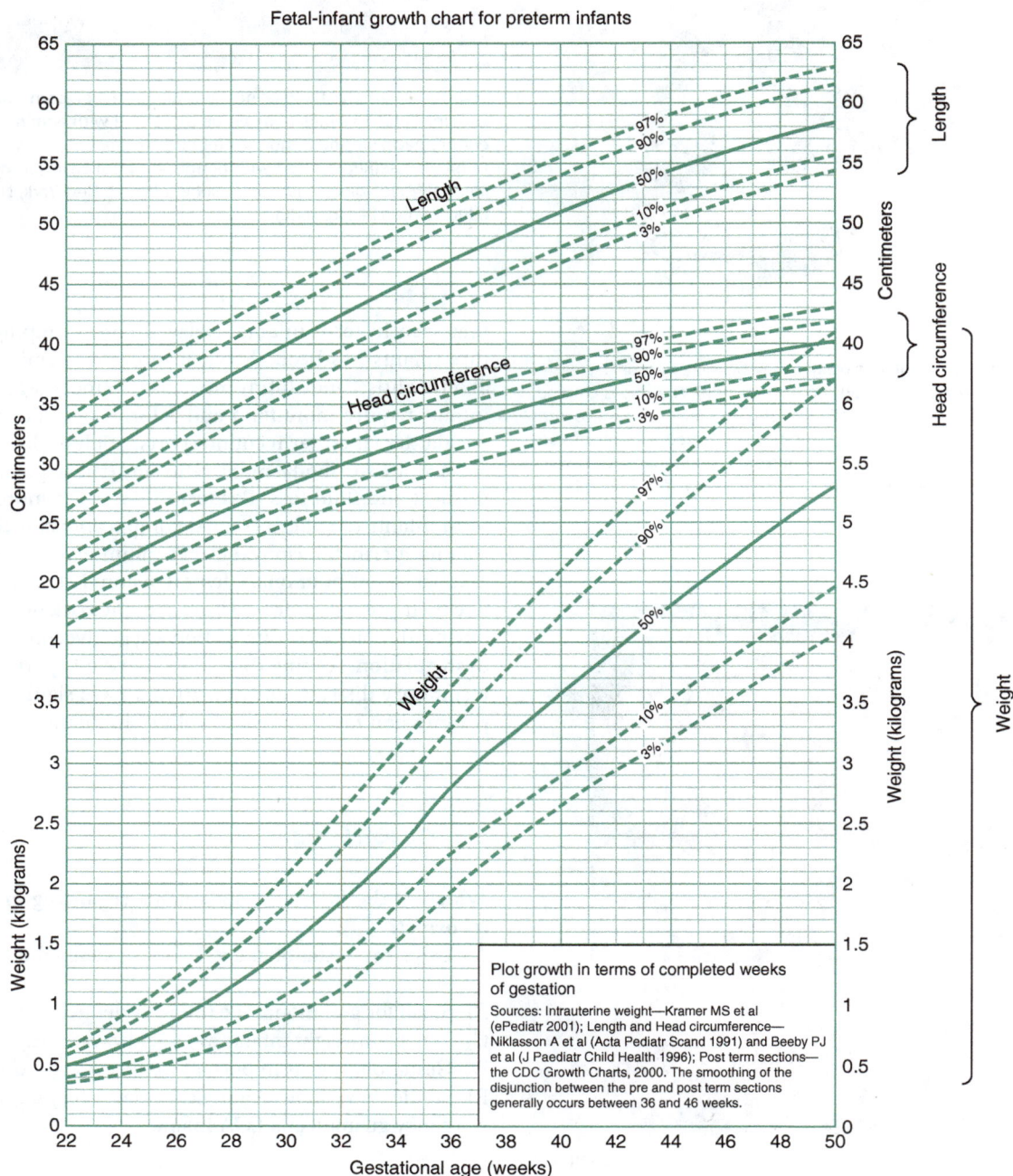

FIGURE 14–5. Neonatal growth chart. The infant's measurements are plotted on the growth curve by gestational age to give a percentile, which is used in classifying the infant as small (SGA), average (AGA), large (LGA) for gestational age. (Reproduced with permission from Fenton TR. A new growth chart for preterm babies: Babson and Benda's chart updated with recent data and a new format, *BMC Pediatr.* 2003;3:13.)

Discussion

The correct answer is "C." IUGR results in impaired fetal growth and the birth of an SGA infant. Not all SGA infants had decreased fetal growth. Some are constitutionally small and healthy. Maternal, placental, or neonatal factors, or a combination of these, are to blame. Growth-restricted SGA infants have more complications, including hypoglycemia, temperature issues, polycythemia, and higher mortality. Think genetic condition or congenital infection when an infant is uniformly small. There is insufficient evidence to support option E but option C is clearly a better choice.

► CASE 4

As you meet with your team in the newborn nursery area before beginning daily rounds, one of the medical students comments on the large size of an infant being weighed by the medical assistant. He asks whether the mother had gestational diabetes, or if the infant is just big.

Question 4-1

Taking this teaching opportunity to discuss how size can relate to either gestational age or intrauterine factors, you could offer the following tidbit:

A) Maternal hyperglycemia is not a risk factor for fetal macrosomia.
B) LGA infants are not at increased risk for birth injuries, such as cephalohematoma or brachial plexus injury.
C) A mother's birthweight can be a predictor that her infant is more likely to be LGA at birth.
D) Maternal prepregnancy weight is not a risk factor for having an LGA infant.
E) The goal of every pregnancy is to have the biggest infant possible.

Discussion 4-1

The correct answer is "C." Excessive fetal growth (macrosomia) is due to a combination of genetic and intrauterine factors. Mothers who themselves were LGA at birth are more likely to deliver an LGA newborn. Maternal obesity, diabetes, and excessive weight gain during pregnancy are predisposing factors. Large parents (not obese) may breed large infants. All oversized infants are at increased risk of birth injuries during delivery. LGA infants are also at increased risk for polycythemia and hypoglycemia. Hyperglycemia exposure in utero increases fetal insulin production. After delivery, the infant's pancreas continues to produce excess insulin despite withdrawal from the previous source of a high glucose load, the placenta. Keeping in mind how infants are born, the mother may disagree with option "E."

The infant's weight plots at the 92nd percentile for his gestational age. Your team correctly identifies this infant as LGA. The resident places the orders for serial glucose levels and asks you why bedside rapid glucose oxidation strips are not utilized for ease and speed of results instead of sending each blood sample to the lab.

Question 4-2

Which of the following responses is correct?

A) Bedside glucose checks require more blood, so parents prefer serial blood tests.
B) Glucose oxidation strips are less reliable in neonates than in older children and adults.
C) Variation in results from test strips is most common at high glucose levels.
D) Heel sticks are never appropriate for monitoring blood glucose levels.
E) Either works fine but insurance reimbursement is lower for bedside glucose checks.

Discussion 4-2

The correct answer is "B." Results of test strip sampling of blood glucose can vary as much as 10 to 20 mg/dL from actual plasma glucose concentrations, and this variance is accentuated at lower glucose concentrations. Both of these considerations make test strips less preferable in neonates, who have normal glucose levels well below the adult norms, for whom the strips were designed. Blood glucose levels may be lower than 30 mg/dL in newborns. Heel sticks are more convenient and less invasive than venous draws and are most accurate when the prewarming technique is used and blood is obtained while free-flowing.

You quiz the resident about neonatal hypoglycemia. You need to be sure she is an independent learner who reads about patient issues. You ask about symptoms of hypoglycemia.

Question 4-3

Which of the following is FALSE?

A) All neonates with hypoglycemia will be jittery.
B) There is no exact definition of hypoglycemia.
C) Polycythemia is a risk factor for hypoglycemia.
D) Respiratory distress may be a clinical sign of hypoglycemia.
E) Neonates utilize fat as an alternative fuel source when hypoglycemic.

Discussion 4-3

The correct answer is "A." Blood glucose levels drop after birth, reaching a low at about 2 to 3 hours of age. During this physiologic process, infants make ketones to use for fuel. The reason this is important is the potential for hypoglycemia to cause neurologic injury (a nicer way of saying brain damage). In asymptomatic infants, the glucose level that should prompt concern is not known. The number picked to define neonatal hypoglycemia is 47 mg/dL. Many infants with hypoglycemia are asymptomatic, and clinical symptoms, when present are nonspecific: jitteriness, lethargy, hypotonia, apnea, respiratory distress, hypothermia, seizures, and poor suck or feeding. Risk factors for neonatal hypoglycemia include polycythemia, sepsis, SGA, LGA, low birthweight, prematurity, and maternal diabetes.

Rounding on day of life (DOL) 1 for this infant, you note that there are no charted stools for him yet. When you speak with his parents and the nurse, you learn that he did have one stool at around 20 hours of life, but the electronic health record has not yet been updated to reflect this. The medical student asks whether it matters when the infant first passes meconium. You would tell him to look it up but you want a good teaching evaluation.

Question 4-4

The most accurate response would be:

A) As long as the infant stools prior to discharge, there are not likely to be any concerns, even if this occurs as late as DOL 3.
B) Meconium should be passed within the first 12 hours; if not, further evaluation is necessary.
C) Any infant who has not passed meconium in the first 24 to 48 hours should be evaluated for Hirschsprung disease or conditions that cause meconium plugs.
D) Now that umbilical cord drug screening is available, the passage of meconium is unnecessary as a prerequisite for discharge as it does not need to be collected for newborn drug testing.
E) As long as the anus is patent, there is no need to worry.

Discussion 4-4

The correct answer is "C." Delayed passage of meconium is defined as no spontaneous passage by 48 hours of life, the time frame by which approximately 99% of normal newborns have passed their first stool (though some sources cite similar rates by 24 hours of life). Failure to pass the first stool within this timeframe should trigger evaluation for potential causes, including Hirschsprung disease, meconium plug syndrome, meconium ileus, small left colon syndrome, or imperforate anus. Intrauterine exposure to narcotics and development of sepsis can also lead to delayed passage of meconium. Contrast enema study, rectal suction biopsy, and abdominal X-rays are some of the most commonly indicated tests, depending on the associated clinical picture and relevant family history. Transition of stool from meconium to the loose, seedy yellow stools (often described as being similar to mustard) of infancy should occur by DOL 4 if feedings are adequate, and delay in this transition should prompt further evaluation of current quality and frequency of feedings.

⏳ QUICK QUIZ

A 5-day-old male infant arrives for his outpatient circumcision appointment. He was born at another hospital, and although you do not have his records, his parents report that he was healthy at birth and that there were no complications of pregnancy or delivery. He is feeding well. The procedure goes well without complications. The nurse checks his diaper 30 minutes postprocedure and notes a significant amount of blood oozing at the site. As the nurse holds pressure, you ask the family for more information that could help you determine the appropriate course of action.

All of the following are high-yield questions to ask the family EXCEPT:

A) Has he received any shots since birth?
B) Is the child fed exclusively with breastmilk?
C) Did he receive phototherapy for jaundice during his birth hospitalization?
D) Was the infant's mother on any medication during the pregnancy?
E) Did you forget to mention that a maternal uncle has hemophilia?

Discussion

The correct answer is "C." All infants should receive a vitamin K injection (0.5-1 mg) at birth, especially those who are breast-fed, as human milk is deficient in vitamin K. Formerly known as hemorrhagic disease of the newborn, vitamin K deficiency bleeding (VKDB) is a preventable cause of coagulopathy in infants. Clotting factors need vitamin K, which is made by intestinal bacteria. Infants are born with insufficient vitamin K stores because their gut is sterile and placental passage of vitamin K is minimal. Presenting signs of VKDB include bleeding at the umbilical cord stump or circumcision site, epistaxis, blood in urine or stool, skin bruising, and even intracranial hemorrhage. Maternal medications taken during pregnancy, particularly antiseizure drugs and warfarin, can predispose to VKDB. Early-onset VKDB occurs from DOL 1 to 14. Late-onset VKDB occurs in infants who are 2 weeks to 2 months old, typically in those who are breastfed and did not receive a vitamin K injection at birth. Vitamin K can be given orally but it is not as effective for preventing late-onset disease. Remind parents that vitamin K has not been proven to cause cancer and brain bleeding is not something to risk.

▶ CASE 5

A newborn infant is admitted to your service at 1 hour of life after an accidental home birth. The labor was precipitous and the child's mother is currently in the operating room for postpartum hemorrhage while the father is in transit from work. The mother was followed by the obstetric team at your hospital, and records indicate this was a healthy and uncomplicated first pregnancy for her. The infant appears robust and healthy on exam.

Question 5-1

Which of the following will occur during the infant's hospitalization?

A) Administration of hepatitis B vaccine.
B) Hearing screen.
C) Ortolani and Barlow maneuvers.
D) Warming of the child, if necessary, and monitoring of vital signs.
E) Screening for hyperbilirubinemia.
F) All of the above.

Discussion 5-1

The correct answer is "F." In general, "all of the above" is usually a safe choice within this book. Newborns are newborns and have the same care requirements regardless of where they were born.

Within 24 hours of birth, newborns should have a full head-to-toe exam while naked. To ensure that you focus on each aspect of the exam, think of your goal as finding a minor defect. Make sure the red reflex is symmetric, present in both eyes, and not white (leukocoria). If not, call ophthalmology to look for cataracts, retinoblastoma or other pathology. Perform Ortolani and Barlow maneuvers when examining the hips to check for developmental dysplasia of the hips (DDH). Risk factors include breech positioning, female sex, and family history. If missed, it can lead to pain and osteoarthritis. Hip "clicks" are benign, common, and not associated with DDH; they are due to ligamentous laxity. All newborns should receive vitamin K injection, erythromycin eye ointment, hepatitis B vaccine, hearing screen, and metabolic screening. Screen for hyperbilirubinemia (jaundice) between 24 and 48 hours of life—obviously earlier is okay if the infant is glowing (yellow). Pulse oximetry screening for critical congenital heart disease should be completed after 24 hours. Risk factors for sepsis should be identified. Although home births in the United States are rare, the number is increasing. Infant mortality appears to be two to three times more prevalent in home births than hospital births in the United States, but small international studies showed no increase in neonatal mortality when a registered midwife or physician was in attendance, as their criteria require, suggesting that the process can be made safer. Considerations in home birth include the following: pregnancy should be uncomplicated, and there should be a certified midwife or physician currently practicing within a regulated health system, and at least one NRP-trained individual in attendance whose primary responsibility following delivery will be the infant. Proximity to a hospital with specialty services is also highly recommended, as travel times greater than 20 minutes have been associated with higher adverse outcomes for the infant, including mortality.

⧗ QUICK QUIZ

Which of the following is FALSE regarding hepatitis B vaccination?
A) Hepatitis B vaccine should be given to all newborns.
B) It is best to wait 24 hours before giving hepatitis B vaccine to exposed infants.
C) If the mother is hepatitis B surface antigen (HBsAg) positive, the infant should receive both the hepatitis B vaccine and hepatitis B immunoglobulin (HBIG).
D) Infants infected perinatally are at risk of liver failure.
E) HBIG can be administered up to 7 days of age.

Discussion

The correct answer is "B." All newborns should get the vaccine. Immunization prevents vertical transmission of hepatitis B from the mother to the infant. It really works! If postexposure prophylaxis is not given, 20% of newborns born to HBsAg-positive mothers will be infected. Infected newborns are at risk for chronic hepatitis and liver failure. If the mother is HBsAg positive, the infant should receive both the hepatitis B vaccine and HBIG at birth. Ensure the injections are given in different thighs. If the mother's status is unknown, the vaccine should be given within the first 12 hours of life. If the mother subsequently tests positive, clinicians have 7 days to give HBIG.

> **Helpful Tip**
> Caregivers, including grandparents, should get yearly influenza vaccination and a one-time booster of diphtheria toxoid and acellular pertussis (Tdap) vaccines to "cocoon" the newborn until he or she can be vaccinated. With *each* pregnancy, mothers should receive a Tdap vaccine between 27 and 36 weeks' gestation.

After finishing rounds on the other infants on your service, the nurse calls you back into the nursery to evaluate an area of scalp swelling on the previously mentioned infant that she had not noticed earlier.

Question 5-2

Which of the following exam finding would you find most concerning?
A) The swelling crosses suture lines.
B) The swelling seems to move toward the dependent areas of the scalp after repositioning.
C) Extensive superficial bruising.
D) Soft tissue swelling concentrated over the highest point of molding.
E) The head looks like a cone.

Discussion 5-2

The correct answer is "B." The point is not to miss a subgaleal hemorrhage, which occurs when the scalp is separated from the periosteum of the skull at the aponeurosis. Although a subgaleal hemorrhage will cross suture lines, caput can do the same. Subgaleal hemorrhages may grow rapidly because there is a large potential space available in which blood can collect, and the swelling can shift under the scalp toward the dependent areas of the infant's head, including near the ears and into the infant's forehead. As there is an almost unlimited potential space available for the blood to fill, a severe subgaleal hemorrhage can lead to hypovolemic shock and death. Careful and frequent monitoring of head circumference and the appearance and location of swelling is imperative, and should be done hourly if there is any concern for such a bleed. Hematocrits should be frequently checked as well. Caput (swelling) and superficial bruising occur within the scalp itself, often at points of highest pressure or trauma during delivery, and do not shift with change in positioning. Cephalohematoma is a collection of blood beneath the periosteum of the skull plate and therefore will have limited potential for blood loss and never cross suture lines. (See Figure 14–6.)

After close examination of the infant, you determine the area of scalp swelling is a cephalohematoma. The next day, the medical student reports the infant's skin appears distinctly yellow on exam today.

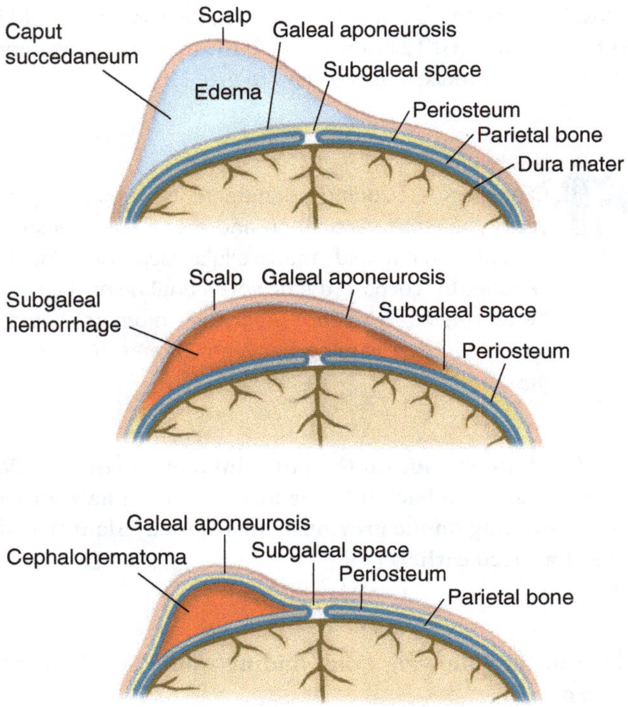

FIGURE 14–6. Extracranial bleeding of the newborn due to birth trauma. (Reproduced with permission from Cunningham FG, Leveno KJ, Bloom SL, et al, eds. *Williams Obstetrics*. 24th ed. New York, NY: McGraw-Hill Education; 2014, Fig. 33-1.)

Question 5-3

Which of the following is NOT considered a major risk factor for developing severe hyperbilirubinemia?

A) Gestational age of 41 weeks.
B) Cephalohematoma.
C) Sibling who required treatment for neonatal jaundice.
D) Exclusive breastfeeding.
E) East Asian race.

Discussion 5-3

The correct answer is "A." Gestational age of 41 weeks or more is actually associated with a decreased risk of severe hyperbilirubinemia, along with exclusive bottle-feeding, neonatal discharge after 72 hours of life, and African-American ethnicity (excluding those with glucose-6-phosphate dehydrogenase [G6PD] or other hemolytic disease). The risk of severe hyperbilirubinemia is directly proportional to the number of risk factors present. Prematurity increases the risk and lowers the threshold for phototherapy. (See Table 14–2.) Additional factors to consider are inherited deficiencies in hepatic conjugation hemolytic disease, and infection.

Question 5-4

Which of the following is the best way to determine the level of concern your team should have regarding this infant's jaundice?

A) Inspect the infant visually to estimate how much of the body appears jaundiced, starting at the head.
B) Ask the mother if the infant has seemed difficult to arouse or had a high-pitched cry.
C) Examine the child for signs of hypotonia, poor suck, or jitteriness.
D) Obtain a transcutaneous bilirubin measurement.
E) Pretend you didn't notice.

Discussion 5-4

The correct answer is "D." The total bilirubin level needs to be measured to determine if phototherapy is indicated to prevent bilirubin-induced neurologic dysfunction (BIND). Infants who are at least 35 weeks' gestational age at birth are typically at risk for BIND at total bilirubin concentration of 25 mg/dL or higher. Options "B" and "C" describe signs of acute bilirubin encephalopathy. Bilirubin is toxic to the central nervous system, causing damage to the basal ganglia and brainstem nuclei that may be irreversible (kernicterus). Visual inspection is important in recognizing jaundice but does not provide a good indicator of

TABLE 14–2 RISK FACTORS FOR DEVELOPING SEVERE HYPERBILIRUBINEMIA[a]			
Risk Factor	**Major**	**Minor**	**Decreased Risk**
Discharge bilirubin level/ zone on nomogram	> 95% (high risk)	> 75% (high intermediate risk)	< 40% (low risk)
Clinically yellow	First 24 hours	Before discharge	None
Gestational age (weeks)	35–36	37–38	≥ 41
Feeding	Breastfed – difficulties, weight loss	Breastfed—going well	Formula
Sibling	Received phototherapy	Jaundiced but no phototherapy	Never
Hemolytic disease	Blood group incompatibility with +DAT, G6PD		
Race	East Asian	Hispanic	African American
Other	Cephalohematoma, bruising	Macrosomic IDM, polycythemia, male gender	Discharged after 72 hours of age

DAT, direct antibody testing; G6PD, glucose-6-phophate dehydrogenase deficiency; IDM, infant of a diabetic mother.

[a]Risk is proportional to the number risk factors present.

concern and is not a reliable method of estimating the actual level of bilirubin in the bloodstream. It is also not acceptable to wait until neurologic symptoms arise before intervening. Measurement of the infant's total bilirubin level may be done by blood test or transcutaneous device. Transcutaneous measurement is noninvasive but does not seem to be as accurate as a total serum or plasma bilirubin in certain settings, particularly following phototherapy, at high levels, or in infants with dark skin pigmentation.

Your transcutaneous bilirubin measurement is 13 mg/dL, which is in the high intermediate risk zone on the nomogram. The level is below the phototherapy threshold for an infant of at least 38 weeks' gestation and without neurotoxicity risk factors.

Question 5-5
Which is NOT a neurotoxicity risk factor when deciding if an infant needs phototherapy?
A) Hemolytic disease.
B) Temperature instability.
C) Sepsis.
D) Hypoalbuminemia.
E) East Asian race.

Discussion 5-5
The correct answer is "E." East Asian race is a risk factor for developing severe hyperbilirubinemia but is not a neurotoxicity risk factor. The Bhutani nomogram is used to the map total bilirubin levels to a risk zone based on the age of the infant at time of collection. This predicts the risk of developing severe hyperbilirubinemia (defined as a serum bilirubin > 95% for age) and determines the urgency for follow-up assessment, which is particularly important when planning for discharge. To determine the threshold for phototherapy, the bilirubin must be plotted on a separate nomogram. The threshold varies based on gestational age and *neurotoxicity* risk factors, which include hemolytic disease, asphyxia, significant lethargy, temperature instability, sepsis, acidosis, and hypoalbuminemia. A third curve is used to determine the threshold for exchange transfusion.

The bilirubin nomogram and treatment threshold curves are not reproduced here. The reader should be aware of their existence, how to read them, and that higher risk babies (those with prematurity, evidence of infection or, concerns for hemolysis) require earlier and more aggressive therapy. It is not useful to memorize the curves or know specific cut off points for treatment.

> **Helpful Tip**
> Any infant with jaundice noted in the first 24 hours of life or whose bilirubin is rapidly rising (> 0.2 mg/dL/h or 5 mg/dL/day) must be evaluated for pathologic cause, often hemolytic disease such as ABO incompatibility. A positive direct antibody test (Coombs test) means hemolysis is present.

The medical student following this infant notes that she has heard of both breast milk and breastfeeding jaundice, and wonders if they are the same thing.

Question 5-6
What of the following best describes breast milk jaundice?
A) Breast milk jaundice typically occurs within the first few days of life before the mother's mature milk is in.
B) Breast milk jaundice may last up to 3 months of age.
C) Supplementation is typically recommended in cases of breast milk jaundice.
D) Breast milk jaundice can be confirmed by an elevated direct bilirubin level.
E) The terms are synonymous.

Discussion 5-6
The correct answer is "B." Breastfeeding failure and breast milk jaundice are both causes of indirect hyperbilirubinemia in infants, resulting in increased enterohepatic circulation of bilirubin. Breast milk jaundice occurs between DOL 5 and 7, usually peaks within the second to third week of life, and gradually decreases over 1 to 3 months. Breast milk is thought to contain an unidentified substance that promotes intestinal absorption of bilirubin. Beta-glucuronidase, an enzyme that deconjugates bilirubin and enhances intestinal reabsorption of bilirubin has been proposed as the causal agent. Although severe hyperbilirubinemia necessitating intervention is unlikely in breast milk jaundice, it is important to monitor for high conjugated bilirubin levels or significant increases over time. If jaundice does not resolve by 12 weeks, pathologic causes should be reevaluated. A simple diagnostic test is to feed the infant formula for a few days. The bilirubin level should rapidly drop, confirming the diagnosis. Resumption of breastfeeding usually does not result in a significant increase in bilirubin. Breastfeeding failure jaundice begins after 24 hours of age, peaks between DOL 3 and 5, and resolves within the first week of life. It is caused by inadequate milk intake, causing hypovolemia through weight and fluid loss, delayed bilirubin excretion, and increased enterohepatic circulation (delayed passage of bilirubin-rich meconium).

> **Helpful Tip**
> All newborns lose weight in the first week of life, with most sources quoting 10% to 12% weight loss as normal.

► CASE 6

A neonatal resuscitation team is called to an impending delivery of a 41-week gestational age male infant. The team is notified of thick meconium-stained fluid and persistent variable heart rate decelerations with slow recovery to baseline for the past 30 minutes. The mother had spontaneous rupture of membranes approximately 20 hours ago. Vacuum-assisted vaginal delivery is being attempted as the team enters the room. The infant is delivered after two pulls on the vacuum device. There was one pop-off of the vacuum device between attempts. The infant is handed to the waiting neonatal intensive care unit (NICU) team for assessment and treatment. He is not crying, has no spontaneous respirations, appears limp and cyanotic, and has a heart rate of 75 bpm.

Question 6-1

What is the first step in the management of this infant?
A) Immediately begin tactile stimulation, including drying and gently rubbing the back to encourage respirations.
B) Apply free-flowing oxygen to the infant's face as he is cyanotic.
C) Suction the mouth followed by the nose with a bulb syringe.
D) Intubate the trachea and suction for meconium.
E) Start positive-pressure ventilation (PPV) as the infant has no spontaneous respirations.

Discussion 6-1

The correct answer is "D." This newborn remains nonvigorous at the time of delivery with meconium present. Therefore, he should be intubated immediately (prior to any stimulation) and the trachea should be suctioned. A vigorous newborn is defined as an infant who has strong respiratory efforts, good muscle tone, and a heart rate greater than 100 bpm. If the newborn is vigorous despite the presence of meconium, suction the mouth and nose only. If the newborn in this case remains nonvigorous after intubation and suctioning of the trachea, then additional resuscitation should be undertaken promptly.

After intubation and suctioning for meconium, the infant's heart rate remains at 80 bpm and he is taking only a few gasping breaths.

Question 6-2

What should the next step be in resuscitation management of this infant?
A) Apply free-flowing oxygen to the infant's face to encourage breathing.
B) Continue to stimulate the infant for several minutes to increase respiratory effort.
C) Provide PPV via bag-mask or T-piece resuscitator.
D) Start chest compressions in response to bradycardia.
E) Apply a pulse oximetry device and only start PPV if oxygen saturations remain less than 75% at 2 minutes of age.

Discussion 6-2

The correct answer is "C." The initial steps of resuscitation include appropriate positioning of the airway into the "sniffing" position and tactile stimulation for not more than 60 seconds. If a newborn has not responded to these efforts and has persistent apnea, then PPV should be started promptly. Chest compressions should only be started after the infant has failed to respond to PPV and the heart rate remains less than 60 bpm. Free-flowing oxygen without PPV should only be used in an infant with adequate respiratory effort. The decisions and actions during newborn resuscitation should be based on respirations, heart rate, and color (oxygenation). Pulse oximetry should be applied when

an infant requires PPV, when central cyanosis is present, when supplemental oxygen is required, or to confirm the perception of cyanosis. Adequate respiratory effort and heart rate will determine the need for PPV, not the pulse oximetry alone. If a newborn is not responding with increased heart rate and saturations, first reassessment of airway position and patency should be completed, followed by continuation of PPV, initiation of chest compressions if the heart rate is less than 60 bpm, and administration of bolus epinephrine, preferably using the intravenous route or endotracheal tube if intravenous access unavailable.

After the initiation of PPV, the newborn's heart rate increased to 165 bpm and the saturation levels increased to 90% on 40% fraction of inspired oxygen (FiO$_2$). The infant is intubated in the delivery room and transported to the NICU for further care. Apgar scores of 1, 3, and 7 are obtained at 1, 5, and 10 minutes of age.

Question 6-3

The newborn is at risk for which of the following consequences?
A) Lactic acidosis due to poor perfusion.
B) Hyperglycemia due to stress counter-regulatory hormones.
C) Increased risk of subgaleal hemorrhage and subsequent hypovolemic shock due to vacuum-assisted delivery.
D) Increased risk of seizures due to initial hypoxia.
E) Respiratory failure due to meconium aspiration.
F) All of the above.

Discussion 6-3

The correct answer is "F." Newborns requiring significant resuscitation at birth are at risk for several metabolic consequences of poor perfusion in the first few minutes of life. They must be observed closely for end-organ damage caused by hypoxemia, including lactic acidosis, liver and kidney damage, cardiovascular instability, and electrolyte abnormalities, especially hypoglycemia and hyperglycemia. Although suctioning of the trachea to remove meconium has been done in this case, a newborn with thick meconium at delivery still remains at risk of the consequences of meconium aspiration syndrome, including persistent pulmonary hypertension of the newborn. The consequences of hypoxia to the brain are the most significant given the nonreversibility of these changes. Prevention of seizures and treatment with therapeutic hypothermia are recommended in moderate and severe cases of hypoxic ischemic encephalopathy. It is important to recognize that the use of vacuum-assist devices in vaginal deliveries is associated with increased risk of subgaleal bleeding. Newborns should be monitored closely by means of serial physical exams and hemoglobin levels if there is any concern for subgaleal hemorrhage. Infants can rapidly decompensate, developing hypovolemic shock in these situations.

▶ CASE 7

A mother is admitted into labor and delivery with a 1-day history of dysuria, fevers to 38.9°C (102°F), and now active contractions every 2 to 3 minutes for about 1 hour. Her fetus has an estimated gestational age of 24-3/7 weeks based on last menstrual period (LMP) and a concordant 8-week ultrasound. The mother had regular prenatal care and an uncomplicated pregnancy until now. On exam, the physician notes that the mother's cervix is dilated to 8 cm with a bulging bag of water. She then has spontaneous rupture of membranes with green-colored, foul-smelling fluid. She rapidly delivers a 575-g male infant prior to maternal administration of betamethasone. The NICU team is present at the delivery.

Question 7-1

Which of these statements is accurate about this infant?

A) The Apgar score can be used to reliably predict asphyxia in a very preterm infant.

B) The Apgar score is composed of five components: heart rate, respiratory effort, blood pressure, color, and oxygen saturation.

C) The Apgar score can be affected by maternal sedation or analgesia as well as neurologic conditions such as muscle disease or cerebral malformations.

D) The Apgar score is composed of five components: heart rate, respiratory effort, oxygen saturation, respiratory distress, and color.

E) None of the above.

Discussion 7-1

The correct answer is "C." The Apgar score is composed of five components—heart rate, respiratory effort, tone, reflex irritability, and color—each of which can be given a score of 0, 1, or 2. Hopefully you remember this from earlier. The scoring provides consistent shorthand for reporting the state of the infant and effectiveness of resuscitation. It is important to recognize, however, that elements of the score, including tone, color, and reflex irritability, are partially dependent on the physiologic maturity of the infant. Thus, normal preterm infants may receive a lower score because of immaturity without evidence of asphyxia. Maternal sedation, neurologic conditions, and cardiorespiratory conditions that interfere with heart rate or tone may alter the Apgar score.

> **Helpful Tip**
> Maternal medications taken during pregnancy, delivery, or both can affect the fetus and neonate. Magnesium or narcotics given during labor may cause neurologic and respiratory depression in the neonate after delivery. Medications taken by breastfeeding mothers may be transmitted through the breastmilk; an example is codeine, which has caused neonatal death from respiratory depression.

Question 7-2

Which of these steps is/are important in the management of this extremely low birthweight (ELBW) preterm infant?

A) Provide thermal support immediately after delivery due to the poor thermoregulation capabilities of preterm infants.

B) Use a bag or plastic covering in the delivery room to minimize heat loss through evaporation or convection.

C) Monitor closely for low blood glucose as this infant will be at risk for hypoglycemia due to gestational age.

D) Monitor closely as this infant will be at risk for apnea due to gestational age.

E) All of the above.

Discussion 7-2

The correct answer is "E." Extremely low and very low birthweight infants are at risk for several medical morbidities beyond the basic resuscitation of airway, breathing, and circulation. The preterm neonate is at high risk for cold stress owing to relatively high surface area with very immature skin. Delivery room practices to minimize hypothermia are important. The infant is also at high risk for hypoglycemia due to poor glycogen stores, relative liver immaturity, and abnormal glucose regulatory hormone pathways. Very preterm infants are at risk of central apnea and may be treated with methylxanthine medications (caffeine) to minimize this risk.

> **Helpful Tip**
> In premature infants, birthweight may be classified as low, very low, or extremely low as follows:
>
> Low birthweight (LBW) < 2500 g
>
> Very low birthweight (VLBW) < 1500 g
>
> Extremely low birthweight (ELBW) < 1000 g

Question 7-3

What prognostic factors in this ELBW infant will improve survival without disability?

A) Singleton gestation.

B) Male sex.

C) Active maternal chorioamnionitis.

D) No betamethasone administration.

E) None of the above.

Discussion 7-3

The correct answer is "A." This ELBW 575-g infant born at 24-3/7 weeks' gestation to a mother with active chorioamnionitis who was unable to receive betamethasone has several risk factors for poor prognosis. Being a single gestation (as opposed to one of multiples) improves risk status, but all of the other options worsen prognosis. Betamethasone is administered to mothers in two doses with 24 hours between dosing. This medication has been found to improve fetal lung maturity and decrease intracranial hemorrhage, which are both major causes of morbidity and mortality in this population. A fetus exposed to active maternal infection (eg, chorioamnionitis) has a worsened probability of survival without disability owing to the high likelihood of fetal infection and multiorgan dysfunction that is associated with infection.

⧗ QUICK QUIZ

Which of the following regarding intraventricular hemorrhage (IVH) is FALSE?
A) IVH is graded I to IV.
B) Hydrocephalus is a complication of IVH.
C) Apnea and seizure are clinical manifestations of IVH.
D) Polycythemia may result from IVH.
E) Premature infants should have routine screening for IVH.

Discussion

The correct answer is "D." The severity of IVH is graded from I to IV based on the location and extent of bleeding, as follows:

- Grade I: germinal matrix
- Grade II: extension of grade I involving the ventricles without ventricular dilation
- Grade III: extension grade II with ventricular dilation
- Grade IV: ventricular dilation with extension into the cerebral cortex

IVH is common in low birthweight and premature infants. The infant may be asymptomatic or have apnea, coma, lethargy, bradycardia, seizures, hypotension, metabolic acidosis, and anemia. Infants at risk should be screened routinely by ultrasound:

> **Helpful Tip**
> Intraventricular hemorrhage (IVH) is a major complication of extreme prematurity. The germinal matrix is a fragile network of blood vessels. It is prone to bleeding with any abrupt change in hemodynamics, especially between the time of delivery until about 1 week of age in preterm infants. Bleeding is most common in those less than 34 weeks' gestation. Intraventricular hemorrhage and hypoxic injury can lead to loss of periventricular white matter (leukomalacia) and subsequent cerebral palsy, one of the major complications of extreme prematurity.

▶ CASE 8

A full-term infant is delivered at 40-2/7 weeks' gestation after a pregnancy complicated by maternal diabetes requiring insulin for blood glucose control. The delivery requires vacuum assistance for a relatively large macrosomic infant. The infant does well in the delivery room, requiring only stimulation and drying. Blood glucose levels are slightly low in the first 6 hours but improve with frequent feeding attempts. The physician caring for the infant receives a call at 24 hours of age that the infant has a transcutaneous bilirubin reading in the high-risk zone and appears well, but somewhat sleepy and quite ruddy in color on exam.

Question 8-1

What evaluation should be completed at this time?
A) Serum bilirubin.
B) Hemoglobin to assess for polycythemia.
C) Infant and maternal blood type.
D) Physical exam to assess for cephalohematoma, caput, and subgaleal hemorrhage.
E) Physical exam to assess hydration.
F) All of the above.

Discussion 8-1

The correct answer is "F." Jaundice in the first 24 hours of life in a neonate is pathologic, most commonly a result of hemolysis. This infant has several risk factors for the development of severe hyperbilirubinemia of the newborn. The transcutaneous bilirubin level should be confirmed with serum bilirubin testing. Infants of diabetic mothers are at higher risk of polycythemia (central hematocrit > 65%), adding to the risk of jaundice. One of the most common causes of severe hyperbilirubinemia is ABO incompatibility, with hemolysis and resultant hyperbilirubinemia. Therefore, screening of mother and infant blood types is important, especially with a blood type O mother. Infants who have been delivered with the assistance of instrumentation such as the vacuum device are at higher risk of cephalohematoma and subgaleal bleeding that can significantly increase bilirubin levels and should be assessed regularly by physical exam. Physiologic jaundice of the newborn is exacerbated by dehydration, manifested by weight loss, poor feeding with decreased stool output, and increased enterohepatic circulation, all leading to increased jaundice. (See Table 14–2.)

The infant undergoes the appropriate evaluation and is found to have a serum unconjugated bilirubin of 13 mg/dL at 24 hours with a conjugated bilirubin of 0.4 mg/dl, a free-flowing hematocrit of 72%, and a small cephalohematoma at the vacuum site. Both mother and infant are blood type A+. The infant has made only marginal breastfeeding attempts due to sleepiness.

Question 8-2

Which is the true statement?
A) This infant does not need phototherapy for increased bilirubin until DOL 3.
B) This infant may need a partial exchange transfusion due to polycythemia with symptoms of hyperviscosity.
C) This infant does not need supplemental feedings or fluids unless the bilirubin continues to rise.
D) This infant can be discharged home as long as parents agree to follow up in 24 hours for another bilirubin check.
E) The conjugated bilirubin is elevated and needs additional evaluation for metabolic disease.

Discussion 8-2

The correct answer is "B." This infant has a bilirubin level above the indicated threshold for treatment with phototherapy and therefore should start inpatient phototherapy immediately. The infant's hematocrit is elevated in a manner consistent with polycythemia. Infants with severe hyperviscosity can have lethargy, tremors, respiratory distress, cyanosis, and even seizures or strokes. This infant needs increased fluid intake and may need a partial volume exchange transfusion (involving removal of blood and replacement with saline or albumin). Infants should not be discharged early if any risk factors for increased jaundice (hemolytic disease, intracranial bleeding, lethargy, sepsis, etc) are present. Kernicterus (irreversible bilirubin encephalopathy) can result from severe hyperbilirubinemia. Infants with bilirubin encephalopathy are lethargic, hypotonic or hypertonic, and have a high-pitched cry. Opisthotonus, seizures, and death may occur if bilirubin is not lowered. Magnetic resonance imaging (MRI) scans shows a high T2 signal in the globus pallidus (part of the basal ganglia). Patients surviving kernicterus have severe permanent neurologic symptoms (choreoathetosis, spasticity, hearing loss, ataxia, and cognitive impairment). Less severe injury is associated with mild neurologic abnormalities, including hearing loss, which may be the only abnormality. This infant has a normal conjugated bilirubin; however, infants who have an increased conjugated fraction of bilirubin need additional evaluation for several serious disorders. The liver and gall bladder anatomy should be assessed for biliary atresia, choledochal cyst, or other anatomic causes of biliary obstruction. Infections, especially viral hepatitis, Ebstein-Barr virus (EBV), cytomegalovirus (CMV), and other neonatal viral infections, should be investigated. Severe sepsis can cause conjugated hyperbilirubinemia. Inborn errors of metabolism should be evaluated. Total parenteral nutrition cholestasis may be the cause in those receiving long-term intravenous nutrition.

QUICK QUIZ

What is the definition of conjugated hyperbilirubinemia?

A) Conjugated bilirubin greater than 1 mg/dL.
B) Conjugated bilirubin greater than 5 mg/dL.
C) Conjugated bilirubin greater than 10 mg/dL.
D) Conjugated bilirubin greater than 10% total serum bilirubin.
E) None of the above.

Discussion

The correct answer is "E." Conjugated hyperbilirubinemia is never normal in a neonate. Its definition is dependent on the total serum bilirubin value, with 5 being the reference value, as follows:

Conjugated bilirubin > 1 mg/dL if the total serum bilirubin is < 5 mg/dL

or

Conjugated bilirubin > 20% of the total serum bilirubin if the serum bilirubin is > 5 mg/dL

▶ CASE 9

A 35-week gestational age infant is born by cesarean delivery to a mother with placenta previa. The infant girl is vigorous after delivery, with Apgar scores of 8 and 8. She is brought to her mother's chest. Fifteen minutes later the NICU team is called because the infant is experiencing worsening respiratory distress with tachypnea, retractions, and mild grunting respirations. She is placed on nasal continuous positive airway pressure (CPAP) and admitted to the NICU. The infant shows clinical improvement on CPAP, requiring approximately 25% FiO_2. Her chest radiograph shows 10-rib expansion with fluid in the fissure and no other focal infiltrates. You are asked to update her family.

Question 9-1

You tell them:

A) This is most consistent with neonatal pneumonia and sepsis. You will start antibiotics immediately and she will recover in several days to a week.
B) This is most consistent with respiratory distress syndrome resulting from surfactant deficiency related to prematurity. She may need to be intubated for surfactant administration.
C) This is most consistent with transient tachypnea of the newborn and fluid retention exacerbated by the cesarean delivery without labor. She will improve in the next 24 hours.
D) This is most consistent with meconium aspiration. She will improve within days to weeks.
E) None of the above.

Discussion 9-1

The correct answer is "C." Transient tachypnea of the newborn is most common in late preterm and term infants who are delivered by cesarean section or precipitous delivery. Chest films demonstrate adequate lung expansion with retained fetal lung fluid. This condition generally improves quickly over hours and affected infants very rarely need intubation and mechanical ventilation.

▶ CASE 10

A 35-week gestational age infant is born by cesarean delivery to a mother with placenta previa. The infant girl is vigorous after delivery, with Apgar scores of 8 and 8. She is brought to her mother's chest. Fifteen minutes later the NICU team is called because the infant is experiencing worsening respiratory distress with tachypnea, retractions, and mild grunting respirations. She is placed on nasal CPAP and admitted to the NICU. The infant continues to be tachypneic, at 80 breaths per minute, has mild retractions, and requires 40% FiO_2 on CPAP. Her chest radiograph shows approximately 7-rib expansion with ground glass opacities throughout all lung fields. You are asked to update her family.

Question 10-1

You tell them:

A) This is most consistent with neonatal pneumonia and sepsis. You will start antibiotics immediately and she will recover in several days to a week.

B) This is most consistent with respiratory distress syndrome resulting from surfactant deficiency related to prematurity. She may need to be intubated for surfactant administration.

C) This is most consistent with transient tachypnea of the newborn and fluid retention exacerbated by the cesarean delivery without labor. She will improve in the next 24 hours.

D) This is most consistent with meconium aspiration. She will improve within days to weeks.

E) None of the above.

Discussion 10-1

The correct answer is "B." Although the clinical scenario is nearly identical to the one described in Case 9, this infant has persistent distress on CPAP with rising oxygen and evidence of respiratory distress syndrome on chest radiograph with decreased lung expansion and findings consistent with surfactant deficiency. (See Figure 14–7.) Although respiratory distress syndrome is most common in very preterm infants, many late preterm infants of less than 37 weeks' gestation have surfactant deficiency, especially those who have not had spontaneous labor. If clinical symptoms continue to worsen, oxygen needs increase, or gas exchange is poor as evidenced by respiratory acidosis on blood gas measurements, then this infant should be intubated and surfactant administered through the endotracheal tube.

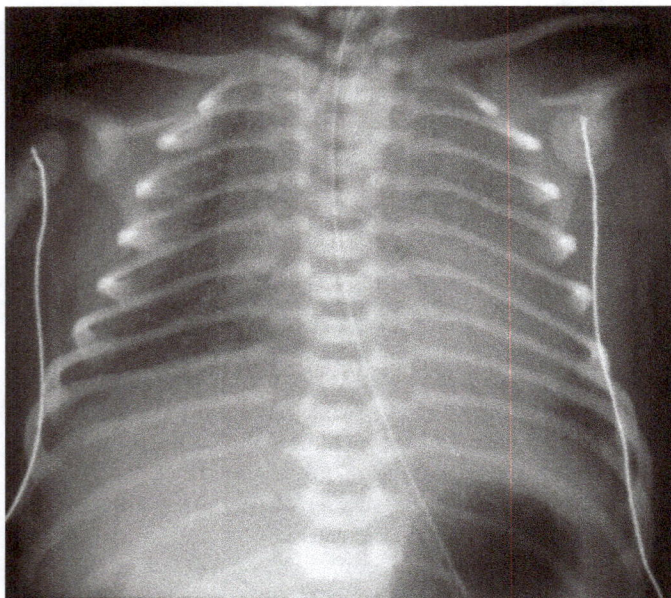

FIGURE 14–7. Respiratory distress syndrome. Bilateral ground glass opacities, poor inflation, and prominent air bronchograms are present on the chest X-ray of this infant with respiratory distress syndrome. (Reproduced with permission from Tintinalli JE, Stapczynski JS, Ma OJ, et al: *Tintinalli's Emergency Medicine: A Comprehensive Study Guide*, 8th ed. McGraw-Hill Education, Inc., 2016. Fig 107-2.)

▶ CASE 11

A 39-week gestational age infant is born after prolonged rupture of membranes. The membranes ruptured 48 hours before admission, and the mother presented to the hospital with a temperature of 39.4°C (103°F), foul-smelling amniotic fluid, and severe abdominal pain. She is started on antibiotics shortly before delivery. The infant is born by cesarean delivery due to persistent fetal tachycardia and concerns for maternal chorioamnionitis. Apgar scores are 8 and 8. The infant is initially vigorous and is placed on the mother's chest for transition. The infant is brought to the NICU for evaluation due to suspected maternal chorioamnionitis and develops respiratory distress within hours of admission. Findings include tachypnea, mild retractions, and grunting respirations. Her chest radiograph has patchy infiltrates bilaterally. You are asked to update her family.

Question 11-1

You tell them:

A) This is most consistent with neonatal pneumonia and sepsis. You will continue antibiotics and she will likely recover in several days to a week.

B) This is most consistent with respiratory distress syndrome resulting from surfactant deficiency. She may need to be intubated for surfactant administration.

C) This is most consistent with transient tachypnea of the newborn and fluid retention exacerbated by cesarean delivery without labor. She will improve in the next 24 hours.

D) This is most consistent with tension pneumothorax.

E) None of the above.

Discussion 11-1

The correct answer is "A." This infant's respiratory distress is most consistent with an infectious cause stemming from prolonged rupture of membranes (PROM) and maternal infection. The most common infectious etiology in the newborn is group B streptococcal (GBS) infection, which can lead to pneumonia, sepsis, or even meningitis. *Escherichia coli* is the next most common cause. The infant is generally infected with vaginal flora bacteria, with higher infection rates associated with PROM. Empiric antibiotic coverage in the newborn period is therefore targeted at these most common organisms, and consists of ampicillin and gentamicin intravenously. (See Figure 14–8.)

> **Helpful Tip**
> Prolonged rupture of membranes (> 18 hours) is associated with neonatal sepsis.

⧗ QUICK QUIZ

What is NOT a risk factor for neonatal sepsis?

A) Rupture of membranes for 20 hours.

B) Maternal chorioamnionitis.

C) Prematurity.

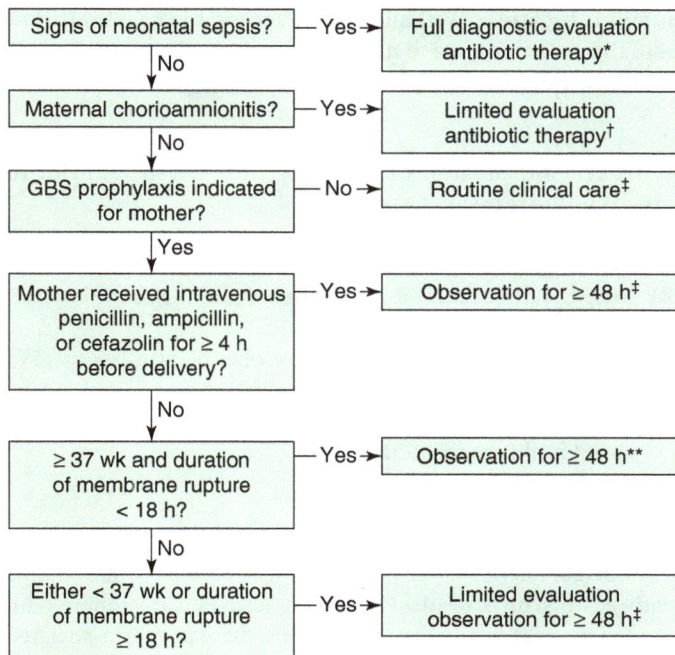

*Full evaluation includes blood culture, a complete blood count (CBC), chest radiograph (if respiratory symptoms present), and lumbar puncture (if infant is stable enough to tolerate procedure).
†Limited evaluation includes blood culture and CBC (at birth and/or 6-12 hours of age).
‡If signs of sepsis develop, perform a full evaluation and start antibiotics.
**CBC at age 6-12 hours of age is recommended.

FIGURE 14–8. Secondary prevention of early-onset group B streptococcal (GBS) disease in newborns. (Reproduced with permission from Verani JR, McGee L, Schrag SJ, et al: Prevention of perinatal group B streptococcal disease—revised guidelines from CDC, 2010, *MMWR Recomm Rep.* 2010 Nov 19;59(RR-10):1-36.)

D) Maternal colonization with GBS.
E) All of the above.

Discussion
The correct answer is "E."

▶ CASE 12

A postterm 42-3/7-week gestational age infant is born after induced vaginal delivery. Meconium-stained fluid was noted after rupture approximately 6 hours before delivery. The NICU team is present at the delivery. The infant's head delivers easily; however, shoulder dystocia is immediately recognized and the infant's body does not deliver for approximately 4 minutes after delivery of the head. The infant is initially apneic, with very poor tone and no spontaneous movements. The NICU team immediately intubates the infant and suctions the airway. The infant is admitted to the NICU with significant hypoxemia that worsens over the first 6 hours of life.

Question 12-1
What is etiology of the respiratory failure in this infant?
A) Respiratory failure resulting from sepsis.
B) Respiratory failure resulting from meconium aspiration syndrome and persistent pulmonary hypertension of the newborn.

C) Respiratory failure resulting from hypoxic ischemic encephalopathy.
D) Respiratory failure resulting from congestive heart failure.
E) All of the above.

Discussion 12-1
The correct answer is "B." This infant likely has hypoxemic respiratory failure resulting from meconium aspiration syndrome and persistent pulmonary hypertension, but this etiology can be complicated by sepsis and hypoxic ischemic encephalopathy. The chest film in meconium aspiration generally shows scattered patchy infiltrates with significant hyperinflation. The hypoxemia associated with these conditions can be extreme, at times requiring high-frequency ventilation or even extracorporeal membrane oxygenation (ECMO).

The infant has been on the ventilator for about 6 hours when you are called to the bedside for a sudden decompensation with decreased saturations as low as 30%, bradycardia, and absent breath sounds on the right.

Question 12-2
What is the most likely problem?
A) The infant has a previously undiagnosed heart problem.
B) The infant has a tension pneumothorax associated with meconium aspiration.
C) The infant needs surfactant.
D) The infant needs antibiotics.
E) None of the above.

Discussion 12-2
The correct answer is "B." Air leak syndrome with pneumothorax is a common serious complication of meconium aspiration syndrome that results from air trapping and the high ventilator needs in this condition. Tension pneumothoraces must be recognized immediately and relieved with needle thoracentesis. Although a ductal-dependent cardiac lesion could lead to severe hypoxemia upon ductal closure, it would be uncommon for a cardiac lesion to suddenly cause absent breath sounds on the right. Although this infant may need surfactant and antibiotics during the course of illness, it would again be uncommon to have a sudden decompensation with these physical findings as a result of those problems.

As the infant improves from a respiratory standpoint, the nurse notices that she does not move her right arm very often and her arm seems to be rotated in toward her body. The nurse asks what you think caused this.

Question 12-3
The most likely cause of this problem would be:
A) The peripheral IV line that was placed in the infant's arm is causing decreased movement.
B) The infant has a brachial plexus injury associated with delivery complicated by shoulder dystocia.
C) The infant had a perinatal stroke.
D) The infant received sedation medication.
E) None of the above.

Discussion 12-3

The correct answer is "B." Stretch injuries to the brachial plexus like this one, which has resulted in an Erb palsy, are associated with difficult deliveries, especially those involving shoulder dystocia and macrosomia. It is important to assess for clavicular fractures as well after delivery. Some brachial plexus injuries are severe enough to require surgery; however, many improve with physical therapy and time.

⏳ QUICK QUIZ

What is NOT true regarding brachial plexus injuries?
A) Brachial plexus injuries may be bilateral.
B) Brachial plexus injuries may cause Horner syndrome if the sympathetic fibers of T1 are affected.
C) Clinical manifestations of a brachial plexus injury depend on the specific nerves involved.
D) The most common brachial plexus injury is associated with the "waiter's tip" posture.
E) Brachial plexus injuries are diagnosed by ultrasound.

Discussion

The correct answer is "E." Brachial plexus injuries are evident clinically but may require electromyography in some cases. The brachial plexus involves cervical nerves C5 to C8 and the first thoracic nerve T1. Brachial plexus injuries may cause arm paralysis, Horner syndrome, or hemidiaphragm paralysis from phrenic nerve involvement. Erb palsy involves injury to C5, C6, and C7. This is the most common injury. The upper arm is adducted and internally rotated; the forearm is pronated and extended; and the wrist and fingers are flexed. This is called the "waiter's tip" posture. Klumpke palsy involves injury to C8 and T1, resulting in isolated hand paralysis and Horner syndrome. It is rare and may represent residual deficit after the upper plexus portion has recovered.

> **Helpful Tip**
> Macrosomia, operative vaginal delivery, maternal pelvic anomalies, breech presentation, and shoulder dystocia are risk factors for birth injuries. Injuries include bruising, scalp bleeding or swelling, brachial plexus injury, cervical spine transection, intracranial hemorrhage, fractures, and intra-abdominal injuries.

▶ CASE 13

An infant is born at 35-5/7 weeks' gestation with a prenatally diagnosed gastroschisis defect. The mother received regular prenatal care at a tertiary care facility throughout the pregnancy. Unfortunately, she developed rapidly progressing preterm labor and was admitted to a small community hospital near her home. The physician on call delivers the infant and requests transport to your center. The physician reports the infant is breathing well and has an acceptable heart rate, but remains slightly pale with prolonged capillary refill time both centrally and peripherally.

Question 13-1

What recommendations do you give this physician prior to arrival of the transport team?
A) Place the infant in a sterile bowel bag to cover the defect and minimize insensible losses.
B) Keep the defect central with minimal kinking of the bowel if possible.
C) Anticipate large insensible losses; obtain intravenous (IV) access and begin IV volume resuscitation.
D) Treat respiratory symptoms if needed, remain aware of apnea in this population.
E) All of the above.

Discussion 13-1

The correct answer is "E." Although it is preferred that infants with gastroschisis be delivered in a tertiary care center with immediate access to pediatric surgeons, there is often associated polyhydramnios in these pregnancies making them high risk for preterm labor. After delivery, many infants with gastroschisis lose a tremendous amount of fluid through insensible losses and require significant volume resuscitation to maintain perfusion to the bowel which is at risk for compromise.

While the transport team is en route to pick up the infant with gastroschisis, labor and delivery calls for another NICU team to attend the delivery of a full-term infant with prenatally diagnosed omphalocele. The infant is delivered via cesarean section and remains vigorous. You note a large abdominal wall defect centrally in the area of the umbilicus that is completely covered with a gelatinous membrane.

Question 13-2

Which of these statements about abdominal wall defects is accurate?
A) Infants with gastroschisis are more likely than those with omphalocele to have associated chromosome problems.
B) The definition of omphalocele is based on the presence of a membrane covering.
C) The definition of omphalocele is based on the location of the defect involving the umbilical ring in contrast to gastroschisis, which is lateral to the umbilicus.
D) Associated cardiac defects and other anomalies are rare in omphalocele, but common in gastroschisis.
E) None of the above.

Discussion 13-2

The correct answer is "C." By definition the defect location assigns the nomenclature of gastroschisis versus omphalocele. Although omphaloceles are generally membrane covered by the umbilicus, these can rupture before or at delivery. Omphalocele is more common in infants born to older mothers and is more often associated with other anomalies, especially aneuploidy. Infants with omphalocele should receive a comprehensive evaluation, including cardiac echocardiogram, karyotyping, and renal ultrasound. Gastroschisis occurs very early in pregnancy. The defect is generally located to the right of the umbilicus, and the amount of intestine outside the body may vary. Gastroschisis is *not* generally associated with other anomalies or chromosome problems. The incidence is higher in adolescent mothers and mothers who smoke cigarettes.

► CASE 14

A preterm infant born at 25 weeks' gestation is now 6 weeks old (31 weeks corrected gestational age). The infant has been stable for the past few weeks, breathing in room air, and receiving full enteral feedings through gavage tube that consist of fortified maternal breastmilk and some formula supplementation. Yesterday the infant had a few large gastric residuals with feeding but otherwise seemed well. You are called to the bedside today because of increased abdominal distention, apneic spells, poor urine output, lethargy, and hypothermia.

Question 14-1

This constellation of findings is most concerning for what condition?
A) Hirschsprung disease.
B) Respiratory viral illness.
C) Jejunal atresia.
D) Necrotizing enterocolitis.
E) Tracheoesophageal fistula.

Discussion 14-1

The correct answer is "D." Necrotizing enterocolitis (NEC) is a disease that is most common in preterm infants who have previously been enterally fed. Early signs of NEC are often systemic signs of illness such as lethargy, apnea, and hypothermia. There are also generally abdominal-specific findings, including increased abdominal distention and high gastric residuals. The disorder may lead to pneumatosis intestinalis with gas present below the serosal surface of the bowel or portal venous gas. Advanced NEC may lead to intestinal perforation, which is a surgical condition requiring immediate assessment and intervention. Laboratory findings including hyponatremia, thrombocytopenia, lactic acidosis, and coagulopathy may also be present. Option "A," Hirschsprung disease, is not correct; this disorder is caused by absence of ganglion cells, generally in the colon, and often presents with severe constipation, abdominal distention, and possibly toxic megacolon in the newborn. Option "C," jejunal atresia, should generally be recognized shortly after birth or prenatally by evidence of significant bowel dilation proximal to the atresia, often with emesis, and poor stooling. Option "E," tracheoesophageal fistula, generally manifests early in life and is characterized by copious oral secretions, respiratory distress, and inability to easily pass an orogastric tube beyond the esophageal defect.

> **Helpful Tip**
>
> Fetuses who are unable to swallow well or have intestinal obstruction in utero may present with polyhydramnios. Examples include infants with tracheoesophageal fistula, intestinal atresias, and neuromuscular conditions. Oligohydramnios can occur with a variety of conditions, including fetal renal anomalies leading to decreased urine output, fetal urinary output obstruction, placental insufficiency, or premature rupture of membranes. Fetuses with severe oligohydramnios may develop pulmonary hypoplasia owing to the role of amniotic fluid in lung development. They may also develop severe contractures due to the inability to move within the uterus. The constellation of IUGR, pulmonary hypoplasia, abnormal facies (low-set ears, micrognathia, flattened nose), and limb abnormalities including club foot are termed *Potter sequence*. This is a consequence of severe oligohydramnios in utero.

► CASE 15

A mother presents to labor and delivery at 39 weeks' gestation for a scheduled induction due to poorly controlled gestational diabetes. She has required insulin since the 29th week and reports that most of her blood glucose readings have been greater than 200 mg/dL over the past 2 weeks. She progresses in labor after oxytocin induction and vaginally delivers a single male infant weighing 4500 g.

Question 15-1

This infant is at increased risk for which of the following problems in the days following delivery?
A) Polycythemia.
B) Respiratory distress syndrome of the newborn.
C) Hypoglycemia.
D) Cardiac defects.
E) All of the above.

Discussion 15-1

The correct answer is "E." Maternal diabetes mellitus causes a variety of complications that can be minimized when mothers maintain good glycemic control during pregnancy. Infants remain exposed to a hyperinsulin state after delivery and can have profound hypoglycemia requiring frequent monitoring after delivery until stable. Infants of diabetic mothers (IDMs) have higher risks of polycythemia due to relative intrauterine hypoxia. Hyperinsulin states also decrease surfactant production and therefore increase the risk of respiratory distress syndrome of the newborn. IDMs are also at increased risk for cardiac defects especially septal wall hypertrophy. These infants should undergo prenatal ultrasound screening for cardiac defects. IDM infants have also been found to have increased rates of iron deficiency and potential neurodevelopmental consequences in iron dependent neuronal processes.

⧗ **QUICK QUIZ**

What is NOT a cause of neonatal polycythemia?
A) Delayed cord clamping.
B) Prematurity.
C) Twin-to-twin transfusion syndrome.
D) Postterm infant.
E) Placental insufficiency.

Discussion

The correct answer is "B." Additional causes include LGA, IUGR, trisomy 21, hypothyroidism, Beckwith-Wiedemann syndrome, and chronic fetal hypoxia.

▶ CASE 16

You are evaluating an infant in the newborn nursery who was born weighing 5 lb, 2 oz at 39-5/7 weeks' gestational age. The infant has small eyes with drooping upper eyelids, a flat philtrum, micrognathia, thin upper lip, and a short upturned nose. The infant fails the first newborn hearing screen.

Question 16-1

During pregnancy, the infant was most likely exposed to what substance?
A) Selective serotonin reuptake inhibitor (SSRI).
B) Oxycodone.
C) Alcohol.
D) Cocaine.
E) Cigarette smoke.

Discussion 16-1

The correct answer is "C." Fetal alcohol syndrome is a spectrum of symptoms involving growth restriction, characteristic facial features, and central nervous system problems that eventually may result in developmental delays, attention deficit hyperactivity disorder (ADHD), and seizures. Infants exposed to narcotics such as oxycodone can have a typical withdrawal syndrome termed neonatal abstinence syndrome, which is characterized by neurologic irritability, poor feeding, gastrointestinal disturbance (diarrhea), and seizures. Infants exposed to stimulants such as cocaine may also experience a withdrawal syndrome. These agents are also associated with poor intrauterine growth and an increased incidence of placental abruption. Cigarette smoking is a major cause of intrauterine growth restriction and also is associated with an increased risk of sudden infant death syndrome (SIDS) postnatally.

> **Helpful Tip**
> Intrauterine growth restriction (IUGR) remains a common cause of small-for-gestational age (< 10% for weight) infants. IUGR is most commonly associated with placental insufficiency. Maternal hypertension is a major cause of placental insufficiency. IUGR can also be associated with congenital infections, chromosome or other fetal anomalies, and severe maternal malnutrition.

▶ CASE 17

A male infant is born at 24 weeks' gestational age after his mother experiences preterm labor. Following a 4-month hospitalization in the NICU, he is discharged at 39-5/7 weeks' corrected gestational age. The infant is feeding well by mouth on fortified maternal breastmilk. He is discharged home on supplemental oxygen at a rate of 1/8 L/min.

Question 17-1

Which statement is true regarding this infant's lung disease?
A) This infant has chronic lung disease of prematurity (bronchopulmonary dysplasia) confirmed by the need for supplemental oxygen beyond 36 weeks' gestational age.
B) This infant's lungs were likely in the canalicular stage of development at the time of birth.
C) This infant's lungs are likely between saccular and alveolar stages of development at the time of discharge.
D) Vitamin A and caffeine are two medications that have been shown to decrease the severity of lung disease of this type.
E) All of the above.

Discussion 17-1

The correct answer is "E." This infant has chronic lung disease of prematurity, also known as bronchopulmonary dysplasia. This disease is most common in infants at the extremes of viability around 23 to 25 weeks' gestation at birth. It is generally defined as the persistent need for oxygen therapy at 36 weeks' corrected gestational age. The fetal lungs go through expected maturation from lung bud to pseudoglandular to canalicular to saccular to alveolar. Preterm infants lack alveolarization until several months of age, adding to difficulties with ventilation and oxygenation. Both vitamin A and caffeine produce modest improvements in chronic lung disease and are administered to many preterm infants.

▶ CASE 18

An infant is born at 38-2/7 weeks' gestation to a mother with immune thrombocytopenia (ITP). The mother's platelet count has averaged 25,000/μL during the pregnancy. She has required platelet transfusions and intravenous immunoglobulin therapy (IVIG). Her platelet count on the day of delivery is 50,000/μL. The infant is born by uncomplicated vaginal delivery. On physical exam he is well without bruising, petechiae, or scalp swelling.

Question 18-1

How should you manage this infant?
A) The infant does not require monitoring of his platelet count as he has no signs of cutaneous bleeding on exam.
B) If the infant's platelet count immediately after birth is normal, no additional monitoring is necessary.

C) The infant's platelet count should be monitored closely over the next few days until it is documented to be stable or increasing.
D) The infant should receive IVIG even if his platelet count is normal.
E) The majority of infants will develop severe thrombocytopenia with platelet counts of less than 50,000/µL.

Discussion 18-1

The correct answer is "C." Maternal ITP is a cause of neonatal thrombocytopenia. Acquired maternal antibodies cause destruction of the infant's platelets. The majority of infants will have safe or normal platelet counts after birth. The maternal platelet count is not predictive of the infant's count and maternal treatment does not decrease the risk of fetal thrombocytopenia. The infant's platelet count will decrease after delivery, reaching a nadir between DOL 2 and 5. The platelet count should be monitored closely after birth until the nadir has been reached. IVIG is given to infants with severe thrombocytopenia. Thrombocytopenia is transient but may last for weeks to months, requiring long-term monitoring.

▶ CASE 19

A term newborn was born by normal vaginal delivery. The mother's pregnancy was uncomplicated. On DOL 2, the infant is noted to be making mouthing movements and appears to be bicycling his legs. He is transferred to the NICU team for management and evaluation. The movements stop during transfer and he is noted to be lethargic.

Question 19-1

What is NOT true regarding neonatal seizures?
A) Neonatal seizures may present as repetitive rhythmic contractions of the arms and legs.
B) Neonatal seizures may present as sustained posturing of one extremity.
C) Neonatal seizures may present as sustained eye deviations or roving eye movements.
D) Neonatal seizures may present as asymmetric arrhythmic body jerks.
E) Neonatal seizures are not associated with changes in vital signs.

Discussion 19-1

The correct answer is "E." Neonatal seizures have a wide variety of clinical presentations, including apnea and fluctuations in vital signs. Seizures may cause coma, lethargy, or both. Seizures may be provoked by stimulation. Seizures may be subtle and difficult to differentiate from jitteriness. Infants typically do not have large motor movements (tonic clonic) as may be seen in an older child.

The infant is intubated and medically stabilized. An MRI brain scan and bedside electroencephalogram (EEG) are ordered. The parents arrive at the bedside.

Question 19-2

You tell them what?
A) Neonatal seizures may be caused by electrolyte disturbances.
B) Neonatal seizures may be caused by infection.
C) Neonatal seizures may be due to a metabolic disorder.
D) Neonatal seizures may be due to intracranial hemorrhage.
E) All of the above.

Discussion 19-2

The correct answer is "E." There are multiple potential etiologies for neonatal seizures. Age at presentation may be helpful in narrowing the differential diagnosis. For example, seizures from hypoxic ischemic encephalopathy typically present in the first 24 hours of life. The differential diagnosis for a lethargic or comatose infant is very similar to that for an infant with seizure.

▶ CASE 20

A term male infant is born vaginally. The NICU team is called to the delivery room to assess the infant due to an abnormality on exam. His right arm is amputated below the elbow with a circumferential depression in the skin. He has normal strength, tone, and movement of the elbow and upper arm. The infant is otherwise well and without dysmorphic features.

Question 20-1

What is the cause of his limb amputation?
A) Amnionic band sequence.
B) Vascular infarct of the distal forearm.
C) Genetic syndrome.
D) Uterine constraint.
E) Birth trauma.

Discussion 20-1

The correct answer is "A." Amnionic band sequence is a group of disorders causing serious structural deformations from early in utero amniotic rupture with bandlike constriction or amputation. The limbs, digits, and craniofacial structures are generally affected. Abnormalities include limb amputation, digit amputation, constriction rings (circle of depressed tissue around a part of the body), encephalocele, and facial clefts.

BIBLIOGRAPHY

American Academy of Pediatrics Committee on Fetus and Newborn. Controversies concerning vitamin K and the newborn. *Pediatrics.* 2003;112(1):191–192.

American Academy of Pediatrics Committee on Fetus and Newborn, American College of Obstetricians and Gynecologists Practice Committee on Obstetrics. The Apgar score. *Pediatrics.* 2006;117(4):1444–1447.

American Academy of Pediatrics Subcommitte on Hyperbilirubinemia, et al. Management of hyperbilirubinemia in the newborn infant 35 or more weeks of gestation. *Pediatrics.* 2004;114(1):297–316.

Anderson MS, Hay WW. Intrauterine growth restriction and the small-for-gestational-age infant. In: Avery GB, Fletcher M, MacDonald M, eds. *Avery's Neonatology: Pathophysiology and Management of the Newborn.* 6th ed. Philadelphia, PA: Lippincott Williams and Wilkins; 2005:490–522.

Chu A, Hageman JR, Caplan MS. Necrotizing enterocolitis: Predictive markers and preventive strategies. *Neoreviews.* 2013;4(3):e113–e120.

de Ungria M Daru J. Delivery room management. In: Zaoutis LB, Chiang VW, eds. *Comprehensive Pediatric Hospital Medicine.* Philadelphia, PA: Mosby; 2007:235–246.

Fanaroff A, Martin R. *Fanaroff and Martin's Neonatal-Perinatal Medicine: Diseases of the Fetus and Infant.* 8th ed. Philadelphia, PA: Mosby Elsevier; 2006.

Gomella T, Cunningham D, Eyal, F. *Neonatology: Management, Procedures, On Call Problems, Diseases and Drugs.* 7th ed. New York, NY: McGraw-Hill; 2013.

Hormann MD. Birth injury. In: Zaoutis LB, Chiang VW, eds. *Comprehensive Pedatric Hospital Medicine.* Philadelphia, PA: Mosby; 2007:255–267.

Kattwinkel J, Bloom R. *Textbook of Neonatal Resuscitation.* 6th ed. Elk Grove Village, IL: American Academy of Pediatrics; 2011.

Keren R. Neonatal hyperbilirubinemia. In: Zaoutis LB, Chiang VW, eds. *Comprehensive Pediatric Hospital Medicine.* Philadelphia, PA: Mosby; 2007:279–285.

Lightdale JR, Gremse DA; Section on Gastroenterology, Hepatology, and Nutrition. Gastroesophageal reflux: Management guidance for the pediatrician. *Pediatrics.* 2013;131(5):e1684–e1695.

Madejczyk K. The well newborn. In: Zaoutis LB, Chiang VW, eds. *Comprehensive Pediatric Hospital Medicine.* Philadelphia, PA: Mosby; 2007:247–254.

Mirkinson LJ. Hypoglycemia and infants of diabetic mothers. In: Zaoutis LB, Chiang VW, eds. *Comprehensive Pediatric Hospital Medicine.* Philadelphia, PA: Mosby; 2007:274–278.

Muller AJ, Marks JD. Hypoxic-ischemic brain injury: Potential therapeutic interventions for the future. *Neoreviews.* 2014;15(5):e177–e186.

Newburger JW, Takahashi M, Gerber MA, et al. Diagnosis, treatment, and long-term management of Kawasaki disease: A statement for health professionals from the Committee on Rheumatic Fever, Endocarditis and Kawasaki Disease, Council on Cardiovascular Disease in the Young, American Heart Association. *Circulation.* 2004;110(17):2747–2771.

Oh W, Blackman LR, Escobedo M, et al. Use and abuse of the Apgar score. *Pediatrics.* 1996;98(1):141–142.

Teramo K. Diabetic pregnancy and fetal consequences. *Neoreviews.* 2014;15(3):e83–e90.

Thebaud B. Chronic lung disease in the neonate: Past, present, and future. *Neoreviews.* 2013;14(5):e252–e258.

Warren JB, Phillipi CA. Care of the well newborn. *Pediatr Rev.* 2012;33(1):4–18.

Fluid and Electrolyte Metabolism

15

Jeff Van Blarcom

▶ CASE 1

A previously healthy 15-month-old girl presents to the emergency department for evaluation for a 3-day history of persistent vomiting and diarrhea. Neither the stool nor the emesis has been bloody, and the emesis has not been bilious. She has had little to drink or eat in the last 24 hours. She has been febrile intermittently and her temperature in triage was 38.6°C (101.5°F). Physically the child appears tired and pale and she has little response to examination. Her heart rate is 140 beats per minute (bpm), her respiratory rate is 28 breaths per minute, and her blood pressure is 95/58 mm Hg. Her peripheral pulses are somewhat difficult to find, her peripheral capillary refill is about 4 seconds, and she has a systolic ejection murmur. Her liver is not enlarged.

Question 1-1

Which answer best describes the status of this child's cardiovascular system?
A) Septic shock.
B) Cardiogenic shock.
C) Compensated hypovolemic shock.
D) Uncompensated hypovolemic shock.
E) Distributive shock.

Discussion 1-1

The correct answer is "C." Shock is defined as a state in which decreased tissue perfusion leads to inadequate delivery of substrate to meet metabolic demands. The tissues are not getting enough oxygen! Shock has many etiologies and can be divided into three main categories depending on the underlying pathophysiologic process: cardiogenic shock, distributive shock, and hypovolemic shock. (See Table 15–1.) Given this child's history of gastrointestinal volume losses and decreased input, it is likely that she is hypovolemic. Whether or not shock is compensated or uncompensated depends on the absence or presence of normal blood pressure. Uncompensated shock is associated with hypotension. (See Table 15–2.) Though our patient is tachycardic and has poor capillary refill, her blood pressure is appropriate for a child of her age, so she has compensated hypovolemic shock. Her fever is likely contributing to her tachycardia, but fever will not contribute to a lengthened capillary refill so it is best to attribute most of her tachycardia to hypovolemia. (See Table 15–3.) The child's murmur is most likely caused by a hyperdynamic cardiovascular state related to her fever, and she has no liver enlargement or past medical history that would suggest significant heart disease, so cardiogenic shock is not likely. Septic shock, which is possible in this child, is a form of distributive shock caused by toxins released by infectious organisms. Differentiating hypovolemic shock from septic shock in an ill-appearing, febrile child can be difficult. It is best to have a high index of suspicion for septic shock, but in this case the child's history is more consistent with hypovolemic shock, which is the most common type of shock seen in children. It is important to keep in mind that several forms of shock can coexist in a patient, although thankfully only on rare occasions. Remember, cardiac output is influenced by preload (blood coming back to heart), afterload (resistance to blood being pumped out of the heart), and contractility (pumping power of the heart). In shock, one or more of these factors is deranged.

> **Helpful Tip**
> A febrile, tachycardic child is most likely not septic, but assuming that the child is septic until proven otherwise is best. The initial interventions for septic shock are readily available in most U.S. hospital settings: intravenous (IV) fluids and antibiotics.

An IV catheter is placed and blood is sent for laboratory studies.

TABLE 15-1 CATEGORIES OF SHOCK

	Pathophysiology	Causes	Signs and Symptoms
Hypovolemic	Decreased preload: 1. Inadequate intake 2. Increased losses 3. Acute blood loss 4. Impaired ability to concentrate the urine	Dehydration Hemorrhage Diabetes insipidus Burns Hyperglycemia Vomiting Diarrhea Adrenal insufficiency Hemorrhage	Tachycardia Decreased urine output[a] Prolonged capillary refill Weak pulses Cool extremities Dry mucous membranes Sunken fontanelle Altered mental status
Cardiogenic	Decreased contractility of the heart	Myocarditis Arrhythmia Cardiomyopathy Congenital heart disease Obstruction (pericardial tamponade, tension pneumothorax, pulmonary embolism) Infarction or ischemia	Heart failure Tachycardia Decreased urine output Weak pulses Cool extremities Prolonged capillary refill Hepatomegaly JVD Pulmonary edema
Distributive	Decreased systemic vascular resistance 1. Vasodilation 2. Capillary leak 3. Third spacing of fluids into interstitial tissues	Sepsis Spinal cord injury Head injury Anaphylaxis Drugs	Tachycardia Decreased urine output Peripheral edema Brisk capillary refill[b] Bounding pulses[b]

JVD, jugular venous distention.

[a]Typically urine output is decreased unless cause is from kidney dysfunction.

[b]Characteristics of early distributive shock.

TABLE 15-2 HYPOTENSION BY AGE AND SYSTOLIC BLOOD PRESSURE

According to the American Heart Association Pediatric Advanced Life Support criteria, hypotension is a systolic blood pressure less than the 5th percentile of normal for age, namely:

< 60 mm Hg in term neonates (0 to 28 days)

< 70 mm Hg in infants (1 month to 12 months)

< 70 mm Hg + (2 × Age in years) in children 1 to 10 years of age

< 90 mm Hg in children 10 years of age or older

Question 1-2

The next best intervention for this child would be to:

A) Administer a 1 g dose of IV ceftriaxone.

B) Administer a 10 mL/kg of body weight IV bolus of normal saline (NS).

C) Administer a 20 mL/kg IV bolus of D_5 ¼ NS.

D) Administer a 20 mL/kg IV bolus of NS.

E) Check the child's fingerstick blood glucose.

TABLE 15-3 CAUSES OF TACHYCARDIA IN A CHILD (IN ORDER OF PREVALENCE)

1. Anxiety
2. Pain
3. Fever
4. Dehydration/hypovolemia
5. Anemia
6. Sepsis
7. Arrhythmia

Discussion 1-2

The correct answer is "D." Giving a 20 mL/kg NS bolus as rapidly as possible is a time-tested intervention that is the initial treatment for any child in shock. This applies to children up to a weight of 50 kg (approximately the weight of an average 14-year-old), over which the initial intervention would be 1 L of NS given as rapidly as possible. If the child were in septic shock, giving a dose of ceftriaxone as rapidly as possible would be an appropriate intervention, though the best first step would be to give IV fluid. As previously mentioned, it is more likely that this child has hypovolemic shock rather than septic shock. A 10 mL/kg NS bolus would not be inappropriate for this child, though there is no indication that a 20 mL/kg bolus would not be tolerated. A 10 mL/kg bolus is considered to be the initial intervention for a child in shock with a cardiac problem, the rationale being to avoid a worsening of congestive heart failure with a larger fluid bolus. Giving a bolus of either a hypertonic or hypotonic solution such as ½ NS is generally felt not to be a good idea, given the possibility of a rapid change in the serum sodium, leading to neurologic issues. Determination of the child's blood glucose level is rarely a bad idea but would not be the initial focus of the child's care in this case. Lactated Ringer's solution can also be given as a bolus in a resuscitation situation.

Question 1-3

Which of the following is the best acute indicator of a child's hydration status?

A) Urine output.
B) Acute change in weight.
C) Acute change in mental status.
D) Clinical signs such as sunken eyes and dry mucous membranes.
E) Input.

Discussion 1-3

The correct answer is "B." An acute change in weight is the best determinant of a person's current hydration status; indeed, our estimates of dehydration are reported in percentages of weight loss. However, previous weights are not often available and are not necessary for decision making in resuscitation scenarios such as in this vignette. If a child just so happens to have had a recent visit for medical care and if the weight measurements were obtained on the same scale, the level of the child's dehydration can be determined accurately. Urine output is a good indicator of hydration status and is used in virtually all inpatient settings, although it is not as reliable a measurement as an acute change in weight and at times can be misleading, such as in a dehydrated child who has diabetic ketoacidosis with an osmotic diuresis. A child's oral input is subject to the interpretation of an anxious parent or frequently is unknown, and thus is a poor indicator of a child's level of hydration. Clinical signs of dehydration may be the only available indicators of a child's hydration status but can be subjective, subtle, or both. If you have time to debate the concavity of an infant's fontanelle, you may not need to act with urgency. (See Table 15–4.)

> **Helpful Tip**
> The fluid deficit of a dehydrated child can be calculated using body weight as follows:
>
> Fluid deficit (in liters) = Baseline body weight (in kg) – Current dehydrated body weight (in kg)

> **Helpful Tip**
> Each 1% of dehydration is equivalent to a fluid deficit of 10 mL/kg. For example, an infant who is estimated clinically to be 6% dehydrated has a fluid deficit of 60 mL/kg that needs to be replaced.

TABLE 15–4 USING CLINICAL SIGNS TO ESTIMATE THE DEGREE OF DEHYDRATION

	Mild	Moderate	Severe
% Dehydration (fluid deficit)			
Child	3% (30 mL/kg)	6% (60 mL/kg)	9% (90 mL/kg)
Infant	5% (50 mL/kg)	10% (100 mL/kg)	15% (150 mL/kg)
Physical Findings			
Skin	Normal	Dry	Cool
Mucous membranes	Tacky	Dry	Parched
Eyes	Normal	Deep set	Sunken
Tears	Present	Reduced	None
Fontanelle	Flat	Soft	Sunken
Mental status	Tired	Irritable	Lethargic/obtunded
Pulses	Normal	Weak	Faint/impalpable
Capillary refill	Normal	2–3 seconds	> 3 seconds
Urine output	Normal/decreased	Decreased	None

Question 1-4

Which of the following statements is FALSE?

A) Dry mucous membranes are consistent with at least 5% dehydration.

B) Sunken eyes are consistent with at least 5% to 10% dehydration.

C) Deterioration in mental status is consistent with at least greater than 10% dehydration.

D) A sunken fontanelle is consistent with at least 5% to 10% dehydration.

E) Increases in blood urea nitrogen (BUN) can be used to accurately estimate the severity of dehydration.

Discussion 1-4

The correct answer is "E." There are too many variables for a direct relationship between BUN and hydration level to be established, although it is true that elevations in BUN are consistent with hypovolemia in most routine cases. Conversely, the lack of an increased BUN should not deter intervention if you believe a child is dehydrated (hypovolemic from water loss, to be more specific). These are by no means all of the clinical signs used to determine a patient's hydration status. Heart rate, for instance, is used to gauge a child's response to rehydration, and therefore can be used as an indicator of hydration status, although tachycardia has a number of confounding causes. (See Table 15–3, earlier.) There obviously is some leeway in the estimation of dehydration based on physical findings, but generally some history is provided when dealing with a patient. Always use all the available information to make an informed decision about what, if any, intervention needs to be undertaken. (See Table 15–4, earlier.)

Question 1-5

What is the best estimate of this child's percentage of dehydration based on her clinical signs?

A) 9%.

B) 5%.

C) 10%.

D) 6%.

E) 15%.

Discussion 1-5

The correct answer is "A." Our patient is 15 months old (not an infant) and estimated to be 9% dehydrated based on her capillary refill of 4 seconds, weak pulses, and lethargy.

After receiving the fluid bolus, the patient's clinical status remains the same, although her capillary refill is marginally better. Her latest blood pressure measure is 90/45 mm Hg. A fingerstick blood glucose reading is reported as 78 mg/dL, and some of her laboratory studies are available. Most notably, sodium is 140 mEq/L, potassium 5.0 mEq/L, bicarbonate 16 mEq/L, creatinine 0.39 mg/dL, BUN 26 mg/dL, and lactate 4.2 mEq/L.

Question 1-6

What is the normal ratio of intracellular volume to extracellular volume?

A) 1:1.

B) 2:1.

C) 5:1.

D) 10:1.

E) 4:3.

Discussion 1-6

The correct answer is "B." Ratio aside, the usual percentages of intracellular volume and extracellular volume in the human body are facts you are just supposed to know. In a healthy, normal subject, intracellular fluid volume represents 67% of total body water; extracellular fluid volume, which includes intravascular fluid and interstitial fluid, represents 33% of total body water: 2:1. The major extracellular cation is sodium (Na^+) and the major intracellular cation is potassium (K^+), but there is no osmotic difference between the two spaces. You will recall that "third-spacing" represents fluid movement within the body from the two useful spaces (the intracellular and extracellular compartments) to a not-so-useful space (the transcellular compartment (ie, the peritoneal space in ascites, the subdural space in subdural hemorrhage), which is as good as volume loss.

Question 1-7

What is the circulating blood volume of a typical 6-year-old child?

A) 75 mL/kg.

B) 50 mL/kg.

C) 65% of body weight.

D) 10 pounds (lb).

E) 100 mL/kg.

Discussion 1-7

The correct answer is "A." The normal amount of circulating blood volume in a child varies with age and is as high as 92 mL/kg in a newborn, as low as 71 mL/kg in an 18-year-old (and even lower in adulthood). An acute drop from "normal" to 50 mL/kg would likely create a state of uncompensated shock, a point which is typically reached when a child loses 30% or so of intravascular volume. The history of the 20 mL/kg bolus is obscure, but it sounds reasonable given that it is in the neighborhood of restoring a symptomatically dehydrated child's intravascular volume back to normal, if only momentarily. Sixty-five percent of total body weight is a good estimate of a 6-year-old's total body water, but not of his or her circulating blood volume. Remember, two thirds of the body is water. As for option D—10 pounds—what kind of answer is that?

Question 1-8

What is the next step in this patient's management?

A) Discuss her case with the intensivist on call at the nearest children's hospital.

B) Initiate an epinephrine drip.

C) Obtain an electrocardiogram (ECG).

D) Administer a bolus of normal saline with 10 mEq/L of potassium bicarbonate.

E) Administer another 20 mL/kg bolus of normal saline.

Discussion 1-8

The correct answer is "E." If you want some hand-holding and possibly a good brow-beating, go ahead and call your local intensivist, who will inform you in some fashion that the child does not, at least up to this point, meet admission criteria for the intensive care unit, nebulous though they may be. The child's blood pressure appears to have decreased some but is still adequate for her age, so an epinephrine drip would not be indicated. The difference in the blood pressure measurements is not likely to be clinically significant and may depend on when, and the manner in which, they were obtained. The pulse pressure (difference between systolic and diastolic pressures) has widened some, which is more common with distributive shock such as occurs with sepsis or anaphylaxis, but not enough to either be alarming or to be an indication for vasopressor medication. A good rule of thumb for pulse pressure is that it should generally be around 40 mm Hg, corresponding to a "normal" adult blood pressure of 120/80 mm Hg. The child's low bicarbonate level is consistent with her history of diarrhea, but it is not low enough to warrant the administration of bicarbonate. Whether or not the bicarbonate level is followed as a marker of the patient's response to therapy is debatable. Obtaining an ECG is not likely to be fruitful; her potassium level is elevated but this should first prompt a further examination of the lab report or a call to the lab itself to determine if there was any hemolysis on the sample. Giving another normal saline bolus is the most appropriate next step. And the next step after that, as well, assuming that her clinical status remains the same. If there is no response thereafter, or if the child is deteriorating despite the administration of fluid, you may well want to discuss the case with an intensivist, this time without fear of a snide response.

> **Helpful Tip**
>
> The history of undertreating patients in need of fluid resuscitation goes all the way back to the beginnings of IV fluid therapy in the early 1800s, which was initially developed for the treatment of cholera. The endpoints of fluid administration are clinical improvement, which is most likely, or pulmonary and peripheral edema, which in a person with normal kidneys is rarely life threatening. If a child in compensated shock proceeds to uncompensated shock (ie, becomes hypotensive), you really ought to call an intensivist, but in the meantime, give more crystalloid.

The child's appearance improves and her mother states that she "has her color back." Her heart rate has decreased to 100 bpm, though it rapidly increases to 140 bpm as she scrambles up her mother's torso whenever you approach. She appears more vigorous but seems to have no interest in drinking or eating. She urinates. You admit her for further treatment.

Question 1-9

Suppose that instead of 140 mEq/L, her sodium level at the time of initial evaluation was 115 mEq/L. Which of the following is a potentially disastrous consequence of correcting a patient's hyponatremia too quickly?

A) Stroke.
B) Osmotic demyelination syndrome.
C) Cardiac dysrhythmia.
D) Cerebral edema.
E) Seizure.

Discussion 1-9

The correct answer is "B." Purists will point out that severe hyponatremia necessitating 3% saline is uncommon in the setting of hypovolemic dehydration from diarrhea. Nonetheless, osmotic demyelination syndrome (ODS) would be possible in patient with a sodium level of 115 mEq/L, so slow correction would be warranted. If that level of hyponatremia had existed in the child for less than 48 hours, rapid correction leading to an occurrence of ODS would not be likely, but generally we cannot know how long a patient's hyponatremia has existed prior to discovery. The brain osmotically adapts to chronic hyponatremia and rapid correction can lead to cellular dehydration and disruption of the blood-brain barrier, which allows immune system factors to damage nerve cells (famously in the pons, as in *pontine*), or so the theory goes. When *hyper*natremia is corrected too rapidly, osmotic flow of water into solute-heavy cells can eventually lead to cerebral edema, which is more than just a headache. Seizures can occur from severe hyponatremia by itself but are not commonly seen in ODS or cerebral edema per se, which both are consequences of overly rapid sodium correction. ODS can produce irreversible neurologic symptoms (usually presenting several days after the correction of the serum sodium level) and cerebral edema can lead to death, so they are best avoided. In this child's case, a rapidly infused 20 mL/kg NS bolus given in the emergency department may well have rectified or lessened the degree of an existing hyponatremia and we may be none the wiser. If you answered "A," you were on the right track with the idea that too-rapid correction of hyponatremia leads to a neurologic problem, but ultimately you were wrong. If you answered "C," you were simply incorrect.

► CASE 2

A 5-day-old infant boy presents to the emergency department 30 minutes after what his mother describes as a seizure. She states that he abruptly stiffened for a few seconds, then "his eyes rolled back." This was followed by a period of sleepiness from which he seems to be recovering. He was born at term, there were no pregnancy or delivery complications, and he has done well since birth. On physical examination, he weighs 4.1 kg and appears to be a healthy infant. He is irritable but consolable. Shortly after an IV catheter is placed and his blood is sent for laboratory studies, he begins to seize. He is given a 0.4 mg IV dose of lorazepam, to no avail. The laboratory technician calls with a critical value: his calcium level is 5.2 mg/dL. There are no other critical values. He continues to seize.

Question 2-1

What is the next most appropriate step in this child's management?

A) Give another 0.4 mg IV lorazepam.
B) Give a 20 mg/kg IV loading dose of fosphenytoin.
C) Give a dose of IV calcium gluconate.
D) Repeat a blood draw for an ionized calcium measurement.
E) Give a dose of IV calcium chloride.

Discussion 2-1

The correct answer is "C." Although giving another dose of lorazepam or a loading dose of fosphenytoin are appropriate therapies for a seizing child, this infant's seizure is most likely caused by hypocalcemia. The treatment of choice for a newborn with symptomatic hypocalcemia (seizing, irritable, or both) is 100 mg/kg of IV calcium gluconate given over a 10- to 20-minute period. Seizures resulting from hypocalcemia are unlikely to stop until the serum calcium level has been normalized. IV calcium chloride would be appropriate if it was more readily available than calcium gluconate, but calcium chloride is less desirable given a greater propensity for venous and local tissue destruction. The ionized calcium level is a more accurate measure of the physiologically active form of calcium in the serum, but given a markedly low calcium level in an actively seizing newborn, the next best step in management would be to administer calcium intravenously in an attempt to stop the seizure. Confirming that the infant's calcium level is indeed low is necessary, but given the presented information it would be reasonable to assume that his measured calcium level was accurate and to proceed accordingly. If the infant was not symptomatic, an ionized calcium measurement would be the next step. Do not forget to investigate why the infant is hypocalcemic after you stop the seizure. (See Table 15–5.) Acute-onset hypocalcemia can cause seizures, as in this infant, along with a range of clinical manifestations. (See Table 15–6.)

TABLE 15–5 CAUSES OF HYPOCALCEMIA AND HYPERCALCEMIA

Hypocalcemia	Hypercalcemia
Vitamin D deficiency	Hypervitaminosis D
Hypoparathyroidism	Hyperparathyroidism
Maternal hyperparathyroidism	Malignancy
Hyperphosphatemia	Thiazide diuretics
Hypomagnesemia	Subcutaneous fat necrosis
Pancreatitis	Williams syndrome
Drugs	Granulomatous disease
Ethylene glycol ingestion	Hyperthyroidism

TABLE 15–6 CLINICAL MANIFESTATIONS OF ACUTE-ONSET HYPOCALCEMIA

Neuromuscular Manifestations (tetany)

Weakness

Paresthesias, particularly perioral and in the extremities

Seizures

Involuntary muscle contractions (twitching, carpal spasm, laryngospasm)

Induced findings:

  Trousseau sign: Carpal spasm following 3 minutes of arm ischemia induced by inflation of a blood pressure cuff

  Chvostek sign: Facial muscle contraction induced by mechanical stimulation of the facial nerve

Cardiac Manifestations

Prolonged QT interval

Arrhythmia

Hypotension

Heart failure

Helpful Tip

Calcium infusion pearls: The child's cardiovascular status must be closely monitored during IV calcium infusion given the possibility of cardiac arrhythmias related to the changing serum calcium level. The infusion should be given slowly, over 10 to 20 minutes. Extravasation of calcium-containing fluids is both mentally and physically traumatic, so close attention must be paid to the IV site. Treatment of such extravasations usually involves subcutaneous or intradermal administration of hyaluronidase to limit the destruction and consultation with plastic surgery.

Question 2-2

Which of the following is most likely to cause a patient's serum calcium measurement to appear falsely low?

A) Hypoalbuminemia.
B) Hyperalbuminemia.
C) Acidosis.
D) Hypermagnesemia.
E) Alkalosis.

Discussion 2-2

The correct answer is "A." About 40% of serum calcium is bound to protein, mostly to albumin. A low level of albumin in the serum will cause the routinely measured serum calcium level to be low but does not affect the ionized calcium level, which is the hormonally regulated form of calcium. A high level of serum albumin, which is usually only seen in children in the setting of severe dehydration, would have the opposite effect. Serum pH has an effect on the binding of calcium to albumin (with alkalosis promoting binding and acidosis decreasing it), so changes in pH affect the ionized calcium level but do not affect the measured serum calcium level. A *low* level of serum magnesium can be associated with hypocalcemia but would not cause the serum calcium measurement to be falsely low. Whenever there is a question about a patient's calcium level, an ionized calcium level should be obtained.

► CASE 3

A mother brings her 2½-week-old daughter for a routine well-child check. Looking at the infant's chart, you see that her heart rate and respiratory rate seem to be normal for her age, and her weight is 3.7 kg. The mother states that the infant is generally doing well, but when you ask about the feeding schedule, she says that the infant has been intermittently vomiting for about a week. The mother has not been particularly concerned about this vomiting because the infant's older brother had reflux when he was an infant, which was messy but did not require any intervention. She notes that her daughter has been breastfeeding readily and most often vomits within a few minutes after finishing a feed, although on occasion the vomiting occurs an hour or so after feeding. The vomit is not bloody or bilious, but occasionally is forceful. The infant has been stooling with less frequency of late. Physically the infant appears well. The mother reports that birth weight was 8 pounds, 11 ounces. The infant's physical examination is unrevealing.

Question 3-1

As the child's pediatrician, you have determined your level of concern with this history. What should you do next?
A) Order a chemistry panel.
B) Order an abdominal radiograph.
C) Reassure the mother that the infant does indeed have reflux and that no intervention is necessary.
D) Order a pH probe.
E) Order an abdominal ultrasound.

Discussion 3-1

The best answer is "E." The infant does not fit the traditional demographic, but this vignette should raise a concern for pyloric stenosis. She is vomiting and remains below her birthweight more than 2 weeks later, which together are bothersome. A lack of physical examination findings does not exclude pyloric stenosis; it would be hard to be absolutely certain that the infant's examination was normal in that regard. Pyloric stenosis is indeed more frequently seen in firstborn males, is frequently associated with projectile vomiting, and presents more frequently at about 1 month of age, but this does not exclude that possibility in this infant. "Projectile" vomiting tends not to be a particularly useful piece of history in many situations given a parental fondness for using the word; its presence or absence should be taken into account

but should not drive an evaluation or the lack of an evaluation. Ordering a chemistry panel might put you on the right track, but why not go directly to a more definitive test if you think you know what the problem is? A normal chemistry pattern would not rule out pyloric stenosis, but a normal ultrasound would. Similarly, an abdominal radiograph would not be helpful, unless you were concerned that a child had a lower obstruction such as duodenal atresia or malrotation with a volvulus, but this infant has no history of bilious vomiting. Pyloric stenosis is much more common as well. A pH probe is usually a hard sell for a gastroenterologist and would not likely be useful in this case, even if the infant did indeed have gastroesophageal reflux, which in many cases need not be objectively substantiated. She could have gastroesophageal reflux, but this history warrants further investigation. You may not be asked to convert a weight from pounds to kilograms on the pediatric board certification test, but as a pediatrician, you will need to do it on a regular basis as long as the English system of measurement persists.

An abdominal ultrasound is obtained and findings are consistent with pyloric stenosis.

Question 3-2

If a chemistry panel were obtained in this dehydrated infant with pyloric stenosis, what pattern would be expected?
A) Hypochloremic metabolic alkalosis.
B) Mixed respiratory and metabolic acidosis.
C) Hyperchloremic metabolic acidosis.
D) Hyperkalemia.
E) Hypernatremia.

Discussion 3-2

The correct answer is "A." Although this is a situation notably associated with pyloric stenosis, persistent vomiting of just about any cause can lead to similar laboratory findings. The main electrolytes lost with vomiting are hydrogen and chloride, as in hydrochloric acid, a product of the stomach essential in the initiation of digestion. Loss of these two substances leads to a hypochloremic metabolic alkalosis. Because of the dehydration, acidosis can also be seen, particularly if the vomiting is rapidly progressive. A hyperchloremic metabolic acidosis can be seen in the setting of diarrhea, given a loss of bicarbonate and other anions in the stool, the hyperchloremia caused by a reaction of the kidneys to the loss of serum anions by retaining chloride. A hyperchloremic metabolic acidosis without a history consistent with bicarbonate loss (most commonly diarrhea) or without a history of exogenous acid input should prompt an investigation for a renal tubular acidosis. By the way, chloride is a player but rarely if ever has the central role in electrolyte disturbances. Hyperkalemia is not often encountered in a child with diarrhea or vomiting unless the blood draw was difficult, in which case the child's potassium level is unlikely to be truly elevated. Hypernatremia certainly can be seen in a dehydrated child, but is not the most frequently encountered metabolic derangement pattern seen in a child with pyloric stenosis.

Back to our patient: Blood for lab studies is drawn, confirming that she does indeed have a hypochloremic metabolic alkalosis. Incidentally, her sodium level is 145 mEq/L, potassium is 4.5 mEq/L, and blood glucose is 62 mg/dL. Her potassium level is normal, but hypokalemia is common in pyloric stenosis. She needs a pyloromyotomy, but first she needs to be hydrated.

Question 3-3

What fluid is most appropriate for this infant's preoperative hydration needs?
A) D_5 ½ NS with 20 mEq KCl per liter.
B) D_{10} ¼ NS with 40 mEq KCl per liter.
C) ½ NS with 20 mEq K acetate per liter.
D) D_5 ½ NS with 40 mEq KCl per liter.
E) Lactated Ringer's.

Discussion 3-3

The correct answer is "D." The choice may be somewhat debatable, but the principles are as follows: (1) She has not been eating well and should be NPO (nil per os, nothing by mouth) prior to her operation; therefore, she needs some glucose in the fluid to keep her brain happy; the choice between D_5 and D_{10} is not straightforward, but her blood glucose level is normal so she probably does not need D_{10}. (2) Although her potassium is normal, children with persistent vomiting from pyloric stenosis usually have a total body potassium deficit, so giving more potassium than the typical maintenance amount (20 mEq KCl/L given at a maintenance rate) would be appropriate. (3) The choice of the NaCl content in the fluid is also not a simple determination, but ½ NS is typical in this situation; ¼ NS has been associated with problematic iatrogenic hyponatremia in hospitalized children and probably should not be used. On the other hand, hypernatremia is more likely when a child with ongoing free water loss is not given an adequate amount of fluid than when an adequate amount of fluid with a higher NaCl content is given, so giving ½ NS and even normal saline is safe. In any case, a high index of suspicion for an electrolyte problem in a hospitalized child who is NPO will likely keep you out of trouble. If the infant appears dehydrated, a 20 mL/kg NS bolus would be appropriate, followed by D_5 ½ NS with 40 mEq KCl per liter. The rationale for not giving a base such as acetate or bicarbonate to a child with an alkalosis should be evident.

Question 3-4

Speaking of IV fluid, what are the components of lactated Ringer's solution?
A) Na^+ 154 mEq/L, K^+ 4 mEq/L, Cl^- 158 mEq/L, lactate 3 g/L.
B) Na^+ 130, K^+ 4, Ca^{2+} 2.7 mEq/L, Cl^- 109, lactate 28 mEq/L.
C) Na^+ 0, K^+ 0, dextrose 50 g/L.
D) Na^+ 154, K^+ 0, Cl^- 154, dextrose 50.
E) Na^+ 130, K^+ 4, Cl^- 109, lactate 28.

Discussion 3-4

The correct answer is "B." Lactated Ringer's does indeed have lactate, calcium, and potassium. Option "C" is D_5W (W = water), option "D" represents the components of D_5NS, option "A" will

not routinely be found in a hospital pharmacy, and option "E" is not possible without involving another anion, in keeping with the law of electroneutrality.

▶ CASE 4

A 6-month-old infant girl is brought to clinic for evaluation after 3 days of progressively worsening vomiting and diarrhea. The vomiting has been increasing to the point that the infant has had very little input today, according to her mother. Her input has consisted of small amounts of formula intermittently. Her mother is not sure of her urine output because of the large amount of stool that the infant has been having. Neither the emesis nor the stool has been bloody, and the emesis has not been bilious. She last vomited about 30 minutes before your exam, and her last stool was shortly thereafter. There are no other bothersome aspects of the infant's present or past medical history. She appears about as tired as her mother but responds to examination as expected for her age; her eyes do not appear to be sunken and her oral mucosa is at worst a little tacky. Her capillary refill is less than 2 seconds. She is holding a bottle with formula in it. She is afebrile, her heart rate is 100 bpm, respiratory rate is about 30 breaths per minute, and blood pressure is 95/65 mm Hg.

Question 4-1

What should be done to help this infant?
A) Begin a trial of a clear liquid such as Pedialyte.
B) Place an IV catheter, order lab studies, and give a normal saline bolus.
C) Begin a trial of formula.
D) Place an intraosseous line and give a normal saline bolus.
E) Give a dose of loperamide.

Discussion 4-1

The correct answer is "A." This is a straightforward case of mild dehydration in a generally healthy infant, of the type that a general pediatrician will see a lot. There certainly are different ways to approach the situation, but in this case a trial of a clear liquid would be the most appropriate. The things that the stomach does not like when it is ailing are mainly (1) anything in large volume, (2) solids, and (3) anything fatty, including milk or formula; so we should avoid those. She is not more than 5% dehydrated according to our previously discussed clinical findings for dehydration, so drastic rehydration measures such as intraosseous fluid and even IV fluid are probably not necessary at this point. What exactly constitutes a large volume is debatable; perhaps starting with a dropperful or an ounce of Pedialyte, depending on the size of the infant, and seeing what happens would be the most appropriate first step. Antidiarrheal drugs such as loperamide are not recommended in routine cases such as this because they are not curative, they can be sedating (not good for a child who needs to drink), and they can, at least in theory, delay the expulsion of the diarrhea-causing agent. You can temporize the infant's diarrhea momentarily, but what's going to come out is going to come out. Placing a nasogastric (NG) tube and slowly administering a liquid such as Pedialyte may also be appropriate, despite a lack of acceptance for this modality in the United States.

Question 4-2

The following are components of oral rehydration therapy (ORT), as specified by the World Health Organization (WHO), EXCEPT:
A) Potassium.
B) Sodium.
C) Zinc.
D) Chloride.
E) Citrate.

Discussion 4-2

The correct answer is "C." While it may not be important to memorize all of the properties of ORT, it is probably useful to have some basic understanding of what those components are and why Pedialyte, the unflavored variety in particular, does not taste very good. Zinc, although commonly lacking in the diets and bodies of children in developing countries, is not a WHO-recommended component of ORT. Although it is similar, Pedialyte is not ORT per se. The sodium and chloride concentrations are lower than in ORT, which makes Pedialyte more palatable. The flavored versions contain the sweetener sucralose, also to increase the palatability. The concentrations of sodium and glucose need to be the same to take advantage of their 1:1 linked transport in the small intestine, which is the speediest method of fluid absorption; the faster the better in an ill, vomiting child. The glucose concentration of ORT needs to be somewhat low so as not to promote an osmotic effect and contribute to the diarrhea. (The child already has enough of that.) Sports drinks and sodas contain much more carbohydrate and much less sodium; it is up to the individual to decide what is more palatable. Dehydrated children will drink Pedialyte or ORT because they are thirsty and not very picky. But any fluid is better than no fluid, so if all a child will drink is a sweetened carbonated soda, let him or her have it. As for our patient, starting with small amounts of Pedialyte and slowly increasing the frequency or the amount is often enough to return the infant to a better hydration status, feeling better, and (somewhat paradoxically) not vomiting. And the hassle and pain of placing an IV line is avoided. Suppose the child appeared to be more ill than our current patient, was tachycardic, and had a prolonged capillary refill (> 3 seconds). Suppose she was known to have cystic fibrosis. Suppose you obtained some laboratory studies.

> **Helpful Tip**
> The WHO-recommended properties of ORT are as follows:
> - Total osmolality between 200 and 310 mOsm/L
> - Equimolar concentrations of glucose and sodium
> - Glucose concentration < 20 g/L (111 mmol/L)
> - Sodium concentration between 60 and 90 mEq/L
> - Potassium concentration between 15 and 25 mEq/L
> - Citrate concentration between 8 and 12 mmol/L
> - Chloride concentration between 50 and 80 mEq/L

Question 4-3

What electrolyte abnormality is more common in dehydrated patients with cystic fibrosis than in otherwise healthy dehydrated patients?
A) Hyponatremia.
B) Hypochloremia.
C) Hypokalemia.
D) Hyperbicarbonatemia.
E) All of the above.

Discussion 4-3

The correct answer is "E." The point is that the evaluation of a dehydrated patient with cystic fibrosis (CF) likely will require more vigilance than that of an average dehydrated patient, but do not ever call your patients "average," at least not to their parents. You will recall that the screening test for CF is the sweat chloride test; high amounts of chloride in the sample are consistent with a diagnosis of CF. Therefore it stands to reason that CF patients lose more chloride (and more sodium) in their sweat, making them more prone to hypochloremia and hyponatremia, especially when they have been exercising in a warm environment. They may even be chronically hyponatremic, which leads to increased aldosterone secretion and further disturbances such as hypokalemia and metabolic alkalosis, otherwise known as hyperbicarbonatemia. Dehydration acutely worsens the chronic stresses on their electrolyte metabolism.

Question 4-4

Which of the following would be an appropriate maintenance IV fluid order for a 23-kg child?
A) We need the child's body surface area to properly determine a fluid rate.
B) D_5 ½ NS with 20 mEq/L KCl at 63 mL/h.
C) D_5 NS with 20 mEq/L KCl at 63 mL/h.
D) D_5 ½ NS with 20 mEq/L at 1000 mL/kg/day.
E) D_5W at 80 mL/kg/day.

Discussion 4-4

The correct answer is "B." Exactly what constitutes a child's "maintenance" IV fluid need is debatable; probably the only true maintenance fluid is total parenteral nutrition (TPN). To maintain hydration, children need to replace the water they lose through urine and stool and the water that is expelled through their skin and lungs, otherwise known as insensible loss. The most prevalent method for determining maintenance fluid needs in children has been with us since at least 1957, when Doctors Holliday and Segar published their seminal paper in *Pediatrics*. They furthered the notion that water needs are best tied to energy expenditure and gave us what has become known as the "4:2:1 rule." Using that rule, a 23-kg child would require 4 mL/kg/h of fluid for his or her "first" 10 kg, 2 mL/kg/h of fluid for the "second" 10 kg, and 1 mL/kg/h for every kilogram beyond those two sets of 10, totaling 63 mL/h for the child in question. The electrolytes added to the water are those that are most important to us, at amounts that were decided upon by Holliday and Segar relative to their concentrations in human and cow milk. Our bodies do require magnesium, but not enough that it needs to be included in the replacement fluid. As noted previously, ¼ NS does not include enough salt. Using normal saline for a maintenance fluid is acceptable, but ½ NS is arguably the best. Five percent dextrose provides just enough calories to keep us from catabolizing ourselves if we are not eating. Option "E" is a good answer for a newborn, but 23 kg is a good birthweight for a dolphin, and who knows what it needs? Other methods of estimating human maintenance IV fluid needs have been developed, such as using body surface area, but none have had the staying power of the 4:2:1 rule. Being precise and using the number 63 is unnecessary, although it is not too hard to program 63 mL/h into an infusion pump. Try it sometime. (See Table 15–7.)

Question 4-5

For our 23-kg patient, which of the following is correct regarding his maintenance needs?
A) His daily sodium needs are 46.8 mEq.
B) His daily sodium needs are 154 mEq.
C) His daily potassium needs are 46.8 mEq.
D) ½ NS provides his exact sodium needs.
E) He needs 1 L of fluid daily.

Discussion 4-5

The correct answer is "A." To determine a "maintenance" IV fluid requirement, you need to calculate the daily water, sodium, and potassium needs. Daily, 3 mEq of Na^+ and 2 mEq of K^+ are needed for every 100 mL of fluid. For our 23-kg patient:

Daily fluid needs: 1500 mL + (20 mL/kg/day × 3 kg) = 1560 mL (see Table 15–7)

Daily Na^+ needs: (3 mEq/100 mL) × 1560 mL = 46.8 mEq

Daily K^+ needs: (2 mEq/100 mL) × 1560 mL = 31.2 mEq

To calculate what fraction of NS is needed, divide the patient's Na^+ need by the Na^+ concentration of NS (46.8/154 = 0.3); ⅓ NS would be perfect. Now add 31.2 mEq KCl/L. A perfect fluid would be D_5 ⅓ NS + 30 mEq KCl/L.

TABLE 15–7 DAILY AND HOURLY FLUID REQUIREMENTS USING THE HOLLIDAY-SEGAR FORMULA

Weight (kg)	24-Hour Calculation	Hourly Calculation
First 10 kg	100 mL/kg/day	4 mL/kg/h
Second 10 kg	1000 mL + 50 mL/kg/day	40 mL + 2 mL/kg/h
Each additional kg > 20 kg	1500 mL + 20 mL/kg/day	60 mL + 1 mL/kg/h

CASE 5

A 12-year-old girl is hospitalized for management of pneumonia with a parapneumonic effusion. Despite being encouraged to eat, she has been eating poorly since admission, although she has been drinking "a lot," despite being on IV fluid. Her mother asks when she is going to get better, especially since her energy level seems to be deteriorating. She largely appears well but is somewhat pale. She appears well-hydrated and has no edema. Her urine output has been steadily dropping since admission. Her vitals have been stable within normal limits for the last several days. The decision is made to start her on parenteral nutrition. Prior to starting TPN, the hospital pharmacist asks for some "baseline" lab tests. Shortly thereafter, you answer a page to the child's nursing unit, and her troublesome lab results are reported to you: Sodium 120 mEq/L, potassium 7.0 mEq/L, albumin 1.9 g/dL, hemoglobin 8 g/dL, and white blood cell count (WBC) 25,000/mm³. There is no record of hemolysis. Her BUN is 16 mg/dL, creatinine 0.65 mg/dL, and glucose 95 mg/dL. The remainder of her chemistry panel is normal.

Question 5-1

What should be rectified first?
A) Sodium.
B) Appetite.
C) Potassium.
D) Albumin.
E) Hemoglobin.

Discussion 5-1

The correct answer is "C." The potassium level is the most bothersome, so deal with that first. A potassium level of 7 mEq/L or higher needs your immediate, undivided attention. Hyponatremia (serum sodium < 135 mEq/L) has variable and nonspecific effects and can certainly make a person tired, but that level of hyponatremia is less urgent than a truly elevated potassium level, which could lead to a fatal arrhythmia, including asystole—fatal, as in death and increased malpractice premiums. Poor appetite, low albumin, low sodium, and low hemoglobin are all commonly seen in this setting, each of which should be addressed in due time, though none of them are emergent issues. These lab results promptly become your first priority, so you drop your donut and proceed to the patient's unit to deal with the situation. When you arrive, she looks no worse than she did in the morning and responds to questions appropriately. The nurse states that she thinks the T waves have been somewhat peaked on the patient's cardiorespiratory monitor tracing. A look at her current tracing shows what appears to you to be a normal sinus rhythm.

Question 5-2

Of the following, which is NOT an appropriate intervention for true hyperkalemia?
A) IV infusion of calcium gluconate.
B) IV infusion of insulin- and dextrose-containing fluid.
C) Sodium polystyrene sulfonate (Kayexalate).

D) An intranasal dose of desmopressin.

E) IV infusion of normal saline and a dose of furosemide.

Discussion 5-2

The correct answer is "D." Calcium gluconate does not lower serum potassium levels per se, but it does lessen the pro-dysrhythmia effect of hyperkalemia and is used in conjunction with interventions that do lower the serum potassium, such as the administration of dextrose and insulin. These together precipitate a shift of potassium from the extracellular compartment to the intracellular compartment, where most of our potassium (~95%) belongs. Fluid administration followed by a dose of furosemide, a non–potassium-sparing diuretic, is also helpful. Sodium polystyrene sulfonate lowers serum potassium by exchanging its sodium ions for a patient's potassium ions while in the intestines. Desmopressin (synthetic antidiuretic hormone) is not a recommended treatment for hyperkalemia.

Question 5-3

What should be the next step in this patient's management?

A) Give an IV dose of calcium gluconate.

B) Repeat the chemistry panel and obtain an ECG.

C) Review her cardiorespiratory tracing for the last 2 hours.

D) Give an oral dose of Kayexalate.

E) Start an insulin drip at 0.1 units/kg/h.

Discussion 5-3

The best answer is "B." Again, a truly elevated potassium level requires urgent attention and steps should be taken to rectify it. The proper thing to do is to assess the totality of the situation first. As far as we have been told, our patient does not have an obvious reason to have hyperkalemia, such as tumor lysis syndrome or a crush injury, but she has been on IV fluid, which can be mixed incorrectly. Laboratory reports are not always perfectly accurate and the sample may well have been hemolyzed, but doing nothing is probably not appropriate in this situation. Repeating the lab draw promptly and obtaining an ECG are the correct first steps. Obtaining an ECG is appropriate not only for confirmation of any suspected cardiorespiratory monitor findings, which are not as sensitive as a 12-lead ECG, but also serves as the best way to later confirm a response to your interventions if there are rhythm abnormalities. A leisurely perusal of the last 2 hours of monitor tracings is unlikely to be fruitful but *is* likely to earn you the ire of the child's nurse, who is a person of action. Sodium polystyrene sulfonate takes time to lower the serum potassium (1–2 hours) and therefore should not be the first intervention for true hyperkalemia. Insulin can be given, although it would be problematic if administered by itself. The hyperkalemia treatment involving insulin should include a glucose infusion, usually 0.5 mg/kg over 30 minutes with a 0.1 unit/kg one-time dose of insulin. The best way to immediately prevent the occurrence of a life-threatening arrhythmia is to give a 0.5 to 1 mL/kg IV dose of 10% calcium gluconate, which stabilizes the myocardium, but usually you have time to sort things out before intervening pharmacologically. The quickest way to

lower the serum potassium is to give a dose of beta-agonist, which promotes potassium uptake into cells. The most readily available beta-agonist in a children's hospital is albuterol, which is a safe intervention even if the patient's potassium is not truly elevated. (See Table 15–8.) Hypokalemia (serum potassium < 3 mEq/L), on the other hand, causes muscle weakness up to the point of paralysis; all sorts of cardiac arrhythmias, including ventricular tachycardia; and renal dysfunction. Hypokalemia in children is most often seen with gastroenteritis or with diuretic use. Levels below 3 mEq/L typically cause symptoms and should be rectified. This is preferably done using oral potassium chloride or with IV doses of 0.25 to 0.5 mEq/kg of K^+ (a "potassium rider") for those who cannot take oral medication. Prunes and chard are high in potassium, if only you could get a child to eat them.

TABLE 15–8 CAUSES OF HYPOKALEMIA AND HYPERKALEMIA

Hypokalemia (K⁺ < 3 mEq/L)	Hyperkalemia (K⁺ > 5.5 mEq/L)
Increased renal excretion	**Decreased renal excretion**
• Hyperaldosteronism	• Kidney disease
• Renal tubular acidosis	• Hypoaldosteronism
• Bartter syndrome	• Addison disease
• Gitelman syndrome	• Congenital adrenal hyperplasia
• Diuretics	• Potassium-sparing diuretics
• Drugs (amphotericin)	• Drugs
	• Aldosterone insensitivity (pseudohypoaldosteronism)
Increased gastrointestinal losses	**Cellular destruction**
• Vomiting	• Tumor lysis syndrome
• Gastric suctioning	• Rhabdomyolysis
• Diarrhea	• Hemolysis
• Laxative abuse	• Transfusion of stored red blood cells
Cellular shifting	**Cellular shifting**
• Metabolic alkalosis	• Metabolic acidosis
• Beta-agonists (albuterol)	• Beta-blockers
• Insulin	• Hyperkalemic periodic paralysis
• Hyperthyroidism	
• Familial hypokalemic periodic paralysis	
Iatrogenic	**Iatrogenic**
• Administration of IV fluids or TPN without K⁺	• Administration of IV fluids or TPN with excess K⁺

The lab is called and the tech apologizes for forgetting to note the hemolysis. To be thorough, a repeat potassium level is drawn and an ECG is obtained, both of which are normal.

Question 5-4

All of the following ECG findings can be seen in a patient with hyperkalemia EXCEPT:

A) Peaked T waves.
B) Prolonged PR interval.
C) Prominent U waves.
D) Absent P waves.
E) Asystole.

Discussion 5-4

The correct answer is "C." U waves can be a normal finding but also can be indicative of hypokalemia, not hyperkalemia. As previously discussed, hyperkalemia can cause asystole, and asystole is pretty close to death, so the answer is not option "E." Hyperkalemia is known to produce all of the other findings, which are listed in order of their occurrence as the potassium level increases.

Now it is time to deal with the patient's hyponatremia. She reportedly has been drinking *a lot*, iatrogenic hyponatremia is common in the inpatient setting, and hyponatremia and syndrome of inappropriate antidiuretic hormone secretion (SIADH) are solidly linked in your impressionable mind, despite the rare occurrence of SIADH in children.

Question 5-5

How can you determine the cause of the patient's hyponatremia?

A) Check her urine output for the last several days.
B) Measure her antidiuretic hormone (ADH) level.
C) Measure her serum osmolality, urine osmolality, and urine sodium.
D) Give a fluid bolus and check her serum sodium level thereafter.
E) Check her cortisol level.

Discussion 5-5

The correct answer is "C." The first step is to assess her hydration status, which is essential in determining the cause of the hyponatremia (Na^+ < 135 mEq/L). She is reportedly well hydrated and not *overly* hydrated (hypervolemic), as is suggested by the lack of edema, which together limit the possible causes of her hyponatremia. Her lung pathology puts her at risk for SIADH, so it is reasonable to be leaning toward that diagnosis. Her urine output alone would not provide all the required information, but a low urine output would be consistent with SIADH. Psychogenic polydipsia is not common in otherwise healthy children but is not out of the question. Establishing a diagnosis of SIADH, and then acting appropriately, first requires a comparison between urine osmolality and serum osmolality and a look at the urine sodium, so the answer to the above question is option "C." The serum osmolality can be ordered separately and measured directly, but it also can be *estimated* by the following equation, conveniently using laboratory tests that in most cases have already been obtained:

$$(2 \times Na^+) + (BUN/2.8) + (Glucose/18)$$

The 2.8 and the 18 in this equation are mg/dL-to-mmol/L conversion factors to make terms agree, and the multiplication of the Na^+ by 2 accounts for the anions (other osmoles) associated with the sodium cations. In SIADH, the urine osmolality will be inappropriately high (> 100 mOsm/kg) in comparison to the serum osmolality. If the urine sodium is in the range of 20 to 30 mEq/L or higher in a euvolemic, hyponatremic patient with an inappropriately high urine osmolality, the main considerations are SIADH, hypothyroidism, and glucocorticoid deficiency. It will, of course, be 25 mEq/L when you order it. Measurement of ADH levels, though intuitive, has not been shown to be clinically useful. (See Figure 15–1.) Tracking down the cause of hyponatremia in a patient with a complex set of findings is not always straightforward (eg, in a patient with meningitis who has heart failure and is taking diuretics). If we learn the principles we should be able to figure things out. Sometimes a fluid bolus followed by repeated lab values is the most appropriate intervention. Our patient's calculated serum osmolality is 251 mOsm/kg, her measured urine osmolality is 220 mOsm/kg, and her urine sodium is 34 mEq/L. She is not simply drinking too much, which would give her a low urine osmolality. In the proper setting (eg, this previously healthy child with a parapneumonic effusion), these results, at least initially, are most consistent with a diagnosis of SIADH. The urine is concentrated with elevated sodium while the serum is dilute.

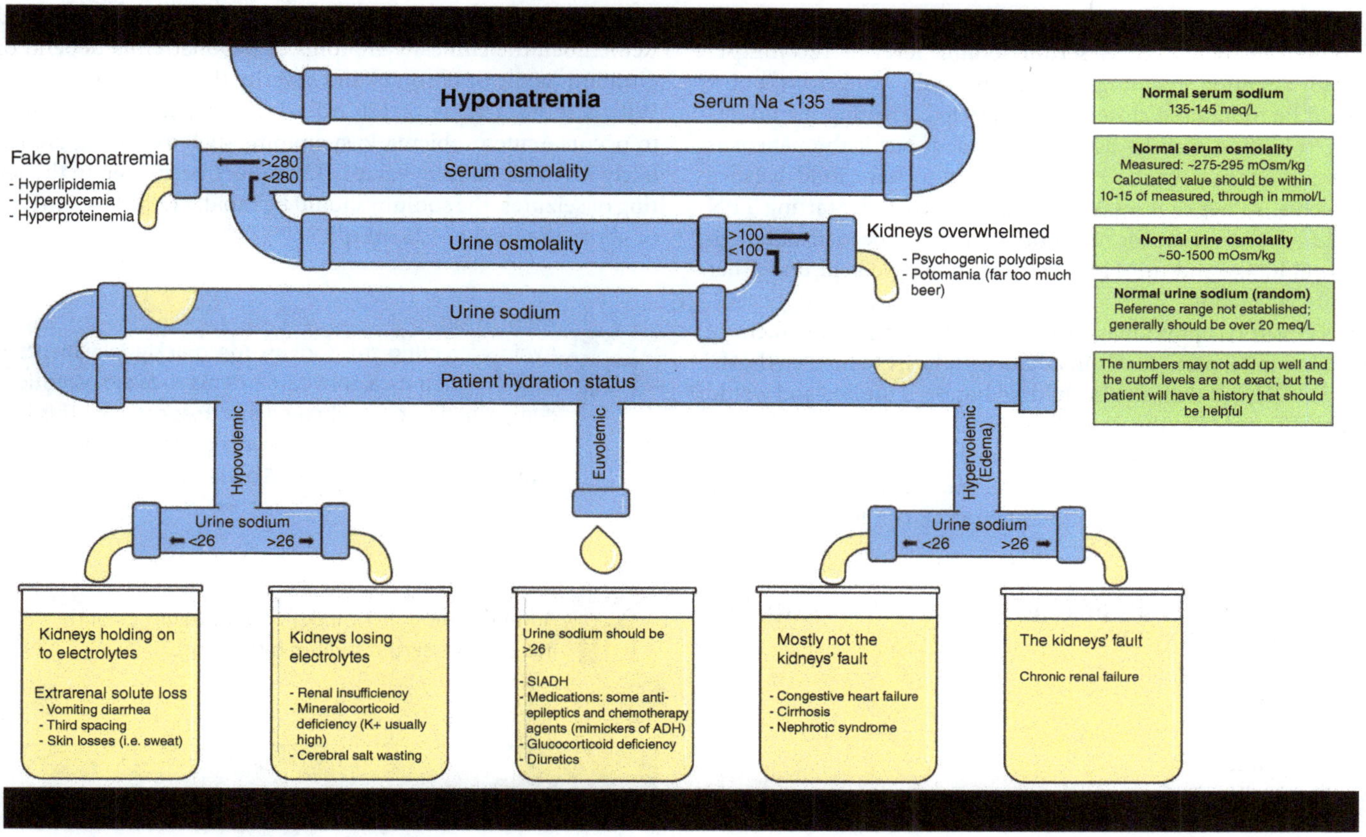

FIGURE 15–1. Causes of hyponatremia.

Hyponatremia   Serum Na <135

Fake hyponatremia   >280
- Hyperlipidemia   <280
- Hyperglycemia
- Hyperproteinemia   Serum osmolality

Urine osmolality   >100
<100   Kidneys overwhelmed
- Psychogenic polydipsia
- Potomania (far too much beer)

Urine sodium

Patient hydration status

Hypovolemic   Euvolemic   Hypervolemic (Edema)

Urine sodium   <26   >26   Urine sodium   <26   >26

Normal serum sodium
135-145 meq/L

Normal serum osmolality
Measured: ~275-295 mOsm/kg
Calculated value should be within
10-15 of measured, through in mmol/L

Normal urine osmolality
~50-1500 mOsm/kg

Normal urine sodium (random)
Reference range not established;
generally should be over 20 meq/L

The numbers may not add up well and
the cutoff levels are not exact, but the
patient will have a history that should
be helpful

Kidneys holding on to electrolytes

Extrarenal solute loss
- Vomiting diarrhea
- Third spacing
- Skin losses (i.e. sweat)

Kidneys losing electrolytes
- Renal insufficiency
- Mineralocorticoid deficiency (K+ usually high)
- Cerebral salt wasting

Urine sodium should be >26
- SIADH
- Medications: some anti-epileptics and chemotherapy agents (mimickers of ADH)
- Glucocorticoid deficiency
- Diuretics

Mostly not the kidneys' fault
- Congestive heart failure
- Cirrhosis
- Nephrotic syndrome

The kidneys' fault
Chronic renal failure

QUICK QUIZ

Why are urine and serum osmolality reported in mOsm/kg while the calculated estimate of serum osmolality is in mmol/L?

A) I don't know.
B) Do I need to know this?
C) I will feel like an expert after this question.
D) Is this relevant?
E) I don't like chemistry.

Discussion

The best answer is "C," or at least we hope it will be after reading the explanation that follows. Millimoles per liter of solution and milliosmoles per kilogram of solvent are measures of osmolarity and osmolality, respectively. Osmolality and osmolarity can differ, depending on the solvent. One liter of water, by definition, equals 1 kg, but 1 L of serum does not. Confusing as this may be, the difference is small enough not to be clinically relevant. In solving the earlier equation, we are technically calculating a serum osmolarity, but let's not get hung up on the words. The most common laboratory testing methodology for osmolality utilizes the difference in freezing temperatures between two solutions of different osmolality; it does not distinguish between osmoles such as sodium,

glucose, and so on. The laboratory testing for sodium, glucose, and BUN relies on different methods; therefore, it is expressed in different units. The difference between the measured serum osmolality and our calculated serum osmolarity is referred to as the "osmolal gap," which if elevated in a patient without an acidosis points to an alcohol ingestion, usually isopropyl alcohol or ethanol.

> **Helpful Tip**
> Think alcohol ingestion if the plasma osmolal gap is elevated! If ethanol is ruled out, consider isopropyl alcohol, methanol, or ethylene glycol. Remember, drinking rubbing alcohol, antifreeze, or deicing solutions is not recommended.

Question 5-6

The most appropriate intervention for this patient with SIADH should be:

A) Administer a dose of tolvaptan (vasopressin receptor antagonist).
B) Postpone starting TPN.
C) Start a 3% sodium infusion.
D) Give an IV NS bolus.
E) Restrict fluid intake.

Discussion 5-6

The best answer is "E." A serum sodium level of 120 mEq/L, though attention grabbing, is not universally dangerous, but it should be monitored closely and corrected. Treating the underlying condition may be all that is needed, but if the patient is drinking excessively she could continue to have fluid balance problems, so her oral intake should be restricted. Starting TPN would be appropriate for nutritional support if needed; although her oral intake and the TPN together should be kept under her maintenance fluid need (60% of maintenance is suggested). Vasopressin receptor antagonists have a role in the treatment of hyponatremia, particularly in adults with heart failure, cirrhosis, and SIADH, but their use in children has been limited and would not be warranted in this case. A 3% NaCl solution would also not be warranted. This patient has too much free water not too little salt. Since we think we know what the problem is, giving a fluid bolus also would not be the most appropriate intervention.

Question 5-7

Of the following, all are predisposing factors for the development of SIADH EXCEPT:
A) Head trauma.
B) Pneumonia.
C) Lithium use.
D) Lung cancer.
E) Meningitis.

Discussion 5-7

The correct answer is "C." Certain medications, most notably in pediatrics the antiseizure medications carbamazepine and oxcarbazepine and selective serotonin reuptake inhibitors such as fluoxetine and sertraline, are known to alter ADH metabolism and cause SIADH, but lithium is not among them. Lithium has in fact been associated with the development of nephrogenic diabetes insipidus and was at one time used as a treatment for SIADH. Pneumonias, malignancies (small cell lung cancer, in particular), and central nervous system disturbances such as head trauma, meningitis, and neurosurgical procedures are all known to cause SIADH. Persistence of hyponatremia is, at best, unpleasant and should be rectified. How this is rectified depends on the situation, but if a child has seizures or altered mental status attributable to hyponatremia, the best treatment is to give 3 to 5 mL/kg of 3% NaCl solution over a short interval (~30 minutes), check the sodium thereafter, and repeat the infusion if the symptoms do not abate. For further, or less urgent, sodium replacement, an initial 3% NaCl solution infusion rate can be estimated by multiplying the patient's body weight in kilograms by the desired rate of increase in serum sodium in milliequivalents per liter per hour. For example, a 10 kg child whose serum sodium you would like to increase at a rate of 0.5 mEq/L/h requires an infusion of 3% NaCl at 5 mL/h. A conservative rate of change of no more than 8 mEq/L in a 24-hour period is recommended, although disagreement about the rate exists. In any case, changes in serum sodium can be unpredictable, so frequent lab draws are warranted, perhaps as frequently as every 2 hours. An appropriate therapeutic end point is a sodium level of 120 to 125 mEq/L, which assumes that the underlying mechanism of the hyponatremia is being addressed. Remember, the clinical symptoms of hyponatremia depend on duration (acute or chronic) and severity (how low the value is). With a sodium value of 120 mEq/L or less, seizures are likely to occur. Acute problematic symptoms such as seizing are less likely when the sodium value is 125 mEq/L or greater. In the setting of seizures, the sodium should be rapidly raised by 5 mEq/L or above the level of 125 mEq/L.

> **Helpful Tip**
> Avoid correcting the sodium too quickly in patients with hyponatremia or hypernatremia to avoid osmotic demyelination or cerebral edema, respectively. This is especially true if the condition is chronic. A general rule is to correct no faster than 0.5 mEq/L/h.

> **Helpful Tip**
> Administration of 1 mL/kg of 3% sodium chloride will increase the serum sodium by 1 mEq/L.

▶ CASE 6

It is a blustery November Sunday evening in Maine, and you are passing through the emergency department (ED) to the physician's parking lot after rounding in the nursery when the ED physician waves you down for some help. A 2½-year-old boy has just been brought in by his father because "He's acting funny, kind of like he's drunk." As far as dad knows, the child has not been sick lately and he apparently was fine when he woke up this morning before the mother left for work. The father figured there was something wrong when he found the boy on the floor of the living room at about 6 PM drooling, with a "glassy look in his eyes." In addition to babbling slowly and insensibly on the way to the hospital, the boy vomited once. He is mildly tachycardic but otherwise appears well, aside from being a little unsteady on his feet and mostly oblivious to the world about him in a happy sort of way. The father seems to have all his wits about him.

Question 6-1

The child was brought to the ED, so he is almost certainly going to undergo *some* lab studies, but which ones would you advocate? What labs should be obtained?
A) Chemistry panel.
B) Serum alcohol level.
C) Blood gas.
D) Serum drug screen.
E) All of the above.

Discussion 6-1

The correct answer is "E." The patient is not of childbearing age, so he probably does not need a serum beta-hCG test, but he needs all of those listed above, plus some more. The history strongly suggests an ingestion of some sort. Short of being tied to their children during all waking hours, parents cannot know what they are up to all the time. Sometimes parents need to attend to other needs, and toddlers are curious and always ready to put just about anything into their mouths, particularly liquids in colorful cups. The father's thought that his son is acting as if he is drunk points us in certain directions, as well it should.

Question 6-2

Which test is least likely to be helpful in the initial evaluation of a child with a suspected methanol or ethylene glycol ingestion?

A) Urinalysis.
B) Serum methanol or ethylene glycol concentration.
C) Blood gas.
D) Chemistry panel.
E) Serum osmolality.

Discussion 6-2

The correct answer is "A." All of these are useful tests in establishing, or ruling out, a methanol or ethylene glycol exposure in a child, but a urinalysis is least helpful given that oxalate crystals are not specific to ethylene glycol ingestions and are a late finding. Serum methanol and ethylene glycol tests are not readily available in many hospital labs, which limits their usefulness, so we often need to rely on some old-school, readily available testing to point us in the right direction so we can limit the damage from such ingestions. If you are thinking anion gap, you are on the right path. Methanol and ethylene glycol are not acids, but their metabolites in the body are, which can and do cause an increased anion gap metabolic acidosis. The elevated osmolal gap was discussed above. Let's hope you were paying attention.

Helpful Tip

Why is the CO_2 (carbon dioxide) on a metabolic profile interpreted as HCO_3 (bicarbonate)? The simple answer is, that is the way it is reported. The more complicated answer stems from the lack of a readily available system for the direct measurement of serum HCO_3. The CO_2 reported on a basic metabolic profile is the total amount of CO_2 produced from the acidification of a serum sample, which converts all of the HCO_3, CO_2, and H_2CO_3 present (95% of which is HCO_3) into CO_2, which *can* be measured and is what is reported. The HCO_3 reported on a serum blood gas analysis is also not a direct measure of serum HCO_3; the value is calculated from the serum pH and pCO_2 using the Henderson-Hasselbach equation, which you may recall from undergrad biochemistry (and which is where it will stay for our purposes). Both of these methods introduce an error into the measurement of HCO_3.

Question 6-3

The anion gap represents:

A) The number of measured serum anions minus the unmeasured serum anions.
B) The discrepancy between the number of serum cations and serum anions.
C) 12.
D) The number of unmeasured serum anions minus the unmeasured serum cations.
E) A number that increases with a decrease in serum osmolality.

Discussion 6-3

The correct answer is "D." Not many things are as exciting as a big anion gap, unless it is your child who has it. The number of serum anions must always equal the number of serum cations, so option "B" is incorrect. The "unmeasured" cations are calcium, magnesium, and potassium. These frequently *are* measured, but the anion gap traditionally is calculated from the lab values reported on a standard basic metabolic profile. The K^+ can be used in the calculation, but the number is small and does not vary to a large degree, so it is usually left out. The normal, "unmeasured" serum anions are phosphate, sulfate, and various proteins and organic acids. The number 12 is a fine number that coincidentally is within the realm of a normal anion gap, but that is only a number and we need some lab values in an actual patient to calculate an anion gap. If the K^+ is ignored, the value of a normal anion gap can range from 8 to 16, but in the question we are being asked what the value actually represents, which technically is the number of unmeasured anions minus the number of unmeasured cations.

An increased anion gap without an acidosis is not a common pediatric scenario; therefore, we can focus on situations in which an increased anion gap is associated with a metabolic acidosis. An increased anion gap clues us in to the presence of abnormal anions, which are a subset of the unmeasured serum anions. Where did they come from?

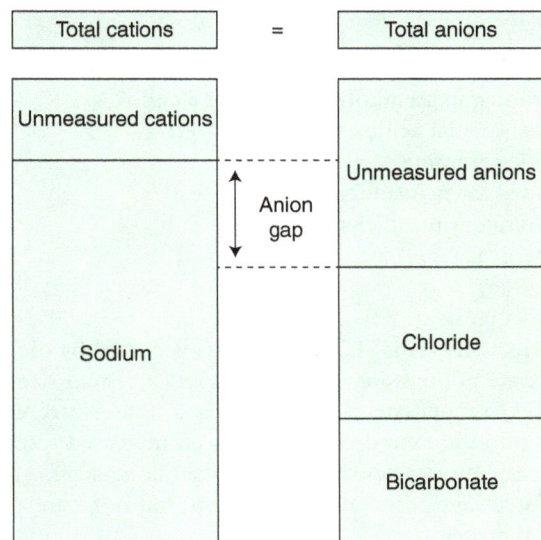

For those who like lists, the mnemonic MUDPILES captures most of the possibilities:

M – Methanol

U – Uremia (isocyanic acid and uric acid)

D – **D**iabetic ketoacidosis (acetoacetic acid and beta-hydroxybutyric acid)

P – Paraldehyde, paracetamol

I – Inborn errors of metabolism, isoniazid

L – Lactic acidosis

E – Ethylene glycol

S – Salicylates

Paracetamol is what acetaminophen is called in most countries outside of the United States and paraldehyde is a sedative, mainly used to stop seizures, that is not available in the United States. For those who like processes, consider this: An increased anion gap with an acidosis, not surprisingly, represents a gain of acid in the blood. The H^+ is buffered in large part by HCO_3, causing the laboratory-reported HCO_3 to drop, and the associated abnormal anions are left to wreak havoc. Where did the rogue acid come from? Perhaps from the body itself: lactate, ketoacids (diabetic ketoacidosis, DKA), or the acids that build up when the kidneys fail. Perhaps not from the body: methanol, ethylene glycol, paraldehyde, toluene (the breakdown products of which are toxic acids), and medications such as isoniazid, aminoglycosides, and salicylates, including aspirin, bismuth subsalicylate (the active ingredient in Pepto-Bismol), and methyl salicylate (the active ingredient in Bengay and oil of wintergreen, which is a source of highly concentrated salicylate). Other than a gain in acid, the other main category of metabolic acidosis (non–anion gap) results from either a loss of, or a failure to generate, HCO_3. This can occur through net base loss, as in gastrointestinal losses from diarrhea or with renal losses from diuretic use or proximal renal tubular acidosis, or from a failure of the kidney to excrete normally produced acids, as in renal insufficiency and distal renal tubular acidosis.

Question 6-4

Of the following, which is the most common cause of a non–anion gap metabolic acidosis in a child?
A) Renal tubular acidosis.
B) Cholestyramine.
C) Acute kidney insufficiency.
D) Respiratory insufficiency.
E) Diarrhea.

Discussion 6-4

The correct answer is "E." The acidosis is caused by the loss of bicarbonate in the stool. The body prefers a pH close to 7.4, so the lungs compensate rapidly for this loss of bicarbonate by stepping up the excretion of CO_2 via an increased respiratory rate. A respiratory acidosis is not a metabolic acidosis. All of the other listed items can cause an acidosis, but none are as common as diarrhea.

Question 6-5

Speaking of diarrhea, what is a normal stool output for a human?
A) 15 g/kg/day.
B) 15 mL/kg/h.
C) 30 g/kg/day.
D) Up to 200 g/day in an adult.
E) Two stools a day.

Discussion 6-5

The correct answer is "D." Anything looser than a child's normal output is interpreted by most parents as diarrhea, but we need to know what normal is so we can either be reassuring or not reassuring, as the situation requires. There is quite a bit of variability in the consistency, frequency, and volume of what can be considered to be normal, but infants typically have 5 to 10 g/kg/day of stool output and an adult will have up to 200 g/day. Two stools a day may be "normal," but what about the volume and consistency? Some practitioners consider diarrhea to be a stool output of greater than 15 g/kg/day, so 30 g/kg/day is enough to be considered abnormal. Urine output is generally measured in milliliters per kilogram per hour, and a normal urine output in a fully hydrated child is 1 to 2 mL/kg/h, although it can be considerably more in a normal, overly hydrated child.

Remember our patient? Let's say his anion gap is indeed elevated at 24 (> 20 is usually worthy of attention). His blood gas shows a metabolic acidosis: pH 7.28, PCO_2 38, HCO_3 18. You start running down the list of possibilities with his father. He admits to putting some antifreeze in the car yesterday, though he is not willing to say that he left any in a location that was accessible to his child. There is no aspirin or alcohol in the home. Some of the lab reports are still pending.

Question 6-6

What is the most appropriate intervention for this child?
A) Intravenous fomepizole.
B) Ethanol infusion.
C) Peritoneal dialysis.
D) Ritualistic bloodletting.
E) Intravenous fluid at 1.5 times the maintenance rate.

Discussion 6-6

The correct answer is "A." Ethanol can be used, but fomepizole is the preferred treatment for suspected ingestion of antifreeze. Both are competitive inhibitors of alcohol dehydrogenase, and therefore keep ethylene glycol from being metabolized into toxic compounds. The parent compounds cause central nervous system depression but are otherwise relatively nontoxic. It is the acids produced from metabolism that are toxic. Sodium bicarbonate and dialysis are also used. Peritoneal dialysis would not, however, be the preferred method. Bloodletting still exists in "Western" medicine; we just call it a partial exchange transfusion, which is a treatment for polycythemia in a newborn. Whether or not it is performed as a ritual is a matter of preference and interpretation.

► CASE 7

A 29-day-old previously healthy infant has had nasal congestion and a cough for about a week. He is diagnosed with respiratory syncytial virus (RSV) bronchiolitis and admitted because he is hypoxic. Several hours after arrival, his nurse tells you that he now has retractions, nasal flaring, and an increasing supplemental oxygen need. A blood gas measurement is obtained, revealing the following: pH 7.29, PCO$_2$ 66, HCO$_3$ 30.4.

Question 7-1

Which of the following statements is FALSE?
A) For each acute 10 mm Hg uncompensated increase in PCO$_2$, there is a 0.08 point decrease in pH.
B) For each acute 10 mm Hg increase in PCO$_2$, there is a 1 mmol/L increase in HCO$_3$.
C) For each chronic 10 mm Hg increase in PCO$_2$, there can be up to a 4 mmol/L compensatory increase in HCO$_3$.
D) The kidneys compensate for a respiratory acidosis by excreting H$^+$.
E) The lungs can rapidly and completely compensate for any metabolic alkalosis.

Discussion 7-1

The correct answer is "E." Functional though they are, the lungs cannot always "fully" compensate for a metabolic alkalosis, given that we can only lower our respiratory rate so much and continue to live. Perhaps this keeps the body aware that whatever fishy is going on needs to be rectified.

Question 7-2

Our patient's blood gas results are consistent with what metabolic circumstance?
A) An uncompensated respiratory acidosis.
B) An uncompensated respiratory alkalosis.
C) A compensated metabolic alkalosis.
D) A partially compensated respiratory acidosis.
E) A mixed metabolic and respiratory acidosis.

Discussion 7-2

The correct answer is "D." Metabolic disturbances are found in patients who have histories of illness, and we have been presented with a child with respiratory difficulty. As we are aware, respiratory difficulties can lead to hypoxia, hypercarbia, or both, so most likely we are looking at a respiratory acidosis in this scenario, which will get you off on the right foot. (See Figure 15–2.) Extrapolating from the commonly used relationships in the options listed above, an acute, uncompensated increase of 1 mm Hg of PCO$_2$ causes a decrease of 0.008 points on the pH scale and a 0.1 mmol/L increase in HCO$_3$. The HCO$_3$ and PCO$_2$ increase together based on their natural balance in the blood. If you note more than the spontaneous increase in HCO$_3$ you know that the kidneys have been compensating. To begin to answer questions such as the one above, you must know what normal is for all of these values. Keeping it simple, a

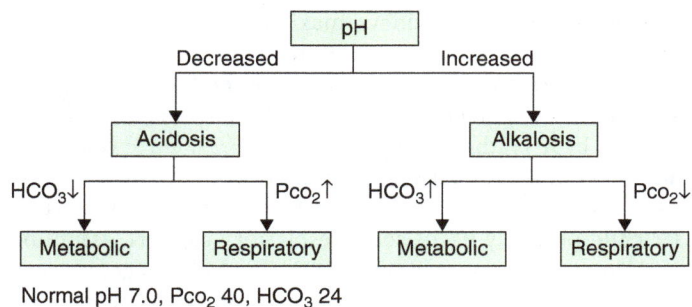

FIGURE 15–2. Acid-base status.

normal, average pH is 7.40; a normal, average HCO$_3$ is 24; and a normal, average PCO$_2$ is 40. In the current scenario, the pH is lower than the normal 7.40, so the child has an acidosis. Easy enough. His PCO$_2$ is higher than normal, which is characteristic of a respiratory acidosis, and his history is consistent with the development of a respiratory acidosis. His HCO$_3$ is higher than normal at 30.4. If the child had a pure, uncompensated respiratory acidosis, his pH should have decreased by approximately 0.21 (0.008 × [66 – 40]), resulting in a pH of 7.19 (7.40 – 0.21) and his HCO$_3$ should have increased spontaneously by 2.6 ([66 – 40] × 0.1) to 26.6. But his pH is 7.29 and his HCO$_3$ is 30.4, so his kidneys must have compensated, which they do by excreting H$^+$ (functionally increasing the serum HCO$_3$). He may have lost H$^+$ or gained HCO$_3$ somewhere else, but we can keep it simple. (See Table 15–9.) This child has a partially compensated respiratory acidosis. The chronic change in HCO$_3$ quoted in the answer choices for Question 7-1 (0.4 mmol/L per 1 mm Hg increase in

TABLE 15–9 SOME ACID-BASE RULES

Respiratory Acidosis

Acute respiratory acidosis, no renal compensation: For each 1 mm Hg increase in PCO$_2$, there will be a 0.1 mmol/L increase in HCO$_3$.

Chronic respiratory acidosis, maximum renal compensation: For each 1 mm Hg increase in PCO$_2$, there will be a 0.4 mmol/L increase in HCO$_3$.

Respiratory Alkalosis

Acute respiratory alkalosis, no renal compensation: For each 1 mm Hg decrease in PCO$_2$, there will be a 0.2 mmol/L decrease in HCO$_3$.

Chronic respiratory alkalosis, maximum renal compensation: For each 1 mm Hg decrease in PCO$_2$, there will be a 0.5 mmol/L decrease in HCO$_3$.

Metabolic Acidosis

For each 1 mmol/L decrease in HCO$_3$, there will be a 1.2 mm Hg decrease in PCO$_2$.

Metabolic Alkalosis

For each 1 mmol/L increase in HCO$_3$, there will be a 0.7 mm Hg increase in PCO$_2$.

PCO_2) represents the kidneys' maximal compensating power, which could change his HCO_3 by 10 ([66 – 40] × 0.4) up to a total of 34. He's at 30.4, which tells you he has compensated some but not as much as is theoretically possible, as might be guessed by his rather unfavorable pH of 7.29. Once you figure all of this out, the next step is to figure out what, if anything, can be done to get his values back to normal. This particular child probably needs some respiratory support, assuming that no one has invented "anti-RSV." The kidneys get to work soon after a disturbance in the force is detected but exercise their compensatory power judiciously over a period of 3 to 5 days. The lungs are able to compensate for a metabolic acidosis much faster, on the order of several minutes, if allowed to do their job without hindrance. The lungs work fast enough that we rarely, if ever, need to worry about whether they have compensated appropriately for a metabolic disturbance. We are all compensating for something, no? Perhaps you did not get accepted to medical school on the first try, or your dad is famous, or some such.

> **Helpful Tip**
>
> In acid-base disturbances, the CO_2 and HCO_3 follow each other. They go up or down together.

Question 7-3

Which of the following is FALSE?
A) Capillary blood gas measurement gives an accurate measure of PO_2.
B) Capillary blood gas PCO_2 and pH measurements are comparable to arterial blood gas measurements.
C) The HCO_3 measure on a blood gas measurement, regardless of source, is a calculated value.
D) Venous blood gas PCO_2 is regularly 5 mm Hg higher than arterial blood gas PCO_2.
E) Capillary and venous blood gas measurements can be used to accurately delineate an acid-base disorder.

Discussion 7-3

The correct answer is "A." All of the other responses are true.

▶ CASE 8

An anxious 3-year-old girl with asthma is brought in for evaluation of a cough and nasal congestion that has been worsening for 3 days. Her mother also states that the child has not been drinking well nor urinating as much as usual over the past several days. She appears somewhat dehydrated and is mildly tachycardic at about 120 bpm. She is mildly febrile at 38.4°C (101.1°F). Her work of breathing appears to be increased, although her level of anxiety and squirminess make it hard to determine just how significant it is. Her respiratory rate is in the upper 20s. After some trouble obtaining the sample, a basic chemistry panel and venous blood gas measurement are completed, the results of which are as follows: pH 7.48, PCO_2 30, HCO_3 22.

Question 8-1

What is the nature of this patient's acid-base disturbance?
A) A compensated respiratory alkalosis.
B) An uncompensated respiratory alkalosis.
C) A metabolic alkalosis.
D) A compensated metabolic alkalosis.
E) A mixed metabolic and respiratory alkalosis.

Discussion 8-1

The correct answer is "B." Again, the first step is to determine whether the pH is high or low. This child's pH is high, so she has an alkalosis. Her HCO_3 and PCO_2 are not normal, but her HCO_3 is pretty close. As usual, knowing something of the child's history is helpful. The concern here is the child's respiratory status, given her past and present histories. Most likely we were looking to see if a respiratory acidosis accompanied the child's respiratory distress. This is obviously not the case, so just what is going on here? Her bicarbonate level is lower than 24, which is not out of what could be considered the normal range. To say that she had a metabolic alkalosis would be an overstatement. Putting that together with her low PCO_2 of 30, she appears to have a respiratory alkalosis, which could make sense given the stated difficulty in obtaining the sample and some resultant screaming and yelling, loosely translated into medicalese as hyperventilation. But is that the only disturbance? Probably, but to be sure you can utilize some grade school arithmetic. The change in her PCO_2 from an assumed baseline of 40 is –10, which would be accompanied by an anticipated change in her HCO_3 of 0.2 multiplied by the change in the PCO_2 which is –2. Her HCO_3 is at the anticipated value of 22 (24 – 2). Therefore you can be confident that she has an acute, uncompensated respiratory alkalosis, which would not be unanticipated with the history. Some blood gas patterns, of course, can represent multiple derangements, which will require some thought to decipher. Examples include acute-on-chronic respiratory acidosis, acute respiratory acidosis with a metabolic acidosis, metabolic acidosis with an acute respiratory acidosis, and so on. To arrive at a correct blood gas interpretation, a guess may need to be made regarding the likely derangement followed by some math to determine if that interpretation is correct.

Question 8-2

What common household substance, if ingested, can produce a metabolic acidosis with an accompanying respiratory alkalosis?
A) Ice melter.
B) Baking soda.
C) Baking powder.
D) Aspirin.
E) Drain cleaner.

Discussion 8-2

The correct answer is "D." Aspirin is acetylsalicylic acid, one of the most commonly encountered salicylates, which we considered in an earlier question. Although acetylsalicylic acid is a weak acid, it is able to cause a lactic acidosis by disruption of cellular metabolism, as are all medicinal salicylates. Salicylates also tend to (1) stimulate the respiratory center to produce a respiratory alkalosis, (2) produce some interesting blood gas results, and (3) participate in the development of Reye syndrome. Here is a characteristic blood gas pattern, which you can play around with in your head: pH 7.48, PCO₂ 22, HCO₃ 14. Baking soda is sodium bicarbonate and is most commonly stored in yellow boxes. Baking powder is sodium bicarbonate, monocalcium phosphate, and sodium aluminum sulfate and is most commonly stored in red cans. Each could cause an alkalosis, but not the pattern in question. Drain cleaners usually contain strong bases, which cause local tissue damage but are rarely ingested in amounts able to cause significant systemic acid-base disturbances; apparently they are mostly buffered by the esophagus. Ice melter, depending on the brand, contains sodium chloride, potassium chloride, magnesium chloride, urea, calcium magnesium acetate, or a combination of these chemicals, none of which would cause an acidosis. Whether or not you knew the content of some of these substances may be immaterial, but you should know the effects of aspirin in an overdose situation, because you may well encounter such circumstances on the board exam or in practice, and you want what is best for your patients, even the hypothetical ones.

▶ CASE 9

An 8-year-old boy is brought to your office for evaluation of a 6-day history of gradually worsening cough, loss of energy, and loss of appetite, which put a damper on his family's visit to Disneyland. He has had a fever for the past several days and has been drinking some, but his mother is not sure how much. His brother had a similar flu-like illness of late. You see in the chart that the patient was diagnosed by your partner with type 1 diabetes 6 months ago, in December, after an emergency department visit for vomiting and diarrhea, which turned out to be diabetic ketoacidosis (DKA). You also see that his weight at that visit was 41 kg. It is 37 kg today. At first glance, he does indeed appear tired. He is tachycardic, but his blood pressure is within normal limits. A blood glucose level is obtained and is too high to be measured. He is promptly sent to the emergency department for further evaluation. Once there, a fluid bolus is given and blood is obtained for laboratory studies. The fluid bolus is repeated. His blood glucose is confirmed to be quite high at 642 mg/dL. Interestingly, the CO₂ on his metabolic panel is 21 mEq/L. His blood gas measurement shows a comparable HCO₃ of 20 mEq/L. His pH is 7.37 with a PCO₂ of 41. He does not have DKA, but you wonder if he is suffering from hyperosmolar hyperglycemic state (HHS).

Question 9-1
Which of the following is NOT a common laboratory finding in a patient with HHS?

A) Blood glucose greater than 600 mg/dL.
B) Increased serum ketones.
C) Elevated serum osmolality.
D) Pseudohyponatremia.
E) Normal pH.

Discussion 9-1
The correct answer is "B." This is one of the distinguishing factors between HHS and DKA. HHS is not associated with an acidosis, which in DKA is caused by serum ketoacids, more commonly referred to as serum ketones. HHS is a rare entity that most commonly occurs in type 1 diabetic patients in the setting of another illness, usually something severe such as sepsis or a significant bacterial pneumonia—the type that you can see without the help of a radiologist. The exact pathophysiology has not been worked out, but it can occur when a diabetic patient has not been receiving insulin and has been drinking a lot of sugar-containing drinks, not unlike our little friend in the vignette. Pseudohyponatremia is a result of hyperglycemia, which occurs in both HHS and DKA. Since the serum glucose contributes to serum osmolality, the blood glucose should be lowered slowly so that cerebral edema does not ensue. Even if the serum potassium is elevated, patients with HHS very likely will have a total body potassium deficit, and insulin will drive K⁺ into the intracellular space, so hypokalemia should be anticipated. Aiming to rectify the serum glucose and the fluid deficit over 48 hours is appropriate, but probably should not occur without the presence and input of an endocrinologist and an intensivist.

▶ CASE 10

It is August in Arizona, and a 9-day-old girl is brought to an urgent care facility for evaluation because she has not been feeding well for several days. She has solely been breastfed. There is no other bothersome history: No fever, no rash, no exposure to ill persons, no concerning information. The urgent care physician is worried when she sees the neonate and sends her to the emergency department (ED) for treatment. In the ED she appears tired but not truly lethargic in the medical sense; an IV line is placed, blood is obtained for laboratory studies, and she is given a 20 mL/kg normal saline bolus. After obtaining the history, the ED physician decides that the neonate would be best served by admission, and you, as the pediatrician on call, agree to take over her care. She improves following fluid administration in the ED, but when you arrive shortly thereafter, you are told that her serum sodium is 165 mEq/L. She appears well and her vital signs are within normal limits; the only other exam finding of note is mild jaundice. Her mother tells you that her birthweight was 3.5 kg, and you notice that her weight in triage was 3.0 kg. The child's mother also asks if it is normal for the child to sweat while feeding, as she has done occasionally since birth.

Question 10-1

What most likely is the principal cause of this child's hypernatremia (serum sodium > 145 mEq/L)?

A) Lack of supplemental water.
B) Diabetes insipidus.
C) Poor feeding leading to dehydration.
D) Neglect or abuse.
E) Excessive sweating and insensible fluid losses.

Discussion 10-1

The correct answer is "C." Hypernatremia (serum sodium > 145 mEq/L) is not common in children, but a general pediatrician may encounter this scenario. Presenting signs include irritability, lethargy, fever, vomiting, and seizures. Additionally, these infants can have a high-pitched cry and tachypnea. We know from this neonate's weights that she is not optimally hydrated; a healthy 9-day-old should be somewhat close to birthweight. Her weight plus the mother's concern about feeding should alert you to the presence of a problem. The amount of breast milk that the child is ingesting, or *not* ingesting in this case, is the most likely issue. If the mother appears reasonably healthy, the breast milk will also be reasonably healthy, but in some cases of breastfeeding failure the sodium content of breast milk has been known to be high. Some component of increased insensible losses would be expected for an infant in a warm environment, but it is unlikely that this neonate's inadequate weight could be accounted for by insensible losses alone. Sweating during feeding can be a tip-off to the presence of heart disease in infants but is not a specific finding; all infants have the capacity to sweat. Normal infants also have an intact thirst mechanism but are dependent on caregivers for their fluid intake. Neglect or abuse is, and should be, on the differential for just about any medical issue in a child, but is not the most likely issue with our patient, given a plausible history that is consistent with the findings. There is no American Academy of Pediatrics (AAP) recommendation for a breastfed infant to receive supplemental

water, although it is not an uncommon practice. Given a history of inadequate oral intake, as in this case, it is most likely that the neonate simply has hypernatremic dehydration caused by poor intake and possibly an abnormal breast milk sodium concentration. It is not possible to eliminate diabetes insipidus as a possibility in this patient without adequate testing, starting with urine and serum osmolalities, but diabetes insipidus is rare and this history represents somewhat of a classic scenario for simple hypernatremic dehydration. (See Figure 15–3.)

Question 10-2

What findings would be expected if the child had hypernatremia due to diabetes Insipidus (DI)?

A) High serum osmolality, low urine osmolality.
B) Low serum osmolality, low urine osmolality.
C) High serum osmolality, high urine osmolality.
D) Low serum osmolality, high urine osmolality.
E) Her serum sodium will always be abnormal.

Discussion 10-2

The correct answer is "A." Serum osmolality is mainly determined by the serum sodium level, as reflected in the equation by which a serum osmolality is calculated, and would be expected to be high in any hypernatremic individual. The problem in DI is a lack of antidiuretic hormone or the lack of a proper response to antidiuretic hormone from the kidneys, so a person with DI will urinate an excessive volume that will give them a tendency toward hypernatremic dehydration. For reference, urine osmolality most frequently is between 300 and 800 mOsm/kg but can range from 50 to 650 mOsm/kg in a neonate (infant younger than 1 month of age), the upper limit of which increases to 1500 mOsm/kg in older children. In a dehydrated child, the kidneys should be holding onto whatever water they can, producing a concentrated urine with a high osmolality, but a lack of ADH or a lack of a response to ADH makes that impossible. Children with DI who can drink enough to overcome a lack of ADH can have a normal serum

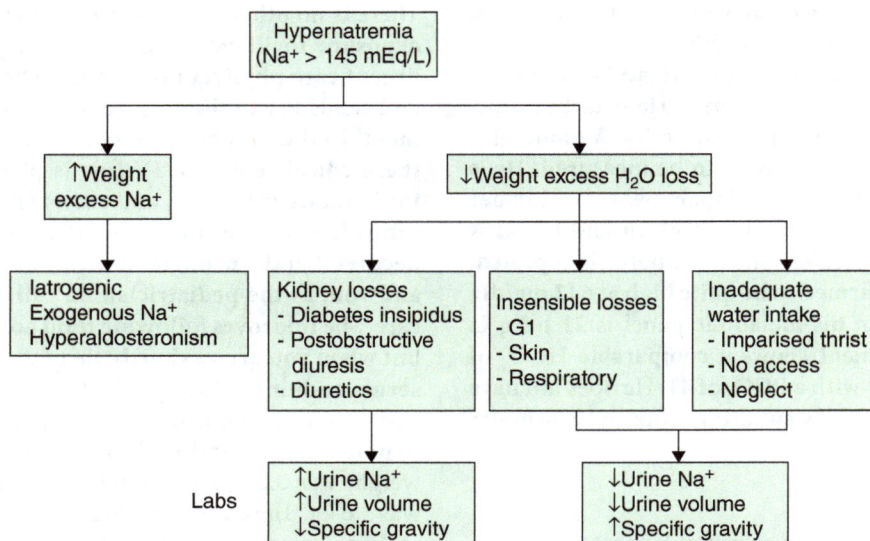

FIGURE 15–3. Causes of hypernatremia.

sodium level. And, of course, children who are given a properly prescribed ADH analog such as desmopressin (DDAVP) will most often also have a normal serum sodium.

Question 10-3

What should be the next step in this patient's medical management?
A) Give another NS bolus.
B) Calculate the child's free water deficit.
C) Give her a ½ NS bolus.
D) Check the sodium content of the mother's milk.
E) Start her on IV fluid at 1.5 times the maintenance amount.

Discussion 10-3

The best answer is "B." It is hard to deny the diagnostic and therapeutic utility of an NS bolus, but in this case, with its limited differential, we first need to figure out how much water the child needs to attain euvolemia and eunatremia, so the best option is "B." An elevated milk sodium level has been associated with insufficient lactation, but this is not routinely evaluated. There is no rationale for option "E."

Question 10-4

Roughly what percentage of a person's body weight is accounted for by water?
A) 75% in a newborn, 65% in an adult.
B) 75% in an 8-year-old, 45% in an adult.
C) 90% in a newborn, 65% in an adult.
D) 55% in a newborn, 70% in a teenager.
E) It is too variable to accurately say, and we do not really need to know.

Discussion 10-4

The correct answer is "A." However, option "E" certainly is a tempting answer. It may not come up very often, but the number is used to calculate the free water deficit in a hypernatremic dehydrated patient in need of IV fluid, so it is a good number to keep in mind. The estimates vary by age, situation, fitness level (ie, body fat), and by your informational source, but we need to start somewhere. Let's say 60%. Here is the salient equation:

$$\text{Free water deficit} = \text{Current total body water} \times ([\text{Current plasma Na}/140] - 1)$$

There is no way to avoid some mental gymnastics in the determination of the fluid needs of a hypernatremic patient. You need to figure out how much electrolyte free water is needed to dilute the patient's sodium to the point that the serum sodium is normal, or 140 mEq/L, as in the equation. Then you give them the water they need, but in the form of an available IV fluid, without forgetting to provide their ongoing maintenance needs and to replace their ongoing losses. But first, answer the next question.

Question 10-5

Which of the following IV fluid concoctions is not isotonic?
A) Lactated Ringer solution (LR).
B) D_5W.
C) D_5 ½ NS.
D) Normal saline.
E) D_5 ¼ NS.

Discussion 10-5

The correct answer is "C." LR has an osmolality of 275 mOsm/kg, D_5W has an osmolality of 277, normal saline has an osmolality of 308 and D_5 ¼ NS has an osmolality of 354, all of which can be considered isotonic because they have an osmolality that is reasonably close to normal serum osmolality, which is 275 to 295 in a healthy, normal child. D_5 ½ NS has an osmolality of 431, which is sufficiently hypertonic that we can call it hypertonic. The upper limit of fluid osmolality acceptable for peripheral IV infusion is generally considered to be 900 mOsm/kg. For reference, standard TPN has an osmolality of over 1800, which is why TPN should not be given through a peripheral IV catheter. Now, back to our hypernatremia quagmire. Isotonic also means "no solute free water," which is a good notion to remember, given that ½ NS contains 50% solute free water, and ¼ NS contains 75% solute free water. This makes our calculations somewhat less taxing. A child with a 500 mL solute free water deficit would need 1 L of ½ NS or 750 mL of ¼ NS to replace the solute free water deficit. The initial rate should give the child half the deficit in 24 hours plus maintenance needs. Losses in addition to the usual insensitive losses, such as with a drainage tube (eg, extraventricular drain or chest tube), will need to be replaced as well. The type of fluid to be used is a matter of opinion and depends on the situation. A sensible approach is the following: D_5 ½ NS for hypernatremia associated with Na^+ and water loss such as with gastroenteritis, and D_5 ¼ NS for hypernatremia associated with free water loss alone such as with breastfeeding failure or DI. The sodium level probably should not be changed by more than 0.5 mEq/L/h. Experiments to determine the most rapid safe rate of correction are not likely to get past a well-intentioned institutional review board (IRB), so the optimal rate will probably never be known. Using a child's dehydrated weight underestimates his or her water deficit, but our calculations are estimates based on estimates, rife with opportunity for error, so calculate a starting rate then set forth and measure the child's sodium frequently. It is late and we are tired, so let's not work through an example.

> **Helpful Tip**
>
> Replacing the fluid deficit in a dehydrated child takes longer that you might think if you follow the book. For isonatremic and hyponatremic dehydration: replace half the deficit over the first 8 hours, then the remaining half over the next 16 hours. In hypernatremic dehydration: replace half the deficit over the first 24 hours, then the remaining half over the next 24 hours.

▶ CASE 11

Being the unfortunate recipient of the night shift, you accept a patient from the emergency department (ED) with the modicum of enthusiasm that you can garner at 02:15. Just adopted from a mother in a neighboring state, the patient is a male infant who is 30 days old, had a fever of 38.3°C (101°F) earlier that day at home, and was dutifully brought to the ED for evaluation. According to the ED physician, the infant appears well and has no other notable history, other than not feeding as well as the day before and having fewer wet diapers. In the ED, blood, urine, and cerebrospinal fluid (CSF) were obtained for laboratory analysis. You discuss the lab results with the ED physician, who details the CBC result: WBC 11,200/mm³, hemoglobin 15.4 g/dL, and platelet count 240,000/mm³. The differential shows 56% neutrophils and 37% lymphocytes and a smattering of other uninteresting white cells. The ED physician reports that the metabolic profile was unremarkable with the exception of mildly elevated liver enzymes. The CSF shows a WBC count of 15,000 and a red blood cell (RBC) count of 1432, and the ED physician comments that the spinal tap was not his smoothest effort. The urinalysis was unremarkable. An IV line was placed and the infant was given a dose of IV cefotaxime and a normal saline bolus, followed by IV fluid at a maintenance rate. You, apparently more aware of your hospital's febrile infant protocol, are somewhat alarmed by the elevation of the liver enzymes (AST 145 units/L, ALT 192 units/L), and you inquire about the possibility of herpes simplex virus (HSV) exposure. The biologic mother's history is not known to the adoptive parents in detail, but they were told that the mother was healthy and the delivery was an uncomplicated caesarian section. The newborn required supplemental oxygen for "several hours" but was able to leave the nursery within 2 days. No cold sores are known to have been in proximity to the infant, but you recommend adding an HSV polymerase chain reaction (PCR) test to the patient's CSF testing as well as starting the infant on a course of acyclovir. These items are accomplished and the infant later arrives on the floor in good shape. The vitals are normal, the infant is vigorous, and you are unable to locate any skin or mucosal lesions consistent with an HSV infection. After discussing your thoughts with the parents, the infant is set on medical autopilot and you head off to the call room.

Fast forward 36 hours. The infant has done well with the exception of not feeding very well. He was given acetaminophen for fever early in his stay, but he has not had a fever for about 12 hours. The blood, urine, and CSF cultures are showing no growth to date. There was a slight snafu with the spinal fluid HSV PCR, which was not set up until the day after his admission, so the result is still pending. The infant is still being given acyclovir and cefotaxime. He appears well and has essentially returned to his usual self, with the exception of suboptimal feeding. His urine output over the last 24 hours is 2.4 mL/kg/h and his weight has increased from 3.24 to 3.27 kg. Given his continued need for IV fluid and your curiosity about the value of his liver enzymes, you order a metabolic profile. Lo and behold, everything, including his liver enzymes, is normal with the exception of a BUN of 42 mg/dL and creatinine of 1.2 mg/dL. Yikes! What have you done?

Question 11-1

What is the most likely cause of the child's elevated BUN and creatinine?

A) HSV interstitial nephritis.
B) Prerenal acute kidney injury.
C) Nephrotoxic acute kidney injury.
D) Hypoxic/ischemic acute kidney injury.
E) Obstructive uropathy.

Discussion 11-1

The best answer is "C." This is a case of acute kidney injury (AKI), which is an acute loss of kidney function, in this case manifested by an acute rise in BUN and creatinine, although AKI covers the spectrum from relatively simple issues such as the one presented here all the way to the necessity for dialysis. All of the options would be good answers for the differential diagnosis list during morning report, but when a patient has received a medication known to be nephrotoxic and has no other obvious historical suggestion of an offending process, it is reasonable to point a finger at the medication. Acyclovir is just such a medication. Therefore the most reasonable answer is nephrotoxic AKI. Just for record, however, prerenal processes are the most common form of acute renal insufficiency in children, in which the kidneys are intrinsically functional. We have been told that the infant's urine output is a robust 2.4 mL/kg/h, which further helps us in our quest for medical truth. Nephrotoxic AKI usually is a nonoliguric process; normouric, we could say. Obstructive uropathy in a child most commonly manifests with a resultant urinary tract infection (UTI), which is not the case for this infant, although without sufficient testing (ie, imaging), it could not absolutely be ruled out. Rapid elevation of the creatinine and BUN, as in this case, argues strongly against an obstructive uropathy, which would more likely have a more insidious course or be found after a UTI. This, and a more obvious offending agent, should be enough to avoid further testing at this point. As for the other potential answers, HSV interstitial nephritis is uncommon and is simply not the best of the given options, and the infant's history, though not known in detail, does not heartily support a diagnosis of hypoxic/ischemic AKI, which is much more commonly seen in premature or critically ill infants and children.

Question 11-2

What should the next step in the infant's management be?

A) Fluid restriction to two thirds of the maintenance level.
B) Pester the lab for the result of the HSV PCR.
C) Lower the dose of the acyclovir.
D) Give a dose of furosemide.
E) Genetic testing to further determine susceptibility to worsening renal injury.

Discussion 11-2

The correct answer is "B." What we are getting at here is a common theme for medicine in general: removal of the offending agent. The child's AKI, as discussed, is most likely due to the acyclovir, so the question becomes: "Do we really need the medication?" Consequently, the next step in this case is to determine the necessity of the medication. Lowering the dose of the offending medication, particularly with acyclovir, is an appropriate measure if the medication is deemed essential to the care of the child and the kidneys are not catastrophically failing, but in our case the acyclovir is probably no longer necessary. Whether it was truly necessary from the beginning is a convoluted story, which is covered in another chapter of this book. In a case such as this, stopping the medication and increasing the infant's fluid intake would be appropriate. Nonsteroidal anti-inflammatory drugs are also common AKI offenders, but this little guy is younger than 6 months old so its acetaminophen for him should his fever return. Let us say that the lab has completed the study by the time you call and that it is negative, so you are able to discontinue the acyclovir. As for option "A" and fluid restriction, you are running the risk of adding a prerenal confounder to the infant's problem, so that is not a good answer. For prerenal AKI, increasing the infant's fluid intake would be appropriate. Diuretics such as furosemide may play a role in severe, oliguric renal failure but are not likely to be beneficial in this case. Genetics probably does play a role in a child's susceptibility to the development of AKI, but genetic testing to further define that susceptibility is unlikely to be of benefit here. Say, for the sake of argument, that despite an appropriate input of fluid the infant's urine output for the previous 24 hours had been 0.3 mL/kg/h, and that was the reason that you wanted to check chemistries, as well you should. Say the BUN and creatinine results were the same as previously mentioned and the infant's weight had increased to 3.4 kg (a gain of 730 g). Now it would be imprudent to increase his fluid intake, unless you would like to add pulmonary edema, hyponatremia, hypertension, or any mixture of these to the problem list. Detailed and frequent assessments of the infant's weight, blood pressure, input, output, and electrolytes, and frequent physical examinations would be in order. The most important of these is the infant's weight, which should perhaps be taken more than once a day, much to the nursing staff's chagrin. And, oh yes—you probably should get a nephrologist involved if you have gotten this far.

QUICK QUIZ

Common physiologic derangements seen in acute renal failure include all of the following EXCEPT:

A) Hyponatremia.
B) Hyperkalemia.
C) Anemia.
D) Metabolic acidosis.
E) Hypocalcemia.

Discussion

The answer we seek is "C." Anemia is the result of a decrease of renally excreted erythropoietin, which is a feature of chronic renal failure—as is osteodystrophy, while we are on the subject.

All of the other options are seen in both acute and chronic renal failure, as a result of the kidneys not doing what they normally do. If the kidneys do not or cannot excrete acid, metabolic acidosis results; if they cannot excrete water, fluid overload and hyponatremia result; and if they cannot excrete potassium? Well you get the idea. Ultimately, as we should all know, the go-to intervention for severe renal failure is dialysis.

Question 11-3

Speaking of dialysis, which of the following is NOT an indication for dialysis?

A) Serum bicarbonate persistently below 10 mEq/L.
B) Persistent azotemia.
C) Clinically significant electrolyte disturbance refractory to other management.
D) Serum creatinine in excess of 10 mg/dL.
E) Intractable fluid overload leading to, in particular, cardiac compromise.

Discussion 11-3

The correct answer is "B." Dialysis should occur when the kidneys have sufficiently demonstrated an inability to perform their usual functions to a degree that is potentially life-threatening. In keeping with that idea, persistent azotemia, that being a high BUN without symptoms, is not specifically an indication for dialysis. Though it is not difficult to state absolute indications for dialysis, in reality the decision is a bit more nuanced and frequently based on a combination of factors. Constitutional factors such as fatigue and anorexia also play a role in the initiation of dialysis, although in less of an acute sense.

BIBLIOGRAPHY

Awad S, Allison SP, Lobo DN. The history of 0.9% normal saline. *Clin Nutr.* 2008;27(2):179–188.

Brenkert TE, Estrada CM, McMorrow SP, Abramo TJ. Intravenous hypertonic saline use in the pediatric emergency department. *Pediatr Emerg Care.* 2013;29:71.

Moritz LM, Ayus JC. Disorders of water metabolism in children: Hyponatremia and hypernatremia. *Pediatr Rev.* 2002;23(11):371–380.

Moritz ML, Ayus JC. Preventing neurological complications from dysnatremias in children. *Pediat Nephrol.* 2005;20:1687–1700.

Riley AA, Arakawa Y, Worley S, Duncan BW, Fukamachi K. Circulating blood volumes: A review of measurement techniques and a meta-analysis in children. *ASAIO J.* 2010;56(3):260–264.

Sarnaik AP, Meert K, Hackbarth R, Fleischmann L. Management of hyponatremic seizures in children with hypertonic saline: A safe and effective strategy. *Crit Care Med.* 1991;19(6):758–762

Verbalis JG, Goldsmith SR, Greenberg A, et al. Diagnosis, evaluation, and treatment of hyponatremia: Expert panel recommendations. *Am J Med.* 2013;126(10 suppl 1):S1–4.

Pediatric Gastroenterology

Dina Al-Zubeidi and Elizabeth Utterson

16

▶ CASE 1

You are evaluating a child younger than 2 years of age with acute abdominal pain, fever, and peritoneal signs.

Question 1-1

Which of the following is high on your differential diagnosis list?
A) Intussusception.
B) Hirschsprung disease.
C) Henoch-Schönlein purpura (HSP).
D) Incarcerated hernia.
E) Perforated appendix.

Discussion 1-1

The correct answer is "E." All of the listed options can cause severe acute abdominal pain, but a perforated appendix causes peritoneal signs. Creating an age-appropriate differential diagnosis is the most important step in making the right diagnosis and planning the diagnostic evaluation. This avoids the "shotgun" approach. The chief complaint of abdominal pain may seem overwhelming but a few key details can help in narrowing the differential: (1) acute or chronic pain, (2) age of the patient, (3) presence or absence of fever, (4) degree of impairment, and (5) presence of peritoneal signs. Peritoneal signs of a perforated appendix include guarding and rebound tenderness. The patient often lays still and winces with the slightest movement. A good test is to inconspicuously bump the bed to see if it causes pain. Peritoneal signs are never normal or good. You must rule out an acute surgical abdomen! (See Table 16–1.)

An ultrasound is performed, which confirms the diagnosis of a ruptured appendix with abscess formation. Appendicitis usually presents with periumbilical abdominal pain that moves to the right lower quadrant in less than 24 hours.

Question 1-2

This typical presentation may be absent in all of the following EXCEPT:
A) Children younger than age 2 years.
B) Retrocecal appendix.
C) Perforated appendix.
D) Fecalith-impacted appendix.

Discussion 1-2

The correct answer is "D." Typically, an appendicitis results from obstruction of the appendiceal lumen by a fecalith. The appendix becomes inflamed, irritating the peritoneum. As the peritoneum becomes inflamed, the pain localizes to the right lower quadrant (McBurney point) with rebounding, guarding, and a positive Rovsing sign (palpating the left lower quadrant hurts the right lower quadrant). The child may have vomiting and fever. He or she will prefer to lie still. The parents may tell you that going over bumps on the car ride caused pain. Ask the child to hop; he or she will not, as it is painful. Recognizing a classic presentation is easy; it is the atypical presentations that will burn you. Less than 2% of cases of appendicitis occur in children younger than age 2; however, more than 70% of cases present with perforation. Toddlers and infants present with diffuse abdominal pain accompanied by guarding, vomiting, and diarrhea that is frequently misdiagnosed as gastroenteritis. A child with a retrocecal appendix presents with generalized abdominal pain. A positive iliopsoas sign (pain with right hip extension) is associated with retrocecal appendicitis. The rectal exam will be painful as you push on the inflamed appendix. With perforation, the pressure in the appendix is released and the abdominal pain suddenly improves for a short time period. It is a clinical diagnosis, but in equivocal or typical presentations imaging may be needed. In children, computed tomography (CT) scan has a sensitivity of greater than 90% and a specificity of 85% to 90%. Ultrasound has a sensitivity of 88% and specificity of 94%. For an ultrasound scan to be useful, the appendix must be seen, which is very operator dependent.

TABLE 16–1 DIFFERENTIAL DIAGNOSIS OF ACUTE ABDOMINAL PAIN BY AGE

Organ System	Infant	Child	Adolescent
Surgical	Appendicitis	Appendicitis	Appendicitis
	Intussusception	Intussusception	Trauma
	Malrotation with midgut volvulus	Incarcerated inguinal hernia	
	Incarcerated inguinal hernia	Trauma with perforation, hematoma	
		Omental infarction or torsion	
Gastrointestinal			Acute cholecystitis
			Gallstones
			Pancreatitis
			Hepatitis
			Inflammatory bowel disease
Renal		Hemolytic uremic syndrome	Pyelonephritis
		Kidney stone	Kidney stone
Genitourinary	Testicular torsion	Urinary tract infection	Testicular torsion
	Urinary tract infection		Urinary tract infection
Gynecologic	Ovarian torsion		Ovarian torsion
			Ectopic pregnancy
			Pelvic inflammatory disease
			Ruptured ovarian cyst
Pulmonary		Pneumonia	Pneumonia
Endocrine		Diabetic ketoacidosis	Diabetic ketoacidosis
Infectious	Gastroenteritis	Gastroenteritis	Gastroenteritis
		Colitis	Colitis
		Streptococcal pharyngitis	Psoas abscess
		Mesenteric adenitis	
Rheumatologic		Henoch-Schönlein purpura	
Hematologic/Oncologic	Malignancy	Vaso-occlusive crisis	Vaso-occlusive crisis
		Porphyria	Porphyria
		Malignancy	Malignancy
Psychiatric		Somatic or functional	Somatic or functional
			Conversion disorder

Helpful Tip

The mnemonic PANT—**P**ain, **A**norexia, **N**ausea, **T**emperature—describes the symptoms of an acute appendicitis.

► **CASE 2**

A 13-year-old African American girl presents with acute right upper quadrant pain radiating to the shoulder. She had one episode of nonbloody, nonbilious emesis and is nauseated. She has no fever or diarrhea. On exam, she is afebrile, obese, and uncomfortable. She has tenderness in the right upper quadrant. Her direct bilirubin, GGT, and transaminase levels are elevated.

Question 2-1

Of the list below, the most likely diagnosis is:

A) Gastroenteritis.
B) Choledocholithiasis.
C) Splenic rupture.
D) Pancreatitis.

Discussion 2-1

The correct answer is "B." Choledocholithiasis refers to gallstones in the common bile duct. Pain, or "biliary colic," arises when a stone temporarily obstructs the biliary tree. Children and adolescents present with right upper quadrant pain, vomiting, and sometimes jaundice. The stone should be removed surgically. Stone removal by endoscopic retrograde cholangiopancreatography (ERCP) is becoming more common.

A right upper quadrant ultrasound is performed, which shows a thickened gallbladder wall. The nurse calls you to report that your patient has a new fever of 38.5°C (101.3°F). The technician notes that when she pushed the transducer into the right upper quadrant, the patient caught her breath.

Question 2-2

What is the next step in her management?
A) ERCP.
B) Cholecystectomy.
C) Intravenous (IV) antibiotics.
D) IV opioids.
E) IV fluids.

Discussion 2-2

The correct answer is "B." The patient has acute cholecystitis, infection, and inflammation of the gallbladder, with a positive Murphy sign. Acute cholecystitis is usually associated with gallstones. Acalculous cholecystitis (no gallstones) occurs in ill patients with serious infections such as streptococcal sepsis. Both present with prolonged right upper quadrant pain that radiates to the back or right shoulder, fever, and leukocytosis. Although options "C," "D," and "E" are important, this patient needs an urgent cholecystectomy. "Biliary colic" can be seen with biliary stones and acute cholecystitis. With stones the pain typically resolves within 6 hours, but it is more persistent with acute cholecystitis. Fever, abnormal laboratory tests, peritoneal signs, or a combination of these findings, are more typical of cholecystitis.

> **Helpful Tip**
> Biliary colic from cholecystitis lasts longer and is accompanied by fever and peritoneal signs, which are not characteristic of biliary colic from cholelithiasis.

Question 2-3

What is NOT a complication of cholelithiasis/choledocholithiasis?
A) Cholangitis.
B) Pancreatitis.
C) Sepsis.
D) Gastritis.

Discussion 2-3

The correct answer is "D." Cholangitis is a bacterial infection of the gallbladder and biliary tree (intrahepatic or extrahepatic

TABLE 16–2 BILIARY TRACT DISEASE[a]

Disease	Symptoms
Cholelithiasis	Gallstones within gallbladder
	May be asymptomatic
	Biliary colic < 6 hours
Choledocholithiasis	Gallstone in common bile duct
	Jaundice
	Abnormal laboratory tests
	Urgent removal of stone
Cholecystitis	Inflammation and infection of gallbladder
	Biliary colic > 6 hours
	Fever, peritoneal signs
	Not jaundiced
	Urgent cholecystectomy
Cholangitis	Bacterial infection of gallbladder *and* biliary tree
	Fever, peritoneal signs
	Jaundiced
	Antibiotics and urgent ductal decompression

[a]Right upper quadrant pain that may radiate to the back or right shoulder is common to all.

ducts, or both) from obstruction of the bile ducts (stones, stenosis, choledochal cyst). Signs include right upper quadrant pain, fever, and jaundice. Blood cultures are frequently positive. Treatment includes IV antibiotics, IV fluids, and relief of the obstruction. (See Table 16–2.)

> **Helpful Tip**
> Consider the gallbladder lazy in hydrops of the gallbladder. It is distended and contracts poorly but is not infected, inflamed, or filled with stones. The condition is self-limited, caused by a systemic illness, and does not require removal of the gallbladder. A classic example is Kawasaki disease.

⧖ QUICK QUIZ

Which is NOT a risk for gallstones in pediatric patients?
A) Obesity.
B) Family history of gallstones.
C) Inflammatory bowel disease.
D) Sickle cell disease.
E) Parenteral nutrition.

Discussion

The correct answer is "C." In a young child who is not obese or with strong family history of choledocholithiasis, consider the underlying hematologic process (hemolytic anemias). Pigmented stones are associated with hemolysis. Cholesterol stones are common in children who are school-aged and older.

The laboratory results for your patient with acute cholecystitis keep rolling in as the afternoon ticks away. Her lipase is elevated at 300 units/L. You recognize that she also has pancreatitis.

Question 2-4

All the following are highly suggestive of acute pancreatitis in children EXCEPT:

A) Acute-onset epigastric pain with radiation to the back or left scapula.
B) Elevation of amylase and lipase more than three times the upper limit of normal.
C) Abdominal ultrasound findings of choledocholithiasis and dilated pancreatic duct with edema.
D) History of episodic suprapubic abdominal pain.

Discussion 2-4

The correct answer is "D." Diagnosis of acute pancreatitis requires at least two of the following three criteria: (1) Abdominal pain consistent with pancreatitis, (2) elevation of amylase and lipase at least three times the upper limit of normal, and (3) radiographic evidence of pancreatitis. Too bad you did not order an abdominal ultrasound at the same time as the right upper quadrant one.

You do a quick mental check to make sure you are not missing another problem. Could gallstones be the common denominator of everything? You start to formulate yet another differential diagnosis list.

Question 2-5

Which of the following is the most common cause of acute pancreatitis?

A) Viral infection.
B) Hyperlipidemia.
C) Cholelithiasis.
D) Medications.
E) Burns.

Discussion 2-5

The correct answer is "A." Viral etiologies include influenza, enterovirus, Epstein-Barr, cytomegalovirus, mumps, and varicella-zoster viruses. Remember, patients with acute pancreatitis can get really sick and develop sepsis, shock, third spacing/capillary leak, multisystem organ failure, and pleural effusions. Options "B" through "E" are also causes of acute pancreatitis. (See Table 16–3.)

> **Helpful Tip**
> Did you know that scorpion bites can cause acute pancreatitis? Now you do.

TABLE 16–3 CAUSES OF ACUTE PANCREATITIS

Anatomic	Annular pancreas
	Pancreatic divisum
Metabolic	Hypercalcemia
	Hyperlipidemia
	Hypertriglyceridemia
	Inborn errors of metabolism
Biliary tract	Cholelithiasis
	Choledocholithiasis
	Bile duct stenosis
Drug/toxin	Antiseizure medications
	Antipsychotics
	Ketogenic diet
	Alcohol
Infectious	Viral (Epstein-Barr, cytomegalovirus, enterovirus, influenza, mumps)
Autoimmune/ rheumatologic	Autoimmune disease
	Kawasaki disease
	Lupus erythematosus
	Henoch-Schönlein purpura
	Inflammatory bowel disease
Hereditary	*PRSS1*, *SPINK1*, and *CFTR* gene mutations
Other	Cystic fibrosis
	Hemolytic uremic syndrome
	Trauma
	Burns
	Idiopathic

⧗ QUICK QUIZ

True or False: Chronic pancreatis is reversible.
A) True.
B) False.

Discussion

The correct answer is "B." Acute pancreatitis is reversible. Chronic pancreatitis causes progressive, irreversible, inflammatory destruction of the pancreas, eventually leading to pancreatic insufficiency (endocrine and exocrine). Call a GI specialist. Reoccurrence is not a good sign. (See Table 16–4.)

> **Helpful Tip**
> Chronic pancreatitis may be the presenting sign of alcohol abuse in adolescents.

TABLE 16–4 CAUSES OF CHRONIC PANCREATITIS

Anatomic	Annular pancreas
	Pancreatic divisum
Metabolic	Hypercalcemia
	Hyperlipidemia
	Inborn errors of metabolism
Biliary tract	Choledocholithiasis
	Bile duct stenosis
Drug/toxin	Alcohol
	Smoking
Autoimmune/ rheumatologic	Autoimmune
	Sjögren syndrome
	Lupus erythematosus
	Inflammatory bowel disease
Hereditary	*PRSS1*, *SPINK1*, and *CFTR* gene mutations
Other	Chronic renal failure
	Cystic fibrosis
	Idiopathic

▶ CASE 3

The mother of a 3-week-old infant calls the office to report the following: Thirty minutes ago the infant started vomiting; it looks "grass green"; she cries if you touch her belly and is starting to get sleepy. You tell her to drive immediately to the emergency department: this is an emergency. You are worried about malrotation with volvulus.

Question 3-1

Most patients with malrotation present at what age?
A) After 1 year of age.
B) In the first month of life.
C) In adolescence.
D) Immediately after birth.

Discussion 3-1

The correct answer is "B." This infant has malrotation with volvulus—a surgical emergency. Rotational anomalies may become symptomatic at any age; however, more than 80% present in the first month of life, often in the first week. Risk of acute volvulus is highest in the neonatal period. In malrotation, the intestine fails to rotate in utero and fixate in the correct position. It is adhered by a narrow pedicle of mesentery, which allows the intestine to twist around itself. The cecum ends up in the right upper quadrant. The risk is volvulus, most often at midgut. This occurs when the intestine strangulates by twisting, cutting off the blood supply and blocking the flow of fecal contents and gas through the tract. Bad outcomes (perforation, infarction) ensue if it is not surgically corrected. (You may have heard the term *Ladd bands* used.

These are tissue bands that cross and obstruct the duodenum). Any infant who presents with bilious emesis is an emergency case. There is also an atypical presentation. (Are you surprised?) Intermittent twisting with pain and vomiting may occur in older children. It is frequently misdiagnosed as cyclic vomiting.

The infant arrives. She appears ill, with a distended abdomen that is tender to the touch. She is tachycardic with cool extremities. An IV is placed and she receives fluid resuscitation. You call the surgeons.

Question 3-2

The best modality for diagnosis of malrotation with midgut volvulus is:
A) Barium enema.
B) Upper gastrointestinal (UGI) series.
C) Abdominal ultrasound.
D) Upper endoscopy (esophagogastroduodenoscopy [EGD]).

Discussion 3-2

The correct answer is "B." A UGI series diagnoses malrotation without volvulus. Anytime you think volvulus, your heart rate should increase. Time is bowel. Call the surgeons. Do not wait. Look for a beak or corkscrew sign with volvulus. For malrotation, check the location of the duodenal jejunal flexure (ligament of Treitz). It will be on the right with malrotation. (See Figures 16–1 and 16–2.)

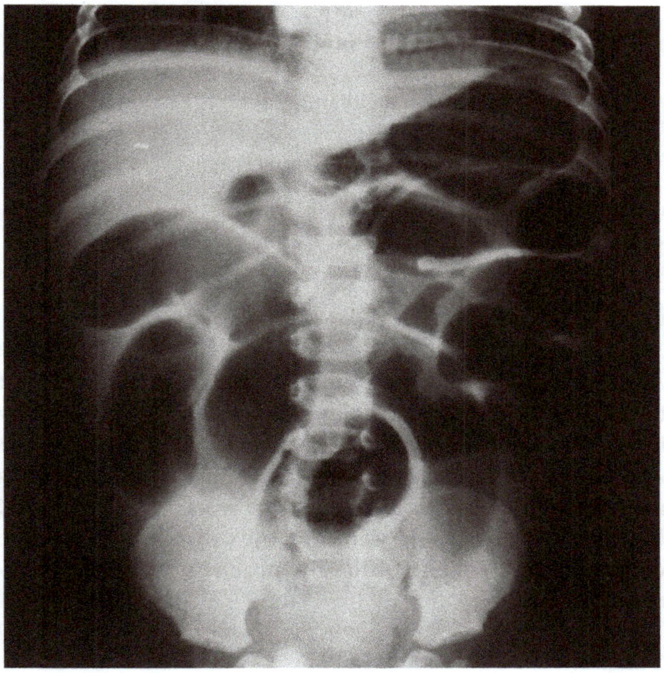

FIGURE 16–1. Malrotation. In utero the intestine fails to rotate and fixate in the correct positions, resulting in the cecum in the right upper quadrant and the third part of the duodenum and jejunum to the right of the midline. Bands of tissue (Ladd bands) adhere to the cecum, crossing the duodenum, and may cause obstruction. (Reproduced with permission from Tintinalli JE, Stapczynski JS, Ma OJ, et al: *Tintinalli's Emergency Medicine: A Comprehensive Study Guide*, 7th edition. McGraw Hill Education, Inc; 2011. Figure 124-4, Pg 843.)

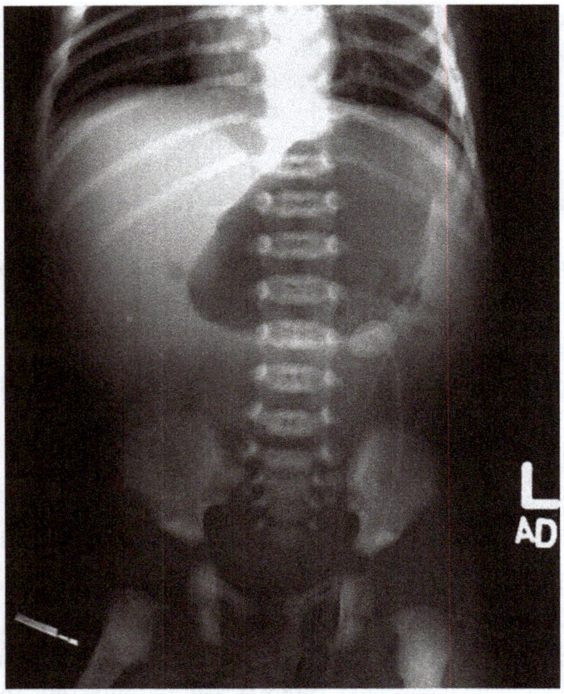

FIGURE 16–2. Volvulus. This 10-day-old infant presented with bilious emesis. Her abdominal X-ray shows a dilated proximal bowel with minimal gas past that point, consistent with volvulus. (Reproduced with permission from Brunicardi FC, Andersen DK, Billiar TR, et al, eds. *Schwartz's Principles of Surgery*. 10th ed. New York, NY: McGraw-Hill Education; 2015, Fig. 39-16.)

> **Helpful Tip**
> Bilious emesis in an infant, especially a newborn, is an emergency. If due to volvulus, emergency surgery is needed. If due to intussusception, emergent reduction with air contrast enema is needed.

▶ CASE 4

A 12-month-old boy is brought to the clinic with a chief complaint of abdominal pain. He appears to be a healthy infant. His mother reports that he had a slight cough last week. Today he has had repeated bouts during which he cries inconsolably and pulls his legs up. He has vomited twice. Between episodes he is well, but the episodes seem to be increasing in frequency. There is no history of fever, diarrhea, or rash.

Question 4-1

What is NOT a presenting sign associated with this condition?
A) Rash.
B) Vomiting.
C) Lethargy.
D) Abdominal pain.
E) Abdominal mass.

Discussion 4-1

The correct answer is "A." Intussusception causes acute intestinal obstruction in children younger than age 2 years. Telescoped bowel causes obstruction, blockage of blood flow, and eventual necrosis, perforation, and peritonitis. Most cases occur in infants (ie, before 12 months of age). There may a history of preceding viral respiratory illness or gastroenteritis. The classic presentation is colicky abdominal pain, vomiting, "sausage-shaped" abdominal mass, and hematochezia ("currant jelly" poop), although rarely does this occur. The vomiting progresses from nonbilious to bilious. Infants may present with lethargy concerning for sepsis. Sometimes intussusception is found incidentally on imaging.

Question 4-2

Most cases of intussusception involve what region?
A) Ileocecal (ileocolic).
B) Colocolic.
C) Jejunojejunal.
D) Ileoileal.
E) Ileo-ileocolic.

Discussion 4-2

The correct answer is "A." The ileocecal or ileocolic region is most commonly involved. Small bowel intussusception is less common.

....

Pretend for a moment that the patient is 7 years old. In a child of that age, you should consider a lead point causing intussusception.

Question 4-3

Which is NOT a lead point?
A) Mekel diverticulum.
B) Polyp.
C) Bowel wall hematoma.
D) Duplication cyst.
E) Meconium plug.

Discussion 4-3

The correct answer is "E." Intussusception is most commonly idiopathic. Less than 10% of cases involve a pathologic lead point. Children and infants outside the typical age range (3 months to 3 years) are more likely to have a lead point. The lead point acts to drag the bowel inside a distal segment of bowel. Tumors, vascular malformations, and lymph nodes are other lead points.

> **Helpful Tip**
> Fecal occult blood testing is positive in 75% of cases of intussusception. The currant jelly stool in intussusception is a late—and bad—finding. It indicates bowel wall ischemia and necrosis.

....

You have your diagnosis and call the interventional radiologist.

Question 4-4

In the management of intussusception all of the following statements are true EXCEPT:

A) Air (pneumatic) enema is safe and fast and uses less radiation, with a success rate of 75% to 95%.

B) Hydrostatic reduction with liquid contrast or saline has a high success rate.

C) Enema reduction is indicated in children with shock and signs of peritonitis.

D) Open surgical reduction is indicated when air/hydrostatic reduction is unsuccessful.

Discussion 4-4

The correct answer is "C." If you strongly suspect an intussusception, go for the air enema. Air reduction is safe and successful in the majority of cases. It diagnoses and treats the condition—a two-for-one deal! If unsure, consider an ultrasound, looking for the target sign or bull's eye. If bad findings are present (shock, perforation, peritonitis), do not squirt anything into the rectum. This includes air. Call the surgeon ASAP!

Question 4-5

Abdominal mass was mentioned as a sign of intussusception. It was even compared to food, as is everything in pediatrics. If the mass is not a "sausage-shaped" intussusception, what else could it be?

A) Distended bladder.

B) Testicular torsion.

C) Neuroblastoma.

D) Ovarian cyst.

E) Choledochal cyst.

Discussion 4-5

The correct answer is "B." Surprise, surprise! The differential diagnosis of abdominal masses depends on the patient's age. The big one not to miss is malignancy, which may present as a child of any age with an abdominal mass. Here is a partial list of pediatric abdominal masses: Wilms tumor, constipation, intussusception, gastric distention, hydronephrosis, cystic kidney disease, splenomegaly, hepatomegaly, distended bladder, Ewing sarcoma, rhabdomyosarcoma, neuroblastoma, ovarian cyst, ovarian torsion, enlarged uterus (pregnancy, hydrometrocolpos), choledochal cyst, and lymphoma. Just think of all the structures in the abdomen, then start running through a list of possibilities based on each structure. For example, kidney masses include Wilms tumor, multicystic dysplastic kidney, hydronephrosis, ureteropelvic junction obstruction, and so on.

⌛ QUICK QUIZ

Which condition is associated with intussusception?

A) Cystic fibrosis.

B) Henoch-Schönlein purpura.

C) Hemolytic uremic syndrome.

D) Celiac disease.

E) All of the above.

Discussion

The correct answer is "E."

⌛ QUICK QUIZ

In the management of acute intestinal obstruction all the following steps are indicated in your initial management EXCEPT:

A) Bowel decompression using a large-bore nasogastric (NG) tube.

B) Fluid resuscitation.

C) Early surgical intervention in cases of malrotation.

D) Correction of electrolyte abnormalities.

E) All of the above.

Discussion

The correct answer is "E." The management depends on the etiology. If the cause is not a surgical emergency, a trial of conservative management is reasonable in partial obstruction, including options "A," "B," and "D." In patients with malrotation, early surgical intervention (Ladd procedure) is important to prevent volvulus. Patients with volvulus need emergent surgery, fluid resuscitation, and IV antibiotics. Those with intussusception require enema reduction. You need to know what is causing the obstruction.

▶ CASE 5

A 12-year-old girl is referred to the gastroenterology clinic for evaluation of chronic abdominal pain. She cannot describe the pain and vaguely rubs the center of her abdomen when asked where it hurts. You ask her to point with one finger and she says she can't. She reports the pain as continuous and 10 out of 10. She has missed school. She denies vomiting, fever, diarrhea, or weight loss. The pain is not associated with eating and does not wake her from sleep. On exam, she appears well but claims to be in pain. She is not tachycardic. She winces in pain when you lightly palpate her abdomen but the pain is distractible. She has no oral ulcers or arthritis, and the rectal exam is normal, with no perianal skin tags or fissures. You suspect functional abdominal pain.

Question 5-1

Functional abdominal pain is typically associated with which of the following findings?

A) Involuntary weight loss.

B) Significant vomiting.

C) Nocturnal symptoms.

D) Periumbilical location.

E) Fever.

Discussion 5-1

The correct answer is "D." The symptoms of functional gastrointestinal (GI) disorders (irritable bowel syndrome, function abdominal pain, abdominal migraine) cannot be explained by an organic cause. Diagnosis of functional abdominal pain can often be made without any specific laboratory testing based on a good history and a thorough physical exam in the absence of red flags, which include abnormal exam, involuntary weight loss, significant vomiting, nocturnal symptoms, growth retardation, delayed puberty, GI blood loss, unexplained fevers, family history of inflammatory bowel disease, and consistent right upper or lower quadrant pain. Between episodes of pain the child is well. The pain is poorly defined and periumbilical or poorly localized. Ask about a family history of irritable bowel syndrome, fibromyalgia, chronic fatigue syndrome, and constipation. Patients have often undergone extensive testing. Testing only reenforces the belief that there is something wrong. Parents may have a hard time accepting that the pain is not due to a medical disorder but rather is psychologic. Remember, the pain in functional abdominal pain is real and symptoms are not created intentionally, as in malingering or factitious disorder. Avoid medicalizing patients with these complaints.

> **Helpful Tip**
> Diagnostic criteria for functional abdominal pain include (1) chronic pain, (2) no red flags, (3) normal exam, and (3) negative fecal occult blood test.

The fecal occult blood test is negative. You discuss the diagnosis and treatment.

Question 5-2

What is NOT an effective treatment for functional abdominal pain?
A) Acid-suppressive medications.
B) Education and reassurance.
C) Hypnotherapy.
D) Cognitive behavioral therapy.

Discussion 5-2

The correct answer is "A." Children need to get back to living. This does not mean they will be pain free. Step one is creating a strong relationship with the child. The current literature does not support dietary restriction of fructose or lactose, fiber supplementation, or probiotics to treat functional abdominal pain. Data support the use of cognitive behavioral therapy and hypnotherapy. There is limited evidence to support the use of medications, including selective antispasmodics, cyproheptadine, acid-blocking medications, gastric motility agents, loperamide, herbal supplements, and antibiotics, to treat functional GI disorders. Low-dose antidepressants may be useful in children with underlying psychiatric illness, such as anxiety.

TABLE 16–5 IRRITABLE BOWEL SYNDROME CRITERIA IN CHILDREN

Recurrent abdominal pain/discomfort:
- 3 days per month for the past 3 months, *and*

Two or more of the following:
- Improved with pooping
- Started after a change in pooping frequency (diarrhea, constipation)
- Started after a change in the poop's appearance

⧗ QUICK QUIZ

Currently the best clinical definition of irritable bowel syndrome (IBS) includes all the following EXCEPT:
A) Recurrent abdominal pain at least 3 days per month in the last 3 months.
B) Daily abdominal pain occurring at night.
C) Pain associated with improvement after defecation.
D) Onset of pain associated with changes in stools.

Discussion

The correct answer is "B." IBS is a clinical diagnosis. The symptoms cannot be explained by an alternative medical diagnosis such as malignancy or an inflammatory process. Definitions vary but the Rome III criteria are most often cited. (See Table 16–5.)

▶ CASE 6

A 15-year-old boy presents with a history of abdominal pain occurring twice a week for the past 6 months. The pain is more of a dull ache and it is not related to eating. The unpleasant feeling in his gut improves after he poops. He denies vomiting, fever, rash, mouth ulcers, joint symptoms, or weight loss. He is on polyethylene glycol 3350 (Miralax) for hard "poop balls." His exam and vital signs are normal.

Question 6-1

All of the following may be helpful in your management of this patient EXCEPT:
A) Serologic testing for celiac disease.
B) Hydrogen breath test (lactose, fructose, or lactulose intolerance).
C) Dietary recall/diary.
D) Colonoscopy.

Discussion 6-1

The correct answer is "D." This adolescent meets the Rome III criteria for IBS. The American College of Gastroenterology (ACG) IBS Task Force recommends that routine diagnostic testing not be performed in patients with typical symptoms of IBS. However, inflammatory bowel disease (IBD) may coexist with celiac disease, with a fourfold increase in IBS symptoms in patients with celiac disease. Lactose or fructose intolerance (or both) in IBS patients may cause IBS-like symptoms. Colonoscopy is not recommended unless alarming symptoms and signs are present.

Question 6-2

Peptic ulcer disease, often caused by *Helicobacter pylori* infection, usually presents with:

A) Abdominal pain located in the epigastric, right upper quadrant, or left upper quadrant area.
B) History of bloating and early satiety.
C) Pain worse after ingestion of a fatty meal.
D) Chronic arthralgias and back pain.
E) Mouth ulcers.

Discussion 6-2

The correct answer is "A." The two most common causes of peptic ulcer disease (PUD) are *H. pylori* infection and nonsteroidal anti-inflammatory drugs (NSAIDs). PUD is uncommon in children. Note that *H. pylori* gastritis is different from *H. pylori* PUD. The role of *H. pylori* in abdominal pain without ulcer disease is unclear. The ESPGHAN (European Society for Paediatric Gastroenterology, Hepatology and Nutrition) and the NASPGHAN (North American Society for Pediatric Gastroenterology, Hepatology and Nutrition) guidelines for *H. pylori* infection recommend that initial diagnosis be made by gastric biopsy histopathology plus a positive rapid urease test *or* positive culture. Serology is not reliable. Treatment includes a proton pump inhibitor and antibiotics. After treatment, the stool antigen test or urea breath test should be checked to ensure eradication. Each of the options listed above is consistent with a diagnosis other than *H. pylori*. Option "C" is seen with gallstones. Option "E" is seen with celiac disease and IBD. Option "D" is seen with Crohn disease. Option "B" may be seen with lactose intolerance.

▶ CASE 7

A previously healthy 14-year-old girl is complaining of daily bloating, gassiness, loose stools, and occasional nonbloody, nonbilious vomiting. There has been no recent travel or dietary changes. She has a family history of Crohn disease. Her growth, findings on physical exam, and lab results are normal.

Question 7-1

All the following steps are appropriate steps in management EXCEPT:

A) Dietary lactose restriction.
B) Endoscopy and colonoscopy.
C) Stool ova and parasite culture.
D) Gluten-free diet.

Discussion 7-1

The correct answer is "D." The differential diagnosis for her symptoms include a parasitic GI infection, such as giardiasis, and celiac disease. Dietary lactose restriction if suspicion is high for lactose intolerance can be a good initial step, and further testing with

a lactose breath hydrogen test may not be needed if the patient improves on a lactose-free diet. Clinical symptoms of lactose intolerance include diarrhea, abdominal pain, and flatulence after the ingestion of milk or milk-containing products. These symptoms have been attributed to low intestinal lactase levels (hypolactasia), which may be due to mucosal injury or, much more commonly, reduced genetic expression of the enzyme lactasephlorizin hydrolase (ie, lactase). African Americans and Asians are most frequently affected. In some Asian countries more than 95% of population is lactase deficient after 5 years of age. Empiric placement on a gluten-free diet is not indicated unless celiac serology is obtained and is abnormal, and results of small intestinal biopsies are consistent with celiac disease.

⌛ QUICK QUIZ

What is the most common cause of chronic abdominal pain in children and adolescents?

A) Functional Abdominal Pain
B) Pancreatitis
C) Celiac Disease
D) Gallstones
E) Renal Colic

Discussion

The correct answer is "A." Functional abdominal pain is the number one cause of chronic abdominal pain in children and adolescents. (See Table 16–6.)

TABLE 16-6 CAUSES OF CHRONIC ABDOMINAL PAIN

Gastrointestinal	Constipation
	Inflammatory bowel disease
	Gastritis
	Esophagitis
	Peptic ulcer disease
	Celiac disease
	Food allergy
	Lactose intolerance
	Gastroparesis
	Gallstones
	Pancreatitis
Renal	Renal colic
Genitourinary	Obstructive uropathy
Gynecologic	Endometriosis
	Dysmenorrhea
	Mittelschmerz
	Hematocolpos
Hematologic	Malignancy
Psychiatry	Somatic/functional disorder
	Conversion disorder

> **Helpful Tip**
> Visceral abdominal pain may be sensed as coming from a different location; this is called *referred pain*. For example, pain from gallbladder disease may be felt in the right shoulder and pain from pancreatic disease in the back.

▶ CASE 8

An 8-year-old girl presents to the clinic with pain in the middle of her abdomen that began last night and has gotten progressively worse. She asked not to go to the movies today with her family because it was so bad. She has had two prior episodes in the past, each lasting a few hours. Between episodes she is well. The mother denies fever, weight loss, diarrhea, nocturnal symptoms, vision changes, seizure, trauma or rash. On exam, the girl is uncomfortable. When you look in her eyes with the ophthalmoscopic, she winces and grabs her head. The disc margins are crisp. Her exam, including neurologic exam, is normal. Her laboratory tests are normal, including a complete blood count, liver function tests, electrolytes, creatinine, urinalysis, and inflammatory markers. A rapid streptococcal antigen test is negative.

Question 8-1

What is the most likely diagnosis?
A) Cyclic vomiting syndrome.
B) Functional dyspepsia.
C) Abdominal migraine.
D) Functional abdominal pain.
E) Constipation.

Discussion 8-1

The correct answer is "C." All the listed options are possible causes of recurrent, acute abdominal pain, but the most likely diagnosis is best teased out by a good history and physical exam. Options "A" through "D" fall under the umbrella of functional GI disorders. In this patient, there are no red flags present. A family history of migraines would be helpful. The diagnosis of abdominal migraines using the Rome III criteria requires (1) intermittent episodes of severe, acute periumbilical pain; (2) episodes lasting 1 hour or more; (3) weeks to months between separate episodes during which the child is well; (4) pain that interferes with activities; (5) associated anorexia, nausea, vomiting, headache, photophobia, or pallor (need two or more); (6) inability to explain the findings by another diagnosis; and (7) two or more episodes in the preceding year. Functional dyspepsia must cause persistent or recurrent pain in the upper abdomen, show none of the bowel changes seen in IBS, and not be explained by a different diagnosis.

▶ CASE 9

An 8-year-old girl has a history of stereotypical episodes of nausea and vomiting that have occurred at least six times in the past year. Vomiting lasts for 2 hours and then completely subsides, with normal health in between these severe episodes. Her parents recall having to bring their daughter to the emergency department for IV rehydration when she was younger.

Question 9-1

The diagnostic approach may include:
A) UGI series.
B) Complete metabolic panel.
C) Dietary recall.
D) Upper endoscopy.
E) All of the above.

Discussion 9-1

The correct answer is "E." The most likely diagnosis is cyclical vomiting syndrome. Cyclic vomiting syndrome is just that: abrupt recurrent episodes of repeated barfing that are short lived. Diagnosis requires three or more episodes in the prior year with vomiting-free intervals in between. A family history of migraines may be present. No single test is diagnostic. Many experts recommend a minimal workup and, if symptoms fit criteria, therapy may be initiated.

National guidelines for children and adolescents state that all of the diagnostic criteria below must be met for a diagnosis of cyclic vomiting syndrome:

- At least five attacks in any time interval, *or* a minimum of three attacks during a 6-month period
- Episodic attacks of intense nausea and vomiting lasting 1 hour to 10 days and occurring at least 1 week apart
- Stereotypical pattern and symptoms in the individual patient
- Vomiting during attacks occurs at least four times per hour for at least 1 hour
- Return to baseline health between episodes
- Not attributed to another disorder

▶ CASE 10

A 6-week-old breastfed male infant presents with nonbilious, nonbloody projectile emesis with progressive worsening and recent weight loss. He has been afebrile without diarrhea. He eats voraciously then vomits, only to want to eat again.

Question 10-1

The most likely diagnosis is:
A) Gastroesophageal reflux disease (GERD).
B) Infantile hypertrophic pyloric stenosis (IHPS).
C) Malrotation with volvulus.
D) Vascular ring.
E) Formula intolerance.

Discussion 10-1

The correct answer is "B." IHPS occurs in approximately 2 to 3.5 newborns per 1000 live births. It is more common in males than females (4:1 to 6:1) and in premature infants. It may run in families. Approximately 30% of cases occur in first-born children (approximately 1.8-fold increased risk). The etiology is unknown. Symptoms usually begin between 3 and 5 weeks of age, and very rarely occur after 12 weeks of age. Vomiting in IHPS is typically forceful and nonbilious, and tends to occur immediately after feeding. The force and timing can help to distinguish IHPS from physiologic gastroesophageal reflux, in which most episodes of vomiting are not forceful and may occur 10 minutes or more after the meal. A history of bilious vomiting does not exclude IHPS but should raise concern about more distal intestinal obstruction, such as malrotation with volvulus or Hirschsprung disease. Vascular rings typically have associated respiratory symptoms such as stridor. Option "E" is incorrect as the case clearly says the newborn is breastfed. Here's a tip if you missed that: slow down, speedy reader! IHPS is diagnosed by ultrasound and treated surgically after rehydration and correction of electrolyte abnormalities.

QUICK QUIZ

Speaking of electrolyte abnormalities, what is NOT an electrolyte derangement seen with pyloric stenosis?
A) Hypokalemia.
B) Hypochloremia.
C) Metabolic alkalosis.
E) Hyperkalemia.

Discussion

The correct answer is "D." In early cases, electrolytes may be normal.

► CASE 11

A 2-month-old male infant has effortless nonbilious, nonbloody emesis (which can on occasion be forceful), occurring 10 to 30 minutes after each meal. He has been tracking at the 15th percentile for weight and height since birth. He has been started on anti-acid therapy without any change in symptoms. He is mostly content and continues to feed well despite these episodes.

Question 11-1

The most likely diagnosis is:
A) Gastroesophageal reflux.
B) Malrotation with volvulus.
C) Pyloric stenosis.
D) Vascular ring.

Discussion 11-1

The correct answer is "A." This is a classic "happy spitter." Key clues include good growth, no cyanotic or apneic spells, no irritability, nonforceful emesis, nonbilious emesis, and a reassuring exam. Management is focused on reassurance and parental education about the natural history of gastroesophageal reflux (GER) and the difference between GER and GERD. D equals

disease. In diagnosing the latter, look for irritability, poor growth, apnea, or a combination of these findings.

Question 11-2

How should you evaluate this patient?
A) Obtain a UGI study.
B) Change formulas.
C) Order a pH probe study.
D) Start an H_2-receptor antagonist.
E) None of the above.

Discussion 11-2

The correct answer is "E." In the majority of infants, a focused history and physical examination will confirm that the reflux is uncomplicated, and little further evaluation or intervention is required. The first step in the evaluation is to determine whether the infant has any warning signs that would suggest an underlying disorder other than GER. The second step is to determine if the infant has secondary complications of the reflux, such as esophagitis, respiratory symptoms, or failure to thrive. This step is guided by whether the infant has associated problems with weight gain, feeding refusal, irritability, apnea, or gross or occult blood in the stool.

► CASE 12

A 2-month-old male infant presents to the emergency department with acute onset of bilious emesis and a history of poor feeding and abdominal distention. His last bowel movement was over 3 days ago. The most likely diagnosis is malrotation with volvulus.

Question 12-1

The best diagnostic test in this case is:
A) Abdominal ultrasound.
B) UGI series.
C) Upper endoscopy.
D) Barium enema.

Discussion 12-1

The correct answer is "B." A limited upper gastrointestinal (UGI) contrast series is the best examination to visualize the duodenum and assess for malrotation and midgut volvulus. It should be performed, whenever possible, under fluoroscopy and by an experienced pediatric radiologist. Sensitivity of a limited UGI series in infants with signs of malrotation is approximately 96%. Do you feel a sense of déjà vu?

QUICK QUIZ

Which is NOT associated with duodenal atresia?
A) Bilious emesis.
B) Polyhydramnios.
C) "Double bubble" sign.
D) Trisomy 21.
E) All of the above.

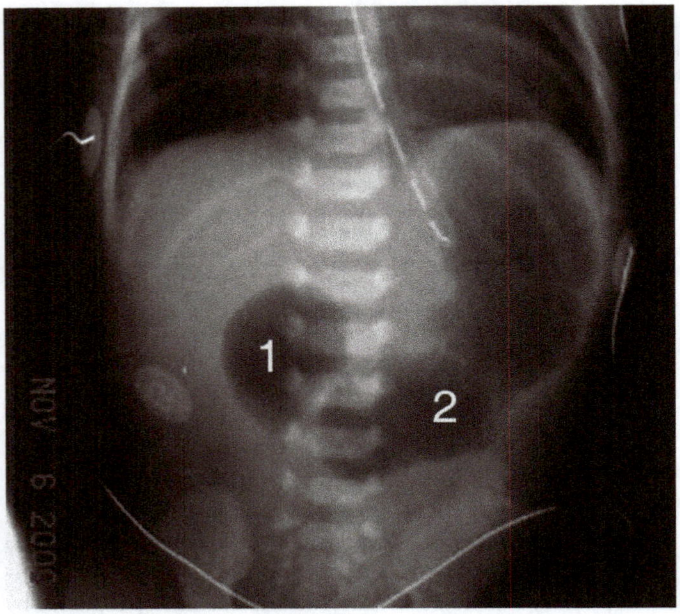

FIGURE 16–3. Double Bubble. Abdominal X-ray showing the "double bubble" sign in a newborn with duodenal atresia. Bubble 1 is the dilated proximal duodenum. Bubble 2 is the dilated stomach. Note the absence of distal bowel gas. (Reproduced with permission from Brunicardi FC, Andersen DK, Billiar TR, et al, eds. *Schwartz's Principles of Surgery.* 10th ed. New York, NY: McGraw-Hill Education; 2015, Fig. 39-13.)

Discussion

The correct answer is "E." On abdominal X-ray, the stomach and proximal duodenum are dilated ("double bubble" sign) and there is no gas distally. Approximately, 25% of infants with duodenal atresia have trisomy 21. Other anomalies including congenital heart disease may also be present. (See Figure 16–3.)

> **Helpful Tip**
>
> Signs of intestinal obstruction include abdominal distention, bilious emesis, and lack of stooling or failure to pass meconium in newborns. If you suspect obstruction, get an abdominal X-ray.

► CASE 13

A 2-year-old boy with a 2-day history of nonbilious vomiting and nonbloody diarrhea is brought to the clinic by his mother. She reports that he has thrown up 12 times in the past 24 hours and cannot keep anything down. He last peed 12 hours ago. The mother received a notice this week that another child at the daycare he attends was sick with a "stomach bug." On exam, the boy appears ill but not toxic. He is slightly tachycardic, has tears, and has normal capillary refill.

Question 13-1

Recommendations include all the following EXCEPT:
A) Start an oral rehydration solution.
B) Give ondansetron by mouth as needed.
C) Consider and IV fluid bolus if moderately dehydrated.
D) Instruct that he is to be NPO (no eating or drinking).

Discussion 13-1

The correct answer is "B." In patients with clinically significant vomiting, the use of antiemetics, particularly serotonin (5-HT$_3$) receptor antagonists such as ondansetron, has facilitated the administration of oral rehydration therapy by reducing vomiting. In children with vomiting due to gastroenteritis, only a single oral dose of ondansetron is needed to reduce vomiting, facilitate the administration of oral rehydration therapy, and reduce the need for intravenous fluids. It is a useful adjunct to oral rehydration therapy and may be used to reduce vomiting in children with gastroenteritis. Maybe slip a little ondansetron in Pedialyte? Administration of 5-HT$_3$ receptor antagonists also prevents nausea and vomiting such as occurs with chemotherapy.

⧖ QUICK QUIZ

True or False: The differential diagnosis for vomiting is short.
A) True.
B) False.

Discussion

The correct answer is "B." The American Board of Pediatrics expects you to formulate an age-appropriate differential diagnosis of vomiting. If we made a chart, it would take up at least 2 pages. Work through each case systematically. Start by determining the following (not all-inclusive): (1) bilious or nonbilious, (2) bloody or nonbloody, (3) age of patient, (4) diarrhea or no diarrhea, (5) febrile or afebrile, (6) peritoneal or nonperitoneal signs, and (7) recurrent, chronic, or acute. The presence of peritoneal signs suggests a surgical process. Bilious emesis suggests obstruction distal to the stomach. You get the rest. You need a differential to guide your workup and begin the journey toward finding the pot of gold at the end of the rainbow (a diagnosis)—or concluding that it is reflux and moving on. Remember to think about every organ system, not just the GI tract. Vomiting is a common player for all.

► CASE 14

A 13-year-old female patient presents with daily regurgitation witnessed by parents. During or after eating, swallowed food it brought back up, chewed, and reswallowed without vomiting or pain.

Question 14-1

The most likely diagnosis is:
A) GERD.
B) Rumination syndrome.

C) Malrotation.
D) Celiac disease.
E) Gastritis.

Discussion 14-1

The correct answer is "B." Rumination disorder is the recurrent effortless regurgitation of food that is rechewed and either swallowed or spit out. It is a habit that serves as self-stimulation, similar to biting nails. In patients of normal intelligence, it is voluntary but not intentional. Rumination can be habitually reversed using diaphragmatic breathing to counter the urge to regurgitate. Alongside reassurance, explanation, and habit reversal, patients are shown how to breathe using their diaphragms prior to and during the normal rumination period. A similar breathing pattern can be used to prevent normal vomiting. Breathing in this method works by physically preventing the abdominal contractions required to expel stomach contents. Regurgitation is bringing up swallowed food or secretions into the mouth not out of habit or pleasure. It is typically involuntary, except in the case of eating disorders.

▶ CASE 15

A 12-year-old boy has a history of intermittent epigastric pain and heartburn with worsening nocturnal cough. Symptoms improved but have not resolved on histamine H_2 blocker therapy.

Question 15-1

All the following are appropriate steps in management except:
A) Start a proton pump inhibitor (PPI).
B) Avoid spicy meals.
C) Avoid late meals before going to bed.
D) Start a prokinetic agent.
E) Obtain a GI specialist consult and upper endoscopy.

Discussion 15-1

The correct answer is "A." The symptoms described are classic for GERD—epigastric pain after eating, substernal burning, and nocturnal symptoms (lying flat). H_2 blocker failure is an indication for a PPI trial (step-up therapy) and referral to a gastroenterologist for further evaluation and follow up. PPIs are superior to H_2 blockers for the relief of GERD symptoms. Prokinetic therapy is not indicated in the management of simple GERD. Lifestyle modifications, including no smoking, avoidance of late-night eating, and dietary changes are reasonable to consider in addition to medications. However, some might choose a little heartburn over a diet devoid of coffee, caffeine, or chocolate.

Question 15-2

What evaluation is necessary to diagnosis GERD?
A) Endoscopy.
B) pH probe study.
C) Patient history.

D) Upper GI series.
E) All of the above.

Discussion 15-2

The correct answer is "C." In older children and adolescents, the patient history and physical exam are adequate to diagnose GERD and rule out other diagnoses. An upper GI series does not rule GERD out or in. If you were looking for a structural issue, then an upper GI would be useful. A pH probe study does not detect nonacidic reflux. It is useful to correlate reflux with symptoms. If the diagnosis of GERD is in question, the patient refractory to medical treatment, red flags are present, or you are looking for a complication then endoscopy with biopsy sampling is indicated.

> **Helpful Tip**
> Use of acid-blocking medication should be judicious as the risk of gastroenteritis and pneumonia is increased in infants and children treated with histamine H_2-receptor antagonists, proton pump inhibitors, or both.

You discuss the patient's symptoms and talk about GERD with him. You explain the treatment. Astutely, the 12-year-old asks, "What does this mean for me when I am old like you?"

Question 15-3

Which is NOT a complication of GERD?
A) Esophagitis.
B) Tonsil hypertrophy.
C) Esophageal stricture.
D) Dental erosions.

Discussion 15-3

The correct answer is "B." Patients who are neurologically impaired, obese, or have anatomic abnormalities of the upper GI tract are at risk for severe, chronic GERD. Complications include esophagitis, esophageal strictures, and Barrett esophagus (metaplastic changes in the mucosa of the esophagus).

⧗ QUICK QUIZ

Which is NOT a symptom of GERD?
A) Wheezing.
B) Dental erosions.
C) Posturing.
D) Cough.
E) All of the above.

Discussion

The correct answer is "E." GERD may present in ways other than regurgitation and heartburn. Laryngospasm, aspiration, apnea, failure to thrive, oral aversion, dysphagia, and nocturnal cough are few examples. GERD can worsen wheezing and respiratory symptoms in asthmatic patients with moderate to severe disease. Sandifer syndrome (opisthotonic posturing and arching) is a sign of reflux and may be confused with a seizure.

▶ CASE 16

A 4-year-old boy returns to clinic for follow-up of chronic nonbilious vomiting and failure to thrive. He has been treated with a PPI for the past 6 months with ongoing weight loss. He has a significant past medical and family history of mild asthma, seasonal allergies, and moderate to severe eczema.

Question 16-1

The most likely diagnosis is:
A) Eosinophilic esophagitis.
B) GERD.
C) Celiac disease.
D) Malrotation with volvulus.

Discussion 16-1

The correct answer is "A." A personal or family history of atopy, nonresponse to adequate PPI therapy, and failure to thrive are concerning for eosinophilic esophagitis. However, diagnosis is still clinicopathologic, so endoscopy with esophageal biopsy sampling is needed to confirm diagnosis before further therapy. Eosinophils are not present in the esophagus unless there is pathology. Food impaction, dysphagia, vomiting, and abdominal pain are typical signs and symptoms. Treatment includes dietary modification (removal of allergic foods), acid suppression, and topical steroids. Steroid inhalers such as fluticasone are sprayed into the mouth without a spacer and swallowed. Esophageal dilation is needed if strictures develop.

▶ CASE 17

A 5-year-old previously healthy male patient has daily watery diarrhea of 3 weeks' duration associated with intermittent abdominal pain. There is no history of vomiting, fever, or bloody stools and he has not taken antibiotics recently. His parents note that the family went on a backpacking trip, but that was 5 weeks ago. The boy is otherwise healthy, has been growing well, and has a normal appetite. His vital signs and exam are normal, including a rectal exam.

Question 17-1

Stool testing is likely to be consistent with:
A) Giardiasis.
B) *Clostridium difficile* colitis.
C) Rotavirus infection.
D) Enterotoxigenic *Escherichia coli* (ETEC).
E) Normal.

Discussion 17-1

The correct answer is "A." Presence of daily diarrhea with abdominal pain suggests an infectious etiology or inflammatory bowel disease. Rotavirus is not a cause of chronic diarrhea. ETEC causes acute bloody diarrhea, and patients appear ill. *C. difficile* colitis is possible, but without presence of blood and prior history of antibiotics exposure it is less likely than *Giardia intestinalis*. The wilderness adventure is a giveaway, as would be travel to a developing country. Giardiasis is a parasitic infection of the small intestine known to cause daycare outbreaks and infect international travelers. It is spread through water, food, and fecal-oral routes. This is why campers are advised to boil, filter, or treat fresh water when in the wilderness. Asymptomatic infection is common. Symptom development is delayed by 1 to 2 weeks. Acute infection causes diarrhea with smelly, fatty stools and abdominal cramps. Fever is uncommon. Diarrhea may last up to 1 month. Chronic infection may cause malabsorption, diarrhea and weight loss.

His ova and parasite stool microscopy is positive for *Giardia*.

Question 17-2

What is the treatment of choice?
A) Antidiarrheal medication.
B) Probiotics.
C) Amoxicillin.
D) Metronidazole.
E) Albendazole.

Discussion 17-2

The correct answer is "D." Metronidazole, tinidazole, or nitazoxanide are first-line treatment. Tinidazole is approved for children over the age of 3 and is given as a single dose. Albendazole and mebendazole are alternative options for children and have fewer side effects. Asymptomatic infection and carriers should not be treated.

> **Helpful Tip**
> Acquired lactose intolerance is common after giardiasis.

The boy's father asks about using loperamide, which he read about on the Internet. He tells you, "International travelers use it all the time."

Question 17-3

What do you recommend?
A) Loperamide
B) Diphenoxylate.
C) Morphine.
D) None of the above.

Discussion 17-3

The correct answer is "D." Antimotility agents, options "A" and "B," are not recommended for patients with acute diarrheal illnesses accompanied by fever or bloody diarrhea as the clearance of the pathogen is delayed and may cause more severe disease. These medications do not treat the infection. In infants and children, use of an antimotility agent to treat gastroenteritis increases the risk of serious adverse effects.

▶ CASE 18

A 22-month-old girl who was recently hospitalized for recurrent febrile urinary tract infection presents with a 5-day history of bloody stools. Her mother made sure she completed her 14-day course of antibiotics. Her stool testing is consistent with *C. difficile* colitis.

Question 18-1

What is the best initial treatment option?
A) Oral vancomycin.
B) Intravenous vancomycin.
C) Oral metronidazole.
D) Intravenous metronidazole.
E) Oral fidaxomicin.

Discussion 18-1

The correct answer is "C." Isn't it funny that an antibiotic-associated infection is treated with antibiotics? Oral metronidazole remains first-line treatment. Metronidazole may be repeated for the initial reoccurrence. Oral vancomycin is used for a second recurrence, and often a pulsed taper dosing regimen is utilized. Fidaxomicin is approved for patients older than 18 years. This is a reminder to prescribe antibiotics wisely, and to choose the narrowest spectrum of activity and the shortest course possible.

Question 18-2

Which of the following is true with regard to *Clostridium difficile*?
A) It primarily causes bloody diarrhea.
B) If present, it always indicates active infection.
C) Prevalence decreases with age.
D) Retesting should be done 1 week after treatment.

Discussion 18-2

The correct answer is "A." Generally retesting is recommended at least 6 weeks or more after treatment, if needed, and generally is not required. Asymptomatic colonization is present in 30% to 40% of some populations (eg, infants), and the prevalence of true infection increases with age.

▶ CASE 19

A 17-year-old boy comes to the clinic with ascending weakness in his lower extremities as well as facial muscle weakness. He had presented 2 weeks earlier with moderately severe abdominal pain and diarrhea.

Question 19-1

Which of the following was the most likely cause of his GI symptoms?
A) *Campylobacter* gastroenteritis.
B) *Clostridium difficile* colitis.
C) Ulcerative colitis.
D) Autoimmune enteropathy.

Discussion 19-1

The correct answer is "A." The patient has Guillain-Barré syndrome, acute immune-mediation polyneuropathy causing ascending paralysis. *Campylobacter jejuni* infection has been established as a trigger of Guillain-Barré syndrome. Diarrhea is self-limited and lasts for a mean of 7 days. Abdominal pain may persist after resolution of diarrhea, and weight loss of 5 kg or more may be observed. It has been estimated that in 30% to 40% of cases Guillain-Barré syndrome is attributable to *Campylobacter* infection, which typically occurs between 1 and 2 weeks before the onset of neurologic symptoms. The infection is most often acquired from preparing and eating undercooked or raw chicken. (Wash that cutting board!) Other sources include unchlorinated fresh water and raw milk—a reminder of why pasteurization of milk is a good thing. *Campylobacter* infections also may cause reactive arthritis (postinfectious).

> **Helpful Tip**
>
> *Campylobacter* and *Yersinia* infections can present with symptoms similar to appendicitis (pseudoappendicitis), with abdominal pain that occurs before the diarrhea.

▶ CASE 20

A 2-year-old boy presents with a 3-month history of diarrhea described as daily blow outs with pieces of raw vegetables visible in the bowel movement. He has as many of four bowel movements per day, with stools that become looser throughout the day. Despite these ongoing episodes of diarrhea, he is growing and thriving. His physical exam is normal, but as you watch him he guzzles 3 cups of juice in 15 minutes.

Question 20-1

The best initial step in your management is:
A) Limit excessive fluid intake.
B) Order upper endoscopy with biopsy sampling.
C) Order screening lab tests for malabsorption.
D) Perform stool studies.
E) Order sweat chloride testing.

Discussion 20-1

The correct answer is "A." The key here is a toddler with diarrhea. Functional diarrhea is defined as the painless passage of three or more large, unformed stools during waking hours for 4 weeks or more, with onset in infancy or the preschool years, and without failure to thrive or a specific definable cause. This common, benign disorder has also been termed *chronic non-specific diarrhea of childhood* or *toddler's diarrhea*. Children with functional diarrhea usually pass stools only during waking hours. Early-morning stools typically are large and semi-formed, and then stools become progressively looser as the

TABLE 16–7 DIAGNOSTIC CRITERIA FOR FUNCTIONAL DIARRHEA

Three or more large, loose, nonbloody stools per day

Painless to pass

Stools occur during the day or awake time

Present for > 1 month

Onset between the ages of 6 to 36 months

No failure to thrive or red flag symptoms

day progresses. (See Table 16–7.) In some cases, the diarrhea is associated with excessive intake of fruit juice or other osmotically active carbohydrates and improves when intake of these foods is moderated. Other than this precaution, restrictions to the diet or other interventions are neither necessary nor helpful. In particular, restriction of dietary fat may be counterproductive. Make sure no red flags are present before making this diagnosis (ie, bloody diarrhea, fever, weight loss, poor growth, etc—you get the picture). If the evaluation suggests functional diarrhea, the following dietary changes should be trialed: (1) Reduce or eliminate fruit juice or other osmotically active carbohydrates; (2) liberalize the fat content of the diet to 35% to 50% of total calories.

▶ CASE 21

A 2-month-old exclusively breastfed male infant has a history of intermittent bloody stools for 3 days. He is afebrile, gaining weight, and thriving without any other concerns. On exam, he is happy with a soft belly with good bowel sounds.

Question 21-1

You are most likely to recommend:
A) Soy-based formula.
B) Amino acid–based formula.
C) Maternal dietary dairy restriction.
D) Stool testing for *Clostridium difficile*.

Discussion 21-1

The correct answer is "C." Clinical findings of cow's milk allergy frequently appear during the first few months of life, often within days or weeks after the introduction of a cow's milk–based formula into the diet, although symptoms may also occur with exclusive breastfeeding if the mother ingests cow's milk. Signs and symptoms may include vomiting, fussiness, failure to thrive, diarrhea with or without blood, and positive fecal occult blood test. Patients with cow's milk allergy present with a wide range of immunoglobulin E (IgE)- and non–IgE-mediated clinical syndromes. Dietary elimination of suspected culprit (milk protein) is the first step in management. Formula-fed babies should be switched to a protein hydrolysate formula.

▶ CASE 22

A 3-week-old full-term healthy breastfed infant girl presents with a 3-day history of blood in the stool. She has been eating well, acting normal, and has gained weight appropriately since birth. There has been no history of fever or sick contacts. On exam, she is a well-nourished newborn with a soft abdomen. No anal fissures are seen on the external anus. There is no bruising or petechiae. You review her newborn record to verify that she received intramuscular vitamin K after birth.

Question 22-1

The initial step in management should be:
A) Stool analysis for *Clostridium difficile* infection.
B) Abdominal X-ray, with two views.
C) Complete blood count and coagulation profile.
D) Maternal dietary exclusion of cow's milk protein.

Discussion 22-1

The correct answer is "D." This is a classic scenario for a patient with allergic proctocolitis resulting from allergy or intolerance to cow's milk protein. It classically presents around 4 weeks of age with bright red blood from the rectum. The key clue is that the newborn is healthy, gaining good weight, and looks well on exam. Specialized testing—including flexible sigmoidoscopy with biopsy sampling, often done at the bedside without sedation—will confirm the diagnosis but is not necessary if the history is classic and exam is reassuring. Infants are frequently colonized with *C. difficile*, and this infant has no risk factors for infection. An abdominal X-ray would look for necrotizing enterocolitis, which can occur in term infants, but again her exam is reassuring. A CBC and coagulation studies would screen for a coagulopathy, but this infant has no other signs of bleeding or bruising and received postpartum vitamin K.

▶ CASE 23

A 5-year-old boy presents with a 6-day history of diarrhea, which has become bloody in the past 48 hours. He is admitted to the hospital, and his laboratory results reveal leukocytosis with reduced hemoglobin and platelet counts. His creatinine and blood urea nitrogen (BUN) are elevated at 0.8 mg/dL and 35 mg/dL, respectively. His urine output is decreased, and he has had severe abdominal cramps. On exam, he is tachycardic, hypertensive, and mildly pale. He is uncomfortable and has mild tenderness to palpation. Bowel sounds are present. No bruising, edema, or petechiae are noted.

Question 23-1

The most likely organism is:
A) *Yersinia*.
B) *Clostridium difficile*.
C) *Salmonella*.
D) *Escherichia coli*.

Discussion 23-1

The correct answer is "D." Acute bloody diarrhea with abdominal cramps and fever is suggestive of bacterial gastroenteritis or colitis. Pathogens include *Salmonella, Shigella, Yersinia, Campylobacter,* and *Clostridium difficile*. Bloody stools and evidence of early renal dysfunction are consistent with hemolytic uremic syndrome (HUS) associated with Shiga-toxin–producing *E. coli* (STEC) or *Shigella* infection. Most cases of HUS are caused by *E. coli* O157:H7 (STEC strain).

⏳ QUICK QUIZ

What is the most common cause of diarrhea in children worldwide?
A) *Salmonella*.
B) Norwalk virus.
C) Rotavirus.
D) Enterotoxigenic *E. coli*.

Discussion

The correct answer is "A." Rotavirus is the leading cause of severe acute gastroenteritis (vomiting and severe diarrhea) among children worldwide. Two different rotavirus vaccines are currently licensed for infants in the United States. The vaccines are RotaTeq (RV5) and Rotarix (RV1). Before being licensed, both vaccines were tested in clinical trials and shown to be safe and effective. In these studies, during approximately the first year of an infant's life, rotavirus vaccine was found to prevent 85% to 98% of rotavirus illness episodes that were severe, and to prevent 74% to 87% of all rotavirus illness episodes.

▶ CASE 24

A 5-day-old formula-fed neonate presents with severe, life-threatening diarrhea. Her diarrhea is watery and continuous. With fasting the diarrhea stops. Her stool is positive for reducing substances. On exam, the neonate is dehydrated and listless.

Question 24-1

What is the most likely cause?
A) Congenital lactase deficiency.
B) Sucrase-isomaltase deficiency.
C) Fructose malabsorption.
D) Improperly mixed formula.

Discussion 24-1

The correct answer is "A." Congenital lactase deficiency is extremely rare and manifests in newborns. Sepsis is always the number one diagnosis to rule out in an ill newborn. Let's stay on the topic of diarrhea rather than being sidetracked by the toxic newborn differential. Congenital diarrheas are rare causes of chronic diarrhea and are either secretory or osmotic

(malabsorptive). Patients present with life-threatening diarrhea in the newborn period. Osmotic diarrheas (malabsorptive) stop when fasting or the problem carbohydrate is eliminated from the diet. There are several types, including glucose-galactose malabsorption, congenital lactase deficiency, congenital sucrase-isomaltase deficiency, and enteric anendocrinosis. Both sucrase-isomaltase deficiency and fructose malabsorption manifest in infants after 3 to 6 months of life when fruit is introduced in the diet. Concentrated formula (ie, fortified) may cause an osmotic diarrhea, but it is not life-threatening and is easy to identify from the history.

▶ CASE 25

A 10-day-old female infant presents with protracted severe diarrhea for the past week. She is down 15% from birthweight. The mother is unsure when she last peed. She continues to have diarrhea even if not eating. Her albumin is 2 g/dL. Her chloride and sodium levels are normal. She has a metabolic acidosis and elevated BUN and creatinine. On exam, she is dehydrated and listless.

Question 25-1

The most likely diagnosis is:
A) Microvillus inclusion disease.
B) Congenital chloride diarrhea.
C) Autoimmune enteropathy.
D) Tufting enteropathy.
E) Enterocyte heparan sulfate deficiency.

Discussion 25-1

The correct answer is "E." All of the options are congenital secretory diarrheas. Option "E," enterocyte heparan sulfate deficiency is a type of congenital protein-losing enteropathy (PLE). The other choices do not typically involve severe enteric protein loss. PLE is a type of secretory diarrhea that leads to massive stool protein loss with subsequent hypoalbuminemia. It may be congenital or acquired. Stool alpha-1 antitrypsin is positive. Acquired causes include severe cow's milk allergy, celiac disease, inflammatory bowel disease, post–Fontan procedure (congenital heart disease surgery) with right-sided heart failure, and giardiasis. Acquired forms result from mucosal injury or increased lymphatic pressure in the gut. The molecular basis of congenital PLE is unknown. However, it has been shown that sulphated glycosaminoglycans may be important in regulating vascular and renal albumin loss. Congenital secretory diarrheas begin at birth with profuse watery diarrhea even when fasting. It may be impossible to distinguish the watery diarrhea from urine. There are several types, including congenital chloride diarrhea, congenital sodium diarrhea, microvillus inclusion disease, and tufting enteropathy. As a nongastroenterologist, knowing the details of each type of congenital diarrhea seems impractical. It is probably enough to (1) recognize that diarrhea in the newborn period may be congenital,

(2) distinguish if diarrhea is secretory or osmotic through a fasting challenge, and (3) support the newborn's hydration and nutrition status while calling your GI colleagues. In infants with profuse insensible fluid losses from diarrhea, it is important to monitor urine output. If urine cannot be distinguished from poop, you should place an indwelling urinary catheter.

⏳ QUICK QUIZ

True or False: The differential diagnosis of diarrhea is long.
A) True.
B) False.

Discussion

The correct answer is "A." Like vomiting, diarrhea raises a laundry list of possibilities. Diarrhea can be classified as secretory or malabsorptive, acute or chronic, or bloody or nonbloody. Ask about nocturnal symptoms. A simple first test is to have the child fast. Secretory diarrhea will continue despite the child being NPO and occurs at night. For malabsorptive diarrhea to continue the child needs to eat. The next simple test is a fecal occult blood test. What is the time frame—acute or chronic? Finally, is the patient a neonate, infant, toddler, child, or adolescent? Now you can start thinking about the exhaustive list of causes of diarrhea, but at least the differential has been narrowed some. (See Table 16–8.)

TABLE 16–8 CAUSES OF DIARRHEA

Category	Example
Infectious	Viral
	Bacterial
	Parasitic
Congenital	Congenital lactase deficiency
	Autoimmune enteropathy
Malabsorptive	Celiac disease
	Cystic fibrosis
	Inflammatory bowel disease
	Pancreatic insufficiency
Allergic	Cow's milk protein allergy or intolerance
Endocrine	Hyperthyroidism
	Hormone-secreting tumors
Miscellaneous	Functional diarrhea (toddler's diarrhea)
	Antibiotics
	Laxative abuse
	Constipation with encopresis

▶ CASE 26

A 4-day-old male infant presents with constipation since birth and abdominal distention in the past 24 hours. He has had no vomiting or fever. He was born at term after an uncomplicated pregnancy. There is no history of polyhydramnios.

Question 26-1

You are mostly concerned about:
A) Functional constipation.
B) Ectopic anus.
C) Spinal dysraphism.
D) Hirschsprung disease.

Discussion 26-1

The correct answer is "D." Hirschsprung disease is caused by failure of the ganglion cells to migrate to the colon. The "aganglionic" segment cannot relax to allow contents to pass normally. Consider it a functional obstruction. More than 95% of infants with Hirschsprung disease fail to pass meconium in the first 24 hours. The diagnosis is best made by rectal suction biopsy; examination shows absence of ganglion cells in the submucosa. Barium enema may still be normal but should be obtained. On rectal exam, the rectum is not dilated and empty; gas and poop may squirt out. Be aware that newborns with Hirschsprung disease may develop an acute life-threatening intestinal obstruction resulting in bilious vomiting and abdominal distention with rapid clinical deterioration.

▶ CASE 27

A 2-month-old male infant presents with fever, bloody diarrhea, and feeding intolerance. His history is notable for short-segment Hirschsprung disease status post–anorectal resection and pull-through on day of life 5.

Question 27-1

The best step in management is:
A) Administer IV antibiotics and perform gastric decompression by means of a nasogastric tube.
B) Administer IV antibiotics and perform rectal irrigation.
C) Send stool for *Clostridium difficile* testing and start an empiric course of oral metronidazole.
D) Perform flexible sigmoidoscopy with biopsy sampling.

Discussion 27-1

The correct answer is "B." Acute enterocolitis is a life-threatening emergency associated with Hirschsprung disease. Enterocolitis can be the initial presentation for a patient with Hirschsprung disease, but even after surgical resection of aganglionic bowel, patients are at risk for enterocolitis for months. Before you dismiss vomiting, fever, explosive diarrhea, abdominal pain, and distention in a patient with a history of Hirschsprung disease make sure you are not missing enterocolitis. Abdominal X-rays will show intestinal obstruction. The pathophysiology of

Hirschsprung-associated enterocolitis is not clear. Rectal irrigation with saline cleans out (decompresses) the colon, potentially making the infection less severe.

QUICK QUIZ

Which of the following is true about Hirschsprung disease?
A) It is more commonly diagnosed in females.
B) In most patients it is associated with other congenital anomalies.
C) Surgery is performed between the ages of 3 and 4 years.
D) Enterocolitis can occur before or after surgical correction.

Discussion

The correct answer is "D." Short segment Hirschsprung disease (the common form) is diagnosed more often in males. Total colonic/intestinal forms occur in females and are often familial. Surgery is rarely performed after first few months of life, unless the diagnosis was initially missed.

> **Helpful Tip**
> Most newborns should pass meconium within the first 48 hours of life. If not, consider Hirschsprung disease and obtain a rectal suction biopsy.

▶ CASE 28

A 3-month-old male infant who was born with a single umbilical artery, vertebral anomalies, radial agenesis, and a single kidney presents with a history of intermittent constipation for the past 2 months.

Question 28-1

The best next step is:
A) Daily stool softener and follow-up in 6 months.
B) Barium enema study.
C) Screening laboratory studies for hypothyroidism.
D) Surgical referral for possible anorectal malformation.

Discussion 28-1

The correct answer is "D." The presence of vertebral and limb anomalies is concerning for VACTERL association (**V**ertebral, **A**norectal, **C**ardiac, **T**racheo**E**sophageal fistula, **R**enal, **L**imb anomalies), also known as VATERR association. It is not a syndrome but rather a group of malformations that occur together. Anorectal abnormalities include imperforate anus and anal atresia. A thorough physical exam and possible surgical evaluation should be top priority. Hypothyroidism can cause constipation. Although the newborn screen has likely ruled out (> 95% likelihood) congenital hypothyroidism, checking levels of thyroid-stimulating hormone (TSH) and free thyroxine (T_4) is reasonable. Barium enema can be done at this age to assess whether the rectosigmoid index is reversed in Hirschsprung

disease or other etiologies such as small left colon are the cause. A history of delayed passage of meconium would be expected in such disorders but is absent in this case.

▶ CASE 29

A 5-year-old girl has a history of large-caliber infrequent bowel movements for 9 months, and more recently developed fecal incontinence. She has frequent streaks of poop in her underwear. Her stools are hard and have clogged the toilet several times. She has intermittent periumbilical abdominal pain. Her neurologic exam is normal, including reflexes in her lower extremities. She has no sacral dimple or hair tuft. Her abdomen is soft but slightly full. Her rectal exam is normal except for palpation of a "poop ball."

Question 29-1

The best initial management is:
A) Prescribe an osmotic daily stool softener and scheduled toilet sitting.
B) Recommend increased daily fiber and fluid intake.
C) Perform stool testing for pH and fecal fat.
D) Order an abdominal X-ray with both supine and upright views.

Discussion 29-1

The correct answer is "A." The diagnosis in this case is functional constipation with overflow fecal incontinence (encopresis). This is the most common cause of constipation and results from voluntary stool withholding with retention. The best management is a combination of stool softener (osmotic stool softener is one of the best choices) and timed toilet sitting. Testing is not usually indicated as long as the history and exam do not raise any red flag signs (ie, delayed passage of meconium, abnormal reflexes, abnormal rectal tone, sacral dimple, vomiting, fever, poor weight gain). Increasing fiber and fluid intake is a good idea; however, once chronic constipation and incontinence is established, a clean-out dose of the stool softener with scheduled timed toilet sitting is needed, followed by maintenance therapy. (See Table 16–9.)

> **Helpful Tip**
> Excessive intake of cow's milk (> 32 ounces per day) is a common cause of constipation in toddlers. Approximately 24 ounces per day is adequate to meet the body's needs.

▶ CASE 30

A 6-year-old boy with a 2-year history of constipation is currently on polyethylene glycol 3350 (Miralax) therapy daily but continues to have daily fecal incontinence.

TABLE 16–9 MEDICATIONS TO TREAT CONSTIPATION

Medication Class	Example	Mode of Action	Route
Laxatives	Senna	Irritates the smooth muscle; stimulates the intestine to contract	Oral
	Bisacodyl		Rectal
	Glycerin		
Osmotic stool softeners	Polyethylene glycol 3350 (Miralax)	Softens stool consistency by pulling fluid into stool; increases stool frequency; nonstimulant	Oral
	Lactulose		
	Magnesium hydroxide		
Lubricants	Mineral oil	Makes stool slick so it is easier to pass	Oral

Question 30-1

The most likely cause is:

A) Lack of scheduled daily toilet sitting.
B) Presacral mass.
C) Ectopic anus.
D) Nonretentive fecal soiling.

Discussion 30-1

The correct answer is "A." Stool softener use without scheduled toilet sitting (every morning and after every meal for 3 to 5 minutes, with properly supported feet) often does not correct constipation problem. Detailed history on daily toilet sitting (or lack thereof) usually gives you the diagnosis. Make sure the neurologic exam is normal, with an anal wink, and there is no sacral dimple to suggest underlying spinal cord pathology such as a tethered cord.

⧗ QUICK QUIZ

Which is NOT a cause of constipation?

A) Hypercalcemia.
B) Tethered cord.
C) Insufficient water intake.
D) Hyperthyroidism.

Discussion

The correct answer is "D." Hypothyroidism causes constipation. Constipation may be (1) functional (withhold stool)—for example, forced potty training or sexual abuse; (2) anatomic—for example, imperforate anus or anteriorly displaced anus; or (3) physiologic—for example, cystic fibrosis or spinal cord pathology.

▶ CASE 31

A newborn girl is noted to be jaundiced on the first of life. Her total bilirubin level is 15 mg/dL, with a direct bilirubin of 1 mg/dL, and the direct antiglobulin testing is positive. She is started on phototherapy.

Question 31-1

The primary source of bilirubin production is:

A) Hepatocytes.
B) Gallbladder.
C) Hemoglobin.
D) Platelets.
E) Skin.

Discussion 31-1

The correct answer is "C." Neonatal jaundice is a common occurrence and is most often nontoxic and transient. However, complications can occur if the total bilirubin level is too high or there is an elevated conjugated bilirubin level. Bilirubin is formed from the degradation of heme compounds. Heme is converted to biliverdin by heme oxygenase, and biliverdin is converted to bilirubin by biliverdin reductase in the reticuloendothelial cells of the spleen and liver. The water-insoluble unconjugated bilirubin is transported to the liver primarily bound to albumin. It is taken up by hepatocytes and conjugated by uridine diphosphoglucuronate (UDP)-glucuronosyltransferases (UGT), enzymes in the glucuronidation pathway. Conjugated bilirubin is secreted in bile by a specific transporter. In the small intestine, some of the conjugated bilirubin is hydrolyzed to unconjugated bilirubin. Most of the unconjugated bilirubin is then excreted in the stool, but some is reabsorbed into the bloodstream and returned to the liver in a process known as enterohepatic circulation. Therefore, if an infant has hemolytic anemia, the hyperbilirubinemia is more severe.

Question 31-2

In differentiating indirect from direct hyperbilirubinemia, a fractionated bilirubin analysis is necessary. When is the level of direct bilirubin abnormal?

A) When the direct bilirubin level is greater than 0.5 mg/dL or the percentage of direct bilirubin is less than 10% of the total bilirubin, or both.
B) When the direct bilirubin level is greater than 2 mg/dL or the percentage of direct bilirubin is greater than 20% of the total bilirubin, or both.

C) When the direct bilirubin level is greater than 1 mg/dL or the percentage of direct bilirubin is 5% of the total bilirubin, or both.
D) When the direct bilirubin level is greater than 1 mg/dL or the percentage of direct bilirubin is 15% of the total bilirubin, or both.

Discussion 31-2

The correct answer is "B." High total bilirubin levels often are associated with a slightly elevated direct bilirubin level—even when the problem is indirect hyperbilirubinemia. These parameters help to distinguish pathologic from nonpathologic direct bilirubin levels.

> **Helpful Tip**
> For a total bilirubin of 5 mg/dL or less, the direct component should be less than 2 mg/dL. For a total bilirubin greater than 5 mg/dL, the direct component should be less than 20% of the total.

TABLE 16–10 CAUSES OF INDIRECT HYPERBILIRUBINEMIA

Increased production	Hemolysis
	Polycythemia
	Extravasation of blood into tissues (cephalohematoma, bruising)
	Concealed hemorrhage (adrenal gland)
	Enterohepatic circulation
	Breastmilk jaundice
	Physiologic jaundice of the newborn
Decreased hepatic uptake	Medications
Decreased conjugation	Gilbert syndrome
	Crigler-Najjar syndrome
	Hypothyroidism

► CASE 32

A 14-year-old boy presents to your office with complaints of fatigue, upper respiratory symptoms, fever, and "yellow eyes." A multiplex nasal swab confirms influenza A infection. Laboratory analysis includes the following pertinent results: total bilirubin 3.5 mg/dL; direct bilirubin 0.4 mg/dL; and normal AST, ALT, albumin, PT, and glucose levels. Direct antiglobulin testing for hemolysis is negative.

Question 32-1

What is the most likely etiology of the hyperbilirubinemia?
A) Gallstone obstruction.
B) Liver failure in the setting of systemic viral infection.
C) Hemolytic anemia.
D) Gilbert syndrome.

Discussion 32-1

The correct answer is "D." Gilbert syndrome is an autosomal dominant condition characterized by mild indirect hyperbilirubinemia resulting from impaired bilirubin conjugation with otherwise normal liver function tests and absence of hemolysis. It most often presents in pubertal boys. During stress or illness, mild scleral icterus or jaundice is often observed. Children with Gilbert syndrome have a mutation in *UGT1A1*, which encodes for bilirubin-UGT. Bilirubin-UGT conjugates bilirubin into a water-soluble form excreted in bile. Gilbert syndrome is benign and is not associated with negative implications for long-term health. (See Table 16–10.)

> **Helpful Tip**
> When investigating indirect hyperbilirubinemia, order a direct antiglobulin test (DAT) to rule out hemolysis.

Suppose the 14-year-old had a total bilirubin of 3.5 mg/dL, with a direct component of 2.5 mg/dL, consistent with a direct hyperbilirubinemia. On exam he is febrile, toxic, and has right upper quadrant abdominal pain.

Question 32-2

Which diagnostic test should be ordered?
A) Right upper quadrant ultrasound.
B) Sweat chloride testing.
C) Cytomegalovirus (CMV) serology.
D) Urinalysis.
E) Prothrombin and partial thromboplastin times (PT, PTT).

Discussion 32-2

The correct answer is "A." Liver function tests, including a gamma glutamyl transferase (GGT) level and a fractionated bilirubin analysis, are the first tests ordered when evaluating a child who is jaundiced. The direct bilirubin level is the fork in the road. Indirect hyperbilirubinemia points to red blood cell hemolysis. Direct hyperbilirubinemia points toward cholestatic liver disease. Elevated transaminases (ALT, AST) indicate hepatocellular damage. Elevated alkaline phosphatase (AP) and GGT indicate cholestasis. The second round of testing depends on the individual scenario and the most likely diagnosis. In this case a right upper quadrant ultrasound will look for suspected gallbladder pathology (cholecystis, cholangitis). (See Table 16–11.)

► CASE 33

A 16-year-old previously healthy girl presents to your office with pharyngitis, fever, cervical lymphadenopathy, and fatigue. Her throat swab is negative for group A streptococcal

TABLE 16-11   CAUSES OF DIRECT HYPERBILIRUBINEMIA

Infectious	Cholangitis	Hereditary disorders of bilirubin transport	Dubin-Johnson syndrome
	Viral hepatitis		Rotor syndrome
	Cytomegalovirus	Drugs	Medications (acetaminophen, rifampin, oxacillin)
	Epstein-Barr virus		
	Herpes simplex virus		Alcohol
	Varicella-zoster virus		Parenteral nutrition
	Congenital infections	Metabolic disorders	Galactosemia
	Histoplasmosis		Tyrosinemia
	Liver abscess		Niemann-Pick disease
	Sepsis		Glycogen storage disease
	Urinary tract infection		
	Bacterial infections		Mitochondrial disorders
Immune mediated	Autoimmune hepatitis		Wilson disease
	Primary sclerosing cholangitis		Cystic fibrosis
	Primary biliary cirrhosis		Alpha-1-antitrypsin deficiency
	Graft-versus-host disease		Hemochromatosis
Extrahepatic biliary obstruction	Biliary atresia	Endocrine	Hypothyroidism
	Choledochal cyst		Hypopituitarism
	Gallstones	Other	Vascular anomalies
	Inspissated bile syndrome		Budd-Chiari syndrome
	Malignancy		Sinusoidal obstruction syndrome (veno-occlusive disease)
Intrahepatic biliary disease	Biliary atresia		
	Alagille syndrome (intrahepatic duct paucity)		Cardiac insufficiency and hypoperfusion
	Caroli disease (congenital hepatitic fibrosis)		
	Malignancy		Trisomies 21, 18

infection. Initial biochemical evaluation is remarkable for a white blood cell count of 3000/mm³ with some atypical lymphocytes, normal hemoglobin and platelet count, and mild transaminase elevation (AST 88 units/L, ALT 92 units/L). Monospot is negative.

Question 33-1

What is the most likely cause of her hepatitis?
A) Epstein-Barr virus (EBV) infection.
B) Hepatitis B infection.
C) Cytomegalovirus (CMV) infection.
D) Autoimmune hepatitis.
E) Alcohol toxicity.

Discussion 33-1

The correct answer is "D." This adolescent girl has viral hepatitis. Elevated transaminases indicate hepatocellular injury or inflammation. Her clinical presentation is most consistent with acute infectious mononucleosis caused by EBV or CMV. A teenager, pharyngitis, and reactive lymphocytosis—who cares about a negative Monospot, which can be negative early in infection (and in young children). Liver transaminases are transiently elevated in 80% of cases. You could consider sending serology testing for EBV and CMV or prescribe watchful waiting. She is healthy, not jaundiced, and with only mild elevations of her transaminases.

⏳ QUICK QUIZ

What is NOT a cause of viral hepatitis?
A) Epstein-Barr virus (EBV).
B) Herpes simplex virus (HSV).
C) Respiratory syncytial virus (RSV).
D) Varicella-zoster virus.
E) Cytomegalovirus.

Discussion

The correct answer is "C." Viral causes include EBV; CMV; hepatitis A, B, C, D and E; HSV; human herpesviruses; measles; rubella; varicella; adenovirus; and human immunodeficiency virus (HIV).

► CASE 34

A 19-year-old male adolescent presents to the student health center for evaluation of acne. On exam, you note he has hepatomegaly. You order blood work; his ALT is 95 units/L and AST 70 units/L. He is not taking any medications. He denies weight loss, vomiting, fever, odd-colored stools, or jaundice. He drinks on the weekends but no more than two to three drinks per weekend. He tests positive for hepatitis C. With additional questions, he admits to IV drug use.

Question 34-1

Which is not a cause of chronic hepatitis?
A) Alcohol abuse.
B) Hepatitis B infection.
C) Nonalcoholic fatty liver disease.
D) Infectious canine hepatitis.
E) Autoimmune hepatitis.

Discussion 34-1

The correct answer is "D." The question should have specified in humans. Consider this a reminder to read questions carefully. Chronic hepatitis is most often infectious. Initial diagnostic evaluation should focus on viral testing; if negative, workup for autoimmune and metabolic processes should occur. The history should include risk factors for hepatitis B and C and HIV infection, including sexual activity, history of transfusion, and illicit drug use. Symptoms of chronic hepatitis may be mild or absent. Chronic hepatitis of any etiology may progress, leading to the development of liver failure, cirrhosis, and possible need for liver transplant.

► CASE 35

An 18-year-old female adolescent returns from her first semester of college and presents to your office with fatigue and yellow skin and eyes. Her mother accompanies her to this visit and informs you that her daughter has been acting "paranoid" and "different than usual" since she returned home for winter break. Last night, she had epistaxis that persisted for several hours. You are concerned about synthetic liver dysfunction in this setting. On exam, her liver is enlarged and she has mild jaundice with scleral icterus. Her mental status appears compromised. You begin the process of hospital admission. You need to give report to the inpatient GI team.

Question 35-1

In addition to tests to assess liver synthetic function, you would recommend:
A) Alpha-1-antitrypsin phenotype.
B) Ophthalmology exam with slit lamp.
C) Hepatobiliary iminodiacetic acid (HIDA) scan.
D) Ceruloplasmin and 24-hour urine copper level.
E) Both B and D.

Discussion 35-1

The correct answer is "E." Wilson disease is an autosomal recessive disease with impaired copper transport. The excess copper accumulates in the liver and brain. It often manifests in the second decade of life with a primary hepatic presentation (hepatitis, jaundice, cirrhosis, liver failure). Psychiatric features can also result from the impaired biliary copper excretion, which leads to copper accumulation in the liver and other organs (brain). Ophthalmologists can confirm the presence of Kayser-Fleischer rings with slit lamp. Lifelong treatment is necessary and aimed at chelating the stored copper and thus removing it from affected organs.

Your young colleague looks at you in confusion and asks, "What liver synthetic function tests?"

Question 35-2

Which of the following tests do you tell him to order?
A) PT and PTT.
B) Sodium.
C) Hemoglobin.
D) 1,25-dihydroxyvitamin D.
E) Glucose.

Discussion 35-2

The correct answer is "A." (See Table 16–12.)

TABLE 16–12 LIVER FUNCTION TESTS

Synthetic function	Prothrombin time (PT), partial thromboplastin time (PTT); international normalized ratio (INR)
	Albumin
	Ammonia (NH_3)
Hepatocellular injury	Alanine aminotransferase (ALT) and aspartate aminotransferase (AST)
	Lactate dehydrogenase (LDH)
Cholestasis	Bilirubin—direct component
	Gamma glutamyl transferase (GGT)
	Alkaline phosphatase (AP)
	Urobilinogen

► CASE 36

A 2-month-old male infant presents with jaundice. Initial exam is remarkable for jaundice, scleral icterus, and hepatomegaly without a palpable spleen. Initial laboratory results were remarkable for AST 150 units/L, ALT 300 units/L, GGT 82 units/L, and normal PT, INR, albumin, and glucose. His total bilirubin was 6 mg/dL, with a direct bilirubin of 3.2 mg/dL. The workup was negative for infectious etiologies, and an ultrasound showed mild hepatomegaly with a homogenous liver without signs of portal hypertension or sonographic evidence of biliary obstruction. Subsequently, a HIDA scan showed good excretion of bile into the intestine.

Question 36-1

What are the next steps in the care of this patient?
A) Alpha-1-antitrypsin level and phenotype.
B) Liver biopsy.
C) Bronchoscopy.
D) Both A and B.

Discussion 36-1

The correct answer is "D." Infants with alpha-1-antitrypsin (AT) deficiency may present with liver involvement (direct hyperbilirubinemia) between 1 and 2 months of age. Older children may present with portal hypertension after a period of "unexplained" neonatal jaundice. The classic alpha-1-AT phenotype is homozygous "PiZZ"; however, we often recommend obtaining an alpha-1-AT level in addition to the phenotype to guide the diagnostic evaluation since the phenotype result may take 10 to 14 days. Although the alpha-1-AT level is an acute phase reactant, deficient levels at baseline often do not increase substantially in the setting of illness. According to the current literature, heterozygous individuals (alpha-1-AT phenotype = PiMZ) may or may not develop liver disease. Lung disease (emphysema) in alpha-1-AT deficiency typically occurs in adults. In alpha-1-AT–deficient individuals, cigarette smoking reduces mean survival by more than 20 years. The pathogenesis of alpha-1-AT deficiency involves a mutant protein (single amino acid substitution) that is trapped within cells and, thus, deficient in the blood and body fluids. The histopathology of alpha-1-AT deficiency in hepatocytes reflects the "buildup" of the mutant protein within hepatocytes. (See Figure 16–4.) Of course, certain etiologies of cholestasis in infants are time sensitive and if surgery is needed, this should be done as quickly as possible. The normal HIDA scan ruled out biliary atresia for this infant.

► CASE 37

A 1-month-old infant girl who is breastfed presents for routine well-infant evaluation and is noted to have jaundice. Her exam is normal otherwise and her growth is good. Initial laboratory evaluation is remarkable for the following: comprehensive metabolic panel with AST of 66 units/L, ALT 78 units/L, total bilirubin 7 mg/dL, and a CBC with normal white blood cell, hemoglobin, and platelet counts.

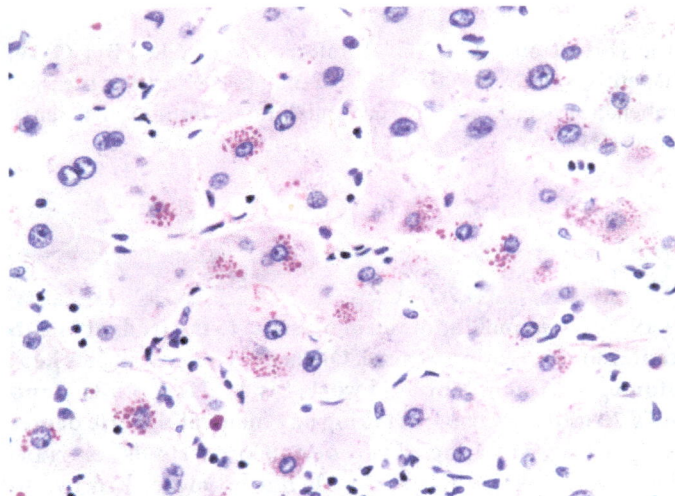

FIGURE 16–4. Alpha-1-Antitrypsin Liver Biopsy. In alpha-1-antirypsin deficiency, mutant proteins (pink globules) cannot exit the hepatocyte due to protein mutation. (Reproduced with permission From, Kasper DL, Fauci AS, Hauser SL, Longo DL Jameson JL, Loscalso J (Eds) *Harrison's Principles of Internal Medicine*, 19ed. McGraw-Hill Education, Inc., 2015. Fig 366E-19.)

Question 37-1

Which of the following blood tests would you ask the laboratory to add first in this setting?
A) EBV serologies.
B) Alpha-1-AT level.
C) Fractionated bilirubin.
D) PT and INR.
E) Albumin.

Discussion 37-1

The correct answer is "C." Breastmilk jaundice may cause prolonged neonatal jaundice but after 4 weeks you need to know if the hyperbilirubinemia is indirect or direct. Direct hyperbilirubinemia in infancy is a sign of cholestasis due to extrahepatic biliary obstruction, defects in bile synthesis, other metabolic etiologies, Alagille syndrome, and infections. (See Table 16–11, earlier.)

....

The direct bilirubin is elevated at 3 mg/dL. You are worried about biliary obstruction, especially biliary atresia. You recognize the need for an urgent evaluation as the clock is ticking if surgical intervention is needed.

Question 37-2

In the setting of extrahepatic biliary atresia, which might you see?
A) Small, atrophic, or absent gallbladder on liver ultrasound.
B) Butterfly vertebrae on X-ray.
C) Kayser-Fleischer rings on slit lamp examination.
D) Pulmonary atresia identified on echocardiogram.
E) Gallstones on liver ultrasound.

Discussion 37-2

The correct answer is "A." Extrahepatic biliary atresia is a progressive, idiopathic disorder. Patients develop biliary obstruction in the neonatal period, presenting with jaundice and acholic stools (pale, chalk, or clay colored). Parents may not notice the funny-colored poop. Fortunately stool color cards and free smartphone applications are available that can help determine whether the poop is normal colored. Another nuclear medicine study that is used to assess biliary function in this setting is a HIDA scan (to see if bile is excreted into the small intestine). Often, a liver biopsy is necessary to assess for bile duct proliferation histopathologically.

The ultrasound is consistent with extrahepatic biliary atresia. You sit down to tell the mother that her infant will need urgent surgery. She is tearful and asks when it will be done as her baby is so tiny.

Question 37-3

In the setting of extrahepatic biliary atresia, what is the optimal age for a Kasai (hepatoportoenterostomy) procedure?
A) At 6 months of age after the infant has grown and developed (to guard against surgical complications).
B) At 4 months of age, because the infant can begin to transition to solid foods after recovering from surgery.
C) At 3 months of age, because the bile ducts are better visualized.
D) Before 2 months of age to have the greatest success in obtaining bile flow.

Discussion 37-3

The correct answer is "D." With respect to the Kasai procedure, the timing of surgery correlates with outcome. In the Kasai procedure, a loop of small intestine is directly anastomosed to the liver. Infants younger than 60 days have a greater than 80% chance of reestablishing bile flow. If the Kasai procedure is performed after age 90 days, the percentage of patients successfully reestablishing bile flow drops to less than 20%. Therefore, it is very important to see infants in your office at 1 month of age for checkup. If the infant is yellow, do not ignore it.

> **Helpful Tip**
> An infant presenting with direct hyperbilirubinemia must have extrahepatic biliary obstruction—specifically, biliary atresia—ruled out as timely surgical intervention is required to save the liver.

Let's say, instead, that the same 1-month-old who presented to her well-infant check with a direct hyperbilirubinemia and elevated transaminases had different findings on ultrasound. This time, cystic dilation of the common bile duct is seen.

Question 37-4

Which is NOT a potential clinical presentation of a choledochal cyst?
A) Fetal abdominal cystic mass.
B) Indirect hyperbilirubinemia.
C) Cholangitis.
D) Direct hyperbilirubinemia.
E) Pancreatitis.

Discussion 37-4

The correct answer is "B." Choledochal cyst is congenital anomaly with cystic dilation of the biliary tree. The classic triad is abdominal pain, jaundice, and right upper quadrant mass, but presentation varies by age. The presentation in infants is similar to biliary atresia, with obstructive jaundice, acholic stools, and hepatomegaly. Children and adolescents present with abdominal pain, cholangitis, jaundice, or pancreatitis. The cyst causes obstruction of bile flow causing a *direct*, not indirect, hyperbilirubinemia.

▶ CASE 38

A 14-year-old girl presents with elevated transaminases. Over the last month, she has had fever and fatigue. She has gotten progressively weaker and can no longer lift her arms above her head. On exam, she appears to have faint purple eyeshadow on and scaling over her knuckles. She is unable to keep her leg lifted off the bed for more than 10 seconds. Her AST is 500 units/L and is ALT 250 units/L. Bilirubin, gamma glutamyl transferase (GGT), lactate dehydrogenase, albumin, alkaline phosphatase, and coagulation studies are normal.

Question 38-1

What is the cause of her elevated transaminases?
A) Myositis/rhabdomyolysis.
B) Muscular dystrophy.
C) Hemolysis.
D) Alcohol.
E) All of the above.

Discussion 38-1

The correct answer is "A." Elevated liver transaminases may originate from the liver, muscle, and red blood cells. Typically in liver pathology outside of alcohol toxicity, the ALT is greater than the AST. Extrahepatic sources should be considered when the pattern is reversed. In this case our patient has dermatomyositis. Her creatine kinase was elevated at 4000 units/L. Of note, alkaline phosphatase is also found in bone. Elevated GGT supports a liver source.

▶ CASE 39

A 13-year-old previously healthy boy faints at a basketball game and is taken to your office for evaluation. The history is remarkable for recent passage of black stools, and the exam is remarkable for pale skin and conjunctiva, and tachycardia. You suspect upper GI bleeding.

Question 39-1

Another historical element that could go with this picture is:
A) Recent pseudoephedrine (Sudafed) administration.
B) Recent ibuprofen administration.
C) Recent bismuth subsalicylate (Pepto Bismol) administration.
D) Recent diphenhydramine (Benadryl) administration.
E) Both B and C.

Discussion 39-1

The correct answer is "E." Nonsteroidal anti-inflammatory drugs (NSAIDs) are known to cause gastric ulcers. Pepto Bismol in the original (not children's) formula contains bismuth subsalicylate, which is an aspirin derivative that can also cause gastric ulcers. Bleeding originating from the upper GI tract (before the ligament of Treitz) may present as hematemesis (including coffee ground) or melena (black stools). Lower GI tract bleeding typically presents as hematochezia or bright red blood from the rectum. *Warning:* A brisk upper GI bleed may present as hematochezia if the blood travels quickly through the intestinal track. Either may cause a positive fecal occult blood test. The etiology of a GI bleed is dependent on the child's age and history, as well as the location (upper or lower). (See Table 16–13.)

You push the patient in a wheelchair to the lab for blood-work. You want the results fast and don't want him sitting in the waiting room forever. His coagulation studies and platelet count were normal. The lab is working on his blood type and cross match; hemoglobin was not normal.

TABLE 16–13 CAUSES OF UPPER AND LOWER GASTROINTESTINAL BLEEDING

Upper GI Bleeding	Lower GI Bleeding
Swallowed maternal blood	Anal fissure
Swallowed nasopharyngeal blood (epistaxis)	Malrotation with volvulus
Esophagitis	Necrotizing enterocolitis
Gastritis	Allergic proctocolitis
Peptic ulcer disease	Crohn disease
Esophageal varices	Ulcerative colitis
Crohn disease	Meckel diverticulum
Coagulopathy	Intussusception
Mallory-Weiss tear	Infectious colitis
	Intestinal polyps
	Henoch-Schönlein purpura
	Coagulopathy
	Hemorrhoids
	Lymphoid hyperplasia
	Malignancy

Question 39-2

What would you expect the hemoglobin value to be based on his clinical presentation?
A) 12 mg/dL.
B) 11.5 mg/dL.
C) 10 mg/dL.
D) 6 mg/dL.

Discussion 39-2

The correct answer is "D." Most often, there is a precipitous drop in hemoglobin when the body has not been able to compensate (ie, fainting occurs). This occurs with acute blood loss. With chronic GI blood loss, the body is able to compensate to maintain a normal blood pressure. Patients are more likely to present with fatigue and pallor rather than syncope.

> **Helpful Tip**
> Iron deficiency anemia is a sign of occult GI bleeding.

Question 39-3

You nearly faint when you read his hemoglobin value. The most appropriate next step is:
A) Emergent upper endoscopy (EGD) for likely upper GI bleed.
B) Surgery consult.
C) Hemodynamic stabilization with a large-bore IV catheter placement and fluid bolus.
D) Repeat of the lab test; it has to be a lab error.
E) Transfer to the emergency department.

Discussion 39-3

The correct answer is "C." The key to this question is the *first* step to take. Remember your ABCs—"C" is for circulation. With acute blood loss, you should resuscitate with IV fluids. Once stabilized, the patient should be transferred to the emergency department by ambulance to be transfused with packed red blood cells and have an EGD to find and fix the source of bleeding. In a patient with anemia due to chronic blood loss, go gingerly with fluid resuscitation to avoid putting the patient into heart failure. With acute hemorrhage, go for it. When a critical lab value returns, it is always good to stop and ask, is it plausible? In this case, the answer is yes.

The patient is at the emergency department receiving a blood transfusion when he is wheeled to the endoscopy suite for EGD.

Question 39-4

The most likely finding on an EGD in this setting is:
A) Nothing; the bleeding source is more distal.
B) Esophagitis.
C) Gastritis.
D) Larger gastric ulcer with visible vessel.
E) Esophageal varices.

Discussion 39-4

The correct answer is "D." Options "B" through "D" can all cause hematemesis. This patient does not have signs of portal hypertension, so varices are unlikely. Esophagitis and gastritis are more indolent conditions that do not present with acute hemorrhage. A large gastric ulcer would fit with this scenario. The visible vessel predicts a significant increased risk of rebleeding if no endoscopic intervention is performed.

Question 39-5

Which is a cause of peptic ulcer disease in adolescents?
A) Alcohol.
B) *Helicobacter pylori* infection.
C) Medications.
D) Critical illness.
E) All of the above.

Discussion 39-5

The correct answer is "E." Consider binge drinking in adolescents with gastritis. Common medications include NSAIDs and steroids. *H. pylori* infection should be considered in the absence of another risk factor such as NSAID use. The infection is treated with antibiotics.

> **Helpful Tip**
> Teenagers who swallow pills without water risk having the pill become lodged in the lower esophagus. Prolonged contact with the pill causes irritation of the mucosa, referred to as pill esophagitis. This has been reported with tetracyclines (doxycycline, minocycline), which are often prescribed for acne.

Question 39-6

After the results of the EGD are reviewed with the team, the most appropriate treatment is:
A) Discharge home with an oral proton pump inhibitor (PPI).
B) Admit the patient overnight for additional IV fluids.
C) Discharge home with sucralfate.
D) Admit for IV PPI therapy, serial monitoring of lab values, and observation for rebleeding.

Discussion 39-6

The correct answer is "D." There is always a risk of rebleeding, even after an endoscopic intervention, so the patient must be monitored closely.

⧖ QUICK QUIZ

What is not a cause of coffee ground emesis?
A) Mallory-Weis tear.
B) Esophagitis.
C) Dental trauma.
D) Epistaxis.
E) All of the above.

Discussion

The correct answer is "A." Vomited blood may be bright red or have a coffee ground appearance. Stomach acid breaks down hemoglobin, giving it a coffee-ground color. Bright red vomit indicates a brisk or acute bleeding source (eg, esophageal varices, large ulcer). Coffee ground emesis is typical of gastritis, esophagitis, or swallowed blood.

▶ CASE 40

A 2-month-old healthy term breastfed infant presents with streaks of bright red blood in an otherwise normal-appearing stool. She is happy, and her abdominal exam is benign. She has been growing well.

Question 40-1

The most likely etiology is:
A) Lymphoid hyperplasia.
B) Cow's milk protein intolerance.
C) Meckel diverticulum.
D) Intestinal polyp.
E) Intussusception.

Discussion 40-1

The correct answer is "A." Lymphoid hyperplasia is very common in infants and should resolve spontaneously without necessary interventions. Intussusception causes colicky abdominal pain, emesis, and dark maroon-colored poop (late finding). Options "C" and "D" are discussed later, in Cases 42 and 43.

Question 40-2

The best management advice for this problem is:
A) Have the breastfeeding mother remove all cow and soy protein from her diet.
B) Stop breastfeeding.
C) Reassurance without changes.
D) Prescribe PPI medication.

Discussion 40-2

The correct answer is "C." Removal of cow's milk proteins from the maternal diet has not been shown to change the course of benign lymphoid hyperplasia and may decrease maternal milk supply if her calorie intake is not sufficient in the setting of dietary elimination.

▶ CASE 41

A 5-year-old white male child presents with painless rectal bleeding. His vital signs and exam are normal. His hemoglobin is 12 mg/dL. The child drinks his bowel preparation like a champ, and a colonoscopy is performed.

Question 41-1

What is most likely to be found?
A) Juvenile polyp.
B) Lymphoid hyperplasia.

C) Severe colitis.
D) Internal anal fissure.
E) Malignancy.

Discussion 41-1

The correct answer is "A." The most common cause of painless rectal bleeding in this age group is a juvenile polyp. An intestinal polyp is a benign hamartoma that causes painless GI bleeding. The polyp may fall off with increased bleeding. Multiple intestinal polyps (> 10) with a family history of polyps is consistent with juvenile polyposis syndrome. Due to the increased risk of malignancy, coloscopies should be performed every few years in patients with this syndrome. Peutz-Jeghers syndrome is an inherited condition characterized by multiple pigmented spots on the lips and inside of the cheeks and multiple GI hamartomatous polyps. When investigating a lower GI bleed, key questions relate to whether the bleeding is (1) painless or painful, (2) bright red or tarry, and (3) stool consistency. For example, a patient with an infection may present with loose stools mixed with bright red blood and mucus associated with cramping.

⏳ QUICK QUIZ

What is NOT a cause of a positive fecal occult blood test?
A) Crohn disease.
B) Gastritis.
C) Horseradish.
D) Swallowed blood.
E) Iron supplements.

Discussion

The correct answer is "E." The question did not differentiate between false and true positive results. False-positive fecal occult blood tests may be caused by eating meat, tomatoes, fresh cherries, turnips, and horseradish. Iron supplements do not cause false-positive tests. True positives detect hidden bleeding somewhere in the digestive tract that is not visible to the human eye. The bleeding may be anywhere along the GI tract. It is commonly positive with smoldering processes such as Crohn disease, peptic ulcer disease, malignancy, and cow's milk protein intolerance. Current iron deficiency anemia from chronic GI blood loss is common.

▶ CASE 42

A 13-year-old boy presents with rapid red blood per rectum that is painless. His hemoglobin is 5 mg/dL. An IV line is placed and he is given fluids and transfused with packed red blood cells.

Question 42-1

The next best step in investigating the source of bleeding is:
A) Colonoscopy to diagnosis and treat the bleeding source.
B) Upper endoscopy (EGD) since the rapid bleeding must be gastric in origin.
C) Meckel scan.
D) Liver biopsy.

Discussion 42-1

The correct answer is "C." A Meckel diverticulum often contains gastric mucosa, which secretes acid and can cause an ulceration of the adjacent ileal mucosa, resulting in significant bleeding. The bleeding is often brisk (therefore, it may be bright red in color despite the source being proximal to the colon) and painless. Remember the Rule of 2s: affects 2% of the population, males 2 times more likely than females, 2 inches long, 2 feet from the ileocecal valve, and contains 2 types of tissue (gastric and intestinal).

> **Helpful Tip**
> Intussusception and Meckel diverticulum may present with dark maroon-colored stool described as "currant jelly."

▶ CASE 43

A 2-year-old boy passed a bowel movement in his diaper with some bright red blood mixed within the soft stool substance. He did not cry or display discomfort during or after defecation. When wiping him, you see a small mass protruding from the left side of the anal orifice. This spontaneously reduces into the rectum when you try to examine it further. The family history is negative for polyposis syndromes.

Question 43-1

The most likely cause of this finding is:
A) Vascular malformation.
B) Juvenile polyp.
C) Rectal prolapse.
D) Both B and C.

Discussion 43-1

The correct answer is "B." Painless rectal bleeding in a 2-year-old is most commonly due to a solitary rectal juvenile polyp. A rectal prolapse is characterized by the protrusion of concentric rings of rectal mucosa and is not typically described as unilateral in position. A rectal prolapse can be easily reduced and is most common in infants. Finding the underlying cause of prolapse is important. Rectal prolapse may occur in patients with cystic fibrosis, constipation, pertussis (increased abdominal pressure with coughing), and infectious enteritis. Often, a picture of the finding helps to distinguish between the two entities.

After confirmation of your clinical suspicion (both endoscopically and histologically) and removal of the polyp, this child will need to return to the GI clinic:

Question 43-2

A) Only if rectal bleeding recurs and persists.
B) Annually.
C) In 6 months.
D) In 1 month, when you will recheck his hemoglobin.

Discussion 43-2

The correct answer is "A." Solitary juvenile polyps are benign and do not warrant further follow-up.

▶ CASE 44

A 13-year-old girl presents to your clinic with new-onset hematochezia for 1 week. She is currently passing two soft, formed stools per day, each with blood mixed throughout the stool substance. Her history is otherwise unremarkable. Her family history is remarkable for fatal colon cancer in her paternal grandfather at 38 years, colon cancer in her father at age 26 years (treated with chemotherapy and colectomy), and colon cancer in her 19-year-old brother, who is currently undergoing chemotherapy after colectomy. Her exam is normal, without evidence of tachycardia or other signs of significant anemia.

Question 44-1

You recommend colonoscopy to better define the source of bleeding and find the following endoscopically:

A) A single mass in the rectum that has polypoid features.
B) Gardens of small, sessile polyps throughout the colon.
C) Nothing in the colon; the bleeding must be more proximal.
D) Endoscopic features of chronic colitis.

Discussion 44-1

The correct answer is "B." The most likely etiology is familial adenomatous polyposis (FAP) due to the significant colon cancer affecting family members at very young ages. FAP is an autosomal dominant condition that causes hundreds to thousands of colon polyps and eventual colon cancer if untreated. It is due to a mutation in a tumor suppressor gene (APC, adenomatous polyposis coli).

Question 44-2

After the results of the colonoscopy are reviewed (including histopathology of the biopsy samples obtained during the procedure), you recommend the following:

A. Watchful monitoring with serial hemoglobin measurements.
B. Surgical consultation for colectomy.
C. Chemotherapy.
D. Radiation therapy.

Discussion 44-2

The correct answer is "B." The treatment for FAP is colectomy in an attempt to avoid colon cancer.

▶ CASE 45

A 3-year-old boy presents for a well-child check-up with a distended liver edge palpable 4 cm below the right costal margin. The history is remarkable for recent increases in soft abdominal girth without other problems. He is growing and developing normally. His parents have not witnessed any excessive bleeding or bruising.

Question 45-1

The next step in evaluation should include:

A) Laboratory testing, including complete liver function panel, serum glucose, and CBC.
B) Abdominal ultrasound.
C) Abdominal ultrasound and the following laboratory tests: AST, ALT and albumin.
D) Abdominal ultrasound and the following laboratory tests: complete liver hepatic function panel, serum glucose, PT, INR, and CBC.

Discussion 45-1

The correct answer is "D." In this setting, sonographic evidence is necessary as is confirmation of normal liver synthetic function. PT, INR, albumin, and ammonia are markers of synthetic function. Altered synthetic function indicates liver failure. Hepatomegaly is never normal and results from congestion, hepatitis, or a tumor. It may be part of a viral illness or represent malignancy. It is important to take a careful history and perform a thorough exam looking for signs of portal hypertension and splenomegaly. Portal hypertension results from obstruction of portal blood flow and is most often caused by cirrhosis. It most commonly presents as esophageal variceal bleeding. Splenomegaly may be caused by a liver process (cirrhosis, portal, or hepatic vein thrombosis) or a manifestation of the same systemic process (viral infection, malignancy). The history and physical exam will guide your workup. For example, hepatosplenomegaly in a girl with classic infectious mononucleosis does not require additional evaluation. Incidental hepatomegaly, as described in this patient, is a different story.

The abdominal ultrasound shows a mass in the liver. Which of the following etiologies is less likely in this setting?

Question 45-2

A) Hepatoblastoma.
B) Fibroadenoma.
C) Hemangioma.

Discussion 45-2

The correct answer is "B." Fibroadenoma occurs in females in their 20s and 30s, especially in those patients taking oral contraceptive pills. Liver hemangiomas are associated with multiple skin hemangiomas and may be asymptomatic. Infants with a large liver hemangioma may develop high output heart failure. Hepatoblastoma is malignant tumor of the liver primarily affecting children younger than 2 years of age. Children with Beckwith-Wiedemann syndrome, trisomy 21, and familial adenomatous polyposis are at increased risk for developing hepatoblastoma.

The liver mass takes up more than 75% of the liver itself. A biopsy of the mass confirms a neoplastic process.

Question 45-3

Which is the best treatment option in this setting?
A) Liver transplant and subsequent chemotherapy.
B) Chemotherapy.
C) Radiation.
D) Watchful monitoring.

Discussion 45-3

The correct answer is "A." The child has a hepatoblastoma. He is the right age, and most often children present with abdominal distention, as he did. Complete resection is the mainstay of treatment. In this setting, a liver transplant will be necessary due to the large size of the mass.

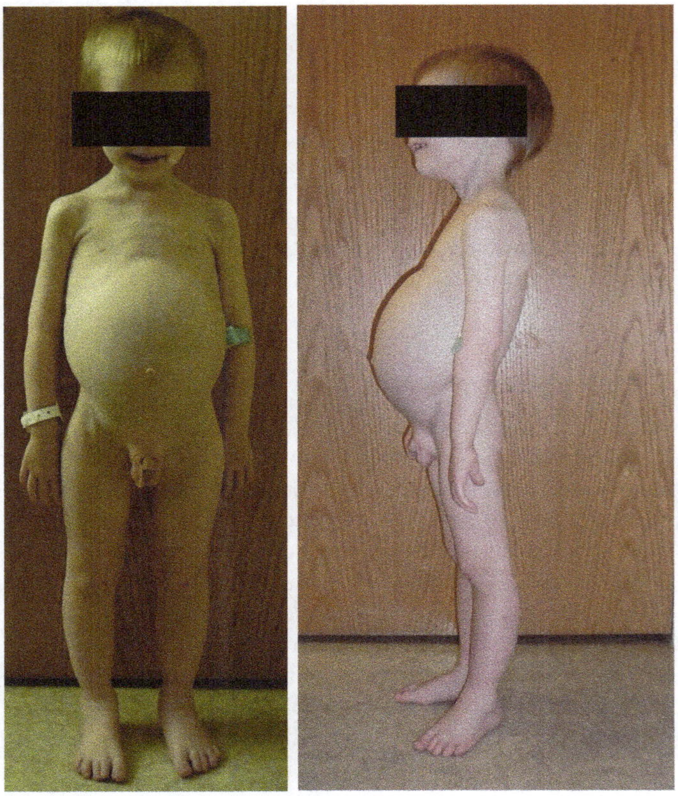

▶ CASE 46

A 2-year-old girl presents to your clinic with diarrhea of 6 weeks' duration, a distended abdomen, and weight loss. When fasting, the diarrhea resolves. You are concerned about malabsorption in this setting.

Question 46-1

Which is NOT an initial diagnostic stool test to obtain?
A) Stool cultures.
B) Microscopy for ova and parasites.
C) Fecal occult blood test.
D) Rotavirus stool antigen.
E) Stool alpha-1-antitrypsin.

Discussion 46-1

The correct answer is "D." The pooping stops with fasting, so think malabsorption. Malabsorption results from either (1) failure to absorb nutrients (ie, problem with the intestinal mucosa) or (2) failure to digest the nutrients for absorption (ie, problem with pancreatic function). Malabsorption can be general (multiple nutrients) or selective (isolated fat, protein, carbohydrates, vitamins). Symptoms include diarrhea, abdominal distention, and poor weight gain. Signs include muscle wasting (toothpick extremities, flat buttocks) and loose skin for loss of underlying fat. In older children, stunting may occur. Edema suggests protein-losing enteropathy (PLE). Bloating suggests carbohydrate malabsorption. Greasy, fatty stools suggest fat malabsorption. (See Figure 16–5.) Bacterial etiologies are less likely in the setting of chronic diarrhea without other features (bloody diarrhea, cramping). Infectious diarrhea is typically secretory, with the exception of chronic diarrhea from *Giardia*. Chronic giardiasis can cause severe malabsorptive diarrhea with significant weight loss, so parasite testing (O&P) is a must. Stool cultures and parasite testing should make the first round of testing. Tests of nutrient malabsorption are also in the first

A   **B**

FIGURE 16–5. Celiac Disease (Anterior and Profile). This young boy has celiac disease with significant protein energy malnutrition. He shows the classic appearance of abdominal distention, hanging skinfolds, loss of subcutaneous fat, and muscle wasting (thin arms and legs, flat buttocks). (Used with permission from Eyad M. Hanna, MD, University of Iowa.)

round of testing and include fecal alpha-1-antitrypsin to test for protein malabsorption, stool-reducing substances for carbohydrate malabsorption, fecal fat for fat malabsorption, and fecal elastase to assess pancreatic exocrine function. A low level of fecal elastase means the pancreas is out of gas. Malabsorption in cystic fibrosis is due to pancreatic insufficiency, so fecal elastase would be low in this patient population.

> **Helpful Tip**
>
> Any time you are asked about a diagnostic workup, always start with a thorough history and physical exam. When done well, these will point you toward the right diagnosis which guides the diagnostic workup.

Question 46-2

The appropriate blood tests to order for this patient should include the following:
A) CBC.
B) Peripheral smear.
C) Tissue transglutaminase antibody and total IgA.
D) Peripheral blood smear.
E) All of the above.

Discussion 46-2

The correct answer is "E." A CBC with differential will detect anemia, neutropenia (Shwachman-Diamond syndrome), and lymphopenia (lymphatic issues, severe combined immunodeficiency). Option "C" screens for celiac disease (gluten-sensitive enteropathy). To recap, the initial diagnostic testing for malabsorption should include:

- Bacterial stool cultures
- Microscopy for ova and parasites
- Fecal occult blood test
- Stool leukocytes: marker of inflammatory process
- Stool alpha-1-antitrypsin: protein malabsorption
- Fecal fat: fat malabsorption (duh!)
- Stool-reducing substances and pH: carbohydrate malabsorption
- Stool elastase: pancreatic exocrine function
- CBC with differential
- Peripheral blood smear
- Tissue transglutaminase (TTG)-IgA antibody level and total IgA: screen for celiac disease
- Comprehensive metabolic panel
- Vitamin D (25-hydroxyvitamin D)

This list is not set in stone but rather a framework to work from. Once you get the results, you can determine your next steps.

The child's TTG-IgA level is greater than 100 units, which is strongly positive.

Question 46-3

The next step in management should include:
A) Colonoscopy.
B) Bone marrow biopsy.
C) Abdominal ultrasound.
D) Upper endoscopy with duodenal biopsy.
E) Trial of a gluten-free diet.

Discussion 46-3

The correct answer is "D." This child's TTG-IgA antibody level needs to be confirmed by biopsy. Celiac disease is an immune-mediated sensitivity to gluten. The mucosa of the small bowel villi is damaged, leading to malabsorption. TTP-IgA antibody level is one of the best screening tools for celiac disease. However, its use is complicated by the fact that it is an IgA antibody, and there is a significant percentage of the population for whom IgA deficiency is a reality. Therefore, assessment of the total IgA level is often obtained in conjunction with the TTG-IgA level. Celiac disease is unlikely if TTG-IgA antibody testing is negative with a normal total IgA level but it is not ruled out completely as testing can be falsely negative. The TTG-IgG antibody test is also utilized, especially in the setting of a low total IgA level; however, it is less specific and sensitive overall. The gold standard for the diagnosis of celiac disease continues to be histopathologic assessment of the duodenal mucosa.

Helpful Tip

IgA anti-TTG antibody is the preferred screening test for celiac disease in children over the age of 2 years.

Endoscopy is performed, and multiple biopsies of the duodenum are obtained for the pathologist to review.

Question 46-4

The most likely histopathologic features found by the pathologist include:
A) Goblet cells.
B) Mastocytes and atypical white blood cells.
C) Blunting of the villi with intraepithelial lymphocytes.
D) Melanocytes.
E) Granulomas.

Discussion 46-4

The correct answer is "C." This is the typical histopathologic picture of celiac disease. Duodenal villous atrophy can be seen with small bowel bacterial overgrowth, Crohn disease, eosinophilic enteritis, giardiasis, and malnutrition. This is why diagnosis requires more than one element—signs and symptoms, serology, and biopsy.

Question 46-5

When the child returns for follow-up and review of the test results to date, you recommend the following treatments:
A) Chemotherapy.
B) Gluten-free diet.
C) Soy-free diet.
D) Stopping all laxatives.
E) Metronidazole.

Discussion 46-5

The correct answer is "B." Dietary elimination of gluten (ie, a protein found in wheat, barley, and rye) is the treatment for celiac disease. The treatment is lifelong and needs to be followed strictly in an attempt to avoid complications of celiac disease, which are most often caused by chronic malabsorption of vital nutrients.

The mother forgot to mention that she has celiac disease. She remarks, "Oops, was that an important detail?" You politely ask how she did not remember to bring this up earlier.

Question 46-6

Which of the following conditions places patients at an increased risk for celiac disease?
A) Trisomy 21.
B) Type 1 diabetes mellitus.
C) Autoimmune thyroiditis.
D) IgA deficiency.
E) All of the above.

Discussion 46-6

The correct answer is "E." Children and adolescents with an affected first-degree relative, Williams syndrome, Turner syndrome, alopecia areata, type 1 diabetes mellitus, autoimmune hepatitis, autoimmune thyroiditis, and Addison disease are at increased risk for celiac disease. Do you see an autoimmune theme?

> **Helpful Tip**
> Celiac likes friends and is frequently found in patients with other autoimmune diseases such as type 1 diabetes mellitus or autoimmune thyroiditis.

QUICK QUIZ

What is NOT a symptom of celiac disease?
A) Diarrhea.
B) Weight gain.
C) Vomiting.
D) Abdominal distention.
E) Mouth ulcers.

Discussion

The correct answer is "B." Okay, that was too easy. Celiac disease can manifest with the typical features of malabsorption but it has a few tricks as well. Constipation, intussusception, rectal prolapse, mouth ulcers, discolored teeth or enamel, dermatitis herpetiformis (weird rash), peripheral neuropathy, and short stature are also manifestations of celiac disease.

> **Helpful Tip**
> Iron deficiency anemia unresponsive to iron therapy is a manifestation of celiac disease.

▶ CASE 47

A 13-year-old boy who has a history of short bowel syndrome resulting from gastroschisis presents for follow-up with a 2-week history of increased stool frequency including passage of loose stools and abundant malodorous gas.

Question 47-1

The best breath test to choose for assessment of the current problem is:
A) Sucrose.
B) Fructose.
C) Lactulose.
D) Urea.

Discussion 47-1

The correct answer is "C." Small intestinal bacterial overgrowth (SIBO) causes inflammation, fermentation (makes a lot of gas), and polynutrient malabsorption and maldigestion. It may be associated with short gut. The lactulose breath test and d-xylose

test may be used to diagnosis SIBO although they are not perfect. Jejunal aspirate cultures are more sensitive and specific. Lactulose is a sugar that is not absorbed. The excess bacteria in the small intestine should produce a "double peak" phenomena on a breath test, showing an initial peak due to baseline fermentation by the bacteria in the small intestine and a second peak when the lactulose reaches the bacteria who happily reside in the large intestine, releasing more methane as they feast on the unabsorbed sugar. The hydrogen or methane gas is absorbed, excreted in the lungs, and measured in the breath. This fermentation will translate into increased gut motility with associated diarrhea and increased malodorous intestinal gas. The [14C]-d-xylose test is another way to check for SIBO that uses xylose, a sugar metabolized by gram-negative anaerobic bacteria, and urine instead of breath.

Question 47-2

Treatment of SIBO in this case would most often be accomplished with which of the following?
A) Oral antibiotics.
B) Laxatives.
C) Change in diet.
D) IV antibiotics.

Discussion 47-2

The correct answer is "A." Flagyl, neomycin, and rifaximin are popular antibiotics to give orally for bacterial overgrowth.

Question 47-3

Carbohydrate malabsorption is assessed by which of the following methods?
A) d-Xylose test.
B) Lactose breath hydrogen test.
C) Fructose breath hydrogen test.
D) All of the above.

Discussion 47-3

The correct answer is "D." All of these tests assess for carbohydrate malabsorption and thus intolerance. The history is often helpful in selecting which sugar to test. The subject fasts overnight then is fed the assumed "problem" carbohydrate (lactose, sucrose, fructose, glucose). In malabsorption, the sugar is not absorbed and passes to the large intestine, where the bacteria feast upon it producing hydrogen gas. Hydrogen gas is absorbed into the bloodstream and then sent out of the body through the lungs. Increased hydrogen gas in a breath suggests carbohydrate malabsorption. If testing for SIBO, the d-xylose test or lactulose breath test is used, which you just read about in Question 43-1.

> **Helpful Tip**
> If you can neither digest nor absorb carbohydrates, your colonic flora will produce gas when you eat carbohydrate-containing foods causing bloating and flatulence. Neither is beneficial to a romantic relationship.

CASE 48

A 3-month-old infant girl who was born at full term has failed to gain weight appropriately despite formula fortification of breast milk. She is taking 6 ounces of fortified breast milk every 3 hours and does not have any feeding difficulties, tachypnea while eating, or perioral cyanosis. Her length and fronto-occipital circumference are also challenged but are following curves under the standard growth curve. She is admitted to the hospital for observation and additional evaluation.

Question 48-1

Tests done during her hospital stay should include:
A) Colonoscopy.
B) Bone marrow biopsy.
C) Sweat test.
D) Bone mineral density analysis.
E) Echocardiogram.

Discussion 48-1

The correct answer is "C." Even if the newborn screen was normal, a sweat test should be done if there is clinical suspicion for cystic fibrosis. The other tests are either not applicable or should not be done as "first-line" analysis. Cystic fibrosis may cause pancreatic exocrine insufficiency resulting in fat malabsorption. Pancreatic enzymes are needed to metabolize and absorb fat. Signs and symptoms of cystic fibrosis include failure to thrive, poor weight gain, and steatorrhea—big, greasy, fatty stools. Treatment is pancreatic enzyme replacement therapy. (Don't forget about your fat-soluble vitamins!)

QUICK QUIZ

Which is NOT a cause of fat malabsorption?
A) Shwachman-Diamond syndrome.
B) Lymphangiectasis.
C) Lipase deficiency.
D) Amylase deficiency.

Discussion

The correct answer is "D." Fat malabsorption should scream pancreatic exocrine insufficiency or biliary tract disease. Pancreatic lipase digests fats with the help of bile salts, followed by absorption through a normal intestine. In pancreatic insufficiency, fecal elastase is low and fecal fat elevated (quantitative measurement). If you want to get fancy, suck some duodenal juice and analyze it. Treatment is replacement enzymes and fat-soluble vitamin supplementation. It is important to identify the underlying reason for the malabsorption. Additional conditions on the list of fat malabsorption culprits include chronic pancreatitis, protein-energy malnutrition, bile acid deficiency, terminal ileum disease, Johanson-Blizzard syndrome, Pearson syndrome, cystic fibrosis, and lymphangiectasis. The American Board of Pediatrics wants you to know Shwachman-Diamond

syndrome, specifically. It is a genetic condition with characteristics facies, bone dysplasia, neutropenia/cytopenias, and pancreatic exocrine insufficiency.

CASE 49

A 2-month-old infant who was evaluated for direct hyperbilirubinemia was found to have extrahepatic biliary atresia (EHBA) and underwent a Kasai procedure at 62 days of life.

Question 49-1

Considering that a substantial percentage of patients undergoing Kasai for EHBA will experience progressive synthetic liver function and eventually need liver transplantation, which is the most appropriate formula to continue during infancy?
A) Enfamil/Similac.
B) Nestlé Good Start.
C) Alimentum.
D) Pregestimil.

Discussion 49-1

The correct answer is "D." Pregestimil contains medium-chain triglycerides (MCTs). These fats are water soluble and absorbed directly through the intestinal villi without need for bile acids or pancreatic lipase. The consumption of MCTs helps to decrease the amount of fat malabsorption in the setting of liver or pancreas compromise and thus promotes the nutritional status of the infant.

CASE 50

A 5-year-old girl presents with bloody diarrhea of 2 months' duration. Stool studies performed at her local pediatrician's office were negative for bacteria (including *Clostridium difficile*) and parasitic pathogens. Her most recent hemoglobin, checked late last week, was 9 mg/dL. She is passing six to eight bloody stools per day and awakening twice nightly to defecate. She complains of lower abdominal cramping prior to defecation but is otherwise comfortable. She denies nausea, vomiting, or anorexia. Her weight is down 5 pounds. Her vital signs are remarkable for a heart rate of 142 bpm, normal blood pressure, and normal temperature. Her abdominal exam is benign. She has no perianal skin tags, fissures, or fistulas. Her rectal exam is remarkable for gross red blood, which is confirmed guaiac positive.

Question 50-1

Your next step(s) in management should be to:
A) Repeat the hemoglobin measurement today.
B) Schedule a colonoscopy in 2 weeks.
C) Perform an abdominal CT scan today.
D) Admit to the pediatric floor for IV fluids.
E) Both A and D.

Discussion 50-1

The correct answer is "E." The most important first step is to stabilize her hemodynamic status. She may need a blood transfusion and undoubtedly needs some IV fluids while waiting for the repeat hemoglobin measurement. Waiting 2 weeks for a colonoscopy is not appropriate as her clinical colitis is moderately active and may become fulminant without near future intervention. Moderate to severe disease (fever, tachycardia, orthostasis, abdominal tenderness) requires hospitalization. Admission will allow for stabilization, timely completion of a colonoscopy, and likely initiation of treatment. The needed diagnostic test is a colonoscopy with biopsies, not an abdominal CT scan (which would expose her to unnecessary radiation). CT scan would be indicated if you were worried about an acute surgical process. The American Academy of Pediatrics' "Choosing Wisely" campaign would not support your decision to irradiate her without strong conviction. Her clinical picture is consistent with colitis. The differential diagnosis includes bacterial infection, *C. difficile* infection, Henoch-Schönlein purpura, and systemic vasculitis. Stool cultures and colonoscopy are the most important diagnostic tests for this child.

Question 50-2

The patient undergoes a colonoscopy, and the most likely finding is:

A) Pancolitis with histologic evidence of cryptitis, crypt abscesses, and signs of chronic inflammation.
B) *C. difficile* pseudomembranous colitis.
C) A clean colon; the bleeding must be more proximal.
D) Vascular malformations throughout the colon.

Discussion 50-2

The correct answer is "A." The clinical picture best fits a new presentation of ulcerative colitis, which most often presents as pancolitis (involvement of the entire colon) in young children. Symptoms of ulcerative colitis include rectal bleeding, diarrhea, fever, and defecation-associated abdominal pain. Ulcerative colitis and Crohn disease are idiopathic inflammatory diseases of the GI tract. They are collectively referred to as inflammatory bowel disease (IBD). The cause is unknown. They are lifelong disorders and are categorized based on symptoms. Crohn disease can involve any part of the GI tract from the mouth to the anus. Ulcerative colitis affects only the colorectal area. Perianal disease is common with Crohn disease but not ulcerative colitis. GI tract inflammation seen with Crohn disease is not continuous. Areas of inflammation are separated by normal areas of mucosa, so-called skip lesions. On biopsy evaluation, inflammation is transmural (affecting the entire intestinal wall) with noncaseating granulomas. In ulcerative colitis, inflammation is continuous, starting at the rectum. On biopsy evaluation, inflammation is limited to the mucosa. Complications of Crohn disease include fistulas, perforations, abscesses, and strictures.

Question 50-3

The initial treatment that you recommend based on the colonoscopy findings includes:

A) Oral vancomycin.
B) IV metronidazole.
C) Methylprednisolone.
D) Tacrolimus.

Discussion 50-3

The correct answer is "C." IV corticosteroids are helpful "rescue" therapies in the setting of IBD. Corticosteroids should be considered temporary treatments, and evaluation should be ongoing to determine the most appropriate maintenance therapy for this problem. Patients who need corticosteroid rescue often need immunomodulator medications to maintain control of their disease.

▶ CASE 51

A 13-year-old boy presents to his pediatrician for evaluation of anorexia and weight loss. He denies abdominal pain, nausea, and vomiting but does acknowledge early satiety. His mother also mentioned that he is more tired than usual, often napping daily in addition to sleeping for 9 hours each night. The family history is negative for chronic diseases. His vital signs are normal. His weight is at the fifth percentile for age (downward trending from the 25th percentile at his last well-check). His abdomen is soft, with tenderness and a palpable inflammatory mass in the right lower quadrant.

Question 51-1

The most likely etiology to explain this constellation of symptoms and exam findings is:

A) Ruptured appendicitis.
B) Eating disorder.
C) Crohn disease involving the terminal ileum.
D) Parasitic infection (eg, giardiasis).

Discussion 51-1

The correct answer is "C." Crohn disease can cause inflammation anywhere in the GI tract. As such, manifestations depend on the area involved. Crohn disease of the small intestine is often insidious in presentation, leading to weight loss and fatigue without many overt GI symptoms. However, severe abdominal pain with nausea and vomiting occurs in the setting of a complication of Crohn disease; namely, small bowel obstruction. Growth (eg, short stature) and development (eg, going through puberty normally) can all be severely compromised by Crohn disease. (See Table 16–14.)

TABLE 16–14 SIGNS AND SYMPTOMS OF CROHN DISEASE

Gastrointestinal manifestations
Diarrhea
Abdominal pain
Weight loss
Vomiting
Perianal disease (skin tags, fissures, fistulas, abscesses)
Mouth ulcers

Question 51-2

You order blood tests to be drawn and find which abnormalities?

A) Positive blood culture for *Salmonella*.

B) Hemoglobin 10.5 mg/dL with mean corpuscular volume (MCV) 69 fL, albumin 3 g/dL, erythrocyte sedimentation rate (ESR) 26 mm/h, and C-reactive protein (CRP) 40 mg/dL.

C) Hemoglobin 16 mg/dL with MCV 105 fL, albumin 5 g/dL, and normal ESR and CRP.

D) Hemoglobin 11 mg/dL with MCV 90 fL, albumin 3.7 g/dL, normal ESR, and CRP 12 mg/dL.

Discussion 51-2

The correct answer is "B." Patients with new-onset Crohn disease most often have microcytic anemia due to iron deficiency. Because Crohn disease is a type of IBD, inflammatory indices are often elevated in the setting of active disease. Due to active intestinal inflammation, there is often a component of malabsorption which is confirmed by hypoalbuminemia (protein malabsorption due to damaged mucosa with impaired absorption).

Question 51-3

What test(s) should be ordered next to help you make your suspected diagnosis?

A) Capsule endoscopy.

B) Upper and lower endoscopy with biopsies to confirm histologic evidence of chronic intestinal inflammation.

C) Abdominal/pelvic magnetic resonance enterography (MRE).

D) Hydrogen breath test.

E) Both B and C.

Discussion 51-3

The correct answer is "E." The gold standard for diagnosing Crohn disease continues to be upper and lower endoscopy with biopsy sampling to confirm characteristic histologic features. However, the area affected in small bowel Crohn disease may not be reached with a typical endoscope or colonoscopy; in such cases, imaging of the remaining small intestine is needed. As noted earlier, in children CT scan is reserved for surgical signs with or without fever in an attempt to spare radiation exposure. A capsule or PillCam is a useful tool for examining the small intestinal mucosa; however, this should not be performed without recent imaging (eg, MRE, CT, UGI small bowel follow-through) to ensure safe passage of the capsule, especially through areas of active intestinal inflammation (which narrows the intestinal lumen). The main risk of capsule endoscopy is capsule retention, which could necessitate emergency surgery.

Question 51-4

What histopathology is pathognomonic for Crohn disease?

A) Mucosal granulomas with features of cryptitis, crypt abscess formation, and chronic inflammation.

B) Low-grade dysplasia in the colon.

C) Intestinal metaplasia.

D) Villous blunting with intraepithelial lymphocytosis.

TABLE 16–15 EXTRAINTESTINAL MANIFESTATIONS OF INFLAMMATORY BOWEL DISEASE

Oral ulcers or stomatitis

Fever

Arthritis

Short stature

Delayed puberty

Iron deficiency anemia

Arthritis or arthralgias

Uveitis

Erythema nodosum

Vasculitis

Thrombosis

Primary sclerosis cholangitis

Hepatitis

Osteoporosis

Nephrolithiasis

Pancreatitis

Discussion 51-4

The correct answer is "A." Option "D" is pathognomonic for celiac disease—remember the earlier discussion? Villous blunting can be seen in the setting of Crohn disease; however, one does not typically see intraepithelial lymphocytosis, too.

⧗ QUICK QUIZ

Which is NOT an extraintestinal manifestation of IBD?

A) Purpura.

B) Ankylosing spondylitis.

C) Thrombosis.

D) Cholelithiasis.

Discussion

The correct answer is "A." (See Table 16–15.) Purpura are seen with Henoch-Schönlein pupura.

▶ CASE 52

An 8-year-old girl presents with her mother, who reports that her daughter has had discharge on her underwear for the past week. Prior to this finding, the girl found it difficult to sit at her desk at school due to pain near her anal orifice. Once the discharge started, her pain resolved. Her family history is remarkable for ulcerative colitis (father).

Question 52-1

On exam, you find the following abnormality:

A) Vaginal candidiasis.

B) Folliculitis in the perineal region.

C) Apparent fistula tract to the left of the anal orifice, which releases white, purulent material from the orifice when the area is manipulated.

D) Cellulitis of the perianal skin.

Discussion 52-1

The correct answer is "C." A perianal fistula involving her vagina is the most likely etiology in this setting. This is often the presentation of perianal Crohn disease. Perianal findings are common with Crohn disease and may include skin tags, anal fissures, abscesses, or fistulas.

Next, blood tests and upper endoscopy and colonoscopy are arranged.

Question 52-2

You should also include which of the following when making the colonoscopy reservation?

A) An exam (of the perianal skin) under anesthesia with a pediatric surgeon.

B) A gynecologic exam with a pediatric gynecologist.

C) A bone marrow biopsy with a pediatric oncologist.

D) A perineal ultrasound with a pediatric radiologist.

Discussion 52-2

The correct answer is "A." Pediatric gastroenterologists and surgeons should work in conjunction for these problems. If a fistulous tract is found, a pediatric surgeon may prefer placement of a Seton drain to allow correct healing of the fistula tract over time. A perineal ultrasound will not provide enough information about a possible fluid collection in the pelvis.

A perianal fistula is found, and you need to decide the best treatment for this problem.

Question 52-3

You should complete the following tests before starting treatment in this setting:

A) Bone marrow biopsy.

B) PPD (a test for tuberculosis).

C) Pelvic imaging in the form of MRI or CT scan.

D) Both B and C.

Discussion 52-3

The correct answer is "D." You need to ensure the absence of a pelvic fluid collection (ie, abscess) before starting potent anti-inflammatory treatments aimed at perianal fistulae. Often, biologic therapies (eg, infliximab) are the most helpful treatments for perianal fistulae. Testing for tuberculosis exposure is necessary before starting these treatments.

Question 52-4

You complete your testing and are ready to begin treatment. The therapy with the most efficacy in the scientific literature for this problem is:

A) Corticosteroids (eg, prednisone).

B) Biologic or anti-TNF agents (eg, infliximab).

C) Immunomodulators (eg, azathioprine).

D) Antibiotics (eg, metronidazole).

Discussion 52-4

The correct answer is "B." Biologic medications have been shown to be efficacious in treating perianal Crohn disease.

► CASE 53

A severely malnourished 16-year-old girl presents to her pediatrician for evaluation. Her mother has not been able to get her to eat more than 500 kcal/day for several weeks. Despite losing 15 kg and having a BMI of 16, the girl says she does not want to eat because she is already fat. Her heart rate is 56 bpm. You admit her to the hospital. The adolescent medicine service is consulted.

Question 53-1

When starting nasogastric feedings, what is the most significant concern with respect to the patient's electrolytes?

A) Hyperkalemia.

B) Thiamine deficiency.

C) Hypophosphatemia.

D) Vitamin D deficiency.

Discussion 53-1

The correct answer is "C." The concern is for refeeding syndrome. The pathogenesis includes depleted phosphate stores during starvation. When the patient is fed carbohydrates, phosphate moves into the cells under the influence of insulin and the serum phosphate level is depleted, causing tissue hypoxia and associated complications. The risk of potassium alteration in patients with anorexia nervosa and other malnourished states is typically low potassium, which can lead to weakness.

Question 53-2

The risk of electrolyte abnormalities persists for how long in this setting?

A) 2 days.

B) 2 weeks.

C) 6 weeks.

D) 8 weeks.

Discussion 53-2

The correct answer is "B." The concern regarding electrolyte abnormalities in the setting of refeeding syndrome persists for 2 weeks after feedings are started; therefore, these patients must continue to be monitored closely during this period. The key is starting slow, monitoring electrolytes frequently, and supplementing (phosphorus) as needed. Some patients may require telemetry monitoring as hypophosphatemia may result in bad cardiac outcomes—arrhythmias or heart failure. The heart can atrophy, too.

BIBLIOGRAPHY

Baumgart DC, Sandborn WJ. Crohn's disease. *Lancet.* 2012;380(9853):1590–1605. doi: 10.1016/S0140-6736(12)60026-9.

Bishop WP. *Pediatric Practice Gastroenterology.* McGraw-Hill Education, Inc., New York, NY: 2010.

Catassi C, Fasano A. Coeliac disease. The debate on coeliac disease screening—are we there yet? *Nat Rev Gastroenterol Hepatol.* 2014;11(8):457–458. doi: 10.1038/nrgastro.2014.119.

Centers for Disease Control and Prevention. Provider information: Rotavirus VIS. http://www.cdc.gov/vaccines/hcp/vis/vis-statements/rotavirus-hcp-info.html. Accessed March 9, 2015.

Chiou E, Nurko S. Management of functional abdominal pain and irritable bowel syndrome in children and adolescents. *Exp Rev Gastroenterol Hepatol.* 2010;4(3):293–304. doi: doi:10.1586/egh.10.28.

Chitkara DK, van Tilburg M, Whitehead WE, Talley N. Teaching diaphragmatic breathing for rumination syndrome. *Am J Gastroenterol.* 2006;101(11):2449–2452.

Cohen GM, Albertini LW. Colic. *Pediatr Rev.* 2012;33(7):332–333. doi: 10.1542/pir.33-7-332.

Committee on Infectious Diseases; American Academy of Pediatrics; Kimberlin DW, Brady MT, Jackson MA, Long SS. *Red Book. 2015 Report of the Committee of Infectious Diseases.* 30th ed. http://www.redbook.solutions.aap.org/redbook.aspx. Accessed June 14, 2015.

Däbritz J, Mühlbauer M, Domagk D, et al. Significance of hydrogen breath tests in children with suspected carbohydrate malabsorption. *BMC Pediatr.* 2014;14:59. doi: 10.1186/1471-2431-14-59.

Daneman A. Malrotation: The balance of evidence. *Pediatr Radiol.* 2009;39(suppl 2):S164–S166.

Egan LJ, Sandborn W. Taking a closer look at IBD. *Gut.* 2014;63(2):e1. doi: 10.1136/gutjnl-2013-305424.

Gorsche JR, Vick L, Boulanger SC, Islam S. Midgut abnormalities. *Surg Clin North Am.* 2006;86(2):286–299.

Harb, R, Thomas, DW. Conjugated hyperbilirubinemia: Screening and treatment in older infants and children. *Pediatr Rev.* 2007;28(3):83–91.

Koletzko S, Jones NL, Goodman KJ, et al. Evidence-based guidelines from ESPGHAN and NASPGHAN for *Helicobacter pylori* infection in children. *J Pediatr Gastroenterol Nutr.* 2011;53(2):230–243. doi: 10.1097/MPG.0b013e3182227e90.

Munck A, Gargouri L, Alberti C, et al. Evaluation of guidelines for management of familial adenomatous polyposis in a multicenter pediatric cohort. *J Pediatr Gastroenterol Nutr.* 2011;53(3):296–302. doi: 10.1097/MPG.0b013e3182198f4d.

Murch SH, Winyard PJ, Koletzko S, et al. Congenital enterocyte heparan sulphate deficiency with massive albumin loss, secretory diarrhoea, and malnutrition. *Lancet.* 1996;347(9011):1299–1301.

Nachamkin I, Allos BM, Ho T. *Campylobacter* species and Guillain-Barré syndrome. *Clin Microbiol Rev.* 1998;11(3):555.

Ohhama Y, Shinkai M, Fujita S, Nishi T, Yamamoto H. Early prediction of long-term survival and the timing of liver transplantation after the Kasai operation. *J Pediatr Surg.* 2000;35(7):1031–1034.

Ordás I, Eckmann L, Talamini M, Baumgart DC, Sandborn WJ. Ulcerative colitis. *Lancet.* 2012;380(9853):1606–1619. doi: 10.1016/S0140-6736(12)60150-0.

Park T, Wassef W. Nonvariceal upper gastrointestinal bleeding. *Curr Opin Gastroenterol.* 2014;30(6):603–608. doi: 10.1097/MOG.0000000000000123.

Rome Foundation. Rome III disorders and criteria. http://www.romecriteria.org/criteria. Accessed June 13, 2015.

Rubio-Tapia A, Hill ID, Kelly CP, Calderwood AH, Murray JA. ACG clinical guidelines: Diagnosis and management of celiac disease. *Am J Gastroenterol.* 2013;108(5):656–676; quiz 677. doi: 10.1038/ajg.2013.79.

Sandborn WJ. Crohn's disease evaluation and treatment: Clinical decision tool. *Gastroenterology.* 2014;147(3):702–705. doi: 10.1053/j.gastro.2014.07.022.

Sandborn WJ, Hanauer S, Van Assche G, Panés J, Wilson S, Petersson J, Panaccione R. Treating beyond symptoms with a view to improving patient outcomes in inflammatory bowel diseases. *J Crohns Colitis.* 2014 Sep 1;8(9):927-35. doi: 10.1016/j.crohns.2014.02.021. Epub 2014 Apr 6.

Sondheimer JM and Hurtado CW, (Eds). The NASPGHAN Fellows Concise Review of Pediatric Gastroenterology, Hepatology and Nutrition. 2011

Srinath, Arvind I., & Lowe, Mark E. (2013). Pediatric Pancreatitis. *Pediatrics in Review,* 34(2), 79-90. doi: 10.1542/pir.34-2-79

Suchy, Sokol and Balistreri. Liver Disease in Children Third Edition. 2007

Thakkar K, Fishman DS, Gilger MA. Colorectal polyps in childhood. *Curr Opin Pediatr.* 2012 Oct;24(5):632-7. doi: 10.1097/MOP.0b013e328357419f.

Theander G, Trägårdh B. Lymphoid hyperplasia of the colon in childhood. *Acta Radiol Diagn* (Stockh). 1976 Sep;17(5A):631-40.

Walker, A. et al. Pediatric Gastrointestinal Disease. Fourth Edition, 2004.

Genetics and Dysmorphology

17

Greg Rice

▶ **CASE 1**

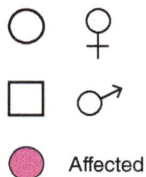

○ ♀

□ ♂

🌑 Affected

A

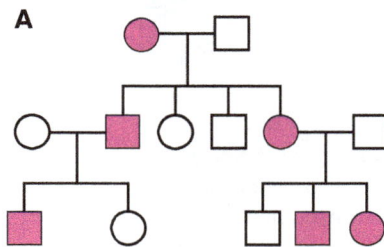

Question 1-1

What is the inheritance pattern shown in this pedigree?
A) Autosomal dominant disorder with complete penetrance.
B) Autosomal dominant disorder with incomplete penetrance.
C) Autosomal recessive disorder.
D) X-linked recessive disorder.
E) X-linked dominant disorder.
F) Mitochondrial disorders.

Discussion 1-1

The correct answer is "A." With autosomal dominant disorders, heterozygotes are affected. Males and females are equally affected. With complete penetrance, all individuals with one dominant mutant allele will be affected. An affected individual will have an affected parent, and 50% of offspring of an affected parent will be affected. Male-to-male transmission distinguishes this from X-linked dominant disorders.

▶ **CASE 2**

B

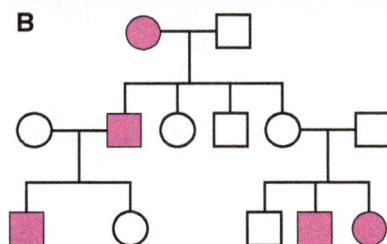

Question 2-1

What is the inheritance pattern shown in this pedigree?
A) Autosomal dominant disorder with complete penetrance.
B) Autosomal dominant disorder with incomplete penetrance.
C) Autosomal recessive disorder.
D) X-linked recessive disorder.
E) X-linked dominant disorder.
F) Mitochondrial disorders.

Discussion 2-1

The correct answer is "B." In autosomal dominant disorders with incomplete penetrance, not all heterozygotes are affected. An individual can have the dominant mutant allele but not express it. Yet, he or she can still pass it to offspring who are then affected. Variable expression of autosomal dominant disorders is different. All individuals with the dominant allele are affected, but symptoms vary from person to person.

▶ **CASE 3**

C

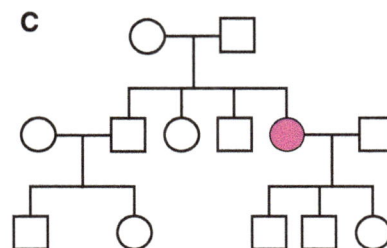

Question 3-1

What is the inheritance pattern shown in this pedigree?
A) Autosomal dominant disorder with complete penetrance.
B) Autosomal dominant disorder with incomplete penetrance.
C) Autosomal recessive disorder.
D) X-linked recessive disorder.
E) X-linked dominant disorder.
F) Mitochondrial disorders.

Discussion 3-1

The correct answer is "C." With autosomal recessive disorders, homozygotes are affected. Heterozygotes are carriers for the trait. Males and females are equal affected. All individuals with two recessive mutant alleles will be affected. An affected individual will not have an affected parent who is a carrier. Twenty-five percent of offspring of parents who are both carriers will be affected whereas 50% of offspring will be carriers.

► CASE 4

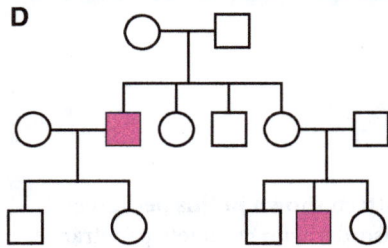

Question 4-1

What is the inheritance pattern shown in this pedigree?
A) Autosomal dominant disorder with complete penetrance.
B) Autosomal dominant disorder with incomplete penetrance.
C) Autosomal recessive disorder.
D) X-linked recessive disorder.
E) X-linked dominant disorder.
F) Mitochondrial disorders.

Discussion 4-1

The correct answer is "D." With X-linked recessive inheritance, only males are affected and females are carriers. Transmission is female to male (ie, mother to son), and 50% of sons born to mothers who are carriers will be affected. X-linked genes are never passed male to male (ie, father to son).

► CASE 5

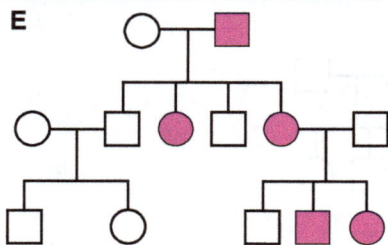

Question 5-1

What is the inheritance pattern shown in this pedigree?
A) Autosomal dominant disorder with complete penetrance.
B) Autosomal dominant disorder with incomplete penetrance.
C) Autosomal recessive disorder.
D) X-linked recessive disorder.
E) X-linked dominant disorder.
F) Mitochondrial disorders.

Discussion 5-1

The correct answer is "E." With X-linked dominant inheritance, males and females may be affected. Male-to-female transmission (ie, father to daughter) may occur. Male-to-male transmission (ie, father to son) of X-linked genes does not occur. One hundred percent of daughters born to affected fathers will be affected. All sons born to affected fathers are normal. Males are typically more affected than female, and the trait may be lethal in males.

► CASE 6

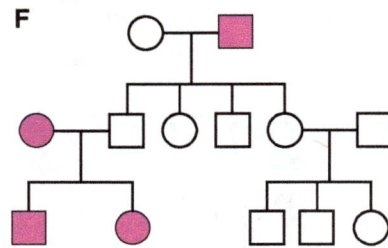

Question 6-1

What is the inheritance pattern shown in this pedigree?
A) Autosomal dominant disorder with complete penetrance.
B) Autosomal dominant disorder with incomplete penetrance.
C) Autosomal recessive disorder.
D) X-linked recessive disorder.
E) X-linked dominant disorder.
F) Mitochondrial disorders.

Discussion 6-1

The correct answer is "F." Mitochondrial disorders are inherited from the mother as nearly all mitochondria come from the mother. One hundred percent of offspring of an affected mother are affected. Affected fathers produce no affected offspring.

> **Helpful Tip**
> Multifactorial disorders (cleft lip or palate, spina bifida) and traits (height, intelligence) are caused by the action of multiple genes or gene-environmental effects.

► CASE 7

You are covering pediatrics at a large community hospital and receive a call on a Saturday night from the labor and delivery nurse who is concerned that a recently born term infant might have trisomy 21. The nurse reports that newborn is stable, feeding well, and has normal pulse oximetry. He was born following an uncomplicated pregnancy to a healthy 28-year-old woman. There is no family history of pregnancy loss or aneuploidy. In the morning your evaluation of the newborn reveals a flatted midface, upslanting palpebral fissures, small low-set ears, nuchal redundancy, and borderline microcephaly.

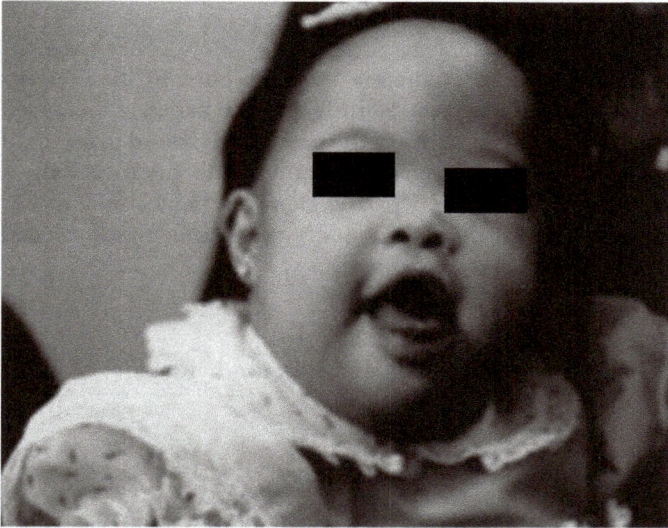

FIGURE 17–1. This 8-month-old has trisomy 21 with the typical facies, including upslanting palpebral fissures, epicanthal folds, large tongue, flat face, low-set ears and brachycephaly. (Reproduced with permission from Valle D, Beaudet AL, Vogelstein B et al: *The Online Metabolic and Molecular Bases of Inherited Disease*, 8ed. McGraw-Hill Education, Inc; 2014. Fig. 63-1.)

(See Figure 17–1.) The cardiac exam is normal. The newborn's hands are small and there are single palmar creases. Based on the typical facial features you make a clinical diagnosis of trisomy 21 and discuss your findings with the family. The parents were not expecting this news and become upset. They wonder how this could have happened because the mother had a normal ultrasound and is only 28 years old.

Question 7-1

Which of the following tests does NOT need to be performed for this newborn before discharge?
A) Karyotype of the newborn.
B) Echocardiogram.
C) Thyroid-stimulating hormone (TSH) level.
D) Newborn hearing screen.
E) CBC.
F) All of the above tests should be performed within the newborn period in a child with suspected trisomy 21.

Discussion 7-1

The correct answer is "F." The newborn has typical physical manifestations of trisomy 21 or Down syndrome. Other physical features include a sandal gap between the first and second toes, hypotonia, and large tongue. Down syndrome is usually due to an extra copy of chromosome 21 (trisomy 21), which is usually the result of maternal nondisjunction. All infants with suspected trisomy 21 should have a karyotype performed, even if the physician is confident of the diagnosis. This is because 4% of cases of trisomy 21 are due to an unbalanced robertsonian translocation (2 chromosomes join) between chromosome 21 and another acrocentric (centromere near one end rather than the center) chromosome (eg, 14 or 15). The recurrence risk for parents who are carriers of the balanced form of the translocation is higher;

it is therefore important for them to be aware of this information for future family planning. Additionally, a small percentage of children with trisomy 21 are mosaic, meaning they have both a normal cell line and a trisomy 21 cell line. The developmental outcomes in these children are more variable and in some cases can be better. Infants with trisomy 21 are at high risk of having congenital heart disease. Approximately 40% of affected infants have an abnormal echocardiogram, endocardial cushion defects (also known as atrioventricular [AV] canal defects) are classic, but isolated atrial and ventricular septal defects also occur frequently. Individuals with trisomy 21 are at increased risk for hypothyroidism and hearing loss. Some infants with trisomy 21 have a leukemoid reaction in which the white blood cell count becomes transiently elevated with the presences of blasts. These infants are at increased risk of developing leukemia later in childhood.

Question 7-2

Which of the following conditions is/are more common in children with trisomy 21?
A) Refractive errors of the eye and amblyopia.
B) Leukemia.
C) Cognitive disability.
D) Duodenal atresia.
E) Atlantoaxial (cervical spine) instability.
F) Celiac disease.
G) All of the above.

Discussion 7-2

The correct answer is "G." All of these conditions are more common in children with trisomy 21. This list helps to guide trisomy 21–specific anticipatory guidance for the pediatrician. Infants with trisomy 21 are more likely to have one or more of the following medical conditions: intestinal obstructions such as duodenal atresia or stenosis, imperforate anus, tracheoesophageal fistula, and Hirschsprung disease. (See Figure 17–2.)

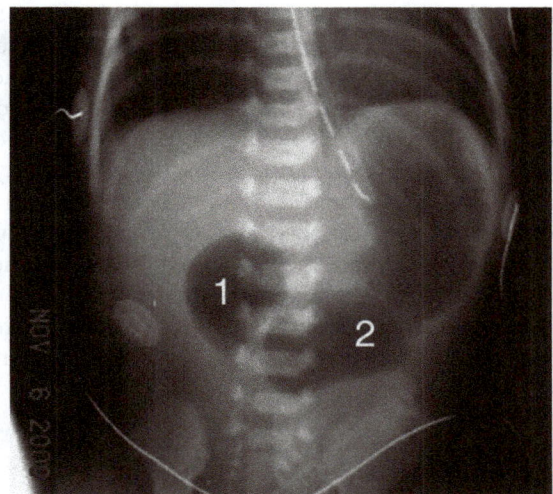

FIGURE 17–2. The "double bubble" sign is suggestive of duodenal atresia, which is associated with trisomy 21. (Reproduced with permission from Brunicardi FC, Andersen DK, Billiar TR, et al, eds. *Schwartz's Principles of Surgery*. 10th ed. New York, NY: McGraw-Hill Education; 2015, Fig. 39-13, p. 1615.)

It is very important that children with trisomy 21 be engaged in early intervention therapies as soon as possible. All children with trisomy 21 have cognitive disability; however, the spectrum is broad and can range from borderline to severe cognitive disability. In recent years some high-functioning young adults with trisomy 21 have attended college. It is important to inform parents about the complete range of outcomes while at same time not giving false hope for "normal" development.

The parents of this newborn were surprised that they could have a child with trisomy 21 because the mother was young and the ultrasound normal.

Question 7-3

Which of the following statements is true regarding the risk of having a child with trisomy 21?

A) Prenatal ultrasound is highly sensitive in detecting a fetus with trisomy 21.

B) Most children with trisomy 21 are born to mothers of advanced maternal age.

C) If a mother carriers a balanced robertsonian translocation between chromosomes 14 and 21, her risk of having a child with trisomy 21 is 50%.

D) Most children with trisomy 21 are born to mothers who are not of advanced maternal age.

Discussion 7-3

The correct answer is "D." Although advanced maternal age (AMA) increases the risk of having a child with trisomy 21, most women who have children with this genetic disorder are not AMA. In fact, although the absolute risk of having a child with Down syndrome increases with age, more children with trisomy 21 are still born to younger women. The risk of having a child with trisomy 21 at age 40 years is around 1%; the risk at 28 is much lower. Parents are often surprised to find out at delivery that their newborn has trisomy 21; therefore, empathic and accurate counseling is critical at this time. Some parents find the diagnosis difficult to accept. In these cases the confirmatory karyotype can be helpful in the process of acceptance. When used alone, a 20-week prenatal ultrasound will detect trisomy 21 in only 50% of the cases. Prenatal screening tests such as the quad screen can increase that sensitivity, but this is still only a screening test. High-risk results would need to be confirmed by examination of the fetal karyotype following amniocentesis or chorionic villus sampling (CVS). The risk of having a child with trisomy 21 for a mother (of any age) who carries a balanced 14:21 robertsonian translocation is around 14%, which is much higher than her age-related risk but still nowhere near 50%.

> **Helpful Tip**
> The facies of trisomy 21 may be subtle in a newborn and may be more pronounced with crying or as the infant grows.

▶ CASE 8

You are called to evaluate a term newborn in the delivery room. The mother received little prenatal care and measured small for dates. At delivery the newborn is found to be small for gestational age and dysmorphic, with microcephaly, a unilateral cleft lip and palate, clenched hands, and rocker bottom feet. The infant has a loud systolic murmur, weak cry, and recurrent episodes of apnea.

Question 8-1

What is the most likely diagnosis in this newborn?

A) Trisomy 18.

B) Trisomy 13.

C) Cornelia de Lange syndrome.

D) CHARGE syndrome.

Discussion 8-1

The correct answer is "A." This newborn has the classic features of trisomy 18 (Edwards syndrome). Affected children are small and thin and often have cleft lip and palate. Congenital heart and renal anomalies are common. The most recognizable features are clenched hands with overlapping fingers (see Figure 17–3) and rocker bottom feet. Prognosis is grim; most infants die in the first several months of life without aggressive support. Apnea, seizures, severe feeding problems, and aspiration are common. Survivors have profound developmental delays. Infants with a mosaic form of trisomy 18 may be less severely affected. It is important to distinguish this condition from trisomy 13 (Patau syndrome). Infants with trisomy 13 often have midline cleft lip and palate, which is often associated with midline brain anomalies (holoprosencephaly), and hypotelorism (eyes close together).

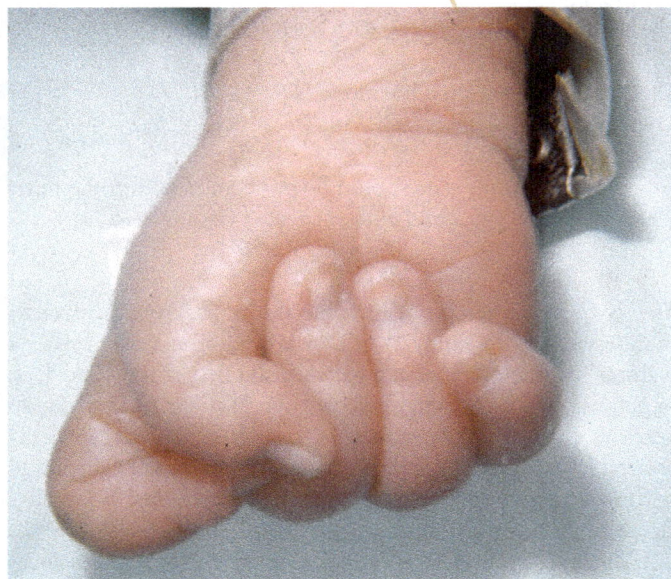

FIGURE 17–3. Distinguishing characteristics of trisomy 18 include rocker bottom feet and clenched hands with overlapping fingers. (Reproduced with permission from Fuster V, Walsh RA, Harrington RA, eds. *Hurst's The Heart.* 13th ed. New York, NY: McGraw-Hill Education; 2011, Fig. 14-13.)

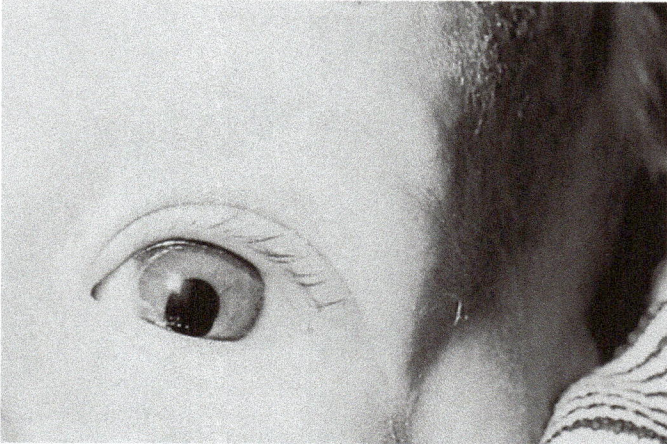

FIGURE 17–4. An iris coloboma is typical of CHARGE syndrome. (Reproduced with permission from Hay WW, Levin MJ, Deterding RR, Abzug MJ, eds. *Current Diagnosis and Treatment Pediatrics.* 22nd ed. New York, NY: McGraw-Hill Education; 2014, Fig. 16-20, p. 469.)

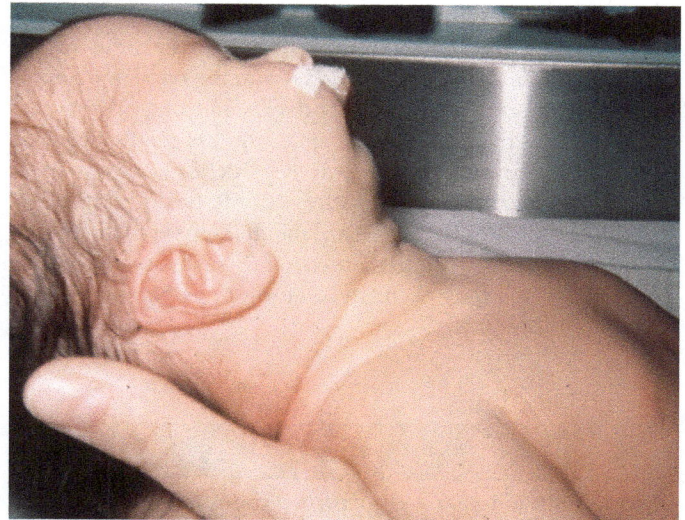

FIGURE 17–5. This newborn has Pierre Robin syndrome with micrognathia and a hypoplastic mandible. (Reproduced with permission from Fuster V, Walsh RA, Harrington RA, eds. *Hurst's The Heart.* 13th ed. New York, NY: McGraw-Hill Education; 2011, Fig. 14-7.)

Scalp defects (cutis aplasia), polydactyly, and congenital heart disease are also common features. The prognosis is similar to that for trisomy 18. Cornelia de Lange syndrome (CDLS) also results in multiple congenital anomalies and small size, but the findings in this case are not suggestive of CDLS. CDLS leads to typical dysmorphic characteristics that are present in the newborn, including synophrys (high-arched and connected eyebrows), long eyelashes, and a long philtrum. Most affected individuals are short statured, with microcephaly and small hands. Reduction defects of the hands and forearms can occur. Renal and cardiac anomalies also occur. CHARGE syndrome results in multiple congenital anomalies but in a predictable pattern: **C**oloboma (see Figure 17–4), **H**eart defects, **A**tresia choanae, **R**etardation of growth, **G**enital anomalies, and **E**ar anomalies.

associated with 22q11.2 deletion syndrome. Paucity of bile ducts is typically associated with Alagille syndrome. Deletion of 22q11.2 is the most common chromosomal microdeletion syndrome and is associated with conotruncal cardiac malformations such as tetralogy of Fallot. Hypoplasia of the thymus can result in immunodeficiency owing to abnormal lymphocyte maturation and function. The parathyroid glands may also be hypoplastic, which leads to hypoparathyroidism and subsequent hypocalcemia, tetany, and seizures. Around 40% of individuals have cognitive delays. Pierre Robin syndrome can occur secondary to the micrognathia (small jaw). (See Figure 17–5.)

▶ CASE 9

A newborn is noted to have a cyanosis and respiratory distress. A chest X-ray shows absence of the thymic silhouette and several vertebral anomalies. A follow-up echocardiogram shows tetralogy of Fallot. The newborn is small for dates and also has mildly dysmorphic facial characteristics, including micrognathia, bulbous nasal tip, and round face.

Question 9-1

The newborn in this case is at risk for all of the following health issues EXECPT:

A) Pierre Robin syndrome.
B) Hypocalcemia secondary to hypoparathyroidism.
C) Cognitive delays.
D) Immunodeficiency.
E) Direct hyperbilirubinemia secondary to a paucity of bile ducts.

Discussion 9-1

The correct answer is "E." The child in the case has 22q11 deletion syndrome (also known as DiGeorge syndrome). All the issues except the one listed as option "E" are commonly

Helpful Tip

Use the mnemonic CATCH-22 to remember the features of 22q11.2 deletion or DiGeorge syndrome:

C – Cardiac defects
A – Abnormal facies
T – Thymus hypoplasia
C – Cleft palate
H – Hypocalcemia/hypoparathyroidism
22 – 22q11.2 deletion

⧗ QUICK QUIZ

Which is a feature of Pierre Robin sequence?
A) Cleft lip.
B) Prognathia.
C) Glossoptosis.
D) Proptosis.
E) Maxillary hypoplasia.

Discussion

The correct answer is "C." Pierre Robin syndrome results from mandibular hypoplasia. It is characterized by micrognathia, glossoptosis (posteriorly displaced tongue), and cleft soft palate. As the mandible is small, the tongue is displaced posteriorly causing upper airway obstruction. Treatment of the airway obstruction may include prone positioning, nasal pharyngeal airway (trumpet), labioglossopexy (tongue-lip adhesion), mandibular distraction, and tracheostomy. Pierre Robin syndrome may occur in isolation or as part of another genetic syndrome.

▶ CASE 10

You evaluate a 4-year-old girl for developmental delay and hyperactivity. She is very social and has good expressive language skills despite her other cognitive deficits. She has short stature and mildly dysmorphic facial characteristics, including a long but well-formed philtrum and puffy periorbital region. She had a history of hypercalcemia in infancy. On physical exam you notice a 2/6 systolic murmur. A follow-up echocardiogram reveals supravalvular aortic stenosis.

Question 10-1

The child in the case has which of the following condition?

A) Fetal alcohol syndrome.
B) Prader-Willi syndrome.
C) Angelman syndrome.
D) Williams syndrome.
E) Rett syndrome.

Discussion 10-1

The correct answer is "D." Williams syndrome is due to a chromosomal microdeletion at 7q11 and is associated with cognitive delays and relatively preserved expressive language. Affected children are described as having elfin facies. Some individuals have an outgoing "cocktail party" personality and may have proclivity toward music. The deletion results in the loss of the elastin gene, which is responsible for the pathognomonic cardiac lesion, supravalvular aortic stenosis. Renal artery stenosis, short stature, and infantile hypercalcemia also occur. Fetal alcohol syndrome (FAS), results in mildly dysmorphic facial characteristic, neurodevelopmental delays, and poor growth. The typical facial features of FAS include a smooth philtrum (area between the nose and upper lip) and small palpebral fissures (eye openings). (See Figure 17–6.) Children often struggle in school, particularly with attention. Prader-Willi syndrome (PWS) results from imprinting abnormalities on chromosome 15, usually due to deletion of the paternal copy of 15q11-13 or maternal uniparental disomy (UPD, which occurs when both chromosome copies come from one parent) for chromosome 15. The maternal copy is imprinted and thus not expressed, so either a paternal deletion or maternal UPD will result in no functional copy of the critical genes. Children with PWS are hypotonic at birth and this

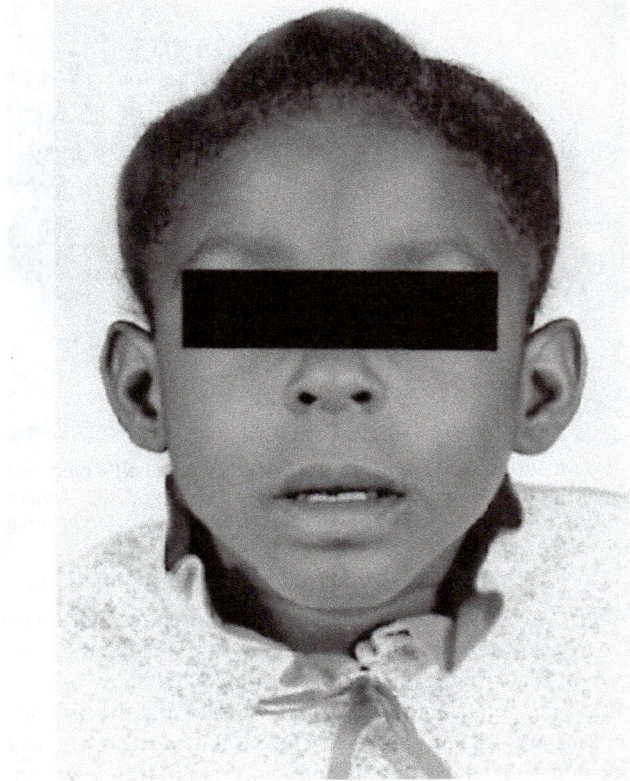

FIGURE 17–6. Children with fetal alcohol syndrome have a smooth philtrum, short palpebral fissures, and a thin upper lip. Notice the long, smooth philtrum in this child. (Reproduced with permission from Fuster V, Walsh RA, Harrington RA, eds. *Hurst's The Heart.* 13th ed. New York, NY: McGraw-Hill Education; 2011, Fig. 14-15.)

often leads to poor feeding. Many affected infants develop failure to thrive and require gastrostomy feedings. Boys may have a small phallus. At age 2 or 3 years the children begin to gain excessive weight due to absent satiety controls, which leads to overeating. Food-seeking behaviors are common, and families may have to lock cupboards. Without aggressive intervention most children with PWS will become obese. Growth hormone administration can be helpful in building lean muscle mass. Most children have mild to moderate cognitive disability and short stature. Angelman syndrome (AS) usually results from deletion of the maternal copy of chromosome 15q11-13 or paternal UPD. The paternal copy is imprinted and thus not expressed, leaving no functional copy of the critical region secondary to either of these mechanisms. Children with AS have global developmental delays, cognitive disability, wide-based gait (ataxia), happy demeanor, inappropriate laughter, microcephaly, and seizures. Children with AS have been described as "happy puppets." Most affected individuals develop little expressive language. Rett syndrome is an X-linked dominant condition that classically affects girls. Girls with Rett syndrome often develop normally for the first 4 to 6 months, then have regression of motor and language skills along with progressive microcephaly and seizures. Most classically affected girls are cognitive disabled and have little expressive language. Midline hand-wringing behaviors are common.

▶ CASE 11

You see a 7-year-old girl who is new to your practice for a well-child exam. You notice that she has borderline short stature and mildly unusual facial characteristics, including downslanting eyes, low-set ears, and a broad neck. Her father has similar facial features and short stature. The father remarks that he struggled in school. The child's cognitive development has been normal. The physical exam also reveals a pectus carinatum of the chest and a cardiac murmur. A follow-up echogram shows mild pulmonic stenosis.

Question 11-1

What syndrome is the girl most likely affected with?

A) Turner syndrome.
B) Achondroplasia.
C) Noonan syndrome.
D) Russell-Silver syndrome.

Discussion 11-1

The correct answer is "C." The child and the father both have Noonan syndrome. In a girl with short stature it is important to distinguish Noonan syndrome (see Figure 17–7) from Turner syndrome (see Figure 17–8). Both conditions have the physical hallmarks of lymphedema, including low-set ears and nuchal webbing. Noonan syndrome is inherited in an autosomal dominant fashion and therefore can affect both males and females.

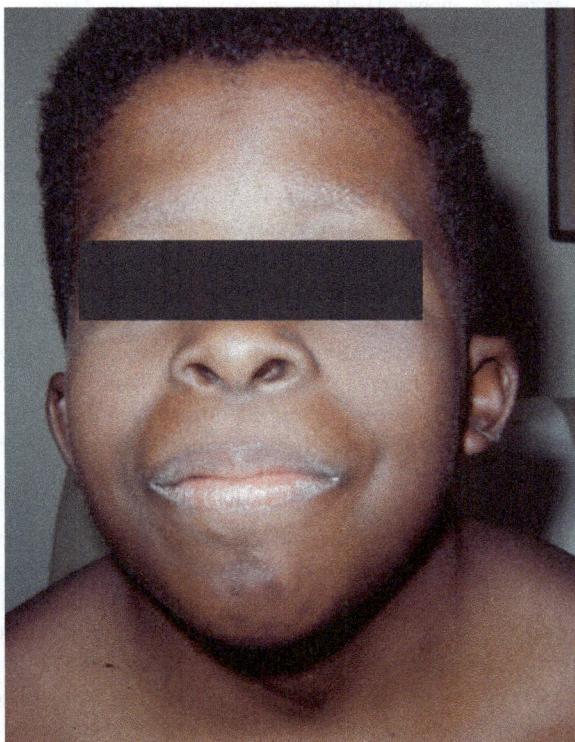

FIGURE 17–7. This child has Noonan syndrome. Notice the low-set ears and broad neck. (Reproduced with permission from Fuster V, Walsh RA, Harrington RA, eds. *Hurst's The Heart*. 13th ed. New York, NY: McGraw-Hill Education; 2011, Fig. 14-17.)

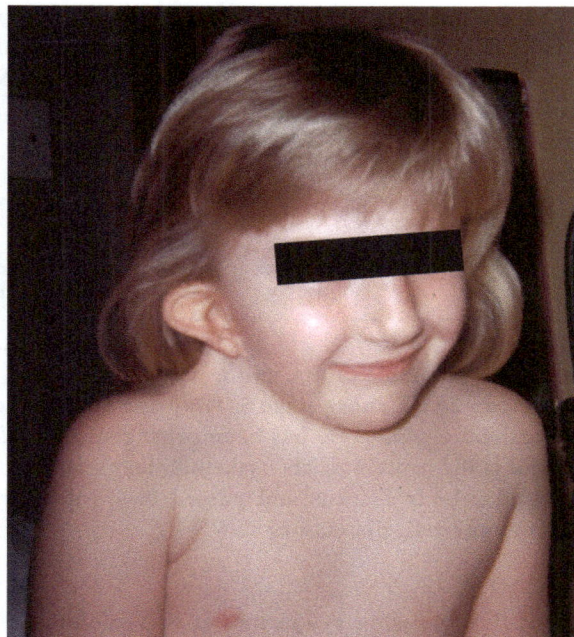

FIGURE 17–8. This girl has Turner syndrome. Again, notice the low-set ears and broad neck. (Reproduced with permission from Fuster V, Walsh RA, Harrington RA, eds. *Hurst's The Heart*. 13th ed. New York, NY: McGraw-Hill Education; 2011, Fig. 14-14.)

Turner syndrome results from monosomy X (45,X), is not inherited, and only affects females. Girls with Turner syndrome have primary ovarian insufficiency (hypogonadism), resulting in lack of development of the secondary sexual characteristics and infertility. Other features include short stature, shield-shaped chest, widely spaced nipples, and increased risk of coarctation of the aorta. Some girls with Turner syndrome have a mosaic karyotype. Girls who have a mosaic karyotype, with the presence of a Y chromosome (45,X +46,XY), are at risk for developing gonadoblastoma and should have their primitive gonads removed. Girls with Turner syndrome have normal cognitive development. Individuals with Noonan syndrome often have short stature, dysmorphic facial features (as described above), pulmonary valve stenosis, and chest wall abnormalities (pectus excavatum or carinatum). Other features include cognitive delays in 40% of affected individuals, bleeding diathesis, and cardiomyopathy. Noonan syndrome is secondary to heterozygous mutations in several genes that use the RAS pathway, including *PTPN11*. Mutations in the genes that cause Noonan syndrome can be inherited from an affected parent in a dominant fashion (as in this case) or can occur de novo. Achondroplasia is the most common skeletal dysplasia. It is secondary to mutations in the gene *FGFR3*, which can be inherited from an affected parent in a dominant fashion or can occur de novo. This condition results in disproportionate (short-limbed) dwarfism, with rhizomelic (upper segment) foreshortening of the limbs. Affected individuals have short stature and macrocephaly, with typical facial features including midface hypoplasia and frontal bossing. The fingers are short and splayed. Intelligence in normal. Russell-Silver syndrome (RSS) also results in short stature; however, these individuals have proportionate short stature (no rhizomelia) with a normal head size.

The body mass index is often very low. Infants with RSS are born very small and grow poorly. Their bodies are very tiny while their head size is normal, with a triangular-shaped face (broad forehead, narrow chin). Fifth finger clinodactyly is present. RSS also increases the risk of hypoglycemia. Some individuals with RSS have development delays.

▶ CASE 12

You are evaluating a 16-year-old boy for a sports physical. He has tall stature, flexible joints, and a pectus excavatum. On physical exam he is Tanner stage 5. His arms and legs seem disproportionately long. He has been getting straight A's in school and is the captain of his basketball team. His mother had a similar body habitus and passed away suddenly at age 35 from an aortic dissection.

Question 12-1

Which of the following syndromes is this adolescent boy most likely affected with?
A) Klinefelter syndrome.
B) Classical homocystinuria.
C) Marfan syndrome.
D) Ehlers-Danlos syndrome.
E) Fragile X syndrome.

Discussion 12-1

The correct answer is "C." Marfan syndrome is a connective tissue disorder that results in a disproportionate body habitus with long arms and legs (arachnodactyly), leading to tall stature. (See Figure 17–9.) Pectus excavatum is common. Progressive aortic root enlargement can result in aortic dissection and death if not recognized and treated early. Ocular manifestations include ectopia lentis (dislocation of the lens). Cognitive development is

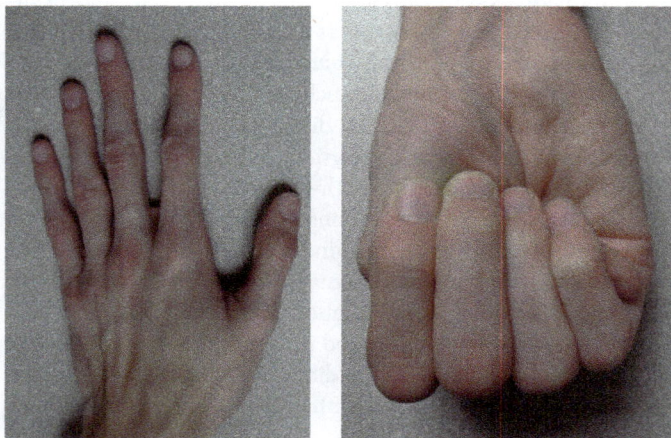

FIGURE 17–10. Klinefelter syndrome (47,XXY) causes primary hypogonadism. Affected males are tall, with small testes and gynecomastia. This male also has sparse body hair with a female pubic hair pattern. (Reproduced with permission from Gardner DG, Shoback D, eds. *Greenspan's Basic & Clinical Endocrinology*. 9th ed. New York, NY: McGraw-Hill Education; 2011, Fig. 12-7.)

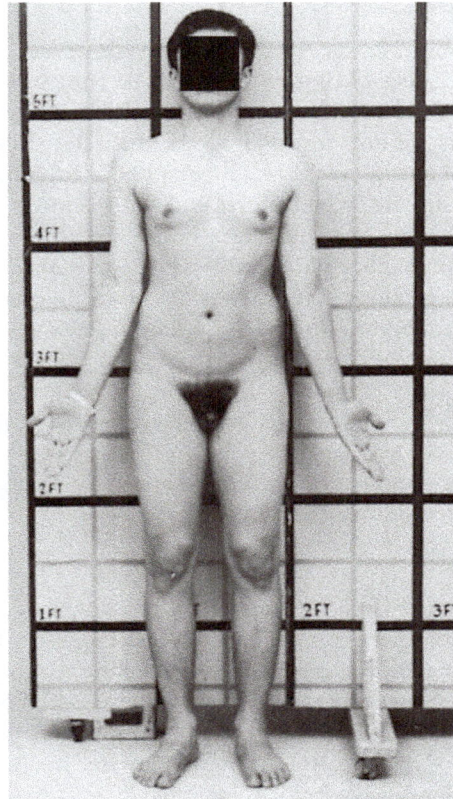

FIGURE 17–9. Typical manifestations of Marfan syndrome include ectopia lentis, tall stature, and arachnodactyly (shown). The thumb sign is positive (thumb extends past the fifth finger when bent into the hand). (Reproduced with permission from LeBlond RF, Brown DD, Suneja M, Szot JF, eds. *DeGowin's Diagnostic Examination*. 10th ed. New York, NY: McGraw-Hill Education; 2015, Plate 29.)

normal. Mutations in the *fibrillin-1* gene cause Marfan syndrome, and it can be inherited from an affected parent (as in this case) in a dominant fashion or can occur de novo. It is important to distinguish Marfan syndrome from classical homocystinuria, which is a metabolic disorder resulting in markedly elevated plasma and urine homocysteine. These individuals can have tall stature and ectopia lentis but are not at increased risk for aortic dilation and often have development delays. Classical homocystinuria also increases the risk of coronary artery disease and stroke due to the atherosclerotic effects of homocysteine. Klinefelter syndrome results from the presence of an extra copy of the X chromosome in a male (47,XXY). Males with Klinefelter syndrome are relatively tall and have small testes. (See Figure 17–10.) Testosterone deficiency can result in delayed puberty. Infertility is common. Most boys have normal intelligence quotient (IQ) but specific learning disabilities can be seen. Ehlers-Danlos syndrome (EDS) is a connective tissue disorder that results in joint hypermobility; soft, stretchy "doughy" skin; and abnormal wound healing. (See Figures 17–11 and 17–12.) Joint dislocations and subluxations are common in EDS. There are several forms of the condition, identified as classic, hypermobile, vascular, arthrochalasia, dermatosparaxis, and kyphoscoliosis types. Individuals with classic-type EDS (formerly EDS 1 and EDS 2) have the typical skin and joint features. Those with vascular-type

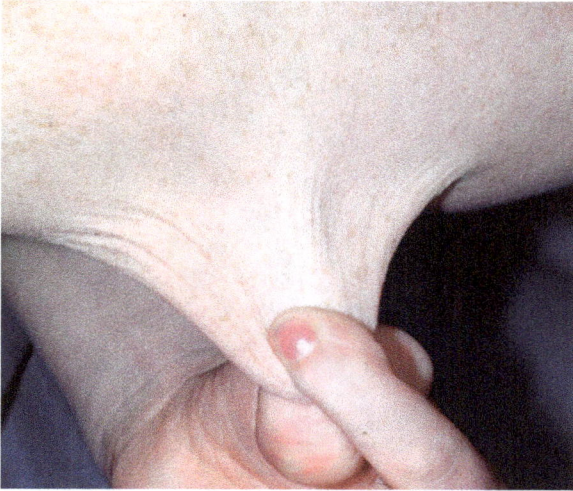

FIGURE 17–11. In Ehlers-Danlos syndrome, the skin is elastic, soft, and heals poorly. (Reproduced with permission from Goldsmith LA, Katz SI, Gilchrest BA, Paller AS, Leffell DJ, Wolff K, eds. *Fitzpatrick's Dermatology in General Medicine*. 8th ed. New York, NY: McGraw-Hill Education; 2012, Fig. 137-1.)

EDS (formerly EDS 4) are at increased risk for arterial rupture. Fragile X syndrome is the most common inherited cause of cognitive disability. It is an X-linked disorder, but both boys and girls can be affected. The condition is due to the expansion of trinucleotide (CGG) repeats in the *FMR1* gene when passed from a carrier mother to offspring. Boys with a large CGG repeat expansion (> 200 repeats) will have cognitive disability. Around 50% of girls with a large CGG repeat expansion will have cognitive disability due to skewing of X chromosome inactivation. Therefore, it is important to perform fragile X molecular testing on all

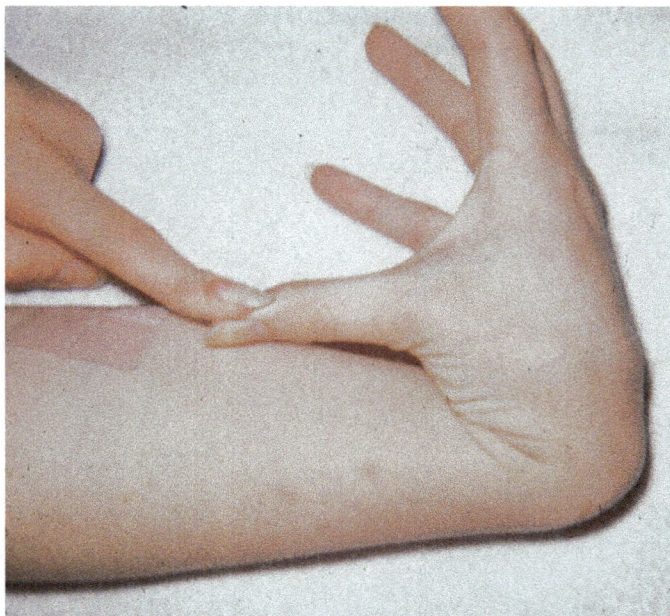

FIGURE 17–12. Joint laxity and hypermobility is associated with Ehlers-Danlos syndrome. (Reproduced with permission from Fuster V, Walsh RA, Harrington RA, eds. *Hurst's The Heart*. 13th ed. New York, NY: McGraw-Hill Education; 2011, Fig. 14-8 B.)

children (boys and girls) with cognitive disability. Other features include macrocephaly, large ears, and male macro-orchidism in adulthood. Anticipation may occur with fragile X syndrome and other trinucleotide repeat disorders. In genetic anticipation, the signs and symptoms of the disorder present earlier and become more severe with each successive generation.

Helpful Tip
Fragile X syndrome is the most common inherited cause of cognitive disability that may affect boys and girls despite being inherited in an X-linked fashion.

► CASE 13

You are evaluating a male infant for his 9-month health supervision visit. You find that he is near the 95th percentile for height, weight, and head circumference. His mother tells you that he was large for gestational age and had several episodes of neonatal hypoglycemia. On physical exam you notice that he has a large tongue and one of his legs is larger than the other in both girth and length. The abdominal exam is unremarkable.

Question 13-1
Which of the following screening tests should be performed?
A) Lead level.
B) Abdominal ultrasounds.
C) Bone age.
D) Serum alpha-fetoprotein (AFP).
E) Both B and D.

Discussion 13-1
The correct answer is "E." This infant likely has Beckwith-Wiedemann syndrome (BWS). Children with BWS are often large, with macroglossia and have distinctive earlobe creases. Hemihypertrophy of a limb, omphalocele, and diastasis recti are common. Neonatal hypoglycemia can occur but is usually transient. Children with BWS or isolated hemihypertrophy are at increased for developing embryonal tumors such as Wilms tumor and hepatoblastoma. The outcomes for children with the tumors are improved through early detection. Therefore, all children with BWS should have abdominal ultrasounds performed every 3 to 6 months until age 8 years, and serum AFP levels every 3 months until age 4 years. The same screening also applies to children with isolated hemihypertrophy.

► CASE 14

A 3-year-old girl with a history of autism and cognitive delays presents to the emergency department with a generalized seizure. On physical exam you notice several white patches on her skin. A computed tomography (CT) scan of the head reveals several calcified subependymal nodules in the brain.

FIGURE 17–13. Hypomelanotic macule, also known as an ash-leaf spot, is common in tuberous sclerosis complex. These spots are more obvious under Wood lamp examination. (Reproduced with permission from Wolff K, Johnson RA, Saavedra AP, eds. *Fitzpatrick's Color Atlas and Synopsis of Clinical Dermatology.* 7th ed. New York, NY: McGraw-Hill Education; 2013, Fig. 16-2 A, B.)

This girl likely has which of the following conditions?
A) Neurofibromatosis type 1.
B) Congenital toxoplasmosis.
C) Tuberous sclerosis complex.
D) Klippel-Feil syndrome.
E) Neurofibromatosis type 2.

Discussion 14-1

The correct answer is "C." This child has classic features of tuberous sclerosis complex (TSC). This condition results in benign central nervous system (CNS) tumors, including subependymal nodules and cortical tubers. However, malignant transformation can lead to subependymal astrocytoma. Seizures are common and some children have autism and developmental delay. Nonetheless there is a large degree of variability within this condition, and some individuals are very mildly affected. Characteristic skin lesions called hypomelanotic macules (also known as ash-leaf spots) are lightly pigmented and ovoid. (See Figure 17–13.) Tumors of the retina and kidney can also occur. Screening consists of monitoring for malignant transformation with cranial and renal imaging and developmental programing. Neurofibromatosis type 1 (NF1) is associated with skin lesion and CNS tumors; however, the skin lesions, known as café-au-lait spots, are hyperpigmented rather than hypopigmented. (See Figure 17–14.) Cutaneous neurofibromas and hamartomas (Lisch nodules) of the iris are common. Optic glioma can occur in childhood, and malignant nerve sheath tumors and pheochromocytoma are more common in adulthood. Around 40% to 50% of affected individuals have developmental or cognitive delays. Both NF1 and TSC may be inherited in an autosomal dominant fashion from an affected parent or may occur de novo. Owing to the extreme variability of both conditions, it is possible that a parent could be mildly affected and previously undiagnosed; this may lead to the false assumption that the disorder was secondary to a de novo event. Klippel-Feil syndrome is associated with a low posterior hairline and fusion of the cervical vertebrae, resulting in a short neck and torticollis. Malformations of the scapula (Sprengel deformity) can also occur. Neurofibromatosis type 2 (NF2) is largely associated with vestibular schwannoma occurring in adulthood and results in hearing loss and vertigo.

▶ CASE 15

A newborn infant boy is noticed at delivery to have absence of the left thumb and hypoplasia of the right thumb, with bowing of forearms. A loud systolic murmur is heard on exam. X-rays of the arms reveal bilateral radial hypoplasia. A chest X-ray is normal.

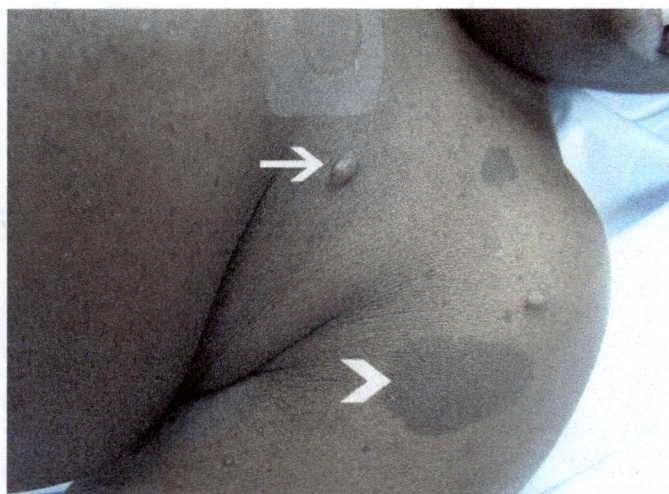

FIGURE 17–14. Café-au-lait spots are associated with neurofibromatosis type 1. The raised lumps in the photo are cutaneous neurofibromas. (Reproduced with permission from Fuster V, Walsh RA, Harrington RA (Eds). *Hurst's The Heart*, 13ed. McGraw-Hill Education, Inc., 2011. Fig 14-7.)

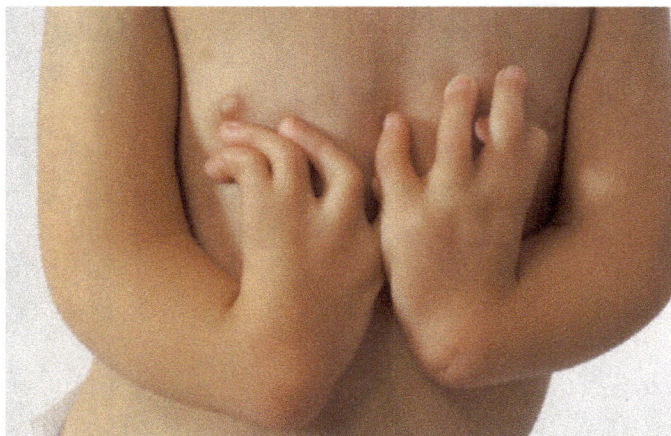

FIGURE 17–15. This child has severe bilateral radial ray hypoplasia. (Reproduced with permission from Lichtman MA, Shafer MS, Felgar RE, Wang N, eds. *Lichtman's Atlas of Hematology*. New York, NY: McGraw-Hill Education; 2007, Fig. XI.A.96.)

Question 15-1

This infant most likely has which of the following disorders?
A) Fanconi anemia.
B) Thrombocytopenia absent radius syndrome.
C) Diamond-Blackfan anemia.
D) Holt-Oram syndrome.
E) VACTERL association.

Discussion 15-1

The correct answer is "D." All of the disorders listed in options "A" through "E" can result in radial ray abnormalities, which are congenital deficiencies of radial bone in the forearm and the thumb. (See Figure 17–15.) It is important to be able to distinguish one from the other. Holt-Oram syndrome results in radial hypoplasia with thumb aplasia or hypoplasia along with an atrial or ventricular septal defect. Fanconi anemia often results in radial ray defects with hypoplastic thumbs and aplastic anemia later in childhood. Other findings may include short stature, café-au-lait spots, and developmental delays. Affected individuals have an increased risk of developing cancer, particularly if exposed to ionizing radiation. Thrombocytopenia absent radius (TAR) syndrome results in neonatal thrombocytopenia with absent or hypoplastic radii; however, the thumb is always present. Diamond-Blackfan anemia results in congenital anemia with thumb and radial hypoplasia. VACTERL association (**V**ertebral anomalies, **A**nal atresia, **C**ardiac defects, **T**racheo**E**sophageal fistula, **R**enal anomalies, and **L**imb deformities) often produces radial hypoplasia and must be included in the differential diagnosis for this infant. However, it is less likely than Holt-Oram to be the cause of this infant's anomalies given the normal chest X-ray.

⧗ QUICK QUIZ

Which syndrome is NOT associated with craniosynostosis?
A) Crouzon syndrome.
B) Trisomy 21.

C) Apert syndrome.
D) Pfeiffer syndrome.
E) Fetal hydantoin syndrome.
F) All of the above.

Discussion

The correct answer is "B." Craniosynostosis results from the premature fusion of one or more cranial sutures. Crouzon, Apert, and Pfeiffer syndromes are all autosomal dominant conditions characterized by craniosynostosis, shallow orbits, proptosis, hypertelorism, and high foreheads. Crouzon syndrome produces a beaked nose, frontal bossing, and midface hypoplasia. Apert syndrome results in a short anteroposterior diameter of the head, flat occiput, syndactyly (mitten hands), and developmental delay. Pfeiffer syndrome causes broad thumbs and great toes. Fetal hydantoin syndrome (also called fetal Dilantin syndrome) is characterized by poor growth, hypoplastic nails and distal phalanges, a broad nasal bridge, wide fontanelle, and metopic ridging. Mothers who take phenytoin (Dilantin) during pregnancy have a 10% of having a fetus with fetal hydantoin syndrome.

> **Helpful Tip**
> Craniosynostosis involving the sagittal, coronal, and lambdoid sutures results in a cloverleaf skull deformity.

⧗ QUICK QUIZ

Which karyotype listed below is associated with tall stature, behavioral problems, and poor school performance?
A) 47,XXX.
B) 47,XYY.
C) 47,XXY.
D) 46,XY.
E) 46,XX.

Discussion

The correct answer is "B." Males with an extra Y chromosome (47,XYY) tend to be tall, have a long face and large ears, and suffer from behavioral problems, including hyperactivity, distractibility, and temper tantrums. Females who are 47,XXX are typically tall, commonly have learning disabilities, and are uncoordinated. Fertility is normal for both 47,XYY and 47,XXX individuals. Option "C" is Klinefelter syndrome, option "D" is a normal male, and option "E" is a normal female.

▶ CASE 16

A 2-year-old boy is being evaluated in the genetic clinic. He has aniridia and hypospadias. He is developmentally delayed and is receiving early intervention services.

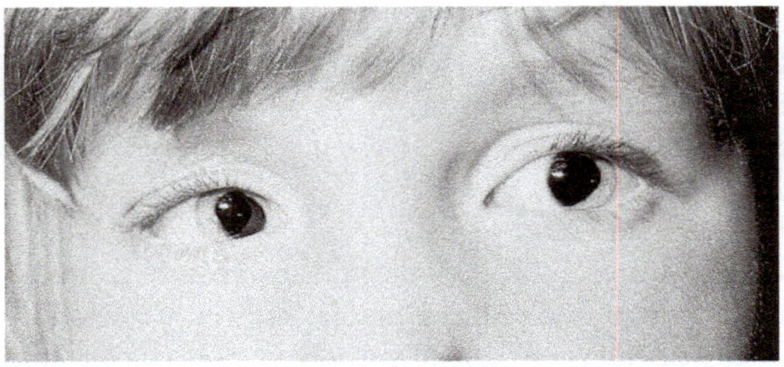

FIGURE 17–16. This child has bilateral aniridia. Small iris remnants are present temporally in each eye. Aniridia is associated with Wilms tumor due to a deletion in contiguous genes. (Reproduced with permission from Hay WW, Levin MJ, Deterding RR, Abzug MJ, eds. *Current Diagnosis and Treatment Pediatrics*. 22nd ed. New York, NY: McGraw-Hill Education; 2014, Fig. 16-21, p. 469.)

Question 16-1

You recommend screening for Wilms tumor. Why?
A) Children with aniridia are at increased risk for Wilms tumor.
B) Aniridia and Wilms tumor may occur together as part of a contiguous gene syndrome.
C) The association results from a deletion affecting a number of neighboring genes, including *PAX6*, the aniridia gene, and *WT1*, the Wilms tumor gene.
D) None of the above.
E) All of the above.

Discussion 16-1

The correct answer is "E." Contiguous gene syndromes result from gene abnormalities (usually deletions) that span more than one neighboring gene. WAGR syndrome (**W**ilms tumor, **A**niridia, **G**enitourinary anomalies, and mental **R**etardation) results from a large deletion of many individual genes that are located contiguously on chromosome 11. (See Figure 17–16.)

▶ CASE 17

A 6-year-old girl is referred to your clinic after failing the school hearing test. The mother has to repeat things to the child but attributes this to her "daydreaming" rather than hearing loss. The girl's face is narrow and flat, with downslanting palpebral fissures. There are clefts over her zygomatic bones. Her auricles are poorly formed, with a small external ear canal opening.

Question 17-1

This child most likely has which of the following disorders?
A) Treacher Collins syndrome.
B) Pierre Robin sequence.
C) Stickler syndrome.
D) Marshal syndrome.
E) Van der Woude syndrome.

Discussion 17-1

The correct answer is "A." Treacher Collins syndrome (mandibulofacial dysostosis) involves abnormal formation of the facial bones. It is characterized by malar and mandibular

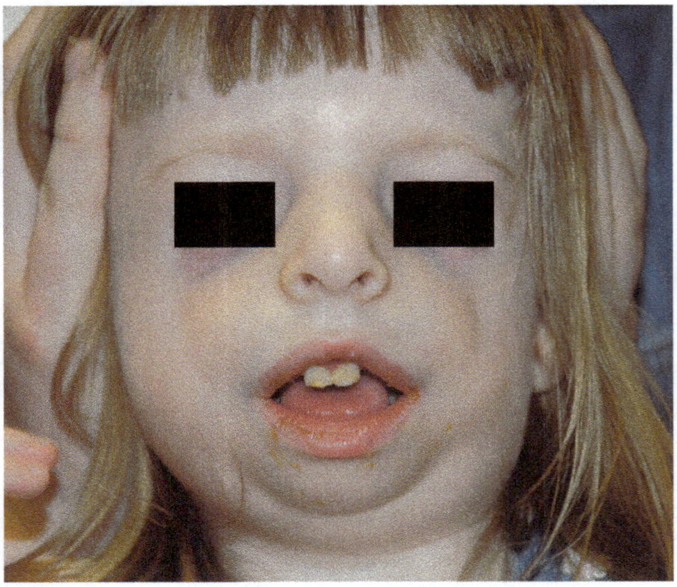

FIGURE 17–17. This girl has Treacher Collins syndrome. Notice the malar hypoplasia, downslanting palpebral fissures, zygomatic bone clefts, micrognathia, and absent lower eyelashes. (Reproduced with permission from Brunicardi FC, Andersen DK, Billiar TR, et al, eds. *Schwartz's Principles of Surgery*. 10th ed. New York, NY: McGraw-Hill Education; 2015, Fig 45-19 A, p. 1847.)

hypoplasia, zygomatic bone clefts, downslanting palpebral fissures, malformed external ears, and absent lower eyelashes. (See Figure 17–17.) Conduction hearing loss is common. The craniofacial anomalies may result in a narrow airway and respiratory distress requiring prone positioning or tracheostomy. Stickler syndrome involves midface and mandibular hypoplasia, high-degree myopia, flattened face with anteverted nares, and arthritis. Marshal syndrome is similar to Stickler syndrome with a flattened face, short depressed nose, anteverted nares, myopia, and eyes that appear to be large. Lower lip pits and cleft lip or palate, or both, are seen in van der Woude syndrome.

▶ CASE 18

A young mother is referred to you for prenatal genetic counseling. She is 20 weeks' pregnant and had a prenatal ultrasound last week that was normal. The fetus is moving well, and her pregnancy has been uncomplicated thus far. Her brother and maternal uncle have Duchenne muscular dystrophy (DMD). Last week at her ultrasound, she found out she is having a boy.

Question 18-1

What is the risk of her son being affected by DMD if the mother is a carrier?
A) 100%.
B) 50%.
C) 25%.
D) 10%.
E) 3%.

Discussion 18-1

The correct answer is "B." DMD is an X-linked recessive disorder. Only males are affected. X-linked traits are never passed from father to son. If a mother is a carrier, then 50% of her sons will be affected and 50% of her daughters will be carriers. This is illustrated by the Punnett square for X-linked recessive inheritance, shown below:

	X^{c} (carrier)	X
X	X^{c} X	X X
Y	X^{c} Y	X Y

The mother asks if there is any testing you can perform now to see if her son will be affected by DMD.

Question 18-2

Of the following, which is NOT an accurate reply to her question?
A) Prenatal ultrasound can identify anomalies and or malformations.
B) Chorionic villi sampling and amniocentesis may result in a spontaneous abortion.
C) The quad screen looks at alterations in serum markers to screen for specific genetic disorders such as trisomy 21.
D) Amniocentesis removes a small amount of amnionic fluid containing fetal cells that cultured for testing.
E) All prenatal screening tests are invasive.

Discussion 18-2

The correct answer is "E." Some prenatal screening tests (ultrasound, quad screen) identify fetuses at increased risk for a genetic condition or birth defect by means of noninvasive testing. Newer testing using cell-free fetal DNA from the mother's blood can screen for fetal aneuploidy, but fetal DNA must be detected. To determine if the disorder is present (yes/no), fetal tissue must be tested. This is called *prenatal diagnosis* and is often done using invasive procedures such as chorionic villi sampling, amniocentesis, or both. If these tests are inconclusive, umbilical cord blood sampling may be performed. This is a high-risk procedure and should be used in limited situations. The quad screen tests the levels of alpha-fetoprotein (AFP), estriol, human chorionic gonadotropin (beta-hCG), and inhibin A in the maternal blood. It is a screening test to identify fetuses at increased risk of having trisomies 21, 18, and 13. An elevated AFP may also indicate an open neural tube defect. Ultrasound may detect an increase in nuchal translucency (marker of chromosomal disorders) and congenital anomalies or malformation such as gastroschisis or clubfoot. In patients who undergo in vitro fertilization, embryos can be tested prior to uterine implantation to identify those free of a specific genetic condition. This is called *preimplantation genetic diagnosis*. No screening test is perfect. False positive test results may occur. To determine with certainty whether a genetic disorder is present, confirmatory fetal testing is required, but this requires invasive means that are not without risk, including fetal loss.

⧖ QUICK QUIZ

Which neuromuscular disorder is NOT correctly paired with its mode of inheritance?
A) Juvenile myotonic muscular dystrophy; autosomal dominant.
B) Spinal muscular atrophy; autosomal recessive.
C) Becker muscular dystrophy; X-linked dominant.
D) Congenital myotonic dystrophy; maternal transmission.
E) Mitochondrial myopathy; maternal transmission.

Discussion

The correct answer is "C." Becker's muscular dystrophy and Duchenne muscular dystrophy share a common genetic defect but Becker is a milder phenotype; therefore, both are X-linked recessive conditions. Congenital myotonic dystrophy is almost exclusively transmitted from the mother. Often the mother is unaware she has the disorder until after the newborn is diagnosed. Mitochondrial myopathies are maternally transmitted except those involving nuclear DNA, which follows autosomal dominant or recessive inheritance patterns.

▶ CASE 19

You see a 2-year-old boy in clinic because his mother has been concerned about his poor language development. At 27 months he uses three words that all pertain to his favorite talking train show and does not form sentences. He gets his mother attention by pulling her hand and does not point or use other gestures. He is unable to follow single-step commands and rarely turns in response to his name. During your evaluation you notice that he has poor eye contact, is self-directed, and is fascinated with turning the handle of the door. His motor skills are within the normal range and he is normally grown. On physical exam he is a handsome toddler with no dysmorphic features. There is no family history of pregnancy loss, autism, or developmental delay. An earlier audiogram was normal. You suspect that the child has autism.

Question 19-1

Following a formal diagnosis of autism, which genetic test would be most indicated?
A) Fluorescent in situ hybridization (FISH) for 7q11 deletion.
B) Microarray comparative genomic hybridization (CGH).
C) Molecular testing for fragile X syndrome.
D) Karyotype.
E) DNA sequencing of the *PTPN11* gene.
F) Next-generation sequencing panel for autism.
G) Whole exome sequencing.
H) Both B and C.
I) Both D and A.
J) None of the above.

Discussion 19-1

The correct answer is "H." This autistic child is normally grown and has no dysmorphic features; therefore, he has nonsyndromic autism. The standard care of care for the genetic diagnosis of nonsyndromic autism or intellectual disability, or both, is the combination of microarray CGH and fragile X molecular testing (polymerase chain reaction [PCR] and Southern blot). This combination of testing is used when a specific condition is not strongly suspected by history or physical exam. Both males and females should undergo fragile X testing as 50% of females with a full expansion will have intellectual disability. Microarray CGH is a new technology that surveys the entire genome for copy number variation (chromosomal deletions and duplications). This technology has completely replaced karyotype as the diagnostic method of choice for the following indications: autism, intellectual disability, syndromic short stature, dysmorphic features, and congenital anomalies. Microarray CGH will only detect unbalanced genomic abnormalities; therefore, karyotype still has a role in the prenatal and preconception settings looking for balanced rearrangements that would predispose a carrier parent to having a child with an unbalanced karyotype. These balanced rearrangements include translocations and inversions. Karyotype is also used to confirm the common trisomy disorders (21, 18, 13) when suspected clinically. These aneuploidies can be detected by microarray CGH but karyotype is more cost effective for this indication. FISH for 7q11 would look for Williams syndrome; however, nothing in this case suggests that specific syndrome. FISH has a very limited role in the genetic diagnosis of children; this technology should only be used to

TABLE 17–1 CONSIDERATIONS IN GENETIC TESTING

Test	Pros	Cons
Karyotype	Whole genomic approach Can detect balanced abnormalities that may predispose that carrier to pregnancy loss or an unbalanced offspring Used in the prenatal setting for detection of aneuploidy	Very low resolution, so only large structural rearrangements are seen
Microarray comparative genomic hybridization (CGH)	Whole genomic approach High resolution; can detect small copy number variants, including all known chromosomal microdeletion and duplication syndromes New arrays can detect exon-level deletions/duplications	Will not detect balanced rearrangements Small variants may have unknown significance May detect normal variation Only detects copy number variation; will not detect DNA point mutations
Fluorescent in situ hybridization (FISH) for specific locus	Looks in high resolution at specific disease-associated regions (eg, Williams syndrome) Should not give variants of unknown significance	Only assays a single chromosomal region Only detects copy number variation; will not detect DNA point mutations
DNA sequencing	Looks for specific point mutations in a suspected gene Used when a specific gene is suspected clinically	May miss small non–sequence-based DNA changes such as small deletions or trinucleotide repeats Only looks at a single gene at a time Will not detect copy number variations
Next-generation DNA sequencing panels	Can look for DNA sequence changes in many genes at the same time based on phenotype (eg, autism)	May miss small non–sequence-based DNA changes such as small deletions or trinucleotide repeats Will not detect copy number variations Expensive
Whole exome sequencing	Can assay all known genes in one test Excellent test for difficult cases in which other tests have been negative	Relatively low sensitivity to specific DNA changes Difficult bioinformatics and interpretation May miss small non–sequence-based DNA changes such as small deletions or trinucleotide repeats Will not detect copy number variations Expensive

confirm a chromosomal microdeletion or duplication syndrome when a specific syndrome such as Williams or 22q11 deletion is strongly suspected. Microarray CGH will also diagnose these conditions as well as many others and therefore is a better first-line test in most cases. DNA sequencing of *PTPN11* would test for Noonan syndrome; again, nothing in this vignette is suggestive of that condition. DNA sequencing of a specific gene is performed when a condition that is suspected is caused by a DNA point mutation. Recently, next-generation DNA sequencing panels have become available. These panels allow for the sequencing of many genes (in some cases hundreds) at the same time. This approach is useful when the condition has many separate genetic causes that are indistinguishable clinically, such as autism, hearing loss, or epilepsy, or when many genes all cause the same syndrome, as in Noonan syndrome. An autism panel might be a good second step but the initial testing should be microarray CGH and fragile X syndrome molecular testing as these tests have higher yield. Finally, whole exome sequencing allows for sequencing of the entire protein coding areas (exons) of the genome. This technology is used when a specific condition or syndrome is not suspected clinically and other tests such as microarray CGH are negative. Table 17–1 describes commonly performed genetic tests.

BIBLIOGRAPHY

Allanson JE, Roberts AE. Noonan syndrome. (2001 Nov 15 [Updated 2011 Aug 4].) In: Pagon RA, Adam MP, Ardinger HH, et al, eds. *GeneReviews* [Internet]. Seattle, WA: University of Washington, Seattle; 1993–2015. http://www.ncbi.nlm.nih.gov/books/NBK1124/

Bondy CA. Care of girls and women with Turner syndrome: A guideline of the Turner Syndrome Study Group. *J Clin Endocrinol Metab.* 2007;92(1):10–25.

Bull MJ. Health supervision for children with Down syndrome. *Pediatrics.* 2011;128(2):393–406.

Dean JCS. Marfan syndrome: Clinical diagnosis and management. *Eur J Hum Genet.* 2007;15(7):724–733.

Friedman JM. Neurofibromatosis 1. (1998 Oct 2 [Updated 2014 Sep 4].) In: Pagon RA, Adam MP, Ardinger HH, et al, eds. *GeneReviews* [Internet]. Seattle, WA: University of Washington, Seattle; 1993–2015. http://www.ncbi.nlm.nih.gov/books/NBK1109/

Hoyme HE, May PA, Kalberg WO, et al. A practical clinical approach to diagnosis of fetal alcohol spectrum disorders: Clarification of the 1996 Institute of Medicine criteria. *Pediatrics.* 2005;115(1):39–47.

Jones KL. *Smith's Recognizable Patterns of Human Malformation.* 6th ed. Philadelphia, PA: Elsevier; 2006.

McDonald-McGinn DM, Emanuel BS, Zackai EH. 22q11.2 deletion syndrome. (1999 Sep 23 [Updated 2013 Feb 28].) In: Pagon RA, Adam MP, Ardinger HH, et al, eds. *GeneReviews* [Internet]. Seattle, WA: University of Washington, Seattle; 1993–2015. http://www.ncbi.nlm.nih.gov/books/NBK1523/

Miles JH. Autism spectrum disorders—a genetics review. *Gen. Med.* 2011;13(4):278–294.

Saul RA, Tarleton JC. FMR1-related disorders. (1998 Jun 16 [Updated 2012 Apr 26].) In: Pagon RA, Adam MP, Ardinger HH, et al, eds. *GeneReviews* [Internet]. Seattle, WA: University of Washington, Seattle; 1993–2015. http://www.ncbi.nlm.nih.gov/books/NBK1384/

Solomon BD, Muenke M. When to suspect a genetic syndrome. *Am Fam Physician.* 2012;86(9):826.

Online Resources

GeneReviews: http://www.ncbi.nlm.nih.gov/books/NBK1116

Online Mendelian Inheritance in Man (OMIM): http://www.ncbi.nlm.nih.gov/omim

Genital System Disorders

Kathleen Kieran

18

▶ CASE 1

An 8-month-old girl presents with a 2-day history of increasing fussiness, fevers (the highest is 39.8°C [103.6°F]), and decreasing oral intake. Her parents note that she has been feeding less frequently and in smaller volumes, and she has had fewer wet diapers than usual. They also report that she has had several febrile episodes in the past and has been treated for ear infections. Her urine has also been quite foul-smelling over the last day. On examination, she is crying loudly and warm to the touch. Her blood pressure is normal, and perfusion is fine. She does not have tears. She is very uncooperative with the examination, but appears to have more discomfort when the right flank is palpated. You suspect a urinary tract infection.

Question 1-1

Which of the following is the most appropriate method to use in collecting urine for a sample?
A) Voided urine into a bag adhered to the perineum, because the child is not toilet trained.
B) Midstream urine collection, because the female urethra has commensal microorganisms.
C) Catheterized urine sample, because a voided sample may be contaminated.
D) Suprapubic aspirate, because catheterization may be traumatic for the child.
E) No urine collection is needed prior to initiation of therapy, because the child is oliguric and ill.

Discussion 1-1

The correct answer is "C." Bag urine specimens, while convenient, may be associated with false positive urinalyses if the perineum is not well cleansed prior to specimen acquisition. Cultures from bag specimens are only helpful if negative. Midstream urine collections, while feasible in older children, would require knowledge of when the child would void, an ability to clean the urethra, and an ability to catch midstream urine, which would be challenging in a non–toilet-trained child. The parents would win an award if able to catch a pee sample from an infant. Catheterization, when performed correctly, is associated with a low risk of contamination and is not traumatic for the child (particularly before the age of genital awareness). Suprapubic aspiration (SPA) is the method least likely to be associated with contamination, but this procedure is not commonly performed and some practitioners may not be facile or comfortable with it. Urine cultures should be collected by SPA or catheterization. Unless the child has clear signs of hemodynamic instability (not present in this scenario), urine should be collected prior to the initiation of antimicrobial therapy to confirm the suspected diagnosis of urinary tract infection (UTI) and to guide antimicrobial therapy. Although antibiotic susceptibility panels may not return until 72 hours after the urine is cultured, community prevalence of certain bacterial species and antibiograms showing local antibiotic resistance patterns are usually available within institutions.

> **Helpful Tip**
> In, 2011 the American Academy of Pediatrics (AAP) published clinical practice guidelines for diagnosis and management of the *first* UTI in febrile infants and children aged 2 to 24 months old. If a UTI is suspected, a clinician has two choices: (1) obtain urine for culture and urinalysis via SPA or catheterization, or (2) obtain a bag urine specimen for urinalysis. If abnormal (positive for leukocyte esterase, microscopic pyuria, or positive for nitrites), a catheterized or SPA culture should be collected. A bag urine specimen should never be sent for culture.

Question 1-2

Which is NOT a risk factor for a UTI?
A) African American race.
B) Fever ≥ 39°C (102.2°F).
C) Uncircumcised.
D) Fever without an alternative source of infection.
E) Female gender.

Discussion 1-2

The correct answer is "A." Five percent of febrile infants with no identified fever source will have a UTI. Nonblack or white race is a risk factor. Girls are at higher risk than boys. Uncircumcised boys are at higher risk than those who are circumcised. Age younger than 12 months is also a risk factor.

A catheterized urine sample is collected.

Question 1-3

Assuming this infant has a UTI, which of the following urinalyses is most likely to be seen when her urine is evaluated?

A) Specific gravity 1.010, 2+ leukocyte esterase, negative nitrites, negative ketones; microscopy shows 2–3 white blood cells (WBCs)/high-power field (hpf) and 5–10 RBCs/hpf.

B) Specific gravity 1.015, negative leukocyte esterase, negative nitrites, negative ketones; microscopy shows 2–3 WBCs/hpf and 1–2 RBCs/hpf.

C) Specific gravity 1.020, 2+ leukocyte esterase, negative nitrites, 3+ ketones; microscopy shows 5–10 WBCs/hpf and 5–10 RBCs/hpf.

D) Specific gravity 1.025, 2+ leukocyte esterase, positive nitrites, negative ketones; microscopy shows 3–5 WBCs/hpf and 0–3 RBCs/hpf.

E) Specific gravity 1.025, 3+ leukocyte esterase, positive nitrites, 3+ ketones; microscopy shows 30–50 WBCs/hpf and 15–20 RBCs/hpf.

Discussion 1-3

The correct answer is "E." The vignette describes a child who is dehydrated, with poor oral intake and decreased urine output; this would be consistent with a higher urine specific gravity and the presence of ketones in the urine. Leukocyte esterase is an enzyme produced by WBCs; thus, its presence would be associated with WBCs on microscopy. Pyuria (defined as 5 or more WBCs/hpf), rather than hematuria, is the most sensitive and specific marker for UTI. Gram-negative bacteria, which are the most common etiologic agents for UTIs, convert nitrates to nitrites. Although a urinalysis for a child with a UTI may not show nitrites, typically this occurs when the causal organism is not a gram-negative bacterium or when the urine is collected quickly after the suspicion of a UTI has been established (conversion of nitrates to nitrates can take up to 4 hours).

Question 1-4

What is NOT a diagnostic criterion for a UTI in a febrile infant or child aged 2 to 24 months?

A) Diagnosis of a UTI requires an abnormal urinalysis.

B) A positive urine culture is ≥ 50,000 colony-forming units of a single, urinary pathogen.

C) Urine culture must be obtained by adequate means.

D) Urine does not need to be fresh to perform a urinalysis.

E) Smelly urine is all that is needed.

Discussion 1-4

The correct answer is "D." Urine specimens need to be freshly collected (< 1 hour at room temperature or < 4 hours if refrigerated) and processed. To diagnosis a UTI, both pyuria or bacteruria on urinalysis and a positive urine culture are required. This avoids unnecessary treatment of asymptomatic bacteruria. One would imagine that most practitioners are not routinely trained in urine sniffing.

Question 1-5

The organism that is associated with most UTIs in otherwise healthy children is:

A) *Escherichia coli.*

B) *Pseudomonas aeruginosa.*

C) *Enterococcus faecalis.*

D) *Streptococcus pneumoniae.*

E) *Streptococcus viridans.*

Discussion 1-5

The correct answer is "A." *E. coli* remains the most common organism causing UTIs.

The girl undergoes a voiding cystourethrogram (VCUG) after her UTI has been appropriately treated. The images show grade V vesicoureteral reflux.

Question 1-6

What is the next step in management?

A) Observation.

B) Trimethoprim-sulfamethoxazole 2 mg/kg once daily.

C) Amoxicillin 20 mg/kg three times daily.

D) DMSA renal scan.

E) Surgical correction.

Discussion 1-6

The correct answer is "B." Reflux is graded on a scale from I to V, with I being reflux into the ureter alone, II being reflux into the calyces with preservation of the calyceal architecture, III being reflux into the calyces with blunting of the calyces, IV being mild ureteral tortuosity, and V being severe ureteral tortuosity. More recent publications have suggested that other radiographic findings, such as distal ureteral diameter, and timing of reflux during the micturition cycle, may refine the predictive value of reflux grade for spontaneous resolution. A meta-analysis cited in the AAP recommendations noted that antibiotic prophylaxis was associated with a decreased risk of UTI recurrence in children with grade V reflux. Among children with a lower grade of reflux, no significant differences in UTI recurrence rates were observed in children prescribed antibiotic prophylaxis compared with those who were not, but factors such as compliance may account for these findings. Amoxicillin is typically used for antibiotic prophylaxis in children younger than 2 months of age, since the immature neonatal liver may be unable to conjugate trimethoprim-sulfamethoxazole (Bactrim) for elimination, resulting in jaundice. The volume of distribution for amoxicillin is the entire body, whereas trimethoprim-sulfamethoxazole concentrates in the urine, allowing a lower dose to be given in order to achieve a locally active antibiotic concentration. DMSA (dimercaptosuccinic acid) renal scans are not endorsed as part of the routine evaluation of a child with vesicoureteral reflux but

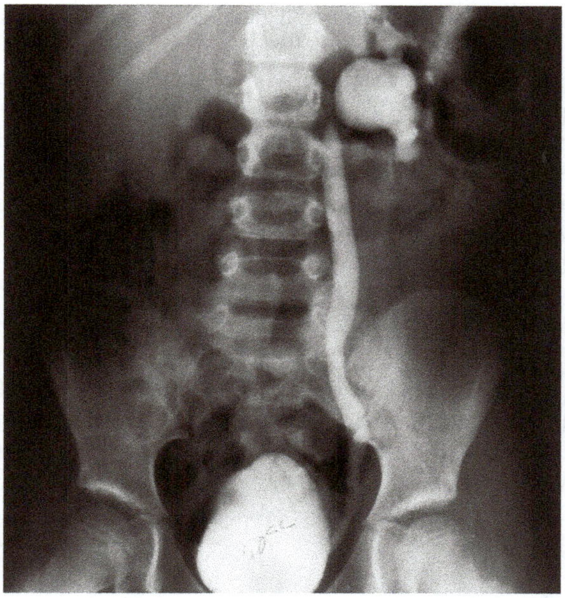

FIGURE 18–1. Vesicoureteral reflux, urine moving from bladder into the upper urinary tract, is evaluated with a voiding cystourethrogram (VCUG). It is graded by level of urinary reflux and dilation as follows: Grade I—reflux into ureter only; grade II—reflux into ureter and renal pelvis; grade III—reflux with dilation of the ureter and renal pelvis; grade IV—reflux with dilation of the ureter and renal pelvis with blunting of the calyces; and grade IV—massive reflux with tortuous dilation of the ureter. Left-sided grade IV vesicoureteral reflux is shown in this image. (Reproduced with permission from Doherty GM, ed. *Current Diagnosis & Treatment: Surgery*. 14th ed. New York, NY: McGraw-Hill Education; 2015, Fig. 38-7.)

may be helpful to identify children with renal scars or decreased renal function. Surgical correction is generally reserved for children who have failed conservative management (ie, those who develop breakthrough UTIs on antibiotic prophylaxis or are unable to comply with antibiotic prophylaxis), or who show signs of renal damage; it is not first-line therapy for the management of vesicoureteral reflux. (See Figure 18–1.) Make note that according to the AAP, a VCUG is not routinely needed. After the *first* UTI, a renal ultrasound should be performed. If abnormal, then a VCUG should be obtained.

Question 1-7

Parents of children with vesicoureteral reflux should be counseled that:

A) VCUGs should be performed in all siblings as there is a 75% prevalence of reflux in first-degree relatives of children with reflux.

B) Surgical correction of the reflux will prevent the child from getting another UTI until at least adulthood.

C) Prophylactic antibiotics will not change the risk of renal scarring.

D) Optimized elimination habits are associated with fewer UTIs and a higher rate of reflux resolution.

E) Resolution rates in secondary vesicoureteral reflux reflect the reflux severity and laterality as well as the age and gender of the child.

Discussion 1-7

The correct answer is "D." When discussing the management of vesicoureteral reflux with parents, it is important to differentiate between UTIs and vesicoureteral reflux. In many cases, particularly in toilet-trained children, UTI risk can be decreased markedly by managing constipation, increasing fluid intake, and promoting frequent urination. Although poor elimination habits (holding it) have been associated with persistence of vesicoureteral reflux, only very high-grade reflux has been shown to be independently associated with an increased risk of UTI. If these habits persist, the child will continue to be at risk for lower tract UTIs even after correction of the reflux. Prophylactic antibiotics are associated with the same or decreased risk of UTI (depending on the reflux grade), and since renal scarring has been shown to occur only in the presence of infected urine, may protect kidneys from the development of new scars. Between 25% and 33% of siblings of children with reflux have been found to have reflux as well; the variation in prevalence reflects children who were screened without symptoms compared with those who underwent imaging based on infection or other symptoms. Presently, a renal ultrasound is recommended for siblings of children with reflux, with a VCUG to follow if renal anatomic abnormalities are identified. Siblings with no renal structural abnormalities who develop UTIs should be managed according to current AAP guidelines. Children with reflux should be carefully evaluated for secondary reflux, in which lower urinary tract abnormalities (eg, neurogenic bladder related to myelomeningocele, or myogenic bladder secondary to posterior urethral valves), rather than an anatomic abnormality at the ureterovesical junction, is the underlying causal factor. Most cases of low-grade primary vesicoureteral reflux resolve spontaneously.

> **Helpful Tip**
> Voiding dysfunction has been associated with an increased risk of UTIs and delayed (and decreased) resolution rates for vesicoureteral reflux. Be sure to ask toilet-trained children about their elimination habits.

> **Helpful Tip**
> Recurrent UTIs are associated with renal scarring. Early antibiotic treatment is better than late. Caregivers need to seek immediate care for future febrile illnesses to evaluate for a repeat UTI.

► CASE 2

A 28-year-old G1P0 (now 1) mother has just given birth to a 6 pound, 7 ounce infant at 39-4/7 weeks' gestation. The pregnancy was uncomplicated and the labor progressed appropriately. The mother underwent several prenatal ultrasounds, all of which showed normal levels of amniotic fluid and no fetal anomalies, but chose not to be informed

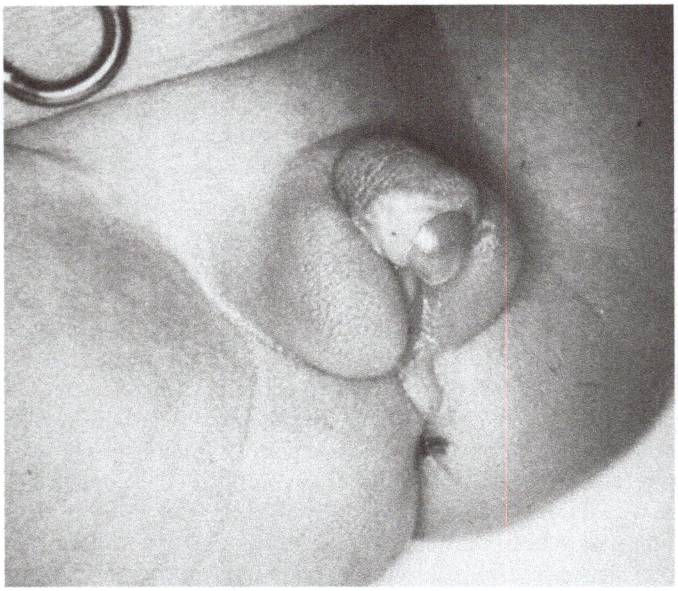

FIGURE 18–2. Ambiguous genitalia in congenital adrenal hyperplasia. The girl in this picture has congenital adrenal hyperplasia with ambiguous external genitalia resulting from excess adrenal androgens. The scrotolabial folds are fused, the clitoris is enlarged, and a penile urethra has formed. No testes will be palpable, suggesting a disorder of sexual differentiation. Males with congenital adrenal hyperplasia have normal external genitalia. (Reproduced with permission from Brunicardi FC, Andersen DK, Billiar TR, et al, eds. *Schwartz's Principles of Surgery*. 10th ed. New York, NY: McGraw-Hill Education; 2015, Fig. 39-36.)

of her baby's gender. On examination, the infant has a good cry and Apgar scores of 8 at 1 minute and 9 at 5 minutes. The abdomen is soft. The genitalia are not clearly male or female. (See Figure 18–2.)

Question 2-1

What is the primary concern when evaluating this infant?
A) Blood pressure.
B) Electrolyte levels.
C) Urine output.
D) Oral intake.
E) Respiratory distress.

Discussion 2-1

The correct answer is "B." In any infant with external genitalia that cannot be definitively categorized as male or female, congenital adrenal hyperplasia (CAH) must be excluded. CAH is the most common cause of disorders of sexual differentiation in newborns. There are several different enzyme deficiencies that may be associated with CAH; in the most common, 21-hydroxylase deficiency, a lack of the 21-hydroxylase enzyme results in a relative excess of 17-hydroxyprogesterone (17-OHP) and shunting of the intermediate products into the sex steroid pathway, resulting in masculinization. Cortisol and aldosterone production are decreased while androstenedione and dehydroepiandrosterone (DHEA) production are increased. Secretion of adrenocorticotropic hormone (ACTH) increases in response to

low cortisol, resulting in adrenal gland enlargement. Inadequate mineralocorticoid production results in salt-wasting crisis with hyponatremia, hyperkalemia, hypovolemia, and cardiovascular collapse if untreated. Classic CAH (no enzyme activity) presents at birth while nonclassic milder forms (partial enzyme activity) present later in childhood. Because of the frequency of CAH and its potentially severe consequences, CAH testing is included on newborn panels for early identification. (See Figures 18–2 and 18–3.)

> **Helpful Tip**
> Newborn boys with classic CAH have normal genitalia. Without newborn screening, they are undiagnosed until presenting with a salt wasting crisis at 1 to 2 weeks of age with significant weight loss, dehydration, hyponatremia, and hyperkalemia.

Question 2-2

What is the inheritance pattern of the most common form of this condition?
A) Autosomal dominant.
B) Autosomal recessive.
C) X-linked dominant.
D) X-linked recessive.
E) Sporadic.

Discussion 2-2

The correct answer is "B." The gene encoding 21-hydroxylase is on chromosome 6p, adjacent to the human leukocyte antigen (HLA) genes, and 21-hydroxylase deficiency is inherited as an autosomal recessive trait. Some rare cases are transmitted as a new mutation or as mutations on chromosomes other than chromosome 6.

Question 2-3

How is CAH diagnosed?
A) Elevated blood 17-hydroxyprogesterone.
B) ACTH stimulation test.
C) Newborn screening.
D) Elevated amnionic 17-hydroxyprogesterone.
E) All of the above.

Discussion 2-3

The correct answer is "E." A very high level of 17-OHP in the blood is diagnostic of CAH. If 17-OHP is only mildly elevated, an ACTH stimulation test should be performed. The level of 17-OHP will increase and cortisol will remain low. In children with salt-wasting, serum renin will be elevated and aldosterone low.

Question 2-4

11-beta-hydroxylase deficiency is associated with:
A) Hypertension.
B) Hypokalemia.
C) Hyperglycemia.
D) Hypotonia.
E) Elevated transaminases.

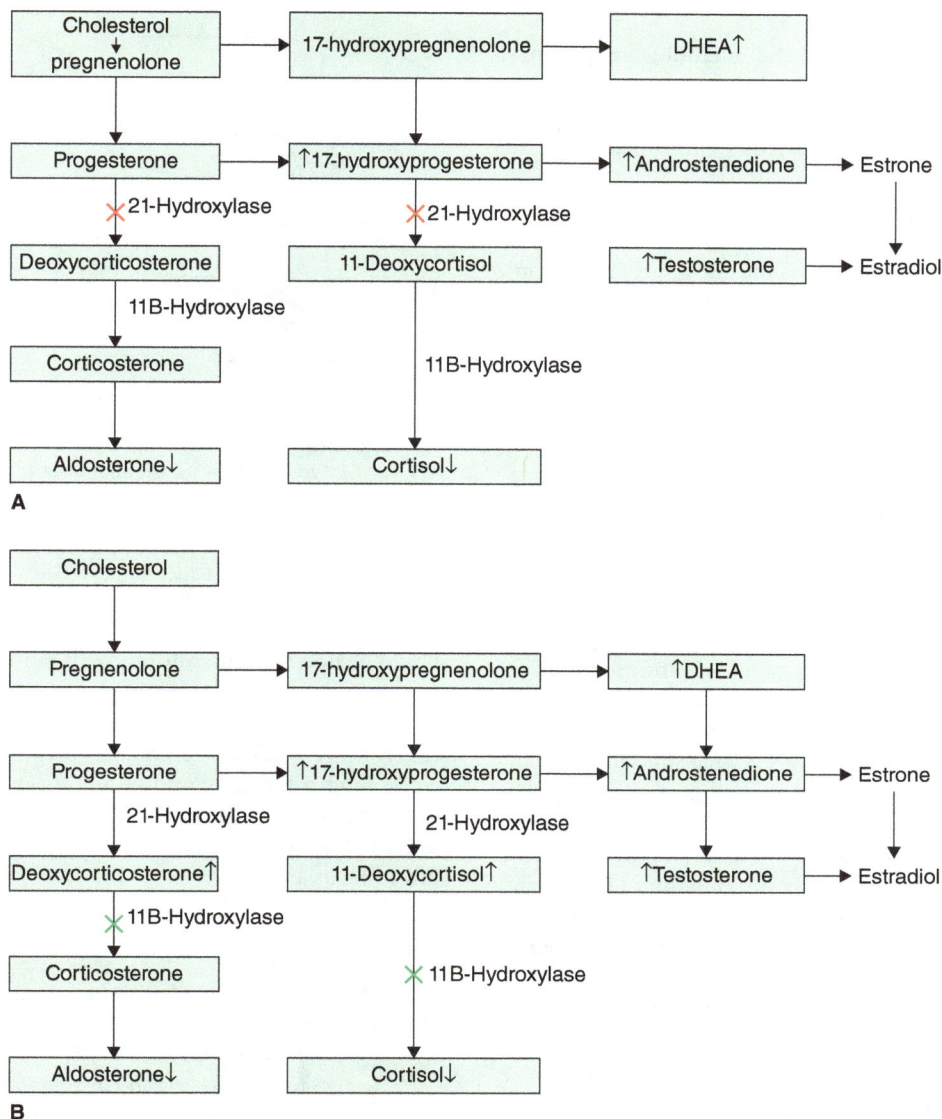

FIGURE 18–3. Depicted is the pathway of adrenal synthesis of mineralocorticoids, glucocorticoids, and adrenal androgens and changes seen in congenital adrenal hyperplasia (CAH). (A) Classic CAH is due to 21-hydroxylase deficiency (*red X*) with excess adrenal androgens and deficiency of cortisol and aldosterone. (B) Less commonly, CAH is due to 11-beta-hydroxylase deficiency (*green X*) with excess adrenal androgens, cortisol deficiency but preserved mineralocorticoid function from high levels of deoxycorticosterone. DHEA, dehydroepiandrosterone.

Discussion 2-4

The correct answer is "A." 11-Beta-hydroxylase deficiency is the second most common cause of congenital adrenal hyperplasia, resulting in cortisol deficiency, excess adrenal androgens, and preserved mineralocorticoid function. In 11-beta-hydroxylase deficiency, corticosterone cannot be synthesized from 11-deoxycorticosterone owing to the missing enzyme. Deoxycorticosterone is a weak mineralocorticoid, but when present in large amounts, contributes to salt and water retention as well as high blood pressure. In 11-beta-hydroxylase deficiency, 17-OHP levels are normal and 11-deoxycortisol and deoxycorticosterone are elevated. Children with 11-beta-hydroxylase deficiency are also at risk for *hypo*glycemia since glucocorticoid synthesis cannot be completed. (See Figure 18–3, earlier.)

▶ CASE 3

A twin newborn male is born after a dichorionic, diamniotic pregnancy that was otherwise uncomplicated. He and his brother were born at 36 weeks' gestation following an uncomplicated normal spontaneous vaginal delivery. He weighs 5 pounds, 3 ounces, and his brother weighs 7 pound, 5 ounces. His Apgar scores were 8 at 1 minute and 9 at 5 minutes. On examination, he is found to have a dorsal hooded foreskin and the urethral meatus is noted at the ventral midshaft. The testes are bilaterally descended and palpably normal and there are no hernias or hydroceles. His brother has normal Tanner 1 male external genitalia with a circumferentially intact foreskin. The parents request that both boys be circumcised.

Question 3-1

Which of the following should be included in parental counseling?

A) Prior to circumcision, he should undergo a renal ultrasound and VCUG to exclude any coexisting abnormalities of the genitourinary tract.

B) Circumcision should be deferred in boys with hypospadias.

C) The AAP recommends neonatal circumcision for all boys (unless there is a religious or cultural contraindication), because this significantly reduces the risk of penile cancer and transmission of viruses such as human immunodeficiency virus (HIV) and human papillomavirus (HPV).

D) Neonatal circumcision can be safely performed without anesthetic as newborns do not feel pain and the benefits of anesthesia are outweighed by the risks.

E) He should undergo hormonal testing prior to circumcision to rule out a disorder of sexual differentiation.

Discussion 3-1

The correct answer is "B." Hypospadias is seen in approximately 0.33% of newborn boys (although this proportion may be variable since mild forms may not be captured, and home births may not be included). It is a congenital anomaly in which the urethral meatus is located on the ventral penile shaft rather than the tip of the glans. Don't forget that in anatomic position the penis is erect. In most cases, hypospadias occurs as a sporadic disorder. There are several theories regarding its development, including failure of the glanular urethra to recanalize and failure of the ventral glans and prepuce to close. Hereditary factors and endocrine disruptors may be associated with an increased risk of hypospadias. The phallus forms at 10 weeks and the remainder of the genitourinary tract at 6 weeks; because the external genitalia and the remainder of the genitourinary system form at different times, evaluation for coexisting abnormalities is not necessary in the absence of findings such as prenatal hydronephrosis. Similarly, evaluation for disorders of sexual differentiation is undertaken when there is an abnormality of the gonad (eg, undescended testis), severe hypospadias, or evidence of other hormonal abnormalities. In particular, children with bilateral undescended testes with a phallic structure should be evaluated for possible congenital adrenal hyperplasia, regardless of whether or not hypospadias is also present. (See Figure 18–4.) The exact method used to repair hypospadias is dependent on many factors, including the tissue quality, meatal location, and coexisting abnormalities (eg, chordee), but circumcision is generally deferred in order to preserve the prepuce for possible repair should this tissue be needed. (Prepuce is a fancy way of saying foreskin.) As neonatal circumcision is associated with a decreased risk of HPV and HIV transmission later in life and the risk of penile cancer is substantially lower in circumcised males, the AAP feels the benefits outweigh the potential risks and that families should have access to the procedure, including insurance coverage. However, the AAP has stopped short of routine endorsement of circumcision for all infants. When neonatal circumcision is performed, local anesthetic with a penile block should be employed; sugar water alone may be an adjunct to but is not a substitute for anesthesia. Circumcision

A. Phimosis   **B. Paraphimosis**

C. Hypospadias   **D. Epispadias**

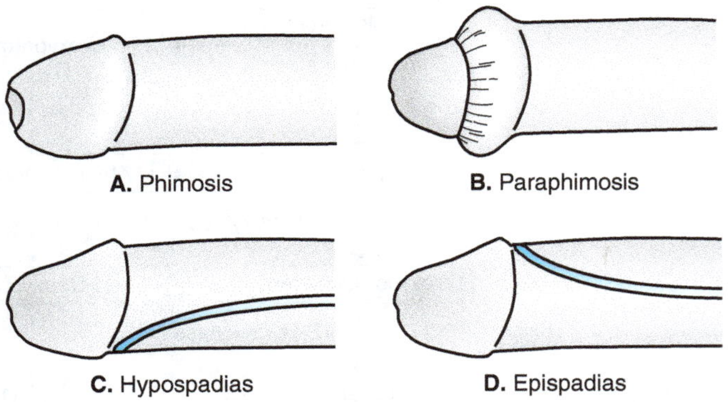

FIGURE 18–4. Abnormalities of the Foreskin. (A) Phimosis—the foreskin is tight and cannot be retracted over the glans penis. (B) Paraphimosis—the foreskin has been retracted over the glans and cannot be reduced, causing swelling. (C) Hypospadias—the urethral meatus opens on the ventral side (underside) of the penis. (D) Epispadias—the urethral meatus opens on the dorsal side (top) of the penis. (Reproduced with permission from LeBlond RF, Brown DD, Suneja M, Szot JF, eds. *DeGowin's Diagnostic Examination*. 10th ed. New York, NY: McGraw-Hill Education; 2015, Fig. 12-7A-D.)

should be deferred in children with penile abnormalities that may necessitate reconstructive surgery, such as chordee, buried penis, micropenis (a penis that, when stretched, had a length more than two standard deviations below the mean penile length for age), and penile torsion. Boys with micropenis should also be assessed for endocrine abnormalities, particularly hypopituitarism, and the position of the testes should be assessed.

> **Helpful Tip**
>
> Not all hypospadias repairs require the foreskin for reconstruction. However, generally the prepuce is left in place so that it is available for urethral reconstruction or skin coverage at the time of repair. Rarely, the foreskin may be circumferentially intact and the meatus located abnormally ventrally; this is called a megameatus with intact prepuce.

▶ CASE 4

A 4-year-old girl has a history of daytime urinary incontinence for the last 6 months. The incontinence has waxed and waned, and some days she is able to stay completely dry but has never been dry for more than a day or two at a time. She also has nocturnal enuresis every night and has never been dry at night. Her parents state that she was toilet trained at 2.5 years old. They report that she often is seen squatting with her heel in her perineum. Her daytime wetting is associated with urinary urgency, and she often runs to the bathroom when she has to void, only to leak urine as she is pulling down her pants. Her parents are quite frustrated because some of the other children have started to make fun of her at school when the wetting accidents occur.

Question 4-1

Which of the following is the most appropriate next step in evaluation and treatment?

A) Renal ultrasound.
B) Voiding cystourethrogram.
C) Voiding diary.
D) Initiation of anticholinergic therapy.
E) Initiation of pelvic floor physical therapy.

Discussion 4-1

The correct answer is "C." Imaging studies are indicated in children who have suggestion of anatomic abnormalities or a failure to improve after a reasonable interval on appropriate treatment. Intermittent incontinence in children is most commonly associated with abnormal voiding habits and, in many cases, constipation or otherwise abnormal stool habits. A voiding diary is helpful in obtaining accurate and more objective data than historical reporting alone. A careful history and physical examination should be performed to assess for possible neurologic causes. Although both anticholinergic therapy and pelvic floor physical therapy have been successfully employed to treat children with urinary incontinence, treatments are most effective when they are symptom-directed, again making the voiding diary helpful. Initiation of therapy in the absence of an understanding of the underlying etiology may result in ineffective therapies being tried and the family becoming increasingly frustrated.

On further questioning, you learn that the girl voids infrequently, using the school restroom only once daily. She has a large, hard stool every third or fourth day, and has fecal leakage once or twice weekly.

Question 4-2

Which of the following is most likely to be true regarding her stool habits?

A) She likely has an inadequate intake of fruits and vegetables.
B) She should undergo evaluation for a neurologic disorder given the coexisting urinary incontinence.
C) The severity of constipation should be evaluated periodically with abdominal X-rays.
D) The Bristol stool scale provides an objective means of assessing stool habits and the success of therapies.
E) Enemas are first-line treatment for this condition as oral therapies result in unpredictable results.

Discussion 4-2

The correct answer is "D." Although many factors have been implicated in the etiology of childhood constipation, many children with constipation have healthy, well-balanced diets that include fruits and vegetables. Limited diets have, however, been associated with an increased risk of developing constipation. Constipation has been associated with a decreased quality of life. Most constipation in children is functional constipation, meaning that it is not associated with an underlying anatomic or physiologic disorder; most commonly, it is due to holding behaviors that allow increased reabsorption of water from stool in the colon. Although stool can be seen on abdominal films, X-rays have not been found to consistently independently correlate with the objective or subjective

Bristol Stool Chart

Type 1		Separate hard lumps, like nuts (hard to pass)
Type 2		Sausage-shaped but lumpy
Type 3		Like a sausage but with cracks on the surface
Type 4		Like a sausage or snake, smooth and soft
Type 5		Soft blobs with clear-cut edges
Type 6		Fluffy pieces with ragged edges, a mushy stool
Type 7		Watery, no solid pieces. **Entirely Liquid**

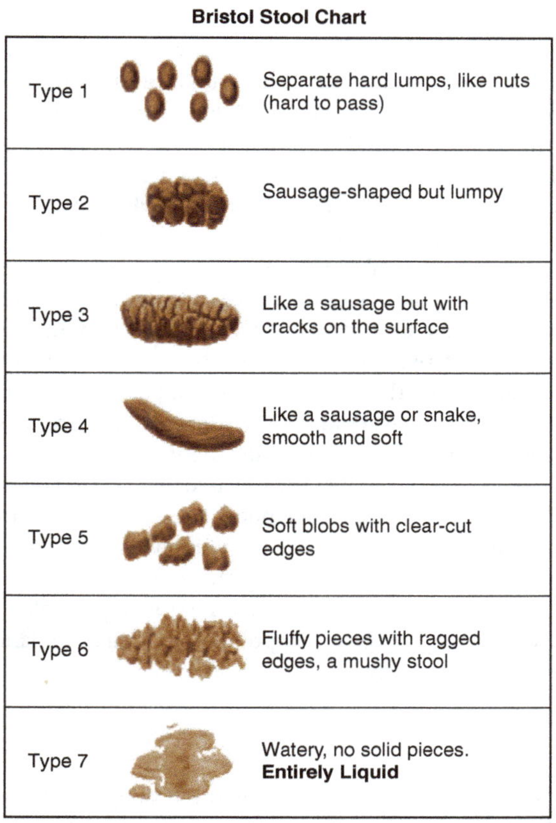

FIGURE 18–5. Bristol stool chart. (Reproduced with permission from Henderson MC, Tierney LM Jr, Smetana GW, eds. *The Patient History: An Evidence-Based Approach to Differential Diagnosis.* 2nd ed. New York, NY: McGraw-Hill Education; 2012, Fig. 32-1.)

severity of constipation. The Bristol stool scale provides a standardized measure of stool appearance and consistency that can be used by both providers and patients. (It also reinforces pediatricians' love of food references.) Management of constipation is multimodal, with scheduled toilet sitting, increased fluid intake, and intake of agents to soften the stool (eg, polyethylene glycol). Enemas may be required to assist in regular stooling but are generally not employed as first-line therapy. (See Figure 18–5.)

Continuous urinary incontinence in girls should raise concern for an ectopic ureter.

Question 4-3

Parental counseling regarding ureteral ectopia should include which of the following statements?

A) Boys and girls are at equivalent risk of urinary incontinence with ureteral ectopia.
B) Ureteral ectopia is typically associated with dysplastic changes in the most caudal portion of the ipsilateral kidney.
C) Excision of the renal parenchyma drained by the ectopic ureter is necessary to reduce the risk of pyelonephritis and future development of hypertension.
D) Ureteral ectopia may be associated with an increased risk of epididymitis.
E) Duplicated ureters occur in 25% of the population.

Discussion 4-3

The correct answer is "D." An ectopic ureter does not enter the trigonal area of the bladder. When duplication is present, the upper pole ureter is ectopic. Ureteral duplication occurs in about 1% of the population, and arises when the ureteric bud (a derivative of the wolffian system) divides. The more caudal and medial orifice drains the upper pole of the kidney, while the lower pole of the kidney is drained by the more cranial and lateral orifice. The upper pole (cephalad portion) may be dysplastic. In some cases, the upper pole ureter can move so caudally that it remains attached to other derivatives of the wolffian system draining into the vas deferens or epididymis. Boys do not present with incontinence like girls but rather manifest pain and infection of the affected organs (ie, epididymitis) In girls, the ectopic ureter may drain from the perineum into the vagina, uterus, or rectum. In boys, ectopic ureters are not associated with continuous incontinence. Surgical management is required when ureteral ectopia is associated with infections, pain, or hypertension, with the first two reasons being much more common than the third. Management options include excision of the upper pole moiety or altered drainage of the upper pole via ureteral reimplantation or ureteroureterostomy.

> **Helpful Tip**
> When treating daytime enuresis, physical therapy to assist in optimizing pelvic floor function may be helpful as an adjunct to improvement of voiding and defecation habits. Biofeedback and physical therapy using visual cues to assist in isolating targeted muscle groups have been associated with higher improvement rates.

▶ CASE 5

You are seeing an 8-year-old-girl who has never been dry at night for more than 2 nights at a time. She goes to bed at 8 PM and wakes at 6 AM. She does not awaken during the night. She voids three to four times during the day and has a bowel movement every other day. The bedwetting is beginning to become bothersome as she does not want to take part in sleepovers because she is embarrassed.

Question 5-1

Which of the following is true when counseling her parents?
A) Approximately 10% of children have nocturnal enuresis at the age of 8.
B) Approximately 20% of children have nocturnal enuresis at the age of 8.
C) Approximately 30% of children have nocturnal enuresis at the age of 8.
D) Approximately 40% of children have nocturnal enuresis at the age of 8.
E) Approximately 50% of children have nocturnal enuresis at the age of 8.

Discussion 5-1

The correct answer is "A." Nocturnal enuresis, or bedwetting, is diagnosed when a child older than 5 years of age is incontinent of urine at night. Although the true prevalence of nocturnal enuresis may be underreported owing to factors such as embarrassment, between 5% and 10% of children have bedwetting at age 7. About 10% to 15% of children experience resolution of their bedwetting every year without additional therapy. To keep it simple, think 8% of 8-year-olds.

On examination, the girl is found to have an unremarkable cardiopulmonary examination, a soft and nontender abdomen, and no weakness in the bilateral lower extremities. Her back is straight, with no tufts of hair, discoloration, or dimples. She has Tanner 1 female genitalia and her labia minora are connected by a thin vertical line of tissue blocking part of the vaginal opening.

Question 5-2

Which of the following is true regarding the treatment of this condition?
A) Hormone levels should be assessed to evaluate for a disorder of sexual differentiation.
B) Topical estrogen cream (enough to cover the parent's index fingertip) should be applied twice daily.
C) Formal labioplasty is needed.
D) Topical anesthetic and incision may be performed in the clinic but is often unsuccessful.
E) Treatment may be deferred if the patient is asymptomatic.

Discussion 5-2

The correct answer is "E." Labial adhesions occur in up to 2% to 3% of girls and should be treated if the child is symptomatic. Common associated symptoms include dysuria and daytime incontinence (often from urine pooling behind the adhesions). If treatment is desired, topical estrogen cream is typically the first-line therapy, although combination creams containing estrogen and betamethasone have also been shown to be successful. Steroid cream of any type should be applied with an applicator to avoid potential systemic administration to the administrator. In cases where conservative treatment has failed, lysis of adhesions in the office with topical anesthetic or under general anesthetic may be required; the decision to perform the procedure in a particular location is generally made based on the demeanor of the child, not the technical difficulty of the procedure. Although many girls experience resolution of the labial adhesions with increased estrogen levels at puberty, estrogen levels do not seem to differ between girls with and without labial adhesions. Though the precise etiology of labial adhesions remains unknown, local irritation is a likely factor, and avoiding perineal irritants and practicing good hygiene is recommended. (See Figure 18–6.)

Despite compliance with timed elimination, fluid restriction, and use of a bed alarm, the girl continues to have wetting every night. She and her parents have instituted a program

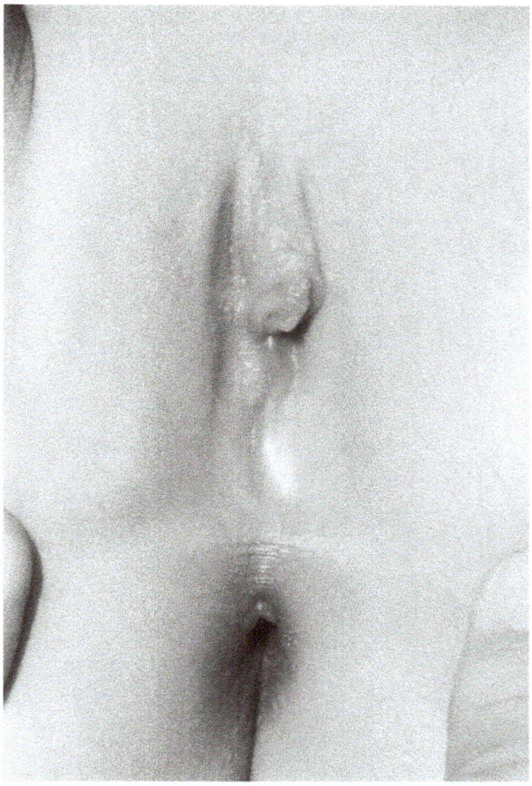

FIGURE 18–6. This young girl has labial adhesions. A thin vertical line is visible in the center where the labia have fused together. (Reproduced with permission from DeCherney AH, Nathan L, Laufer N, Roman AS, eds. *Current Diagnosis & Treatment: Obstetrics & Gynecology.* 11th ed. New York, NY: McGraw-Hill Education; 2013, Fig. 37-16.)

where she is able to change her sheets herself at night, and her parents are not angry with her for the bedwetting. The girl is doing well in school and is growing appropriately. The bedwetting, however, is limiting her participation in activities such as sleepovers and scout camp. Her mother has asked if there is any other option to manage the nocturnal enuresis for "special occasions."

Question 5-3

Pharmaceutical therapy for nocturnal enuresis:

A) Is useful for children with high nocturnal urine production secondary to diabetes or renal concentrating defects.

B) Generally results in resolution of the enuresis more quickly than if pharmaceutical agents were not used.

C) Will allow the child to sleep through the night.

D) Is most useful in conjunction with increased fluid intake before bedtime.

E) May be associated with significant side effects.

Discussion 5-3

The correct answer is "E." Further discussion follows after Question 5-4.

The girl's parents are trying to decide if pharmaceutical therapy is right for them.

Question 5-4

During counseling about DDAVP (desmopressin), they should be told:

A) DDAVP should be given before bed, and the girl may continue to drink water until bedtime.

B) The intranasal administration method is considered safer than the oral route.

C) The girl should have an electrocardiogram (ECG) prior to initiation of therapy.

D) Up to three pills (0.2 mcg each) may be used to achieve dryness, and instructions given to titrate the dose up every 2 to 3 nights until dryness is achieved.

E) The girl may be more difficult to awaken in the morning as she will likely sleep more soundly.

Discussion 5-4

The correct answer is "D." Pharmaceutical agents used for the treatment of enuresis include DDAVP (desmopressin) and imipramine (a tricyclic antidepressant). DDAVP works by decreasing water secretion in the kidney, while the mechanism of imipramine is unknown. In general, pharmacologic therapy of enuresis masks, but does not resolve, the enuresis. Children may sleep through the night if they do not need to awaken to change their clothes and sheets, but there is no evidence that either medication directly impacts sleep duration or quality. Administration of DDAVP should be oral (the intranasal formulation, which is no longer available in the United States, is associated with an increased risk of hyponatremia), and fluid intake should be limited to avoid hyponatremia and fluid overload. Up to three pills at a time may be used; titration is generally encouraged every 2 to 3 days to allow for nightly variations in fluid intake that may affect dryness.

> **Helpful Tip**
>
> The DDAVP nasal spray has a black box warning for hyponatremia. Parents must be carefully counseled on the potential side effects of DDAVP and imipramine, and children taking these medications must be followed closely. Given the risk of QT prolongation with imipramine, an ECG is recommended before starting therapy.

▶ CASE 6

A 26-year-old G1P0 (now 1) mother gave birth to a boy (Apgar scores of 9 and 9 at 1 and 5 minutes, respectively) at 39-3/7 weeks' gestation. At the 20-week ultrasound, the fetus was noted to have left hydronephrosis with slight thinning of the parenchyma. The right kidney had no hydronephrosis and normal sonographic parenchymal echotexture. The bladder was visualized. The amnionic fluid level was normal. The pregnancy had otherwise been progressing well, without complications. During the pregnancy, the mother had no problems with blood pressure, and no significant swelling of the face or hands. The newborn has been feeding well and has had multiple wet diapers since delivery 16 hours earlier.

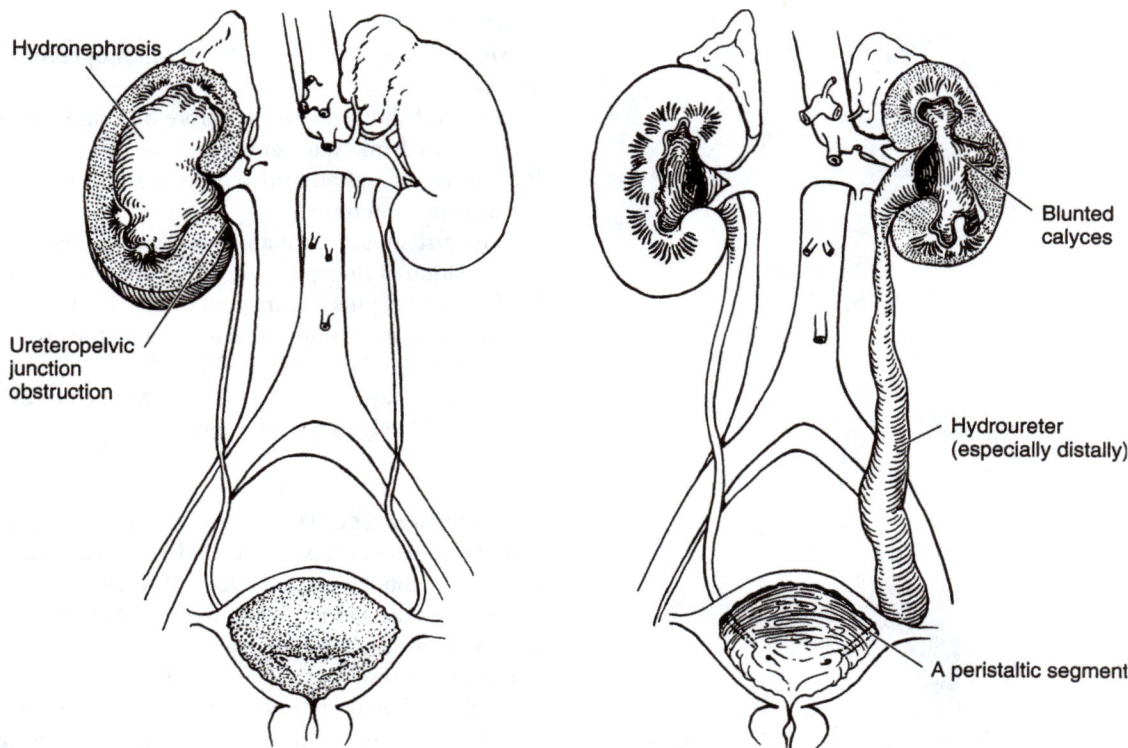

FIGURE 18–7. Congenital ureteral obstruction. Causes of prenatal hydronephrosis include ureteropelvic junction (UPJ) obstruction, ureterovesical junction (UVJ) obstruction, vesicoureteral reflux, or posterior urethral valves. The image at left shows right-sided UPJ obstruction with hydronephrosis. The image at right shows left UVJ obstruction with hydroureteronephrosis. (Reproduced with permission from McAninch JW, Lue TF, eds. *Smith & Tanagho's General Urology*. 18th ed. New York, NY: McGraw-Hill Education; 2013, Fig. 37-9.)

Question 6-1

The first step in postnatal evaluation of the newborn is:

A) Placement of a urethral catheter.
B) Measurement of serum creatinine.
C) Renal ultrasound.
D) Voiding cystourethrogram (VCUG).
E) MAG-3 renal scan.

Discussion 6-1

The correct answer is "C." A renal ultrasound will provide a non-invasive assessment of the renal anatomy. As newborns may be relatively dehydrated in the early postnatal period, it is important to recognize that an ultrasound early in life (particularly on day of life 1) will often underestimate the degree of hydronephrosis. If there is sonographic suspicion for upper tract abnormalities (eg, persistent postnatal hydronephrosis, abnormal parenchymal echogenicity), then consideration of further radiographic studies is reasonable. A VCUG is performed by inserting a catheter into the bladder, filling the bladder with contrast, and then having the infant void. The VCUG will assess for abnormalities such as vesicoureteral reflux, bladder diverticula, incomplete bladder emptying, and outlet obstruction (eg, posterior urethral valves). A MAG-3 scan will quantify the relative function of each renal unit and will also demonstrate any points of obstruction (eg, ureteropelvic junction [UPJ] obstruction, ureterovesical junction [UVJ] obstruction). Renal scans are generally deferred until 1 month of age, unless there is an extenuating circumstance such as suspicion for bilateral UPJ obstructions, because the neonatal kidney has relatively poor concentrating ability. If the newborn is voiding spontaneously and there is no clinical suspicion for bladder outlet obstruction, then catheter placement is not required. Serum creatinine in the early postnatal period is more reflective of maternal rather than neonatal renal function, although in cases of severe renal dysfunction in an infant, it may be elevated. (See Figure 18–7.)

▶ CASE 7

An 11-year-old boy presents to the emergency department following a fall from an all-terrain vehicle (ATV). Vital signs are temperature of 37°C (98.7°F), heart rate 92 beats per minute (bpm), respirations 12 breaths per minute, and blood pressure 126/75 mm Hg. He has bruising around the left flank and is very tender to palpation in this area. He is alert and oriented, has some pain on deep inspiration, and is moving all extremities. He is able to void and has grossly bloody urine. Computed tomography (CT) scan of the abdomen and pelvis shows a left UPJ disruption.

Question 7-1

The grade of the renal injury is:

A) 1.
B) 2.
C) 3.
D) 4.
E) 5.

Discussion 7-1

The correct answer is "D." Grade 1 renal injuries are subcapsular hematomas. Grade 2 renal injuries are lacerations into the superficial renal parenchyma. Grade 3 injuries are lacerations into the deep renal parenchyma. Grade 4 renal injuries include damage to segmental vasculature as well as entry into the collecting system. In this case, the UPJ is disrupted. Grade 5 renal injuries include main renal artery thrombosis and shattered kidney.

Question 7-2

Management of this injury includes all of the following EXCEPT:
A) Bedrest.
B) Serial hematocrit measurement.
C) Drainage of the collecting system.
D) Repeat imaging of kidneys.
E) Exploratory laparotomy.

Discussion 7-2

The correct answer is "E." Most renal injuries can be managed with bedrest and serial hematocrit measurement. Collecting system entry should be managed with internal (ureteral stent) or external (percutaneous nephrostomy tube) drainage. Although repeat imaging is not always performed for low-grade injuries, it is routine for high-grade injuries in order to ensure viability of the renal parenchyma and delineate the anatomy following an injury. Emergent surgical repair is performed only rarely, when bleeding from the kidney cannot be controlled or when the patient is undergoing surgical intervention for other injuries. In the latter case, the risks and benefits of surgical repair versus conservative management should be carefully considered, because bleeding can often be controlled by tamponade within the retroperitoneum, and release of a retroperitoneal hematoma (from the kidney or from an injury to the liver or spleen) may be difficult to control.

Question 7-3

When counseling parents and patients, which of the following is true regarding renal trauma?
A) Children with a history of solitary kidney should not be allowed to take part in sports given the increased risk of renal injury in this population.
B) Renal units with underlying structural abnormalities are at increased risk of damage with renal trauma.
C) Hypertension may be seen for the first several years after renal injury and typically reflects damage to the large renal vessels.
D) Children are at decreased risk of UPJ disruption and renal pedicle avulsion compared with adults.
E) In children with a history of trauma, microscopic hematuria is an indication for cross-sectional imaging to exclude renal trauma as the cause.

Discussion 7-3

The correct answer is "B." Children with a solitary kidney or abnormal renal anatomy may be at increased risk of injury compared with the general population when participating in contact sports, but much of this risk can be controlled with use of patient education and appropriate padding. Patients with a history of renal trauma are at an increased risk for development of late hypertension, which is most commonly caused by local scarring causing compression of the renal unit with resulting increase in renin and angiotensin levels (Page kidney). Children are actually at increased risk for avulsion injuries caused by sudden deceleration when compared with adults, perhaps owing to the relative decrease in adipose tissue surrounding the kidney in the pediatric population. Finally, although microscopic hematuria (> 5 RBCs/hpf) alone is an indication for cross-sectional imaging in adults, in children microscopic hematuria plus a plausible mechanism of injury is needed before cross-sectional imaging is undertaken.

> **Helpful Tip**
> Renal injuries should always be suspected in the setting of injuries to nearby organs (spleen, liver, spine), or when the mechanism of injury could potentially cause renal injury (eg, sudden deceleration). In children, there is less perinephric fat to cushion the kidney, so they are at increased risk for renal injuries compared with adults.

► CASE 8

A 3-day-old boy was born at term after an uncomplicated pregnancy. His mother has brought him to the clinic because at his postnatal examination he was noted to have a descended left testicle and a nonpalpable right testicle. The mother does not recall being told anything about the genitalia being abnormal at birth, and also does not recall seeing the right testis in the scrotum during warm baths. On examination, the boy has Tanner 1 male external genitalia with a circumcised phallus and orthotopic meatus, and a palpably normal descended left testicle. The right testicle is nonpalpable. No hernia or hydrocele is palpable on either side.

Question 8-1

Which of the following is the most appropriate course of action at this point?
A) Observation.
B) Ultrasound of the inguinal canal and scrotum.
C) Intramuscular human chorionic gonadotropin (hCG) therapy.
D) Referral to a pediatric urologist for exploration and possible orchidopexy.
E) Intramuscular testosterone therapy.

Discussion 8-1

The correct answer is "A." Approximately 2% of male infants are born with an undescended testicle, the vast majority of which descend by 3 months of age. Early in gestation the testes descend from the abdomen to the inguinal ring. Later, at 25 to

30 weeks' gestation, the testes move through the inguinal canal to the scrotum. Although the exact factors governing descent are not known, abdominal pressure, gubernacular location, and hormone responsiveness appear to play a role (although to different degrees in different people). There is a postnatal testosterone surge at 2 to 3 months in term infants (occurring later in premature infants); therefore, observation to determine whether the testicle remains undescended after this time period is warranted. Hormone therapy (hCG and testosterone) has not been shown to be effective in promoting testicular descent. Inguinal and scrotal ultrasounds have not been shown to be cost-effective in identifying the presence and location of a nonpalpable gonad. An undescended testis is a risk factor for torsion. In contrast, retractile testes are those that can be brought down to the scrotum and stay in place following cremasteric fatigue, but which may have a strong cremasteric reflex and thus may reside higher in the scrotum, or on occasion, in the inguinal canal much of the time. Approximately 30% of retractile testes may ascend over time; thus, annual examinations should be performed by a skilled provider. Care should be taken to relax the child and to provide adequate time for the cremasteric reflex to fatigue.

> **Helpful Tip**
> Cryptorchidism is associated with prematurity and low birthweight. The testes move into the scrotum through the inguinal canal at 25 to 30 weeks' gestation.

Question 8-2

When counseling parents regarding the need to consider surgical intervention for an undescended testicle, which of the following is true?

A) Surgery should be performed no sooner than 6 months corrected age given anesthetic considerations.
B) Fertility parameters may be abnormal with undescended testes, but typically normalize provided that surgery is performed before the age of 2 years.
C) Undescended testes are at an increased risk for development of neoplasia, but this risk normalizes when orchidopexy is performed before the age of 1 year.
D) Boys who have undergone orchidopexy should wear a cup when playing contact sports.
E) Testicular atrophy occurs in up to one third of boys undergoing open inguinal orchidopexy.

Discussion 8-2

The correct answer is "A." Many testes that are undescended at birth descend by 2 to 3 months of age, in conjunction with the postnatal testosterone surge. In boys with testes that remain undescended, surgery is planned after the age of 6 months given anesthetic considerations (although more recent literature suggests that elective surgery as early as 4 months of age is safe). There is an increase in the risk of neoplasia in both testes in the setting of cryptorchidism (even if only one is

undescended), with the risk increasing with more proximal testicular location and later orchidopexy. The most recent studies have recommended orchidopexy earlier than 1 year of age to achieve maximal fertility benefit. It is recommended that boys with a solitary functioning testicle wear a cup for contact sports. Testicular atrophy has been estimated to occur in 20% to 30% of orchidopexies for intra-abdominal testes, and an inguinal approach for staged procedures has been associated with a lower risk of atrophy.

> **Helpful Tip**
> Routine sonography to locate an undescended testicle does not change surgical management in most cases, and is not cost effective.

> **Helpful Tip**
> Newborns with male-looking external genitalia but bilateral nonpalpable testes should undergo evaluation for disorders of sexual differentiation, as a female infant with severe CAH can be morphologically identical to a male infant with bilateral nonpalpable gonads.

► CASE 9

A 7-year-old boy presents with a 3-hour history of right testicular pain arising acutely without associated history of trauma. He has associated nausea and vomiting. On examination, the right hemiscrotum is swollen, tender, and erythematous. The testis is very tender to palpation and is higher than the left. You suspect testicular torsion.

Question 9-1

The next appropriate step is:

A) Emergent scrotal exploration for testicular detorsion.
B) Cord block and manual detorsion in the emergency department.
C) Scrotal ultrasound with Doppler.
D) Measurement of serum tumor markers (AFP, beta-hCG, LDH).
E) Administration of ketorolac for pain relief.

Discussion 9-1

The correct answer is "A." Testicular torsion often presents as abrupt onset of testicular or scrotal pain, but patients may also have referred abdominal pain and systemic symptoms such as nausea and vomiting (the embryologic origin of the testes is in close proximity to the kidneys, along the gonadal ridge). The exact symptoms are dependent on the severity of the torsion, the duration of the torsion, and the patient's pain threshold, and so providers must have a high index of suspicion. Testicular torsion has a bimodal distribution, with infants and teenagers most commonly affected, although torsion has been reported in all age groups, including adults. Teenagers are most commonly affected. The increasing weight of the testis during puberty is thought to play a role. The testis twists around the spermatic cord, interrupting blood flow. If testicular torsion is suspected, maneuvers to institute detorsion should be promptly instituted. Surgical exploration is the standard of care for testicular torsion, as it allows visual confirmation of both the viability of the testis and the success of detorsion maneuvers. When surgical exploration cannot be performed promptly, manual detorsion may be attempted; the testicle is gently rotated outward as if one were opening a book. In many cases, the testicle has twisted more than one full rotation, and so manual detorsion should be considered an adjunct to, rather than a substitute for, operative intervention. Pain medication, including a cord block or narcotic medications, may be helpful in relaxing the cord and limiting pain so that this can be accomplished. Ketorolac and other anti-inflammatories that inhibit platelet function are not recommended in the preoperative patient, given the increased risk of bleeding. Scrotal ultrasound with Doppler should be used to confirm the presence of blood flow in patients in whom the examination is equivocal, and in no case should delay surgical intervention. Testicular torsion is generally not associated with testicular masses, and so measurement of tumor markers before surgery is unnecessary unless other signs of a testicular mass are present. Torsion of the appendix testis (a remnant of the müllerian system) or the appendix epididymis (a remnant of the wolffian system) typically manifests with testicular and scrotal pain and swelling, and a blue dot (the infarcted appendage) may be seen through the scrotal skin. Systemic symptoms are much more rare with appendix torsion. Appendix torsion can be managed conservatively, with anti-inflammatory medications, ice, and scrotal support. (See Figures 18–8 and 18–9.)

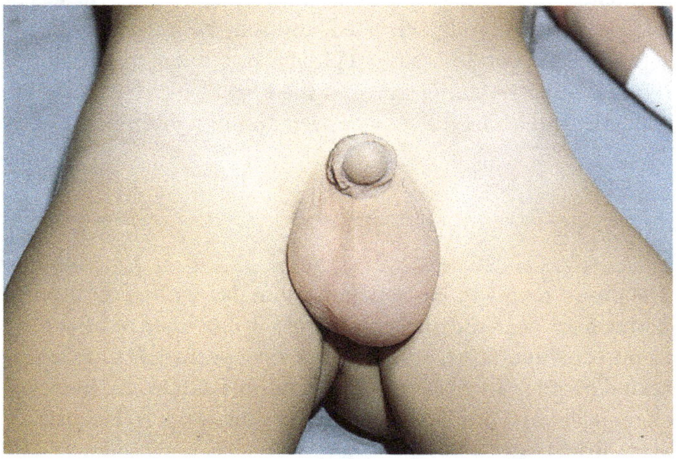

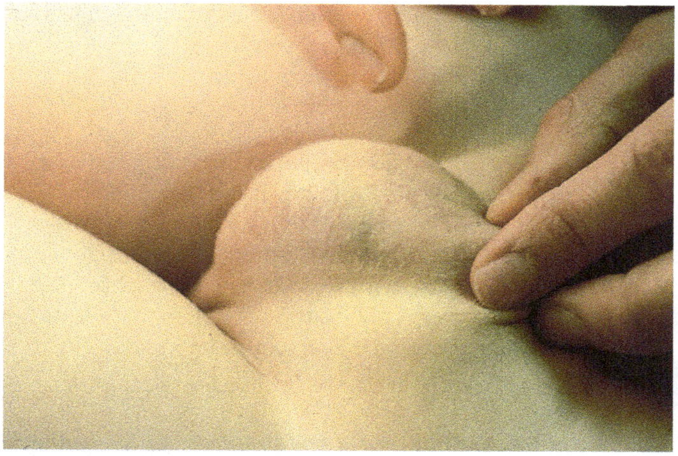

FIGURE 18–9. Blue Dot Sign. In torsion of a testicular appendage, the infarcted appendage may be seen under the scrotal skin, appearing as a blue dot. (Reproduced with permission from Knoop KJ, Stack LB, Storrow AB, Thurman RJ (Eds). *The Atlas of Emergency Medicine*, 3ed. McGraw-Hill Education, Inc., 2010. Photo contributor: Javier A. Gonzalez del Rey, MD.)

> **Helpful Tip**
> The cremaster reflex (elevation of the testis when the inner thigh is touched) can help differentiate between torsion of the testis and torsion of a testicular appendage. It is absent in the former but present in the latter condition.

Question 9-2

Which of the following is true of neonatal testicular torsion?
A) Risk factors include large birthweight infants and those who have been delivered after their due dates.
B) Most torsions occur after birth rather than in utero.
C) Operative salvage rates are approximately 50%.
D) The testicle is typically twisted externally and intravaginally.
E) Most cases of neonatal torsion are associated with testicular tumors.

Discussion 9-2

The correct answer is "A." Neonatal torsion affects approximately 2.5% of newborns. Risk factors include infants who are large for gestational age, those delivered after their estimated due date or after a prolonged labor, and those born to mothers with a history of diabetes. Tumors are not typically seen in association with neonatal torsion. Although the exact etiology is unknown, torsion is thought to arise when the testicle twists as a result of comparatively poor fixation of neonatal tissues. In comparison to testicular torsion in older children, neonatal torsion is typically extravaginal (outside the tunica vaginalis), rather than intravaginal. It is suspected that most "neonatal" torsions actually occur antenatally. Considerable debate remains concerning the best treatment for neonatal torsion; owing to the low operative salvage rate and the risks of anesthesia in the neonate, some urologists advocate conservative management. However, in the first 30 days of life, an increased risk of contralateral torsion has

FIGURE 18–8. Testicular Torsion. The boy has torsion of his left testicle. The hemiscrotum is swollen, red, and tender. On exam, the testis would be elevated in the scrotum and tender, and the cremaster reflex would not be present. (Reproduced with permission from Knoop KJ, Stack LB, Storrow AB, Thurman RJ (Eds). *The Atlas of Emergency Medicine*, 3ed. McGraw-Hill Education, Inc., 2010. Photo contributor: Patrick McKenna, MD.)

been observed; thus others have endorsed operative intervention for fixation of the contralateral testis.

> **Helpful Tip**
> Intravaginal (inside the tunica vaginalis) testicular torsion is associated with the "bell clapper" deformity, which occurs when the testis is not attached normally in the scrotum. Instead, the testis hangs in the scrotum in a horizontal position and is more mobile. The deformity is typically bilateral; therefore, both testes should be corrected during surgery for torsion.

The patient's 9-year-old cousin had presented to his pediatrician recently with a 1-day history of scrotal pain and swelling, as well as low-grade fever. On examination, the scrotum was swollen and erythematous, particularly over the left side, the testis was nontender, and a tender mass was felt over the upper pole of the testis.

Question 9-3

The structure most likely responsible for this presentation is derived from the same embryologic origin as the:

A) Pyramidalis.
B) Lower third of the vagina.
C) Uterus.
D) Ureter.
E) Parasympathetic nerves.

Discussion 9-3

The correct answer is "C." In a child of this age, the most likely cause of this presentation is torsion of the appendix testis, which is a remnant of the müllerian system. The müllerian system also gives rise to the uterus and upper third of the vagina. The lower third of the vagina develops from the genitourinary sinus. The ureters are derivatives of the wolffian system. Nervous tissues are not involved in this presentation. (See Figure 18–10.)

Question 9-4

What is the most appropriate management?

A) Emergent surgical exploration.
B) Anti-inflammatory medication.
C) Ciprofloxacin.
D) Trimethoprim-sulfamethoxazole.
E) Scrotal ultrasound with Doppler.

Discussion 9-4

The correct answer is "B." Torsion of the appendix testis is managed conservatively, with ice, scrotal support, and oral anti-inflammatory agents. Antibiotics are not indicated (and in any event, ciprofloxacin is not recommended for children given the risk of tendon rupture). Although scrotal ultrasound with Doppler may be used to demonstrate blood flow to the testis, clinical examination is generally adequate for the diagnosis of both testicular torsion and torsion of the appendix testis. In both conditions, the scrotum may be erythematous, swollen,

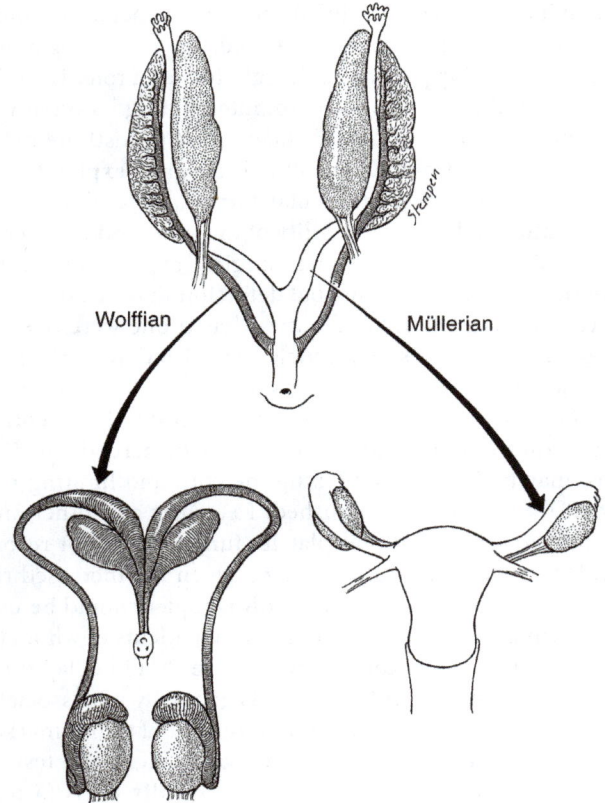

FIGURE 18–10. Formation of the Male and Female Internal Genitalia. A fetus is born with the embryologic precursors for both genders' internal genitalia. In males, the wolffian ducts form the epididymidis, vas deferens, seminal vesicles, and ejaculatory ducts. The testis secretes müllerian-inhibiting substance causing the müllerian ducts to regress. In females, the müllerian ducts form the female internal genitalia: fallopian tubes, uterus, cervix, and upper part of the vagina. Without testosterone, the wolffian ducts do not differentiate. (Reproduced with permission from McAninch JW, Lue TF, eds. *Smith & Tanagho's General Urology*. 18th ed. New York, NY: McGraw-Hill Education; 2013, Fig. 43-2.)

and tender. In testicular torsion, the cremaster reflex is absent and the testis is tender, elevated, and may be horizontal in the scrotum. In appendix testis or epididymis torsion, the cremaster reflex is intact, a tender mass on the upper pole of the testis is palpable, and a blue dot may be seen on the scrotum.

▶ CASE 10

The clinic seems to be besieged by males with scrotal pain. Today a 15-year-old presents with a 4-day history of aching in his scrotum, fever, and burning with peeing. He has a new sexual partner and does not use condoms. On exam, his testis exam is normal but he has tenderness posteriorly. His urinalysis shows pyuria.

Question 10-1

Which of the following is the most likely cause of his symptoms?

A) *Chlamydia trachomatis*.
B) Adenovirus.

C) *Escherichia coli.*
D) *Neisseria gonorrhoea.*
E) Mumps.

Discussion 10-1

The correct answer is "A." The epididymis serves as a sort of sperm storage shed located on the posterior side of the testis. This adolescent boy has bacterial epididymitis. In a sexually active male, the most common cause is chlamydia. In addition to the organisms listed, other possible causes include *Mycoplasma pneumoniae*, adenovirus, and enterovirus. Pain may be acute or subacute, with possible urinary symptoms and or fever. On exam, tenderness is localized to the epididymis, the cremaster reflex is present, and elevation of the testis may relieve the pain (Prehn sign). The Prehn sign is absent in torsion but it is not sufficiently reliable to differentiate between epididymitis and torsion. If in doubt, order a Doppler ultrasound. Management includes obtaining cultures, treating the infection, and reminding the boy to use condoms. Reflux of sterile urine or ectopic insertion of a ureter resulting in noninfectious inflammation is the most common cause of epididymitis in younger children. Mumps is the most common cause of orchitis. Orchitis is most commonly caused by a viral infection but may be bacterial. If epididymitis is present, the etiology is more likely bacterial.

> **Helpful Tip**
> The differential diagnosis of scrotal pain includes testicular torsion, testicular appendage torsion, epididymitis, Henoch-Schönlein purpura, orchitis, trauma, and incarcerated hernia.

> **Helpful Tip**
> Many children with testicular torsion retrospectively recall prior episodes of similar pain, typically of shorter duration, that resolved spontaneously ("intermittent torsion"); thus, children with repeated episodes of severe but self-limited pain without other apparent etiologies may benefit from evaluation by a urologist.

► CASE 11

A 14-year-old girl presents with acute onset of severe abdominal pain localized to the left lower quadrant. She feels sick to her stomach and has vomited several times. She denies trauma, fever, or vaginal discharge. Her last menstrual period was 1 week ago. On exam, she is very uncomfortable and cannot lie still. Her external genitalia are normal, no cervical motion tenderness is present, her abdomen is diffusely tender, and a mass is palpable in her left adnexa.

Question 11-1

What is the most likely cause of her pain?
A) Ovarian torsion.
B) Tuboovarian abscess.
C) Ectopic pregnancy.
D) Ruptured ovarian cyst.
E) Hematocolpos.

Discussion 11-1

The correct answer is "A." In torsion, the adnexa twist, cutting off the blood supply to the ovary and fallopian tube. An ovarian cyst may cause torsion. Early recognition and surgery is important to save the ovary. Tuboovarian abscess, ectopic pregnancy, and ruptured ovarian cyst should be ruled out. A pelvic ultrasound with Doppler is the imaging study of choice. Physiologic ovarian cysts are common in fetuses and neonates as a result of maternal hormones and in adolescent pubertal females as a result of failure of the follicle to ovulate. Rupture causes acute onset of pain and bleeding. An imperforate hymen blocks the drainage of menstrual products, resulting in the accumulation of blood and fluid in the uterus called hematocolpos. A bulging bluish hymen is present on exam. Girls present with amenorrhea and cyclical abdominal or pelvic pain. The contents can be secondarily infected (pyometra). Our patient's presentation is acute, and she told you her period was 1 week ago.

► CASE 12

A 4-year-old girl presents with a 1-week history of vaginal itching and redness. The child is potty trained and wears cotton underwear. She loves bubble baths and dance. She has had no fever, abdominal pain, urinary symptoms, or bleeding. On exam, she has normal external genitalia with erythema and irritation of the labial majora.

Question 12-1

It is important to tell parents or caregivers:
A) Her dance leotards should be tight fitting.
B) Bubble baths are fine, especially with scented soap.
C) It doesn't matter which way she wipes.
D) She should wear cotton underwear.
E) Keeping her vaginal area moist will help.

Discussion 12-1

The correct answer is "D." Vulvovaginitis in the prepubertal child is due to local irritation and associated with poor hygiene, bubble baths, scented soaps, obesity, tight-fitting clothes, and foreign bodies. Look for retained toilet paper. Patients should wear cotton underwear, avoid tight-fitting clothes, keep the area dry, wipe front to back, minimize moisture, and avoid bubble baths or scented bath products, Warm soaks in clean bath water may help but it is important to dry the genital area afterward before putting on underwear. If symptoms do not improve, consider a foreign body or infectious cause.

Question 12-2

Which is NOT an infectious cause of vulvovaginitis?
A) *Streptococcal pyogenes*.
B) *Candida vaginalis*.
C) Pinworms.
D) *Yersinia*.
E) All of the above.

Discussion 12-2

The correct answer is "E." If symptoms are persistent or discharge is purulent, cultures should be obtained. *Candida* is associated with antibiotics, immunosuppression, and wet diapers. Abuse should be suspected if vulvovaginitis is caused by a sexually transmitted pathogen in young girls.

▶ CASE 13

A male fetus was noted at the 20-week ultrasound to have bilateral hydronephrosis and a thickened bladder wall. He was delivered at 32 weeks' gestational age weighing 2690 g. The delivery was uncomplicated, but shortly after birth the newborn developed respiratory distress and was intubated. Examination shows a palpable bladder and normal Tanner 1 male external genitalia with bilateral descended testes. Chest X-ray shows a right-sided pneumothorax. After stabilization a voiding cystourethrogram is performed and shows a dilated posterior urethra and a thickened bladder.

Question 13-1

Initial management of this condition is which of the following?
A) Urethral catheter placement.
B) Cystoscopy.
C) Postnatal renal ultrasound.
D) Measurement of serum electrolytes and creatinine.
E) Vesicostomy.

Discussion 13-1

The correct answer is "A." Posterior urethral valves affect male infants, causing bladder outlet obstruction. (See Figure 18–11.) Typically newborns present with delayed voiding, but some void normally. Although serum creatinine and electrolytes should be assessed, and a renal ultrasound should be obtained, the most urgent matter is obtaining adequate drainage of the lower urinary tract, which is blocked by the posterior urethral valves. Subsequently pressure increases in the bladder then the upper urinary tract, resulting in development of hydroureteronephrosis. The renal parenchyma may be irreversibly damaged from the high pressure in the upper tract. If obstruction is severe enough to cause oligohydramnios, respiratory distress and pneumothoraces may develop from lung hypoplasia. Remember, voided urine enters the amnionic fluid. Normal amnionic fluid is required for lung development. Prior to undergoing surgery to ablate the valves, pulmonary function should be optimized since ventilators utilize positive-pressure ventilation (which can worsen pneumothoraces), and serum electrolytes should be normalized.

> **Helpful Tip**
> When evaluating a newborn for hydronephrosis or other urinary tract pathology, renal ultrasound may be falsely negative if obtained on the first few days of life before urine production has increased. It is okay to order but keep in mind you should repeat it at 1 to 2 weeks of age.

Question 13-2

In this case, optimal initial surgical management of the posterior urethral valves is best achieved by:
A) Prolonged catheter drainage.
B) Transurethral ablation of the valves.
C) Vesicostomy.
D) Bilateral ureterostomy.
E) Bilateral pyelostomy.

Discussion 13-2

The correct answer is "B." While initial catheter drainage should be performed, prolonged catheter drainage may increase the risk of urethral pressure necrosis and UTIs. Transurethral resection of the valves is an option in children in whom the urethra is large enough to accommodate the scope. In most very small or premature infants, the initial procedure is a vesicostomy since transurethral resection cannot be safely performed. In infants and children with tortuous ureters in whom an adequate decline in serum creatinine cannot be achieved with vesicostomy alone, ureterostomy or pyelostomy (bringing the ureter and renal pelvis to the skin, respectively), or both, may be needed to optimize drainage.

> **Helpful Tip**
> Posterior urethral valves may manifest in older male children as problems with daytime continence or with bedwetting, although this presentation is less common with the increased use of prenatal imaging.

▶ CASE 14

A 2-year-old girl is brought into clinic today because her mother felt an abdominal mass while she was giving the child a bath. The girl is otherwise healthy and was delivered at term after an uncomplicated pregnancy. Her family history is significant for two cousins with Wilms tumor. A renal ultrasound shows a large echogenic renal mass on the right.

Question 14-1

All of the following should be included in the evaluation of this mass EXCEPT:
A) Mesoblastic nephroma.
B) Renal cell carcinoma.
C) Wilms tumor.

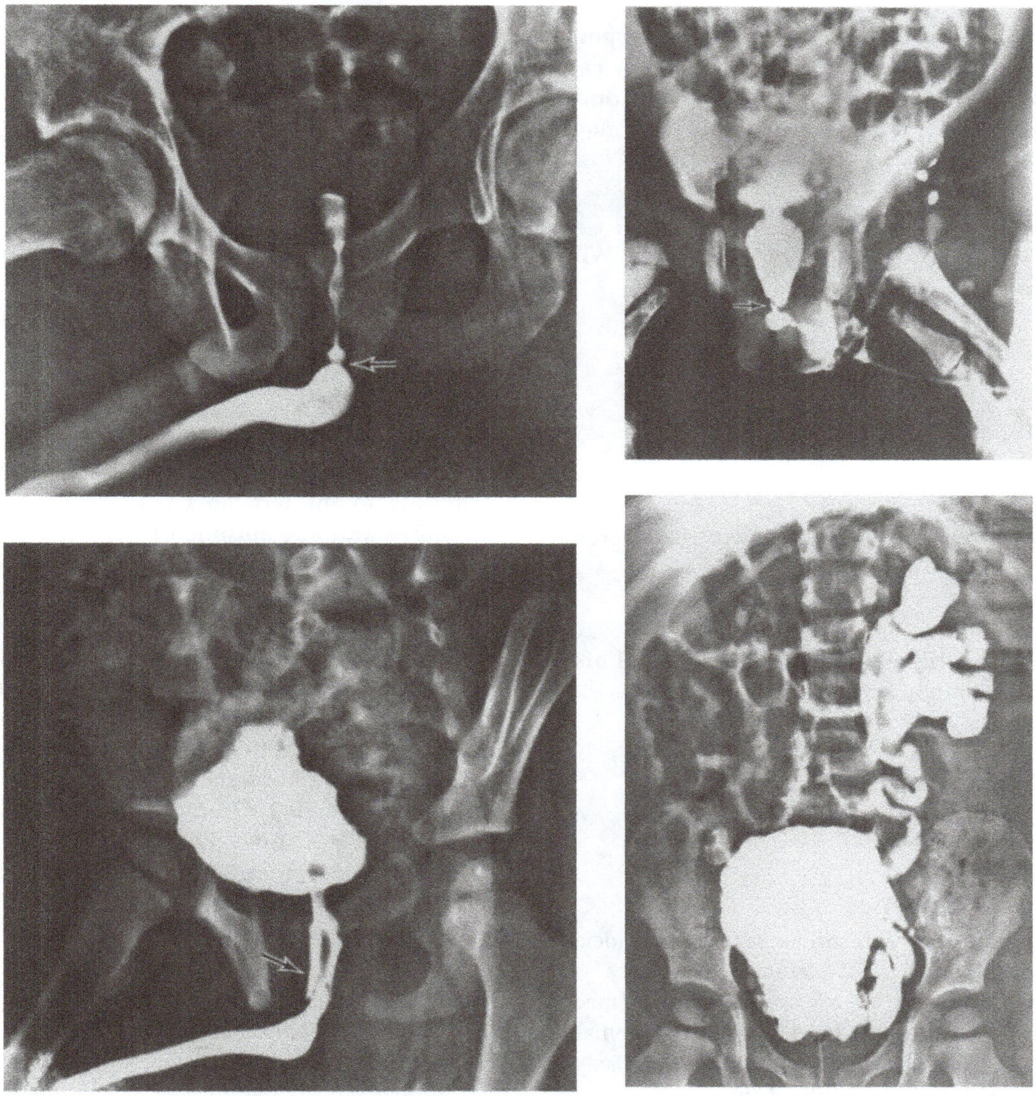

FIGURE 18–11. The posterior urethra is enlarged on voiding cystoureterogram in this boy with posterior urethral valves. (Reproduced with permission from McAninch JW, Lue TF, eds. *Smith & Tanagho's General Urology*. 18th ed. New York, NY: McGraw-Hill Education; 2013, Fig. 41-1.)

D) Neuroblastoma.

E) Hypertrophied column of Bertin.

Discussion 14-1

The correct answer is "E." A hypertrophied column of Bertin is a column of renal cortical tissue that extends to the renal sinus; since it is normal renal parenchyma, it has normal uptake and excretion of contrast compared with the remainder of the kidney. Mesoblastic nephroma, renal cell carcinoma, Wilms tumor, and neuroblastoma are all abnormal findings. Neuroblastoma may develop from any neural tissue, including the adrenal gland, whereas the other masses are seen in the kidney. Mesoblastic nephroma is most commonly seen in newborns and young infants, Wilms tumors in toddlers, and renal cell carcinoma (typically translocation-type) in older children. However, these age ranges are not strict, and so physicians should be aware of the differential diagnosis for all renal masses. (See Figure 18–12.)

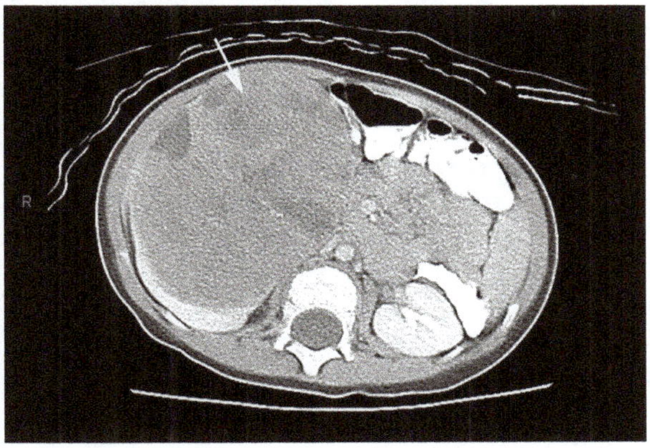

FIGURE 18–12. This 3-year-old has a Wilms tumor of the right kidney (*white arrow*), a malignant tumor that presents as an asymptomatic abdominal mass in toddlers. (Reproduced with permission from Brunicardi FC, Andersen DK, Billiar TR, et al, eds. *Schwartz's Principles of Surgery*. 10th ed. New York, NY: McGraw-Hill Education; 2015, Fig. 39-37.)

This toddler has a Wilms tumor, a malignant tumor of the kidney. Wilms tumors are the most common cause of a renal mass. It typically presents as an asymptomatic abdominal mass. Hematuria, hypertension, or both may be present.

Question 14-2

The chromosome on which the gene responsible for Wilms tumor resides is:
A) 1p.
B) 3p.
C) 11p.
D) 17p.
E) 22q.

Discussion 14-2

The correct answer is "C." The *WT1* gene is located on chromosome 11p13-15.

Question 14-3

Syndromes associated with Wilms tumor include all of the following physical examination findings EXCEPT:
A) Café-au-lait spots.
B) Macroglossia.
C) Hypospadias and undescended testes.
D) Aniridia.
E) Hemihypertrophy.

Discussion 14-3

The correct answer is "A." Café-au-lait spots are associated with neurofibromatosis. The most common syndromes associated with Wilms tumor are Beckwith-Wiedemann (macroglossia), WAGR (**W**ilms tumors, **A**niridia, **G**enital anomalies, mental **R**etardation), and Denys-Drash. Associated isolated anomalies include aniridia, hypospadias, hemihypertrophy, and cryptorchidism.

The tumor is excised and the pathology returns as 475 g, favorable histology, negative margins. There was no intraoperative tumor spill. The girl does well and is discharged from the hospital.

Question 14-4

The most appropriate further treatment is:
A) Surveillance with periodic cross-sectional imaging.
B) Surveillance with renal ultrasound.
C) Chemotherapy with vincristine, doxorubicin, and cyclophosphamide.
D) Flank radiotherapy.
E) Total abdominal radiotherapy.

Discussion 14-4

The correct answer is "A." In the United States, Wilms tumors are generally treated according to the Children's Oncology Group protocols. For children 2 years of age and younger, with favorable histology tumors, negative margins without spill, and

tumors weighing less than 550 g, additional therapy is not recommended. These children are followed on the surveillance protocol. Children with favorable histology tumors receive chemotherapy with vincristine and dactinomycin or with vincristine, doxorubicin, and dactinomycin. Cyclophosphamide is not used as an initial chemotherapeutic agent in Wilms tumor. Radiation therapy is reserved for children with anaplastic histology, positive margins, extensive intraperitoneal disease, or intraoperative tumor spill.

▶ CASE 15

An 11-year-old girl presents to the emergency department complaining of a 3-day history of increasing left flank pain radiating to the left labia majora. She had one episode of emesis and one episode of pink urine. She has had no fevers, and her urine does not have a foul odor. She is otherwise healthy. She has a family history of kidney stones in multiple relatives. On examination, she is afebrile, alert and interactive, in obvious pain, and has left flank and abdominal tenderness to palpation. She has no rebound tenderness or guarding on abdominal exam. Urinalysis shows 3 to 5 WBCs/hpf, 11 to 20 RBCs/hpf, negative nitrites, and no bacteria. Complete blood count shows a WBC count of 10.2 K/mm^3, hematocrit 38.4%, and platelet count 375 K/mm^3. The basic metabolic panel shows sodium of 137 mEq/L, potassium 4.6 mEq/L, chloride 112 mEq/L, bicarbonate 26 mEq/L, BUN 13 mg/dL, and creatinine 0.5 mg/dL.

Question 15-1

The initial imaging test should be:
A) Renal ultrasound.
B) Intravenous pyelogram (IVP).
C) Computed tomography (CT) scan of the abdomen and pelvis with oral and intravenous contrast.
D) Magnetic resonance imaging (MRI) of the abdomen and pelvis with gadolinium.
E) KUB (kidney, ureter, bladder) X-ray.

Discussion 15-1

The correct answer is "A." Renal ultrasound has been shown to accurately diagnose renal stones but not ureteral stones in at least 90% of children when employed as the initial imaging modality. This reduces radiation exposure, which is especially important for children who may develop multiple stones. The AAP's "Image Gently" campaign urges clinicians to consider whether a test with ionizing radiation is necessary, or whether the same clinical information can be gleaned from a test without ionizing radiation. The most sensitive imaging study is a noncontrast helical CT, which can show ureter, radiolucent, and small stones that may be missed with other imaging modalities. KUB is useful to demonstrate radiopaque stones, but these may be obscured by overlying bowel gas. IVP and CT scan with contrast can demonstrate delayed drainage from

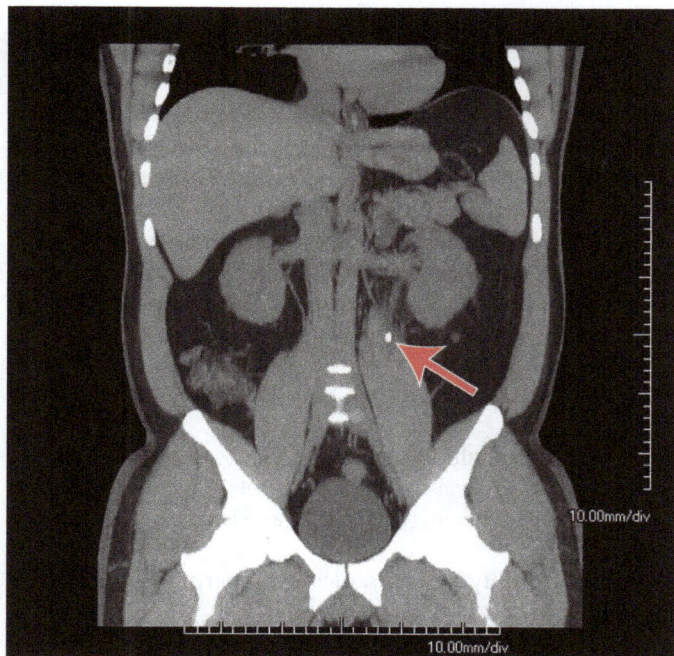

FIGURE 18–13. Ureter Stone. A 6-mm stone (*red arrow*) is present in the proximal left ureter on noncontrast helical CT. (Reproduced with permission from Tintinalli JE, Stapczynski JS, Ma OJ, Yealy DM, Cline DM, Meckler GD, eds. *Tintinalli's Emergency Medicine: A Comprehensive Study Guide*. 8th ed. New York, NY: McGraw-Hill Education; 2016, Fig. 94-1.)

a stone, but the contrast may obscure smaller stones. MRI is not a useful modality to demonstrate renal and ureteral stones. (See Figure 18–13.)

Question 15-2

Which is NOT a presenting sign of nephrolithiasis in children?
A) Microscopic hematuria.
B) Asymptomatic.
C) Irritability.
D) Abdominal pain.
E) All of the above.

Discussion 15-2

The correct answer is "E." Microscopic hematuria is present in nearly all cases of nephrolithiasis. Gross hematuria, while important to ask about, is not always present. Some patients may have a concurrent urinary tract infection.

Ultrasound reveals the girl has a left-sided renal stone.

Question 15-3

Further management in the emergency department should include:
A) Tamsulosin.
B) Trimethoprim-sulfamethoxazole.
C) Nephrology consultation for acute kidney injury.
D) Urology consultation for ureteral stent.
E) Admission for pain control.

Discussion 15-3

The correct answer is "E." Management includes pain control, hydration, and antibiotics if a concurrent urinary tract infection is present. Tamsulosin (Flomax) is a selective alpha-1 blocker used to help with stone passage; these receptors are located in the distal ureter and the bladder trigone as well as in the prostate in males. In adults, medical expulsive therapy has been associated with decreased cost and increased rate of spontaneous stone passage. There is limited experience with tamsulosin in children; early reports suggest that it may be successfully employed to encourage stone passage in the pediatric population as well, but the benefit has not been fully established. Indications for a ureteral stent include suggestion of infection behind an obstructing stone, acute kidney injury, obstruction of all functional renal units, immunocompromise (eg, chemotherapy, diabetes mellitus, immunosuppressive medications), or failure to achieve adequate pain control.

> **Helpful Tip**
> Kidney stones should be collected and analyzed to help identify an underlying cause and prevent future stones.

On hospital day 2, she passes the stone. She is pain free and has no complaints.

Question 15-4

The stone composition is most likely:
A) Calcium oxalate dihydrate.
B) Calcium phosphate.
C) Uric acid.
D) Ammonium acid urate.
E) Struvite.

Discussion 15-4

The correct answer is "A." Calcium oxalate (monohydrate or dihydrate) stones are most common; calcium phosphate stones are seen less commonly. Uric acid stones typically arise in patients with conditions associated with an increase in purine byproducts (eg, Lesch-Nyhan syndrome, gout). Ammonium acid urate stones are associated with diarrhea and laxative use. Struvite stones arise in the presence of infected urine and are often seen in patients with chronic UTIs from urea-splitting bacteria (eg, *Proteus, Klebsiella*). Large struvite stones that fill the renal pelvis and calyces are called staghorn calculi. A diagnostic workup is important to identify underlying metabolic conditions (eg, hypercalciuria) predisposing to stone reoccurrence. Testing should include stone analysis, 24-hour urine collection, urinalysis with culture, basic metabolic panel, and phosphate, magnesium, and uric acid levels. Check parathyroid hormone and vitamin D levels if the calcium or phosphate levels are elevated.

She is asked to complete a 24-hour urine collection.

Question 15-5

The abnormality most likely to be seen on this test is:

A) Hypercalciuria.
B) Hypomagnesemia.
C) Low total urine volume.
D) Hypercitraturia.
E) Elevated urine pH.

Discussion 15-5

The correct answer is "C." The most common abnormality seen on 24-hour urine collection performed for urolithiasis is decreased total urine volume. Low urine volume, high urine solute levels (eg, calcium, oxalate, uric acid), and decreased urine inhibitors are risk factors for stone formation. Although abnormalities of calcium metabolism (eg, hyperparathyroidism) may be associated with stone formation, hypercalciuria is uncommon in the absence of these conditions. Both magnesium and citrate are considered inhibitors of lithogenesis; thus, decreased urinary concentrations of these ions may be observed. Hypomagnesemia would not be detectable on a urine test. An alkaline urine pH is associated with the development of calcium phosphate stones or struvite stones.

Question 15-6

Dietary recommendations to prevent stone recurrence in this patient should include all of the following EXCEPT:

A) Limited sodium intake.
B) Limited calcium intake.
C) Low oxalate diet.
D) Increased fluid intake.
E) Lemonade.

Discussion 15-6

The correct answer is "B." Inhibitors of stone formation include magnesium and citrate, while increased urinary oxalate and sodium have been shown to predispose to stone formation. In many calcium stones, increased urinary sodium serves as the nidus for crystallization; decreased sodium intake has been associated with a lower rate of stone recurrence, while decreasing calcium levels has not. A low-oxalate diet, while challenging to follow, can be effective in decreasing the urinary oxalate, although the majority of urinary oxalate is endogenously produced. Increased fluid intake increases urine output and not only provides more solvent in which solute might dissolve, but also reduces urinary stasis. All children with stones should increase their daily fluid intake. Lemonade is an excellent source of citrate in the form of citric acid.

Helpful Tip

Urolithiasis is becoming increasingly common in children, although the exact etiologic factors have not been well described. Children may pass larger stones more easily than adults because their ureters are more distensible.

► CASE 16

A 17-year-old boy presents for evaluation of a "lump" in the right testicle that he noticed in the shower 2 days ago. It has not changed in size since then and is not painful. He has had no abdominal pain, no cough, no recent illnesses, and states that he is not sexually active. On examination, the left testicle is descended and palpably normal, but on the right side, there is a firm area at the superior pole of the testis. A scrotal ultrasound is obtained showing a testicular mass. (See Figure 18–14.)

Question 16-1

Which of the following is the LEAST appropriate next step in management?

A) Repeat scrotal ultrasound in 2 weeks.
B) Check serum levels of alpha-fetoprotein, beta-human chorionic gonadotropin (beta-hCG), and lactate dehydrogenase (LDH).
C) Discuss fertility concerns, including sperm banking.
D) Obtain a chest X-ray.
E) Referral to a urologist.

Discussion 16-1

The correct answer is "A." A solid testicular mass is an indication for exploration and surgical resection. Testicular cancer is the

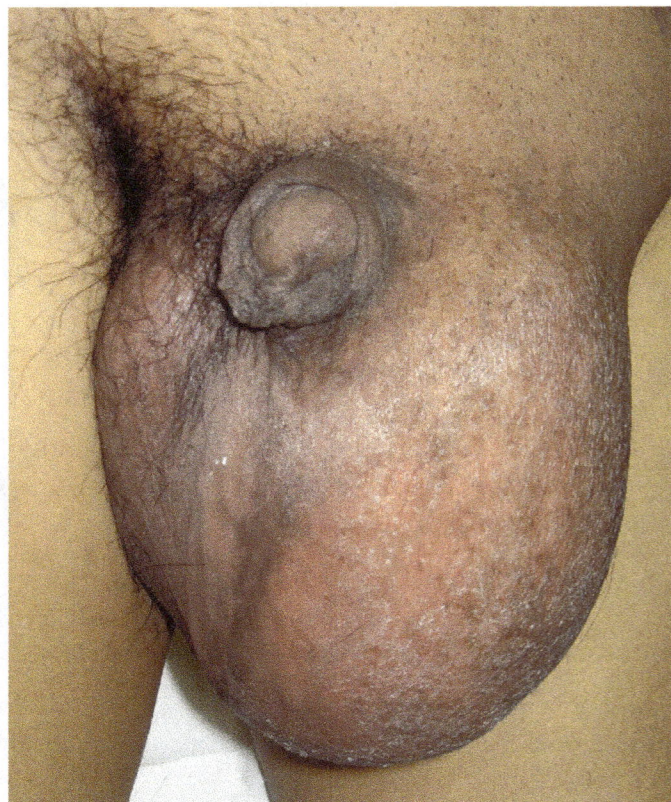

FIGURE 18–14. Testicular Cancer. This patient has a large mass in his left hemiscrotum. Despite often being slow-growing tumors, testicular cancer often presents quite late. (Reproduced with permission from Brunicardi FC, Andersen DK, Billiar TR, et al, eds. *Schwartz's Principles of Surgery*. 10th ed. New York, NY: McGraw-Hill Education; 2015, Fig. 40-1.)

most common solid neoplasm in older adolescent boys and young men. Workup includes measurement of tumor markers (alpha-fetoprotein, LDH, and beta-hCG). Once a neoplasm is confirmed, further therapy is dictated by staging of the tumor, including surgical pathology and the results of a metastatic workup.

> **Helpful Tip**
> Not all solid masses are testicular neoplasms. Testicular hamartomas, testicular microliths, and epidermoid cysts have also been described. Partial orchiectomy may be appropriate for benign processes. In younger children, yolk-sac tumors are the most common testicular neoplasm, but teratomas may also occur. Leydig cell tumors, which are hormonally active, may present in patients with precocious puberty, including increased muscle mass and a deepened voice.

► CASE 17

A 10-month-old infant boy is brought for evaluation by his mother after she noticed a bulge in his groin. She tells you that he was crying at the time, and when he stopped crying, the bulge was no longer there. He has not been irritable nor has he had a fever. She did not notice any redness in the groin area. On exam, a reducible mass is noted in the inguinal canal consistent with an indirect hernia.

Question 17-1

What is NOT a cause of inguinal swelling?
A) Indirect hernia.
B) Spermatic hydrocele.
C) Lymphadenopathy.
D) Retractile testis.
E) None of the above.

Discussion 17-1

The correct answer is "E." Other causes include lymphadenitis, malignancy, and even an appendicitis if the appendix is inside the hernia sac. In the abdomen, the process vaginalis is created from peritoneum. The testes descend through the inguinal canal, pushing the process vaginalis into the scrotum. Once the testes are home safe and sound, the process vaginalis obliterates. If the process vaginalis remains wide open, an indirect inguinal hernia forms, allowing organs to move into the inguinal canal. If it remains open but narrows, a communicating hydrocele filled with peritoneal fluid forms. If it remains open in the middle but closes on both ends, a hydrocele of the spermatic cord develops.

> **Helpful Tip**
> A hernia that cannot be reduced is called *incarcerated*. This is an emergency and requires immediate treatment to avoid strangulation at the point where blood flow to the hernia contents is compromised.

► CASE 18

A 16-year-old boy was found on routine physical examination to have a left testicular mass. He notes that the mass is associated with an occasional "aching" feeling in the left testicle, but no nausea. The mass enlarges when he lifts heavy objects or strains, and decreases in size when he lies down. He has no other complaints. On examination, both testicles are approximately 5 × 3 × 2 cm and of normal consistency, and he has a palpable plexus of veins in the left scrotum that reduces in the supine position.

Question 18-1

Management of this condition includes:
A) Endovascular injection of sclerosing agents.
B) Observation.
C) Ligation of the spermatic cord.
D) Microscopic denervation of the spermatic cord.
E) Orchiectomy.

Discussion 18-1

The correct answer is "B." Varicoceles are dilated veins of the pampiniform plexus that surrounds the spermatic cord in the scrotum and may feel like a "bag of worms." The management of varicocele in adolescents remains a matter of debate, but most experts agree that surgery should be performed in children with severe pain, significant (> 10–15%) and persistent discrepancy in testicular size, and those engaged in activities likely to promote progression of the varicocele (eg, varsity sports, entry into the armed forces). When varicocelectomy is undertaken, first-line options for surgical management include laparoscopic clipping of the gonadal vessels, open inguinal approach, or subinguinal microscopic varicocelectomy. Each approach has benefits and drawbacks: the laparoscopic approach is easy, but ligation of lymphatics and the testicular artery may be associated with testicular atrophy and hydrocele formation, respectively. The inguinal approach is familiar to most surgeons and there are often fewer veins and an increased ability to spare the testicular artery at this location, but this approach requires significant activity limitations postoperatively given the risk for hernia, and may be more painful. Subinguinal microscopic varicocelectomy is associated with the best artery- and lymphatic-sparing results as well as an earlier return to activities. Endovascular management is generally reserved for surgical failures, and denervation of the spermatic cord is appropriate for refractory orchalgia. There is no indication for orchiectomy if the testicle is otherwise healthy.

Question 18-2

If no palpable varicocele were found on physical examination, but retrograde flow was seen in the veins of the left pampiniform plexus on the scrotal ultrasound, the boy and his family should be counseled that:
A) Endovascular repair is less likely to be successful.
B) Prolonged observation is not recommended as the varicocele may progress to become symptomatic.
C) Monthly testicular examinations with a clinician are necessary to ensure adequate testicular growth.
D) He likely has decreased sperm motility on semen analysis.
E) Surgical repair is not undertaken for subclinical varicoceles.

Discussion 18-2

The correct answer is "E." Given the indications for consideration of surgical repair of a varicocele, subclinical varicoceles should not be repaired. Annual examination (unless there is a change in symptoms or anatomic findings) is generally adequate to assess for progression, although testicular self-examinations are recommended in all pubertal boys and postpubertal men to assess for testicular cancer. There are no data to suggest that subclinical varicoceles adversely affect sperm motility.

Question 18-3

If this mass were located on the right side rather than the left side, additional evaluation would include:
A) Retroperitoneal ultrasound.
B) CT scan of the abdomen and pelvis.
C) Measurement of serum follicle-stimulating hormone and luteinizing hormone.
D) Scrotal ultrasound with Doppler.
E) Measurement of serum testosterone.

Discussion 18-3

The correct answer is "A." Varicoceles are more common on the left than on the right, owing to the insertion of the gonadal vein into the left renal vein at a 90-degree angle. On the right side venous flow is more continuous as the gonadal vein drains directly into the inferior vena cava (IVC). Isolated left varicoceles and bilateral varicoceles generally do not require additional evaluation. However, in the case of isolated right-sided varicoceles, retroperitoneal imaging should be undertaken to rule out a mass or other pathology causing increased local venous pressure (IVC or right renal vein thrombosis). Initial evaluation can be performed with a retroperitoneal ultrasound, with cross-sectional imaging reserved for patients in whom the ultrasound does not provide good-quality images and those in whom additional characterization of the mass is necessary. Scrotal ultrasound may be used to determine the absolute size of both testes, although it has not been shown to be more accurate than physical examination by an experienced clinician. Serum hormone levels are not indicated in the absence of clinical evidence of an endocrinopathy.

► CASE 19

A 4-year-old boy who was not circumcised at birth owing to parental preference has difficulty completely retracting the foreskin, and he has "whitish" material that comes from under the foreskin on occasion. He has not had urinary tract infections (UTIs) and has no ballooning of the foreskin with voiding. His parents would prefer to keep him uncircumcised.

Question 19-1

When counseling the boy and his family, which of the following is true?
A) He should undergo circumcision because the AAP now encourages circumcision for all boys unless there is a religious or cultural objection.
B) He should undergo circumcision because phimosis at this age is abnormal.
C) He should not undergo circumcision because this will increase his risk of UTIs.
D) He should not undergo circumcision until he is treated with antibiotics and the white discharge stops.
E) None of the above.

Discussion 19-1

The correct answer is "E." Although the AAP has issued a 2012 statement saying that circumcision may be associated with a decreased risk of UTIs, penile cancer, and sexually transmitted infection, the procedure was not recommended for all male infants. Phimosis, the failure of the foreskin to retract, may be present even in older children and is not problematic in the absence of infections, irritation, or pain. The phimosis is normal or physiologic. As the child grows the foreskin separates from the glans becoming retractable. Some children will have smegma (dead skin cells) expressed from under the foreskin, but this alone is not an indication for circumcision. Topical steroid cream (betamethasone) may be used to release adhesions in children whose parents wish to preserve the foreskin. Paraphimosis is a condition that occurs when the retracted foreskin becomes edematous and cannot be reduced, resulting in a subsequent decrease in blood flow to the glans. It is a urologic emergency and should be treated by prompt reduction of the foreskin, or incision of the foreskin to relieve the pressure. (See Figure 18–4B, earlier.)

BIBLIOGRAPHY

Acker A, Jamieson MA. Use of intranasal midazolam for manual separation of labial adhesions in the office. *J Pediatr Adolesc Gynecol.* 2013;26:196–198.

American Academy of Pediatrics, Task Force on Circumcision. Circumcision policy statement. *Pediatrics.* 2012;130:585–586.

Amerstorfer EE, Haberlik A, Riccabona M. Imaging assessment of renal injuries in children and adolescents: CT or ultrasound? *J Pediatr Surg.* 2015;50:448–455.

Ammenti A, Cataldi L, Chimenz R, et al. Febrile urinary tract infections in young children: Recommendations for the diagnosis, treatment and follow-up. *Acta Paediatr.* 2012;101:451–457.

Best SL, Sivalingam S, Penniston KL, Nakada SY. Radiographic and laboratory data ("the Megaprofile") can accurately guide medical management in the absence of stone analysis. *J Endourol.* 2015;29:357–361.

Bisogni S, Olivini N, Festini F. Undertreated and untreated pain should be considered an adverse event of neonatal circumcision. *JAMA Pediatr.* 2014;168:1076–1077.

Bleeker MC, Heideman DA, Snijders PJ, et al. Penile cancer: Epidemiology, pathogenesis and prevention. *World J Urol.* 2009;27:141–150.

Boettcher M, Bergholz R, Krebs TF, et al. Differentiation of epididymitis and appendix testis torsion by clinical and ultrasound signs in children. *Urology.* 2013;82:899–904.

Brioude F, Lacoste A, Netchine I, et al. Beckwith-Wiedemann syndrome: Growth pattern and tumor risk according to molecular mechanism, and guidelines for tumor surveillance. *Horm Res Paediatr.* 2013;80:457–465.

Bulum B, Özçakar ZB, Ustüner E, et al. High frequency of kidney and urinary tract anomalies in asymptomatic first-degree relatives of patients with CAKUT. *Pediatr Nephrol.* 2013;28:2143–2147.

Burgers RE, Mugie SM, Chase J, et al. Management of functional constipation in children with lower urinary tract symptoms: Report from the Standardization Committee of the International Children's Continence Society. *J Urol.* 2013;190:29–36.

Butler RJ, Heron J. The prevalence of infrequent bedwetting and nocturnal enuresis in childhood. A large British cohort. *Scand J Urol Nephrol.* 2008;42:257–264.

Byrd RS, Weitzman M, Lanphear NE, Auinger P. Bed-wetting in US children: Epidemiology and related behavior problems. *Pediatrics.* 1996;98:414–419.

Canavese F, Mussa A, Manenti M, et al. Sperm count of young men surgically treated for cryptorchidism in the first and second year of life: Fertility is better in children treated at a younger age. *Eur J Pediatr Surg.* 2009;19:388–391.

Casanova NC, Johnson EK, Bowen DK, et al. Two-Step Fowler-Stephens orchiopexy for intra-abdominal testes: A 28-year single institution experience. *J Urol.* 2013;190:1371–1376.

Cost NG, Bush NC, Barber TD, et al. Pediatric testicular torsion: Demographics of national orchiopexy versus orchiectomy rates. *J Urol.* 2011;185:2459–2463.

Dahlstrom K, Dunoski B, Zerin JM. Blunt renal trauma in children with pre-existing renal abnormalities. *Pediatr Radiol.* 2015;45:118–123.

Davidoff AM. Wilms tumor. *Adv Pediatr.* 2012;59:247–267.

DeFoor W, Clark C, Jackson E, et al. Risk factors for end stage renal disease in children with posterior urethral valves. *J Urol.* 2008;180:1705–1708.

de Grauw AM, den Dekker HT, de Mol AC, Rombout-de Weerd S. The diagnostic value of routine antenatal ultrasound in screening for congenital uropathies. *J Matern Fetal Neonatal Med.* 2014:1–5.

Diamond DA, Gargollo PC, Caldamone AA. Current management principles for adolescent varicocele. *Fertil Steril.* 2011;96:1294–1298.

Dickson PV, Sims TL, Streck CJ, et al. Avoiding misdiagnosing neuroblastoma as Wilms tumor. *J Pediatr Surg.* 2008;43:1159–1163.

Downs SM. Technical report: urinary tract infections in febrile infants and young children. The Urinary Tract Subcommittee of the American Academy of Pediatrics Committee on Quality Improvement. *Pediatrics.* 1999;103:e54.

Ellison JS, Kaufman SR, Kraft KH, et al. Underuse of 24-hour urine collection among children with incident urinary stones: A quality-of-care concern? *Urology.* 2014;84:457–461.

Eroglu E, Yip M, Oktar T, et al. How should we treat prepubertal labial adhesions? Retrospective comparison of topical treatments: Estrogen only, betamethasone only, and combination estrogen and betamethasone. *J Pediatr Adolesc Gynecol.* 2011;24:389–391.

Faurschou S, Mouritsen A, Johannsen TH, et al. Hormonal disturbances due to severe and mild forms of congenital adrenal hyperplasia are already detectable in neonatal life. *Acta Paediatr.* 2015;104:e57–62.

Freedman SB, Thull-Freedman J, Manson D, et al. Pediatric abdominal radiograph use, constipation, and significant misdiagnoses. *J Pediatr.* 2014;164:83–88.

Friedlander JI, Moreira DM, Hartman C, et al. Comparison of the metabolic profile of mixed calcium oxalate/uric acid stone formers to that of pure calcium oxalate and pure uric acid stone formers. *Urology.* 2014;84:289–294.

Gandhi V, Khosravi M, Burns A. Page kidney in a 17-year-old renal allograft. *BMJ Case Rep.* 2012;2012.

Gaspari L, Sampaio DR, Paris F, et al. High prevalence of micropenis in 2710 male newborns from an intensive-use pesticide area of Northeastern Brazil. *Int J Androl.* 2012;35:253–264.

Gessler M, Thomas GH, Couillin P, et al. A deletion map of the WAGR region on chromosome 11. *Am J Hum Genet.* 1989;44:486–495.

Giel DW, Noe HN, Williams MA. Ultrasound screening of asymptomatic siblings of children with vesico-ureteral reflux: A long-term followup study. *J Urol.* 2005;174:1602–1604.

Glazener CM, Evans JH, Peto RE. Tricyclic and related drugs for nocturnal enuresis in children. *Cochrane Database Syst Rev.* 2003;3:CD002117.

Godbole P, Wade A, Mushtaq I, Wilcox DT. Vesicostomy vs primary ablation for posterior urethral valves: Always a difference in outcome? *J Pediatr Urol.* 2007;3:273–275.

Goldman RD. Child health update: Estrogen cream for labial adhesion in girls. *Can Fam Physician.* 2013;59:37–38.

Green DM, Breslow NE, Beckwith JB, et al. Treatment with nephrectomy only for small, stage I/favorable histology Wilms' tumor: A report from the National Wilms' Tumor Study Group. *J Clin Oncol.* 2001;19:3719–3724.

Guven A, Kogan BA. Undescended testis in older boys: Further evidence that ascending testes are common. *J Pediatr Surg.* 2008;43:1700–1704.

Haleblian GE, Leitao VA, Pierre SA, et al. Assessment of citrate concentrations in citrus fruit-based juices and beverages: Implications for management of hypocitraturic nephrolithiasis. *J Endourol.* 2008;22:1359–1366.

Holland JM, Graham JB, Ignatoff JM. Conservative management of twisted testicular appendages. *J Urol.* 1981;125:213–214.

Hollingsworth JM, Rogers MA, Kaufman SR, et al. Medical therapy to facilitate urinary stone passage: A meta-analysis. *Lancet.* 2006;368:1171–1179.

Hunziker M, Colhoun E, Puri P. Renal cortical abnormalities in siblings of index patients with vesicoureteral reflux. *Pediatrics*. 2014;133:e933–e937.

Hunziker M, Puri P. Familial vesicoureteral reflux and reflux related morbidity in relatives of index patients with high grade vesicoureteral reflux. *J Urol*. 2012;188:1463–1466.

Jamieson MA, Ashbury T. Flavored midazolam elixir for manual separation of labial adhesions in the office. *J Pediatr Adolesc Gynecol*. 1999;12:106.

Johnson EK, Faerber GJ, Roberts WW, et al. Are stone protocol computed tomography scans mandatory for children with suspected urinary calculi? *Urology*. 2011;78:662–666.

Kaye JD, Levitt SB, Friedman SC, et al. Neonatal torsion: A 14-year experience and proposed algorithm for management. *J Urol*. 2008;179:2377–2383.

Keys C, Heloury Y. Retractile testes: A review of the current literature. *J Pediatr Urol*. 2012;8:2–6.

Koenig JF, McKenna PH. Biofeedback therapy for dysfunctional voiding in children. *Curr Urol Rep*. 2011;12:144–152.

Koff SG, Paquette EL, Cullen J, et al. Comparison between lemonade and potassium citrate and impact on urine pH and 24-hour urine parameters in patients with kidney stone formation. *Urology*. 2007;69:1013–1016.

Kolon TF, Herndon CD, Baker LA, et al. Evaluation and treatment of cryptorchidism: AUA guideline. *J Urol*. 2014;192:337–345.

Korets R, Woldu SL, Nees SN, et al. Testicular symmetry and adolescent varicocele—does it need followup? *J Urol*. 2011;186:1614–1618.

Krone N, Arlt W. Genetics of congenital adrenal hyperplasia. *Best Pract Res Clin Endocrinol Metab*. 2009;23:181–192.

Kumar M, Thakur S, Puri A, et al. Fetal renal anomaly: Factors that predict survival. *J Pediatr Urol*. 2014;10:1001–1007.

Ladi-Seyedian S, Kajbafzadeh AM, Sharifi-Rad L, et al. Management of non-neuropathic underactive bladder in children with voiding dysfunction by animated biofeedback: A randomized clinical trial. *Urology*. 2015;85:205–210.

Lemmens AS, Mekahli D, Devlieger R, et al. Population-specific serum creatinine centiles in neonates with posterior urethral valves already predict long-term renal outcome. *J Matern Fetal Neonatal Med*. 2014:1–6.

Leung AK, Robson WL, Tay-Uyboco J. The incidence of labial fusion in children. *J Paediatr Child Health*. 1993;29:235–236.

Lev M, Ramon J, Mor Y, et al. Sonographic appearances of torsion of the appendix testis and appendix epididymis in children. *J Clin Ultrasound*. 2015;43(8):485–489.

Lewis SJ, Heaton KW. Stool form scale as a useful guide to intestinal transit time. *Scand J Gastroenterol*. 1997;32:920–924.

Lukong CS, Ameh EA, Mshelbwala PM, et al. Role of vesicostomy in the management of posterior urethral valve in Sub-Saharan Africa. *J Pediatr Urol*. 2014;10:62–66.

Malkan AD, Loh A, Bahrami A, et al. An approach to renal masses in pediatrics. *Pediatrics*. 2015;135:142–158.

Mano R, Livne PM, Nevo A, et al. Testicular torsion in the first year of life—characteristics and treatment outcome. *Urology*. 2013;82:1132–1137.

Marks A, Vasquez E, Moylan S, et al. Definition of reliable, objective criteria by abdominal radiography to identify occult constipation in children with lower urinary tract symptoms. *J Urol*. 2013;189:1519–1523.

Matsubara K, Kataoka N, Ogita S, et al. Uniparental disomy of chromosome 8 leading to homozygosity of a CYP11B1 mutation in a patient with congenital adrenal hyperplasia: Implication for a rare etiology of an autosomal recessive disorder. *Endocr J*. 2014;61:629–633.

Matsuo N, Ishii T, Takayama JI, et al. Reference standard of penile size and prevalence of buried penis in Japanese newborn male infants. *Endocr J*. 2014;61:849–853.

McLeod DJ, Alpert SA, Ural Z, Jayanthi VR. Ureteroureterostomy irrespective of ureteral size or upper pole function: A single center experience. *J Pediatr Urol*. 2014;10:616–619.

Meyrier A, Rainfray M, Lacombe M. Delayed hypertension after blunt renal trauma. *Am J Nephrol*. 1988;8:108–111.

Monga M, Scarpero HM, Ortenberg J. Metachronous bilateral torsion of the testicular appendices. *Int J Urol*. 1999;6:589–591.

Morey AF, Brandes S, Dugi DD 3rd, et al. Urotrauma: AUA guideline. *J Urol*. 2014;192:327–335.

Mori R, Yonemoto N, Fitzgerald A, et al. Diagnostic performance of urine dipstick testing in children with suspected UTI: A systematic review of relationship with age and comparison with microscopy. *Acta Paediatr*. 2010;99:581–584.

Motzer RJ, Agarwal N, Beard C, et al. NCCN clinical practice guidelines in oncology: Testicular cancer. *J Natl Compr Canc Netw*. 2009;7:672–693.

Nguyen HT, Benson CB, Bromley B, et al. Multidisciplinary consensus on the classification of prenatal and postnatal urinary tract dilation (UTD classification system). *J Pediatr Urol*. 2014;10:982–998.

Park JM. Normal development of the genitourinary tract. In: McDougal WS, Wein AJ, Kavoussi LR, et al, eds. *Campbell's Urology*. 10th ed. Philadelphia, PA: Elsevier; 2011: 2975–3002.

Park S, Song SH, Lee C, et al. Bacterial pathogens in first febrile urinary tract infection affect breakthrough infections in infants with vesicoureteral reflux treated with prophylactic antibiotics. *Urology*. 2013;81:1342–1345.

Pastuszak AW, Kumar V, Shah A, Roth DR. Diagnostic and management approaches to pediatric and adolescent varicocele: A survey of pediatric urologists. *Urology*. 2014;84:450–455.

Pearle MS, Calhoun EA, Curhan GC; Urologic Diseases of America Project. Urologic diseases in America project: Urolithiasis. *J Urol*. 2005;173:848–857.

Pelletier J, Bruening W, Kashtan CE, et al. Germline mutations in the Wilms' tumor suppressor gene are associated with abnormal urogenital development in Denys-Drash syndrome. *Cell*. 1991;67:437–447.

Plaire JC, Pope JC 4th, Kropp BP, et al. Management of ectopic ureters: Experience with the upper tract approach. *J Urol*. 1997;158:1245–1247.

Pulido JE, Furth SL, Zderic SA, et al. Renal parenchymal area and risk of ESRD in boys with posterior urethral valves. *Clin J Am Soc Nephrol*. 2014;9:499–505.

Rittig N, Hagstroem S, Mahler B, et al. Outcome of a standardized approach to childhood urinary symptoms-long-term follow-up of 720 patients. *Neurourol Urodyn.* 2014;33:475–481.

Saini AK, Regmi S, Seth A, et al. Outcome analysis of tumors in undescended testes—a single center experience of 15 years. *Urology.* 2013;82:852–856.

Sansom SL, Prabhu VS, Hutchinson AB, et al. Cost-effectiveness of newborn circumcision in reducing lifetime HIV risk among U.S. males. *PLoS One.* 2010;5:e8723.

Sarhan OM, Helmy TE, Alotay AA, et al. Did antenatal diagnosis protect against chronic kidney disease in patients with posterior urethral valves? A multicenter study. *Urology.* 2013;82:1405–1409.

Satoh Y, Nakadate H, Nakagawachi T, et al. Genetic and epigenetic alterations on the short arm of chromosome 11 are involved in a majority of sporadic Wilms' tumours. *Br J Cancer.* 2006;95:541–547.

Seo S, Ochi T, Yazaki Y, et al. Soft tissue interposition is effective for protecting the neourethra during hypospadias surgery and preventing postoperative urethrocutaneous fistula: A single surgeon's experience of 243 cases. *Pediatr Surg Int.* 2015;31:297–303.

Shamberger RC, Anderson JR, Breslow NE, et al. Long-term outcomes for infants with very low risk Wilms tumor treated with surgery alone in National Wilms Tumor Study-5. *Ann Surg.* 2010;251:555–558.

Sharp VJ, Kieran K, Arlen AM. Testicular torsion: Diagnosis, evaluation, and management. *Am Fam Physician.* 2013;88:835–840.

Shnorhavorian M, Jacobs MA, Stearns G, et al. Practice variation and clinical confusion regarding undescended testes and retractile testes among primary care respondents: A multi-regional survey study in the United States. *Pediatr Surg Int.* 2012;28:635–639.

Smith-Bindman R, Aubin C, Bailitz J, et al. Ultrasonography versus computed tomography for suspected nephrolithiasis. *N Engl J Med.* 2014;371:1100–1110.

Smyth A, Collins CS, Thorsteinsdottir B, et al. Page kidney: Etiology, renal function outcomes and risk for future hypertension. *J Clin Hypertens (Greenwich).* 2012;14:216–221.

Snodgrass W, Bush N. Recent advances in understanding/management of hypospadias. *F1000Prime Rep.* 2014;6:101.

Subcommittee on Urinary Tract Infection, Steering Committee on Quality Improvement and Management, Roberts KB. Urinary tract infection: clinical practice guideline for the diagnosis and management of the initial UTI in febrile infants and children 2 to 24 months. *Pediatrics.* 2011;128:595–610.

Tanito K, Ota A, Kamide R, et al. Clinical features of 58 Japanese patients with mosaic neurofibromatosis 1. *J Dermatol.* 2014;41:724–728.

Tasian GE, Copelovitch L. Evaluation and medical management of kidney stones in children. *J Urol.* 2014;192:1329–1336.

Tasian GE, Cost NG, Granberg CF, et al. Tamsulosin and spontaneous passage of ureteral stones in children: A multi-institutional cohort study. *J Urol.* 2014;192:506–511.

Tekgül S, Riedmiller H, Dogan HS, et al. Guidelines on paediatric urology. European Association of Urology, European Society for Paediatric Urology, 2012. Accessed http://uroweb.org/wp-content/uploads/22-Paediatric-Urology_LR.pdf. March 11, 2015.

Tharner A, Jansen PW, Kiefte-de Jong JC, et al. Bidirectional associations between fussy eating and functional constipation in preschool children. *J Pediatr.* 2015;166:91–96.

Tracy CR, Pearle MS. Update on the medical management of stone disease. *Curr Opin Urol.* 2009;19:200–204.

van Gool JD, de Jong TP, Winkler-Seinstra P, et al. Multi-center randomized controlled trial of cognitive treatment, placebo, oxybutynin, bladder training, and pelvic floor training in children with functional urinary incontinence. *Neurourol Urodyn.* 2014;33:482–487.

Varni JW, Bendo CB, Nurko S, et al. Health-related quality of life in pediatric patients with functional and organic gastrointestinal diseases. *J Pediatr.* 2015;166:85–90.

Vicentini FC, Mazzucchi E, Brito AH, et al. Adjuvant tamsulosin or nifedipine after extracorporeal shock wave lithotripsy for renal stones: A double blind, randomized, placebo-controlled trial. *Urology.* 2011;78:1016–1021.

Wallis MC, Khoury AE, Lorenzo AJ, et al. Outcome analysis of retroperitoneal laparoscopic heminephrectomy in children. *J Urol.* 2006;175:2277–2280.

Wayne C, Chan E, Nasr A; The Canadian Association of Paediatric Surgeons Evidence-Based Resource. What is the ideal surgical approach for intra-abdominal testes? A systematic review. *Pediatr Surg Int.* 2015 Feb 8. [Epub ahead of print]

White B. Diagnosis and treatment of urinary tract infections in children. *Am Fam Physician.* 2011;83:409–415.

Williams GJ, Macaskill P, Chan SF, et al. Absolute and relative accuracy of rapid urine tests for urinary tract infection in children: A meta-analysis. *Lancet Infect Dis.* 2010;10:240–250.

Growth and Development

Erin Howe

19

▶ CASE 1

At a health maintenance exam, a 13-year-old girl and her mother note that she has not started to show any signs of puberty. They are wondering if this is normal. Her growth chart reveals that she is in the 25th percentile for weight and the 15th percentile for height. On physical exam, you note that she is Tanner stage 1 for breast and pubic hair. You decide to obtain a bone age, which reveals a skeletal maturity of 10 years.

Question 1-1

Her upper-to-lower segment ratio would be expected to be closest to which of the following?

A) 0.80.
B) 1.0.
C) 1.2.
D) 1.4.
E) 1.6.

Discussion 1-1

The correct answer is "B." This bone age for this child indicates that her skeletal maturity is approximately 10 years, which would suggest that her body proportions are closer to those of a 10-year-old rather than her chronological age of 13 years. The upper-to-lower segment ratio is useful for evaluating tall or short stature and differentiating disproportionate growth from immaturity. To obtain the upper-to-lower segment ratio, first obtain the lower segment measurement, which is the distance between the symphysis pubis and the plantar surface of the foot. The upper segment is calculated by subtracting the lower segment measurement from the child's height. At birth, the head and trunk are large relative to the length of the limbs, resulting in an upper-to-lower segment ratio of around 1.7. This gradually declines to approximately equal proportions at age 10 years, with a ratio close to 1.0. Following puberty, the upper-to-lower segment ratio in most adults is less than 1.0.

Question 1-2

For this child, which of the following is appropriate advice in counseling the parents on linear growth rate in childhood and into puberty?

A) Linear growth is approximately 25 cm/y from birth to 1 year, 10 cm/y from ages 1 to 4 years, 5 cm/y until puberty, and then is between 8 and 10 cm/y during the pubertal growth spurt.
B) Linear growth is approximately 15 cm/y from birth to 1 year, 7.5 cm/y from ages 1 to 4 years, 5 cm/y until puberty, and then is between 8 and 10 cm/y during the pubertal growth spurt.
C) Linear growth is approximately 25 cm/y from birth to 1 year, 7.5 cm/y from ages 1 to 4 years, 3 cm/y until puberty, and then is between 8 and 10 cm/y during the pubertal growth spurt.
D) Linear growth is approximately 25 cm/y from birth to 1 year, 7.5 cm/y from ages 1 to 4 years, 3 cm/y until puberty, and then is between 10 and 12 cm/y during the pubertal growth spurt.
E) Linear growth is approximately 25 cm/y from birth to 1 year, 10 cm/y from ages 1 to 4 years, 5 cm/y until puberty, and then is between 10 and 12 cm/y during the pubertal growth spurt.

Discussion 1-2

The correct answer is "A." It lists the correct combination of linear growth rates in childhood and adolescence. The average girl begins a pubertal growth spurt around age 11.5 years and grows at a peak of 8.3 cm/y, which then slows to a stop around age 16 years. The average boy begins a pubertal growth spurt around age 13.5 years and grows at a rate of 9.5 cm/y before slowing to a stop by the age of 18 years. Remember, girls have an earlier growth spurt than boys. (Think about junior high school dances; it is normal for girls to be taller than boys.)

> **Helpful Tip**
> In children younger than 2 years of age, length not height should be measured. Length is obtained with the child lying down rather than standing up (as for height measurement).

A family presents with their breastfed newborn for a weight check at 8 days of life. They are concerned that she still has not regained her birthweight and are wondering what constitutes a normal rate of weight gain during infancy.

Question 2-1

Which of the following statements correctly describes changes from birthweight during the first 12 months of life?

A) Birthweight is regained by 7 days of life, doubles by 4 months, and triples by 12 months of age.

B) Birthweight is regained by 10 days of life, doubles by 3 months, and triples by 10 months of age.

C) Birthweight is regained by 14 days of life, doubles by 6 months, and triples by 12 months of age.

D) Birthweight is regained by 14 days of life, doubles by 4 months, and triples by 12 months of age.

E) Birthweight is regained by 21 days of life, doubles by 6 months, and triples by 10 months of age.

Discussion 2-1

The correct answer is "D." It is expected that normal term newborns will have a decrease in as much as 10% of birthweight in the first week of life but then will regain, if not surpass, birthweight by 2 weeks of age. Compared with breastfed neonates, formula-fed newborns lose less weight and regain their birthweight sooner. During the first 12 months of life, weight gain typically follows the pattern indicated in option "D," with birthweight doubling by 4 months and tripling by 12 months of age.

....

The same child is now 3 years old and is again in clinic for a routine health maintenance exam. Her parents are wondering if she is gaining adequate weight. They note that some days she eats what they consider to be an adequate amount of food and other days she barely eats anything.

Question 2-2

Of the following, what is the most appropriate recommendation for the child's parents regarding weight gain in childhood?

A) Between the ages of 1 and 5 years, a child typically gains 2 pounds per year.

B) Weight gain gradually increases by 1 pound per year from the age of 2 years until peaking in adolescence.

C) A toddler should continue to gain approximately 10 pounds per year until age 5 years when weight gain slows down until adolescence.

D) After the age of 2 years and until adolescence, normal weight gain is approximately 5 pounds per year.

E) Children typically do not gain weight until puberty.

Discussion 2-2

The correct answer is "D." Weight gain slows down after a child reaches 2 years and increases at a fairly steady rate of 5 pounds per year throughout childhood until adolescence.

The feeding pattern of the 3-year-old in this question is typical of toddler and preschool-aged children. Although it can be quite frustrating for parents and caregivers, such fluctuations in food intake do not typically require intervention as the child continues to take in appropriate calories for growth.

A family in your practice brings their 9-month-old son for a well-baby exam. At birth, the infant was in the 95th percentile for both weight and length, but starting at his 6-month visit he has shown a decline in percentiles for both weight and length. He was at the 85th percentile for weight and length at 6 months and is now at the 75th percentile. His head circumference has been consistently in the 90th percentile since birth. The parents recall that their older daughter (who is currently a healthy 5-year-old) showed a similar pattern in growth starting at around 6 months of age, and she leveled off at the 50th percentile for weight and the 25th percentile for length, where she has remained. The mother reports that her height is 5 feet, 1 inch, and the father's height is 5 feet, 7 inches.

Question 3-1

Of the following, what is the next most appropriate thing to tell the parents regarding this infant's growth pattern?

A) The infant should have lab tests to evaluate renal function given his recent decline in growth percentiles and concern for failure to thrive.

B) The parents should consider boosting the infant's caloric intake by fortifying breast milk and offering table foods higher in calories and fat to make up for his decline in weight percentile.

C) The infant's weight and length at birth most likely reflected the intrauterine environment, and now he has started tracking toward his genetic potential.

D) The family should be screened for an underlying genetic condition that is causing this failure to grow along a consistent curve.

E) As long as the head circumference maintains its growth percentile, changes in percentiles for weight, length, or both are not worrisome.

Discussion 3-1

The correct answer is "C." It is fairly common for an infant who was at the top of the growth charts at birth to begin to track toward his or her genetic potential during the later stages of infancy. The measurements at birth reflect the intrauterine environment more than genetic potential. In this case, given that the genetic potential of this infant is to not be particularly tall and that an older sibling had a similar pattern, it is reasonable to not be too concerned about an underlying cause of failure to thrive at this point. Nonetheless, it would be a good idea to keep potential causes for delayed growth in mind as you follow this child's growth curves, and if he continues to show significant declines or other signs of developmental delay or chronic illness, consider further workup for an underlying cause of poor growth.

Question 3-2

For this same infant, what is the predicted midparental height?
A) 5 feet, 7 inches,
B) 5 feet, 6.5 inches.
C) 5 feet, 5.5 inches.
D) 5 feet, 4 inches.
E) 5 feet, 8 inches.

Discussion 3-2

The correct answer is "B." Calculation of midparental height is a useful tool when evaluating a child for short stature, particularly if there has been a decline in percentile for length since birth and you are trying to decide if it is due to genetic potential or another underlying cause that would require further investigation. The formula for midparental height calculation in inches for boys is:

$$[(\text{Maternal height} + 5) + \text{Paternal height}]/2$$

In the case described above, the mother is 5 feet, 1 inch, and the father is 5 feet, 7 inches tall. The midparental height would thus be calculated as: $[(61 + 5) + 67]/2 = 66.5$ inches.

Question 3-3

What would the predicted midparental height be if this infant was female?
A) 5 feet, 4 inches.
B) 5 feet, 5.5 inches.
C) 5 feet, 1 inches.
D) 5 feet, 3 inches.
E) 5 feet, 1.5 inches.

Discussion 3-3

The correct answer is "E." The formula for midparental height calculation for girls is:

$$[\text{Maternal height} + (\text{Paternal height} - 5)]/2$$

Adult target height is then expected to be midparental height ± 2 inches.

▶ CASE 4

Parents of a 3-month-old girl express concern that she still does not lift her head while prone and does not socially smile or show interest in visual stimulation. You note on physical exam that her head circumference is less than the second percentile, and review of her growth charts shows it has been between the third and fifth percentile since birth. Also on exam, the infant is hypotonic but does not have any other abnormal findings.

Question 4-1

What is the next most appropriate step in diagnosing the underlying cause of the infant's symptoms?
A) Head ultrasonography.
B) Brain magnetic resonance imaging (MRI).
C) Electroencephalography (EEG).
D) Plain films of the skull.
E) Both C and D.

Discussion 4-1

The correct answer is "B." When head circumference is found to be more than 2 standard deviations below the mean for associated age and sex, a child is considered to have microcephaly. Microcephaly may be primary or secondary. In secondary or acquired microcephaly, the head circumference is normal at birth. Primary causes are predominantly genetic and may be associated with certain syndromes such as trisomy 21, cri-du-chat, or Smith-Lemli-Opitz. Secondary microcephaly is nongenetic and may be due to an infectious or other harmful insult during periods of rapid brain growth. Infections such as cytomegalovirus, rubella, and toxoplasmosis are known to cause secondary microcephaly. Additionally, a child exposed to alcohol in utero or who experiences a hypoxic-ischemic event in the perinatal period is more likely to have microcephaly. Of the listed options, a brain MRI would be the most useful study as it may identify structural brain abnormalities as an underlying cause of the microcephaly. If the microcephaly is due to premature fusion of the fontanelles, a head ultrasound would not be feasible as patent fontanelles are required. An EEG is a useful tool in characterizing and quantifying seizure activity, but at this point in your evaluation, you do not have a history of concern for seizures in this infant. Additionally, plain skull radiographs or films may be useful in the initial workup of craniosynostosis (premature fusion of the cranial sutures) but would not identify underlying brain abnormalities.

⏳ QUICK QUIZ

What is the average frontal-occipital head circumference of a newborn born at 40 weeks' gestation?
A) 25 cm.
B) 30 cm.
C) 35 cm.
D) 40 cm.
E) 45 cm.

Discussion

The correct answer is "C." The average head circumference of a term newborn is 35 cm. Frontal-occipital head circumference should be measured at each health supervision visit from birth to 24 months of age.

As part of your examination of the infant, you check for the "soft spot" on the infant's head.

Question 4-2

Which of the following statements most accurately describes the timing of the closure of the anterior and posterior fontanelles?

A) The anterior and the posterior fontanelles typically close by 2 months of age.

B) The anterior fontanelle closes by 4 months of age, but the posterior fontanelle can still be palpated in most 9-month-olds.

C) The anterior and posterior fontanelles both close at approximately 12 months of age.

D) The anterior fontanelle may be closed starting at 10 months of age, and the posterior fontanelle closes around 2 months of age.

E) The anterior fontanelle may close as late as 18 months of age, and the posterior fontanelle closes around 4 months of age.

Discussion 4-2

The correct answer is "D." The anterior fontanelle is palpable where the metopic, sagittal, and coronal sutures meet, and the posterior fontanelle is palpable at the juncture of the lambdoid and sagittal sutures. Usually the posterior fontanelle is smaller than the anterior fontanelle and typically is no longer palpable after 2 months of age. The anterior fontanelle has a wider window of closure that spans the period between 10 and 24 months of age. (See Figure 19–1.)

> **Helpful Tip**
> The bones of the newborn skull are not fused but are separated by sutures. This mobility is important for (1) birth, as the skull can be transiently molded to allow for delivery; and (2) accommodation of rapid brain growth during infancy and childhood.

Question 4-3

What is the normal growth rate of an infant's head?

A) Head circumference increases on average 0.5 cm per month for the first year of life.

B) Head circumference increases on average 1 cm per month for the first year of life.

C) Head circumference increases on average 1.5 cm per month for the first year of life.

D) Head circumference increases on average 2 cm per month for the first year of life.

Discussion 4-3

The correct answer is "B." It is expected that an infant's head will grow on average 1 cm per month for the first year of life. More specifically, this is broken down further into 2 cm per month from birth to 3 months, 1 cm per month from 3 to 6 months, and then 0.5 cm per month from 6 to 12 months.

> **Helpful Tip**
> The frontal-occipital circumference reflects brain growth. If the brain is not growing the skull with not grow, so a small head typically equals a small brain. A large head may be caused by a number of things, including a big brain, hydrocephalus, or a tumor or mass.

▶ CASE 5

At a 9-month well-baby exam, the infant's frontal-occipital circumference is at the 97th percentile. She has been at the same percentile since birth. Her weight and length are normal. She is meeting all developmental milestones. Her fontanelle is soft, cranial nerves are intact, and her tone is normal.

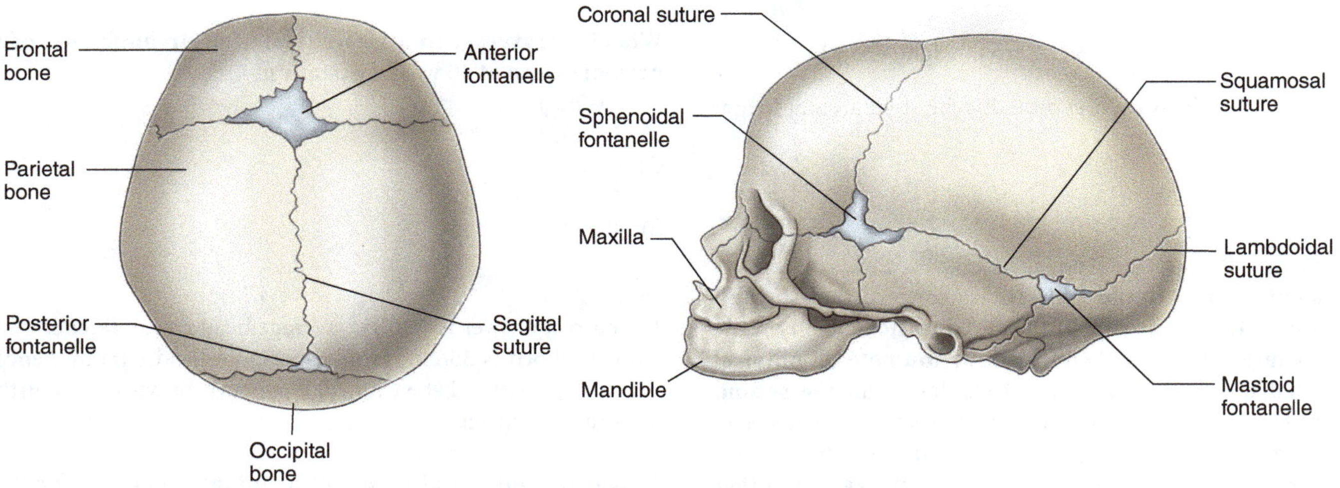

FIGURE 19–1. Cranial sutures. Memorize this drawing. It is high yield for the Pediatrics Board Exam.

She is not dysmorphic nor does her head look big. There is no family history of developmental delay or hydrocephalus. The father notes that he has a big head and cannot wear fitted hats as they are not available in a large enough size.

Question 5-1

Of the following, what should you do next?
A) Order a brain MRI.
B) Order a head ultrasound.
C) Refer the child to a neurologist.
D) Tell the father that her head size is normal.
E) Measure the father's and mother's head circumferences.

Discussion 5-1

The correct answer is "E." Macrocephaly is defined as a frontal-occipital circumference greater than 2 standard deviations above the mean for age, sex, and gestation (≥ 97%). It is important to evaluate head growth over time by looking at serial measurements plotted on a growth curve. A growth rate that is faster than normal or a head circumference that has crossed 2 or more percentiles is concerning. Head imaging should be obtained to look for hydrocephalus or a mass lesion. Normal development is reassuring. During the exam, attention should be paid to signs of increased intracranial pressure or features of a genetic syndrome.

The father's and mother's head circumferences are measured and plotted on the Weaver curve. The infant's frontal-occipital circumference falls within the expected range.

Question 5-2

What do you tell the family about the infant's macrocephaly?
A) It is familial condition.
B) It is a benign condition.
C) No additional workup is necessary at this time.
D) Her brain cells are increased in size and number.
E) All of the above.

Discussion 5-2

The correct answer is "E." Megalencephaly is enlargement of the brain parenchyma. It results from an increase in the number or size of neurons or from deposition of substances (eg, storage disorders) within the brain tissues. In benign familial megalencephaly, infants are born with large heads and normal body size. Their neurologic exams and development are normal. There is typically a history of large heads in the family. The parents' head circumferences should be measured and plotted on the Weaver curve to confirm the diagnosis.

⏳ QUICK QUIZ

Which is NOT a cause of macrocephaly?
A) Hydrocephalus.
B) Lissencephaly.
C) Subdural hematoma.

D) Arteriovenous malformation.
E) Osteopetrosis.

Discussion

The correct answer is "B." Macrocephaly can be caused by hydrocephalus, intracranial mass lesions (tumors, subdural effusions), a big brain (megalencephaly), or a thickened or enlarged skull (skeletal dysplasias). Megalencephaly is seen in neurocutaneous syndromes (ie, neurofibromatosis), Soto syndrome, achondroplasia, leukodystrophies, and mucopolysaccharidosis. It can also occur in families as a benign trait. Osteopetrosis results in uncontrolled growth of the bones of skull due to impaired osteoclast function. Lissencephaly results from abnormal formation of the brain cortex and is associated with microcephaly.

▶ CASE 6

You are seeing a 4-month-old male infant for a routine health maintenance visit. On physical exam you notice that he has a midline palpable vertical ridge running along the forehead and his head appears to be triangular in shape. You note on the growth chart that his head circumference is normal and he is otherwise growing and developing as expected.

Question 6-1

Of the following, you are most likely to tell the infant's mother that his head shape is due to:
A) Premature fusion of the metopic suture.
B) Premature fusion of the sagittal suture.
C) Positional plagiocephaly.
D) Premature fusion of the coronal suture.
E) Premature fusion of the bilateral coronal suture.

Discussion 6-1

The correct answer is "A." Craniosynostosis is due to premature fusion of any of the cranial sutures. Up to 20% of cases are associated with a genetic syndrome (Apert, Crouzon), but most often the cause is unknown. The four major sutures are sagittal, coronal, lambdoid, and metopic. Fusion of any one suture restricts the perpendicular growth of the skull to the affected suture. The infant in this case most likely has premature closure of the metopic suture, which has resulted in trigonocephaly, characterized by a pointed forehead with a midline vertical ridge and hypotelorism. (See Figure 19–2.)

Question 6-2

What would be next stage in workup for this patient?
A) Obtain a head ultrasound.
B) Refer the infant for a genetic evaluation.
C) Obtain a brain MRI.
D) Obtain a three-dimensional head computed tomography (CT) scan.
E) Obtain plain films of the skull.

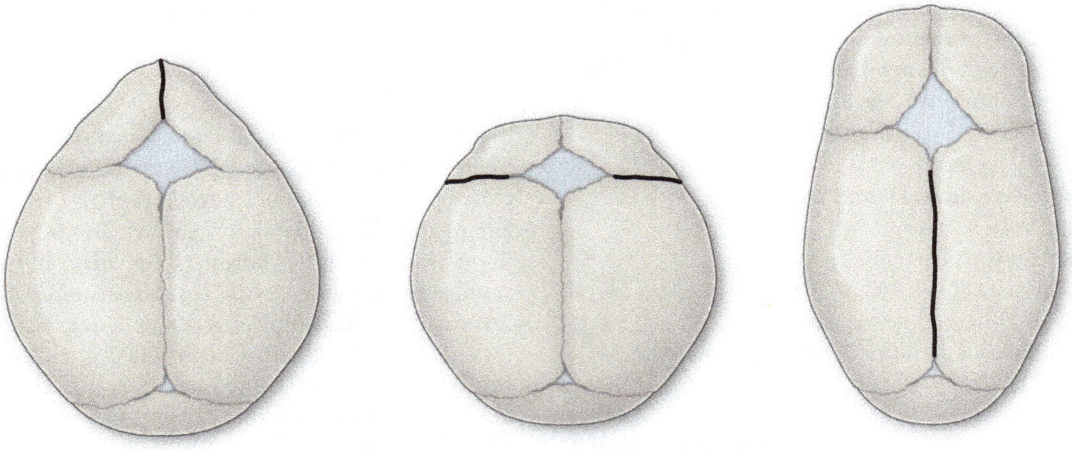

Metopic craniosynostosis (Trigonocephaly)   **Bicoronal craniosynostosis (Brachycephaly)**   **Sagittal craniosynostosis (Scaphocephaly)**

FIGURE 19–2. The most common variations of congenital craniosynostosis.

Discussion 6-2

The correct answer is "D." In the diagnosis of craniosynostosis, a three-dimensional (3D) CT scan of the head is considered the gold standard test. A brain MRI would be indicated in the investigation of brain structures, but in this case we are more interested in the bony structure of the skull. Plain skull films may be used in the initial workup for a child with suspected craniosynostosis, but for full characterization of premature suture closure a 3D head CT is recommended. Finally, although this patient may end up requiring a referral to a geneticist if it is suspected that the craniosynostosis is due to an underlying syndrome, this would not be the first step in diagnostic workup. Once diagnosed, the infant should be referred to a surgical specialist for surgical correction.

Question 6-3

What is the most common form of premature suture closure?
A) Brachycephaly resulting from bilateral premature fusion of the coronal sutures.
B) Plagiocephaly resulting from unilateral premature fusion of the lambdoid sutures.
C) Scaphocephaly resulting from premature fusion of the sagittal suture.
D) Trigonocephaly resulting from premature fusion of the metopic suture.
E) Trigonocephaly and brachycephaly occur most frequently at approximately equal rates.

Discussion 6-3

The correct answer is "C." Scaphocephaly (boat-shaped head) due to premature closure of the sagittal suture is the most common form of craniosynostosis. Affected children have frontal bossing with a prominent occiput. The head circumference is normal but biparietal diameter is reduced. In bilateral coronal suture synostosis (brachycephaly), there is a broad flattened forehead. In unilateral coronal suture synostosis (anterior plagiocephaly), the forehead on the affected side is flat with a raised eyebrow and the nose and chin deviate toward the normal side. Posterior plagiocephaly results from unilateral premature fusion of the lambdoid suture, with resultant flattening of the occiput and bulging of the ipsilateral forehead. There is also a form of nonsynostotic plagiocephaly known as positional plagiocephaly, which occurs as a result of malpositioning in utero or after birth. Trigonocephaly, described in Question 6-1, is characterized by a triangle-shaped head with a pointed forehead and a midline vertical ridge along the forehead. A cloverleaf skull is a form of craniosynostosis involving premature fusion of multiple sutures.

⧖ QUICK QUIZ

Which of the following is NOT an associated complication of uncorrected craniosynostosis?
A) Facial asymmetry.
B) Intracranial hypotension.
C) Hydrocephalus.
D) Strabismus.
E) Dental malocclusion.

Discussion

The correct answer is "B." Intracranial hypertension not hypotension is a complication of craniosynostosis. Neurologic complications are more likely to occur when two or more sutures are involved. Strabismus may develop from asymmetry of the orbits. The treatment of craniosynostosis is surgical correction.

▶ CASE 7

While examining a 4-month-old girl at her health maintenance exam her parents ask you to inspect the shape of her head as they are worried that it appears abnormal. You note that there is some flattening over the occiput on the left side but no other abnormal findings on head or neck exam.

Question 7-1

Which of the following descriptions is most consistent with benign posterior positional plagiocephaly?

A) Trapezoid-shaped head with ipsilateral occipitoparietal flattening, posterior displacement of the ipsilateral ear, and contralateral frontal bossing.

B) Triangle-shaped skull with midline vertical ridge running along forehead.

C) Flattened occiput, prominent and flattened frontal bone, and anterior displacement of the vertex.

D) Parallelogram-shaped head with ipsilateral occipitoparietal flattening, ipsilateral anterior displacement of the ear, and ipsilateral frontal bossing.

E) Long and narrow-shaped head.

Discussion 7-1

The correct answer is "D." When evaluating a flat occiput, it is important to differentiate unilateral lambdoid synostosis from the more common benign positional plagiocephaly. In positional plagiocephaly, the skull is flattened from prolonged periods of lying supine. It has become more common since the "back to sleep" campaign was initiated to help prevent sudden infant death syndrome. To differentiate the two, view the infant's head from above. Remember to look closely at the ears. In benign positional plagiocephaly, you would expect the ipsilateral ear to be displaced anteriorly. The skull is sometimes noted to have a parallelogram shape with frontal prominence noted ipsilateral to the occipitoparietal flattening. In contrast, the ipsilateral ear is displaced posteriorly in unilateral lambdoid synostosis, with frontal prominence contralateral to the occipitoparietal flattening. This has been described as a trapezoidal shape. (See Table 19–1 and Figure 19–3.)

TABLE 19–1 POSITIONAL PLAGIOCEPHALY VERSUS UNILATERAL LAMBDOID SYNOSTOSIS

	Positional Plagiocephaly	Unilateral Lambdoid Synostosis
Head shape from above	Parallelogram	Trapezoid
Ipsilateral occipitoparietal flattening	Yes	Yes
Ipsilateral ear displacement	Anterior	Posterior and inferior
Frontal bossing (forehead)	Ipsilateral	None or contralateral
Palpable suture ridge	No	Sometimes
Incidence	Common	Rare

Used with permission from Erin Howe, MD.

Question 7-2

What is appropriate counseling for this family regarding positional plagiocephaly?

A) Recommend placing the infant prone as much as possible while awake and supervised, and alternating the point of contact between occiput and crib mattress while sleeping.

B) Recommend use of a side-positioning device to alternate sleep positions in the crib.

C) Recommend physical therapy.

D) Advise that the degree of skull flattening due to positional plagiocephaly should peak at around 12 months of age.

E) Recommend surgical consultation.

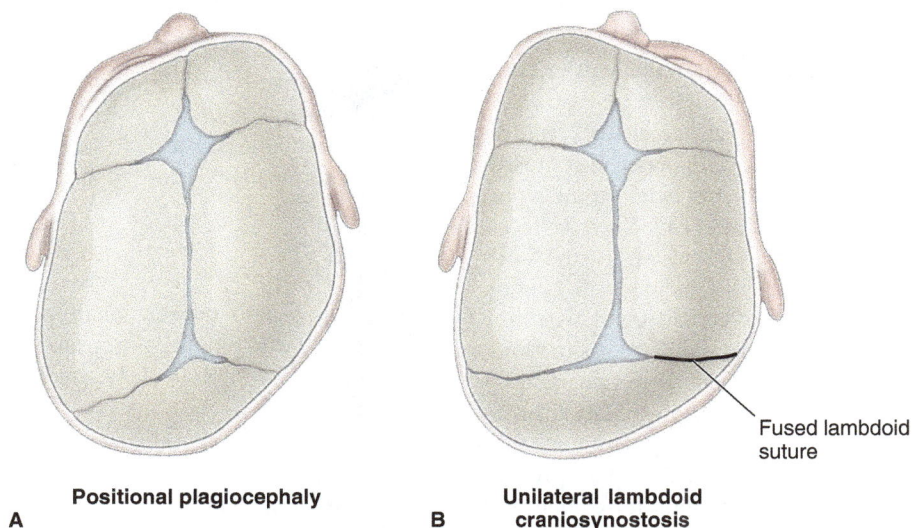

Positional plagiocephaly
A

Unilateral lambdoid craniosynostosis
B

Fused lambdoid suture

FIGURE 19–3. Plagiocephaly. Differentiating plagiocephaly that is positional from that due to premature fusion of the lambdoid suture is challenging. (A) Positional plagiocephaly is characterized by a parallelogram-shaped head, unilateral flattened occiput, anterior displaced ear, and frontal bossing on the ipsilateral side. (B) Unilateral lambdoid synostosis is characterized by a trapezoid-shaped head, unilateral flattened occiput, posterior displaced ear on the ipsilateral side, and frontal bossing on the contralateral side.

Discussion 7-2

The correct answer is "A." For an infant with benign positional plagiocephaly, conservative management is recommended such as placing the infant prone ("tummy time") while awake and supervised, and alternating the orientation in the crib when he or she is put to bed, as infants tend to want to face away from the wall and will turn their head accordingly. Infants should always sleep on their backs even if they have a flat head. It is not recommended that any positioning devices be used in the infant's sleep environment. Unless the infant has torticollis on exam, physical therapy is unlikely to improve the plagiocephaly. The degree of plagiocephaly should peak between 4 and 8 months and then begin to improve as the infant becomes more mobile and spends less time in the supine position. (See Figure 19–3, earlier.)

► CASE 8

A 21-month-old boy presents to your clinic for a late 18-month health maintenance exam. You note that his last well-child exam was at age 6 months at a different clinic and you do not have access to those records at this time. He is in the fifth percentile for weight and the third percentile for weight-for-length.

Question 8-1

What else do you want to know from the history of this child?
A) Details about the environmental setting in which meals are offered.
B) Whether there is any history of maternal depression.
C) Growth pattern for the first 6 months of life, including birth history.
D) Detailed diet history.
E) Midparental height calculation.
F) All of the above.

Discussion 8-1

The correct answer is "F." When a child presents with findings that are concerning for poor growth, the first step is usually to inspect the growth chart for length, weight, and head circumference starting at birth to evaluate trends. While evaluating growth curves, it may be useful to plot midparental height to help predict genetic potential. After growth charts have been assessed, a detailed diet history is warranted, including when new foods were introduced. The history should also include information about feeding behaviors, such as who feeds the child, when the child eats, whether he or she eats better in different situations, and the dining environment (highchair, television on, distractions, etc). A complete review of systems to evaluate for gastrointestinal, respiratory, or other constitutional symptoms may reveal an underlying organic cause for the child's poor growth. During the physical exam, it is helpful to look for evidence of developmental delay, abnormal social interaction, or dysmorphic features while also evaluating for signs of malnutrition, such as hair or skin changes and body fat stores. Also, be sure to observe the caregiver's interaction with the child.

TABLE 19–2 EXPECTED WEIGHT GAIN FROM BIRTH TO 3 YEARS OF AGE

Age Group	Minimum Weight Gain
Infants 0–3 months	≥ 20 g/day
Infants 3–6 months	≥ 15 g/day
Infants 6–12 months	≥ 10 g/day
Toddlers 1–3 years	≥ 7 g/day

Question 8-2

All of the following are common definitions of failure to thrive EXCEPT:
A) Weight less than the third percentile.
B) Weight-for-height less than the fifth percentile.
C) Weight gain of less than 30 g/day for an infant from birth to 3 months of age.
D) Weight 20% or more below ideal weight for height.
E) Weight gain of less than 15 g/day from 3 to 6 months of age.

Discussion 8-2

The correct answer is "C." Failure to thrive has a number of different definitions and is typically used to describe infants and toddlers younger than 3 years of age who are not growing as expected. It is not a diagnosis. The definition includes weight for age below the third percentile, weight crossing two or more percentile lines on the growth curve, or weight less than 80% of ideal weight for age. All of the listed choices are common definitions of failure to thrive except option "C." Actually, weight gain of less than 20 g/day, not 30 g/day, from birth to 3 months of age is considered a definition of failure to thrive. If a child has normal weight for length and normal growth velocity, consider other options such as short stature or constitutional growth delay instead of failure to thrive. (See Table 19–2.)

> **Helpful Tip**
> In premature infants, weight is corrected for gestational age until 2 years of age. After 2 years of age, standard World Health Organization (WHO) growth curves may be used to track growth.

> **Helpful Tip**
> In certain genetic syndromes, such as trisomy 21 or achondroplasia, specialized growth curves are available and should be used.

⧖ QUICK QUIZ

Which is NOT a cause of symmetric failure to thrive?
A) Chronic malnutrition.
B) Growth hormone deficiency.

C) Genetic syndrome.
D) Congenital infection.
E) Teratogen exposure.

Discussion

The correct answer is "B." In acute malnutrition, head circumference is generally preserved. Protecting the brain is important! Weight decreases first, followed by length (stunting), and finally head circumference if malnutrition is longstanding. This pattern is called *asymmetric failure to thrive*. In symmetric failure to thrive, all three growth measurements are equally affected and suggest one of the etiologies listed in the answer choices. If a child is stunted and short but not wasted, consider an endocrine disorder (eg, hypothyroidism or growth hormone deficiency). Chronic diseases, including inflammatory bowel and celiac disease, can cause stunting. Sometimes slowed linear growth is the first manifestation.

Question 8-3

What is the most common cause of failure to thrive in developed countries?
A) Gastroesophageal reflux.
B) Inadequate caloric intake in the setting of psychosocial influences.
C) Tuberculosis.
D) Chronic renal failure.
E) Thyroid disease.

Discussion 8-3

The correct answer is "B." The social environment for the infant or child plays a key role in weight gain and growth. Substance abuse, domestic violence, parental intellectual disability or mental illness, and poverty are all risk factors for a child failing to thrive. Therefore, failure to thrive in developed countries is most commonly found to be due to inadequate caloric intake in the setting of a complex social situation at home. In addition to considering inadequate intake, one should also consider impaired nutrient absorption such as that seen in infants with cystic fibrosis and greater than normal energy needs as experienced by some infants with chronic medical conditions such as congenital heart disease. Gastroesophageal reflux is a known cause of failure to thrive, but not more common than inadequate caloric intake. In developing countries with a higher prevalence of tuberculosis, this infection can certainly contribute to failure to thrive. Another infectious cause of failure to thrive that should be considered is human immunodeficiency virus. Finally, chronic renal or endocrine diseases should be considered in the workup of failure to thrive. (See Table 19–3.)

> **Helpful Tip**
> Causes of failure to thrive vary by age and can be broken down into three main categories: (1) inadequate intake, (2) malabsorption, and (3) increased metabolic demand.

TABLE 19–3 DIFFERENTIAL DIAGNOSIS OF FAILURE TO THRIVE BY ORGAN SYSTEM

Congenital	**Cardiovascular**
Genetic syndromes (eg, trisomy 21, Turner)	Congenital heart disease
Intrauterine growth retardation	
Craniofacial malformation (eg, cleft palate)	
Congenital infection	
Endocrine	**Gastrointestinal**
Hypothyroidism	Malabsorption syndromes
Hyperthyroidism	Celiac disease
Type 1 diabetes mellitus	Inflammatory bowel disease
Adrenal insufficiency	Gastroesophageal reflux
	Hepatobiliary disease
Respiratory	**Renal**
Cystic fibrosis	Chronic kidney disease
Poorly controlled asthma	Renal tubular disease
Airway anomaly (eg, upper airway obstruction)	
Immunology/Infectious Disease	**Psychosocial**
Immunodeficiency	Poverty
Food protein allergy	Maternal depression
Chronic infection (eg, tuberculosis, HIV)	Physical or emotional abuse
Hematology/Oncology	**Metabolic**
Chronic anemia	Inborn errors of metabolism
Malignancy	
Neurologic	**Environmental**
Cerebral palsy	Sucking or swallowing dysfunction
Neuromuscular disorders	Improper mixing of formula
	Underfeeding
	Improper mealtime environment

Question 8-4

What is the most appropriate next step in investigating the cause of failure to thrive in this child?
A) Immunodeficiency workup.
B) Skeletal survey to investigate for signs of physical abuse.
C) Admission to the hospital for observation of feeding.
D) Detailed history and complete physical exam.
E) Sweat chloride test to evaluate for cystic fibrosis.

Discussion 8-4

The correct answer is "D." While all of the answer choices in this question may elicit an underlying cause of failure to thrive for this child, you should always start with a detailed history and a complete physical exam, including development screening. The information gained will guide your laboratory investigation. Not all children will require hospital admission for observation of feeding, but if after counseling about caloric intake and close follow up the child does not demonstrate adequate weight gain, inpatient admission should be considered for an extended diagnostic evaluation and observation of feeding.

► CASE 9

During a health supervision visit for a 9-year-old boy, you note that his body mass index (BMI) has been gradually increasing in percentile over the last 3 years and today is above the 95th percentile. His mother and father are obese as is his 15-year-old sister. On further review of the family history, you note that his paternal grandmother has type 2 diabetes mellitus and his maternal grandfather had a myocardial infarction at the age of 47 years.

Question 9-1

You are most likely to recommend that the child have which of the following laboratory investigations?
A) Fasting glucose.
B) Fasting lipid profile.
C) Liver function tests.
D) Hemoglobin A_{1c}.
E) All of the above.

Discussion 9-1

The correct answer is "E." All children aged 9 to 11 years should be screened for high cholesterol with a fasting lipid panel, but given this child's obesity and family history, it is recommended that fasting glucose, lipid panel, liver function tests (ALT, AST), and hemoglobin A_{1c} be obtained to screen for dyslipidemia, type 2 diabetes mellitus, and nonalcoholic fatty liver disease.

Helpful Tip
In children 2 years of age and older, BMI should be used to detect overweight and obesity. Weight for height should be used for children younger than 2 years of age.

QUICK QUIZ

A 9-year-old boy weighs 100 pounds (45 kg) and is 54 inches (137 cm) tall.
What is his BMI?
A) 24 kg/m².
B) 20 kg/m².
C) 21.5 kg/m².
D) 19.2 kg/m².
E) None of the above.

Discussion

The correct answer is "A." To calculate BMI, body weight in kilograms is divided by height in meters squared. For this patient:

$$BMI = 45 \text{ kg} \div (1.37 \text{ m})^2 = 24 \text{ kg/m}^2.$$

In children, the BMI percentile for age and sex—not the absolute value—is used to define weight status, as follows:

Underweight: BMI < 5%
Healthy weight: BMI ≥ 5% and < 85%
Overweight: BMI ≥ 85% and < 95%
Obese: BMI ≥ 95%

You begin to counsel the 9-year-old boy and his mother on lifestyle modifications for obesity. His mother admits that he eats fast food three times per week and drinks at least two energy drinks per day. However, she would like to know if, rather than simply modifying his lifestyle and diet, he should undergo further testing for a disorder that could be the underlying cause of his obesity.

Question 9-2

All of the following may be findings on physical examination of this child that would indicate the need for further assessment of an underlying cause of obesity EXCEPT:
A) Violaceous striae.
B) Acanthosis nigricans.
C) Short stature.
D) Developmental delay.
E) Micropenis.

Discussion 9-2

The correct answer is "B." When considering an underlying cause of childhood obesity for the boy in this case, it is important to keep in mind medical conditions that secondarily cause obesity. These include endocrine diseases such as hypothyroidism or growth hormone deficiency, which may be present in an obese child, especially if stunting (low height percentile) is present. Additionally, violaceous striae may indicate hypercortisolism due to adrenal hyperplasia or a pituitary tumor leading to Cushing syndrome. A buffalo hump or moon facies may also be present. Striae from rapid weight gain are not violaceous. An example of a syndromic cause for obesity is Prader-Willi syndrome (caused by a partial deletion on chromosome 15), which produces small hands and feet, mental retardation, and hypogonadism. Children with Prader-Willi syndrome binge eat and parents may need to lock cupboards to minimize access to food. Finding an undiagnosed genetic syndrome as the cause of obesity is rare, but consider a genetics referral for an obese child with developmental delay and short stature. For the child in this case, a finding of acanthosis nigricans (dark pigmented skin at places such as the nape of the neck or axilla) is consistent with obesity and may indicate associated insulin resistance.

Question 9-3

The most common health problem that this 9-year-old obese child is at risk for is:
A) Asthma.
B) Slipped capital femoral epiphysis.
C) Type 2 diabetes mellitus.
D) Nonalcoholic fatty liver disease.
E) Psychosocial problems.

Discussion 9-3

The correct answer is "E." Although the boy in this case is susceptible to all of the health problems listed above, the most common sequelae of childhood obesity are psychosocial dysfunction and social isolation. Negative societal messages about obesity have an impact on the self-esteem of both male and female adolescents. Obese children are more likely to experience peer discrimination and teasing. Anxiety, depression, and discrimination in social settings and in the workplace have been found to be obesity-associated comorbidities even into adulthood. While psychosocial problems are most common, the other conditions listed do occur more frequently in obese children. Children with obesity tend to have a higher prevalence of asthma and are also at increased risk for developing obstructive sleep apnea. Slipped capital femoral epiphysis is more common in obese children and adolescents than in their nonobese peers. Additionally, obese children are more susceptible to Blount disease due to increased weight-bearing on cartilaginous bone, leading to overgrowth and bowing of the tibia. Children who are obese also are more susceptible to fractures as they have lower bone area and bone mass compared with their body weight. Owing to impaired glucose tolerance and insulin resistance, children who are obese are more likely to develop type 2 diabetes mellitus. Other risk factors for type 2 diabetes include evidence of acanthosis nigricans (indicating insulin resistance) on exam, a family history of type 2 diabetes mellitus, and female sex. Obese children are at increased risk for hepatobiliary and gastrointestinal disorders, with the most likely being nonalcoholic fatty liver disease. Obese girls more frequently have reproductive system complications (eg, early onset menarche and irregular menstrual periods as well as polycystic ovarian disease) than their nonobese peers.

Question 9-4

For children with obesity, all of the following interventions are suggested in initial therapy EXCEPT:
A) Change in family food habits, such as eating breakfast, eating meals together as a family, and avoiding eating while watching television.
B) Improving access to recreational spaces and play equipment.
C) Metformin therapy.
D) Removal of the television from the child's bedroom.
E) Reduction in sweetened beverage consumption.

Discussion 9-4

The correct answer is "C." All of the listed options except initiation of metformin therapy are considered first-line interventions for childhood obesity. Changing family food habits plays a significant role in the success of the child's treatment and also involves changing what foods are purchased and available for consumption around the house. For children who live in environments that do not provide easily accessible and safe outdoor space, finding a way to allow them regular access to a recreational area will help increase physical activity level. Children should be active for at least 60 minutes per day. Finally, time spent watching television (TV) and in front of screens in general has contributed to the obesity epidemic. Not only does a TV in the bedroom contribute to poor sleep hygiene, but it also is associated with increased time spent watching TV, and lack of monitoring of TV programs the child watches. Total screen time should be limited to 2 hours per day or less.

▶ CASE 10

You are seeing an 18-month old male toddler for his first health maintenance exam in your clinic as his family just moved to your community from out of state. His mother notes that because of their recent move, she has been delayed in bringing him for health maintenance exams. The last time he had a clinic visit was at 12 months of age. This is her only child. Recently the boy began attending daycare and his teachers have expressed concern that he does not always answer when his name is called, repeats questions that are asked of him, and rarely makes direct eye contact with care providers. His mother states that she noticed this as well but was not sure how concerned to be as he has a wide vocabulary (speaks at least 50 words) and seemed to be meeting fine and gross motor developmental milestones without delay throughout infancy. You obtain a hearing screen in the office, and the results are normal.

Question 10-1

What is the next most appropriate step for this child?
A) Administer a standardized developmental screening tool in the office and review answers and scoring with the child's mother.
B) Immediately refer to a developmental pediatrician for a workup of autism spectrum disorder.
C) Reassure the mother and plan for follow-up in 3 months.
D) Order baseline electroencephalography.
E) Refer the child to a geneticist for evaluation of an underlying genetic syndrome causing intellectual disability.

Discussion 10-1

The correct answer is "A." It is recommended that a formal developmental screening tool such as the Ages and Stages Questionnaire (ASQ) be performed at 9-, 18-, and either 24- or 30-month visits. Additionally, screening for autism specifically with a tool such as the Modified Checklist for Autism in

Toddlers (M-CHAT) is advised at 18 and 24 months of age. So, the first step in evaluating the concerns expressed by this child's mother and daycare teachers is this formal development assessment with screening questionnaires. If answers indicate developmental delay or behavior concerning for autism, a referral to a developmental pediatrician is definitely warranted.

> **Helpful Tip**
> A good reference for preventive care, including which screening tests to perform and at what age, is the *Recommendations for Preventive Pediatric Health Care* published by the American Academy of Pediatrics (AAP) and Bright Futures.

You identify areas of concern on the personal-social and communication sections of the ASQ, as well as on the M-CHAT, and decide to refer the child to a developmental pediatrician. You also refer him for early intervention services so that he may start receiving services before his formal evaluation with the developmental pediatrician. The medical student who has been shadowing you in clinic during the visit asks you about the use of screening and surveillance tools for developmental assessment.

Question 10-2

Which of the following is true regarding developmental screening and surveillance tools?
A) Both screening and surveillance are important components in the routine health maintenance exam of children.
B) A good screening test may have low sensitivity, but must have a high specificity.
C) Parents are generally not very reliable in their assessment of their child's developmental progress.
D) Early intervention services are not typically helpful for children until after the age of 2 years.
E) All of the above.

Discussion 10-2

The correct answer is "A." Both screening and surveillance should be integrated into the routine health maintenance exams of infants, children, and adolescents. While some screening tools are tedious, it has been shown that when administered at regular intervals, they play a key role in identifying children at risk for developmental delay. Additionally, regular surveillance as reported by parents, who tend to be quite reliable about the child's developmental progress, is useful in assessment of a child's developmental stage. It is important that a screening tool be highly sensitive as you want to detect nearly all children with problems. It is also nice to have fairly high specificity in order to avoid labeling healthy children as developmentally delayed. Early intervention services have been shown to have positive and improved outcomes for children with developmental delay, and there is no lower limit to the age at which these are helpful for a child.

▶ CASE 11

Accompanied by a medical student, you are seeing a 2-day-old term neonate on rounds in the newborn nursery. You take advantage of this teaching opportunity to begin a discussion of newborn reflexes while examining the neonate.

Question 11-1

Which one of the following reflexes will you NOT be able to demonstrate to the medical student while examining this neonate?
A) Palmar grasp.
B) Parachute.
C) Moro.
D) Tonic neck.
E) Rooting.

Discussion 11-1

The correct answer is "B." The parachute reflex is the last of the infant reflexes to appear; it typically is seen first between 7 and 9 months of age and then is present throughout life. To demonstrate this reflex, hold the infant facing away from you above a table or other surface and then simulate a fall by moving the infant suddenly forward toward the ground. As a protective mechanism the infant will extend the upper extremities as if to break the fall. The other reflexes listed as answer choices are present at birth. The palmar grasp, in which the infant grasps a finger or other object placed in the open palm, is present at birth and typically disappears by 4 months of age. The Moro or startle reflex is also seen in newborn infants and lasts until approximately 6 months of age. To elicit this reflex, hold the infant in a supine position and gently allow the head to fall back slightly. In response, the infant will extend and abduct the upper extremities. The tonic neck reflex is present at birth and persists until approximately 6 months of age. If the infant is lying supine and the examiner turns the head to one side, the infant with a normal tonic reflex will extend the leg and arm on the same side as the direction of the face with flexion of the contralateral extremities (fencing posture). Finally, the rooting reflex is present at birth and persists for approximately the first 2 months. To elicit the rooting reflex, stroke the infant's cheek. In response the infant will turn the head toward the side that is being stroked.

▶ CASE 12

An infant boy that you followed in the newborn nursery is now at your office for a health maintenance exam. You observe that he can lift his head to approximately 45 degrees while in the prone position, has a social smile, holds his hands briefly at midline while lying supine, and has minimal head lag.

Question 12-1

What would you expect the age of this infant to be?
A) 2 weeks.
B) 1 month.

C) 2 months.
D) 4 months.
E) 6 months.

Discussion 12-1

The correct answer is "C." All of the milestones the infant is displaying are consistent with an age of 2 months. A newborn infant will be able to lift the head momentarily while in the prone position, but 2-month-olds can consistently lift their heads to a 45-degree angle. Additionally, the social smile develops around 2 months of age, along with bringing hands to the midline position. There should no longer be head lag by the time the infant reaches 4 months of age, but it may still be present to varying degrees in a 2-month-old.

You are seeing the same infant at 4 months of age. His parents ask if it is normal that he does not show any concern when they drop him off at daycare in the morning.

Question 12-2

What is the minimum age at which you would expect this infant to first experience stranger anxiety?
A) 4 months of age.
B) 6 months of age.
C) 8 months of age.
D) 10 months of age.
E) 12 months of age.

Discussion 12-2

The correct answer is "B." At 6 to 7 months of age, infants begin to develop stranger anxiety with unfamiliar situations or people; this typically peaks around 2 years of age. Therefore, it is normal for the infant at this point not to show significant signs of distress when parents drop him off at daycare, but parents can expect more concern at their departure to develop in the next couple of months. Additionally, daycare is likely considered to be a familiar place for this infant, so once he develops stranger anxiety, it may be more pronounced in unfamiliar settings or with an unfamiliar care provider.

Question 12-3

Which of the following is a developmental milestone that would be expected for the 4-month-old at this age?
A) Rolls front to back.
B) Sits well without support.
C) Babbles.
D) Grasps an object using the whole hand.
E) Crawls.

Discussion 12-3

The correct answer is "A." Rolling from front to back occurs at 4 months and back to front at 5 months of age. A 6-month-old is expected to sit well, and crawling starts around 8 months. A 3-month-old infant coos, a 4-month-old laughs, a 5-month-old razzes, and a 6-month-old babbles. A 5-month-old holds

objects in the center of the hand without using the thumb (palmar grasp). A 7-month-old rakes the objects up into the hand (raking grasp). A 9-month-old uses the underside of the first two fingers and thumb to hold and pick up objects (radial digit grasp). A 12-month-old uses the fingertips of the index finger and thumb to pick up and hold objects (mature pincher grasp).

▶ CASE 13

A father brings his daughter into your clinic for a routine health supervision visit. The infant is babbling to her father when you enter the room and eyes you cautiously as you sit down. As she warms to your presence, you are able to engage her in a game of "pat-a-cake," and when you offer her a small book, she easily transfers it from her left hand to her right hand. The father tells you that he has been child-proofing the house as his daughter is pulling up on furniture and starting to get into things around the house.

Question 13-1

The developmental milestones demonstrated by this girl are most typical for a child whose age is:
A) 4 months.
B) 6 months.
C) 9 months.
D) 12 months.
E) 15 months.

Discussion 13-1

The correct answer is "C." The infant in this case demonstrates typical behavior for a 9-month-old, including some stranger anxiety when the examiner enters the room, the ability to play "pat-a-cake," and mastery of the ability to transfer objects between hands (which most infants begin to develop around age 6 months). Additionally, the gross motor development of becoming mobile and the ability to pull to stand, which the father has mentioned as necessitating child-proofing at home, are also characteristic of a 9-month-old.

Question 13-2

What other developmental milestone might the infant be displaying at this age?
A) Walking.
B) Building a tower with two cubes.
C) Using a cup well for drinking.
D) Saying first words.
E) Scribbling.

Discussion 13-2

The correct answer is "D." Of the above milestones, the only one a 9-month-old might display is saying first words. The range for beginning to say first words spans the period from 9 to 12 months. We would not expect her to begin walking until closer to 12 months. Most children begin to use a cup well between

15 and 18 months of age, which coincides with scribbling and building a tower of two cubes around 15 months.

When the girl returns at age 12 months for a health supervision exam, her parents have questions about whether or not she is meeting developmental milestones appropriately.

Question 13-3

At 12 months of age you would expect that this normally developing child should be able to do all of the following EXCEPT:
A) Make a tower of four cubes.
B) Participate in symbolic play.
C) Say "mama" and "dada" specifically.
D) Use fingertip and distal thumb to pick up a small item (mature pincher grasp).
E) Wave "bye-bye."

Discussion 13-3

The correct answer is "A." At 12 months of age, the child should be able to do all the listed actions except build a tower of four cubes. A 15-month-old may be able to build a tower of two cubes but will not advance to four cubes until closer to 18 months of age. Children advance to building towers of six blocks at around 24 months of age, and eight blocks at approximately 30 months.

▶ CASE 14

During a health supervision visit, parents of an 18-month-old boy express concern that he has not started speaking words yet. They were told by the child's paternal grandmother that since he is a boy and has three older sisters, this delay in speech is expected. The boy has been developing normally and has been otherwise healthy, except for a few episodes of acute otitis media diagnosed in the last 6 months.

Question 14-1

Of the following, the most appropriate next step in management is:
A) Obtain cytogenetic chromosome testing.
B) Reassure and follow up in 3 months.
C) Refer the child to a developmental pediatrician.
D) Obtain a hearing screen.
E) Refer to an otolaryngologist to assess for structural problems of the respiratory tract and mouth.

Discussion 14-1

The correct answer is "D." The fact that this child is not speaking any words at the age of 18 months is concerning and obtaining a hearing screen is always the first step in the evaluation of a child who has a language disorder, even if you would also consider sending this child for further evaluation by a developmental pediatrician and otolaryngologist. Reviewing the prenatal and newborn history and assessing the home environment for this child also would be important in a thorough evaluation of this expressive language delay.

Question 14-2

What would be considered normal speech development for a child of this age?
A) Uses two-word sentences.
B) Speech is 50% understandable by a stranger.
C) Vocabulary of 10 to 50 words.
D) Uses plurals.
E) Names seven body parts.

Discussion 14-2

The correct answer is "C." It is expected that an 18-month-old will have a vocabulary of 10 to 50 words and be able to follow simple verbal commands. The use of two-word sentences and speech that is 50% understandable by a stranger is not expected until approximately 2 years of age. A 30-month-old child can name around seven body parts, and the use of plurals begins at about 36 months.

Before you send the child to have his hearing screened, you decide to do a formal developmental assessment to see if any other delays are noticed.

Question 14-3

Which of the following behaviors is most consistent with a normally developing 18-month-old?
A) Goes up and down stairs, one foot per step each way.
B) Throws a ball standing.
C) Buttons large buttons.
D) Uses a fork well.
E) Jumps with both feet off the floor.

Discussion 14-3

The correct answer is "B." The only option considered to be a milestone that should be reached at 18 months is throwing a ball while standing. Going up and down stairs, one foot per step each way, is something a 4-year-old will have mastered. A 2-year-old can walk up and down stairs but will use two feet on each step. A 3-year-old can button large buttons, and while an 18-month-old may be able to use a spoon, the use of a fork is not mastered until age 4 years. Jumping with two feet off the floor is expected of a child 2½ to 3 years old.

▶ CASE 15

You are seeing a 2-year-old girl for her routine health supervision visit and are discussing with her parents the milestones you expect her to have achieved at this point. Her parents note that when they bring her to the park or story time at the library where other small children are present, she is always excited to see the other children but does not play interactively with them. They have seen children participating in pretend play together and are wondering if it is abnormal that their daughter has not started displaying this play behavior.

Question 15-1

What is the most appropriate response to the concerns these parents have expressed about their daughter?
A) Explain that it is typical for children to still be displaying parallel play at this age; parents can expect that she will begin to play cooperatively over the next year.
B) Reassure them that playing alongside but not with other children will continue until she is ready for kindergarten.
C) Recommend a full developmental evaluation because although 1-year-olds may show this play behavior, we would expect her to have started to participate in cooperative play by now.
D) Explain that because the child does not have older siblings, she has not seen cooperative play modeled often enough at this point; however, she will begin to pick up this behavior if they bring her to more social events.

Discussion 15-1

The correct answer is "A." Children begin to engage in cooperative play around age 3 years. Before that time, they participate in parallel play characterized by enjoying playing alongside other children but not actually cooperatively playing. Therefore, the play behavior this child is displaying is completely normal for a 2-year-old and only reassurance is recommended.

Question 15-2

All of the following are expected of a normally developing 3-year-old EXCEPT:
A) Able to dress self.
B) Pedals a tricycle.
C) Balances on one foot for 2 to 3 seconds.
D) Speaks in 3- to 4-word sentences.
E) Hops on one foot.

Discussion 15-2

The correct answer is "E." All of the options except hopping on one foot are expected of a typically developing 3-year-old. The age at which a child can hop on one foot is 4 years. A 3-year-old can dress independently, which includes buttoning large buttons. Additionally, although they cannot hop yet, 3-year-olds can balance on one foot for 2 to 3 seconds at a time. Speech development at age 3 years is expected to have advanced to speaking in 3- to 4-word sentences, and speech is 75% understandable to a stranger.

▶ CASE 16

A child can copy a circle, a cross, and a square for you, but cannot copy a triangle.

Question 16-1

Which of the following is the most likely age of this child?
A) 2 years of age.
B) 3 years of age.
C) 4 years of age.

D) 5 years of age.
E) 6 years of age.

Discussion 16-1

The correct answer is "C." Three-year-olds should be able to copy a circle and then develop the ability to draw a cross between the ages of 3 and 4 years. Four-year-olds can copy a square, but not until 5 years will most children have the ability to copy a triangle.

This same child now can hop, skip, tie his own shoelaces, write his first name without assistance, and his speech is 100% understandable to a stranger. When you ask him to draw a picture of himself on the chalkboard in the exam room, he easily draws a person with six body parts. When you ask him about bike riding, he states that he is still working on learning how to ride without training wheels.

Question 16-2

This child's age is most likely closest to:
A) 3 years.
B) 4 years.
C) 5 years.
D) 6 years.
E) 7 years.

Discussion 16-2

The correct answer is "C." A typical 5-year-old can do all of the listed tasks. Four-year-olds can hop but not yet skip or tie shoelaces. By the time a child reaches age 6 years, he or she will be able to ride a bicycle without training wheels and participate in games with rules. When a 7-year-old is asked to draw a person, you would expect more than six body parts.

Question 16-3

Which of the following would be consistent with this child's current stage of development?
A) Demonstrate the ability to sustain attention in the classroom for more than 45 minutes at a time.
B) Use concrete logic to solve problems.
C) Ability to differentiate fantasy from reality.
D) Both B and C.
E) All of the above.

Discussion 16-3

The correct answer is "C." At the age of 5 years, a child can differentiate fantasy from reality. Although the boy in this example may still be quite fascinated by superheroes, he would not think it likely that any human he knows possesses the powers of Superman. The other options describe children older than 5 years. Typically children who are older than 7 years begin to use concrete logic to solve problems and understand the concept of conservation (ie, that an object remains the same in quantity despite whatever shape it assumes). You would not expect a 5-year-old to be able to sustain attention in the classroom for 45 minutes, but by the time he is in third grade, this is expected. (See Table 19–4.)

TABLE 19–4 DEVELOPMENTAL MILESTONES

Age	Gross Motor	Visual Motor	Language	Social
1 mo	Raises head slightly from prone, makes crawling movements, lifts chin up	Has tight grasp, follows to midline	Alert to sound (eg, by blinking, moving, startling)	Regards face
2 mo	Holds head in midline, lifts chest off table	No longer clenches fist tightly, follows object past midline	Smiles after being stroked or talked to	Recognizes parent
3 mo	Supports on forearms in prone, holds head up steadily	Holds hands open at rest, follows in circular fashion	Coos (produces long vowel sounds in musical fashion)	Reaches for familiar people or objects, anticipates feeding
4–5 mo	Rolls front to back and back to front, sits well when propped, supports on wrists, and shifts weight	Moves arms in unison to grasp, touches cube placed on table	Orients to voice; 5 mo: orients to bell (localized laterally), says "ahgoo," razzes	Enjoys looking around environment
6 mo	Sits well unsupported, puts feet in mouth in supine position	Reaches with either hand, transfers, uses raking grasp	Babbles; 7 mo: orients to bell (localizes indirectly); 8 mo: "dada/mama" indiscriminately	Recognizes strangers
9 mo	Creeps, crawls, cruises, pulls to stand, pivots when sitting	Uses pincer grasp, probes with forefinger, holds bottle, finger-feeds	Understands "no," waves bye-bye; 10 mo: "dada/mama" discriminantly; 11 mo: one word other than "dada/mama"	Starts to explore environment, plays pat-a-cake
12 mo	Walks alone	Throws objects, lets go of toys, hand release, uses mature pincer grasp	Follows one-step command with gesture, uses 2 words other than "dada/mama"; 14 mo: uses 3 words	Imitates actions, comes when called, cooperates with dressing
15 mo	Creeps upstairs, walks backward	Builds tower of 2 blocks in imitation of examiner, scribbles in imitation	Follows one-step command without gesture, uses 4–6 words and immature jargon (runs several unintelligible words together)	Indicates some simple needs by pointing, hugs parents
18 mo	Runs, throws toy from standing without falling	Turns 2 or 3 pages at a time, fills spoon and feeds self	Knows 10-50 words, knows 1 body part, uses mature jargon (includes intelligible words in jargon)	Copies parent in tasks (eg, sweeping, dusting), plays in company of other children
21 mo	Squats in play, goes up steps	Builds tower of 5 blocks, drinks well from cup	Points to 3 body parts, uses 2-word combinations, has 20-word vocabulary	Asks to have food and to go to toilet
24 mo	Walks up and down steps without help	Turns pages one at a time; removes shoes, pants, etc; imitates behavior of others	Uses 50 words, 2-word sentences, uses pronouns (I, you, me) inappropriately, points to 5 body parts, understands 2-step command	Parallel play

(continued)

TABLE 19-4   DEVELOPMENTAL MILESTONES (*CONTINUED*)

Age	Gross Motor	Visual Motor	Language	Social
30 mo	Jumps with both feet off floor, throws ball overhand	Unbuttons, holds pencil in adult fashion, differentiates horizontal and vertical lines	Uses pronouns (I, you, me) appropriately, understands concept of "one," repeats 2 digits forward	Tells first and last names when asked, gets drink without help
3 y	Pedals tricycle, can alternate feet when going up steps	Dresses and undresses partially, dries hands if reminded, draws a circle	Uses 3-word sentences, plurals, and past tense. Knows all pronouns. Minimum of 250 words, understands concept of "two"	Group play, shares toys, takes turns, plays well with others; knows full name, age, sex
4 y	Hops, skips, alternates feet going downstairs	Buttons clothing fully, catches ball	Knows colors, says song or poem from memory, asks questions	Tells "tall tales," plays cooperatively with a group of children
5 y	Skips, alternating feet, jumps over low obstacles	Ties shoes, spreads with knife	Prints first name, asks what a word means	Plays competitive games, abides by rules, likes to help in household tasks

Reproduced with permission of Erin Howe, MD.

BIBLIOGRAPHY

Barlow SE, Expert Committee. Expert committee recommendations regarding the prevention, assessment, and treatment of child and adolescent overweight and obesity: Summary report. *Pediatrics.* 2007;120(suppl 4):S164–S192.

Berkowitz CD. *Pediatrics: A Primary Care Approach.* 2nd ed. Philadelphia, PA: Saunders; 2000.

Bronfin DR. Misshapen heads in babies: Position or pathology? *Ochsner J.* 2001;3:191–199.

Carey WB, Crocker AC, Elias ER, Feldman HM, Coleman WL 2nd, eds. *Developmental-Behavioral Pediatrics.* 4th ed. Philadelphia, PA: Elsevier Saunders; 2009.

Kliegman RM, Stanton BM, St Geme J, Schor NF, Behrman RE, eds. *Nelson Textbook of Pediatrics.* 20th ed. Philadelphia, PA: Elsevier Saunders; 2011.

Linz C, Collman H, Meyer-Marcotty P, et al. Occipital plagiocephaly: Unilateral lambdoid synostosis versus positional plagiocephaly. *Ach Dis Child.* 2015;100:152–157.

Mackrides P, Ryherd SJ. Screening for developmental delay. *Am Fam Physician.* 2011;84(5):544–549.

Mei Z, Grummer-Strawn LM, Thompson D, Dietz WH. Shifts in percentiles of growth during early childhood: Analysis of longitudinal data from the California Child Health and Development Study. *Pediatrics.* 2004;113(6):617–627.

South M, Isaacs D. *Practical Paediatrics.* 7th ed. Philadelphia, PA: Elsevier; 2012.

Infectious Disease

20

Nathan Price

► CASE 1

A term female infant has just been born vaginally to a mother who had no prenatal care. The mother has no known medical problems. She has another child at home who is 6 years old. As you are examining the patient, the obstetrician calls you and informs you that the mother's human immunodeficiency virus (HIV) antibody test is positive, but that the Western blot result is pending and will not be back for another 24 hours.

Question 1-1

You determine:
A) PCP prophylaxis should be started.
B) Nothing can be done at this point to prevent vertical transmission.
C) Zidovudine should be started immediately.
D) Nevirapine is contraindicated.
E) Cesarean delivery is always indicated for infants being born to HIV-positive mothers.

Discussion 1-1

The correct answer is "C." HIV can be transmitted from mother to child en utero, during delivery, and after delivery if the fetus or infant is exposed to the virus. The most common form of exposure is during vaginal delivery. Risk of maternal-to-child transmission is highest when the maternal viral load is high but can occur even if viral load is suppressed on antiviral therapy. This infant is at high risk for acquiring HIV because its mother likely has a new infection. With a new infection viral load is often high for a time before reaching the lower virologic "set point." Anything that exposes this infant to infectious fluids will increase the risk of transmission. Mothers with high viral loads are often delivered by cesarean section to decrease this risk. However, cesarean delivery is not recommended if the maternal

viral load is less than 1000 on antiretroviral medications. All infants born to mothers with HIV should receive immediate prophylaxis to prevent HIV infection. Usually this requires zidovudine. Infants born to mothers with high viral loads, or who have not received antiretroviral therapy during pregnancy, should have a 3-dose series of nevirapine added to their regimen. Fortunately prophylaxis has reduced maternal-to-child transmission of HIV from 25% to less than 5%. Because waiting for confirmation of maternal testing would lead to delay in starting prophylaxis, and because zidovudine is well tolerated in the infant, it is recommended that the infant start therapy before confirmatory testing is back for the mother. *Pneumocystis jiroveci* (PCP, formerly named *Pneumocystis carinii*) pneumonia prophylaxis is not indicated.

The newborn is started on zidovudine. The mother asks if she can still breastfeed even though she is HIV positive.

Question 1-2

What should you tell her?
A) Breastfeeding is acceptable.
B) HIV transmission through breastmilk has not been documented.
C) It depends on her viral load.
D) Access to safe water is an important consideration.
E) Breastfeeding is always contraindicated.

Discussion 1-2

The correct answer is "D." Postpartum transmission through breast milk has been documented. In the United States, breastfeeding is contraindicated. In developing countries, where the water supply is not safe, breastfeeding is still recommended because the risk of HIV transmission through breast milk is much less than acquiring life-threatening infection from unsafe water used to mix formula.

Question 1-3

Which of the following is true regarding HIV testing in this infant?

A) Positive HIV antibody in the infant confirms the infant is infected.

B) Infants should have DNA or RNA PCR (polymerase chain reaction) testing.

C) The infant only needs to be tested once for HIV.

D) The infant is considered infected and does not need testing.

E) None of the above.

Discussion 1-3

The correct answer is "B." HIV testing in infants can be tricky due to transplacental passage of maternal antibody. A positive antibody test in the infant may simply indicate the presence of maternal IgG, rather than neonatal infection. To test for HIV in infants, either DNA or RNA PCR should be done. These tests are repeated at regular intervals (at 2–3 weeks, 1–2 months and 4–6 months of age) to rule out infection in the case of a previously negative test. After 18 months of age, maternal antibody likely is no longer present, making it acceptable to use antibody testing in that age group. It is important to remember that at any age, early HIV infection can cause fever, pharyngitis, and lymphadenopathy, during which time the patient may not have seroconverted, leading to a false-negative HIV antibody result. A patient suspected of having acute HIV should have either an RNA or DNA PCR test done.

> **Helpful Tip**
> In acute HIV, or when trying to diagnose HIV in an infant, use PCR testing, not antibody testing. In acute HIV the patient may not have seroconverted. In infants, the antibody detected may be maternal rather than infant antibody, leading to a false-positive result.

> **Helpful Tip**
> Think of HIV (especially AIDS) when an infant, child, or adolescent has an infection that you would not expect in an immunocompetent individual; for example, thrush in an adolescent who is not taking steroids or antibiotics. Failure to thrive in an infant should prompt inclusion of HIV on the differential. Patients with AIDS have low CD4 counts and are thus ill equipped to fight off infections that healthy people should have no problem dealing with, including severe cytomegalovirus (CMV), ocular toxoplasma, *Pneumocystis* pneumonia, disseminated fungal infections (*Coccidioides*, *Histoplasma*, *Cryptococcus*), and disseminated mycobacterial disease.

▶ CASE 2

A mother brings her 4-year-old child for you to evaluate because he has a red eye that has crusting and mucoid drainage. You diagnose him with conjunctivitis. His mother is frustrated because it seems he always has some illness for which the daycare sends him home. She asks you what illnesses should preclude him from attending daycare.

Question 2-1

You answer:

A) Cough and runny nose.

B) Conjunctivitis without fever.

C) Rash with fever.

D) Diarrhea.

E) Head lice.

Discussion 2-1

The correct answer is "C." Out-of-home child care is a common source of infection. Think of a room full of snotty-nosed kids running around touching everything. Infection prevention among young children is difficult because they have not yet developed good hygiene skills. How many toddlers ask for a tissue and cover their mouths every time they cough? There is a tendency of care providers to want to exclude children with upper respiratory tract infection (URI) symptoms from child care settings. However, viral respiratory infections are likely transmitted during the asymptomatic rather than the symptomatic period. Though it is common practice in some child care centers, excluding children with conjunctivitis who do not have fever is unnecessary unless there is an outbreak at the care center. Rash with fever is typically indicative of a communicable disease, and the child should be excluded until improvement of symptoms. Diarrhea itself is not a reason for exclusion unless it is unable to be contained in the diaper in infants and toddlers, or if toilet-trained children have accidents. Discouraging swimming in public pools is a good idea. Certain pathogens such as *Escherichia coli* 0157:H7 or *Salmonella typhi* pose a risk of serious morbidity and mortality if transmitted. Asymptomatic children with these organisms should not return to care until there is documented clearance of the pathogen from their stool. Criteria for return in this situation may vary from state to state. Other reasons for exclusion from daycare include draining skin lesions that cannot be adequately covered and contagious oral lesions in a child. The following specific diseases require the child's exclusion from daycare until considered no longer contagious: measles, mumps, rubella, varicella, pertussis, group A streptococcal pharyngitis, tuberculosis, and scabies. Fifth disease caused by parvovirus B19 is not a reason for exclusion since by the time the rash develops, patients usually are no longer contagious. Head lice, while a nuisance and cause of considerable concern among parents and caregivers, are not a reason for exclusion as infestation is not associated with any severe morbidity or mortality.

▶ CASE 3

A 17-year-old girl presents with a 2-week history of fever, runny nose, cough, sore throat, fatigue, and some abdominal pain. She was seen by another provider 1 week ago, at which time she had enlarged, erythematous tonsils, with bilateral anterior cervical adenopathy. She had a positive rapid streptococcal antigen throat swab, a negative Epstein-Barr virus (EBV) heterophile antibody test, and positive cytomegalovirus (CMV) IgG antibody test. She was prescribed amoxicillin, which she has taken faithfully. She now has developed a generalized maculopapular rash that is somewhat pruritic. Her exam is relatively unchanged from last week, but you notice her spleen tip is palpable. She is non-toxic appearing, although she appears ill.

Question 3-1

The most likely explanation of her symptoms is:
A) She has scarlet fever caused by *Streptococcus pyogenes*.
B) She has *Arcanobacterium haemolyticum* infection.
C) She has infectious mononucleosis caused by EBV.
D) She has infectious mononucleosis caused by CMV.
E) Drug reaction to amoxicillin.

Discussion 3-1

The correct answer is "C." Viral illness is the most common cause of pharyngitis in children. Etiologies include EBV, CMV, adenovirus, enteroviruses, herpes simplex virus (HSV), rhinoviruses, parainfluenza virus, and rarely HIV. A monospot negative mononucleosis syndrome would make one suspect a virus such as CMV. This patient's CMV IgG was positive, which would be indicative of prior illness, rather than acute CMV infection. CMV seropositivity can be high, ranging from 50% to 80% depending on age, ethnicity, and socioeconomic status. Splenomegaly is not a common finding in mononucleosis caused by CMV in a normal host. This patient has EBV mononucleosis with a false-negative heterophile antibody test. The heterophile antibody test (ie, monospot) is a useful, rapid test for diagnosing acute EBV infection. However, it can be negative up to 10% to 20% of the time. EBV can have a broad range of symptoms, including pharyngitis, lymphadenopathy, URI symptoms, and hepatosplenomegaly. Other organ systems can be involved as well, although this is rare in immunocompetent patients. Chronic active infection can occur in immunocompromised patients. Other rare complications include encephalitis, hemophagocytic syndrome, cancer (Burkitt lymphoma), and post-transplant lymphoproliferative disease. Rash is common when amoxicillin is used. It can be pruritic and typically begins 5 to 10 days after starting the antibiotic. It is not considered an allergy and will resolve after cessation of the offending antibiotic. Mycoplasma may cause pharyngitis as can gonorrhea in sexually active patients or in the setting of sexual abuse. *A. haemolyticum* can cause pharyngitis that can have associated scarlatiniform rash. It can cause gray membranes on the tonsils, reminiscent of diphtheria. It typically affects adolescents and young adults. It can be detected on culture and usually is susceptible to penicillins as well as a broad range of other antibiotics often used to treat pharyngitis. Group A beta-hemolytic *Streptococcus* (GAS, *S. pyogenes*) only accounts for 15% to 30% of pharyngitis in children. Additionally, up to 20% of children can have asymptomatic carriage of GAS, leading to misinterpretation of rapid tests and throat cultures in the setting of pharyngitis. There has never been a case of GAS resistant to penicillin, and symptoms typically improve within 24 to 48 hours of initiation of appropriate therapy in the setting of simple pharyngitis. Interestingly, up to 40% of children with GAS pharyngitis still have positive throat cultures despite successful treatment with antibiotics. Other symptoms such as cough, runny nose, and splenomegaly are not associated with strep pharyngitis.

> **Helpful Tip**
> A heterophile antibody test (ie, monospot) is not a reliable test in children younger than 4 years of age. EBV serologies are more reliable in that age group.

> **Helpful Tip**
> Patients with mononucleosis and splenomegaly should avoid high-risk activities (contact sports, etc) until symptoms have improved and splenomegaly has resolved, due to risk of splenic rupture.

You decide to get EBV serologies.

Question 3-2

You would expect:
A) Positive viral capsid antigen (VCA) IgM, negative VCA IgG, negative EBV nuclear antigen (EBNA).
B) Negative VCA IgM, positive VCA IgG, positive EBNA.
C) Negative VCA IgM, negative VCA IgG, negative EBNA.
D) Positive VCA IgM, positive VCA IgG, positive EBNA.

Discussion 3-2

The correct answer is "A." EBV is a virus that typically establishes lifelong infection by becoming latent. EBV serologies can be useful in determining if infection is acute or if the patient was infected in the past. EBV VCA IgM typically becomes positive first by the time of onset of symptoms. It remains positive for several weeks, then wanes and disappears over the course of a few months. VCA IgG often is negative initially but becomes positive after a few weeks and often persists for life. EBNA does not become positive in acute infection. It becomes positive several months after infection and can persist for life. IgM can occasionally be positive in the setting of relapse. In that case the VCA IgM and EBNA would both be positive. (See Table 20–1.)

> **Helpful Tip**
> A positive result for EBNA antibody means the patient was infected more remotely. This test is very unlikely to be positive in the setting of acute infection in a normal host.

TABLE 20–1 OVERLY SIMPLIFIED INTERPRETATION OF EBV SEROLOGIES[a]

	Acute Infection	Recent Infection	Past Infection	Reactivation	Naïve
VCA IgM	Pos	Pos/Neg	Neg	Pos	Neg
VCA IgG	Neg	Pos	Pos	Pos	Neg
EBNA	Neg	Pos/Neg	Pos	Pos	Neg

EBNA, EBV nuclear antigen; Pos, positive; Neg, negative; VCA, viral capsid antigen.

[a]Variations may still exist.

► CASE 4

During a busy morning in the newborn nursery you notice that you have four term infants born to mothers with a history of various infections: (1) a mother with chronic hepatitis C, (2) a mother with chronic hepatitis B, (3) a mother with a history of CMV and HSV, and (4) a mother with a positive tuberculin skin test (TST) who is asymptomatic and has a negative chest X-ray, but has never received antituberculosis therapy. All the mothers would like to breastfeed their infants.

Question 4-1

You decide:
A) None of the mothers should breastfeed.
B) The hepatitis C mother should not breastfeed.
C) The mother with a history of CMV and HSV should not breastfeed.
D) The mother with hepatitis B should not breastfeed.
E) The mother with the positive TST may breastfeed.

Discussion 4-1

The correct answer is "E." There are few true contraindications to breastfeeding in the United States. A mother with active tuberculosis (TB) should not breastfeed due to risk of transmission associated with close contact to the infant who has a poorly developed immune system. However, latent TB infection, as in this mother, is not contagious. There is no risk of transmission to the infant. CMV can be intermittently shed in breast milk. However, the benefit of breast milk outweighs the potential risk of postnatal infection in a term infant. Hepatitic C virus has been detected in human milk; however, there has not been any known transmission from mother to child attributed breastfeeding. Breastfeeding in this setting is not an absolute contraindication, but a theoretical risk. Hepatitis B surface antigen can be detected in breast milk, but transmission risk is not increased in this group. In hepatitis B or C, breastfeeding in the setting of cracked and bleeding nipples is not advised. Mothers with a history of HSV can breastfeed as long as there are no active lesions (vesicles) on the breast. Although human T-lymphotropic virus (HTLV) 1 and 2 is rare in the United States, mothers who are seropositive also should not breastfeed.

Helpful Tip

Contraindications to breastfeeding in the United States include maternal HIV, HTLV, active TB, active HSV vesicles on the breast, and cracked or bleeding nipples in the setting of hepatitis B or C.

► CASE 5

A term infant was born vaginally to a mother who was positive for group B *Streptococcus* (GBS, also known as *Streptococcus agalactiae*). She received intravenous antibiotics during delivery.

Question 5-1

GBS intrapartum antibiotic prophylaxis is indicated in all the following situations EXCEPT:
A) GBS-positive screening test with prior pregnancy.
B) Another daughter developed GBS meningitis as a newborn.
C) Positive GBS culture during current pregnancy.
D) GBS bacteriuria during current pregnancy.
E) Active labor with unknown GBS status and rupture of membranes for 20 hours.

Discussion 5-1

The correct answer is "A." All pregnant women should be screened for GBS colonization at 35 to 37 weeks' gestation. If positive, intravenous (IV) prophylactic antibiotics should be given during labor to decrease the risk of neonatal infection. Indications for intrapartum antibiotic prophylaxis:

- Mother with prior infant who developed GBS disease
- Maternal GBS bacteriuria during this pregnancy
- Maternal GBS positive screening during pregnancy
- Unknown maternal GBS status if infant is preterm, rupture of membranes occurred 18 hours or more before delivery, or maternal intrapartum temperature of 38°C (100.4°F) or higher.

Question 5-2

Regarding neonatal GBS disease, which of the following is FALSE?

A) Maternal colonization with GBS is the biggest risk factor for neonatal GBS disease.
B) Intrapartum antibiotics prevent late-onset GBS disease.
C) Maternal testing may be falsely negative.
D) Infected neonates with early-onset disease will develop signs of infection within the first few days of life.
E) Early-onset GBS infections are vertically transmitted.

Discussion 5-2

The correct answer is "B." Approximately, 10% to 30% of women are colonized with GBS in their genitourinary or gastrointestinal tracks. During delivery, GBS is transmitted from the mother's vagina to the infant. Risk factors for early-onset disease include maternal colonization, prematurity, prolonged rupture of membranes, and chorioamnionitis. Intrapartum antibiotic prophylaxis prevents early-onset (< 1 week old) not late-onset (1 week to 3 months old) disease. Signs of disease usually present within the first 48 hours of life. Sepsis and pneumonia are the most common early-onset infections but meningitis may occur.

► CASE 6

You are trying to see all of the new infants born in the nursery overnight. It seems every infant was born to a GBS-positive mother. None had the same intrapartum antibiotic prophylaxis.

Question 6-1

Which of the infants received adequate intrapartum antibiotic prophylaxis?

A) A term infant born to a GBS-positive mother who received IV penicillin 4 hours before delivery.
B) A premature infant born to a mother with unknown GBS status who received IV clindamycin 2 hours before delivery.
C) A term infant born to a GBS-negative mother who received IV vancomycin 1 hour before delivery and has a history of a prior infant with GBS pneumonia.
D) A premature infant born to a mother who had GBS bacteriuria in the first trimester treated with oral penicillin but received no intrapartum antibiotics.
E) None of the above.

Discussion 6-1

The correct answer is "A." Adequate prophylaxis is considered to be IV administration of a beta-lactam antibiotic (penicillin, ampicillin, or cefazolin) at least 4 hours before delivery with repeated dosing until delivery. Penicillin is the preferred drug. Penicillin-allergic mothers should receive cefazolin (if allergy was not anaphylaxis) or vancomycin. Clindamycin should be considered only if maternal GBS isolate has been proven to be susceptible to clindamycin since resistance is increasing.

Treatment with a non–beta-lactam antibiotic is considered inadequate as efficacy data are lacking. Oral therapy is not considered adequate, and prior antibiotic therapy in pregnancy does not ensure eradication of colonization. Infants born by cesarean section before the onset of active labor or spontaneous rupture of membranes do not require maternal intrapartum GBS prophylaxis.

► CASE 7

You evaluate a term infant delivered vaginally with rupture of membranes near the time of delivery who did not receive adequate maternal intrapartum prophylaxis for GBS despite having risk factors. He has a normal exam and is acting appropriately for a newborn infant.

Question 7-1

You decide to:

A) Observe for 24 hours then discharge home.
B) Observe for 48 hours then discharge home.
C) Obtain a CBC with differential and a blood culture.
D) Start IV ampicillin.
E) Both C and D.

Discussion 7-1

The correct answer is "B." A healthy term infant with rupture of membranes at delivery, but with risk factors for GBS disease, who did not receive adequate maternal intrapartum GBS prophylaxis, does not need workup and therapy if he or she has a normal exam. This infant should be observed for 48 hours and then can be discharged home if clinically well. Healthy-appearing preterm infants or infants who had rupture of membranes 18 or more hours before delivery and who did not receive adequate prophylaxis should have a complete blood count (CBC) with differential and blood culture obtained and should be observed for signs and symptoms of infection according to current Centers for Disease Control and Prevention (CDC) guidelines. Empiric antibiotics are not necessary if the infant continues to appear well. The CDC further recommends that all infants born to a mother with chorioamnionitis be treated empirically with antibiotics after having a CBC with differential and blood culture obtained. Length of therapy will depend on the clinical course. Any infant with signs of sepsis should have a full evaluation, including lumbar puncture, and be treated with antibiotics.

► CASE 8

A 7-year-old boy living in the northeastern United States presents in August with a 1-day history of fever, pain, erythema, and swelling of his right knee. He tells you that he fell on his knee a couple of days ago while playing but did not notice any significant pain until yesterday. He is febrile to 40°C (104°F),

tachycardic, tachypneic, and appears systemically ill. He is refusing to bear weight and the right knee is warm, tender, erythematous, and swollen. He does not have any other rash on exam. You are concerned for bacterial infection and initiate a diagnostic workup and plan for immediate therapy.

Question 8-1

The most likely cause of his infection is:

A) *Borrelia burgdorferi.*
B) *Streptococcus pyogenes.*
C) *Staphylococcus aureus.*
D) *Kingella kingae.*
E) *Neisseria gonorrhea.*

Discussion 8-1

The correct answer is "C." This patient has acute bacterial or septic arthritis with classic symptoms of fever and joint erythema, swelling, and tenderness. Often there is a history of preceding minor trauma. Joint aspiration should be performed for cell count and culture and usually shows neutrophil-predominant leukocytosis, often with cell counts of 50,000/mm³ or greater. Typical bacteria that cause septic arthritis are the same that typically cause bacteremia in this age group since most bone and joint infections are due to hematogenous spread of infection. *S. aureus* is the most common cause of bone and joint infections in children. Other common bacteria include *Streptococcus pyogenes* and *S. pneumoniae*. Before widespread vaccination *Haemophilus influenzae* type B was common as well. *K. kingae* should be suspected in preschool-aged children, but such children usually have milder disease. This child has rapid onset of symptoms with progression to systemic illness suggesting bacteremia and should be managed aggressively. Lyme disease should be suspected in a child with arthritis who presents during the summer in the northwestern United States, where *B. burgdorferi* is endemic, but it usually is a more indolent and mild course of low-grade pain and swelling. The knee is most often affected. Rarely are there such severe systemic symptoms as in this patient. Gonorrhea should be considered in a sexually active patient, or if sexual abuse is suspected.

Question 8-2

Which is NOT consistent with a diagnosis of acute bacterial or septic arthritis?

A) Fever.
B) Refusal to bear weight or walk on the affected joint.
C) Limited range of motion of the affected joint.
D) Improvement without treatment.
E) Joint erythema.

Discussion 8-2

The correct answer is "D." This is an acute process with an acute presentation. The joint is inflamed with redness, warmth, and swelling. The joint hurts. The child will not want to move it or bear weight. This is a systemic process with fever, leukocytosis, and elevated serum inflammatory markers. Without antibiotics, the joint will not improve. Delayed treatment results in more joint damage.

> **Helpful Tip**
> Bacterial or septic arthritis of the hip is a surgical emergency. It requires surgical drainage, not just aspiration. Swelling in the hip can compromise blood flow to the femoral head, causing avascular necrosis. Children will keep the infected hip flexed, abducted, and externally rotated. Internally rotating the hip is painful.

▶ CASE 9

A 3-week-old boy is brought to the emergency department seizing. His seizures abate after administration of phenobarbital. He is noted to be febrile and sleepy after his seizure. Upon further questioning you find out he was born at term by vaginal delivery to a mother who received normal prenatal care and had no complications and no prior history of sexually transmitted or other diseases. The neonate is somnolent, has a bulging fontanelle, and is somewhat hypertonic. You decide to get blood, urine, and cerebrospinal fluid (CSF) analyses including cultures and start antibiotics. The medical student asks if you should start acyclovir to empirically treat neonatal HSV disease.

Question 9-1

You correctly tell him:

A) This boy does not have neonatal HSV disease because he has no rash.
B) Neonatal HSV disease commonly occurs in the setting of negative maternal HSV history.
C) This boy has a high risk of neonatal HSV disease only if his mother has a history of genital HSV.
D) Central nervous system (CNS) involvement can be ruled out with a negative CSF HSV PCR.
E) Infants do not die from neonatal HSV infection.

Discussion 9-1

The correct answer is "B." Neonatal HSV disease is relatively uncommon, occurring in 1 in 3000 to 1 in 20,000 live births, but has high rates of morbidity and mortality, often even with antiviral therapy. Symptoms can be mild in the setting of skin, eye, and mouth disease (SEM), but can be severe in disseminated and CNS disease. Infants usually present before 6 weeks of age, most commonly at about 2 to 3 weeks of age. They very rarely have infection at birth. Symptoms include rash, fever, lethargy, seizures, or mucous membrane lesions depending on site of infection. Liver function tests are commonly elevated in disseminated disease. It is important to note that some infants with HSV never develop vesicular skin lesions and some may not have fever. Also important to remember is that initially well-appearing infants with skin vesicles may have more disseminated disease. A neonate who has a seizure should always have HSV infection on the differential diagnosis list. (See Figures 20–1 and 20–2.) Transmission most likely occurs during vaginal

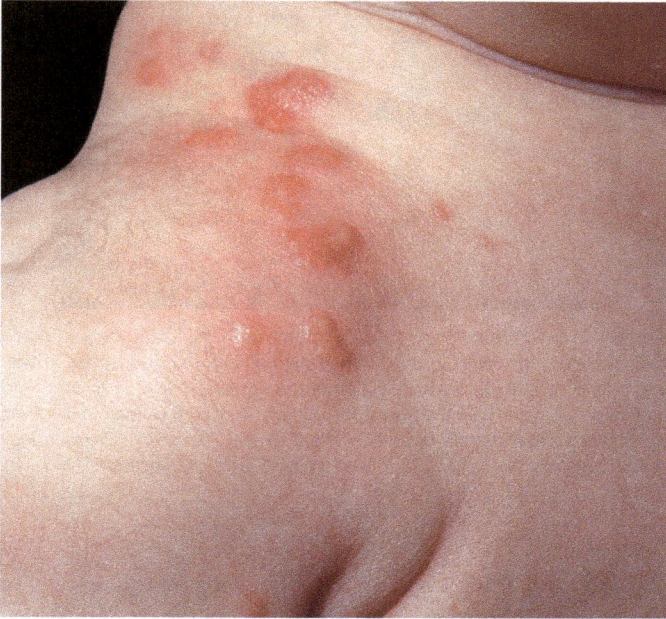

FIGURE 20–1. Neonatal Herpes Simplex Virus Disease—Skin. A cluster of erythematous vesicles are present on the shoulder of this 2-week-old with skin, eye, and mouth disease. Untreated it may progress to disseminated disease. (Reproduced with permission from Wolff K, Johnson RA, Saavedra AP, eds. *Fitzpatrick's Color Atlas and Synopsis of Clinical Dermatology.* 7th ed. New York, NY: McGraw-Hill Education; 2013, Fig. 27-40.)

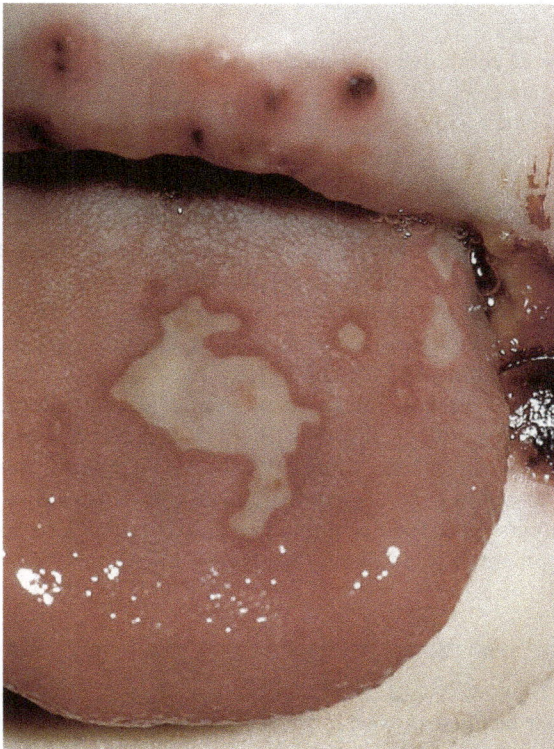

FIGURE 20–2. Neonatal Herpes Simplex Virus Disease—Mouth. Vesicles are present on the tongue and lips along with ulcerations of the tongue and crusted erosions on the lips of this 3-week-old with neonatal herpes involving the mouth. (Reproduced with permission from Wolff K, Johnson RA, Saavedra AP, eds. *Fitzpatrick's Color Atlas and Synopsis of Clinical Dermatology.* 7th ed. New York, NY: McGraw-Hill Education. 2013, Fig. 27-39.)

delivery but can occur postnatally as well (such as a person with a cold sore that kisses the neonate's broken skin at the previous site of a scalp electrode). Rupture of membranes more than 4 hours before delivery increases risk in infants born vaginally and via cesarean section. Neonates born to mothers with first-time active genital lesions at time of delivery have about a 60% chance of developing neonatal HSV disease. This is thought to be due to lack of protective maternal antibodies. Such infants should be delivered by cesarean section to decrease this risk. Neonates born to mothers with history of prior genital HSV infection but no active lesions at the time of delivery have only a 2% chance of developing neonatal HSV disease. HSV can be shed intermittently in vaginal secretions without active lesions present. The majority of infants with neonatal HSV disease are born to mothers with no known history of HSV. Neonates with suspected HSV disease should be evaluated immediately and empiric acyclovir started pending results of testing. Acyclovir decreases mortality, but in the setting of disseminated and CNS disease there can still be significant morbidity despite therapy. Testing should include viral cultures of skin and mucous membranes, liver function tests, CSF indices, as well as PCR of blood, CSF, and lesion if present. CSF PCR can be falsely negative early in the disease and should be interpreted with caution. CSF PCR often remains positive for several days after the initiation of acyclovir, so administration of acyclovir should not be delayed to obtain a lumbar puncture if neonatal HSV disease is suspected. Imaging of the brain can be useful in the setting of CNS abnormalities such as seizures, altered mental status, or other related symptoms.

QUICK QUIZ

HSV infection can cause all of the following clinical illnesses EXCEPT:
A) Gingivostomatitis.
B) Encephalitis.
C) Genital infections.
D) Herpangina.
E) Herpetic whitlow.

Discussion

The correct answer is "D." Herpangina is caused by coxsackievirus, which is part of the enterovirus family. It causes fever and painful ulcers in the posterior oropharynx. (See Figure 20–3.) HSV causes a number of different infectious illnesses. It likes the skin and mucous membranes. Most infections are caused by herpes simplex virus type 1 (HSV-1), although genital infections are more often caused by type 2 (HSV-2). After the initial or primary infection, the virus lives in the nerve ganglia cells and can reactivate. This is why someone with cold sores (herpes labialis) keeps getting lesions over and over. If you have a history of cold sores, stay calm as stress triggers reactivation. The virus never is eradicated from the body. Consider it the gift that keeps on giving. In children, primary HSV-1 mouth infection causes gingivostomatitis and pharyngitis resulting in fever, swelling of

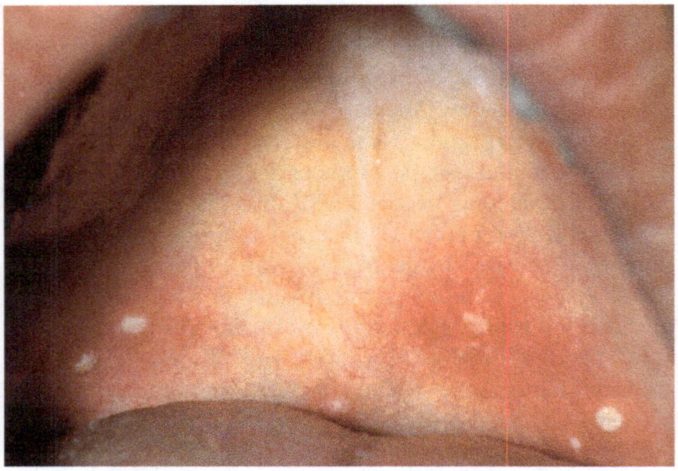

FIGURE 20–3. Herpangina is a caused by coxsackievirus. It presents with multiple erythematous vesicles and erosions primarily in the posterior oropharynx but may occur anterior in the mouth, including the lips. Herpes gingivostomatosis looks similar but gingivitis is present. (Reproduced with permission from Wolff K, Johnson RA, Saavedra AP, eds. *Fitzpatrick's Color Atlas and Synopsis of Clinical Dermatology.* 7th ed. New York, NY: McGraw-Hill Education; 2013, Fig. 27-27.)

the gums, and vesicular lesions of the mouth and pharynx. The gums are friable and bleed easily. This is very painful. Children may require hospitalization for hydration and pain control. Herpetic whitlow is an infection of the finger. (See Figure 20–4.) It results from autoinoculation of the virus through a break in the skin such as when a child with oral herpes sucks on his or her finger. In herpes gladiatorum, wrestlers pass skin lesions back and forth. HSV can cause keratitis, encephalitis, meningitis,

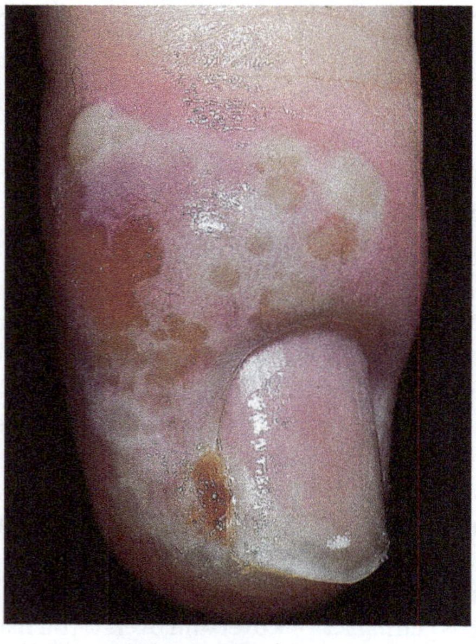

FIGURE 20–4. Herpetic whitlow is a painful herpes simplex infection of the finger. It is often mistaken for a bacterial infection and treated with antibiotics. (Reproduced with permission from Goldsmith LA, Katz SI, Gilchrest BA, Paller AS, Leffell DJ, Wolff K, eds. *Fitzpatrick's Dermatology in General Medicine.* 8th ed. New York, NY: McGraw-Hill Education; 2012, Fig. 193-7.)

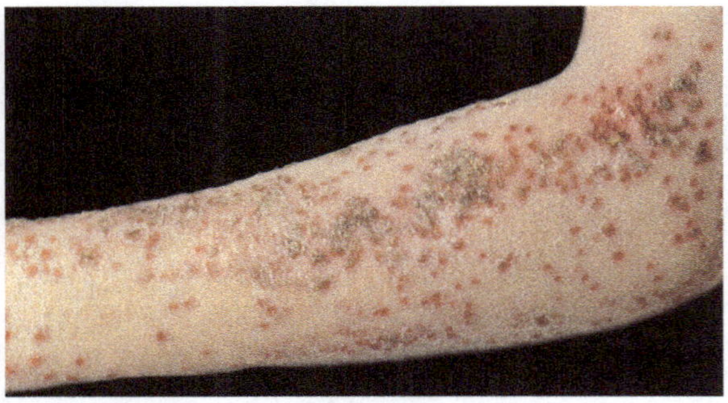

FIGURE 20–5. Eczema Herpeticum. Eczema may be commonly infected by herpes simplex virus, a condition known as eczema herpeticum. Fever and irritability may proceed development of vesicles, crusted erosions, and punched-out lesions. (Reproduced with permission from Goldsmith LA, Katz SI, Gilchrest BA, Paller AS, Leffell DJ, Wolff K, eds. *Fitzpatrick's Dermatology in General Medicine.* 8th ed. New York, NY: McGraw-Hill Education; 2012, Fig. 14-12.)

hepatitis, and Bell palsy. Treatment depends on the severity of infection, host immune status and timing of the onset of symptoms. Ideally, treatment is started within 72 hours of onset.

⧗ QUICK QUIZ

What is NOT a risk factor for severe HSV infection?
A) HIV.
B) Burns.
C) Severe combined immunodeficiency (SCID).
D) Eczema.
E) All of the above.

Discussion

The correct answer is "E." To fight HSV you need a functioning cellular immune system. Any cause of immunodeficiency, either congenital or acquired, increases the risk for severe, recurrent, and or disseminated infection. Examples include HIV, malnutrition, malignancy, organ transplant, chronic steroids, and congenital immunodeficiencies. HSV likes the skin, especially if the skin is disrupted from burns, atopic dermatitis (eczema), or other dermatologic disorder. The skin of children with atopic dermatitis can become infected with HSV (eczema herpeticum). The skin becomes erythematous, with clustered vesicles and punched-out lesions. Irritability and fever may precede the development of skin lesions. (See Figure 20–5.)

▶ CASE 10

A father has just moved to the area and brings his 1-month-old son, 3-year-old daughter, and 7-year-old son for their well-child checks. It is May and all are healthy and doing well. He has heard from neighbors that there are ticks and mosquitos in the area that harbor infectious diseases. He asks you for advice on how to prevent both tick- and mosquito-borne infections.

Question 10-1

You suggest that he should:
A) Avoid letting the children play outside in the evening time.
B) Apply DEET to exposed skin of all the children before they go outside.
C) Apply permethrin to exposed skin of all the children before they go outside.
D) All of the above.
E) None of the above.

Discussion 10-1

The correct answer is "E." A broad range of bacterial, viral, and parasitic infections in the United States have tick and mosquito vectors. The type of infection depends on geography, but examples include Rocky Mountain spotted fever, ehrlichiosis, Lyme disease, babesiosis, Colorado tick fever, West Nile virus, and La Crosse virus. Diseases thought to be more associated with tropical locales, such as dengue and chikungunya, are now starting to appear in some parts of the southern United States. In the United States mosquitoes often are more active at dawn and dusk, so avoiding outside activities at this time may decrease risk of infection. However, many species of mosquitoes are active and bite during the day, making transmission of infection possible at any time. Avoiding evening activity would not prevent tickborne infection. There are multiple repellants available for use to decrease tick and mosquito exposure. Permethrin can be used to impregnate clothing and will repel ticks and mosquitoes, but should not be applied directly on the skin due to risk of absorption. DEET (N,N-diethyl-meta-toluamide) is available in various concentrations and repels both ticks and mosquitoes. It should be applied to exposed skin. As a general rule, the higher the concentration of DEET, the longer lasting the effect, and the greater the risk of systemic absorption and toxicity. DEET is not recommended for use in children younger than 2 months of age. For children 2 months of age and older, DEET concentrations of 10% to 30% are recommended. Picaridin is also available for use as a tick and mosquito repellent. The Environmental Protection Agency (EPA) does not recommend its use in children younger than 3 years of age. Oil of lemon and eucalyptus may repel ticks and mosquitoes, but neither has undergone formal evaluation and their use is not recommended for children younger than age 3. Repellents should not be applied to the hands as children often put their hands in their mouth, increasing the risk of systemic absorption. Tick exposure can be limited by exercising care in tick-prone areas such as woods and heavy brush. Long sleeves and pants can limit exposure. Children should be regularly checked for ticks after playing in these areas. One solution might be to avoid the outdoors and take supplemental vitamin D to offset the lack of sunlight exposure.

CASE 11

A 3-year-old girl with sickle cell disease is brought by her parents to your office to establish care. Her parents have not been very good at arranging health care visits in the past, and you realize that she has not received any vaccines recommended for children.

Question 11-1

Which of the following vaccines is/are recommended for this patient to optimally protect her from future infection?
A) Hib vaccine.
B) Pneumococcal conjugate vaccine.
C) Meningococcal conjugate vaccine.
D) Pneumococcal polysaccharide vaccine.
E) Both A and B.
F) Options A, B, and C.
G) All of the above vaccines should be given at the recommended time and intervals.

Discussion 11-1

The correct answer is "G." This question may have too many choices but with vaccines more is usually better. Children with sickle cell anemia develop functional asplenia. The spleen is an important site for antigen processing and antibody production. Any child with asplenia is at risk for invasive infection with encapsulated organisms such as *Haemophilus influenzae* type B, *Streptococcus pneumoniae,* and *Neisseria meningitidis.* Less commonly such children can have invasive infection with *Staphylococcus aureus*, streptococcal species, and gram-negative organisms such as *Escherichia coli, Klebsiella, Salmonella,* and *Pseudomonas* species. They are also at risk for severe malaria and babesiosis. Efforts should be made to mitigate the risk of invasive infection in children with asplenia. If possible, immunization should occur before surgical splenectomy because of poorer response to vaccines postsplenectomy. Pneumococcal conjugate vaccine (PCV13), pneumococcal polysaccharide vaccine (PPSV23), meningococcal conjugate vaccine, and Hib vaccine are all recommended for asplenic patients to prevent invasive infection with those encapsulated organisms. It is important to note that several meningococcal conjugate vaccines are approved for various ages and indications. PPSV23 should not be administered at the same time as PCV13, but should be given 8 weeks after finishing the PCV13 series. Additionally, penicillin prophylaxis is generally recommended in young asplenic patients to prevent invasive pneumococcal disease. Length of prophylaxis or decision to initiate prophylaxis in older children depends on the clinical scenario.

CASE 12

A 6-year-old girl is brought by her mother for evaluation of a new rash in August. Her mother noted an approximately 2-cm red circular lesion a week ago. It has increased in size slowly over the last week and now has central clearing. (See Figure 20–6.) The girl has been outside a lot this summer but does not remember any tick bites. She is afebrile and has no other symptoms. You suspect Lyme disease.

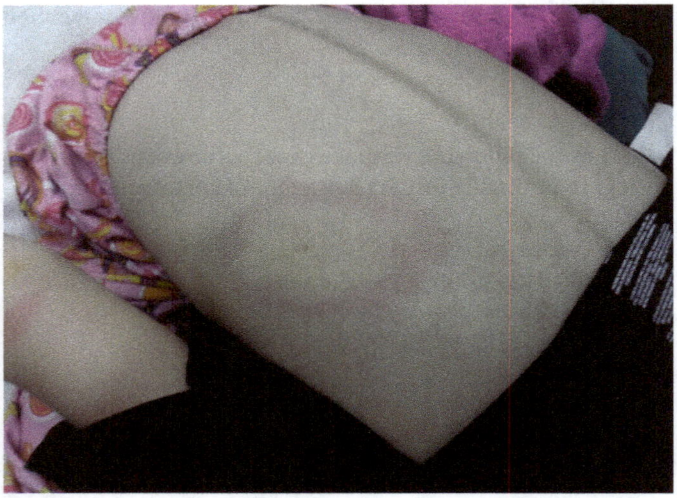

FIGURE 20–6. Erythema migrans is the hallmark of Lyme disease. It starts as a small red bump then grows to form a large annular erythematous lesion. Central clearing may occur to form the classic "bull's eye". (Used with permission from Nathan Price, MD.)

Question 12-1

Your next step should be to:
A) Obtain Lyme serologies.
B) Prescribe amoxicillin.
C) Prescribe doxycycline.
D) Observe, only, since she is otherwise asymptomatic and has no reliable history of tick exposure.
E) Perform a lumbar puncture.

Discussion 12-1

The correct answer is "B." Lyme disease is caused by the bacterium *Borrelia burgdorferi*. It is transmitted by ticks, predominantly by the *Ixodes scapularis* or deer tick, though other *Ixodes* species can transmit the organism. Geographic distribution in the United States tends to follow the *Ixodes* habitat, which is more common in the Northeastern United States. The disease is named for Lyme, Connecticut, the town nearby to where multiple early cases were described. The tick generally needs to feed for 36 hours for the bacteria to be transmitted. A large proportion of patients with Lyme disease have no recollection of a tick bite. This is likely due to the fact that bites are painless and the tick can feed in areas not easily observed such as the back or scalp. In addition the nymph, which has a higher likelihood of transmitting Lyme disease than the adult tick, can be very small, about the size of the tip of a ball point pen. Typically after the tick bites, a small macule appears within a few days. The macule then increase in size to several centimeters (cm) in diameter. The lesion may not have the classic bull's eye appearance and it is often missed because it can be asymptomatic. It then fades over the next days to weeks. Fever can occur, especially with the multiple erythema migrans that occur in the setting of dissemination of the organism. Other symptoms such as arthritis, cranial nerve palsies (especially facial nerve), meningitis, encephalitis, heart block, and fatigue are possible as well.

Early disease such as erythema migrans in this patient is a clinical diagnosis. Serologies in early disease are not recommended due to poor sensitivity and specificity. Antibiotics should be prescribed even if symptoms are mild because treatment can prevent the development of arthritis, which is fairly common in children. Doxycycline is generally the oral drug of choice but is usually not used in children younger than 8 years of age due to the potential for staining of permanent teeth. Amoxicillin is used to treat younger children with Lyme disease. Other drugs that may be used are ceftriaxone (especially if there are severe symptoms, including CNS involvement) and cefuroxime. It is reasonable to use doxycycline prophylaxis after a tick bite in areas of high endemicity if the patient is aged 8 years or older and the tick is an *I. scapularis* species that was attached for at least 36 hours. Prophylaxis with amoxicillin is not recommended.

▶ CASE 13

A 15-year-old girl is evaluated in the emergency department (ED) for abdominal pain and fevers. The fevers started about 3 weeks ago and have not resolved despite intermittent treatment with acetaminophen and ibuprofen. The girl has had some right upper quadrant pain for the last several days and had a small bump on her right arm a few weeks ago that has since resolved. She cannot remember any other symptoms. Because of no improvement in symptoms her family brought her in to be evaluated. On exam you note her to be febrile to 38.5°C (101.3°F) with a heart rate of 110 beats per minute, but she is non–toxic appearing. She has a somewhat tender right axillary lymph node that feels like it is approximately 3 cm in diameter. She has some tenderness in the right upper quadrant and the liver edge is palpable about 2 cm below the right costal margin. Her lab results are remarkable for a mildly elevated white blood cell count of 13,000 with neutrophil predominance and normal liver function tests. A computed tomography (CT) scan with contrast is ordered and shows a normal appendix and gallbladder but some mild hepatomegaly with multiple scattered small abscesses.

Question 13-1

You explore the history further and are most likely to find that:
A) She recently went to rural Mexico.
B) She has a kitten at home.
C) She had *Staphylococcus aureus* bacteremia a few months ago that was treated with IV antibiotics.
D) She drinks unpasteurized milk.
E) None of the above.

Discussion 13-1

The correct answer is "B." This patient has cat-scratch disease caused by *Bartonella henselae*. Cats, especially kittens, are known to carry the bacteria in their blood. Infection usually occurs after being scratched, but often patients cannot remember a specific scratch occurring. Typically a couple of weeks after the scratch, a red papule forms near the area of inoculation. The lesion then resolves and lymphadenopathy occurs somewhere along the chain of lymph nodes that drain the skin where the lesion occurred. Because scratches often occur on the arm, axillary and epitrochlear lymphadenopathy is common. Fever, though not always present, can develop and last for weeks. The lymph nodes may suppurate and drain or may require surgical drainage to improve pain. The disease often resolves spontaneously (may take months), though antibiotics may help symptoms to improve. In some cases, more systemic involvement may occur, and liver and splenic lesions often are seen on CT scan or ultrasound. These lesions typically are small and scattered in the liver or spleen. They can calcify after disease resolution. The CNS and eye (neuroretinitis) may be involved as well. Infectious organisms can reach the liver by several mechanisms such as bacteremia, contiguous spread of intra-abdominal infection, or traumatic inoculation. Organisms such as *S. aureus* are common owing to their propensity to cause bacteremia leading to their deposition in the liver. Gram-negative enteric organisms are common as well, due to spread from intra-abdominal infection such as appendicitis or cholangitis. Rarer causes include *Brucella,* which should be suspected if the patient has been exposed to livestock or unpasteurized dairy products. Travel to undeveloped countries should prompt inclusion of amebic abscess, such as *Entamoeba histolytica,* on the differential diagnosis. In these situations the abscess is often solitary, but a few smaller or larger abscesses may be present. Multiple small abscesses would be more likely in the setting of *Bartonella* infection.

► CASE 14

It is a busy time of year on the inpatient pediatric ward in the hospital. The nurses ask about several patients who have been admitted. They would like to know what kind of isolation precautions should be taken to prevent spread of infection.

Question 14-1

In addition to standard precautions you tell them:
A) The infant admitted with respiratory syncytial virus (RSV) should be on droplet precautions, only.
B) The child admitted with pertussis should be on contact and droplet precautions.
C) The child admitted with chickenpox should be on contact and droplet precautions.
D) The child with measles should be on airborne precautions.
E) The infant with pulmonary tuberculosis and a right middle lobe infiltrate on chest X-ray should be on airborne precautions.

Discussion 14-1

The correct answer is "D." Isolation precautions should be taken in certain situations to prevent spread of infection among hospital patients, visitors and employees. Droplet precautions are implemented when there is risk of transmission in the air within

3 feet of the patient. Airborne precautions are necessary when transmission occurs by means of droplet nuclei, which are small particles that can be suspended in the air for long periods of time and can travel farther from the bedside than organisms that require droplet precautions. Some organisms require a combination of contact and droplet or airborne precautions depending on mode of spread. Though counterintuitive, RSV is transmitted through contact rather than inhalation of virus. Pertussis requires droplet precautions. Chickenpox can be spread by droplet nuclei in addition to contact and requires both contact and airborne precautions. Measles requires airborne precautions, only. In adults and older children, tuberculosis requires airborne precautions. However, young children with pulmonary disease usually are not contagious and so do not necessarily need airborne isolation. This is because their infection is usually paucibacillary (few bacteria present) and they are unable to generate aerosols due to relatively weaker strength of cough. The exception to this is if they have cavitary lesions (which have a much higher bacterial load), laryngeal infection, disseminated pulmonary infection, acid-fast bacteria (AFB) positive sputum smears, or are undergoing aerosol-generating procedures such as bronchoscopy or pulmonary function testing. (See Table 20–2.)

► CASE 15

While his family is setting the table for dinner a 2-year-old pulls a hot-off-the-stove bowl of soup, spilling it over his body. His father takes him to the emergency department immediately, and he is found to have partial thickness burns on his arms and chest. As you are discussing medical history with the family, you find out that he received three tetanus immunizations as an infant.

Question 15-1

You decide that regarding tetanus:
A) He is adequately immunized.
B) He is not adequately immunized, but does not need tetanus prophylaxis for this wound.
C) He needs tetanus immune globulin.
D) He needs a tetanus booster.
E) Both C and D.

Discussion 15-1

The correct answer is "D." Tetanus is a terrible disease caused by the bacterium *Clostridium tetani.* It is an anaerobe that produces spores that are ubiquitous in the environment, especially in soil. Once in the body, the organism produces a neurotoxin that causes muscular rigidity and spasms notably of the masseter muscle, hence its common name of "lockjaw." Prior to widespread immunization tetanus was a fairly common disease. Despite modern medicine and intensive care, mortality is still 10% to 30%. Determining prophylaxis for tetanus in the setting of a new injury can be tricky as it involves the answers to three questions: (1) Is this a tetanus-prone wound? (2) How many, if

TABLE 20–2 RECOMMENDED PRECAUTIONS FOR VARIOUS ORGANISMS OR SYNDROMES

Precaution Type

Contact	Droplet	Airborne
Chickenpox, zoster	Mumps	Chickenpox
Syphilitic skin lesions	Influenza	Tuberculosis
Herpes simplex virus, if mucocutaneous lesions	*Haemophilus influenzae*	Measles
Adenovirus conjunctivitis	Adenovirus pneumonia	
Human metapneumovirus	Parvovirus B19 (before rash)	
Parainfluenza	Diphtheria	
Salmonella or *Shigella*	Pertussis	
Escherichia coli 0157:H7 or shiga toxin producing *E. coli*	*Streptococcus pyogenes* (GAS) pharyngitis, pneumonia, scarlet fever	
Viral hemorrhagic fevers	Viral hemorrhagic fevers	
Enteroviruses	Rhinovirus	
Rotavirus	Rubella	
Hepatitis A		
Clostridium difficile		
Lice		
Scabies		
Draining wounds that cannot be covered		
Diarrhea thought to be infectious		
Skin, wound or urinary tract infection caused by a multidrug resistant organism		

any, tetanus vaccinations have been given? (3) How long ago was the last tetanus vaccine dose? Tetanus-prone wounds are any wound that could be contaminated with spores, or wounds amenable to infection with an anaerobe—in other words, any wound that is deep or has devitalized tissue. Even seemingly minor wounds may have some potential for tetanus infection. High-risk wounds, such as puncture wounds, crush wounds, avulsions, burns, frostbite, or wounds contaminated by soil, feces, or saliva, require tetanus prophylaxis in a more aggressive

manner than clean, minor wounds. Tetanus prophylaxis is based on a three-dose vaccine backbone with additional boosters given based on age and time since last dose. The key to remembering whether tetanus immune globulin (TIG) is needed in high-risk wounds is based on whether or not a patient received the three-dose backbone. If the patient has received the three doses, then TIG is not needed. Regardless of wound type a booster may need to be given based on timing of the last dose, both to boost current protection and provide longer term immunity. A patient who received the three-dose series and was otherwise up to date with a high risk wound will need a booster if the last dose was given 5 or more years ago. A clean minor wound in that same scenario would require a booster if the last dose was given 10 or more years ago. A patient who is not considered up to date should receive a booster provided the correct interval has passed since the last tetanus immunization. The 2-year-old child received his initial three-dose series at 2, 4, and 6 months, but also should have gotten a booster at 15 to 18 months of age. Since he is not up to date on his tetanus immunization, he should receive a booster dose now. He does not need TIG even though he has a high-risk wound (burn) since he had his three-dose initial series. If an infant younger than 6 months of age presents with a tetanus-prone wound, then the same principles apply, but the mother's tetanus status is taken into account. In other words, a 4-month old with a tetanus-prone wound does not require TIG if the mother received her three-dose series with the last dose given less than 5 years ago. The infant should be immunized according to the tetanus schedule for infants.

Helpful Tip

Test writers love to ask about tetanus prophylaxis. Know this backward and forward. Remember:

- Tetanus-prone wound without prior 3-dose vaccine series = TIG + Vaccine dose (if age appropriate)
- Clean, minor wound or prior 3-dose series + High-risk wound = No need for TIG
- Prior 3-dose series + Clean minor wound + ≥ 10 years since last booster = Boost now
- Prior 3-dose series + High risk wound + ≥ 5 years since last booster = Boost now
- Not up to date at time of wound + Correct minimum interval since last dose = Boost now

▶ CASE 16

A 5-day-old term male infant is being seen in clinic for follow up after discharge from the newborn nursery. He has been breastfeeding appropriately and is vigorous and afebrile, but you note on exam that he has bilateral purulent conjunctivitis. Upon further review of his chart and discussion with his mother, you determine that she had normal newborn care, with negative sexually transmitted diseases (STDs) screening early in pregnancy, but she had several new sexual partners later in the pregnancy.

Question 16-1

You decide to:

A) Perform a lumbar puncture.
B) Obtain blood cultures.
C) Start IV ceftriaxone.
D) Obtain cultures of the eye exudate.
E) All of the above.

Discussion 16-1

The correct answer is "D." This newborn has conjunctival injection with discharge consistent with ophthalmia neonatorum. This condition is often caused by maternal sexually transmitted infection such as gonorrhea or chlamydia, but other non–sexually transmitted organisms such as *Staphylococcus aureus, Haemophilus* species, *and Streptococcus pneumoniae* are possible as well. Viral etiologies such as HSV should also be considered, but usually do not cause a purulent conjunctivitis. Historically gonorrhea was the most common cause of neonatal conjunctivitis and blindness, but chlamydia is now a more common etiology of ophthalmia neonatorum. All newborns should receive topical prophylaxis to prevent gonococcal ophthalmia neonatorum. In the United States topical erythromycin is typically used. Remember none of the topical prophylactic therapies are effective in preventing chlamydial ophthalmia neonatorum. The use of topical erythromycin may seem counterintuitive as it does not prevent chlamydial eye disease, yet systemic erythromycin is used to treat infant chlamydial infection. The opposite is true for erythromycin and gonorrhea: the topical therapy prevents eye disease, but systemic erythromycin is not used to treat gonorrheal infection due to widespread resistance. Newborns whose mothers have untreated gonococcal infection should receive a prophylactic one-time intramuscular (IM) dose of ceftriaxone. Newborns whose mothers have untreated chlamydial infection are at high risk of development of infection, but systemic prophylactic therapy is not recommended due to unknown efficacy. They should be followed closely for development of disease and treated appropriately. A newborn presenting with conjunctivitis should be evaluated for the usual causes of ophthalmia neonatorum. This evaluation includes a thorough history and exam to assess for signs and symptoms of extraocular disease, as well as cultures and stains of the exudate and conjunctival scrapings. Although not approved by the Food and Drug Administration (FDA) for conjunctival specimens, nucleic acid amplification testing (NAAT) may be available for diagnosis of chlamydia. Ophthalmia neonatorum caused by *Neisseria gonorrhoeae* typically manifests in the first week of life. Inflammation and purulence can be significant and persist for some time despite treatment. Corneal scarring and systemic infection is possible. An otherwise healthy-appearing, afebrile infant without signs or symptoms of extraocular infection does not require blood cultures and lumbar puncture prior to initiation of therapy for gonococcal ophthalmia neonatorum. Diagnosis can be made by Gram stain and culture of exudate. For localized gonococcal ophthalmia neonatorum, a single dose of ceftriaxone may be given if the infant is not hyperbilirubinemic. Alternatively cefotaxime may be given. Chlamydial ophthalmia neonatorum tends to present later than gonococcal infection, typically toward the end of the first week

of life, although there can be overlap of presentation for both illnesses. Inflammatory response in chlamydial infection tends to be less intense compared with gonococcal disease. Healing is usually complete, although scarring is possible with untreated disease. *Systemic* erythromycin or azithromycin should be given to treat both ophthalmologic infection and possible pneumonia. Topical antibiotic therapy is not effective in preventing or treating ophthalmia neonatorum caused by chlamydia. HSV is an uncommon but potentially devastating cause of ophthalmia neonatorum. It typically presents after the first week of life as conjunctivitis with serous discharge. Full examination, including lumbar puncture, HSV cultures of eye, oropharynx, and rectum, as well as blood and CSF HSV PCR and liver function tests, should be obtained to assess for systemic involvement. Treatment with IV acyclovir should be started pending results of testing, and length of therapy depends on type of infection.

> **Helpful Tip**
> Infants younger than 2 weeks of age treated with erythromycin or azithromycin are at increased risk for hypertrophic pyloric stenosis.

▶ CASE 17

A 15-year-old otherwise healthy boy living in Wisconsin presents in September for evaluation of knee swelling. He started having pain about a week and half ago and noted swelling of the knee that started several days ago. He does not remember any trauma and has not been aggressively exercising. He has been afebrile and denies any other symptoms currently, but does remember that several weeks ago he had several days of fever and a rash with multiple large circular lesions on his arms, legs, and trunk that resolved without therapy. On exam he has a left knee effusion, with mild warmth to the touch, and mild tenderness but no overlying erythema.

Question 17-1

You are concerned about joint infection and should:

A) Have the joint aspirated emergently for cell count and culture.
B) Start empiric antistaphylococcal antibiotics.
C) Obtain Lyme enzyme immunoassay (EIA) with reflex IgG Western blot.
D) Obtain a blood culture.
E) Prescribe ibuprofen.

Discussion 17-1

The correct answer is "C." Joint swelling warrants further workup to determine the cause. Septic arthritis with typical virulent organisms such as *Staphylococcus aureus* and *Streptococcus pyogenes* (group A beta-hemolytic *Streptococcus,* GAS), should be suspected in patients with an acute presentation of joint pain, swelling, erythema, and systemic symptoms. In such cases urgent aspiration and empiric antibiotics are indicated when septic arthritis is suspected. In the case of this patient, emergent aspiration of the joint is unlikely to be necessary owing to insidious onset, mild symptoms, and mild findings on exam. Given the time of year and geographic location, Lyme disease should be high on the differential. Arthritis can be associated with other infections either due to acute infection or postinfectious inflammation. Trauma and rheumatologic disease should be considered as well. Arthritis is a late manifestation of Lyme disease, usually occurring 2 to 12 months after the initial infection. This patient had rash and fevers typical of multiple erythema migrans, consistent with earlier infection with the bacteria. Any joint can be affected, but the knee is most common. Often the arthritis has a slow onset with relatively mild symptoms and can resolve and recur intermittently if untreated. Most children will continue to walk and bear weight on the affected joint. Testing for late manifestations of Lyme disease is a two-step approach. The screening lab is an enzyme-linked immunosorbent assay (ELISA) for total antibody to *Borrelia burgdorferi*. Positive or equivocal screens should be confirmed with an IgG Western blot test in the setting of late disease such as arthritis. Blood cultures, while indicated for evaluation of acute bacterial arthritis, are not useful in diagnosing Lyme arthritis.

> **Helpful Tip**
> Acute monoarticular arthritis accompanied by fever is treated as if due to a bacterial infection of the joint until proven otherwise. Aspirate the joint for culture and treat with IV antibiotics right away.

► CASE 18

A 3-year-old otherwise healthy, fully immunized child presents with cough and runny nose of 5 days duration, but has now developed fever to 39°C (102.2°F) and significant left ear pain for 2 days. On exam she has a red, bulging left tympanic membrane that does not move with pneumatic otoscopy. She also has bilateral conjunctivitis. You diagnose acute left otitis media with bilateral conjunctivitis. She has no drug allergies and has not had otitis media in the past.

Question 18-1

Antibiotic treatment is indicated in all of the following scenarios EXCEPT:

A) A 5-month-old with acute otitis media.
B) A 2-year-old with unilateral otitis media and low-grade fever.
C) An 18-month-old with unilateral otitis media and high-grade fever.
D) A 3-year-old with bilateral acute otitis media.
E) All of the above should receive antibiotic treatment.

Discussion 18-1

The correct answer is "B." Acute otitis media (AOM) is a very common diagnosis in children, and one of the most common

reasons for antibiotic prescriptions in the United States. Often patients have a prodrome of viral URI symptoms that can cause inflammation, which leads to bacterial superinfection. Diagnosis is based on clinical exam findings that include erythematous, bulging tympanic membrane with middle ear effusion as determined by pneumatic otoscopy or tympanometry. New-onset otorrhea not caused by otitis externa can be used to diagnose AOM as well. AOM is painful. Regardless of whether antibiotics are used, pain should be addressed and may be treated with either topical or systemic therapy. Antibiotics should be prescribed for all infants younger than 6 months of age with AOM. For those 6 months of age or older, antibiotics should be prescribed for (1) severe symptoms such as moderate to severe otalgia for 48 hours or fever above 39°C (102.2°F), or (2) bilateral AOM. Children older than 6 months with less severe symptoms and unilateral involvement may be managed with observation only, but there should be a plan in place for evaluation or treatment if there is worsening of symptoms or lack of improvement in the next 48 to 72 hours.

You decide she meets treatment criteria.

Question 18-2

Which is the appropriate antibiotic treatment for her AOM?

A) High-dose amoxicillin for 7 days.
B) High-dose amoxicillin for 10 days.
C) High-dose amoxicillin clavulanate for 7 days.
D) High-dose amoxicillin clavulanate for 10 days.
E) Ceftriaxone IM.

Discussion 18-2

The correct answer is "C." Common bacterial etiologies of AOM include *Streptococcus pneumoniae*, nontypeable *Haemophilus influenzae*, and *Moraxella catarrhalis*. First-line therapy should target *S. pneumoniae*, which is the most common cause of AOM in children. *S. pneumoniae* often is resistant to lower dose amoxicillin. This resistance mechanism occurs through alteration of penicillin binding proteins (not beta-lactamase production), and usually can be overcome by increasing the dose of amoxicillin. If the child has concurrent conjunctivitis, then *H. influenzae* is a likely possibility. *H. influenzae* often is resistant to penicillin through beta-lactamase production. Addition of the beta-lactamase inhibitor clavulanate usually is able to overcome this resistance mechanism. Other reasons to consider therapy with amoxicillin clavulanate in a child with AOM include receipt of amoxicillin within the prior 30 days, history of recurrent AOM unresponsive to amoxicillin, and failure of current symptoms to improve while receiving amoxicillin. Third-generation cephalosporins such as cefdinir or IM ceftriaxone can be considered as well for treatment of beta-lactamase-producing organisms. It is important to note that in the United States resistance rates of *S. pneumoniae* are often higher for cefdinir than they are for amoxicillin. Children younger than 2 years of age or children with recurrent AOM or with craniofacial abnormalities should be treated for 10 days. Older children with uncomplicated AOM can receive a shorter 5- to 7-day course of oral antibiotics.

CHAPTER 20 • INFECTIOUS DISEASE

The patient's ear pain and fevers resolve, but 5 days into antibiotic therapy she develops mild abdominal pain and non-bloody diarrhea. She has some perineal erythema from the diarrhea, but otherwise her exam is unremarkable. She is afebrile and vital signs are normal. She is eating and drinking well. A PCR test done on her stool is positive for *Clostridium difficile*.

Question 18-3

You decide to:
A) Treat with oral metronidazole.
B) Treat with oral vancomycin.
C) Stop the amoxicillin clavulanate.
D) Both A and C.
E) Both B and C.

Discussion 18-3

The correct answer is "D." Diarrhea acquired during antibiotic therapy is common. Antibiotics disrupt the normal intestinal flora, making it possible for other organisms to grow and cause diarrhea. The differential diagnosis for diarrhea in the setting of antibiotics includes side effect of the antibiotic (as seen with drugs such as erythromycin and clavulanate), or new infection with a virus, bacteria, or parasite. Infection with *C. difficile* is becoming more common with antibiotic use. It is a spore-forming anaerobic bacterium that can be difficult to eradicate. Because the spores are hardy and can contaminate multiple surfaces, reinfection and relapse are common even if treated appropriately. If possible, any time *C. difficile* infection occurs, offending antibiotics should be discontinued. This patient has received 5 days of antibiotics for uncomplicated AOM and it would be reasonable to stop her antibiotics at this time. First-line therapy in mild to moderate *C. difficile* infection is oral metronidazole. Resistance to metronidazole is rare. More severe infection should be treated with oral vancomycin due to possibility of resistance. The first infection with *C. difficile* usually is treated for 10 to 14 days. The first recurrence of mild to moderate disease should be treated with another course of metronidazole. Further recurrences should be treated with oral vancomycin owing to risk of neurotoxicity with prolonged, repeated courses of metronidazole. Care should be taken when using oral agents if the patient has septic ileus, as the antibiotics may not be able to reach the area of infection. IV metronidazole, rectally administered vancomycin, and colectomy have been used in severe cases. Other treatments (eg, prolonged treatment courses, treatment with other drugs such as fidaxomicin, or fecal microbiota transplant) are less well studied, but show promise.

> **Helpful Tip**
> Infants can be colonized with toxigenic *C. difficile* bacteria and not have disease. Animal data suggest that they do not have the receptor for the toxin. Testing and or treating for *C. difficile* in infants younger than a year of age generally is not recommended.

▶ CASE 19

A 16-year-old boy presents to the clinic with penile discharge. He has had several sexual partners in the past year. He is otherwise healthy. His last clinic visit was for his 11-year-old well-child check, when he received the recommended immunizations. Gram stain of the discharge shows multiple white blood cells with intracellular gram-negative diplococci.

Question 19-1

You recommend:
A) Oral cefixime for treatment of *Neisseria gonorrhea*.
B) Oral azithromycin for treatment of *Chlamydia trachomatis*.
C) HIV testing.
D) All of the above.
E) Both B and C.

Discussion 19-1

The correct answer is "E." This patient has gonococcal urethritis. Typical symptoms include penile discharge and inguinal lymphadenopathy, although infection can be asymptomatic, especially in females. Treatment is important to stop progression of disease and prevent spread of infection to sexual partners. Sexual partners should be treated at the same time, and the patient should abstain from sex until both partners are appropriately treated. Uncomplicated urogenital gonorrhea is treated with 250 mg of IM ceftriaxone. Oral cefixime is no longer recommended due to concerns for resistance. Other oral regimens are not recommended for the same reason. Anytime someone is treated for gonorrhea, empiric therapy for chlamydia should be given as well as coinfection is common, symptoms are similar, infection may be asymptomatic, and chronic infection can have permanent sequelae in certain patients. Chlamydia can be treated with 1 g of oral azithromycin. Alternatively a 7-day course of doxycycline may be used, although potential compliance with this regimen should be considered. HIV testing should be done at least once in every adolescent 13 years of age or older, with more frequent testing if risk factors are present for higher risk of acquiring HIV. Given the fact that this patient has another STD, now would be a good time to test. Syphilis testing should be considered as well.

You try to remember who should have screening for sexually transmitted infections. This is important for your adolescent patients. You decide to review the CDC guidelines.

Question 19-2

Who is NOT at an increased risk for STDs?
A) A sexually active 17-year-old female patient who faithfully uses condoms.
B) A 14-year-old male patient who has been sexually active with other men.
C) A 15-year-old male patient in a juvenile detention center.
D) A 20-year-old pregnant female patient.
E) All of the above.

Discussion 19-2

The correct answer is "E." In the United States, the adolescent population has the highest rate of STDs. During the yearly adolescent visit, sexual activity and risk and prevention of STDs and pregnancy should be discussed. Sexually active females should be screened yearly for gonorrhea and chlamydia. This can be accomplished through urine nucleic acid amplification testing (NAAT). Sexually active males with risk factors (men who have sex with men) or in certain clinical settings (correction centers, STD clinics) should be screened for chlamydia. Pregnant adolescents and young men who have sex with men require expanded screening for infections such as syphilis in addition to gonorrhea and chlamydia. HIV testing should be encouraged for all sexually active adolescents and those who use injection drugs. It is important to remember that STDs can be transmitted even with consistent condom use. An example is human papillomavirus (HPV), as the lesion may be in an area not covered by the condom.

⧗ QUICK QUIZ

What is the most common STD?
A) Chlamydia.
B) Gonorrhea.
C) Human papillomavirus.
D) Syphilis.

Discussion

The correct answer is "C." Human papillomavirus (HPV), which causes anogenital warts, is the most common STD. (Chlamydia is the most common reportable disease but occurs much less often than HPV, which is not reportable.) The virus is acquired by close contact with lesions (ie, sex) but nonsexual transmission can occur. Infants commonly become infected at delivery if the mother has genital infection. (So, just because an infant has lesions consistent with HPV it does not mean the infant is being sexually abused.) Other presentations include common skin warts and recurrent respiratory papillomatosis. Certain HPV types cause various cancers, with cervical cancer being the most common. HPV vaccination and screening have decreased the incidence of cervical cancer, and evidence suggests that vaccination may decrease other related cancers as well (ie, penile cancer). The quadrivalent vaccine contains types 6 and 11, which cause genital warts, and 16 and 18, which cause 70% of cervical cancer. Other vaccines are under development.

> **Helpful Tip**
> Trichomonas should be suspected in sexually active adolescents (or abuse victims) with malodorous yellow-green vaginal discharge or in males with urethral discharge. The infection commonly is asymptomatic and self-limited. Infection can rarely be seen in newborns who acquired it at delivery from the mother. Diagnosis is made by microscopic visualization of organisms on wet prep or by dipstick or nucleic acid point-of-care testing. The infection responds well to metronidazole or tinidazole. Resistance is rare, but reinfection is common. Sexual partners should be treated at the same time.

▶ CASE 20

A 5-year-old boy was playing at his uncle's house at night when he found a hypodermic needle and accidentally punctured his thumb with it. His father brought him immediately to be evaluated by you in the emergency department. The father thinks there was blood on the needle and is concerned that the child's uncle may be an IV drug user. Dad does not know any of the uncle's medical history and he is not available to speak with at this time. The child is otherwise healthy. Dad thinks he has gotten the recommended immunizations but is not sure if he completed his hepatitis B series. His records are not available. Exam shows a small puncture wound in the thumb with some dried blood on the skin.

Question 20-1

You are concerned about preventing transmission of hepatitis B and decide that you should:
A) Immediately give a dose of hepatitis B vaccine.
B) Immediately give a dose of hepatitis B immune globulin.
C) Obtain a hepatitis B surface antibody measurement.
D) Obtain a hepatitis B surface antigen measurement.
E) Both A and B.

Discussion 20-1

The correct answer is "C." Our apologies for not including an option to advise that the child never visit the uncle's house again. Hepatitis B is a DNA virus that is relatively hardy. It can survive for several days in the environment before losing its infectivity. Transmission can occur by means of infected blood and body fluids (semen, vaginal secretions, saliva, and open wounds). Common modes of transmission include sexual activity, IV drug use, and vertical transmission from mother to child. Transmission through transfusion is rare in the United States due to extensive screening of blood products. Transmission between close home contacts has been documented, likely in the setting of open skin wounds such as eczema, or sharing of razors or toothbrushes. Percutaneous needle injury can transmit infection up to 62% of the time if the source is hepatitis B positive. Disease transmission can be prevented by preexposure vaccination as well as postexposure prophylaxis and vaccination, depending on the situation. A child who has been potentially exposed to hepatitis B should be assessed for immunization history and response to vaccination. A child with an up-to-date vaccination record who has regular access to medical care should have received the hepatitis B series as an infant. A hepatitis B surface antibody measurement should be obtained to determine immunity because results usually are rapid and can inform care. A level of antibody that is 10 mIU/mL or greater indicates immunity and no further therapy is needed. If the source is known to be hepatitis B positive, exposed nonimmunized patients or patients who did not respond to initial vaccine series should be given hepatitis B immune globulin (HBIG) and a dose of hepatitis B vaccine. If hepatitis B status of the source is unknown but is high risk, vaccine nonresponders should be treated with HBIG and vaccine. Unimmunized children should start the vaccine series if the hepatitis B status of the source is unknown. HBIG and the hepatitis B vaccine should be administered in different locations. Children with needlestick injuries should also be assessed for risk of hepatitis C, HIV, and tetanus infection.

In a follow-up visit with you, the father provides medical records from the uncle. They show that the uncle recently had hepatitis serologies done, which shows a negative hepatitis B surface antigen (HBsAg), a negative hepatitis B surface antibody (HBsAb), and positive hepatitis B core antibody (HBcAb).

Question 20-2

You determine that:

A) The uncle did not have hepatitis B.
B) The uncle was immunized for hepatitis B, but is a nonresponder.
C) The uncle has hepatitis B infection but is low risk for transmission.
D) The uncle should be tested for hepatitis B e antigen.
E) All of the above.

Discussion 20-2

The correct answer is "C." The uncle has negative HBsAg, negative HBsAb, and positive HBcAb. This can occur as a result of a false-positive HBcAb test but also can occur in the "window period" during which HBsAg is waning and HBsAb is being produced, but neither is able to be detected by the assay. This period occurs as infection is being controlled and the patient is becoming immune. Risk of transmission of infection during this period is very low. Over time the HBsAb level would be expected to become positive. Core antibody would be *negative* if the uncle was not infected, or if he had been immunized, but had not responded to vaccine, since HBcAb is not part of the vaccine. Hepatitis B e antigen (HBeAg) is detectable during active replication and usually is a marker of higher risk of transmissibility, because viral load is usually high during times of e antigen positivity. Conversion of HBeAg to negative and production of hepatitis B e antibody usually signals lower levels of viremia.

QUICK QUIZ

Which serologic marker can be seen without hepatitis B infection?

A) Positive hepatitis B surface antigen (HBsAg).
B) Positive hepatitis B core antibody (HBcAb).
C) Positive hepatitis B surface antibody (HBsAb).
D) Positive hepatitis B e antigen (HBeAg).
E) None of the above.

Discussion

The correct answer is "C." HBsAb can be present from immunization or infection. HBsAg is the classic marker of infection. HBcAb is the only marker of infection during the window period when neither HBsAg nor HBsAb can be detected. HBeAg indicates active viral replication.

> **Helpful Tip**
>
> Hepatitis C is transmitted in a similar fashion as hepatitis B: blood, sexual activity, and mother to fetus or newborn. Like hepatitis B it is usually asymptomatic in early childhood. It can be diagnosed with PCR or antibody (wait until 18 months of age if testing hepatitis C IgG as the results could just indicate presence of maternal antibody before then). Chronic infection is common and, like hepatitis B, can lead to chronic liver inflammation causing cirrhosis, liver failure, and liver cancer. New therapies with high cure rates and few side effects are on the way so keep a lookout for better therapies for children in the near future.

> **Helpful Tip**
>
> While we are on the subject of hepatitis viruses, hepatitis A differs from hepatitis B and C in being transmitted person to person through the fecal-oral route. People tend to acquire the virus in ways that are not surprising—from daycare settings, food handlers, poor sanitary conditions, infected shellfish, and so on. Younger children tend to have milder disease, whereas older children and adults are more likely to develop jaundice and diarrhea. The infection is self-limiting and no antiviral agents are available that effectively treat it. Diagnosis can be made with serology. Fortunately the vaccine works well to prevent disease. Postexposure prophylaxis usually involves vaccination, although immunoglobulin is given to those who are too young or too old to get the vaccine (patients younger than 1 year or older than 40 years of age), and to immunocompromised patients.

▶ CASE 21

You have been placing tuberculin skin tests (TSTs) on various children to screen for tuberculosis (TB).

Question 21-1

Which of the following children should be considered as having a positive TST that requires further evaluation for possible TB disease?

A) A healthy, asymptomatic 6-year-old boy who moved from Virginia and has 5 mm of induration and 20 mm of erythema.
B) A 12-year-old girl with acute lymphocytic leukemia receiving chemotherapy with 5 mm of induration.
C) A 2-year-old afebrile girl with anterior cervical lymphadenopathy that has increased in size over the last few weeks and has not responded to antistaphylococcal antibiotics. She has no other symptoms. Her TST measured 10 mm of induration.
D) All of the above.
E) None of the above.

Discussion 21-1

The correct answer is "B." The TST causes a type IV hypersensitivity reaction (cellular mediated) in patients with prior or current TB infection. Typically the TST is placed on the left forearm and induration is marked and measured 48 to 72 hours later. It should be done by someone with experience as misinterpretation of the test is common (such as measuring erythema instead of induration). Various values are interpreted as positive depending on the situation to increase or decrease sensitivity. A TST measuring 5 mm or greater is considered positive when the risk of TB or consequences of missed TB disease is high, such as children with symptoms or radiographic findings consistent with TB, immunocompromised children, or children who have had direct contact with a contagious case of TB. A TST of 10 mm or greater is considered positive in children who are from or have traveled to areas of the world with high TB endemicity and children with certain diseases (diabetes mellitus, HIV, lymphoma, Hodgkin disease, malnutrition, chronic renal failure). A measurement of 15 mm or greater is considered positive for all patients regardless of risk factors. (See Figure 20–7.) Some nontuberculous mycobacteria can cross-react with the TST and cause induration. Nontuberculous lymphadenitis with organisms such as *Mycobacterium avium-intracellulare* can commonly cause induration with TST placement, as exemplified by the 2-year-old child described in option "C."

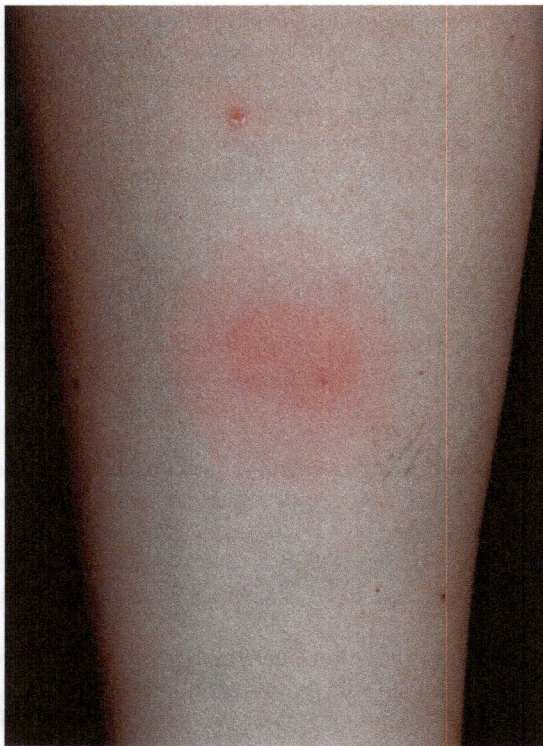

FIGURE 20–7. The tuberculin skin test (TST) for tuberculosis is positive in this patient who recently traveled internationally. There is an elevated area of induration with surrounding erythema. The amount of induration determines the result. (Reproduced with permission from Wolff K, Johnson RA, Saavedra AP, eds. *Fitzpatrick's Color Atlas and Synopsis of Clinical Dermatology.* 7th ed. New York, NY: McGraw-Hill Education; 2013, Fig. 25-72.)

▶ CASE 22

A 7-year-old child was born in India and lived there until 6 months ago. He now presents in clinic for evaluation. He is healthy and up to date on his immunizations. He has a circular scar on the skin overlying his right deltoid muscle. As part of his workup a TST was placed, which showed 10 mm induration. He has no signs or symptoms of infection and a chest X-ray was normal. There is no family history of TB, and no close contacts have symptoms consistent with the disease.

Question 22-1

You determine:

A) He should have an interferon gamma release assay such as Quantiferon Gold or T-SPOT.
B) No further workup is needed since his TST is negative.
C) No further workup is needed because he received a BCG (bacillus Calmette-Guérin) vaccine.
D) He should receive 9 months of isoniazid for latent TB.

Discussion 22-1

The correct answer is "A." As discussed in a Question 21-1, induration of 10 mm in a patient from a country with high rates of TB is considered a positive purified protein derivative (PPD) result, and further investigation to determine if this patient has tuberculosis is warranted. TB is a common infection, affecting an estimated third of the world's population. The organisms associated with TB infection include mycobacteria such as *Mycobacterium tuberculosis, M. africanum, M. bovis,* and *M. canetti.* There is a distinction between infection and disease. Initial pulmonary infection is often asymptomatic and controlled by the body's cellular immune response. Disease occurs when symptoms develop or when the infection spreads beyond the lungs. Almost any organ system can be involved. Symptoms can be insidious or fulminant depending on multiple factors. In developing countries where TB is endemic and risk of severe disease is high, BCG vaccination is standard practice. BCG vaccine is a live attenuated strain of *M. bovis.* Vaccination does not prevent TB infection but does protect against severe disease such as meningitis and miliary pulmonary disease in young children. Evidence of BCG vaccine can often be seen as a scar on skin of the lateral surface of the shoulder. Diagnosis of TB can be problematic because no test has 100% sensitivity. Other than culture, no test has 100% specificity either. The PPD can cross-react with other mycobacteria, notably the BCG vaccine and common nontuberculous mycobacteria such as *M. avium-intracellulare* (MAI). Cross-reactivity resulting from BCG vaccination is most common within the first few years after vaccination. Unfortunately, that generally includes young children, who are the age group at highest risk of progression to severe disease if infection is acquired and not treated. Most positive PPD results in the setting of BCG vaccine are due to TB infection. A positive PPD result several years after receipt of BCG is unlikely to be due to cross-reactivity of BCG vaccine. Interferon gamma release assays (IGRAs) such as the Quantiferon gold and T-SPOT tests are able to determine production of interferon gamma when the patient's lymphocytes are exposed to TB antigens. The antigens are more specific to TB, though a few nontuberculous mycobacteria can still cross-react. Notably, MAI and BCG do not cause a positive IGRA result. For this reason many experts recommend IGRA testing when TB is suspected in a patient who received BCG vaccination. However reliability of IGRA in children younger than 5 years of age is unknown, and IGRA is not recommended by many experts for this age group. Progression of asymptomatic latent TB infection to active disease can occur at any time, but is most common during the first few years after initial infection. Treatment of latent TB with isoniazid monotherapy for 9 months usually prevents disease progression. TB disease requires prolonged multidrug treatment.

> **Helpful Tip**
> A negative PPD or interferon gamma release assay (IGRA) does not rule out TB. False-negative results can occur in young infants, overwhelming TB infection, immunosuppression, and some viral infections such as measles.

> **Helpful Tip**
> The terms *purified protein derivative* (PPD) and *tuberculin skin test* (TST) can be used interchangeably. Both PPD and TST are used in this chapter, mainly to confuse you. Because that is how the world works.

> ► **CASE 23**

A 3-year-old otherwise healthy girl develops irritability, headache, and myalgias shortly after waking up one morning. Later that day she develops fever to 40°C (104°F) and becomes lethargic. In the emergency department she is found to have meningismus, as well as purpuric lesions on her trunk and extremities with scattered petechiae. She has hypotension that requires fluid resuscitation and vasopressor support. She is intubated to protect her airway. Blood cultures obtained are positive and are growing gram-negative diplococci.

Question 23-1

Empiric antibiotics should include:
A) IV ceftriaxone.
B) IV cefepime.
C) IV ampicillin.
D) IV meropenem.
E) Any of the above.

Discussion 23-1

The correct answer is "A." This child has meningitis with purpura fulminans caused by *Neisseria meningitidis*. Onset can be mild, but progression to fulminant disease can be rapid, with a high rate of mortality even with rapid empiric antibiotic treatment. (See Figure 20–8.) *N. meningitidis* appears as a gram-negative diplococcus on Gram stain. Care should be taken

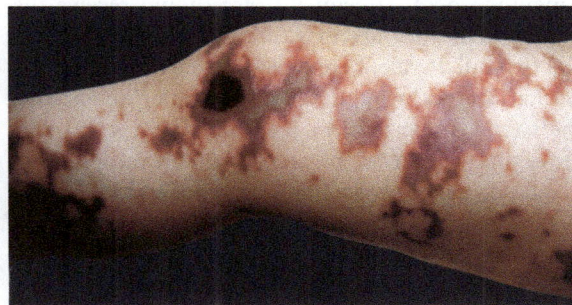

A   **B**

FIGURE 20–8. Acute Meningococcemia. FGC>This child has acute infection with *Neisseria meningitidis* with development of purpura fulminans and disseminated intravascular coagulation. He has petechiae, purpura, and areas of necrosis on his legs consistent with tissue infarction. (Reproduced with permission from Goldsmith LA, Katz SI, Gilchrest BA, Paller AS, Leffell DJ, Wolff K, eds. *Fitzpatrick's Dermatology in General Medicine.* 8th ed. New York, NY: McGraw-Hill Education; 2012, Fig. 180-1A-C.)

when antibiotic therapy is initiated based on Gram stain. Other organisms such as *Streptococcus pneumoniae* could cause meningitis and septicemia. An over-decolorized Gram stain with *S. pneumoniae* could appear as gram-negative diplococci to the untrained eye. A good rule of thumb is to use the Gram stain to broaden therapy rather than narrow it until the culture results are available. When the organism is not known, or if there is potential for resistant *S. pneumoniae* or methicillin-resistant *Staphylococcus aureus* (MRSA)-causing septicemia, vancomycin should be part of the empiric regimen. Ampicillin would not be recommended for empiric therapy because of potential for resistance of *Neisseria meningitidis* to this antibiotic. Cefepime or meropenem would be unnecessary as empiric therapy for *N. meningitidis*. Ceftriaxone (or cefotaxime) has good penetration into the CSF and is the empiric drug of choice for treating infections, including meningitis, caused by *N. meningitidis*.

The child's father tells you that she has always been healthy and that there are no immediate family members with any medical problems. He asks you how she could have gotten this illness and what could or should have been done to prevent it.

Question 23-2
You answer:
A) She should have received a meningococcal vaccine as part of her routine immunizations.
B) Her infection likely was acquired from an asymptomatic carrier of the bacteria.
C) Vaccination would most likely have prevented this infection.
D) She should be tested for complement deficiency.
E) She acquired the infection from a mosquito bite.

Discussion 23-2
The correct answer is "B." Asymptomatic nasopharyngeal carriage of *Neisseria meningitidis* can be common. Disease is thought to occur in nonimmune individuals within 24 to 48 hours after infection is acquired from a colonized person. Vaccination of healthy children for meningococcus is not recommended until 11 years of age. Certain high-risk children (eg, children with complement deficiency, asplenia, travel to an area with high meningococcal endemicity, etc) should receive the vaccine series earlier. The current vaccines approved for children include two quadrivalent conjugate vaccines, a quadrivalent polysaccharide vaccine, and a bivalent conjugate vaccine. None of the vaccines approved in the United States for children the age of this girl provide protection against serogroup B, which is a common cause of meningococcal infection in young children. A new vaccine was recently approved by the FDA for prevention of serotype B infection in children and young adults aged 10 to 25 years. No widespread recommendations have been made yet for its use. Children who are otherwise healthy with no family history of immunodeficiency who have a first episode of meningococcus without chronic meningococcal disease do not need evaluation for complement deficiency. *N. meningitis* is not an arthropod-borne infection.

The pediatric intensive care unit (PICU) nurse taking care of the patient is concerned about her exposure to this contagious, potentially fatal infection. She asks who needs postexposure prophylaxis (PEP).

Question 23-3
You respond:
A) The PICU nurse using droplet and standard precautions does not need PEP.
B) The family does not need PEP.
C) The physician who emergently intubated the patient without droplet precautions should receive PEP.
D) The phlebotomist who used standard precautions, but not droplet precautions, needs PEP.
E) Both C and D.

Discussion 23-3
The correct answer is "C." In addition to standard precautions, droplet precautions should be implemented during the first 24 hours of antibiotic therapy to prevent spread of infection. Close contacts such as household members and daycare contacts exposed to the patient within 7 days of the onset of symptoms should receive PEP. Health care providers with unprotected exposure to respiratory secretions (emergent intubation or suctioning without wearing a mask) prior to 24 hours of appropriate antibiotic therapy should also receive PEP. Antibiotics recommended for PEP include ciprofloxacin, rifampin, and ceftriaxone.

► CASE 24

A 4-year-old is brought to the emergency department in the summertime in Arkansas. His mother is concerned because he has been having fever for a couple of days and has been complaining of headache today. On exam he is tachycardic and you notice a petechial rash on his arms and legs that his mother had not noticed until now. Last week he went fishing with his father at a nearby lake.

Question 24-1
You decide you should:
A) Send serologies for tick-borne infections.
B) Start doxycycline immediately.
C) Start amoxicillin immediately.
D) Biopsy the rash to send for tick-borne infection PCR.
E) Ask the mother how she could have overlooked the rash.

Discussion 24-1
The correct answer is "B." This patient has Rocky Mountain spotted fever (RMSF), which is caused by the bacterium *Rickettsia rickettsii*. That is a fun one to say. RMSF occurs throughout North and South America, but most commonly occurs in several Southern states such as Arkansas. The bacteria are usually transmitted through bites of the American dog tick

or the Rocky Mountain wood tick. Cases usually occur in the spring or summer when the ticks are active but can occur year round where the weather is warm enough. Ticks probably need to feed for up to 6 hours before transmitting infection. Up to half of patients with RMSF do not remember a tick bite. Infection causes a vasculitis leading to fever, headache, rash, with the potential for severe multiorgan involvement if not treated. It is important to remember that early in the course of the illness, headache or rash may not be present, or may not occur at all. (Okay, maybe the mother wasn't unobservant.) The rash starts as red macules and papules, usually on the extremities, and can involve the palms and soles. It typically progresses centrally and often evolves into petechiae. The vasculitis can lead to third spacing and hyponatremia. Thrombocytopenia is often present. Serologies are usually negative early in the disease course; seroconversion occurs about 10 days after transmission, making serologic testing useless early in the disease when therapy should be administered. A biopsy of the rash can be obtained and sent for RMSF PCR, but usually this is unnecessary. Untreated, mortality is 20%. Doxycycline is the drug of choice regardless of age. The short course used to treat RMSF does not increase risk of tooth staining, and most other antibiotics generally are not effective in treating RMSF. (In this situation, I would take funny-colored teeth over the consequences of untreated infection.) Other infections such as ehrlichiosis and anaplasmosis can cause fevers and be transmitted by ticks. There can be significant overlap with areas in which RMSF is endemic. Doxycycline also will treat all three. Fever with petechiae can also be concerning for infection with *Neisseria meningitidis,* and empiric IV ceftriaxone is often started pending results of evaluation for this organism. A world without ticks would be nice.

> **Helpful Tip**
> When evaluating children with rashes, look for involvement of the palms or soles, or both. It narrows the differential a bit, including Rocky Mountain spotted fever, syphilis, hand foot-and-mouth disease, disseminated gonococcal infection, and vasculitis such as Kawasaki disease.

▶ CASE 25

A term female infant is born to a mother who did not receive any prenatal care. As you are evaluating the neonate for the first time a few hours later in the newborn nursery you notice that she is irritable and has extensive peeling of the skin, most prominently on her hands and feet, with some bullae present. Additionally, you notice cracking of the skin at the nares and the presence of white bloody nasal discharge. The neonate has some hepatosplenomegaly and cries when you palpate her legs. She is non–toxic appearing. You are concerned for infection.

Question 25-1

Her symptoms are most likely caused by:
A) CMV.
B) HSV.
C) Syphilis.
D) HIV.
E) None of the above.

Discussion 25-1

The correct answer is "C." This newborn has signs and symptoms consistent with congenital syphilis. Wash your hands and put on gloves! The secretions and rash are very contagious. (See Figure 20–9.) Contact precautions should be used until the neonate has received 24 hours of IV antibiotics. Are you really going to stop wearing gloves? CMV can cause hepatosplenomegaly but usually does not cause bullous lesions or musculoskeletal abnormalities. Congenital infection with HSV is exceptionally rare and an infant usually would be more toxic appearing with this degree of involvement. HIV is usually asymptomatic at birth. Syphilis is caused by the spirochete *Treponema pallidum.* It is a highly contagious STD. It can also be acquired by close, nonsexual contact with someone who has skin lesions due to secondary syphilis. In a healthy adult, adolescent, or child, primary infection involves a painless chancre at the site of inoculation, sometimes with associated painless lymphadenopathy. This lesion then resolves. Owing to the painless nature it is often missed. Secondary syphilis occurs weeks to months later and can manifest as fever, rash (including palms and soles), myalgias, and headaches. The rash is highly contagious. The infection then becomes latent during which time patients are asymptomatic but can still transmit infection through sexual activity. Many years later tertiary syphilis can manifest as granulomatous nodules called gummas. Other late manifestations include neurologic and cardiac abnormalities. All pregnant women should be screened for syphilis early in pregnancy so treatment can be given to prevent transmission to the infant. Mothers at high risk for syphilis should have repeat screening done just prior to or at delivery.

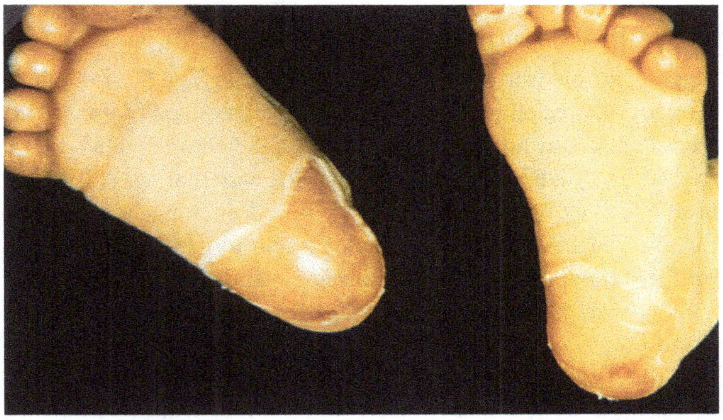

FIGURE 20–9. Congenital Syphilis. Newborns with congenital syphilis have peeling of the skin with bullae, especially on the hands and feet. Here the bullae have ruptured, leaving erosions on the feet of this newborn. (Reproduced with permission from Goldsmith LA, Katz SI, Gilchrest BA, Paller AS, Leffell DJ, Wolff K, eds. *Fitzpatrick's Dermatology in General Medicine.* 8th ed. New York, NY: McGraw-Hill Education; 2012, Fig. 200-32.)

Question 25-2

Which is NOT a manifestation of congenital syphilis?
A) Blueberry muffin rash.
B) Saber shins.
C) Snuffles.
D) Bullous rash.
E) Hepatomegaly.

Discussion 25-2

The correct answer is "A." Congenital syphilis has a broad spectrum of manifestations, but most infants are asymptomatic at birth. These children can develop symptoms later in life if the infection is not detected and treated. Infants with early symptomatic disease can present with hepatosplenomegaly, generalized lymphadenopathy, skin findings such as rash or peeling skin, rhinorrhea (ie, snuffles, which contain viable spirochetes), and limb pain resulting from osteochondritis and periostitis. The lungs, CNS, gastrointestinal tract, and eyes can be involved. Anemia, thrombocytopenia, leukopenia, or leukocytosis may be present on laboratory testing. Forty percent of untreated infants develop late manifestations of congenital syphilis. These include musculoskeletal abnormalities such as frontal bossing, saddle nose, high palatal arch, bowing of the tibiae (saber shins), painless swelling of the joints (Clutton joint); dental abnormalities, including small, widely spaced, notched permanent upper incisors (Hutchinson teeth) and mulberry molars; interstitial keratitis (common); sensorineural hearing loss; fissures and scars around the mouth called rhagades; gummas; and CNS manifestations, including tabes dorsalis and cranial nerve deafness.

Question 25-3

The following confirms the diagnosis of syphilis in an infant:
A) Positive rapid plasma reagin (RPR) in the newborn.
B) Positive RPR in the newborn's mother.
C) Positive fluorescent treponemal antibody absorption (FTA-ABS) test in the newborn.
D) Positive venereal disease research laboratory (VDRL) test in the newborn.
E) None of the above.

Discussion 25-3

The correct answer is "E." Syphilis testing can be a bit difficult to interpret, especially in a newborn. Testing is usually done with treponemal and nontreponemal testing. Screening tests such as the RPR or VDRL are considered nontreponemal tests. They are antibody tests but can cross-react with other spirochetes. Other disease processes (certain types of pneumonia, systemic lupus erythematous) can cause inflammation and false-positive nontreponemal test results. A false-negative nontreponemal test can occur due to the prozone phenomenon, when levels are so high that the assay cannot detect it properly. This can be overcome by diluting the specimen. VDRL or RPR titer will increase with infection and decrease and disappear with treatment and resolution of infection and are used to follow response to therapy. Treponemal tests are more syphilis-specific antibody tests. They become positive with infection and often remain so for life despite treatment. Examples include the FTA-ABS and MHA-TP

(microhemagglutination assay for *Treponema pallidum* antibodies). Many labs are starting to use syphilis IgG/IgM screening EIA in mothers because of cost and technical benefits. Other tests such as PCR or darkfield microscopy are used less often. The typical algorithm for diagnosing syphilis in an older child or adult includes a screening nontreponemal test such as RPR confirmed by a treponemal test such as FTA-ABS. Infants may have positive treponemal or nontreponemal tests as a result of active infection or transplacental passage of maternal antibody. If a mother has a positive nontreponemal and treponemal test concerning for syphilis, then the diagnosis of syphilis should be considered in the infant, even if the infant is asymptomatic. Workup depends on whether the mother was treated before delivery, the antibiotic used, and maternal response to therapy. An asymptomatic infant born to a mother treated for syphilis before pregnancy with negative maternal RPR during pregnancy does not need further evaluation or therapy. If the mother was treated appropriately during pregnancy, then infant and maternal RPR are compared. If the asymptomatic infant's RPR is not fourfold higher than the mother's RPR, then no further workup is needed (probably mom's antibody is just circulating), but an intramuscular (IM) dose of penicillin is given (just in case). Inadequately treated maternal infection, symptomatic infants, or infants with RPR fourfold higher than maternal RPR should be evaluated and therapy initiated with IV penicillin. Evaluation includes CBC with differential, long bone X-rays, and lumbar puncture to evaluate CSF indices and VDRL. Response to therapy should be evaluated over time by following RPR titer (or VDRL, if that was used—just pick one and stick with it so you are comparing apples to apples) and symptoms.

▶ CASE 26

A 4-month-old infant presents to clinic with a history of constipation and poor feeding. On exam, he looks well and is afebrile. His cardiopulmonary exam is normal. His suck is terrible and he does not gag despite sticking tongue depressors into the posterior oropharynx. Oddly, he cannot pick up his head and barely moves his arms. His arms are floppy without reflexes. Everything below that level is neurologically normal.

Question 26-1

Which is true regarding his disease?
A) Infantile disease results from ingestion of preformed toxin.
B) Hypotonia is progressive and ascends caudally to cranially.
C) Respiratory failure may occur.
D) Eating home-canned foods is a cause of this disease.
E) No treatment is available.

Discussion 26-1

The correct answer is "C." Think botulism in the setting of acute onset of bilateral cranial nerve palsies, symmetric descending weakness, and lack of fever. Infantile botulism results from ingestion of *Clostridium botulinum* spores, which become the bacteria, colonize the gastrointestinal tract, and produce a neurotoxin that blocks presynaptic acetylcholine transmission. Smooth muscle, skeletal muscle, and the autonomic systems are affected. Sources of bacteria include ingestion of raw honey, home-canned foods, and environmental dust containing spores. Initial presentation is constipation and poor suck followed by cranial nerve palsies (absent gag, fatigable pupillary response, ptosis, poor suck) and descending cranial-to-caudal hypotonia. Typically, children and adults get sick by ingesting, inhaling, or acquiring the preformed toxin (eg, eating contaminated home-canned foods, infected wounds with *C. botulinum*, or iatrogenic overdose of injectable toxin). Diagnosis is made based on clinical syndrome, isolation of the organism, and detection of toxin which can take weeks. If the diagnosis is suspected, then antitoxin should be given pending results of testing. Antibiotics should not be given to infants as lysis of the bacteria living in the gut will release more toxin to be absorbed. The diaphragm may be affected, causing respiratory failure, so monitor respiratory status closely!

> ### Helpful Tip
> Tetanus and botulism both produce neurotoxins. Botulism affects the peripheral nervous system, causing hypotonia and muscle paralysis. Tetanus affects the central nervous system, causing muscles spasms and rigidity.

► CASE 27

A local family has just returned from a country in sub-Saharan Africa, where they adopted a 3-year-old boy. The orphanage had little documentation about the boy, and his family history is unknown. He did receive some vaccines locally and the family has that documentation with them at today's visit. The boy has a history of malaria and chickenpox in the past but otherwise has been healthy while living at the orphanage.

Question 27-1

As part of your evaluation you decide that:
A) HIV testing should be done.
B) A TST should be placed if not already done.
C) The vaccines will need to be repeated using U.S. vaccines.
D) Both A and B.
E) All of the above.

Discussion 27-1

The correct answer is "D." Children adopted internationally usually undergo an evaluation locally as required by law. However this usually is not an extensive evaluation, so adoptive parents of these children should establish care with a provider shortly upon arrival to the United States to screen for disease as well as update the child's vaccinations. It is important to remember that each country of origin is different with regard to accessibility to prenatal care, screening, treatment, and disease prevention.

TABLE 20–3 DIAGNOSTIC TESTING FOR NEWLY ADOPTED INTERNATIONAL CHILDREN

HIV serologic testing

Syphilis serologic testing

Hepatitis B surface antigen

Hepatitis C antibody

Tuberculin skin test (TST) (or interferon gamma release assay [IGRA] if age appropriate)

Stool ova and parasite testing:
- Obtain 3 samples
- Request *Giardia* and *Cryptosporidium* testing

Stool bacteria culture (if diarrhea present)

CBC with differential

Hemoglobinopathy screening for at risk ethnicities

Lead level

Rickets screening (calcium, phosphorus, alkaline phosphatase, vitamin D level)

Vaccine quality control is fairly reliable in countries outside the United States. Generally vaccines can be accepted as valid if there is written documentation that shows the vaccines were given at the appropriate age and intervals as recommended by the Advisory Committee on Immunizations Practices (ACIP) and World Health Organization (WHO). All international adoptees should have diagnostic testing. Testing completed outside of the United States should be repeated. (See Table 20–3.) A CBC with differential will assess for anemia as well as eosinophilia, which could be indicative of parasitic disease. If the child has eosinophilia and a stool ova and parasite test is negative, serologies for *Strongyloides* and *Schistosoma* (if from an endemic country) should be obtained. Children adopted from countries with *Trypanosoma cruzi* or lymphatic filariasis should be tested for those infections, as well.

► CASE 28

A 15-year-old unimmunized male adolescent presents to clinic with a 5-day history of fever. He began with fever and myalgia and developed some tender swelling at the left angle of his jaw. Over the next day or two he developed similar painful swelling on the other side.

Question 28-1

You discuss with the patient that the most common potentially serious complication of this infection is:
A) Orchitis with the risk of possible infertility.
B) Meningitis.
C) Pancreatitis.
D) Myocarditis.
E) None, other than looking like a chipmunk from his swollen glands.

C) The patient with mumps should not return to school for 5 days after onset of symptoms.

D) The patient with mumps has a high risk of getting mumps again.

E) The patient should not live in the same house as his immunosuppressed sibling.

Discussion 28-2

The correct answer is "C." As previously noted, mumps is spread by respiratory secretions. Droplet precautions should be used with hospitalized patients while deemed contagious. Patients should not return to school until 5 days after onset of symptoms, at which time they are no longer considered contagious. Postexposure IVIG does not prevent infection or ameliorate symptoms once infection occurs. The MMR vaccine is a live virus vaccine recommended for all nonimmune persons aged 12 months and older (though can be given at an earlier age in outbreak situations) who do not have a contraindication to the vaccine (such as immunocompromising illness). Though postexposure immunization will not prevent infection, it should be given to all nonimmunocompromised family members for prevention of future infection with mumps should they not become infected now, and will also provide immunity to measles and rubella. There is no contraindication to vaccinating immunocompetent family members with MMR if there is a household member with an immunocompromising condition. Use this opportunity to point out why vaccines are important! Immunity acquired is usually lifelong, and reinfection is incredibly rare. Most recurrences of parotid swelling are due to infection with another virus such as EBV, CMV, enteroviruses, influenza, parainfluenza, and adenovirus, which can cause clinical syndromes similar to mumps. Keeping the patient away from immunocompromised individuals is not a bad idea, but removing one or the other from the household can be difficult and likely not possible in many cases. In addition, mumps is quite contagious several days before onset of parotid swelling, so the bulk of exposure has already occurred.

► CASE 29

A 2-year-old girl presents to your clinic in southern Arizona in January with a 3-day history of fever to 39°C (102.2°F), runny nose, cough, congestion, and myalgias. She is otherwise healthy and is up to date on all her immunizations. In December she traveled to visit family members in Indiana. She is febrile with some mild tachycardia. Her oxygen saturation is normal. She is mildly tachypneic without retractions. She is well perfused, and is non-toxic appearing. On lung exam, you hear crackles and wheezes. Her chest X-ray shows some increased perihilar haziness and possible interstitial infiltrates.

Question 29-1

The most likely explanation for her illness is infection with:

A) *Coccidioides immitis/posadasii.*

B) *Histoplasma capsulatum.*

C) *Mycoplasma pneumoniae.*

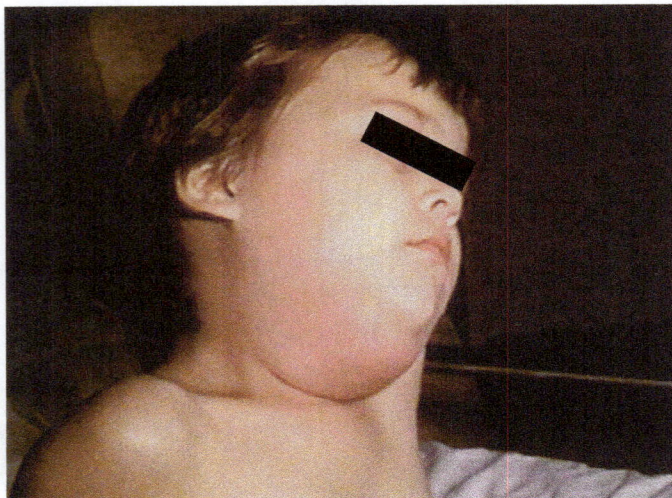

FIGURE 20–10. Mumps. This patient with mumps has classic unilateral parotid gland swelling. (Reproduced with permission from Centers for Disease Control and Prevention.)

Discussion 28-1

The correct answer is "A." This patient has mumps, which is caused by a paramyxovirus. It is highly contagious among unimmunized patients and is spread by respiratory secretions. Symptoms usually include fever and upper respiratory symptoms for several days, with unilateral painful swelling of the parotid gland that often becomes bilateral during the course of illness. (See Figure 20–10.) Infection is self-limiting and patients usually improve within several days after onset of symptoms. Potentially serious complications may occur and include orchitis, meningitis or encephalitis, pancreatitis, and myocarditis. Of these, orchitis is the most common complication, occurring in up to 35% of male adolescents and young adults. Infection can affect most other organ systems causing hepatitis, glomerulonephritis, arthritis, and sensorineural hearing loss. Some patients with mumps are asymptomatic or only have mild upper respiratory symptoms and never develop parotid gland swelling. Acute and convalescent mumps IgG and IgM (antibody titers) can be obtained to help make the diagnosis. These can be a bit difficult to interpret if the patient was previously immunized. Attack rate among immunized individuals is much less when compared to those who are unimmunized. Virus can be detected by PCR from CSF, urine, and swabs of the buccal mucosa at the Stensen duct after parotid massage.

Further discussion reveals that the boy has several other siblings at home aged 4 to 16 years, one of whom has cancer and is receiving chemotherapy.

Question 28-2

Upon learning that none of the family members has been immunized, you tell the parents:

A) All the family members should receive the measles, mumps, and rubella (MMR) vaccine.

B) All the family members should receive intravenous immunoglobulin (IVIG).

D) A respiratory virus.
E) *Streptococcus pneumoniae.*

Discussion 29-1

The correct answer is "D." This child has signs and symptoms of pneumonia. Common things are common, so while the other organisms are possible, the most common cause of pneumonia in a toddler is a respiratory virus such as rhinovirus, coronavirus, influenza, human metapneumovirus, and so on. Coccidioidomycosis is caused by a dimorphic fungus endemic to the southwestern United States. Infection is caused by inhalation of spores and typically causes a self-limiting pneumonia. It is one of the more common causes of community-acquired pneumonia in adults living in endemic areas and is often underrecognized. It can cause extrapulmonary infection, which can affect just about any organ system including bone and CNS. Diagnosis is made with serology, biopsy, and culture when needed. Histoplasma is caused by a dimorphic fungus that is present mostly in the midwestern United States. It also can cause a self-limited pulmonary infection. Extrapulmonary infection is possible as well, although bone infection is unusual. Diagnosis is made using serology, blood, and urine antigen as well as biopsy and culture when needed. Mycoplasma usually causes infection in school-aged children, but there is evidence that it can cause infection in younger children as well. Symptoms of fever, cough, and wheezing are common and can last for weeks. Infection is self-limiting but symptoms are often improved with azithromycin. Mycoplasma can also cause other infections such as encephalitis, hepatitis, pharyngitis, conjunctivitis, lymphadenitis, and so on. It is associated with Stevens-Johnson syndrome. Diagnosis is made using serology and PCR, but interpretation of these tests can be difficult as IgM can be positive for months, and bacteria can be shed in the oropharynx for prolonged periods despite resolution of symptoms.

Helpful Tip
Upper and lower airway infections caused by respiratory viruses such as rhinovirus, respiratory syncytial virus (RSV), human metapneumovirus (hMPV), influenza, and parainfluenza virus often have symptoms that overlap and are indistinguishable from one another. For the majority, treatment is supportive.

▶ CASE 30

A 6-year-old fully immunized, otherwise healthy boy born in the United States has just returned from visiting his extended family in sub-Saharan Africa. He was there for 3 weeks and did not receive any destination-specific pretravel vaccinations or take any medications while on his trip. He developed fever 2 days before returning to the United States and arrived home last night. He has some diarrhea, headache, and has not been drinking very well. His mother has noticed that his eyes are more yellow than usual. His temperature is 40°C (104°F), heart rate 140 bpm, and blood pressure 60/30 mm Hg. He is awake, but appears very tired. He has

scleral icterus, generalized pallor, dry mucous membranes, and splenomegaly on exam. His CBC shows a hemoglobin of 3.5 g/dL with a platelet count of 80,000/mm³. His glucose is 30 mg/dL and creatinine is 3 mg/dL. You are concerned about malaria and order a blood smear, which shows 12% of red blood cells infected with the parasite. You are concerned about severe infection and admit him to start IV antimalarial medications.

Question 30-1

Which of his signs, symptoms, or laboratory findings are indicative of severe malaria?
A) Glucose of 30 mg/dL.
B) Creatinine of 3 g/dL.
C) Hemoglobin of 3.5 g/dL.
D) All of the above.
E) Isn't it enough to say he looks like a ghost with yellow eyes?

Discussion 30-1

The correct answer is "D." Malaria is a parasitic disease transmitted by the *Anopheles* mosquito, which lives in tropical areas. Species of malaria that infect humans include *Plasmodium falciparum, P. ovale, P. vivax, P. knowlesi,* and *P. malariae.* None of these organisms are endemic in the United States. Despite rare occurrence of malaria in the United States, a basic understanding of the disease is important because it can be life threatening in travelers returning home if it is not quickly recognized and treated. This is particularly true with *P. falciparum* as it can have a rapidly progressive course. The other species of parasites causing malaria usually have a less severe course. Mild infections can often be treated with oral therapy, but severe symptoms require parenteral therapy and close monitoring and management of complications. Findings of severe malaria include hypoglycemia, hypotension, obtundation, seizures, severe anemia, high parasitemia (> 5%), acute renal failure, hemoglobinuria, metabolic acidosis, coagulopathy, and acute respiratory distress syndrome. Remember when ordering peripheral blood smears to ask for thick and thin. If available, rapid malaria testing can also be useful when awaiting thick and thin blood smears. Travelers to countries with malaria should take chemoprophylaxis, use insecticides containing DEET, and hang mosquito netting treated with permethrin over their bed at night.

Helpful Tip
In malaria, fevers may occur every 48 to 72 hours corresponding to lysis of infected red blood cells spilling the parasite into the bloodstream. Cyclical fevers are a hallmark of malaria, and different timing often corresponds to different species of the parasite.

▶ CASE 31

A 4-year-old girl is brought to the emergency department in the summer time with a complaint of diarrhea lasting several days. She initially had loose stools several times a day, then developed crampy abdominal pain with some low-grade fevers. Her stools continue to be loose, but she now has blood and mucous in her stool. She lives in Iowa and has not traveled outside the state. She has no known animal exposures and has not been camping or swimming in rivers or lakes. She did visit a water park recently. She attends daycare, but her mother is not aware of any other children with similar symptoms.

Question 31-1

To make the appropriate diagnosis you should test for:
A) *Salmonella.*
B) *Shigella.*
C) *Giardia.*
D) *Cryptosporidium.*
E) *Entamoeba histolytica.*
F) Both A and B.
G) Options A, B, and E.
H) All of the above.

Discussion 31-1

The correct answer is "F." Did you notice the extra answer options? Just making sure you are paying attention. This child has bloody diarrhea and fevers consistent with dysentery. Typical bacteria causing bloody diarrhea include *Salmonella, Shigella, Campylobacter, Yersinia,* and enterohemorrhagic *E. coli* (EHEC). Bloody stools can also be seen with *Clostridium difficile,* which is typically associated with prior antibiotic use. *Entamoeba histolytica* can cause dysentery as well. It is rarely seen in the United States without a history of travel to an endemic area or contact with a returning traveler. Giardiasis is caused by the parasite *Giardia lamblia.* Symptoms include watery diarrhea with flatulence and cramping, but not bloody diarrhea. Transmission is fecal-oral and outbreaks have occurred in daycare settings. It can also be acquired by drinking untreated water. *Cryptosporidium* is a parasite that also is transmitted by the fecal-oral route. It is commonly associated with water exposure, and outbreaks have known to occur at water parks. It can be resistant to usual chlorination and filtration, making it a difficult organism to prevent and eradicate. Symptoms include watery diarrhea. Bloody diarrhea is not seen. Infection is usually self-limiting, except in immunocompromised patients.

> **Helpful Tip**
> Children with infectious diarrhea should not swim for 2 weeks after symptoms resolve. Never drink pool water! Think of infant diapers as tea bags for pool water.

The patient's stool culture is positive for *Salmonella enteritidis.* Her blood culture is negative. She continues to have fevers, but is nontoxic. She has several loose, bloody stools a day but is not dehydrated. Her mother asks if people infected with *Salmonella* get antibiotics and if her daughter should be treated.

Question 31-2

You tell her:
A) Use of antibiotics prolongs the carrier state.
B) Antibiotics are generally recommended in children younger than 1 year old.
C) Treatment with antibiotics usually improves symptoms.
D) All of the above.
E) None of the above.

Discussion 31-2

The correct answer is "A." Nontyphoidal *Salmonella* is a common cause of bloody diarrhea in the United States that is spread by fecal-oral transmission. It is associated with contaminated poultry, beef, and dairy products, but outbreaks have also occurred from contaminated fruits and vegetables. Disease is usually self-limiting and treatment in low-risk patients without invasive infection is not recommended because antibiotics do not decrease symptoms and can prolong the carrier state. Patients younger than 3 months old and those who have hemoglobinopathies, chronic gastrointestinal tract abnormalities, HIV, or an immunocompromised state are at risk for invasive infection. In these patients treatment is warranted to prevent invasive infection. Other bacterial causes of bloody diarrhea may or may not require antibiotic therapy. In the case of EHEC caused by Shiga toxin–producing *E. coli,* there is a risk of precipitating hemolytic uremic syndrome (HUS) with the use of antibiotics. Some meta-analyses suggest this may not be the case, but it is still controversial and antibiotics are not recommended by most experts. *Shigella* infection often is self-limited. Treatment for uncomplicated infection caused by *Shigella* may be beneficial as it can hasten symptom improvement and decrease stool shedding, which is important since transmission can occur with ingestion of only a few organisms. Uncomplicated infections with *Yersinia* and *Campylobacter* are usually self-limited, but treatment with antibiotics may improve symptoms and decrease shedding of bacteria in the stool.

> **Helpful Tip**
> If a child becomes pale or has petechiae 5 to 10 days after having bloody diarrhea, think about HUS—which produces anemia, thrombocytopenia, and acute kidney injury. It is a known complication of infection with Shiga toxin–producing EHEC or *Shigella.* Progression to renal failure requiring dialysis may occur.

⏳ QUICK QUIZ

Which of the following is FALSE?
A) *E. coli* is acquired from eating raw hamburger.
B) *Campylobacter* is acquired from drinking fresh water, such as when camping.
C) *Salmonella* is acquired from undercooked chicken.
D) Unpasteurized milk tastes sour but is safe to drink.
E) *Salmonella* is acquired from infected reptiles and amphibians.

Discussion

The correct answer is "D." This one was too easy. Unpasteurized or raw milk and dairy products can contain and cause infection with *Campylobacter*, Shiga toxin-producing *E. coli*, *Salmonella*, *Yersinia*, *Listeria*, and other bacteria. These are all stool pathogens and can be found in substances that can be contaminated with stool. Do not get hung up on specific animals because outbreaks caused by many of these organisms are associated with beef, chicken, vegetables, and nut processing, as well as other sources. Hamburger is particularly problematic as the bacteria become mixed throughout the meat during the process of making it. That's why a rare burger is never a good thing!

> **Helpful Tip**
> Postinfectious complications of *Campylobacter jejuni* include Guillain-Barré syndrome and reactive arthritis.

> **Helpful Tip**
> The gut is full of fun bacteria that are just fine when they stay put, but problematic when on the loose. *Enterococcus* is one of these. It likes to cause urinary tract infection (one of the common causes of nitrite-negative urinary tract infection), but can infect other areas of the body as well, especially if there are other contributors leading to breakdown of natural barriers such as indwelling central catheters, bed sores, surgery, and so on. Finding enterococci in a stool culture is not worrisome. Finding it on the skin is not terribly surprising, especially if that skin was close to the anus (and especially in a diapered child, whose stool can easily migrate anywhere). Finding it in blood or another sterile site is not a good thing.

► CASE 32

As Fall starts a father of a 7-month-old girl is asking you about RSV and prophylaxis with palivizumab (Synagis). His daughter was born at 30 weeks' gestational age and was in the neonatal intensive care unit (NICU) for 2 months because of feeding difficulty and chronic lung disease requiring oxygen therapy. She is doing well today and requires a quarter liter of oxygen via nasal cannula.

Question 32-1

Regarding RSV and prophylaxis you tell him:
A) Palivizumab prevents infection with RSV.
B) Palivizumab decreases RSV-related mortality.
C) Palivizumab is recommended for his child.
D) Palivizumab is inexpensive.
E) All of the above.

Discussion 32-1

The correct answer is "C." RSV is a common cause of upper and lower respiratory infection in infants and children. Infants are at particular risk for severe disease requiring hospitalization and intervention. Infection is self-limiting and treatment is generally supportive in immunocompetent individuals. Premature infants and infants with chronic lung disease, immunodeficiency, and hemodynamically significant congenital heart disease have a higher risk of severe infection. Palivizumab is a monoclonal anti-RSV antibody. It is quite expensive. Prophylaxis with palivizumab has been shown to decrease hospitalization rates for infants infected with RSV and also has been shown to decrease length of stay in those hospitalized for RSV infection. It is important to remember that palivizumab does not decrease RSV-related mortality rates and does not prevent RSV infection. At-risk patients receive monthly doses for 5 months during the RSV season. Prophylaxis does not prevent infection and does not decrease mortality. Palivizumab also is not useful to treat active infection. Infants born before 29 weeks' gestational age should receive palivizumab if they are younger than 12 months old at the start of RSV season. Older gestational age infants should receive prophylaxis if they have chronic lung disease or hemodynamically significant congenital heart disease. Immunocompromised infants may benefit from prophylaxis as well. New AAP guidelines published in 2015 indicate that if an infant receiving palivizumab is hospitalized for RSV, monthly prophylaxis should be stopped (again, it is effective in preventing hospitalization and decreasing stay, so no reason to continue now).

► CASE 33

An otherwise heathy, fully immunized 4-year-old girl presents with increased urinary frequency, dysuria, fever, and flank tenderness. She has vomited many times in the last 24 hours and appears dehydrated. Urinalysis shows 30 white blood cells per high-power field (WBCs/hpf) and with positive nitrite. You suspect pyelonephritis and start her on empiric ceftriaxone based on your knowledge of the antimicrobial susceptibilities of local urinary pathogens. The next day she is feeling a bit better but still has emesis and fever. Her urine culture is growing *E.coli* susceptible to ampicillin, cefazolin, ceftriaxone, meropenem, ciprofloxacin, and gentamicin. Her blood culture is negative and she shows no signs of other infection at this time. Because she is not tolerating oral intake she requires ongoing IV therapy.

Question 33-1

Her therapy should be continued with:
A) Ampicillin.
B) Cefazolin.
C) Ceftriaxone.
D) Meropenem.
E) Ciprofloxacin.
F) Gentamicin.

Discussion 33-1

The correct answer is "A." Empiric antibiotic therapy should be guided by the type of illness, local rate of antibiotic resistance, and location of infection. Once the organism is identified and susceptibilities are available the antibiotic regimen should be tailored to provide the narrowest coverage possible for the organism provided that antibiotic is safe and effective for the type of infection it is being used to treat. Unnecessary use of antibiotics has led to increasing rates of resistant organisms and superinfection. Areas with careful use of antibiotics tend to have lower rates of infection with drug-resistant bacteria such as vancomycin-resistant enterococci (VRE) and methicillin-resistant *Staphylococcus aureus* (MRSA). Of the choices of antibiotics in the question, ampicillin has the narrowest range of antibacterial activity, has a good side effect profile, and is effective in treating urinary tract infections. Several factors must be considered when choosing an antimicrobial regimen. Though a narrower spectrum drug may be available, it may not be appropriate to treat certain types of infection. For example, cefazolin does not cross the blood-brain barrier well and should not be used to treat meningitis caused by *E. coli* even if it is susceptible in vitro. Other factors to consider include the frequency of administration and the possibility of developing resistance to the antibiotic during the course of therapy.

► CASE 34

A 6-year-old boy with acute lymphoblastic leukemia (ALL) undergoing induction chemotherapy presents with fever and dyspnea. He began with a mild cough 2 weeks ago that has worsened since then. He developed fevers yesterday and now is having difficulty breathing. He has not been compliant with his home medication regimen. He appears acutely ill and has a temperature of 38.7°C (101.6°F), heart rate of 120 bpm, and respirations of 40 breaths per minute with oxygen saturation of 82% on room air. He is tachypneic, has intercostal retractions, and is unable to speak in full sentences. No crackles or wheezes are heard on pulmonary auscultation. The remainder of his exam is unremarkable. His white blood cell count is 2.4 K/mm³, hemoglobin 8 g/dL, and platelets 80 K/mm³. His absolute neutrophil count (ANC) is 900/mm³. PaO_2 is 60 mm Hg. Chest X-ray shows diffuse bilateral ground glass opacities. Silver stain of induced sputum shows small round organisms.

Question 34-1

You determine:

A) His infection could have been prevented with an antibiotic.
B) He may benefit from steroids.
C) He should be started on an IV antibiotic right away.
D) He should be placed in standard precautions.
E) All of the above.

Discussion 34-1

The correct answer is "D." This patient has pneumonia caused by *Pneumocystis jiroveci* (formerly known as *Pneumocystis carinii*).

It was initially thought to be a protozoan, but further research has shown it is more closely related to fungi. Asymptomatic infection is common in immunocompetent hosts, but active disease generally only presents in patients with a compromised immune system. Symptoms can range from rapid, fulminant onset to insidious, progressive disease. Often symptoms begin as mild cough and progress to more severe symptoms. Fever can be present and hypoxia often develops if the infection is untreated. Auscultation is often normal, with rhonchi and wheezing developing after the patient begins improving. Immunocompromised patients at risk should be on a regimen that prevents pneumocystis. Trimethoprim-sulfamethoxazole is usually the drug of choice for prophylaxis. Breakthrough infection on prophylaxis can occasionally occur, especially if the patient is not compliant with the prophylactic regimen. First-line therapy for pneumocystis pneumonia is usually IV trimethoprim-sulfamethoxazole. Severe disease may be caused by inflammation, and steroids are often recommended in severe disease when the PaO_2 is less than 70 mm Hg or the A-a gradient is less than 35 mm Hg. Diagnosis is made by finding the organism, which appears as a small dark cyst on silver stain. Induced sputum can be helpful in making the diagnosis, but often more invasive procedures such as bronchoscopy and occasionally biopsy are necessary as sputum staining is not very sensitive. Patients hospitalized with pneumocystis pneumonia should have standard precautions in place. Not sharing a room with another immunocompromised patient is reasonable.

► CASE 35

A 7-year-old girl is complaining that her butt itches. Her mother is mortified that the child won't stop scratching her bottom. The girl is having trouble sleeping at night. On exam she has perianal excoriations but is otherwise normal.

Question 35-1

You suspect:

A) Enterobiasis.
B) Ascariasis.
C) *Necator americanus.*
D) Toxocariasis.
E) Cysticercosis.

Discussion 35-1

The correct answer is "A." All of the listed options are parasitic infections with some type of worm. We become infected after swallowing the eggs brought to our mouths by our dirty hands. This child has pinworms, or enterobiasis. School-aged children are most commonly affected and present with perianal itching predominately at night. Eggs are deposited on the perianal skin. Eggs get under the fingernails when the child scratches the area. The fingers transfer the eggs to the mouth. After ingestion, the eggs hatch into worms. The tape test involves pressing a piece of tape on the skin around the anus then looking at the tape under a microscope to see if eggs are present. The worms come out of the anus at night to lay eggs, so have the parent look for worms in the middle of the night! A dose of albendazole or mebendazole is given at diagnosis followed by a repeat dose 2 weeks later. Remember to treat the family members and clean the sheets and bedding. Ascariasis is caused by *Ascaris lumbricoides* (giant round worm). The worms can migrate to the lungs or form a bolus within the intestine, causing obstruction. *Necator americanus* is a hookworm infection that can cause infection by penetrating the skin. Toxocariasis is transmitted from dog or cat feces. It causes visceral larva migrans and ocular larva migrans. Cysticercosis is caused by a pork tapeworm, *Taenia solium*, which is acquired from eating infected pork. Cysts can accumulate in any human tissue and frequently affect the CNS (neurocysticercosis).

> **Helpful Tip**
>
> Infected animal bite wounds are often due to bacterial oral flora of the animal. Dogs and cats often have *Pasteurella* spp. Infection usually occurs within a day of the bite. Other invasive infections, such as bacteremia, meningitis, and osteomyelitis, can occur but are rare. Sometimes infection occurs without traumatic contact with animals (eg, getting licked in the face). *Pasteurella* spp can produce beta-lactamases. Amoxicillin-clavulanate is often used as postbite prophylaxis or as treatment of mild wound infection as it has good activity against animal oral flora, including *Pasteurella* spp.

▶ CASE 36

Question 36-1

Which of the following statements about viral rashes is correct?

A) The vesicular rash in chickenpox is typically more prominent on the extremities than on the trunk.
B) Rubella rash starts caudally and progresses cranially.
C) The measles rash starts cranially and progresses caudally.
D) Parvovirus is likely to be transmitted when rash is present on the face.
E) Initial human herpesvirus 6 infection and associated rash most commonly occur in adolescents.
F) Adenovirus does not cause rash.
G) Enteroviruses do not cause vesicular rashes.
H) None of the above.

Discussion 36-1

The correct answer is "C." Warning this answer is long but there are eight response choices. Varicella is caused by the varicella zoster virus. It is extremely contagious and is spread by the airborne route. Its transmission can occur from 2 days prior to onset of rash up until the lesions are crusted over. The vesicular rash typically starts cranially and progresses caudally. Vesicles sit on an erythematous base frequently described as "dew drops on a rose petal." It usually involves the trunk much more than the

extremities. The hallmark of varicella is that the lesions occur in crops, so a couple of days into the rash lesions of varying stages will be seen. This is in contrast to smallpox, where the lesions are all in the same stage and tend to be more prominent on the extremities. Pneumonia, hepatitis, CNS disease, and bacterial superinfection are potential complications. Incomplete varicella can occur in immunized individuals, manifesting as papules and sometimes vesicles, but usually these are few in number and associated symptoms are mild or absent. Two doses of varicella zoster vaccine are extremely effective in preventing mild and severe chickenpox and have been shown to decrease rates of zoster. Acyclovir can be used to treat immunocompromised patients or those at risk for more severe infection (adults and adolescents). Rubella is caused by the rubella virus. Subclinical infection is common, but fever, lymphadenopathy, and rash are the typical presentation of the illness. The rash is maculopapular, starts on the face, and then progresses caudally to become generalized. It can take many forms and can be confused with acne, scarlet fever, and measles. The rash starts to fade by 2 to 3 days. Rubella is contagious from a few days prior to a week after onset of the rash and is spread by droplet route. Complications include arthritis, encephalitis, thrombocytopenia, and congenital infection. It is effectively prevented by two vaccine doses, which has led to its eradication in North and South America (though imported cases still occur). Measles is caused by rubeola virus. Fever and rash are often preceded by Koplik spots in the mouth, although these are often missed as they are asymptomatic at that time. (See Figure 20–11.) The classic symptoms are cough, coryza, and conjunctivitis. The rash starts cranially and moves caudally as well. (See Figure 20–12.) Measles is contagious 4 days prior to 4 days after onset of rash and is spread by the airborne route. Complications include orchitis, encephalitis, pneumonia, and the dreaded, progressive fatal syndrome of subacute sclerosing panencephalitis, which occurs years after infection. Two doses of vaccine are almost 100% effective, but the disease is becoming more common due to unwarranted fear of vaccination. Treatment is supportive. Vitamin A decreases morbidity and mortality in patients from developing countries.

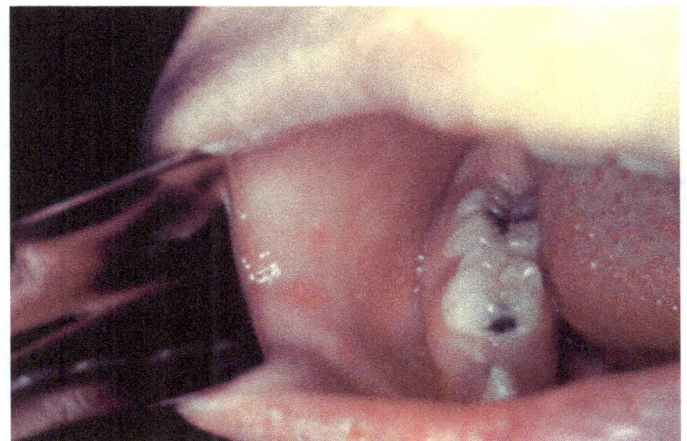

FIGURE 20–11. Koplik spots are white lesions with a surrounding ring of erythema on the buccal mucosa seen in measles. (Reproduced with permission from Centers for Disease Control and Prevention.)

FIGURE 20–12. Measles presents with fever, cough, coryza, and conjunctivitis. Look for an ill-appearing child with a morbilliform rash that rapidly spreads from the head down. (Reproduced with permission from Goldsmith LA, Katz SI, Gilchrest BA, Paller AS, Leffell DJ, Wolff K, eds. *Fitzpatrick's Dermatology in General Medicine*. 8th ed. New York, NY: McGraw-Hill Education; 2012, Fig. 192-3.1A&B.)

Parvovirus B19 causes the classic erythema infectiosum or fifth disease (diseases 1 to 4 are measles, scarlet fever, rubella, and Dukes disease). It can be asymptomatic or have a mild febrile prodrome. The rash on the face ("slapped cheek" appearance) usually occurs later when the patient is no longer contagious. (See Figure 20–13.) A lacy reticular rash can occur on the trunk

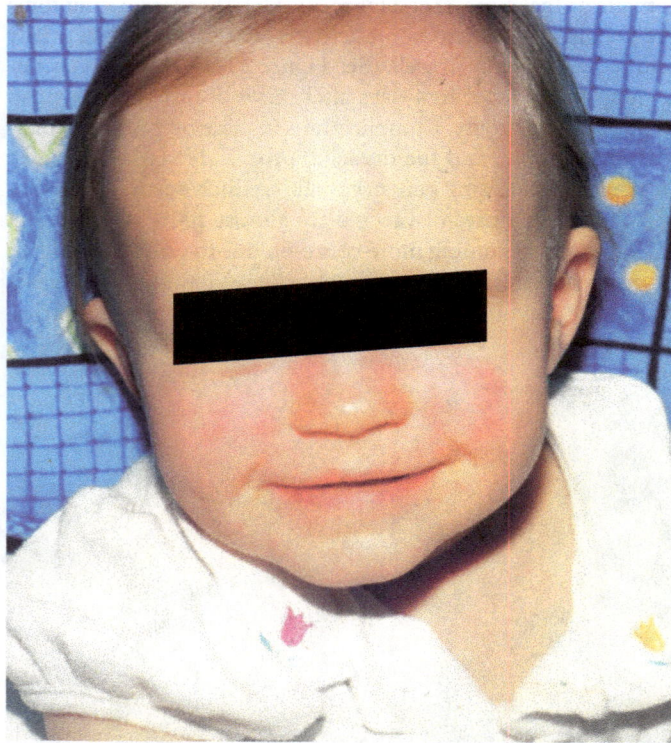

FIGURE 20–13. Erythema Infectiosum—"Slapped Cheeks." Children with erythema infectiosum (fifth disease), caused by parvovirus B19, have a classic "slapped-cheek" appearance. Notice the child looks otherwise well. (Reproduced with permission from Kasper DL, Fauci AS, Hauser SL et al: *Harrison's Principles of Internal Medicine*, 19th ed. McGraw-Hill Education, Inc., 2015. Fig 221-2.)

and move peripherally as well. (See Figure 20–14.) Arthralgias or arthritis can also occur and are thought to be immune mediated. Pure red cell anemia is possible, though rarely other cell lines may be affected. Rarer presentations include papular purpuric gloves and socks syndrome and aplastic crisis. Congenital infection can lead to hydrops fetalis. Treatment is generally supportive as no antiviral agents are available to treat parvovirus. Infection is common and about half the population has been infected by adolescence. Human herpesvirus 6 (HHV-6) causes roseola (exanthem subitum), which often manifests as high fever for several days. It is one of the most common causes of simple febrile seizures in toddlers. The rash is maculopapular and tends to appear as fever resolves. Complications include encephalitis and hepatitis and are more common in immunocompromised patients. Almost every child has been infected with HHV-6 by age 3. Roseola in an adolescent would be very unlikely. Treatment is supportive, though foscarnet or ganciclovir may provide benefit in immunocompromised patients. Adenovirus can have a wide variety of presentations. Common manifestations include upper respiratory infections, exudative or nonexudative tonsillitis, conjunctivitis, otitis, and diarrhea. Its constellation of symptoms can include a maculopapular rash. When present in the setting of fever, conjunctivitis, pharyngitis, and lymphadenopathy, it can be very difficult to distinguish from Kawasaki disease. Other complications include diarrhea, hepatitis, and encephalitis. Immunocompromised patients can have especially severe symptoms. Treatment for immunocompetent hosts is usually supportive, though cidofovir may be useful in treating immunocompromised patients. Non-polio enteroviruses include coxsackievirus, echoviruses, and parechoviruses. They have a broad range of presentations, including fever, rash, diarrhea, conjunctivitis, and encephalitis, and are one of the most common causes of aseptic meningitis in the summer months. Coxsackie viruses tend to cause hand, foot and mouth disease (which can appear vesicular) as well as herpangina and have been implicated in myocarditis. Parechovirus and enteroviruses can cause a severe, sepsis-like syndrome in the

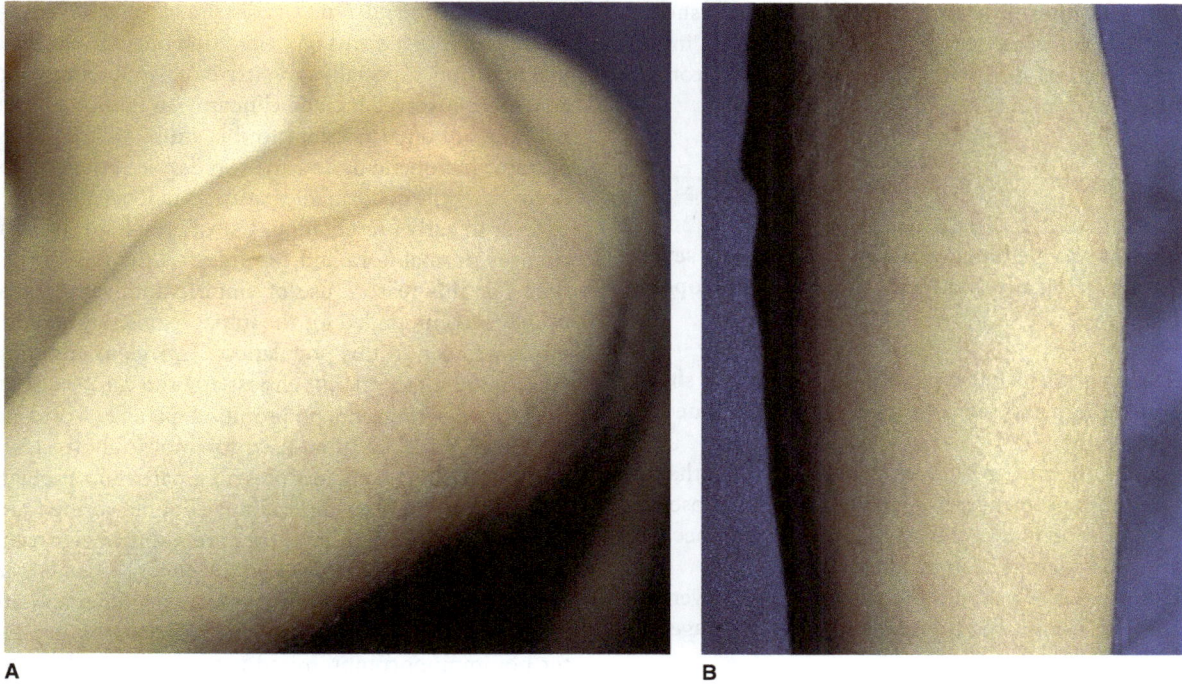

FIGURE 20–14. Erythema Infectiosum—Reticular Rash. A lacey reticular rash may be seen on the trunk and periphery in children with erythema infectiosum (fifth disease). (Reproduced with permission from Goldsmith LA, Katz SI, Gilchrest BA, Paller AS, Leffell DJ, Wolff K, eds. *Fitzpatrick's Dermatology in General Medicine.* 8th ed. New York, NY: McGraw-Hill Education; 2012, Fig. 192-6A, B.)

newborn. Immunocompromised patients, especially those who lack immunoglobulins, can have severe, relapsing infections with enteroviruses. Non–polio enteroviruses tend to circulate more frequently in the summer in temperate climates. Serologies and PCR can be useful in diagnosis. Treatment is generally supportive; however, intravenous immunoglobulin (IVIG) may have benefit in newborns, patients with myocarditis, and immunocompromised patients.

▶ CASE 37

A child with ALL who lives in a commune that does not believe in immunization recently received chemotherapy and is becoming pancytopenic. She just turned 4 years old and her parents decided to invite all her friends from the commune over for a party (probably as much a germ party as it was a birthday party). Unfortunately various members of the party have now come down with chickenpox, measles, mumps, and influenza. The family is worried that their daughter may have been exposed to those infections and calls you to ask if anything can be done at this point to prevent infection.

Question 37-1
You correctly tell the family that:
A) Nothing is available to prevent or ameliorate chickenpox.
B) IVIG should be given to prevent mumps.
C) IVIG should be given to prevent measles.

D) Rimantadine should be given to prevent influenza.
E) MMR and varicella vaccine should be given now to prevent future infection.

Discussion 37-1
The correct answer is "C." This child is at high risk for severe infection should she acquire measles. She has the double misfortune of not being immunized and having a severely immunocompromising condition. Considering how contagious some of these viruses are, she has high risk of becoming infected. Chickenpox can be prevented or at least ameliorated by giving varicella immune globulin (VariZIG). IVIG can be useful as well if VariZIG is not available but the amount of antivaricella antibody varies from lot to lot. Acyclovir may be useful as well, but is third line as far as prevention options go as there are fewer data to support its use. IVIG can prevent or ameliorate measles and should be given in that case, but it will not affect acquisition or severity of mumps infection. Influenza can be effectively prevented by prophylaxis with a neuraminidase inhibitor such as oseltamivir. Additionally, neuraminidase inhibitors may improve symptoms in influenza infection. Treatment should be considered for patients with high risk of severe influenza disease (eg, immunocompromised patients and those with chronic illnesses such as pulmonary disease, cardiac disease, diabetes, etc). Influenza viruses are widely resistant to the adamantines such as rimantadine, so prophylaxis would be useless with this drug. In healthy children, vaccination can be used in certain situations to both prevent infection due to recent exposure and

prevent future infection; however, live virus vaccines such as MMR and varicella vaccine should not be given to an immunocompromised patient due to risk of severe infection from the attenuated vaccine strain.

► CASE 38

You are busy on the pediatric oncology ward with several patients who are being admitted with fever and neutropenia.

Question 38-1

You are thinking about what type of empiric therapy should be given for oncology patients admitted for fever and neutropenia and determine:

A) Initial empiric regimen should include an antibiotic that has broad-spectrum gram-negative activity (including pseudomonas) in addition to an antibiotic that has broad-spectrum gram-positive coverage such as vancomycin.

B) Initial empiric therapy should include antifungal coverage.

C) Initial empiric therapy should have anaerobic coverage.

D) None of the above.

E) All of the above.

Discussion 38-1

The correct answer is "E." Cancer patients receive chemotherapy that cause suppression of the immune system and often present with fever and neutropenia. They are at increased risk for serious invasive infection. Immediate action should be undertaken to evaluate these patients and determine if there is a source of infection causing their fevers. Empiric therapy should be started as soon as possible, especially if a patient appears septic. The empiric regimen depends on the risk factors for each patient. Recent surgery, indwelling catheters, and mucosal barrier breakdown all increase risk of invasive infection in addition to the immunosuppressed state of the patient with cancer. A careful exposure history is important as well to assess what infection a patient may have acquired. Concomitant infection with multiple organisms is not unusual. About one third of children with fever and neutropenia in the setting of cancer have a documented infection. Bacterial causes are common, with bloodstream and lung infections (ie, pneumonia) being the most likely sites, although any site could potentially become infected in this population. Gram-positive infection with organisms such as coagulase-negative staphylococci and viridans group streptococci are most common, but due to low pathogenicity, mortality is lower compared with gram-negative organisms. *Pseudomonas* spp have a particularly high mortality rate in this group. For this reason empiric therapy should target gram-negative organisms including *Pseudomonas* spp, with some degree of gram-positive coverage as well. Addition of agents with broader spectrum gram-positive activity such as vancomycin is not recommended for additional therapy unless there is concern for skin or soft tissue infection or the patient is hemodynamically unstable. The antibiotic chosen will depend on local resistance patterns as well as the individual patient history. Anaerobic infections in children are rare, even in febrile neutropenic patients. Empiric therapy with anaerobic coverage is not usually recommended unless the site of infection is suggestive of an anaerobic organisms (eg, aspiration pneumonia; intra-abdominal infection, especially typhlitis; etc). Antibiotics with potential anaerobic coverage include clindamycin (although gastrointestinal flora are often resistant to this antibiotic), piperacillin-tazobactam, meropenem, and metronidazole. Fungal infection can occur in febrile neutropenic patients but it usually is not the cause of fever in early presentation. Use of broad-spectrum antibiotics changes normal flora and can increase the risk of fungal infection. For this reason, use of empiric antifungal therapy is not usually recommended for the initial regimen. *Candida* is a common pathogen in this population. *Aspergillus* commonly causes pulmonary infection, but almost any site can be affected by this mold in the immunocompromised patient. Voriconazole and amphotericin B are often used to empirically treat mold infections. Indwelling catheters present a particular problem. On the one hand they are an important part of delivering much-needed therapy. On the other hand they are a source of infection. Many organisms such as *Staphylococcus aureus*, *Pseudomonas aeruginosa*, and *Candida albicans* can form biofilms and are difficult to eradicate without removing the catheter (this is often the case for nonimmunocompromised patients with indwelling catheter infections as well). The decision to remove an infected catheter is based on how quickly the patient improves, complications, underlying comorbidities, type of pathogen, and expected response to medical therapy.

Helpful Tip

Coagulase-negative staphylococcus (CONS; eg, *Staphylococcus epidermidis*) isolated from a blood culture is often a skin contaminant due to its low pathogenicity. Obtaining blood cultures from multiple sites before initiation of antibiotics is helpful in determining if it is a contaminant. Some populations are at higher risk of having true invasive infection with CONS. These include immunocompromised patients, premature infants, patients with breakdown of protective barriers, and patients with a foreign body in place (eg, ventriculoperitoneal shunt, orthopedic hardware, etc).

⧖ QUICK QUIZ

Which of the following is NOT transmitted by mosquitos?
A) Dengue fever virus.
B) Yellow fever virus.
C) West Nile virus.
D) Eastern equine encephalitis.
E) Babesiosis.
F) Chikungunya virus.

Discussion

The correct answer is "E." Remember, whether at home or abroad, mosquitos are not your friends. Most mosquito-borne infections tend to be prevalent in warmer, tropical regions, but exceptions occur as in the case of West Nile virus. Dengue virus is transmitted by *Aedes* spp mosquitos in tropical climates. Symptoms include fever and headaches. Pain can be severe, and it has been called "breakbone fever" by some. It can be mild or cause shock with coagulopathy, hemorrhage, and multiorgan failure. Diagnosis is made by serology, PCR, and clinical syndrome. Treatment is supportive. Yellow fever virus is transmitted by *Aedes* and *Haemagogus* spp mosquitos in tropical Africa and South America. Infection often is asymptomatic but can cause severe illness with a high mortality rate. Symptoms include fever, hepatitis, coagulopathy, and shock. Treatment is supportive. A live attenuated vaccine is available for travelers. West Nile virus is transmitted by *Culex* spp mosquitos, which have a broad range throughout the world. Infection can be asymptomatic and often causes a self-limiting flu-like illness in most symptomatic patients. Headache, meningitis, and rash can occur as well. Flaccid paralysis reminiscent of polio is a rare complication. Diagnosis is by serology and treatment is supportive. Eastern equine encephalitis is caused by a virus. Humans and horses can become infected, although this is rare because the mosquito usually feeds on birds rather than humans. Fever, headache, and encephalitis can occur, with death and permanent brain damage being fairly common results. Treatment is supportive. Chikungunya (say that 10 times fast) is starting to spread to the Caribbean and southern United States with potential to spread further. It is transmitted by *Aedes* spp mosquitos. Symptoms include fever, rash, and joint pain so severe that it often causes patients to hunch over while walking (which is what the name chikungunya means). Conjunctivitis and CNS symptoms can occur. Treatment is supportive. Long-lasting arthralgias and arthritis can remain (up to years later) after other symptoms resolve. Babesiosis is a *tick-borne* infection most commonly caused by the parasite *Babesia microti*. It is transmitted by *Ixodes* ticks and is seen in the upper Midwest and northeastern United States. Coinfection with *Anaplasma* and *Borrelia burgdorferi* (Lyme disease) may occur as they share the same vector. Most infections are asymptomatic, but the parasite can infect red cells causing hemolysis and symptoms similar to malaria. Diagnosis is made by blood smear (ie, four organisms characteristically forming a "Maltese Cross" in the red blood cells), serology, and PCR. Treatment is with atovaquone and azithromycin in addition to supportive care.

> ▶ **CASE 39**

Before rounding in the NICU, you review the files of several children who have possible congenital infections.

Question 39-1

As you are thinking of signs, symptoms, and lab abnormalities that are manifestations of the various infections, you tell your medical student that:

A) Congenital CMV is not associated with thrombocytopenia.
B) Congenital toxoplasmosis can be associated with circumferential scarring leading to limb amputation.
C) An ophthalmologic exam should be done on the child suspected of having congenital rubella.
D) Blueberry muffin rash is commonly seen in congenital varicella.
E) Infants with congenital toxoplasma usually present with hepatosplenomegaly and either microcephaly or macrocephaly.
F) All of the above.
G) None of the above.

Discussion 39-1

The correct answer is "C." Congenital CMV affects 1% of newborns. It can range from asymptomatic infection that is only discovered by screening to severe multiorgan disease. Pneumonia, hepatitis, and thrombocytopenia are common in more severe disease. CNS involvement can be severe, with cerebral calcifications. When present, blueberry muffin rash is due to dermal erythropoiesis (also seen in congenital rubella). (See Figure 20–15.) Other physical findings include microcephaly, hepatosplenomegaly, and lymphadenopathy. Ophthalmologic exam may reveal chorioretinitis. Hearing loss can be present initially or manifest later, and can occur even in asymptomatic children. Diagnosis can be made with PCR, culture, or IgM. Treatment of symptomatic newborns with IV ganciclovir or oral valganciclovir for 6 weeks may improve hearing and cognitive outcomes and is often recommended for this purpose. Cats are the definitive host for *Toxoplasma gondii*. Cysts are shed in the stool and for that reason pregnant women are advised to avoid changing the cat litter. Other animal's muscles and organs may become infected by ingested cysts. Consumption of the undercooked meat may cause infection in humans. Typical infection causes a self-limiting flu-like illness with fever, myalgia, and lymphadenopathy in immunocompetent individuals. Immunocompromised patients can have severe disease, including CNS and ocular infection. Congenital infection occurs when the mother acquires primary infection during pregnancy. The majority of congenital toxoplasma

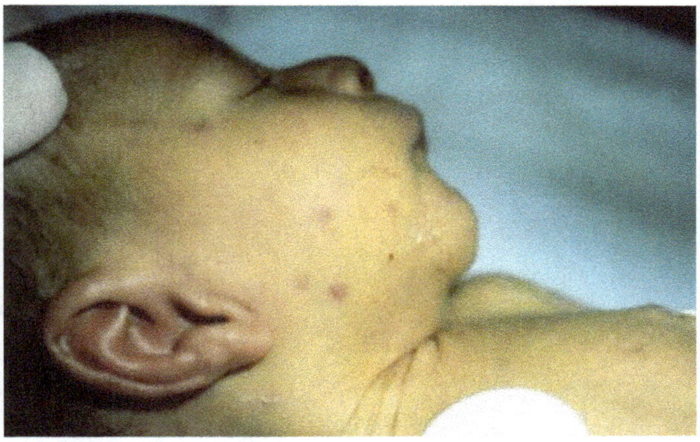

FIGURE 20–15. A blueberry muffin rash may be seen in newborns with congenital rubella or cytomegalovirus (CMV). The lesions, reddish-blue and maculopapular, are sites of dermal extramedullary erythropoiesis. (Reproduced with permission from Lichtman MA, Shafer MS, Felgar RE, Wang N, eds. *Lichtman's Atlas of Hematology*. New York, NY: McGraw-Hill Education; 2007, Fig. XI.A.56.)

infections are asymptomatic. Symptomatic infants can have hepatosplenomegaly, microcephaly or macrocephaly, failure to thrive, chorioretinitis, and hearing loss. Developmental delay and seizures can be severe. As in congenital CMV, cerebral calcifications may be seen on head imaging. Serologies and PCR can be useful in making the diagnosis. Often serology in the infant is compared with serology in the mother to determine if the infant is infected or there has been transplacental transmission of maternal antibody. Treatment of congenital toxoplasma usually involves sulfadiazine and pyrimethamine with leucovorin for at least 1 year. Eye disease can recur despite appropriate therapy. Congenital rubella is acquired when the mother becomes infected with the virus during pregnancy. The classic triad of findings is cardiac defects (eg, patent ductus arteriosus), sensorineural hearing loss, and cataracts. Ophthalmologic exam should be performed to assess for possible eye involvement. Hepatosplenomegaly, blueberry muffin rash, thrombocytopenia, encephalitis, and developmental delay are possible as well. (See Figure 20–15, earlier.) Infants can shed virus for 1 year or more. Fortunately rubella has been eradicated from the United States, but imported cases happen from time to time. Diagnosis can be made by serologies, PCR, and viral culture of urine and oral secretions. Treatment is supportive, and hospitalized infants should be isolated with contact and droplet precautions (often up to 1 year until cleared by testing). Congenital varicella occurs when the mother becomes infected with chickenpox in early pregnancy (it does not occur if an immunocompetent mother gets zoster). Signs and symptoms include cutaneous scarring (which can be circumferential, causing intrauterine limb amputation or hypoplasia), encephalitis, developmental delay, and bone and eye abnormalities. Treatment is supportive. If a mother contracts chickenpox from 5 days before to 2 days after delivery, her infant has a 20% mortality rate from chickenpox infection. These infants should receive VariZIG prophylaxis, which decreases mortality and ameliorates disease if it does not completely prevent infection.

Helpful Tip

CMV is everywhere! Up to 70% of children in daycare shed the virus. Most adults are seropositive. Infants can become infected in utero from the mother and postnatally from breastmilk, exposure to secretions of infected people, and blood transfusions. Pregnant caregivers should wash their hands to prevent infection.

Helpful Tip

Cerebral calcifications are seen in congenital CMV infection and toxoplasmosis. Here is a handy way of distinguishing the two: ToXoplasmosis has an "X" so calcifications are in the cortex. CMV has a "V" so calcifications are periVentricular. (See Figure 20–16.)

► CASE 40

A 4-year-old otherwise healthy girl is brought to your clinic for evaluation of a swollen submandibular lymph node. Her mother noticed the initial swelling about 4 weeks ago. At that time the girl had a mild runny nose and cough with temperature of 38°C (100.4°F). Her URI symptoms and low-grade fever resolved within a few days, but the node has increased progressively in size. It does not seem to be particularly tender, and the girl has not had any fevers. The mother mentions that she had taken her daughter to the urgent care clinic a few times and was given amoxicillin and clindamycin, but this treatment has not improved the lymphadenopathy. The girl has no other symptoms or signs at this time. On exam the node measures 5 cm and is firm without fluctuance. The overlying skin has a somewhat purple hue. The rest of her exam is unremarkable. You send her to the otolaryngology service for lymph node biopsy.

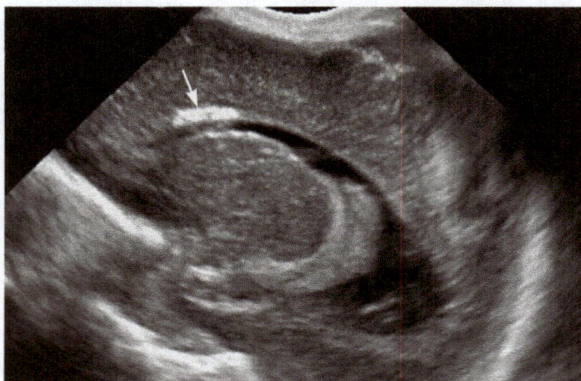 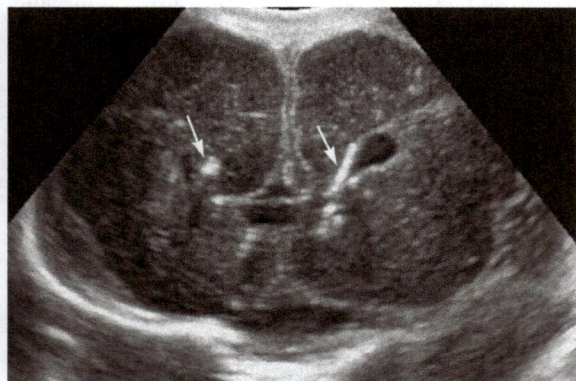

A   B

FIGURE 20–16. Congenital CMV causes periventricular calcifications as seen in these ultrasound photos. Congenital toxoplasmosis causes cerebral cortex calcifications. (Reproduced with permission from Cunningham FG, Leveno KJ, Bloom SL, et al, eds. *Williams Obstetrics*. 24th ed. New York, NY: McGraw-Hill Education; 2014, Fig. 64-3A&B.)

Question 40-1

The results from pathology staining and lab testing are most likely to come back as:

A) Malignant cells.
B) Gram-positive cocci in chains.
C) Gram-positive cocci in clusters.
D) Acid-fast bacilli.
E) Normal reactive lymph node.

Discussion 40-1

The correct answer is "D." You didn't really think we'd put a question about cancer in the infectious disease section did you? This child has classic presentation for nontuberculous mycobacterial lymphadenitis. It often affects children aged 1 to 4 years and presents as a relatively nontender lymph node that continues to slowly increase in size despite therapy with antibiotics targeting typical suppurative bacteria. Associated symptoms are minimal. Untreated, the lymph node can suppurate and can cause scarring. There is often a violaceous hue to the overlying skin, which can have a thin, papery appearance. *Mycobacterium avium-intracellulare* (MAI) is the most common cause although other nontuberculous bacteria are possible as well. Disseminated infection is almost nonexistent in immunocompetent individuals. Diagnosis is made by biopsy and culture identification of the organism. PCR is available in some labs. TST can be reactive, depending on the mycobacterial species (especially with MAI, but it does not cause a positive IGRA). The most effective treatment is complete excision of the lymph node (although this can be difficult if nearby structures such as the facial nerve are in danger of damage from surgery). Therapy with two or three antibiotics (eg, azithromycin or clarithromycin with rifampin and ethambutol in the case of MAI) can be used as well, but failure of this regimen is common. Fortunately these are not aggressive infections in immunocompetent hosts and can resolve without therapy, although unsightly scarring may occur. Gram-positive cocci in chains would be seen in the setting of group A streptococcal infection (GAS, or *Streptococcus pyogenes*). This is a common cause of acute bacterial lymphadenitis but tends to have more rapid onset, with a warm, tender lymph node and systemic symptoms (fever). Therapy involves penicillin or ampicillin, as GAS is not resistant, and surgical intervention if necessary. GAS infections tend to involve skin and soft tissue (eg, necrotizing fasciitis) but may also affect the bone and joint. GAS is also a classic cause of pharyngitis. Diagnosis is usually made by culturing the affected site (although rapid testing in pharyngitis is useful as well). Serologic testing such as anti-streptolysin O (ASO) and anti-DNAse B can be useful in determining if an invasive infection has occurred in the recent past, but usually are not useful in the acute phase. These tests help evaluate noninfectious sequelae, including rheumatic fever, post-streptococcal glomerulonephritis, or postinfectious arthritis. Gram-positive cocci in clusters would be seen in *Staphylococcus aureus* infection, which has a presentation similar to GAS lymphadenitis. It is resistant to amoxicillin and could be resistant to clindamycin, but should cause a more rapid, tender lymphadenopathy, often with systemic symptoms which this patient lacks. *S. aureus* also has a broad range of clinical manifestations and is a nasty bug. It is one of the most common causes of bone and joint infections in children. It has a propensity to cause bacteremia and consequently can infect almost any organ system. Methicillin-susceptible and methicillin-resistant strains (MSSA and MRSA) can cause both mild and severe disease. Some strains produce toxins and can cause toxic shock and staphylococcal scalded skin syndrome. Asymptomatic colonization is common as well. Therapy is based on susceptibility profile and the site of infection. *S. aureus* tends to form abscesses, so surgical debridement is often necessary. Infection is difficult to eradicate with infected foreign bodies in place.

> **Helpful Tip**
>
> Toxic shock syndrome results from toxin production by *Staphylococcus aureus* or *Streptococcus pyogenes*. Findings include rash (erythroderma), hypotension, end-organ damage (liver and kidney), and coagulopathy. Treatment includes antibiotics to treat the bacteria, antibiotics to prevent toxin production (clindamycin), and IVIG in addition to aggressive supportive care and surgical debridement when necessary.

QUICK QUIZ

Which of the following is/are reliable indicators of infection in children with severe burn injury?

A) Fever.
B) Elevated inflammatory markers.
C) Hypotension.
D) Leukocytosis.
E) All of the above.
F) None of the above.

Discussion

The correct answer is "F." Infection in burn victims can be difficult to diagnose owing to the high degree of inflammation, increased metabolic rate, and fluid shifts that occur due to lack of the natural barrier that the skin provides. Fevers, hypotension, leukocytosis, and inflammatory marker elevation can all occur in noninfected patients, making it difficult to distinguish infection from a noninfectious physiologic response. Complicating the diagnosis is the fact that sepsis due to burn wound infection has a mortality rate of 80%. These patients often have indwelling catheters, which also are a potential source of infection. Blood supply may be compromised to injured tissues, making it difficult to prevent and treat infection in those tissues. Careful evaluation and wound management is necessary to both prevent and treat wound infections. Typical organisms causing infection include skin flora such as *Staphylococcus aureus* and *Streptococcus pyogenes* as well as gastrointestinal flora and *Pseudomonas* spp. Fungi such as *Candida* spp can be common as well. All burn victims should be assessed for tetanus immunization status and be managed appropriately since they are at risk for tetanus infection.

Helpful Tip

Candida spp can cause a wide variety of infections. Colonization of the gastrointestinal tract and skin is common. In infants thrush and mild skin infection in the diaper area are common and easily treated with topical agents. Invasive candidal infections can occur as well, especially in immunocompromised patients, premature infants, and patients with indwelling catheters. The organism grows easily using standard culturing techniques. It usually responds well to systemic antifungal therapy, but catheters usually should be removed as it can form biofilms and can be difficult to eradicate when catheters are left in place.

► CASE 41

Question 41-1

Which statement about vaccine preventable infections is true?

A) Markedly elevated neutrophils are associated with *Bordetella pertussis* infection.

B) Bilateral, pitting edema of the lateral neck is associated with diphtheria.

C) Occult bacteremia with *Haemophilus influenzae* type B is common and does not usually progress to invasive infection.

D) The rotavirus vaccine covers all known strains of rotavirus.

E) Brucella should be considered in children with fever of unknown origin who consume unpasteurized dairy products.

Discussion 41-1

The correct answer is "B." *Bordetella pertussis* is the bacterium responsible for pertussis. The illness it causes is called the "100 days cough" for good reason. It is toxin mediated and does not cause invasive infection. Infants can present with apnea, or have cyanosis due to paroxysms. The coughing can be so severe that it causes rib fractures, cerebral hemorrhage, hernia, and rectal prolapse. Diagnosis can be made clinically, but PCR is often used and is more likely to be positive early in the course of infection (remember the three stages: catarrhal, paroxysmal, and convalescence). Young children often do not have the characteristic whoop after coughing paroxysms. A classic finding is lymphocytosis, not neutrophilia. Treatment with azithromycin can prevent spread to other contacts. The pertussis vaccine is fairly effective in preventing spread, but vaccinated close contacts still have a high risk of infection and should receive postexposure prophylaxis. Diphtheria no longer occurs in the United States, but it is just a plane ride away. Symptoms include sore throat with membrane formation and nasal discharge (can be bloody). Fever is often mild or absent. Cervical lymph nodes can swell and cause soft tissue pitting edema that obscures the

mandible (also known as bull neck). Toxins produced can cause neuropathy and cardiomyopathy (often weeks later). Death can occur from airway obstruction or the toxin mediated response. Treatment is with antitoxin and antibiotics (erythromycin). Diagnosis is made by culturing the bacteria (special media are needed, so tell the lab). *Haemophilus influenzae type B* (Hib) used to be widespread before vaccine for this organism was available. The bacterium causes a broad range of severe invasive disease such as epiglottitis, orbital cellulitis, osteomyelitis, meningitis, and pneumonia. Bacteremia with this bug is bad as there is a high risk of meningitis and other severe invasive disease. It is an encapsulated organism, so asplenic patients are at particular risk for severe infection (and should be immunized for Hib regardless of age if not already done). Nontypeable *H. influenzae* strains are less virulent and common causes of upper and lower respiratory tract infection, including sinusitis, otitis media, and pneumonia. Rarely CNS infection can occur with these nontypeable strains, but this is usually in the setting of complications of local infection, or disruption of barriers due to surgery or anatomic abnormalities. Diagnosis is made by culture. Treatment usually involves a third-generation cephalosporin (eg, ceftriaxone) as initial therapy for invasive infection until susceptibilities are known, since Hib and other serotypes can produce a beta-lactamase that renders penicillins ineffective. In the setting of Hib meningitis, administration of steroids before or at the time of initial dosing of antibiotics decreases the risk of hearing loss (the benefit of steroids after this period or with other bacteria is still a matter of debate in children). Postexposure prophylaxis with rifampin should be given to all household members of the index case if there is an under- or unimmunized child younger than age 4 years, or an immunocompromised child of any age in the household. Rotavirus can cause severe diarrhea, leading to dehydration and death if not appropriately managed. Mortality rates due to this virus are high in developing countries where access to supportive care is limited. Two licensed oral, live attenuated vaccines are available for infants. One is monovalent and the other is pentavalent, but there are other strains of rotavirus not covered by the vaccines. There may be a risk of intussusception with rotavirus vaccination, but it is much lower than with a previous vaccine that was withdrawn from the market for that reason. Rotavirus tends to circulate in the winter months in temperate climates. The virus is transmitted by the fecal-oral route and relatively few organisms are required to transmit infection. Symptoms include fever, vomiting, and diarrhea. The vomiting usually lasts a few days, with profuse watery diarrhea lasting as long as a week. Diagnosis is made using stool antigen, but as care is supportive (similar to other viral gastroenteritis infections), diagnostic testing often is not necessary. *Brucella* spp are often transmitted by close contact with livestock, carcasses of animals, and consumption of unpasteurized dairy products. Brucellosis can cause fevers that last for weeks and can lead to invasive infection such as osteomyelitis and bacteremia. The course is often indolent. It should be suspected in children with risk factors and fever of unknown origin. However, it is not a vaccine-preventable illness.

Helpful Tip

Caliciviruses such as norovirus and sapovirus can cause a self-limiting gastroenteritis. Both may cause outbreaks, notably on cruise ships. Norovirus (known as the cruise ship virus) is exceptionally contagious and can last for many days on surfaces. Treatment is supportive.

Question 41-2

Which of the following is true regarding nutrition and infection?

A) Malnourished children have poor wound healing.
B) Malnourished children may have false results on diagnostic testing.
C) Malnourished children should be considered relatively immunodeficient.
D) Malnourished children can have atypical presentation of infection.
E) All of the above.

Discussion 41-2

The correct answer is "E." Malnutrition and infection go hand in hand. Children who are malnourished lack the key nutrients to build and sustain the immune system, making them more prone to infection and less likely to eradicate infection effectively. They also tend to have poor wound healing and increased skin breakdown. Their inflammatory response may be abnormal as well, leading to atypical presentation of disease. Infection itself can cause malnutrition as a result of the increased metabolic rate or poor absorption of nutrients (as can happen with infectious diarrhea). Malnourished children may also have false results on diagnostic testing (eg, a negative TST despite active tuberculosis). Optimizing nutrition is important to both prevent and treat infection.

▶ CASE 42

A 1-week-old infant is admitted for fever. Blood, urine, and CSF cultures are obtained and the infant is placed on empiric IV ampicillin and cefotaxime. The microbiology lab calls to report that the blood culture is growing gram-positive rods from both the aerobic and anaerobic bottles at 19 hours of incubation.

Question 42-1

What do you do next?

A) Disregard the culture as a contaminant.
B) Discontinue ampicillin and start IV vancomycin.
C) Continue the current antibiotic regimen.
D) Add IV gentamicin.
E) None of the above.

Discussion 42-1

The correct answer is "D." This neonate has *Listeria monocytogenes* sepsis. *Listeria* is a rare pathogen outside of neonates, pregnant women, immunocompromised patients, and the elderly. In neonates, the infection is acquired prenatally and presents early as sepsis (first week of life) and later as meningitis. Intravenous ampicillin and an aminoglycoside, usually gentamicin, are recommended for severe infections. Food-borne outbreaks are the norm and may cause self-limited gastroenteritis in immunocompetent hosts. To prevent infection, pregnant women should not consume soft cheeses (eg, blue cheese, queso fresco) or unpasteurized dairy products, and hot dogs and deli meats should be reheated until steaming hot before eating. A positive blood culture, especially involving both bottles, with positivity after less than 24 hours of incubation in a susceptible host with a plausible organism should not be called a contaminant based on the results of the Gram stain only.

⧗ QUICK QUIZ

What is a known pathogen causing neonatal sepsis?

A) *Streptococcus agalactiae.*
B) *Escherichia coli.*
C) *Listeria monocytogenes.*
D) Enterovirus.
E) All of the above.

Discussion

The correct answer is "E." *S. agalactiae* (group B *Streptococcus*, GBS) and *E. coli* are the most common pathogens, but all organisms listed are known causes of neonatal sepsis. If a skin or soft tissue infection is present, *Staphylococcal aureus* should be included as a possible pathogen.

BIBLIOGRAPHY

American Academy of Pediatrics Committee on Infectious Diseases; American Academy of Pediatrics Bronchiolitis Guideline Committee. Policy statement: Updated guidance for palivizumab prophylaxis among infants and young children at increased risk of hospitalization for respiratory syncytial virus infection. *Pediatrics.* 2014;134(2):415–420.

Centers for Disease Control and Prevention. 2010 guidelines for the prevention of perinatal group B streptococcal disease. http://www.cdc.gov/groupbstrep/guidelines/guidelines.html. Accessed October 31, 2015.

Cherry J, Harrison G, Kaplan S, Steinbach W, Hotez P. *Feigin and Cherry's Textbook of Pediatric Infectious Diseases.* 7th ed. Philadelphia, PA: Elsevier; 2014.

Cohen S, Gerding D, Johnson S, et al. Clinical practice guidelines for Clostridium difficile infection in adults: 2010 update by the Society for Healthcare Epidemiology of America (SHEA) and the Infectious Diseases Society of America (IDSA). *Infect Control Hosp Epidemiol.* 2010;31(5):431–455.

Committee on Adolescence, Society for Adolescent Health and Medicine. Screening for nonviral sexually transmitted infections in adolescents and young adults. *Pediatrics.* 2014;134(1):e302–311.

Guidelines for the Use of Antiretroviral Agents in Pediatric HIV infection. [Updated February 12, 2014.] http://aidsinfo.nih.gov/guidelines/html/2/pediatric-treatment-guidelines/0, Accessed February 2, 2015.

Jones VF; Committee on Early Childhood, Adoption, and Dependent Care. Comprehensive health evaluation of the newly adopted child. *Pediatrics.* 2012;129(1):e214–e223.

Leiberthal A, Carrol A, Chonmaitree T, et al. The diagnosis and management of acute otitis media. Clinical Practice Guideline. *Pediatrics.* 2013;131(3):e964–999.

Long S, Pickering K, Prober C. *Principles and Practice of Pediatric Infectious Diseases.* 4th ed. Philadelphia, PA: Elsevier; 2012.

Pickering L, Baker C, Kimberlin D, Long S. *Red Book 2012: Report of the Committee of Pediatric Infectious Diseases.* 29th ed. Grove Village, IL: American Academy of Pediatrics; 2012.

Recommendations for use of antiretroviral drugs in pregnant HIV-1 infected women for maternal health and interventions to reduce perinatal HIV transmission in the United States. [Updated March 28, 2014.] http://aidsinfo.nih.gov/guidelines/html/3/perinatal-guidelines/0. Accessed February 2, 2015.

Remington J, Klein J, Wilson C, Nizet V, Maldonado Y. *Infectious Diseases of the Fetus and Newborn Infant.* 7th ed. Philadelphia, PA: Elsevier; 2011.

Metabolic Disorders

21

Eric T. Rush

▶ CASE 1

An 8-month-old girl is brought to outpatient care for evaluation of developmental delay with poor muscle tone. She was also observed to have a seizure, for which the family brought her to the emergency department. On examination, the infant appears small and listless with patchy development of scalp hair and a rather severe eczemoid rash in several areas about the body, most notably the oral region. There is no family history of a similar condition and the parents are not known to be related, although they state that they recently emigrated to the United States from the same small village in Guatemala. They do not think their daughter had any newborn screening after birth, as the delivery occurred at home with a midwife who was the father's great aunt. A basic metabolic panel performed as part of the evaluation in the emergency department was normal, and serum lactate was slightly elevated at 2.2 mmol/L.

Question 1-1

What is the most appropriate next step in the evaluation of this patient?

A) Magnetic resonance imaging (MRI) of the brain to look for perisylvian cerebral dysgenesis.
B) Referral to developmental-behavioral pediatrics to assist with managing developmental delays.
C) Further metabolic testing, including plasma amino acids, urine organic acids, acylcarnitine profile, and serum biotinidase activity.
D) Low-potency corticosteroid cream for treatment of the patient's severe eczema.
E) Scrapings of exfoliated skin around hair follicles for electron microscopy.

Discussion 1-1

The correct answer is "C." This infant girl has presented with developmental delay, eczema, and alopecia. These findings are typical of a diagnosis of biotinidase deficiency in which the body cannot recycle the vitamin biotin. Additional clues provided in the case history are that the parents are probably distantly related, suggesting an increased risk of autosomal recessive disease. In addition, a clue is provided that the infant did not have newborn screening, suggesting that she may suffer from a disorder that would be detected by a typical newborn screen. Broad metabolic testing would be the most appropriate next step for this patient. MRI of the brain is likely to be of low yield, and perisylvian cerebral dysgenesis can be seen in other disorders, but is not likely to be found in biotinidase deficiency. Referral to behavioral-developmental pediatrics is generally helpful in the management of patients with developmental delay, but it is not appropriate for the evaluation of a patient with evidence of an inborn error of metabolism. Low-potency steroid cream for eczema suggests symptomatic treatment only, which misses the point of the question and in any event is unlikely to be efficacious in a patient who has biotinidase deficiency. Scrapings of exfoliated skin around hair follicles does not pertain to one disorder in particular, but serves as caution to test takers to avoid unusual or unfamiliar foils that sound authoritative. (If only a magic crystal ball of metabolic disorders existed. Who wouldn't pay good money for an easy way to solve the dilemma of the child who has a metabolic disorder—but which one? For a simplified overview of metabolic disorders, see Table 21–1.)

> **Helpful Tip**
> Inborn errors of metabolism result from the absence or abnormality of a necessary enzyme or cofactor that causes either buildup or deficiency of a specific metabolite.

▶ CASE 2

As a newly graduated and board-eligible pediatrician, you are covering for the newborn nursery service at the local university hospital. It is a rather slow day, being slightly before the fall baby season, and you have time to discuss issues of importance with your gaggle of third-year medical students. One of the nursing staff obtains a heel-stick on an 18-hour-old infant for the state

TABLE 21–1 BREAKDOWN OF INBORN ERRORS OF METABOLISM

Disorder	Examples	Pathophysiology	Clinical Manifestations	Laboratory Abnormalities	Maintenance Treatment
Amino acid	Phenylketonuria Maple syrup urine disease	Defect in metabolism of amino acids, resulting in accumulation of amino acids that cannot be metabolized and deficiencies of certain essential amino acids Child gets sick after eating protein	Newborns: • Poor feeding • Lethargy • Vomiting • Encephalopathy • Death Child: • Delayed	Metabolic acidosis Elevated ammonia Hypoglycemia with ketoacidosis Liver dysfunction	Low-protein diet Replacement of essential amino acids
Organic acidemia	Methylmalonic acidemia Propionic acidemia Glutaric acidemia	Defect in metabolism of amino acids Accumulation of abnormal toxic organic acid metabolites Increased urinary excretion of organic acids Child gets sick after eating protein and with illnesses	Newborns: • Poor feeding • Lethargy • Vomiting • Failure to thrive • Hypotonia • Progress to coma/death Child: • Failure to thrive • Delayed • Seizures • Vomiting Recurrent metabolic crises and bone marrow suppression with illnesses	Anion gap metabolic acidosis Elevated ammonia Hypoglycemia Ketosis Liver dysfunction ± Pancytopenia	Low-protein diet L-carnitine supplementation
Urea cycle	Ornithine transcarbamylase deficiency Citrullinemia	Defect in metabolism of nitrogen (NH_3^- ammonia) to urea Child gets sick after eating protein	Newborns: • Somnolence • Poor feeding • Vomiting • Coma Child: • Vomiting • Protein refusal	Elevated ammonia Ketosis Respiratory alkalosis	Protein restriction Ammonia scavengers
Carbohydrate	Glycogen storage disease Galactosemia	Defect in metabolism of glycogen, galactose, and fructose Child cannot handle fasting even for short time periods	Symptoms after fasting: • Lethargy • Encephalopathy ± Hepatomegaly	Fasting hypoglycemia Ketosis ± Urine reducing sugars	Avoidance of fasting Raw corn starch

(Continued)

TABLE 21–1 BREAKDOWN OF INBORN ERRORS OF METABOLISM (*CONTINUED*)

Fatty acid oxidation	MCAD Beta-oxidation defects Transportation defects	Defect in metabolism of fatty acids to ketones and glucose Child cannot handle prolonged fasting	Symptoms after fasting: • Lethargy • Encephalopathy Cardiomyopathy Myopathy	Fasting hypoglycemia No or low ketosis Liver dysfunction	High-carbohydrate, low-fat diet Avoidance of fasting
Mitochondrial	MELAS MERRF Kearns-Sayre syndrome	Defect in mitochondrial production of ATP (cellular energy)	Headache Vomiting Seizure Deafness Myopathy Delayed blindness	Lactic acidosis (blood and CSF) Liver dysfunction Ragged red fibers on muscle biopsy	Supportive
Peroxisomal	Zellweger syndrome	Defect in cellular metabolism in peroxisome	Microcephaly Dysmorphic features Delayed hypotonia Hepatomegaly	Increased phytanic acid Increased very long-chain fatty acids	
Lysosomal	Mucopolysaccharidoses (eg, Hunter syndrome) Sphingolipidoses (eg, Fabry, Gaucher, Tay-Sachs disease) Membrane transport defects (eg, cystinosis)	Defect in lysosomes metabolism Buildup of compounds inside cells	Enlargement of organs Coarse facies Short stature Joint contractures Acroparesthesias		Enzyme replacement therapy for some
Purine and pyrimidine	Purine (eg, Lesch-Nyhan disease, gout) Pyrimidine (eg, hereditary orotic aciduria)	Defect in metabolism of purines and pyrimidine, which are building blocks of DNA and RNA	Varies by disorder Kidney stones Delayed Self-injurious behaviors	Elevated uric acid Anemia	Allopurinol for hyperuricemia

ATP, adenosine triphosphate; CSF, cerebrospinal fluid; MCAD, medium-chain acyl-CoA dehydrogenase deficiency; MELAS, mitochondrial encephalopathy, lactic acidosis, and stroke syndrome; MERRF, myoclonic epilepsy and ragged red fibers.

newborn screening program. You kindly and professionally remind the nurse that collection of the sample before 24 hours of age is not recommended. One of your medical students asks you why the timing is so important for newborn screening.

Question 2-1

How do you respond?

A) The code for insurance billing is different on the second day of life and will result in higher reimbursement.

B) Infants have a more difficult time with temperature regulation over the first day of life, and this can alter the results of newborn screening and increase the false-positive rate.

C) There is no scientific reason for this rule, and it exists only as tradition.

D) Determination of the cutoff point for each analyte is an age-related phenomenon and is always a compromise between values that rise with age and those that decrease with age.

E) In all states, the examination for phenylketonuria is performed with capillary electrophoresis, and performing this test prior to 24 hours will result in falsely low phenylalanine levels.

Discussion 2-1

The correct answer is "D." Determination of the cutoff point for each analyte is indeed age-dependent, with some analytes decreasing and others increasing after birth. Standardized age of testing ensures a minimum of both false-positive and false-negative results. Generally speaking, newborn testing is provided by individual states (within the United States) or similar arrangements in other countries, so insurance coding is not altered by the newborn screening. Although it is true that neonates not infrequently have temperature regulation difficulties in the first 24 hours of life, this is not the deciding factor in the integrity of newborn screening. The supposition that there is no scientific consensus for this rule is incorrect for the reasons stated above, although "received wisdom" in medicine sometimes does exist in the absence of evidence. Lastly, virtually all modern newborn screening tests are performed with tandem mass spectrometry, not with capillary electrophoresis.

> **Helpful Tip**
>
> Newborn screening programs are probably, after vaccination programs, the most important pediatric public health endeavor that we have accomplished. As our testing has become more complex, diseases that we diagnose early have also become more complex to follow and treat. Neonatal ACT sheets have become an important tool for primary care physicians to ensure that they are caring appropriately for their patients. ACT sheets are updated as needed and are freely available through the National Library of Medicine (http://www.ncbi.nlm.nih.gov).

▶ CASE 3

You are on weekend call for your pediatrics group and are woken up from a deep slumber early on a Saturday morning (as these things tend to go) by the coordinator for the state newborn screening program. She tells you that a 3-day-old male infant who was recently discharged from the hospital by one of your partners has an abnormal newborn screen showing significant elevation in C8, suggesting that the infant has a diagnosis of medium-chain acyl-CoA dehydrogenase deficiency (MCADD).

Question 3-1

What is the most appropriate next step to take in the evaluation and management of the patient?
A) Alert the family of the results of testing immediately and enquire as to the well-being of the infant.
B) Make a note to call the family the next morning and suggest follow-up on Monday morning.
C) Reference the American College of Medical Genetics ACT Sheet for MCADD and follow the algorithm.
D) Refer the infant and family to a metabolist when you get back to the clinic on Monday.
E) Both A and C.

Discussion 3-1

The correct answer is "E." The American College of Medical Genetics publishes ACT sheets, which serve as a guide for the

diagnosis and immediate management of patients in whom an abnormal newborn screening results has been found. Certainly in an infant who has suspected MCADD, reference to the ACT sheets absolutely must be coupled with immediate discussion with the family, which concerns avoidance of fasting and what to do if the infant were to fall ill. Waiting until light of day would be inappropriate, as MCADD can be a cause of sudden infant death syndrome (SIDS). Additionally, while referral to a metabolist would be appropriate, it would be terribly cavalier to forgo any meaningful immediate discussion with the family.

▶ CASE 4

A local NICU has been caring for a premature Hispanic male infant who was noted on initial newborn screen to have elevated levels of tyrosine and several other amino acids. Urine succinylacetone was not detected. He was receiving total parenteral nutrition at that time, so it was felt that this was related to the result. A follow-up newborn screen performed several weeks later, after the infant was on full enteral feedings, continued to show an elevated tyrosine level and urine succinylcholine was still not detected. At present, the infant continues to have a typical clinical course for prematurity. The results of his recent chemistry panel, complete blood count (CBC), and hepatic profile are within normal limits. Urine organic acids were tested and are normal. There is no family history of any similar problems.

Question 4-1

What is the most likely diagnosis for this patient, and what is the most appropriate management?
A) No diagnosis is present, and no further management is required.
B) Transient hypertyrosinemia, which should be treated with ascorbic acid.
C) Excessively high-protein diet resulting in hepatocellular damage, which should be treated by referral for orthotopic liver transplant.
D) Tyrosinemia type I, which should be treated with nitisinone.
E) Hawkinsuria, which requires no treatment.

Discussion 4-1

The correct answer is "B." Transient hypertyrosinemia is a relatively common condition that appears to show increased prevalence in premature male infants and is the result of hepatic immaturity, which leads to elevation in tyrosine levels on newborn screening. The treatment is high-dose ascorbic acid, and providers should be careful to continue measuring tyrosine levels to ensure they are falling as expected in response to therapy. It may be tempting to suggest that because the patient is doing well, no diagnosis is present; however, this patient has a sustained abnormal result, which should always prompt additional investigational. An excessively high-protein diet can certainly cause an elevated tyrosine level, but hepatocellular damage should also produce elevation of other amino acids. The patient also shows no sign of hepatocellular damage or coagulopathy, which would make type I tyrosinemia very unlikely. Children with Hawkinsuria generally present with elevated tyrosine level, but also with metabolic acidosis, which this patient does not have. Several abnormal organic acids are also found in the urine of patients with Hawkinsuria. Unlike most metabolic disorders, it obeys an autosomal dominant pattern of inheritance, and the absence of family history in this case would make that unlikely. (If you knew what Hawkinsuria was, you can skip the rest of this chapter.)

▶ CASE 5

The parents of a 10-day-old male infant have come to the clinic for newborn screening follow-up because their son's screening was suggestive of isovaleric academia, an organic acidemia. This was confirmed on second screening, and it was also confirmed that the infant was homozygous for the relatively common c.932C>T mutation in the *IVD* gene. Fortunately, the infant is doing well with no sequelae of the condition at the present time. The parents are incredulous, denying that the condition is real, and breaking into tears at several times during the encounter. They are very concerned that their son is going to die suddenly and are afraid to leave him by himself to sleep.

Question 5-1

Aside from restriction of leucine and education on dietary needs in this condition, which intervention could be most helpful for this patient and family?
A) Give the infant supplementation with ubiquinol, which is proven to decrease the number of metabolic episodes.
B) Follow with the family in 1 month to further investigate their adaptation to the diagnosis.
C) Repeat molecular testing, as it is often unreliable and this may represent a false-positive result.
D) Place the infant on an apnea and bradycardia monitor to decrease parental anxiety about sudden death.
E) Have the parents meet with a genetic counselor to discuss their reaction to this condition and discuss the natural history in greater detail.

Discussion 5-1

The correct answer is "E." All hail the genetic counselor. Unlike pediatricians or geneticists, who receive little to no formal training in counseling, genetic counselors have extensive training in helping patients and their families work through difficult diagnoses from a psychosocial standpoint. Following up with the family in a month is probably a good idea on general principle but does not address the parents' immediate concerns about their child. Repeating genetic molecular testing would not be indicated, as the testing is highly reliable and the result is very unlikely to be incorrect. Placing the infant on an apnea and bradycardia monitor may appear reasonable but does not address root concerns and may end up reinforcing the parents' anxiety

about their child. Did you know that isovaleric acidemia is associated with smelling like sweaty feet?

> **Helpful Tip**
> Management of the sick neonate is one of the most anxiety-producing aspects of the care of children. This is particularly true of metabolic disorders because there are so many of them and they are, individually, rare conditions. However, for practical purposes they can be grouped into a few types and, with few exceptions, the immediate care for these patients is the same. Emergent information must be obtained. This involves assessment of respiratory status, glucose status, and acid-base status. For nearly all inborn errors of metabolism, giving the patient glucose and intravenous (IV) fluids will be helpful and potentially lifesaving, so this should be done as quickly as possible.

▶ CASE 6

A 7-day-old infant girl is brought into the emergency department unconscious. Her parents accompany her and report a history of an uneventful pregnancy and delivery at 39 weeks' gestational age, with no unusual postnatal events, and discharge on day of life 2. The parents report that the infant's behavior was normal during the first 3 days at home, but for the past 2 days she has not wanted to feed as much. They were not terribly concerned until about an hour before admission when she became difficult and then impossible to awaken. Emergency department personnel report that they already have plans to evaluate the infant for a cardiac lesion and infectious disease.

Question 6-1

What are the most important immediate steps in evaluation and treatment of this critically ill infant?
A) Obtain an electrocardiogram (ECG) to look for occult arrhythmia.
B) Measure glucose, lactic acid, and ammonia, and start IV fluids with at least 10% dextrose concentration.
C) Start the infant on ampicillin and gentamicin for presumed sepsis.
D) Await the results of an echocardiogram before making further management decisions.
E) Obtain plasma amino acids and urine organic acids to look for metabolic disease.

Discussion 6-1

The correct answer is "B." When a child presents with a critical illness, it is vitally important to determine acid-base status, ammonia level, and blood glucose, as these will have immediate management implications and results will be quickly available. The usefulness of dextrose-containing IV fluids cannot be overstated, as most inborn errors of metabolism feature some amount of volume depletion and even if hypoglycemia is not present, dextrose provides a ready energy supply and suppresses catabolism. In some metabolic disorders, a further cardiac evaluation is appropriate, but it would be difficult to argue that it should be the most important step. Likewise, although ordering an echocardiogram and placing the patient on antibiotics are both reasonable in the management of a critically ill infant, evaluation for an inborn error of metabolism should not wait. Plasma amino acids and urine organic acids are also indicated for this patient, but in most locations they will need to be sent out to a biochemical laboratory and will not be back for several days. Even those fortunate enough to have an in-house biochemistry lab that performs these tests will have to wait for the results, and it would not be acceptable to wait for results before providing treatment for the patient.

► CASE 7

You are asked to see a formerly premature male infant in the neonatal intensive care unit (NICU) for hypoglycemia. The infant was born at 34 weeks' gestational age, and did not require ventilation, although he was on oxygen for a short period of time. The infant, now 38 weeks' corrected gestational age, has continued to struggle somewhat with feeding. He is rather large for his gestational age and continues to require a rather high rate of glucose infusion. You note that he does not have hepatomegaly. His most recent serum glucose level was 76 mg/dL, and he continues to receive a 12.5% dextrose concentration infusion. If the glucose infusion is stopped, serum glucose levels drift down rather quickly. The NICU providers have started an evaluation for hypoglycemia, and neither ketosis nor lactic acidosis has been seen.

Question 7-1

What class of disorder is most likely the cause of this patient's hypoglycemia?
A) Congenital hyperinsulinism.
B) Glycogen storage disease.
C) Ketotic hypoglycemia.
D) Organic aciduria.
E) Congenital disorder of glycosylation type 1a (CDG1a).

Discussion 7-1

The correct answer is "A." The fact that the infant is large for gestational age and has hypoketotic hypoglycemia in the absence of organomegaly is suggestive of hyperinsulinism. (See Figure 21–1.) Glycogen storage diseases generally present with organomegaly. Ketotic hypoglycemia is excluded by the text of the case study. (Were you reading carefully?) An organic aciduria is unlikely given the infant's prominent hypoglycemia without prominent acidosis. Congenital disorders of glycosylation can cause hypoglycemia, although it is not prominently featured in CDG1a. Fatty acid oxidation disorders present after the neonatal period with hypoketotic hypoglycemia after fasting or during an illness.

► CASE 8

A female neonate is evaluated at 5 days of age for poor feeding and alteration in the level of consciousness. The mother's pregnancy was normal, and the infant was delivered at 39 weeks' gestational age with Apgar scores of 9 and 9 at 1 and 5 minutes, respectively. There were no problems in the immediate postnatal period. The neonate has two older siblings who are healthy. Examination reveals a normally sized and nondysmorphic neonate who is listless with poor tone

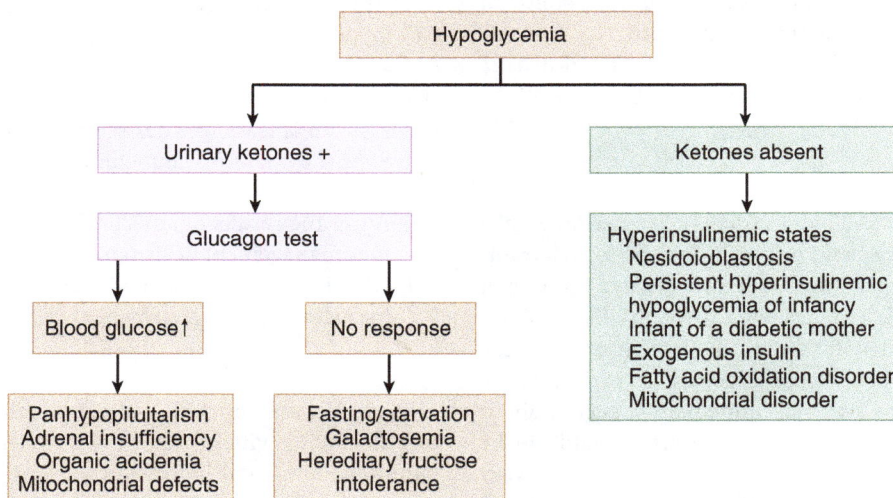

FIGURE 21–1. Simplified diagnostic approach to hypoglycemia. (Reproduced with permission from Tintinalli JE, Stapczynski JS, Ma OJ, Yealy DM, Cline DM, Meckler GD, eds. *Tintinalli's Emergency Medicine: A Comprehensive Study Guide.* 8th ed. New York, NY: McGraw-Hill Education; 2016, Fig. 144-1.)

and prolonged capillary refill. There is no organomegaly, and the cardiac examination is normal.

Question 8-1

What is the most important next step in this neonate's evaluation and management?

A) Evaluation should start with glucose, blood gases, lactic acid level, ammonia level, and serum ketones.

B) Plasma amino acids, urine organic acids, and acylcarnitine profile should be obtained.

C) IV fluids containing 10% dextrose should be started at 1.5 times the maintenance rate.

D) Both A and C.

E) None of the above.

Discussion 8-1

The correct answer is "D." Patients who are critically ill and are suspected of having an inborn error of metabolism should have their acid-base status, glucose level, and ammonia level measured immediately upon presentation. However, one should not wait until those results are available to begin treatment with dextrose-containing IV fluids, which can be lifesaving. Measurement of the plasma amino acids, urine organic acids, and acylcarnitine profile is very important for making a definitive biochemical diagnosis, but those results will be unavailable for some time and it would be inappropriate to wait for treatment.

▶ CASE 9

A 4-month-old girl is brought to the emergency department after an initial seizure. Her serum glucose is low at 37 mg/dL, and lactic acid is moderately elevated. She is noted on examination to have massive hepatomegaly, and her face is described as "doll-like" with rather chubby cheeks. While in the hospital, the infant's glucose level starts to drop after only 2 hours, and administration of glucagon does not improve serum glucose, but does transiently worsen lactic acidosis.

Question 9-1

What is the most likely reason for the infant's clinical findings?

A) A defect in beta-oxidation of medium-chain fatty acids.

B) A defect in phosphatase, which converts glucose-6-phosphate into glucose.

C) A defect in the enzyme that converts phenylalanine into tyrosine.

D) A defect in the myophosphorylase activity in skeletal muscle.

E) A defect in metabolism of sphingolipids.

Discussion 9-1

The correct answer is "B." Defects in glucose-6-phosphatase cause glycogen storage disease type I (GSD I, von Gierke disease), which results classically in hepatomegaly and also

frequently causes hypoglycemia, which can happen after a rather short fast. Glucagon does not raise the blood glucose level as glycogen cannot be utilized. Defects of fatty acid oxidation can certainly cause hypoglycemia with fasting, although typically this occurs after prolonged fasts. Additionally, these defects generally do not cause hepatomegaly to the degree seen in this case. Conversely, disorders of sphingolipids may cause hepatomegaly but do not frequently cause hypoglycemia. Defects in metabolism of phenylalanine to tyrosine cause phenylketonuria and would cause neither hypoglycemia nor hepatomegaly. Lastly, myophosphorylase deficiency causes glycogen storage disease type V (GSD V, McArdle disease), which frequently causes muscle cramping and breakdown, but without hepatomegaly.

▶ CASE 10

An infant with severe hypotonia is referred to the clinic for evaluation. The infant also has failure to thrive, recurrent respiratory infections, and cardiac hypertrophy. Acid alpha-glucosidase level is measured on a dried blood spot and is found to be less than 1% of normal. Molecular analysis of the GAA gene shows that the infant is homozygous for the common p.Arg854Ter mutation, confirming diagnosis of GSD II (Pompe disease). Enzyme replacement therapy (ERT) is the mainstay of treatment in patients with Pompe disease.

Question 10-1

What can be stated about the use or efficacy of ERT in this disease?

A) Timing of therapy has little bearing on the outcomes for patients who are treated.

B) ERT is helpful in reducing cardiac disease burden but does not affect the course of disease for skeletal muscle.

C) Infusion reactions are common and usually require the patient to discontinue therapy.

D) IgG-antibodies to ERT seem to have little bearing on the efficacy of the treatment.

E) Patients who commence treatment in the first 6 months of life have better ventilator-independent survival, cardiac outcomes, and developmental milestones.

Discussion 10-1

The correct answer is "E." Pompe disease in its classic infantile form causes hypertrophic cardiomyopathy, severe generalized hypotonia followed by death from cardiopulmonary failure by 1 year of age. Patients who commence treatment early generally have better responses to therapy, although not all patients respond equally. Therefore, timing is important in treatment. Patients may have improvements in both cardiac and muscle disease. Infusion reactions occur in about half of patients who are being treated, although it is usually possible to continue treatment. High-titer IgG antibodies may reduce the efficacy of enzyme replacement therapy.

► CASE 11

An 16-year-old boy who plays left tackle for his high school football team complains of cramping in his muscles after practice. You, as the team physician, dig a bit further and find that he has experienced a number of such episodes, usually after fairly strenuous practices. Laboratory evaluation shows normal glucose at 97 mg/dL, normal blood urea nitrogen (BUN) of 12 mg/dL, and normal creatinine at 1.0 mg/dL. His creatine kinase (CK) was markedly elevated at 2216 IU/L. The patient denies use of performance-enhancing substances and a urine drug screen is normal. You wonder about a glycogen storage disease as a cause of his problems.

Question 11-1

Which of the following is the most likely cause of this patient's findings?
A) GSD type II.
B) GSD type III.
C) GSD type V.
D) GSD type VI.
E) GSD type VII.

Discussion 11-1

The correct answer is "C." Patients with GSD V (McArdle disease) present with muscle cramping, poor exercise tolerance, and rhabdomyolysis. It would not be uncommon for a patient to present in adolescence during strenuous athletic activities. GSD II (Pompe disease) is a lysosomal storage disease that manifests with skeletal and cardiac findings. Although adult-onset forms of this condition exist, this patient's presentation would be atypical for that condition. GSD III is a liver glycogen storage disease that causes hepatosplenomegaly and myopathy. It would be an unlikely presentation in an otherwise healthy adolescent. GSD VI (Hers disease) and VII (Tarui disease) are rarer GSDs.

> **Helpful Tip**
> Glycogen storage diseases can be challenging to diagnose and have very different presentations. Patients with GSD I (von Gierke disease) present with low blood glucose, fasting intolerance, growth failure, and hepatosplenomegaly. Patients with GSD II (Pompe disease) present with muscle weakness and heart failure, and also hepatosplenomegaly. Enzyme replacement is available for this condition. Patients with GSD III present with hepatosplenomegaly and myopathy. Patients with GSD V (McArdle disease) present with exercise-induced cramps and rhabdomyolysis. Other forms of GSD manifest variably with hepatosplenomegaly, muscle weakness or cramping, hypoglycemia, and growth concerns.

► CASE 12

A 6-day-old girl presents to the emergency department with her parents, who relate a history of decreased level of consciousness that has worsened over the past 48 hours. The parents state that they received a call from the state laboratory about an abnormality the infant's newborn screen but did not understand what the concern was. On examination, the infant has tachypnea and decreased level of alertness with poor capillary refill. She is otherwise nondysmorphic. Laboratory evaluation shows metabolic acidosis, and interestingly the urine shows the presence of reducing sugars. Blood cultures are drawn and broad-spectrum antibiotic therapy is commenced. Within 12 hours, both sets of blood cultures show growth of a pathologic organism.

Question 12-1

Given the presentation of the patient, which organism is most likely to have been found?
A) *Streptococcus pyogenes.*
B) *Escherichia coli.*
C) *Staphylococcus aureus.*
D) *Streptococcus pneumoniae.*
E) *Klebsiella pneumoniae.*

Discussion 12-1

The correct answer is "B." The case history for this patient includes clues to the diagnosis of galactosemia, including evidence of sepsis at presentation, an abnormal newborn screen, and presence of reducing sugars on urinalysis (indicating errors in sugar metabolism). Galactose and glucose form the disaccharide lactose. One important aspect of galactosemia is its association with sepsis in patients who do not have prompt treatment, *E. coli* being the most common organism isolated in such cases. Therefore, for the primary care provider, it is crucial that these patients be placed on galactose-free feeding (no lactose) as soon as a diagnosis is made. Other findings include liver dysfunction and cataracts. Remember, soy formula is the drink of choice in galactosemia.

After stabilization of the patient, you as the diligent pediatrician call the state laboratory to find out exactly what was abnormal on the newborn screen. However, since you studied metabolic diseases extensively in preparing for your examination you already have a pretty good idea of what was found.

Question 12-2

What laboratory abnormality should you suspect in this patient?
A) Elevation of C8 (octanoylcarnitine).
B) Elevation of phenylalanine and decreased tyrosine.
C) Presence of succinylacetone.
D) Reduced activity of galactose-1-phosphate uridyltransferase (GALT).
E) Reduced activity of biotinidase.

Discussion 12-2

The correct answer is "D." Classic galactosemia is caused by mutations in the gene that encodes the galactose-1-phosphate uridyltransferase enzyme (GALT). GALT is part of the enzymatic pathway that metabolizes galactose to glucose for energy utilization. Elevation of octanylcarnitine is typical of a diagnosis of medium-chain acyl-CoA dehydrogenase deficiency (MCADD). Elevation of phenylalanine with decreased tyrosine is seen in patients with phenylketonuria (PKU). Presence of succinylacetone is seen in patients with type I tyrosinemia. Reduced activity of biotinidase would, of course, be seen in biotinidase deficiency.

Your patient has recovered well from her acute health problem and is thriving with the benefit of appropriate dietary intervention. Thus far her growth and development have been normal, to the delight of her parents.

Question 12-3

In addition to providing them advice about the recurrence risk of this condition, what should you tell the parents about long-term sequelae that may not be prevented by diet?
A) All long-term sequelae are preventable by dietary interventions.
B) Learning disability and premature ovarian failure are more common.
C) Liver failure is unavoidable and not prevented by diet.
D) Cataract development occurs in treated and untreated patients at the same frequency.

Discussion 12-3

The correct answer is "B." Patients with classic galactosemia have an increased risk of learning disabilities, speech deficits, and premature ovarian failure, which does not appear to be prevented, even with scrupulous adherence to diet. Liver failure is a complication that is typically seen in patients when treatment is delayed or not commenced. Cataract development appears to be more common in patients who are untreated, but it does not appear that risk of cataract is eliminated in patients who are treated with diet.

> **Helpful Tip**
> Galactosemia is associated with sepsis, particularly *E. coli.*

▶ CASE 13

An 18-month-old girl presents to the clinic with findings of poor linear growth and developmental delay. Her facial features are becoming coarse, and she has developed an inability to fully extend the joints. On further investigation, you note that she has corneal clouding and hepatosplenomegaly.

Question 13-1

What is the most likely diagnosis in this patient?
A) Krabbe disease.
B) Fabry disease.
C) Hurler syndrome (MPS I).
D) Hunter syndrome (MPS II).
E) Morquio disease (MPS IV).

Discussion 13-1

The correct answer is "C." Patients with Hurler syndrome tend to present very early in life with typical features of mucopolysaccharidosis (MPS) such as hepatosplenomegaly, developmental delay, coarse facial features, and limitations in joint movement. (See Figure 21–2). MPS is a lysosomal storage disorder in which glycosaminoglycans accumulate in the lysosomes. Corneal clouding is present in MPS I. Other features include short stature, skeletal dysplasia, hearing loss, hydrocephalus, and persistent nasal drainage. MPS II shares a number of features with MPS I, but it has an X-linked inheritance pattern and does not feature corneal clouding, both of which would be inconsistent with the findings described for this child. Patients with MPS IV may present with short stature but not cognitive delays. The description given is also inconsistent with diagnoses of Krabbe disease and Fabry disease.

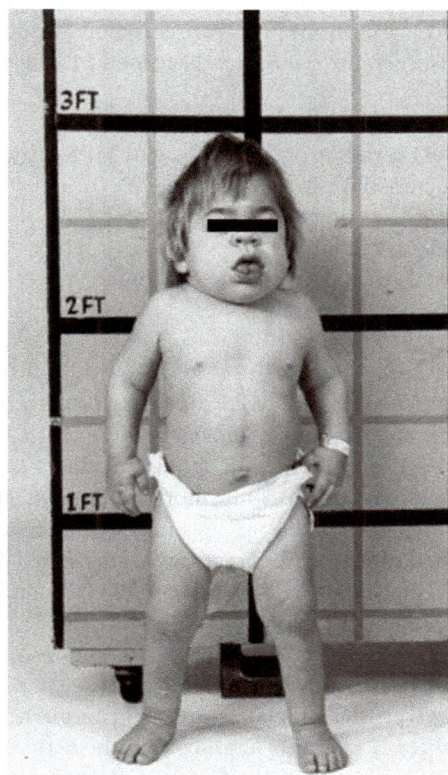

FIGURE 21–2. This child has a mucopolysaccharidosis type I (Hurler syndrome) characterized by short stature, coarse facies, enlarged tongue, joint stiffness, developmental delay, and hepatomegaly. An enzymatic defect results in the accumulation of glycosaminoglycans in the lysosomes. (Reproduced with permission from Valle D, Beaudet AL, Vogelstein B et al: *The Online Metabolic and Molecular Bases of Inherited Disease*, 8ed. McGraw-Hill Education, Inc; 2014. Fig 136-6.)

Helpful Tip

In comparing MPS I and II, remember that a hunter needs clear eyesight, so Hunter syndrome (MPS II) does not have corneal clouding, whereas Hurler syndrome (MPS I) does.

Question 13-2

Which of the following laboratory investigations would be the most likely to provide a definitive diagnosis in this patient?

A) Carbohydrate-deficient transferrin.
B) Very long-chain fatty acids.
C) Acylcarnitine profile.
D) Lactic acid level.
E) Urine glycosaminoglycans.

Discussion 13-2

The correct answer is "E." Patients with mucopolysaccharidoses have characteristic patterns of abnormalities on urine glycosaminoglycan (GAG) profile, and this is likely to make the diagnosis. Carbohydrate-deficient transferrin is used to diagnosis congenital disorders of glycosylation, which are not suspected in this patient. Very long-chain fatty acids are used to diagnose peroxisomal disorder, which we also do not expect here. Lactic acid level and acylcarnitine profile are common tests to screen for metabolic disorders but would not diagnose a patient with MPS I.

Question 13-3

Which is NOT a radiographic finding of MPS disorders?

A) Delayed cranial suture closing.
B) Thick ribs.
C) Hypoplastic flared iliac bones.
D) Metacarpals with narrowing proximally.
E) Coarse trabeculated long bones.

Discussion 13-3

The correct answer is "A." MPS disorders produce characteristic skeletal abnormalities known as dysostosis multiplex. Therefore, diagnostic evaluation should include a skeletal survey. Radiographic signs include short, thick long bones with irregular metaphyses and epiphyses; thick ribs; enlarged skull with thickened calvarium and craniosynostosis; ovoid vertebral bodies; and gibbus deformity (thoracolumbar spine kyphosis). Closure of the sutures is premature, not delayed.

Congenital hyperinsulinism can be a cause of particularly severe hypoglycemia, which requires continuous administration of significant amounts of glucose in the neonatal period.

Question 13-4

Which of the following long-term interventions would be appropriate for this patient?

A) Therapy with diazoxide.
B) Therapy with octreotide.
C) Partial resection of the pancreas.
D) High-carbohydrate diet.
E) All of the above.

Discussion 13-4

The correct answer is "E." Patients with hyperinsulinism may require any of all of these interventions depending on the severity of disease. Pharmacologic therapy and dietary therapy by themselves may not be sufficient to decrease insulin secretion, and in some patients a partial pancreatectomy may be required to reduce the bulk of beta islet cells and insulin secretion.

▶ CASE 14

A 6-year-old child presents with onset of acute abdominal pain, and pancreatitis is diagnosed. This is the second presentation of pancreatitis for this child. His parents report that he is otherwise healthy and takes no medication. On physical exam he also has hepatosplenomegaly and xanthomas on his elbows and Achilles tendons.

Question 14-1

What laboratory investigation is most likely to lead to the correct diagnosis for this patient?

A) Lactic acid.
B) Lipid panel.
C) Fingerstick glucose.
D) Urine organic acids.
E) Carbohydrate-deficient transferrin.

Discussion 14-1

The correct answer is "B." This patient has a disorder of lipoprotein metabolism, in this case familial lipoprotein lipase deficiency. Patients with this disorder present in childhood with severe hypertriglyceridemia, pancreatitis, cutaneous xanthomata, and hepatosplenomegaly. They may also have accumulation of chylomicrons in the blood, giving a milky appearance that may be appreciated with phlebotomy. Although lactic acid and urine organic acids are frequently measured in patients with metabolic disorders, they are unlikely to be helpful in this instance. Patients with pancreatitis may indeed have deviations in their glucose level, but such discovery is unlikely to lead toward a diagnosis. Transferrin isoelectric focusing may show a carbohydrate-deficient pattern in patients with congenital disorders of glycosylation but is unlikely to shed any light on a lipoprotein disorder.

▶ CASE 15

A family presents to the clinic with their two children, aged 2 and 5 years, who are known to be healthy. The father, who is 34 years old, relates a personal history of extremely premature

cardiovascular disease with coronary artery bypass grafting at age 26. He is presently taking three different lipid-lowering agents to control his extremely high low-density lipoprotein (LDL) cholesterol.

Question 15-1

Assuming that the father is homozygous for familial hypercholesterolemia, what should you tell him about the proper next step in management for his children?
A) Begin weekly LDL apheresis.
B) Reassure the father that his children are unlikely to be affected.
C) Commence high-dose HMG-CoA reductase therapy in both children.
D) Commence bile acid sequestrant therapy in both children.
E) Order a lipid panel and institute appropriate lifestyle changes.

Discussion 15-1

The correct answer is "E." If the father in this scenario is a homozygote for familial hypercholesterolemia, his children would be obligate heterozygotes and in this condition heterozygotes also have elevated serum cholesterol and increased risk of disease, with 50% of men and 25% of women affected having coronary artery disease by age 50. In very young children who have heterozygous familial hypercholesterolemia (HeFH), it would be appropriate to start measurement of a lipid panel at age 2 years. However, it would not be appropriate to start definitive therapy such as bile acid sequestrants or statins (HMG-CoA reductase inhibitors) at such a young age. LDL apheresis is used in some cases for patients with homozygous familial hypercholesterolemia (HoFH), but would not be appropriate in such young children. Telling the parent that the children are unlikely to be affected is inappropriate. The proper course of action in this case is for both children to be screened with a lipid panel. Should any lifestyle factors be contributing to risk, those also should be addressed. The present guidelines suggest treatment of children with HeFH using statin medications starting at age 8 years.

⧖ QUICK QUIZ

Type I Gaucher disease is a relatively common disorder of sphingolipid metabolism that leads to health concerns involving multiple organ systems.

Which of the following findings would NOT be consistent with a diagnosis of Gaucher disease type I?
A) Hepatosplenomegaly.
B) Low bone mineral density.
C) Intellectual disability.
D) Thrombocytopenia .
E) Interstitial lung disease.

Discussion

The correct answer is "C." Gaucher disease is a lysosomal storage disease—specifically involving sphingolipidoses—that affects the cell's ability to recycle cellular glycolipids. Lysosomes are the digestive system of the cell. In Gaucher disease, glycolipids build up in the lysosomes of macrophages. The lipid-laden macrophages then accumulate in affected organs (liver, spleen, lungs, bone marrow). Type I Gaucher disease is characterized by a number of conditions, including hepatosplenomegaly, low bone density, and painful bone crises. Patients also may have leukopenia, thrombocytopenia, and anemia in any combination or together. They may suffer from a variety of lung diseases, including interstitial lung disease and pulmonary hypertension. There is some evidence to suggest that monoclonal gammopathies, including multiple myeloma, may be more common in patients with Gaucher disease than in the general population. Intellectual disability would be inconsistent with a diagnosis of Gaucher disease. Gaucher disease is treated by replacement of the missing lysosomal enzyme, glucocerebrosidase.

▶ CASE 16

An adolescent boy presents with the lesions shown in Figure 21–3. He has been suffering from episodic pain in his hands and feet that has not been adequately explained. His mother reports that she also has had tingling in her hands for a number of years, but the pain has never been severe.

Question 16-1

Which of the following choices represents a major risk for early death in this adolescent male patient?
A) Hematologic malignancy.
B) Cirrhosis.
C) Immune deficiency.
D) Cerebrovascular disease.
E) Alzheimer dementia.

Discussion 16-1

The correct answer is "D." This patient presents with a history consistent with Fabry disease, which is an X-linked lysosomal storage (sphingolipidosis) disorder arising from deficient activity of the alpha-galactosidase enzyme. Patients with this disorder frequently suffer from painful acroparesthesia (tingling of the extremities), and a large percentage of them present with angiokeratoma. (See Figure 21–3.) As patients age, their risk for cardiovascular and cerebrovascular disease increases. Patients also frequently have renal involvement and progress to end-stage renal disease. Although the classic findings of this condition have been historically described in males (X-linked), it is understood that females may also have manifestations of the disease, which may be relatively mild but can be as severe as those in affected males.

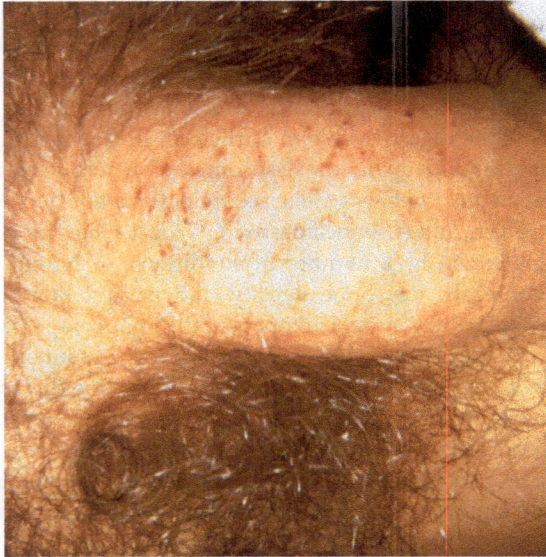

FIGURE 21–3. Patients with Fabry disease develop angiokeratomas such as the one located on the penis in this figure. (Reproduced with permission from Fuster V, Walsh RA, Harrington RA, eds. *Hurst's The Heart*. 13th ed. New York, NY: McGraw-Hill Education; 2011, Fig. 14-11.)

> **Helpful Tip**
> Enzyme replacement therapy (ERT) has revolutionized the treatment of several genetic disorders, and increasing numbers of products are available on the market. The following products are presently available in the United States:
> - For Gaucher disease (lysosomal storage disorder [LSD])—imiglucerase, velaglucerase, taliglucerase
> - For Fabry disease (LSD)—agalsidase beta
> - For Pompe disease (glycogen storage disease [GSD] II)—agalsidase alfa
> - For Hurler disease (mucopolysaccharidosis [MPS] I)—laronidase
> - For Hunter disease (MPS II)—idursulfase
> - For Maroteaux-Lamy disease (MPS VI)—galsulfase
> - For Morquio A disease (MPS IV)—elosulfase alfa

▶ CASE 17

A patient presents in the neonatal period with decreased level of consciousness and inability to feed. The patient has also experienced spells of vomiting and is lethargic on examination. Initial laboratory studies show glucose of 61 mg/dL, a lactic acid level of 3.3 mmol/L, and an ammonia level of 320 mg/dL. The metabolist on call evaluates the patient and tells you that she is concerned for a urea cycle disorder.

Question 17-1

Which of the patient's findings is most specific for a urea cycle disorder?
A) Decreased level of consciousness.
B) Hypoglycemia.

C) Vomiting.
D) Hyperammonemia.
E) Lactic acidosis.

Discussion 17-1

The correct answer is "D." Decreased level of consciousness and vomiting are common signs of a variety of metabolic conditions and are not terribly specific. Likewise, a number of conditions can cause lactic acidosis, particularly mild lactic acidosis. The patient's blood glucose level is also not particularly low, which is often the case in a urea cycle disorder. However, prominent hyperammonemia in a situation such as this is suggestive of a urea cycle disorder as the primary metabolic defect. Early recognition of this significant metabolic disorder is very important for its successful treatment. The longer hyperammonemia is present, the worse the neurologic outcome will be.

Patients with urea cycle disorders may experience symptoms of acute hyperammonemia, but also may experience chronic symptoms if control of the disorder is inadequate. For most patients, this requires daily management of their condition.

Question 17-2

Which of the following treatments is/are indicated for the daily care of a patient with a urea cycle disorder?
A) Carnitine supplementation.
B) Protein restriction.
C) Ammonia scavengers such as sodium phenylbutyrate.
D) Both B and C.
E) Options A, B, and C.

Discussion 17-2

The correct answer is "D." Patients with urea cycle disorders benefit from protein restriction, although the level of protein restriction required varies by patient. Sodium phenylbutyrate is an ammonia scavenger that allows patients with urea cycle disorders to have an alternate pathway for ammonia excretion. Treating patients who have a urea cycle disorder with L-carnitine will probably not harm them, but it is unlikely to be productive.

> **Helpful Tip**
> The urea cycle is responsible for detoxifying ammonia into urea, which can then be easily excreted. (See Figures 21–4 and 21–5.) Ammonia is produced as a byproduct of protein metabolism. The treatment of urea cycle disorders has a few central themes. First, if a person consumes less protein, he or she will also produce less ammonia so protein restriction is recommended. Second, many patients with urea cycle disorders also benefit from amino acid supplements, generally either citrulline or arginine. Third, if dietary therapy and amino acid therapy are not sufficient to control the ammonia level (and they frequently are not), patients will be treated with an ammonia scavenger. The most common oral scavenger is sodium phenylbutyrate, but others exist.

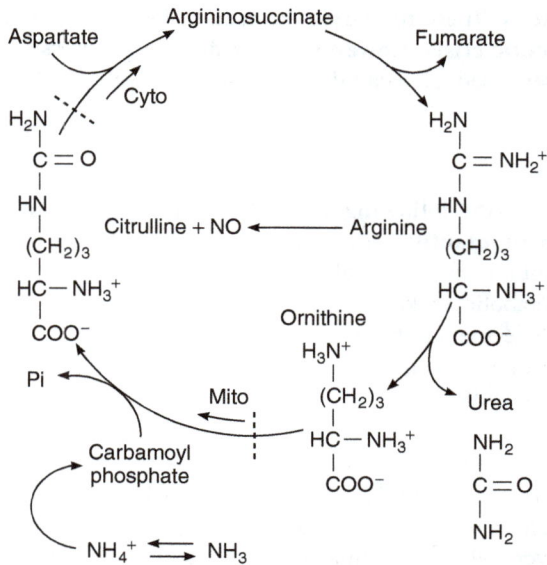

FIGURE 21–4. Urea Cycle. The urea cycle converts ammonia, the byproduct of protein metabolism, into urea for excretion from the body. Disruption of this process results in various degrees of hyperammonemia. Cyto, cytoplasm; Mito, mitochondria. (Reproduced with permission from Barrett KE, Boitano S, Barman SM, Brooks HL, eds. *Ganong's Review of Medical Physiology.* 24th ed. New York, NY: McGraw-Hill Education; 2012, Fig. 1-20.)

▶ CASE 18

A female neonate is brought by her parents to the pediatrics office after 1 day of poor feeding and worsening vomiting over the past few hours. She has a decreased level of consciousness and poor muscle tone. A basic metabolic panel shows a metabolic acidosis with increased anion gap, CBC shows thrombocytopenia and neutropenia, and ammonia is mildly elevated. The neonate was born in a different state and the parents report "there was something wrong with the newborn screening," but since their daughter was doing well they did not follow up on it.

Question 18-1
What is the most likely diagnosis for this neonate?
A) Phenylketonuria.
B) Propionic acidemia.
C) NARP syndrome (neuropathy, ataxia, and retinitis pigmentosa).
D) Medium-chain acyl-CoA dehydrogenase deficiency.
E) Nonketotic hyperglycinemia.

Discussion 18-1
The correct answer is "B." The neonate has findings typical of an organic acidemia, in which patients have a metabolic acidosis

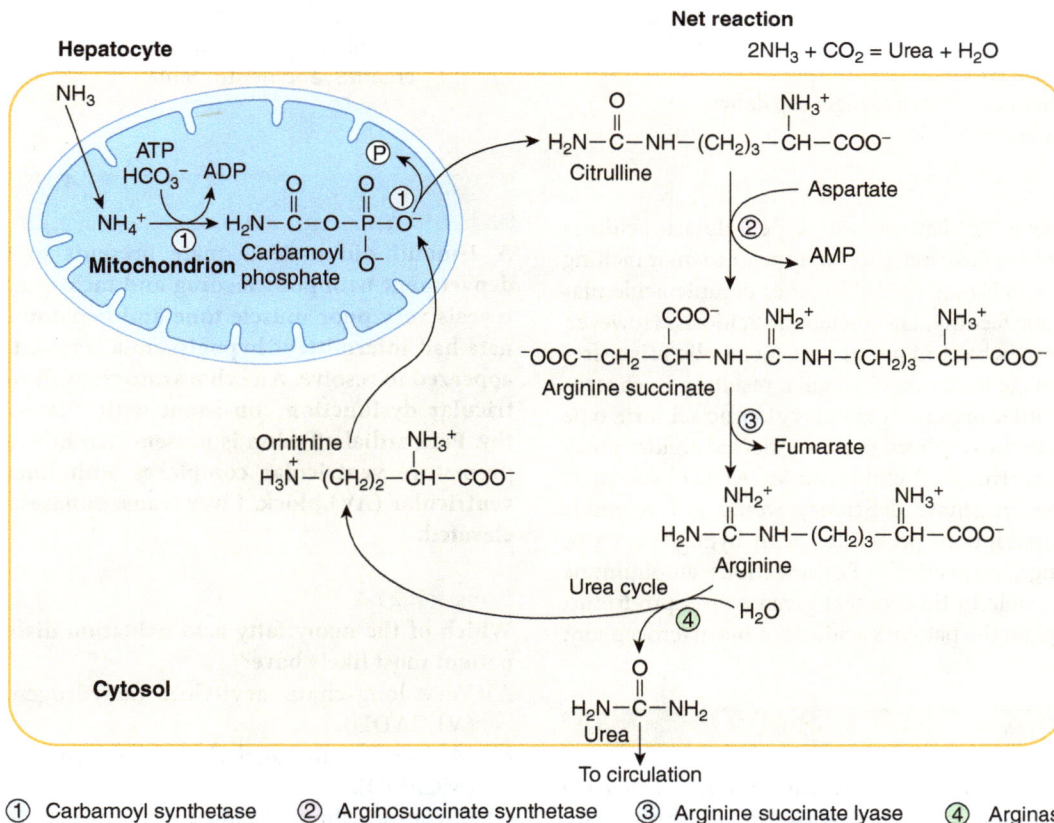

FIGURE 21–5. Urea Cycle. The urea cycle controls the processing of NH_3 to urea for excretion. (Reproduced with permission from Barrett KE, Barman SM, Boitano S, & Brooks HL (Eds). *Ganong's Review of Medical Physiology*, 25th ed. McGraw-Hill Education, Inc., 2016. Fig 1-20.)

and frequently present with poor feeding and vomiting. Patients with organic acidemias also commonly have thrombocytopenia or neutropenia from bone marrow suppression. The history in this case is inconstant with the diagnosis of phenylketonuria, as a neonate with untreated PKU is not likely to have developed symptoms yet. Patients with NARP also likely would not present in the neonatal period, and would not present in this fashion. Patients with MCADD may present early in life with critical illness that is usually caused by hypoglycemia, without prominent acidosis (minimal to no ketones). Nonketotic hyperglycinemia manifests as a neurologic disorder, including encephalopathy and seizures. Acidosis is not a prominent feature.

▶ CASE 19

A 5-year-old boy is brought to the emergency department after 2 days of vomiting and decreased level of consciousness. Laboratory evaluation shows significant metabolic acidosis. He had previously been healthy, but several days before vomiting started had an apparently mild viral illness. The boy has had generally normal growth, but has significant macrocephaly that has not been well-explained. Since admission, he has been medically stable but has developed unusual choreoathetoid movements.

Question 19-1

What disorder best fits the patient's clinical findings?
A) 3-Methylcrotonyl-CoA carboxylase deficiency.
B) Medium-chain acyl-CoA dehydrogenase deficiency.
C) Glutaric aciduria type I.
D) Succinate semialdehyde dehydrogenase deficiency.
E) Postinfectious encephalitis.

Discussion 19-1

The correct answer is "C." Patients with type I glutaric aciduria frequently are noted to have macrocephaly prior to their inciting metabolic crisis, which may resemble other organic acidemias with vomiting, poor feeding, and metabolic acidosis. However, the disorder is somewhat unique in that metabolic crises frequently cause damage to the basal ganglia, resulting in choreoathetosis. Unlike other organic acidemias glutaric aciduria type I rarely manifests in the newborn period. Affected children may have subdural hemorrhages. A child with MCADD or succinate semialdehyde dehydrogenase deficiency would not resemble the boy in this description, presenting with hypoglycemia or neurologic findings, respectively. Postinfectious autoimmune encephalitis is possible in this context given a viral prodrome, but would not explain the patient's acidosis or his macrocephaly.

▶ CASE 20

Patients with methylmalonic academia require intensive long-term management of their disease. In the short term, the focus becomes dietary in nature with implementation of a low-protein diet, and in some patients routine cobalamin

injections. These measures are used to keep the patient out of acidotic crisis. However, as the disease progresses, many long-term sequelae can develop that are problematic for the patient.

Question 20-1

Which of the following is NOT a typical long-term consequence of infantile-onset methylmalonic acidemia?
A) Tubulointerstitial nephritis.
B) Metabolic stroke.
C) Intellectual disability.
D) Cardiomyopathy.
E) Pancreatitis.

Discussion 20-1

The correct answer is "D." Cardiomyopathy is not a typical long-term effect of methylmalonic acidemia, an organic acidemia. However, tubulointerstitial nephritis, metabolic stroke, intellectual disability, and pancreatitis can also be seen in patients with this condition. These can occur even in patients with good dietary control who do not have recurrent metabolic crises.

> **Helpful Tip**
> Patients with organic acidemias can present early in the neonatal period with lethargy, vomiting, hypotonia, irritability, and acidosis. These are nonspecific findings and mimic sepsis, but should always be considered in such a patient. Chronic sequelae of organic acidemia can include metabolic stroke, pancreatitis, and neutropenia.

▶ CASE 21

A 2-month-old male neonate presents to the emergency department with poor feeding and tachypnea. Examination reveals very poor muscle tone and hepatomegaly. The neonate had intermittent hypoglycemia soon after birth, which appeared to resolve. An echocardiogram shows severe biventricular dysfunction consistent with dilated cardiomyopathy. Pericardial effusion is present. An ECG shows frequent premature ventricular complexes with intermittent atrioventricular (AV) block. Liver transaminases are moderately elevated.

Question 21-1

Which of the many fatty acid oxidation disorders does this patient most likely have?
A) Very long-chain acyl-CoA dehydrogenase deficiency (VLCADD).
B) Medium-chain acyl-CoA dehydrogenase deficiency (MCADD).
C) Carnitine palmitoyltransferase 1 (CPT-1) deficiency.
D) Short-chain acyl-CoA dehydrogenase deficiency (SCADD).
E) Long-chain acyl-CoA dehydrogenase deficiency (LCADD).

Discussion 21-1

The correct answer is "A." Patients with VLCADD are at high risk for cardiac manifestations, such as dilated cardiomyopathy with heart failure and arrhythmia, and also may have hypoglycemia and hepatic dysfunction. Patients with long-chain 3-hydroxyacyl-CoA dehydrogenase (LCHAD) deficiency may also have cardiac manifestations. Patients with MCADD, SCADD, or CPT-1 often have other manifestations of disease, but a predominantly cardiac presentation would be unusual. "Long-chain acyl-CoA dehydrogenase deficiency" (LCADD) sounds like a very worrisome disorder, but as far as we know it does not actually exist. Don't confuse LCHAD (real) with LCADD (not real).

⏳ QUICK QUIZ

Which is the most likely diagnosis in a patient presenting in early childhood with hypoglycemia who has excessive amount of total carnitine in an acylcarnitine analysis?
A) Very long-chain acyl-CoA dehydrogenase deficiency (VLCADD).
B) Medium-chain acyl-CoA dehydrogenase deficiency (MCADD).
C) Carnitine palmitoyltransferase 1 (CPT-1) deficiency.
D) Short-chain acyl-CoA dehydrogenase deficiency (SCADD).
E) Long-chain acyl-CoA dehydrogenase deficiency (LCADD).

Discussion

The correct answer is "C." CPT-1 is the rate-limiting step for transport of fatty acids into the mitochondria, and is unique in that it shows elevations in C0, or unesterified carnitine. Patients frequently present early in life with hypoketotic hypoglycemia after fasting. They may also develop liver dysfunction and renal tubular disorders. Patients with VLCADD tend to have elevations in C14, C14:1, and C14:2. Patients with MCADD have elevations in C8. Patients with SCADD have elevations in C4. LCADD does not exist. (Were you paying attention when you read the preceding question?)

Helpful Tip

It is important to understand what tests to order to confirm the diagnosis of a metabolic disorder.
• Order plasma amino acids for urea cycle defects and amino acid disorders
• Order urine organic acids for organic acidemias
• Order an acylcarnitine profile for fatty acid oxidation disorders

---

▶ CASE 22

Worried parents bring their 4-month-old son to the clinic because of motor weakness and low muscle tone, which they feel is getting worse. While you are interviewing the parents, one of your nurses opens the examination room door and then closes it again. You note that the infant startles in an obvious manner, with extension of his arms and legs. On examination you are not able to get the boy to track visually, and a macular cherry red spot is visible on funduscopic examination. On palpation, there is no organomegaly.

Question 22-1

What is the most likely diagnosis in this patient?
A) Krabbe disease.
B) Tay-Sachs disease.
C) Niemann Pick disease type A.
D) Gaucher disease.
E) Metachromatic leukodystrophy sphingolipidoses.

Discussion 22-1

The correct answer is "B." Tay-Sachs disease, a lysosomal storage disorder (sphingolipidosis), is characterized by the early onset of hypotonia and muscular weakness. Often, visual tracking is lost very early in the disease process. Patients have a "cherry red" spot on the macula that is typical of this condition and some other related conditions. (See Figure 21–6.) An exaggerated startle reflex is characteristic as well. Children with Tay-Sachs disease have a relentless clinical course characterized by neurologic deterioration, seizures, and blindness. Average life expectancy for a child with acute infantile Tay-Sachs disease is less than 4 years. Although patients with Gaucher disease or Niemann-Pick type A (which are other sphingolipidoses) can have the cherry red spot, both of those disorders feature prominent hepatosplenomegaly, and patients with neuronopathic forms of Gaucher disease may have neurodegeneration. Patients with Krabbe disease present in infancy with irritability, spasticity, and developmental delay, with regression and evidence of leukodystrophy on neuroimaging. Metachromatic leukodystrophy generally manifests

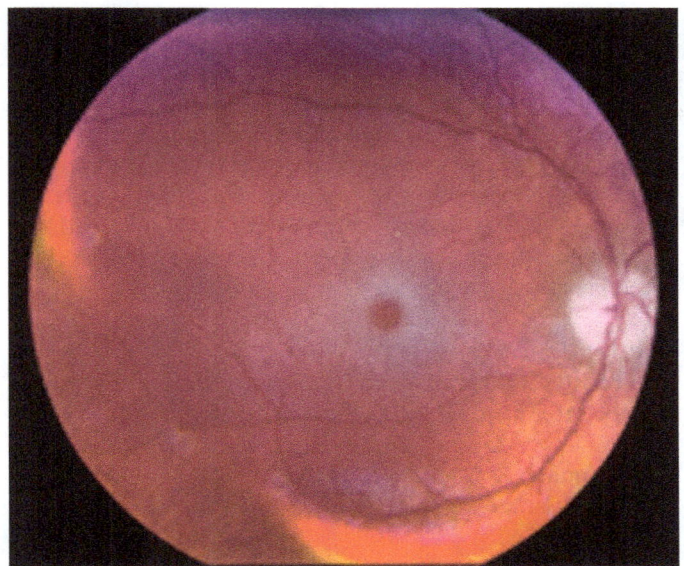

FIGURE 21–6. Tay-Sachs Disease. A cherry red spot is present on the macula in patients with Tay-Sachs, Gaucher, and Niemann-Pick type A diseases, all of which are sphingolipidoses, a type of lysosomal storage disorder. (Reproduced with permission from the National Institute of Health (NIH) and the National Eye Institute.)

after 1 year of age with weakness and hypotonia. Children who have gained speech eventually lose that ability, and vision and hearing are lost. If your patient has an exaggerated startle reflex and a cherry red spot, think Tay-Sachs disease.

The parents have brought their now 12-month-old child with hexosaminidase A deficiency for follow-up care. He has continued to suffer from the effects of the disease, and his mother asks you what interventions are appropriate for his supportive care.

Question 22-2

Which of the following interventions would NOT be appropriate?

A) Ensuring adequate nutrition.
B) Pharmacologic treatment of seizures.
C) Management of airway and respiratory compromise.
D) Treatment of chronic constipation.
E) Enzyme replacement therapy.

Discussion 22-2

The correct answer is "E." Tay-Sachs disease is caused by a deficiency of the enzyme hexosaminidase A. At present, no enzyme replacement therapy exists. Several strategies to treat this disease have been proposed but none is approved at the present time. Supportive care is indicated for children with this condition and includes nutritional support and management of respiratory concerns. Chronic constipation and seizures are also typical problems seen as the disease progresses, and their management is also appropriate. Honest discussion among family members and medical providers regarding the goals of therapy is appropriate to ensure that medical interventions are implemented with the goal of relieving suffering and not merely because the option exists.

▶ CASE 23

A patient presents in the neonatal period with lethargy and hypotonia. The neonate subsequently develops myoclonus and spells of central apnea, and requires mechanical ventilation for 3 weeks before starting to recover spontaneous respiration. An electroencephalogram (EEG) is obtained and shows a burst-suppression pattern. Laboratory studies show a notable absence of ketosis or acidosis.

Question 23-1

What amino acid is likely to be elevated in both the plasma and the cerebrospinal fluid of this neonate?

A) Glycine.
B) Threonine.
C) Phenylalanine.
D) Methionine.
E) Proline.

Discussion 23-1

The correct answer is "A." This neonate has nonketotic hyperglycinemia (also known as glycine encephalopathy), presenting with the typical neurologic findings of this condition, including a classic burst-suppression EEG pattern. The patient does not have ketosis or acidosis, which distinguishes this disorder from other organic acidemias that have been variably described as ketotic hypoglycemias (a somewhat archaic description). Elevations in threonine are exceedingly rare, although at least one case report from 1978 describes this finding in a male infant. Elevations in phenylalanine are typically seen in patients with phenylketonuria (PKU), but these patients are normal at birth with neurologic findings that develop over time. Elevations in methionine can be seen in patients as a reflection of an immature liver or with hepatocellular damage. They can also be seen in patients with cystathione beta-synthetase deficiency (homocystinuria) or methionine adenosyltransferase deficiency. Elevations in proline are seen in patients with hyperprolinemia, which is often asymptomatic but can cause seizures and intellectual disability.

▶ CASE 24

Maple syrup urine disease is a disorder of branched-chain amino acids, and the specific cause is a decrease in the activity in the branched-chain alpha-ketoacid dehydrogenase complex. If untreated, the disease leads to ketonuria, poor feeding, and encephalopathy. Patients with this condition have a maple syrup or burnt sugar smell to their body fluids, particularly the cerumen in the ear canals.

Question 24-1

Which of the following amino acids is not considered a branched-chain amino acid that would be elevated in a patient with maple syrup urine disease?

A) Leucine.
B) Isoleucine.
C) Alloleucine.
D) Histadine.
E) Valine.

Discussion 24-1

The correct answer is "D." Histadine is not a branched-chain amino acid. This is a question you might be able to reason out even if you do not recall any amino acid chemistry. One might assume (correctly) that leucine, isoleucine, and alloleucine share a common chemical structure. This being the case, none of them could be the odd amino acid out. You would only then have to remember either that valine is a branched-chain amino acid or that histadine has an imidazole functional group to arrive at the correct conclusion. If nothing else, you would have a 50-50 shot at guessing right.

▶ CASE 25

Historically phenylketonuria (PKU), an amino acid disorder, has constituted an important share of children with developmental disabilities. The results of untreated PKU can be truly devastating for these individuals. **Although mandatory screening for the disorders means that you are unlikely to manage patients with untreated PKU in your practice, you are very likely to care for a patient who has received treatment for the disorder. Thus it is important to know what the potential complications of untreated PKU could be.**

Question 25-1

All of the following are potential complications in an untreated patient with PKU EXCEPT:

A) Seizure disorder.
B) Cardiomyopathy.
C) Poor pigmentation of the hair and skin.
D) Microcephaly.
E) Severe eczema.

Discussion 25-1

The correct answer is "B." Patients with PKU are not believed to be at risk for cardiomyopathy. Phenylketonuria is an inborn error of metabolism that results from a deficiency of the enzyme phenylalanine hydroxylase, which prevents phenylalanine from being metabolized to tyrosine. The resulting deficiency of tyrosine and buildup of phenylalanine in blood and tissues have widespread effects in the body. Patients with untreated PKU are at risk for severe behavioral problems and intellectual impairments, and can have microcephaly and seizure disorders, with variable structural brain changes visible on MRI. The deficiency in tyrosine results in decreased production of melanin and is also detrimental to the production of dopamine, which contributes to neurocognitive deficits in the brains of patients with untreated PKU. The skin condition and the musty body odor often attributed to the disorder result from excretion of phenylalanine byproducts through alternate means.

....

Treatment of patients with PKU involves the restriction of phenylalanine in the diet and the supplementation of other amino acids to ensure protein sufficiency. However, in many cases additional non–diet-based therapy is appropriate for optimal management.

Question 25-2

Which of the following therapies is approved by the U.S. Food and Drug Administration (FDA) for treatment of PKU?

A) Adeno-associated virus 1 (AAV1)–based gene therapy.
B) Miglustat.
C) IV phenylalanine hydroxylase.
D) Sapropterin hydrochloride.
E) Carglumic acid.

Discussion 25-2

The correct answer is "D." Sapropterin hydrochloride (Kuvan) is FDA-approved for the treatment of PKU. It is a pharmacologic form of the tetrahydrobiopterin cofactor for phenylalanine hydroxylase. Not all patients respond to sapropterin, but those who do can have significant decreases in their blood phenylalanine level. Gene therapy does not yet exist, and IV

phenylalanine hydroxylase is not used, although investigation of enzyme replacement through other pathways is ongoing. Miglustat is substrate reduction therapy for disorders such as Gaucher disease. Carglumic acid is used in a rare urea cycle disorder called NAGS (*N*-acetylglutamate synthase) deficiency.

▶ CASE 26

An 18-year-old patient presents to your practice after a long absence. He is known to have PKU and, after consulting your records, it is clear that he had reasonable adherence to diet at least until age 12, when social problems within his family resulted in poor dietary adherence. Since that time, he has been essentially lost to follow-up. He presents with a case worker as he has recently been released from a brief incarceration for some petty crimes. He now carries diagnoses of bipolar disorder and attention deficient hyperactivity disorder and is being treated with methylphenidate, valproic acid, and sertraline. He is not following a low-phenylalanine diet.

Question 26-1

What is the best next step in his medical management?

A) Measure the patient's intelligence quotient (IQ) to assess level of cognitive functioning.
B) Increase the dosage of sertraline and add a heterocyclic antidepressant.
C) Check the patient's phenylalanine level and restart him on a low-phenylalanine diet.
D) Obtain an MRI of the brain with and without contrast.
E) Refer the patient to psychiatry for evaluation.

Discussion 26-1

The correct answer is "C." Surprisingly, this is not an unheard of scenario. Patients with PKU who are treated throughout the early childhood critical period escape the effects of intellectual impairment that are a well-known consequence of the disorder. However, when the restrictive diet is stopped, patients frequently complain of poor focus, impulsiveness, mood swings, and psychiatric distress. When phenylalanine control is improved, patients report improvement in these symptoms and generally better functioning. Measuring this patient's IQ is unlikely to be helpful in the quest for improving his functioning and well-being as it is likely to be normal, albeit with decreases in attention and perhaps processing speed. Increasing the dosage of sertraline and adding another antidepressant or referral to psychiatry may be reasonable management strategies for a patient with treatment-resistant depression, but would not be the best first step in this case. MRI of the brain in a patient such as this may show white matter changes, but their discovery is unlikely to change management from the prescription for a low-phenylalanine diet. Such white matter changes also commonly resolve when the patient's phenylalanine levels return to better control. The artificial sweetener aspartame contains phenylalanine and must be avoided by patients with PKU, which means no diet soda!

► CASE 27

An 8-year-old boy with previously normal development presents for care after an initial tonic-clonic seizure. He has had a poor appetite and frequent headaches, which have been resistant to conventional therapies. Prior to these episodes, the child had been healthy. The examination is only significant for proximal muscle weakness. Metabolic acidosis is noted, with a lactic acid level of 3.9 mmol/L. Evaluation of a muscle biopsy sample shows ragged red fibers. The family history is significant for mother with type 2 diabetes mellitus and hearing impairment.

Question 27-1

What is the most likely molecular cause of the patient's findings?
A) Deletion located at 1p36.1.
B) Trinucleotide expansion at the *DM2* gene.
C) Missense mutation in the *MT-TL1* gene in the patient's mitochondrial (mt) DNA.
D) Uniparental disomy of chromosome 14.
E) Biallelic loss in the *POLG* gene in the patient's nuclear (n) DNA.

Discussion 27-1

The correct answer is "C." This patient has typical presentation for MELAS (Mitochondrial Encephalopathy, Lactic Acidosis and Stroke) syndrome, a mitochondrial disorder. The mitochondria perform oxidative phosphorylation via their respiratory chain to produce adenosine triphosphate (ATP)—energy. In mitochondrial disorders, the respiratory chain is dysfunctional. This question appears on its face to be impossibly difficult, but there are several important clues in the case description. First, the patient presents with acute onset of neurologic complaints. Second, he has lactic acidosis and ragged red fibers, which are typical of mitochondrial disorders. Third, there is mention that his mother has unusual health concerns, including deafness. Fourth, he has proximal muscle weakness consistent with a myopathy. All of these point toward a mitochondrial disorder, and specifically one that is encoded in the mitochondrial genome as opposed to the nuclear genome. Remember, mtDNA is inherited exclusively from the mother so some disorders are maternally inherited. Others result from nDNA mutations

and can be inherited from either parent. Options "A" and "D" are neurodevelopmental disorders that would be present from infancy; hence, the patient would not have been previously normal. Option "B" describes the typical mutation for type II myotonic dystrophy. Option "E" does describe a mitochondrial disorder, but one that would present differently and most importantly is not consistent with the family history.

► CASE 28

A 17-year-old boy presents to the clinic complaining of bilateral blurring of his central vision. He noted blurring initially in the right eye but did not alert his parents. Over the past week he has noticed onset of blurring in his left eye. He describes no pain with his vision loss. Examination by an ophthalmologist showed disk swelling but was otherwise normal. His maternal grandmother had onset of vision loss in her early 20s and is now legally blind, but no other family members have vision loss.

Question 28-1

What is the most likely natural course for this patient's vision?
A) The patient is unlikely to experience further vision loss.
B) The patient is likely to experience further vision loss acutely, but full recovery is the rule.
C) The patient is likely to experience slow vision loss over the next 10 to 20 years.
D) The patient is likely to experience onset of sensorineural hearing loss along with vision loss.
E) The patient will continue to experience further vision loss and will stabilize only with near-complete vision loss within a few months.

Discussion 28-1

The correct answer is "E." This patient described is experiencing symptoms of Leber hereditary optic neuropathy (LHON), a disorder characterized by painless loss of vision that proceeds to near-complete loss of vision within a few months. This maternally inherited mitochondrial disorder (mtDNA mutation) results in painless bilateral vision loss and typically presents in the teenage years. Most patients experience only vision loss, and males are approximately five times more likely than females to experience vision loss from this condition. It is unlikely that a patient would experience complete or even significant resolution of symptoms, and it is unlikely that hearing loss would be associated with LHON.

► CASE 29

A 2-year-old boy who is developmentally delayed presents with new onset of self-injurious behavior, biting his lips and fingers, sometimes quite severely. He has been hypotonic since shortly after birth and has failed to gain significant motor milestones, with frequent dystonic movements. He was recently diagnosed with choreoathetoid cerebral palsy due to this constellation of findings. His mother notes that her older brother passed away at a young age without diagnosis.

Question 29-1
Overproduction of which molecule could adequately explain this patient's clinical findings?
A) Uric acid.
B) Arginosuccinic acid.
C) Ammonia.
D) Lactic acid.
E) Glycine.

Discussion 29-1
The correct answer is "A." This patient has findings that are typical of Lesch-Nyhan syndrome, including cardinal features of developmental delay, movement disorder such as choreoathetosis or dystonia, and self-injurious behavior, particularly biting behaviors. The latter often start in the second year of life. An X-linked disorder caused by mutations in the *HPRT* (hypoxanthine-guanine phosphoribosyltransferase) gene, Lesch-Nyhan syndrome leads to overproduction of uric acid from impaired purine metabolism. Patients with arginosuccinic aciduria, hyperammonemia, lactic acidemia, or hyperglycinemia generally will not present with movement disorders or self-injurious behavior. Most disorders that would cause these findings would also be autosomal recessive in nature, and the affected maternal uncle is suggestive of an X-linked disorder. Do not forget that biting and self-injurious behaviors are big clues for Lesch-Nyhan syndrome.

▶ CASE 30

An infant with Menkes disease may appear to be normal at birth, with manifestations of neurodegeneration such as seizures and hypotonia only becoming evident by about 3 months of age. However, even at birth if scalp hair (brittle, depigmented) is present it may exhibit the microscopic pili torti that gives Menkes disease its alternate moniker, kinky hair syndrome.

Question 30-1
Disruption of the metabolism of which metal is responsible for this condition?
A) Copper.
B) Cobalt.
C) Zinc.
D) Nickel.
E) Magnesium.

Discussion 30-1
The correct answer is "A." Although a large number of metals have important activities in the human body, Menkes disease is a disorder of copper metabolism. Mutations in the *ATP7A* gene result in failure of intracellular trafficking of copper, which prevents extracellular excretion. This results in decreased copper delivery

to organs including the brain, where copper-requiring enzyme function is impaired. In some patients, parenteral administration of copper has improved functional outcomes although this does not appear to be a universal phenomenon.

> **Helpful Tip**
> Both insufficient and excess metal delivery to end organs can be harmful to humans, and present with different clinical features. Copper is an essential component of a number of important metalloenzymes. Menkes disease involves insufficient copper delivery to tissues such as the brain, where the deficiency leads to neurodegeneration. Wilson disease results from inability to adequately excrete copper into the bile; this causes copper to be stored within tissues such as the liver, brain, and eye. The excess copper can produce movement disorders, psychiatric disease, hepatic failure, and renal tubular dysfunction. Zinc is a cofactor in dozens of important enzymes and has important regulatory functions. Hereditary deficiency of zinc can result from mutations in genes responsible for absorption of zinc from the intestines. One consequence is acrodermatitis enteropathica, which consists of diarrhea, infections, poor growth, and dermatitis occurring around body orifices, particularly perianal. An excess of zinc, as seen in the condition hyperzincuria with hypercalprotectinemia, can present with infections, hepatosplenomegaly, arthritis, anemia, and inflammatory reactions. Magnesium is essential for several chemical reactions within the body, and inborn errors of metabolism that cause hypomagnesemia can result in irritability and seizures. Hypocalcemia can also be variably present and can result in tetany and nephrocalcinosis.

▶ CASE 31

A 6-year-old boy with previously normal growth and development presents with decreasing school performance and onset of erratic behavior over the past 4 months. A screening hearing examination conducted by the school nurse showed hearing loss that was not present on similar screening done 18 months earlier. His parents note that their son has seemed listless with poor weight gain. They also note that he continues to be very tan despite a long winter in Vermont. There is no family history of similar concerns in the family. A MRI scan of the brain is obtained. (See Figure 21–7.)

Question 31-1
What is the most likely diagnosis for this patient?
A) Glutaric aciduria type I.
B) Metachromatic leukodystrophy.
C) Infection with Lyme borreliosis.
D) X-linked adrenoleukodystrophy.
E) Münchausen syndrome by proxy.

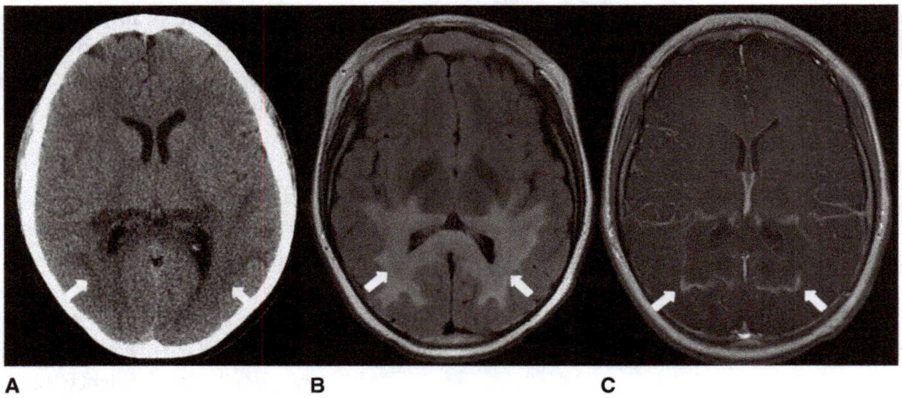

FIGURE 21–7. ALD. White matter changes are seen on this brain MRI of a male patient with adrenoleukodystrophy. There is hyperintensity of the posterior periventricular white matter. The leukodystrophies are a diverse group of neurodegenerative disorders characterized by demyelination of the white matter of the brain. (Reproduced with permission from Kasper DL, Fauci AS, Hauser SL et al: *Harrison's Principles of Internal Medicine*, 19th McGraw-Hill Education, Inc., 2015. Fig 441E-56.)

Discussion 31-1

The correct answer is "D." This patient has presented with neurologic deterioration caused by white matter changes to the brain. Even if nothing else is known about the condition, it could be narrowed to being a leukodystrophy. The leukodystrophies are a diverse group of disorders characterized by degeneration of the white matter of the brain. Disorders include vanishing white matter disease, Krabbe disease, Pelizaeus-Merzbacher disease, and Canavan disease. Patients with X-linked adrenoleukodystrophy (X-ALD) also have adrenal insufficiency, with features that include poor weight gain and bronze skin from increased ACTH secretion. Lastly, the MRI obtained shows posterior periventricular white matter changes, which are typical of patients with X-ALD. Glutaric aciduria type I can present with neurologic changes, but they are more frequently related to movement. Metachromatic leukodystrophy (MLD) can certainly present with cognitive dysfunction, but ataxia is also a common presenting feature. Patients with MLD also do not generally have adrenal insufficiency as a presenting feature. Lyme disease would typically not present in this fashion, and Münchausen syndrome by proxy would be a diagnosis of exclusion in a patient with concerning health problems.

BIBLIOGRAPHY

Adam BW, Flores SR, Hou Y, Allen TW, De Jesus VR. Galactose-1-phosphate uridyltransferase dried blood spot quality control materials for newborn screening tests. *Clin Biochem*. 2015;48(6):437–442.

Antenor-Dorsey JA, Hershey T, Rutlin J, et al. White matter integrity and executive abilities in individuals with phenylketonuria. *Mol Genet Metab*. 2013;109(2):125–131.

Aronica E, van Kempen AA, van der Heide M, et al. Congenital disorder of glycosylation type Ia: A clinicopathological report of a newborn infant with cerebellar pathology. *Acta Neuropathol (Berl)*. 2005;109:433–442.

Baris HN, Cohen IJ, Mistry PK. Gaucher disease: The metabolic defect, pathophysiology, phenotypes and natural history. *Pediatr Endocrinol Rev*. 2014;12(suppl 1):72–81.

Bensend TA, Veach PM, Niendorf KB. What's the harm? Genetic counselor perceptions of adverse effects of genetics service provision by non-genetics professionals. *J Genet Couns*. 2014;23(1):48–63.

Bley AE, Giannikopoulos OA, Hayden D, Kubilus K, Tifft CJ, Eichler FS. Natural history of infantile G(M2) gangliosidosis. *Pediatrics*. 2011;128(5):e1233–e1241.

Bonnet D, Martin D, De Lonlay P, et al. Arrhythmias and conduction defects as presenting symptoms of fatty acid oxidation disorders in children. *Circulation*. 1999;100:2248–2253.

Brunzell JD, Deeb SS. Familial lipoprotein lipase deficiency, apo CII deficiency and hepatic lipase deficiency. In: Scriver CR, Beaudet AL, Sly WS, Valle D, eds. *The Metabolic and Molecular Bases of Inherited Disease*. 8th ed. New York, NY: McGraw-Hill; 2001:2789–2816.

Channon S, Goodman G, Zlotowitz S, Mockler C, Lee PJ. Effects of dietary management of phenylketonuria on long-term cognitive outcome. *Arch Dis Child*. 2007;92:213–218.

Clow CL, Laberge C, Scriver CR. Neonatal hypertyrosinemia and evidence for deficiency of ascorbic acid in Arctic and subarctic people. *Can Med Assoc J*. 1975;113(7):624–626.

Croffie JM, Gupta SK, Chong SK, Fitzgerald JF. Tyrosinemia type 1 should be suspected in infants with severe coagulopathy even in the absence of other signs of liver failure. *Pediatrics*. 1999;103:675–678.

de Sain-van der Velden MG, Diekman EF, Jans JJ, et al. Differences between acylcarnitine profiles in plasma and bloodspots. *Mol Genet Metab*. 2013;110(1–2):116–121.

Dionisi-Vici C, Deodato F, Röschinger W, Rhead W, Wilcken B. 'Classical' organic acidurias, propionic aciduria, methylmalonic aciduria and isovaleric aciduria: Long-term outcome and effects of expanded newborn screening using tandem mass spectrometry. *J Inherit Metab Dis.* 2006;29:383–389.

Fernandes J, Saudubray J-M, van den Berghe G, Walter JH. *Inborn Metabolic Disease.* 4th ed. Heidelberg: Springer; 2006.

Ficicioglu C, Hussa C, Gallagher PR, Thomas N, Yager C. Monitoring of biochemical status in children with Duarte galactosemia: Utility of galactose, galactitol, galactonate, and galactose 1-phosphate. *Clin Chem.* 2010;56(7):1177–1182.

Hennermann JB, Berger JM, Grieben U, Scharer G, Van Hove JL. Prediction of long-term outcome in glycine encephalopathy: A clinical survey. *J Inherit Metab Dis.* 2012;35:253–261.

Hussain K, Aynsley-Green A, Stanley CA. Medications used in the treatment of hypoglycemia due to congenital hyperinsulinism of infancy (HI). *Pediatr Endocrinol Rev.* 2004;2(suppl 1):163–167.

Kaback MM, Desnick RJ. Hexosaminidase A deficiency. (1999 Mar 11 [updated 2011 Aug 11].) In: Pagon RA, Adam MP, Ardinger HH, et al, eds. *GeneReviews* [Internet]. Seattle, WA: University of Washington, Seattle; 1993–2014. http://www.ncbi.nlm.nih.gov/books/NBK1218/.

Kaler SG, Liew CJ, Donsante A, Hicks JD, Sato S, Greenfield JC. Molecular correlates of epilepsy in early diagnosed and treated Menkes disease. *J Inher Metab Dis.* 2010;33:583–589.

Kasapkara ÇS, Cinasal Demir G, Hasanoğlu A, Tümer L. Continuous glucose monitoring in children with glycogen storage disease type I. *Eur J Clin Nutr.* 2014;68(1):101–105.

Lucia A, Ruiz JR, Santalla A, et al. Genotypic and phenotypic features of McArdle disease: Insights from the Spanish national registry. *J Neurol Neurosurg Psychiatry.* 2012;83(3):322–328.

Muenzer J, Wraith JE, Clarke LA. Mucopolysaccharidosis I: Management and treatment guidelines. *Pediatrics.* 2009;123:19–29.

Nesbitt V, Pitceathly RD, Turnbull DM, et al. The UK MRC mitochondrial disease patient cohort study: Clinical phenotypes associated with the m.3243A>G mutation— Implications for diagnosis and management. *J Neurol Neurosurg Psychiatry.* 2013;84:936–938.

Nordestgaard BG, Chapman MJ, Humphries SE, et al; European Atherosclerosis Society Consensus Panel. Familial hypercholesterolaemia is underdiagnosed and undertreated in the general population: Guidance for clinicians to prevent coronary heart disease. *Eur Heart J.* 2013;34:3478–3490.

Orteu CH, Jansen T, Lidove O, et al. Fabry disease and the skin: Data from FOS, the Fabry outcome survey. *Br J Dermatol.* 2007;157:331–337.

Ortiz RG, Newman NJ, Shoffner JM, Kaufman AE, Koontz DA, Wallace DC. Variable retinal and neurologic manifestations in patients harboring the mitochondrial DNA 8993 mutation. *Arch Ophthalmol.* 1993;111:1525–1530.

Parini R, Corbetta C. Metabolic screening for the newborn. *J Matern Fetal Neonatal Med.* 2011;24(suppl 2):6–8.

Parviz M, Vogel K, Gibson KM, Pearl PL. Disorders of GABA metabolism: SSADH and GABA-transaminase deficiencies. *J Pediatr Epilepsy.* 2014;3(4):217–227.

Petraitienė I, Barauskas G, Gulbinas A, et al. Congenital hyperinsulinism. *Medicina (Kaunas).* 2014;50(3):190–195.

Picca S, Bartuli A, Dionisi-Vici C. Medical management and dialysis therapy for the infant with an inborn error of metabolism. *Semin Nephrol.* 2008;28(5):477–480.

Pierro A, Nah SA. Surgical management of congenital hyperinsulinism of infancy. *Semin Pediatr Surg.* 2011;20(1):50–53.

Prater SN, Banugaria SG, Dearmey SM, et al. The emerging phenotype of long-term survivors with infantile Pompe disease. *Genet Med.* 2012;14:800–810.

Robey KL, Reck JF, Giacomini KD, Barabas G, Eddey GE. Modes and patterns of self-mutilation in persons with Lesch-Nyhan disease. *Dev Med Child Neurol.* 2003;45:167–171.

Robinson JG. Management of familial hypercholesterolemia: A review of the recommendations from the National Lipid Association Expert Panel on Familial Hypercholesterolemia. *J Manag Care Pharm.* 2013;19(2):139–149.

Santosh Rai PV, Suresh BV, Bhat IG, Sekhar M, Chakraborti S. Childhood adrenoleukodystrophy—Classic and variant—Review of clinical manifestations and magnetic resonance imaging. *J Pediatr Neurosci.* 2013;8(3):192–197.

Saudubray JM, Martin D, de Lonlay P, et al. Recognition and management of fatty acid oxidation defects: A series of 107 patients. *J Inherit Metab Dis.* 1999;22(4):488–502.

Scarpa M, Almássy Z, Beck M, et al; Hunter Syndrome European Expert Council. Mucopolysaccharidosis type II: European recommendations for the diagnosis and multidisciplinary management of a rare disease. *Orphanet J Rare Dis.* 2011;6:72.

Scriver CR, Kaufman S. Hyperphenylalaninemia: Phenylalanine hydroxylase deficiency. In: Scriver CR, Beaudet AL, Sly SW, Valle D, eds. *The Metabolic and Molecular Bases of Inherited Disease.* 8th ed. New York, NY: McGraw-Hill; 2001:1667–724.

Seashore MR. The organic acidemias: An overview. (2001 Jun 27 [updated 2009 Dec 22].) In: Pagon RA, Adam MP, Ardinger HH, et al, eds. *GeneReviews* [Internet]. Seattle, WA: University of Washington, Seattle; 1993–2014. http://www.ncbi.nlm.nih.gov/books/NBK1134/.

Strauss KA, Morton DH. Branched-chain ketoacyl dehydrogenase deficiency: Maple syrup disease. *Curr Treat Options Neurol.* 2003;5(4):329–341.

Strauss KA, Morton DH. Type I glutaric aciduria, part 2: A model of acute striatal necrosis. *Am J Med Genet.* 2003;121C:53–70.

Summar M, Tuchman M. Proceedings of a consensus conference for the management of patients with urea cycle disorders. *J Pediatr.* 2001;138:S6–10.

Tomatsu S, Shimada T, Mason RW, et al. Establishment of glycosaminoglycan assays for mucopolysaccharidoses. *Metabolites.* 2014;4(3):655–679.

Tuchman M, Lee B, Lichter-Konecki U, et al; Urea Cycle Disorders Consortium of the Rare Diseases Clinical Research Network. Cross-sectional multicenter study of patients with urea cycle disorders in the United States. *Mol Genet Metab*. 2008;94(4):397–402.

Vockley J, Andersson HC, Antshel KM, et al; American College of Medical Genetics and Genomics Therapeutics Committee. Phenylalanine hydroxylase deficiency: Diagnosis and management guideline. *Genet Med*. 2014;16(2):188–200.

Waggoner DD, Buist NR, Donnell GN. Long-term prognosis in galactosaemia: Results of a survey of 350 cases. *J Inherit Metab Dis*. 1990;13:802–818.

Waisbren SE, Potter NL, Gordon CM, et al. The adult galactosemic phenotype. *J Inherit Metab Dis*. 2012;35:279–286.

Wolf B. The neurology of biotinidase deficiency. *Mol Genet Metab*. 2011;104:27–34.

Yu-Wai-Man P, Griffiths PG, Hudson G, Chinnery PF. Inherited mitochondrial optic neuropathies. *J Med Genet*. 2009;46:145–158.

Musculoskeletal Disorders

Natalie Stork and Blaise Nemeth

22

▶ CASE 1

A 14-month-old boy presents with refusal to bear weight on his right leg after falling off the bed. X-rays demonstrate a midshaft femur fracture. Medical records demonstrate prior visits for a wrist fracture and a tibial fracture over the past 3 months. Physical examination reveals multiple bruises. Skeletal survey demonstrates healing right distal radius and right spiral tibial fractures, but no other healing or new fractures. Head magnetic resonance imaging (MRI) does not reveal any intracranial injury and there are no retinal hemorrhages.

Question 1-1
Which of the following findings is least consistent with a possible diagnosis of osteogenesis imperfecta?
A) Blue sclera.
B) Dental caries.
C) Negative family history.
D) Low vitamin D level.
E) Short stature.

Discussion 1-1
The correct answer is "D." Concerns regarding osteogenesis imperfecta are frequently entertained in cases of unusual or frequent fractures and may be mistaken for nonaccidental trauma. Numerous genetic causes have been identified, most commonly in the formation of bone involving collagen (*COL1A1*, *COL1A2*, and others). Vitamin D levels are normal. Inheritance patterns of the genetic abnormalities include autosomal dominant, recessive, and X-linked forms, but current classification remains based on phenotype. Type I, or nondeforming, is the mildest, and patients typically achieve normal height. Type II is lethal in the perinatal period. Type III often presents at birth with frequent fractures and results in progressive deformity, and type IV is the moderate form. Type V involves ossification of the interosseous membrane, hypertrophic callus formation, or both. Blue sclera are common in types I and III, but individuals with type IV often have white sclera. Patients often have

triangular facies and macrocephaly, and may have hearing loss. Short stature, easy bruising, and joint hypermobility may also occur. X-rays often demonstrate osteopenia or wormian bones of the skull.

> **Helpful Tip**
> Although osteogenesis imperfecta is part of the differential diagnosis in the etiology of fractures in infants and children, it is important to remember that children with osteogenesis imperfecta may still be victims of child abuse.

▶ CASE 2

A 6-month-old girl presents as a new patient for a well-child check. Her length is below the third percentile and her weight is at the 10th percentile. Head circumference is greater than the 90th percentile. Her mother is 5 feet, 4 inches tall (50th percentile), and her father is 5 feet, 8 inches (25th percentile). She has normal eyes, a prominent forehead, and a prominent curve to her spine. She also demonstrates mild hypotonia.

Question 2-1
The most likely diagnosis is:
A) Achondroplasia.
B) Osteogenesis imperfecta.
C) Klippel-Feil syndrome.
D) Trisomy 21.
E) Familial short stature.

Discussion 2-1
The correct answer is "A." Achondroplasia is a skeletal dysplasia arising from a defect in *fibroblast growth factor receptor 3* (*FGFR3*). Patients are of short stature with normal height through the trunk but shortening of the extremities. Although fingers may be short, the most pronounced shortening is of the upper

arms and thighs (rhizomelic shortening). Macrocephaly with frontal bossing is often present, and midface hypoplasia predisposes to otitis media and obstructive apnea. Abnormalities at the base of the skull and cervical spine predispose to hydrocephalus, cervical instability, hypotonia, and central apnea. Orthopedic manifestations include excessive thoracic kyphosis, hyperlordosis, spinal stenosis, and bowed legs, often requiring surgical correction. Patients often have ulnar deviation of the fifth digits creating the appearance of a "trident hand." Osteogenesis imperfecta is a genetic syndrome associated with frequent fractures, and while short stature may be present in more severe forms, the other findings are atypical. Klippel-Feil syndrome involves congenital fusion of the cervical spine and a short, webbed neck. Patients with trisomy 21 have short stature, short fingers, and hypotonia but demonstrate other characteristic findings (see Chapter 17). This patient's length is below the fifth percentile, much lower than predicted by midparental height, making familial short stature less likely, especially when taking the other clinical findings into consideration.

> **Helpful Tip**
> Other bone dysplasias, such as multiple epiphyseal dysplasia, spondyloepiphyseal dysplasia, and camptomelic dysplasia, may manifest with short stature, limb bowing, or spine deformities. Genetics evaluation is helpful in making a definitive diagnosis of the specific dysplasia.

▶ CASE 3

A newborn male is found to have hyperextended knees and bilateral clubfeet. Both hips are flexed and have limited abduction; the spine appears straight and without any cutaneous lesions. The pregnancy was unremarkable, other than decreased fetal movement on prenatal ultrasounds.

Question 3-1

All of the following would be consistent with a diagnosis of amyoplasia EXCEPT:
A) Cognitive delay.
B) Lack of flexion creases at joints.
C) Bilateral hip dislocations.
D) Difficulty swallowing.

Discussion 3-1

The correct answer is "A." Arthrogryposis is the presence of congenital joint contractures, usually associated with decreased fetal movement due to either a restricted intrauterine environment or intrinsic muscular or neurologic disorders, and occurs in approximately 1 in 10,000 live births. The most common cause is amyoplasia, an abnormality of muscle development often referred to as arthrogryposis multiplex congenita. Arthrogryposis may also occur in patients with abnormalities of the central nervous system, in the presence of oligohydramnios, or

in certain genetic syndromes, such as diastrophic dysplasia or Larsen syndrome. In addition to the multiple joint contractures, which can include hand and foot deformities as well as dislocate hips, amyoplasia is characterized by cylindrical-shaped limbs with lack of flexion creases, dimpling at joints, and normal cognitive function. Difficulty swallowing and breathing may occur at birth. Abnormal cognitive development would suggest an underlying neurologic abnormality as the cause of multiple joint contractures.

> **Helpful Tip**
> Arthrogryposis is the clinical finding of joint contractures in multiple joints. Identifying an underlying cause is important in determining associated medical issues, prognosis and guiding treatment for the patient and family.

▶ CASE 4

A 4-month-old boy with torticollis returns to clinic for a well-child check. His head is preferentially held in a tilt to the left and rotation to the right. He also has flattening of the right occiput. Shaking keys to the right and left side reveals that he can rotate 90 degrees to the right and 60 degrees to the left. He has a palpable mass within the left sternocleidomastoid muscle. His parents have tried adjustments to his home environment, consisting of laying him in his crib with his right side toward the wall and a music box to his left, to stimulate him to turn more to his left side.

Question 4-1

What is the most appropriate next step in management?
A) Continued home management.
B) Referral for physical therapy.
C) MRI evaluation of the mass.
D) Referral to pediatric orthopedics.
E) Referral to orthotics.

Discussion 4-1

The correct answer is "B." Patients with congenital muscular torticollis have tightness within the sternocleidomastoid muscle thought to be secondary to in utero positioning. This muscle tightness results in a tilt of the head toward the side of tightening and rotation to the contralateral side. Presentation is typically between 2 weeks and 2 months of life. Initially, treatment with modification of the home environment is appropriate. If there is no improvement over 2 to 4 months, then referral to physical therapy is most appropriate. Occasionally infants will have a palpable mass within the sternocleidomastoid muscle; the etiology of this "tumor" is unknown, but since it appears fibrotic on microscopic analysis, theories include arterial occlusion or venous congestion from in utero positioning causing avascularity of the muscle or potentially even primary fibrosis of the muscle. Ultrasound, not MRI, is the preferred initial imaging modality as the mass is in proximity to the skin surface and this modality does not require sedation. Ultrasound should reveal a heterogeneous mass within the sternocleidomastoid muscle; MRI might be warranted if there was an atypical appearance on ultrasound. Presence of a "tumor" may suggest decreased response to physical therapy, but since surgical release of the sternocleidomastoid typically does not occur until after 1 year of age, referral to orthopedics is usually not necessary unless the infant fails to improve with physical therapy over 2 to 4 months. Plagiocephaly often occurs in the presence of torticollis, and cranial remolding orthoses are a consideration, but it can often be prevented with proper physical therapy and resolution of the torticollis.

▶ CASE 5

A mother presents with her 6-month-old son whose head is tilted to the right and rotated to the right. She first noticed this abnormal positioning at 2 months of age, and it has not changed. He has developed some flattening of the right occiput. No esotropia, exotropia, or nystagmus is noted. His neck appears shortened and his hairline low. His right scapula is smaller than the left and slightly elevated. Cervical spine X-rays are as shown. (See Figure 22–1.)

Question 5-1

What is the most likely diagnosis?
A) Congenital muscular torticollis.
B) Klippel-Feil syndrome.
C) Ocular torticollis.

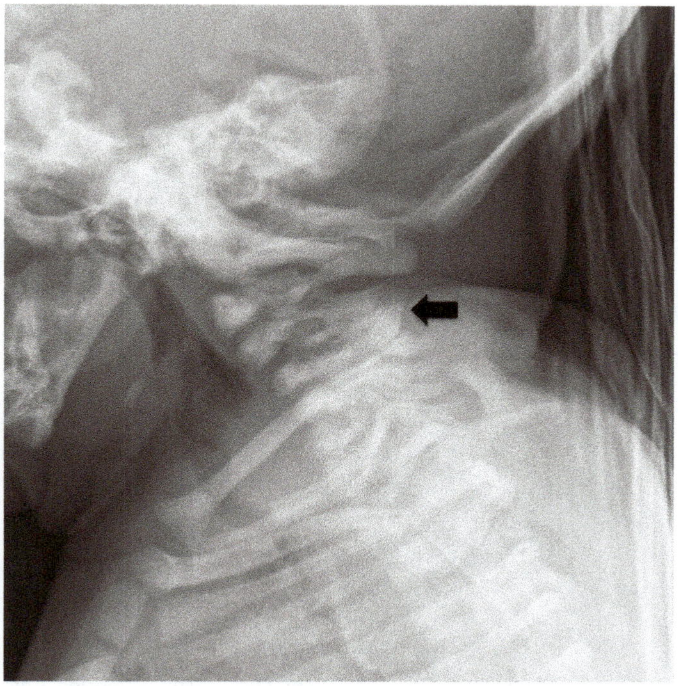

FIGURE 22–1. Lateral cervical spine X-ray. Note fusions at C3-4 posteriorly (*block arrow*). (Used with permission from Blaise Nemeth, MD, MS.)

D) Benign paroxysmal torticollis.
E) Sandifer syndrome.

Discussion 5-1

The correct answer is "B." Klippel-Feil syndrome encompasses the combined findings of shortened neck with low hairline in the presence of cervical vertebral fusions. (See Figure 22–1.) Approximately 20% of patients have Sprengel deformity, with a small, elevated scapula due to incomplete somite migration during fetal development. The typical presentation of congenital muscular torticollis is an infant with a tilted head that is rotated to the contralateral side due to tightness within the sternocleidomastoid muscle on the side of the tilt. In ocular torticollis, children with strabismus or amblyopia tilt their head to reduce the contribution of the eye with abnormal vision. Benign paroxysmal torticollis is a rare cause of torticollis, thought to be a migraine-related disorder based on family history, that occurs every few days to months and resolves completely between episodes. Sandifer syndrome is posturing of the torso and turning of the head related to gastroesophageal reflux disease in the presence of a hiatal hernia. Other causes of torticollis include trauma, malignancy, and inflammation in the soft tissue structures adjacent to the vertebra, such as retropharyngitis or lymphadenitis (Grisel syndrome).

> **Helpful Tip**
> If a patient with torticollis does not improve after 2 to 4 months, obtain anteroposterior (AP) and lateral cervical X-rays to evaluate for vertebral body anomalies of Klippel-Feil. If C1 is not well visualized due to the tilted head from the torticollis, an X-ray of the lateral skull may be helpful.

> **Helpful Tip**
> Cervical spine abnormalities, whether due to fusion or congenital instability, may result in exclusion from certain sports or activities, depending on the abnormality and level of activity.

▶ CASE 6

A 12-month-old girl presents with her parents who are concerned that she is standing "crooked." She has just started walking and they have no concerns regarding her gait. Examination reveals that her spine is curved. X-rays reveal multiple vertebral body anomalies, including hemivertebrae and butterfly vertebrae.

Question 6-1

All of the following should be performed EXCEPT:
A) Renal ultrasound.
B) Echocardiogram.
C) Referral to pediatric orthopedics.
D) Referral to pediatric neurology.

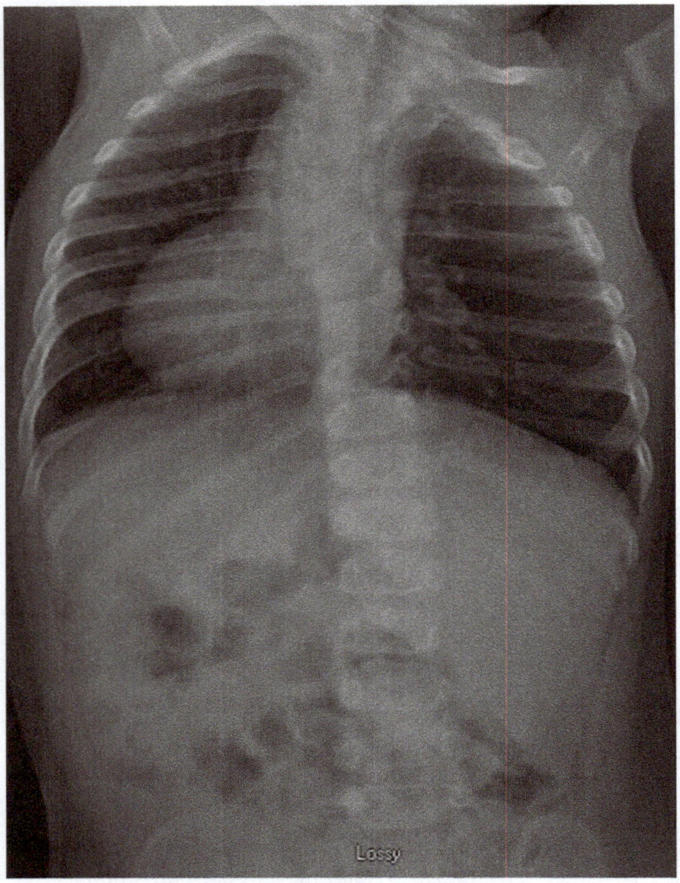

FIGURE 22–2. Posteroanterior (PA) scoliosis X-ray in an infant demonstrating multiple segmentation and fusion abnormalities of the upper thoracic spine in a patient with congenital scoliosis secondary to vertebral malformations. (Used with permission from Blaise Nemeth, MD, MS.)

Discussion 6-1

The correct answer is "D." Congenital scoliosis encompasses curves of the spine associated with vertebral abnormalities due to failures of formation or segmentation of the vertebral bodies. (See Figure 22–2.) Since the renal and cardiac systems develop at the same time as the spine (eg, VACTERL association), patients with congenital scoliosis should undergo evaluation with renal ultrasound and echocardiogram. Spinal dysraphism, such as syrinx or tethered cord, may also occur in the presence of vertebral body anomalies. Referral to neurology is not necessary, but referral to neurosurgery would be appropriate if there are clinical concerns or findings on MRI. MRI may be indicated if there are abnormal neurologic findings; otherwise, necessity may be left to the discretion of the consulting pediatric orthopedist. The curve should be followed for progression necessitating surgery, which may occur at any point during growth.

▶ CASE 7

You are evaluating a new patient in the newborn nursery. The patient is male, born at 38-5/7 weeks' gestational age to a G_2P_2 mother by normal spontaneous vaginal delivery.

She reports the pregnancy was uncomplicated and the delivery went well. Apgar scores were 8 and 9 at 1 and 5 minutes, respectively. The newborn's mother and father are concerned because his feet are turned in. They do not remember their first child's feet looking this way after delivery. Mom states that the night nurse mentioned it was likely caused by the way he was positioned in utero. You begin your newborn exam; as you approach the feet, you notice the toes on both feet point inward.

Question 7-1

Which of the following clinical findings define(s) congenital clubfoot?
A) Metatarsus adductus.
B) Hindfoot varus.
C) Rigid equinus.
D) Cavus.
E) All of the above.

Discussion 7-1

The correct answer is "E." Congenital clubfoot (talipes equinovarus) is a complex deformity affecting the bones and soft tissues of the lower extremity. It is clinically defined by four characteristic findings: cavus, metatarsus adductus, hindfoot varus, and rigid equinus. (See Figure 22–3.) The etiology of clubfoot is not well understood but it is thought to be multifactorial, with both genetic and environmental influences. Clubfoot can be idiopathic or associated with other neuromuscular diagnoses, with an incidence around 1 in 1000 live births. Prenatal ultrasounds have detected the deformity as early as 12 weeks'

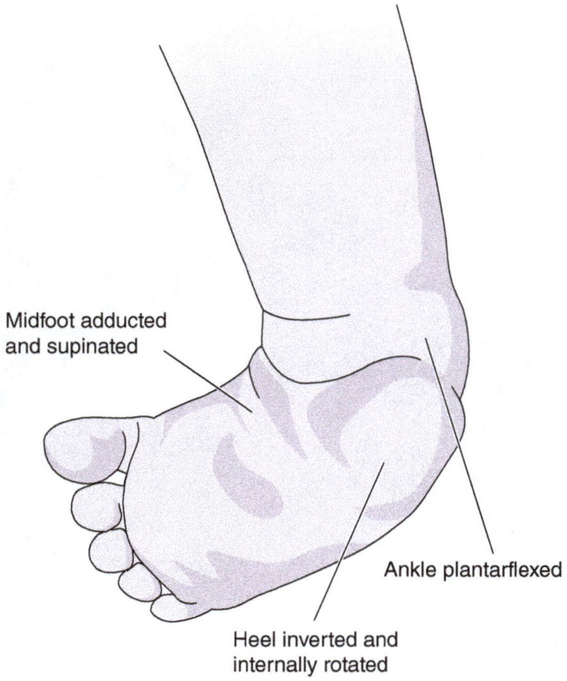

Midfoot adducted and supinated

Ankle plantarflexed

Heel inverted and internally rotated

FIGURE 22–3. Congenital clubfoot. (Reproduced with permission from Skinner HB, McMahon PJ, eds. *Current Diagnosis & Treatment in Orthopedics.* 5th ed. New York, NY: McGraw-Hill Education; 2014, Fig. 10-15.)

gestation. The diagnosis is confirmed with postnatal clinical exam, X-rays are generally not necessary. The treatment goal of idiopathic clubfoot is to shape a painless, flexible, plantigrade foot. Standard treatment of idiopathic clubfoot comprises serial manipulations with long leg cast application. Early initiation of treatment is recommended; however, a delay of several days has not demonstrated a negative outcome with regard to correction. Casts are generally changed every 5 to 7 days. Generally, manipulation and casting is successful in achieving correction of the cavus, metatarsus adductus, and hindfoot varus. However, the majority of patients (90%) require a small surgical procedure (percutaneous Achilles tenotomy) to achieve full correction of the rigid equinus. Once full correction is obtained patients are transitioned into a foot abduction brace to maintain correction. The foot abduction brace is worn full time for 3 months after which the brace is worn part time until about 4 years of age. The foot abduction brace is a key component of treatment, and high rates of recurrence are associated with brace noncompliance. Despite appropriate correction with casting and compliance with the brace, a small group of patients will require another small surgical procedure, to transfer a tendon, in order to maintain correction. This procedure is typically performed around 3 to 4 years.

► CASE 8

The nurse begins telling you about your next patient in the newborn nursery. The patient is a girl born at 39 weeks' gestational age by normal spontaneous vaginal delivery to a G_1P_1 mother. Apgar scores were 6 and 9 at 1 and 5 minutes, respectively. The nurse is concerned the newborn may have a clubfoot. Her exam overall is normal with the exception of her feet. On inspection, the left foot appears normal; however, on the right foot the toes point toward the midline and the lateral border is curved. Additionally, there are multiple creases over the posterior heel with passive dorsiflexion of about 20 degrees. When gentle pressure is applied over the medial aspect of the first ray you are able to gently abduct the forefoot just past neutral. The parents are anxious to know why the right foot turns in so much.

Question 8-1

What is the most appropriate next step?
A) Obtain three views of bilateral feet to assess for bony malalignment.
B) Refer to orthopedics for serial manipulations and long leg cast application.
C) Provide reassurance and gentle stretching techniques, and follow up in 3 to 4 months.
D) Recommend wearing shoes backward and follow up in 3 to 4 months.

Discussion 8-1

The correct answer is "C." This newborn has metatarsus adductus, a condition in which the forefoot is adducted relative to

the hindfoot. Metatarsus adductus is the most common foot deformity referred to orthopedic surgeons. It is more common in male infants, and in preterm and multiple gestation births. Generally, it is diagnosed within the first year of life and can be bilateral in up to 50% of cases. Clinically, the forefoot is adducted with toes pointing medially. Subsequently, there is a convex curve to the lateral border of the foot. The medial border of the foot is concave in shape and a medial crease may be present. In contrast to talipes equinovarus (clubfoot), there is normal motion through the ankle with normal dorsiflexion and multiple creases over the posterior ankle. Metatarsus adductus can be further characterized by the flexibility and severity of the deformity. Flexibility is assessed while gently abducting the forefoot by applying pressure to the medial border of the first ray. If the forefoot is easily corrected past neutral, the deformity is flexible. If the forefoot corrects to neutral, the deformity is partially flexible, and if the forefoot cannot be corrected to neutral, the deformity is rigid. Severity can be described by assessing the heel bisector. The heel bisector intersects the third toe in mild deformities, the third web space in moderate deformities, and the fourth web space in severe deformities. Most patients with metatarsus adductus demonstrate spontaneous correction by around 3 to 4 years of age. The use of splints, braces, or special shoe wear has not been effective in the treatment of metatarsus adductus. Parents can be advised on gentle stretching exercises to perform at home. However, the efficacy of such stretches also has not been demonstrated. Patients with severe or rigid deformities may benefit from treatment with serial stretching casts. Serial casting is typically recommended before 1 year of age. Surgery is generally not necessary.

Helpful Tip

Clubfoot and metatarsus adductus can both be a cause of intoeing in infants. However, they require very different treatment. Clubfoot is a combination of *four* characteristic components in which metatarsus adductus is included. In addition, with clubfoot, there is associated rigid equinus, cavus, and hindfoot varus—none of these are present in metatarsus adductus.

► CASE 9

An 18-month-old boy presents for his well-child check. His parents think he may have attained 6 to 10 words. He walks fairly well but does tend to trip and fall. When he falls he gets up right away and carries on with his activities. He eats a varied diet without any restrictions. Their main concern today is that he looks "bowlegged," especially when ambulating. The father reports that he, too, was a bit bowlegged when he was young but did not receive treatment and "grew out of it." Exam demonstrates mild genu varum, which clinically appears symmetric. Gait demonstrates a wider base, with toes pointing to the midline bilaterally (L > R), and no lateral

thrust, waddling, or antalgia. X-rays demonstrate mild genu varum bilaterally affecting the femur and the tibia, with normal-appearing physes.

Question 9-1

Which of the following statements is/are consistent with the patient's condition?
A) History of delayed walking is common.
B) Maximal deformity is noted around 3 years old.
C) Internal tibia torsion is a common association.
D) Obesity increases the risk of deformity.
E) All of the above

Discussion 9-1

The correct answer is "C." Genu varum and genu valgum are angular variations in alignment, which occur naturally at defined points in development. Each of these angular variations, although part of normal development, can be pathologic. Thus, it is important to be able to differentiate physiologic from pathologic findings. Maximal genu varum occurs between birth and 6 months of age, with a femoral-tibial angle between 10 and 15 degrees. Remodeling occurs naturally, and neutral alignment is typically attained by 15 months of age. The differential diagnosis for persistent genu varum beyond 15 months of age includes physiologic genu varum, tibia vara (early-onset Blount disease), metabolic bone disease, skeletal dysplasia, focal fibrocartilage dysplasia, and growth arrest. Standing AP films of the bilateral lower extremities are helpful in assessing for physiologic versus pathologic causes of genu varum. X-rays are indicated in children with genu varum outside the expected physiologic age range, unilateral deformity or significant asymmetry, pronounced deformity, short stature, or a lateral thrust on exam. Images should be obtained with the patella in a neutral position (pointing straight ahead). Physiologic genu varum is defined as persistent varus beyond 18 months of age, with femoral-tibial angle greater than 10 degrees, and without radiographic findings of other abnormalities. It is characterized by a varus angulation of the entire lower extremity, distributed through the femur and tibia. It is often bilateral but can be asymmetric. Patients often have a history of early independent ambulation. There may be a family history of relatives who were "bowlegged." On exam the genu varum is apparent on inspection. Gait exam often reveals an agile walker with an intoed gait. Internal tibial torsion is also commonly associated with physiologic genu varum. Physiologic genu varum spontaneously resolves by around 2 years of age. Braces and splints have not been shown to be effective in altering the natural course. Referral to orthopedics should be considered when there is concern for pathologic genu varum; that is, severe deformity, unilateral or significant asymmetry, progression of the deformity, pathologic findings on X-ray, or persistence of the deformity beyond 2 years of age. Tibia vara, or early-onset Blount disease (previously infantile Blount disease), is characterized by abnormal endochondral ossification of the medial proximal tibia. This results in varus angulation and medial rotation of the proximal tibia. The etiology is unknown as the disorder is rare, especially in comparison with physiologic varus. It is more common in the African American population and in obese or overweight toddlers. Patients often have a history

of early independent ambulation. Similar to physiologic genu varum, it is often bilateral and also commonly associated with internal tibial torsion. On exam, genu varum is evident on inspection. Gait exam may reveal a lateral thrust (knee thrusts laterally through stance phase), indicating concern for lateral subluxation of the femur on the tibia or ligamentous laxity. On X-rays, it is characterized by varus deformity of the proximal medial tibia. In children younger than 18 months of age, differentiating between physiologic genu varum and tibia vara can be difficult, even with X-rays. Treatment of early-onset Blount disease depends on the age of the patient and the severity of deformity. Bracing may be an option in patients 2 to 3 years old, so patients should be referred to an orthopedic physician for management.

▶ CASE 10

A 10-year-old girl presents for evaluation of her lower extremities. Her mother accompanies her to the visit and is concerned because her daughter appears "knock-kneed," with her left side worse relative to her right side. The mother had noticed this before but believes it has worsened over the past 6 months. The patient denies any significant limitations at this time. She does occasionally have some anterior knee pain bilaterally that is worse with activity. On inspection you notice a knock-kneed appearance to her lower extremities with an intermalleolar distance measuring 14 cm. The left lower extremity has a greater valgus angle relative to the right. You elect to obtain a standing AP lower extremity X-ray for further assessment. While awaiting X-rays you begin to form your differential diagnosis.

Question 10-1

Each of the following could explain the child's clinical findings EXCEPT:
A) Physiologic.
B) Juvenile arthritis.
C) Rickets.
D) History of infectious osteomyelitis.
E) Renal osteodystrophy.

Discussion 10-1

The correct answer is "A." Similar to varus angulation, valgus angulation is part of the natural development of lower extremity alignment. The femoral tibial angle generally reaches peak valgus alignment between 3 and 4 years of age, with an average value between 8 and 10 degrees (range, between 2 and 20 degrees of valgus). This valgus angulation naturally decreases with age, achieving a stable, average "adult" alignment of 0 to 12 degrees of valgus around 6 to 7 years. The differential diagnosis for genu valgum is similar to that for genu varum and includes physiologic, idiopathic, metabolic bone disease, skeletal dysplasia, posttraumatic growth arrest, fibrous cortical defect, and benign bone lesions (multiple hereditary enchondroses). A standing AP X-ray that includes both lower extremities (teleoroentgenogram) is helpful in assessing for pathologic causes of genu

TABLE 22–1 RED FLAGS ASSOCIATED WITH LOWER EXTREMITY ANGULAR DEFORMITIES

Short stature

Persistence beyond expected corrected physiologic age

Unilateral deformity

Severe deformity

Underlying metabolic disease

Abnormal X-ray findings (growth plate changes, lytic/sclerotic lesions)

History of trauma of affected limb

valgum. As with genu varum, X-rays should be obtained with the patella in neutral position, regardless of the placement or appearance of the feet. Indications for obtaining X-rays include severe deformity, unilateral deformity or significant asymmetry, progressive deformity, persistent genu valgum outside expected corrected age, and short stature. Physiologic genu valgum is often bilateral. The intermalleolar distance (distance between the medial malleoli, with the patient lying supine with knees together) can be measured clinically and may fall between 2 and 10 cm. As previously noted, there is wide variation in the femoral tibial angle around the peak valgus age. Physiologic genu valgum spontaneously resolves by 8 to 10 years of age. Braces and splints have not been proven to be effective in altering the natural history of physiologic genu valgum. Genu valgum, defined as a femoral-tibial angle greater than 10 degrees, which persists beyond the expected corrected age should be further investigated and referred to an orthopedic specialist. In addition, referral should be considered in patients with genu valgum and severe deformity, unilateral deformity or significant asymmetry, progressive deformity, pain, short stature, or a combination of these findings.

Helpful Tip

Varus and valgus angular deformities of the lower extremities can be part of normal development that resolve with age and require no further intervention. Red flags for pathologic deformities and indications for referral to an orthopedic specialist are listed in Table 22–1. Surgical intervention using guided growth is a minimally invasive method that may be used in growing children with pathologic valgus or varus. After skeletal maturity, a more extensive corrective osteotomy is required.

▶ CASE 11

You are seeing a 5-year-old child for a new visit due to concern about gait. Both parents accompany the child to the visit and voice the same concern: the child is pigeon-toed. They are concerned because the child is always "W" sitting despite constant reminders and has a "funny" run. They deny any concerns for pain. Watching the child walk in the hallway you notice a negative foot progression angle bilaterally (the feet point toward the midline). In addition, you notice the knees tend to point inward, too. When running, the child tends to swing the legs out to the side bilaterally.

Question 11-1

Which of the following is true about this child's condition?

A) AP and frog-leg films of the pelvis are recommended for initial diagnosis.

B) It occurs more commonly in males than females.

C) It is associated with decreased external rotation of the hips relative to internal rotation.

D) A negative thigh foot angle is the most common clinical measurement for this condition.

E) It is the most common cause of intoeing in children younger than 3 years of age.

Discussion 11-1

The correct answer is "C." Femoral anteversion is the most common cause of intoeing in children (average age between 3 and 6 years old). It refers to the orientation of the femoral neck relative to the axis of the distal femoral condyles. Femoral anteversion is more commonly identified in females. History is often positive for an unusual run (in which the patient swings the legs out to the side, also referred to as an "eggbeater" run) and "W" sitting, with the knees bent and the legs stretched out behind. Exam often demonstrates a fairly symmetric intoeing gait pattern with kneecaps that appear to roll toward the midline through stance phase. A negative thigh-foot angle is seen in tibial torsion, and when walking, the patella typically points straight ahead, or even outward, while the feet point inward. Tibial torsion is the most common cause of in-toeing in a child younger than 3 years old. As with other rotational variations, femoral anteversion generally improves, with around 80% of individuals demonstrating spontaneous resolution by around 8 years of age. Femoral anteversion is generally not associated with any functional limitations in an otherwise typically developing child. Braces or splints have not been effective in treatment. Reassurance and observation is recommended for otherwise typically developing children.

▶ CASE 12

You are evaluating a previously healthy 2-year-old boy for his well-child check. His mother states that she feels that he is doing well overall. He is quite social in daycare. In addition, he has been running without pain or difficulty, but she is concerned because he prefers to walk on his toes. She noticed this when he first started walking and denies any progression. She thinks he spends about 50% to 75% of the time ambulating on his toes. Gait exam reveals predominantly a toe-walking pattern; however, the boy demonstrates the ability to roll onto his heels and will stand with his feet flat on the floor at times. Upon tripping in the hallway, he is able to easily stand up and return to running down the hallway. He has 20 to 25 degrees of passive dorsiflexion bilaterally. Neurologic exam is normal.

Question 12-1

What is the most likely etiology of the patient's clinical findings?
A) Duchenne muscular dystrophy.
B) Tethered cord.
C) Autism.
D) Idiopathic toe walking.

Discussion 12-1

The correct answer is "D." Idiopathic toe walking is a common gait pattern often observed in first-time walkers. The typical heel-toe gait pattern is observed on average about 22.5 weeks after commencement of independent walking or by around 2 years of age. Persistent toe walking beyond 2 to 3 years of age may be the first manifestation of underlying neurologic or neuromuscular pathology and warrants further evaluation. The true prevalence of idiopathic toe walking is not well documented. However, a recent study demonstrated prevalence around 4.8%. About half of these individuals ceased to toe walk by 5.5 years of age, leaving about 2.7% with persistent toe walking beyond 5.5 years. Toe walking is more common in male patients and most patients have a positive family history for a relative with toe walking. Idiopathic toe walking is a diagnosis of exclusion, and other causes of toe walking must first be ruled out. (See Table 22–2.) A thorough history investigating for other causes of toe walking is necessary. Recent toe walking in an older child with a prior history of heel-toe gait raises concern for underlying pathology. Although prevalence of toe walking is higher among individuals with autism and other cognitive delays, not all toe walkers have autism or global developmental delays. There is suggestion for a possible sensory component to the etiology of toe walking in individuals with cognitive delays. In addition, a thorough physical exam, including orthopedic and neurologic exam, should be conducted. Patients with idiopathic toe walking should demonstrate a normal neurologic exam. An associated heel cord contracture may be present. Complications for persistent idiopathic toe walking include the development of heel cord contracture; splaying of the forefoot, making shoe

wear difficult; and progressive external tibial torsion. Treatment of idiopathic toe walking depends on the age of the patient and ankle range of motion. In patients younger than 2 years of age with appropriate range of motion about the ankle, observation is recommended. For patients older than 2 years of age, with appropriate range of motion, continued observation in addition to therapy focusing on maintaining range of motion, with or without the use of stretching splints or stretching casts, may be used. For patients with a fixed equinus contracture, referral for surgical evaluation is recommended as the patient is not likely to respond to physical therapy alone.

> **Helpful Tip**
> Idiopathic toe walking is a diagnosis of exclusion. Persistent toe walking beyond 2 to 3 years of age can be the first manifestation of neuromuscular pathology; thus, a thorough neurologic exam should be conducted. Concern should be raised in an older child without history of toe walking who presents with change in gait and recent toe walking.

▶ CASE 13

Your next new patient is 15-month-old girl who recently moved to your community. Her parents are concerned because she is pigeon-toed. She began walking independently just after her first birthday, which is when they noticed the intoeing. The mother is concerned as her husband wore a brace for a while when he was young because his toes pointed inward. On examination of the patient you notice a wide-based gait with a negative foot progression angle (toes point toward the midline with ambulation). This is more pronounced on the left relative to the right. When you straighten her legs so the kneecaps point straight ahead her feet turn in, more so on the left than on the right. The transmalleolar angle is 0 degrees on the left and about 10 degrees on the right. She has symmetric hip abduction to 75 degrees bilaterally. Internal and external rotation of the hips is 50 degrees, respectively, bilaterally. Neurologic exam is normal.

Question 13-1

What would you include in your discussion with the parents regarding their daughter's condition?
A) It is often associated with "W" sitting.
B) Asymmetry raises concern for underlying pathology.
C) It is more common in females than males.
D) This rotational variation generally improves with growth.
E) Surgery is beneficial if correction has not been obtained by 3 years of age.

Discussion 13-1

The correct answer is "D." Internal tibial torsion is the most common cause of intoeing in toddlers and young children. Often there is a history of an intoeing gait pattern first noticed when

TABLE 22–2 DIFFERENTIAL DIAGNOSIS FOR TOE WALKING
Cerebral palsy
Spina bifida
Muscular dystrophy
Myotonic dystrophy
Tethered cord
Charcot-Marie-Tooth disease
Leg-length discrepancy
Autism or global developmental delay

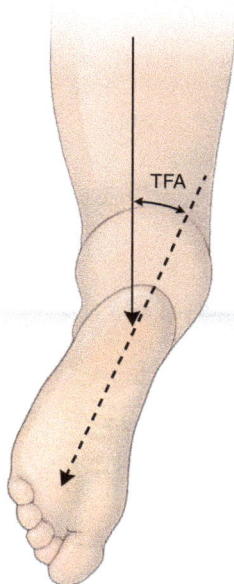

FIGURE 22–4. Thigh-foot angle (TFA).

the child begins walking. Parents may also report that the child trips over the affected foot or feet and falls frequently. Internal tibial torsion occurs equally in males and females. It is bilateral about 66% of the time. Unilateral cases tend to affect the left side more commonly than the right. Clinically, patients demonstrate a negative foot progression angle, consistent with intoeing. In addition, the examiner should assess the thigh-foot angle (TFA) or transmalleolar angle (TMA), or both. The TFA (see Figure 22–4) is measured while the patient is prone and is the angle created between the thigh and an imaginary line bisecting the foot. The TMA is the angle created between the plane of the femoral condyles and the plane of the medial and lateral malleoli. In children with internal tibial torsion, the thigh foot angle will be negative and the TMA will be decreased (average adult TMA is about 15 to 20 degrees). The natural history of internal tibial torsion, as with other rotational variations, is gradual improvement. With growth the tibia will naturally externally rotate. Braces and splints have not been shown to be effective in altering the natural history of this deformity. Gradual improvement occurs on average by around 5 years of age. Functional limitations associated with persistent internal tibial torsion are uncommon. Surgery is rarely necessary and requires a rotational osteotomy. Indications for surgery include persistent deformity after 8 years of age and significant functional limitations.

> **Helpful Tip**
> Internal tibial torsion is the most common cause of intoeing in toddlers and young children and generally improves with growth.

► CASE 14

As you are finishing your rounds in the newborn nursery, the nurse asks you to see one more infant. The patient is a female born at 38-5/7 weeks' gestational age to a G_1P_1 previously healthy mother by normal spontaneous vaginal delivery. Apgar scores were 7 and 9 at 1 and 5 minutes, respectively. On exam, the newborn's head is normocephalic; heart and lung sounds are normal. A bilateral red reflex observed. The spine is straight without evidence of a sacral dimple or cutaneous sacral lesions. On inspection of the patient's feet you notice 5 well-formed toes on the left. On the right however, you notice an extra digit, laterally, next to the fifth toe. This appears well formed, similar in appearance to the other digits. Ortolani and Barlow tests are negative. In talking with the mother, you learn that she had an extra digit, as well, which was removed surgically.

Question 14-1
Which of the following statements regarding polydactyly is true?
A) Surgery is indicated for improved cosmesis or difficulty with shoe fit.
B) Postaxial refers to duplication of thumb or great toe.
C) It occurs most commonly through autosomal recessive inheritance.
D) A family history of polydactyly should raise strong concern for associated anomalies.

Discussion 14-1
The correct answer is "A." Polydactyly can occur as the result of autosomal dominant inheritance (variable penetrance) and commonly is an isolated trait. It occurs bilaterally in about 50% of cases. Preaxial polydactyly refers to duplication of the thumb or great toe. Postaxial polydactyly refers to duplication of the fifth toe or small finger, and central polydactyly refers to duplication of the second, third, or fourth phalange. Polydactyly is more common in the black population. Postaxial polydactyly (79%) is more common than preaxial (15%) and central polydactyly (6%). Associated anomalies occur more commonly with preaxial polydactyly than postaxial polydactyly. Indications for surgical removal include improved cosmesis, persistent skin irritation or breakdown, or intolerance with shoe wear.

> **Helpful Tip**
> Polydactyly commonly occurs as an autosomal dominant isolated trait; thus, family history is often positive. Surgical referral is warranted for cosmesis or persistent intolerance of shoe wear or skin irritation. Anything more than a simple skin tag should be referred to a specialist if removal is indicated.

► CASE 15

You are seeing a 5-month-old boy who was recently placed in foster care. Overall, the foster parents report the placement has been going well and everyone in the home is adjusting well. They report the infant has been feeding well. He recently began rolling over and is rather vocal with his babbling. Their only concern today is that they have noticed one of his lower extremities appears longer than the other. They are not sure whether this had been noticed previously but are working with the case worker to transfer his previous records to your office for further review.

Question 15-1

All of the following would raise concern for an organic etiology of limb-length inequality EXCEPT:
A) A large vascular cutaneous lesion of one lower extremity.
B) Asymmetric girth of the thigh and calf of a lower extremity.
C) Multiple café-au-lait lesions.
D) History of distal femur fracture.
E) None of the above.

Discussion 15-1

The correct answer is "E." Leg-length discrepancy is a rather common occurrence with reports of differences ranging from greater than 0.5 cm to greater than 1 cm in 36% and 25% of the population, respectively. The differential for discrepancy is wide and includes congenital, acquired, and idiopathic etiologies. Idiopathic leg-length discrepancy while common is a diagnosis of exclusion; thus, a thorough history and exam should assess for other pathologic etiologies of leg-length discrepancy. (See Table 22–3.) Given the variety of causes of leg-length discrepancy, the chief complaint for evaluation of leg-length discrepancy can be equally as varied. Clinical exam should include height and weight, assessing for any signs of short stature or growth abnormalities. Inspection should include evaluation for any girth differences in the extremities, limitations in range of motion, or any abnormal skin markings (café-au-lait spots, axillary freckling suggesting neurofibromatosis, vascular cutaneous lesions, or variations in pigmentation suggestive of other syndromes). A thorough neurologic exam should assess for any evidence of neurologic deficit or asymmetry. In addition, exam of the spine should assess for signs of scoliosis. Clinically, the difference can be measured using the apparent and the true leg-length discrepancy. The apparent leg-length discrepancy is determined by measuring the length of each lower extremity, starting at the umbilicus and measuring to the medial malleolus. This accounts for pelvic obliquity or any associated contracture, which may be present about the hip. The true leg-length discrepancy is determined by measuring the length of each limb from the anterior superior iliac spine (ASIS) to the medial or lateral malleolus and determining the difference between either side. Another method for assessing difference includes first assessing the height difference measured between the right and left posterior superior iliac spines, then adding graduated blocks under the short limb until the pelvis is level (the examiner's hands are level).

TABLE 22–3 DIFFERENTIAL DIAGNOSIS FOR LEG-LENGTH DISCREPANCY (LLD)

Congenital

  Proximal femoral focal deficiency

  Congenital short femur or tibia

  Fibular or tibial hemimelia

  Skeletal dysplasias (eg, achondroplasia, osteogenesis imperfecta, etc)

  Fibrous dysplasia

  Pseudoarthrosis of tibia

  Neurofibromatosis

  Ollier disease

  Multiple hereditary exostoses

  Hemi-hypertrophy or hemi-atrophy

  Beckwith-Weidemann syndrome

  Klippel-Trenaunay-Weber syndrome

  Parkes Weber syndrome

  Proteus syndrome

  Russell-Silver disease

  Congenital coxa vara

  Cerebral palsy

  Clubfoot

Acquired

  Hip dysplasia (subluxed or dislocated hip)

  Trauma (fracture complicated by shortening or overgrowth or angular deformity)

  Cerebral palsy (functional LLD due to contracture)

  Myelomeningocele

  Infection (septic arthritis, osteomyelitis)

  Juvenile idiopathic arthritis

  Hemophilia

  Avascular necrosis (Legg-Calvé-Perthes disease)

  Blount disease

  Fixed pelvic obliquity

  Scoliosis

  Neoplastic

  Radiation exposure (growth arrest)

Idiopathic

As with the clinical evaluation, several standard radiographic evaluations exist to assess for leg-length discrepancy. These include teleoroentgenography (single weight-bearing AP view of lower extremities extending from pelvis to ankles with a ruler in between) and orthoroentgenography, also referred to as a scanogram (AP imaging of entire limb with three exposures). Treatment options vary depending on the etiology, severity of the discrepancy, age of the patient, and remaining growth. It is important to determine the projected discrepancy at skeletal maturity as this provides an initial foundation for the development of treatment options. Determining the skeletal age and the projected remaining growth of the child is of similar importance. For leg-length discrepancies of less than 2 cm at skeletal maturity, observation is recommended. In these minor discrepancies a shoe lift can be instituted, correcting for about half of the difference. Shoe lifts up to 1 cm can be comfortably inserted in the shoe; lifts greater than 1 cm generally are not well tolerated within the shoe. Surgical treatment is considered for leg-length discrepancies greater than 2 cm and can include surgical shortening of the longer limb or lengthening procedures of the short limb (generally for discrepancies > 5 cm). Amputation or early prosthetic fitting is considered for severe discrepancies with a projected difference greater than 20 cm.

> **Helpful Tip**
> The differential diagnosis for leg-length discrepancy is quite wide; thus, a thorough history and physical must be conducted to identify potential organic causes. Leg-length discrepancies up to 1 cm are fairly common and often idiopathic. Discrepancies less than 2 cm are fairly well tolerated with a simple shoe lift correcting half the difference (up to a 1 cm shoe lift can be comfortably tolerated inside a shoe).

▶ CASE 16

A 2-year-old boy presents with a limp. His parents first noticed it about 5 days ago, and it has progressively worsened since. He has become increasingly fussy with weight bearing. Today he developed a temperature of 37.9°C (100.2°F). On exam, he has limited flexion of his right knee and is tender over the distal femur. The knee is not swollen or warm to touch. X-rays are unremarkable. CBC reveals a white blood cell (WBC) count of 10,100/mm³ with 70% neutrophils, C-reactive protein (CRP) of 7, and erythrocyte sedimentation rate (ESR) of 29.

Question 16-1

What is the most appropriate next step in management?
A) Observation.
B) MRI scan.
C) Ultrasound.
D) CT scan.

Discussion 16-1

The correct answer is "B." These findings are concerning for possible infection. Children may experience infections of the musculoskeletal system involving bones (osteomyelitis), septic arthritis, or muscle (pyomyositis). With lack of joint swelling,

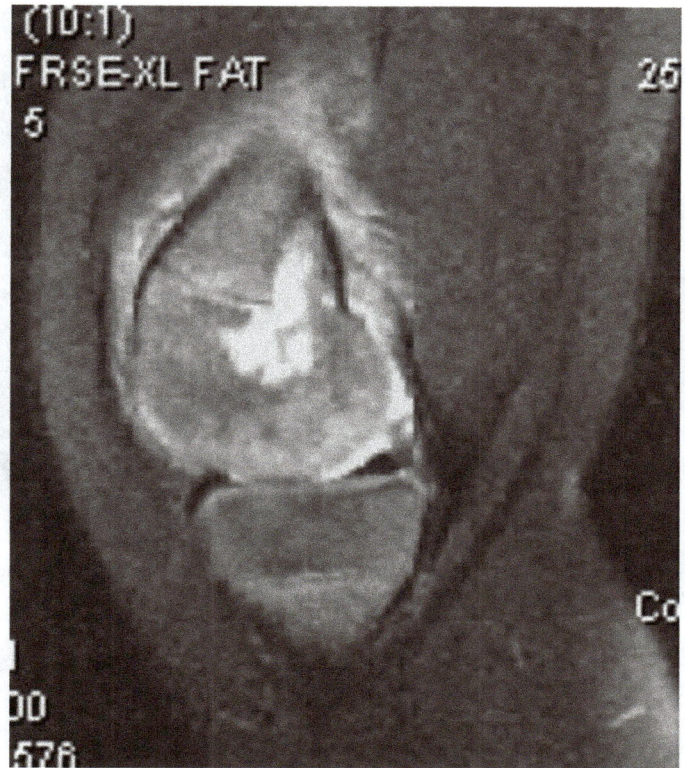

FIGURE 22–5. T2-weighted MRI scan demonstrating edema within the metaphysis and epiphysis of the femur (bright white). (Used with permission from Blaise Nemeth, MD, MS.)

osteomyelitis would be most likely, although early septic arthritis may not present with clinically detectable swelling. Early in the course of osteomyelitis, X-rays may be negative. MRI is the most helpful next imaging tool, if an area of concern can be localized, to identify early osteomyelitis, demonstrating edema and early destruction within the bone. (See Figure 22–5). A bone scan may be helpful if an area of involvement cannot be identified. Ultrasound is useful for imaging soft tissue structures, including evaluation for joint effusions, especially if there is concern for septic arthritis, and to guide aspirations, but is less helpful in evaluating bone. CT scan works well to highlight bone abnormalities but is more helpful in trauma than when infection is suspected. Treatment of osteomyelitis usually requires only antibiotics, initially intravenous (IV), followed by oral therapy, and surgery is required only when there is an area of focal abscess (see Figure 22–6) or associated septic arthritis. Osteomyelitis often involves the metaphysis of the long bones, occurring as the result of hematogenous spread, although eruption into the joint may occur, most commonly in the proximal femur or hip, or in infants. Infectious organisms may be identified by direct culture of the infected area or on blood culture. Resolution of changes on MRI can take weeks to months, so repeat imaging with MRI is not helpful to evaluate for resolution of infection; following declines in WBC and ESR is more helpful, reserving repeat MRI for patients who are clinically worsening, which may raise concern for potential subperiosteal abscess requiring surgical irrigation and debridement.

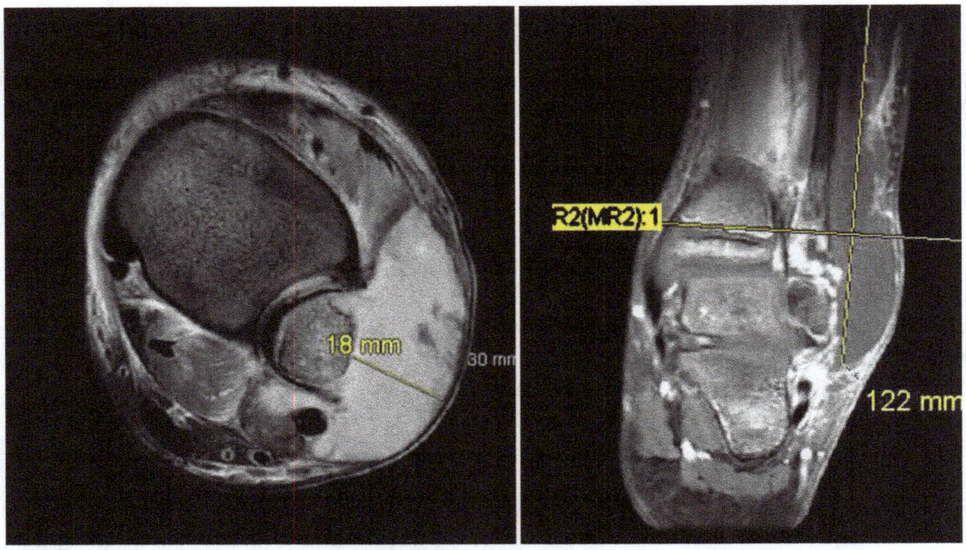

FIGURE 22–6. T2-weighted axial image (left) and T1-weighted coronal image (right) of periosteal abscess related to distal fibular osteomyelitis. (Used with permission from Matthew Halanski, MD.)

Helpful Tip

X-rays are often negative in patients presenting with osteomyelitis. MRI may be necessary for diagnosis if X-rays are negative. MRI abnormalities take months to resolve, so serial MRIs are not indicated in patients with osteomyelitis who are improving based on clinical and laboratory parameters.

► **CASE 17**

A 13-year-old girl presents with a swollen right knee. She first noticed it 2 days ago. She will walk, but she limps and appears uncomfortable. Her temperature is 38°C (100.4°F). Her right knee is swollen and slightly warm to touch. She cries with attempts to flex the knee. X-rays are negative. CBC demonstrates WBC 15,000/mm³ with 82% neutrophils, CRP of 10, and ESR of 45. She is taken to the operating room for suspected septic arthritis.

Question 17-1

What is the most likely causative organism?

A) *Staphylococcus aureus.*
B) *Streptococcus pyogenes.*
C) *Neisseria gonorrhoeae.*
D) *Kingella kingae.*
E) *Salmonella.*

Discussion 17-1

The correct answer is "A." Pyogenic arthritis arises from bacterial infection of the joint. This can result from direct hematogenous seeding of the joint or when osteomyelitis occurs in an intra-articular metaphysis and ruptures through the bone into the joint. Diagnosis is an urgency as joint infection results in joint destruction within 3 to 5 days and permanent long-term sequelae. (See Figure 22–7.) The greatest yield in recovering an organism includes performing blood culture and joint aspirate. Ultrasound may be helpful in identifying joint effusions, especially in the hip, and to guide aspiration. Treatment includes emergent irrigation and debridement of the joint in the operating room and initiation of antibiotic therapy. The most common causative organism in both osteomyelitis and septic arthritis is staphylococcus aureus. Methicillin-resistant strains are increasing in prevalence, so the preferred antibiotic treatment of choice typically varies based on regional prevalence. In areas where methicillin-sensitive strains prevail, initiation of treatment may begin with nafcillin, but in methicillin-resistant areas, vancomycin is preferred, although clindamycin may be reasonable if strains are D-test negative. *S. pyogenes* (group A beta-hemolytic streptococcus) is another common cause of septic arthritis, but less frequent than *S. aureus*. *N. gonorrhoeae* is a potential causative organism in sexually active individuals that is treated with penicillin; patients may experience polyarthralgia before onset of arthritis. *K. kingae* is an emerging cause of septic arthritis, primarily in children under 3 years of age, that may make up many of the reported "culture-negative" cases of septic arthritis as it is a fastidious organism that may be missed on routine cultures; recovery is improved by use of culture bottles. Salmonella is a common cause of musculoskeletal infection in individuals with sickle cell disease. Infections from historically significant organisms, such as *Streptococcus pneumoniae* and *Haemophilus influenza* type b have been reduced by vaccinations but represent important considerations in unimmunized children or infants too young to receive immunizations.

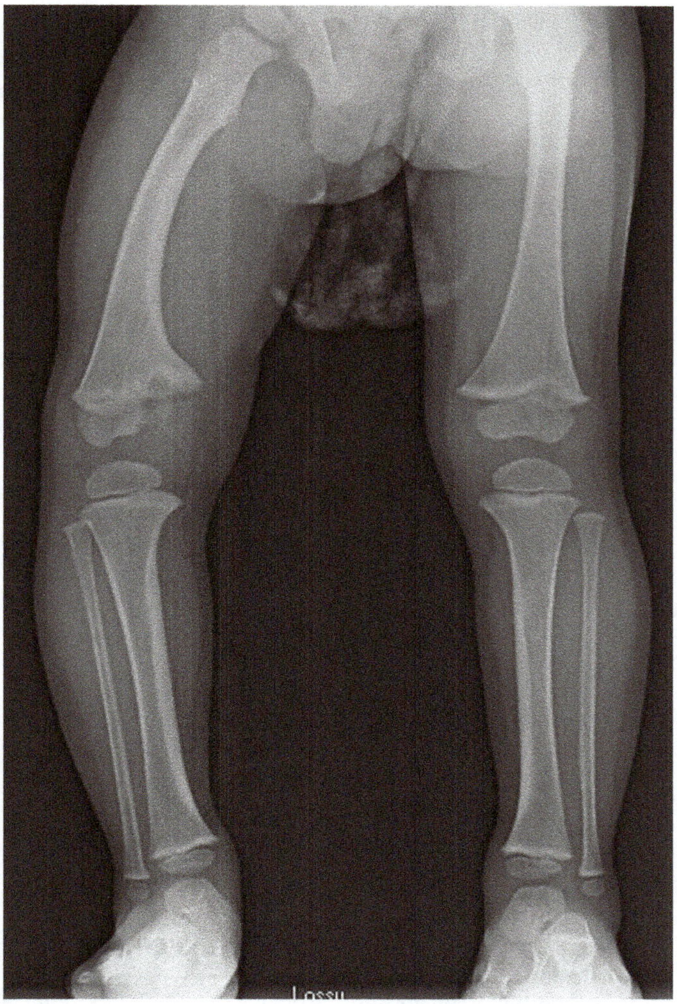

FIGURE 22–7. Full-length orthoroentgenogram of patient with a history of right distal femoral osteomyelitis and subsequent septic arthritis resulting in osteonecrosis of the medial femur. As a result, this patient has developed growth arrest and varus deformity. Fortunately, the patient presented upon development of the septic arthritis and was treated immediately, preventing osteonecrosis of the rest of the joint (lateral femur and proximal tibia). (Used with permission from Blaise Nemeth, MD, MS.)

Helpful Tip

While *S. aureus* is the most common cause of musculoskeletal infections in children, consider other organisms when performing testing and initiating antibiotics to improve detection and coverage in patients with a history of travel, other medical issues, or incomplete immunization status.

► **CASE 18**

A 2-year-old girl presents with a limp and decreased weight bearing on her right leg. This was first noticed by her parents this morning after she awoke. Her parents do not recall any trauma, and she has not had any fevers. They have not noticed any swelling. Physical examination reveals limited motion at her right hip. There is no focal tenderness throughout her thigh, lower leg, or foot. There is no swelling at her knee. X-rays of her femur, tibia, and foot are normal.

Question 18-1

What is the most appropriate next step in evaluation and management?
A) Hip ultrasound with aspiration.
B) Continued observation.
C) Consultation with pediatric orthopedics.
D) CBC with differential and ESR.
E) Lyme titer

Discussion 18-1

The correct answer is "D." Children with a limp present a difficult diagnostic challenge owing to the broad differential diagnosis, which ranges from the benign to the gravely concerning. A systematic approach is helpful in evaluating these patients, starting with a detailed examination to localize the area of involvement. X-rays are helpful in assessing for fractures, tumors, or developmental orthopedic issues, such as Legg-Calvé-Perthes disease or late-presenting developmental dysplasia of the hip, which may manifest with limited hip motion. When X-rays are negative, the two most common causes of hip pain in a child include septic arthritis and transient (ie, toxic) synovitis. The physical exam in both cases is remarkably similar, but differentiation is important as untreated septic arthritis can cause significant destruction of the joint within 4 to 5 days; therefore, timely diagnosis is paramount. Kocher described four findings, originally determined retrospectively but validated prospectively, that help differentiate septic arthritis from transient synovitis: fever (temperature > 38°C [100.4°F]), refusal to walk, WBC count greater than 12,000/mm³ and ESR greater than 40. Patients with none of these criteria were unlikely to have septic arthritis, whereas those with three or four were very likely to have septic arthritis. It is important to remember that the Kocher criteria are only part of the decision-making process, and subsequent prospective studies have shown that patients with none of the criteria may have as much as a 16.9% chance of having septic arthritis. Therefore, the criteria should be used in the context of the remainder of the history, examination, and clinical concern. As a result, CBC would be helpful in guiding decision making in this patient. If septic arthritis is a concern, regardless of Kocher criteria, then ultrasound of the hip with aspiration of any detectable fluid for definitive diagnosis may be indicated. Pyogenic arthritis typically contains greater than 50,000 WBCs/mm³ and requires treatment with irrigation and debridement of the joint, as well as antibiotics. An orthopedist should be consulted emergently for treatment of the infected joint or to assist in diagnosis in the emergency department. Transient synovitis occurs primarily in the hip, and the etiology is unknown. In contrast to reactive arthritis or inflammatory arthritis from juvenile idiopathic arthritis, transient synovitis will resolve spontaneously without any treatment other than supportive measures, so observation may be appropriate once clinical concern for septic arthritis has resolved. Occasionally, initial presentation of Legg-Calvé-Perthes disease may be misdiagnosed as transient synovitis, as X-rays may be negative, but recurrence of limp and subsequent development of radiographic changes of the femoral head ultimately result in diagnosis. Lyme disease, caused by *Borrelia burgdorferi*, transmitted by the *Ixodes* tick, is a consideration in endemic areas; arthritis is a late manifestation occurring months after inoculation and is typically nonpainful.

> **Helpful Tip**
> Kocher criteria (inability to ambulate, T > 38°C [100.4°F], WBC > 12,000, ESR > 40) assist in guiding evaluation but should not dictate decision making in patients with history and exam findings that are concerning for septic arthritis versus transient synovitis. Definitive diagnosis is based on ultrasound identification of effusion, joint aspirate, and results from microscopy and culture of synovial fluid in concerning cases.

▶ CASE 19

You are moonlighting in the emergency department when a 16-year-old boy presents with a left leg injury. He was playing in a football game earlier in the day and ended up at the bottom of the pile. He states his leg was planted while he was twisted underneath a large pile. He heard and felt a large crack and developed immediate onset of pain over the left shin and lower extremity. There was visible deformity and he was unable to bear weight on his left lower extremity. He was transferred by ambulance to the emergency department, where X-rays demonstrated a displaced midshaft tibia and fibula fractures. He is noted to have a fair amount of swelling. Exam demonstrates normal sensation over the dorsal and plantar aspects of his foot. Normal and symmetric pulses are palpated in both lower extremities. He is able to move all of his toes without difficulty. While you await the orthopedist, you begin educating the resident about compartment syndrome.

Question 19-1

Which statement is false regarding acute compartment syndrome?
A) Definitive diagnosis is made by attaining intracompartmental pressure measurements.
B) Pain requiring increasing analgesia is a late finding.
C) Emergent fasciotomy is treatment of choice.
D) It can be a complication associated with fracture or crush injury.

Discussion 19-1

The correct answer is "B." Acute compartment syndrome results from increased interstitial pressure within a finite compartment, leading to vascular compromise of the associated nerves and muscles within that compartment and ischemic injury. Although relatively uncommon in children, acute compartment

syndrome can result in irreversible damage to the associated nerves and muscles. This damage can occur in 4 to 6 hours and thus is a medical emergency. Fractures are the most common injury associated with acute compartment syndrome; other risk factors include crush injury, restrictive splints or casts following a fracture or manipulation of a fracture, and vascular injury. Specifically, supracondylar fractures and tibial shaft fractures are the most common fractures associated with compartment syndrome. Pain out of proportion to the injury or pain requiring increasing analgesia is classically an early symptom and the most sensitive symptom of acute compartment syndrome. Other symptoms include a tense swollen extremity, paraesthesias, pallor, paralysis, and pulselessness. However, many of these are late findings and indicate vascular compromise. Diagnosis requires a high suspicion for acute compartment syndrome and can often be made clinically in the older, alert, reliable patient. However, in younger or obtunded patients, intracompartmental pressures may be required to confirm the diagnosis. Treatment requires emergent fasciotomy of the affected compartment(s).

> **Helpful Tip**
> One should have a high suspicion for compartment syndrome in a child who sustained a supracondylar fracture of the distal humerus, or a tibial shaft or eminence fracture, and is requiring increasing analgesia due to progressive pain. Check the compartments!

▶ CASE 20

Your next patient while moonlighting in the emergency department is a 4-year-old boy who presents after falling on his left arm, which was fully extended, while playing on the monkey bars at school. He developed immediate pain in his left arm, which was initially rather diffuse in nature. However, once the patient was taken to the nurse's office, the pain appeared to concentrate around the elbow. No obvious deformity was noted; however, the elbow began to swell shortly after the fall. Due to the pain and swelling, the family was called and advised to take the patient to the doctor. In the emergency department X-rays were obtained and demonstrated a type II supracondylar fracture of the left distal humerus. While awaiting the orthopedic consultation, you begin to discuss the evaluation and management of pediatric elbow injuries with the resident.

Question 20-1

Which statement is false regarding the patient's injury?
A) The presence of a posterior elbow fat pad can be normal, and comparison views should be obtained.
B) Ulnar nerve function can be checked by asking the patient to cross the index and middle fingers.
C) A fall on an outstretched hand is the most common mechanism of injury.
D) The brachial artery is the most common vascular injury associated with this injury.

Discussion 20-1

The correct answer is "A." Supracondylar fractures are the most common type of elbow fracture in children. This fracture often occurs after a fall on an outstretched hand (FOOSH), with subsequent hyperextension of the elbow. The fracture is commonly classified into three types. Type I is a nondisplaced or minimally displaced fracture. Type I fractures can present as an occult fracture, without a fracture line visible on X-ray. In the absence of a fracture line on X-ray, the presence of a fat pad sign can indicate an occult fracture. Specifically, the posterior fat pad visible on X-ray indicates a joint effusion, raising concern for an occult fracture in the setting of an acute injury in the skeletally immature patient. (See Figure 22–8.) Type I supracondylar fractures generally respond well to non-operative treatment in a long arm cast for about 3 weeks. Type II supracondylar fractures are characterized by obvious disruption of one cortex (often the anterior) with the opposite cortex intact (often posterior). Type II supracondylar fractures also commonly have some degree of associated angulation or extension. Due to the angulation, type II supracondylar fractures often require reduction and surgical stabilization. Type III supracondylar fractures involve disruption of both cortices with complete displacement, requiring reduction and further surgical stabilization. Supracondylar type II and III fractures should be referred urgently to orthopedics. Neurovascular injuries can occur in the setting of supracondylar fractures.

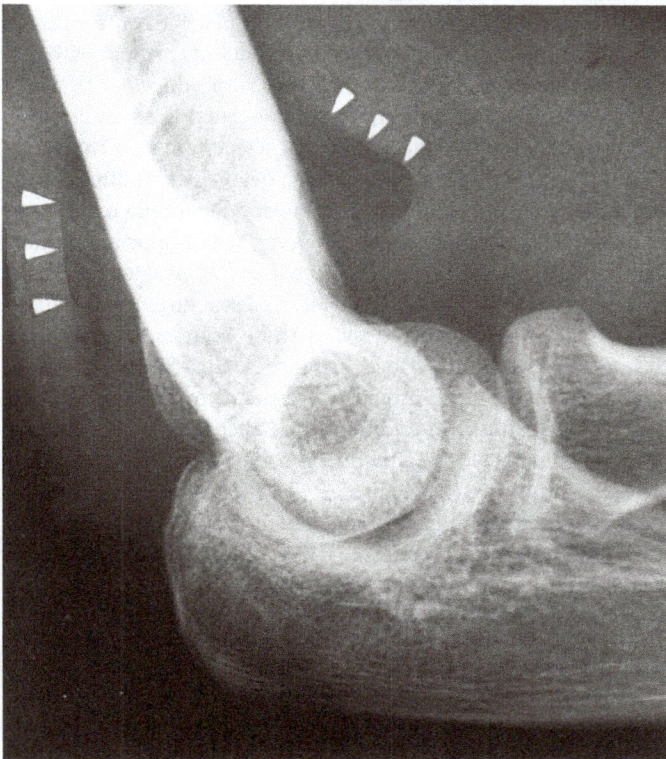

FIGURE 22–8. Supracondylar fracture. Note that the fracture is not visible, but the anterior and posterior fat pad signs are. (Reproduced with permission from Tintinalli JE, Stapczynski JS, Ma OJ, Cline DM, Cydulka RK, & Meckler GD (Eds). *Tintinalli's Emergency Medicine: A Comprehensive Study Guide*, 7th ed. New York, NY: McGraw Hill Education, Inc. Figure 133-12, Pg 898.)

Thus, a thorough neurovascular exam should be conducted on the initial encounter and each subsequent encounter. The median nerve is the most commonly injured nerve. Sensation and function of the median nerve can be checked by assessing sensation along the palmar aspect of the index and long finger and active flexion at the interphalangeal joint (asking the patient to form an "O" with the thumb and index finger). The radial nerve is the second most common nerve injured. Sensation of the radial nerve is assessed along the dorsal first web space. Motor function can be assessed by having the patient extend his or her thumb ("thumbs up"). Distal sensation of the ulnar nerve is assessed along the palmer aspect of the small finger. Motor function can be checked by have the patient actively abduct the fingers ("crossed finger").

> **Helpful Tip**
> Remember the mantra "examine (and image) the joint above and below." Elbow injuries can occur in the context of other upper extremity injuries, so complete evaluation of FOOSH injuries involves examining the wrist, elbow, and shoulder, and imaging may include not only wrist, forearm, and shoulder X-rays, but also elbow X-rays (and vice versa).

▶ CASE 21

In clinic the following day, your first patient is a 20-month-old boy who presents with refusal to bear weight through his right lower extremity. His mother states he was playing in his room and came running to show her something. She heard him fall and went to see if he was okay. He was lying next to a toy on the floor crying. She is unsure what happened, but thinks he may have slipped on the toy. She did not appreciate any swelling or bruising of his leg. However, the patient refused to bear any weight through his right lower extremity and thus she called right away to make an appointment. She reports he has otherwise been well, no fevers, normal appetite, no other joint swelling or erythema. No prior upper respiratory or gastrointestinal symptoms. On exam the patient is well appearing, nontoxic, and afebrile. There is no effusion appreciable throughout his right lower extremity (knee or ankle). He has normal range of motion at the ankle, knee, and hip. He is fairly anxious during the exam making assessment of focal tenderness difficult. X-rays of his femur, tibia, and bilateral hips are negative for any obvious fracture lucency at this time, and there are no signs of effusion on X-rays.

Question 21-1

The most likely diagnosis is:

A) Juvenile rheumatoid arthritis.
B) Occult fracture of the distal tibia.
C) Legg-Calvé-Perthes disease.
D) Transient synovitis.
E) Developmental dysplasia of the hip.

Discussion 21-1

The correct answer is "B." The toddler's fracture was initially described as an occult or obscure fracture of the distal tibia. This type of fracture takes its name from its most common sufferer: a young ambulator (commonly 9 months to 3 years old) who loses balance and twists while falling, causing a low-energy and rather minor torsional injury. Not too uncommonly, the injury is unwitnessed. Often, the presentation includes a new-onset limp or refusal to bear weight. As with any injury, especially fracture, in a child, an appropriate history should be obtained, making sure the fracture pattern fits the mechanism. If not, or if other concerns are present, nonaccidental trauma should be considered; any fracture in a nonambulatory patient should raise concern for nonaccidental trauma. Care should be taken to evaluate signs and symptoms consistent with other etiologies of new-onset limp or refusal to bear weight (eg, transient synovitis, septic arthritis, etc). AP and lateral X-rays of the affected lower extremity should be obtained. Initial films may be negative for fracture lucency. An internal oblique X-ray of the tibia and fibula may be beneficial in these cases, providing another view. However, these too may be negative in some cases. If X-rays are negative, but history and exam are consistent with concern for an occult fracture, treatment should be instituted. Treatment often consists of cast immobilization in a long leg cast. In cases where initial X-rays are negative for fracture lucency, follow-up X-rays 10 to 14 days after injury may help to confirm the diagnosis. Treatment consists of cast immobilization for about 3 to 4 weeks.

> **Helpful Tip**
>
> Fractures in children may not always be readily apparent on initial X-rays; thus, suspicion for an occult fracture should be raised in the setting of an acute injury. Children with type I supracondylar fractures may present with refusal to use the affected arm following a FOOSH injury. X-rays may be negative for a fracture line; however, care should be taken to assess for the fat pad signs indicating an effusion and subsequently an occult fracture. Toddler's fractures are another common injury in young children that may present with limited clinical and radiographic signs. These fractures do not occur in the nonambulatory patient and thus should raise concern if seen in this population. Additionally, fractures are concerning for child abuse when the injury mechanism does not fit the type of fracture or other historical or physical findings are present.

▶ CASE 22

A 9-year-old girl presents for evaluation of a right ankle injury she sustained over the weekend in a basketball game. She went up for a rebound and "landed funny" on her right foot and ankle. She had difficulty ambulating afterward and had to be helped off the court. An athletic trainer, volunteering at the tournament, evaluated the patient shortly after the injury. Her mother is unsure what the diagnosis from the trainer was but knows that rest, ice, and wrapping the ankle with an elastic bandage were advised. She was also advised to follow up with the doctor this week. On exam the patient has mild swelling over the lateral aspect of the ankle. Sensation is intact and she has appropriate pulses. Motor function is intact, with ability to wiggle her toes. Movement at the ankle is limited and painful. With palpation, the point of maximal tenderness is over the lateral malleolus at the level of the joint line. No significant tenderness extends anterior to the lateral malleolus. There is no significant translation when cupping the heel and attempting translation of the talus on the tibia. X-rays demonstrate a skeletally immature patient, with no obvious fracture or dislocation, but with mild soft tissue swelling over the lateral ankle.

Question 22-1

What is the most likely diagnosis?
A) Septic arthritis.
B) Lateral ankle sprain.
C) Tendinopathy.
D) Salter-Harris I fracture of the distal fibula.

Discussion 22-1

The correct answer is "D." The physis is made up of different zones of cartilaginous cells, which provide longitudinal growth of long bones. This structure is inherently weaker relative to the associated ligaments. Thus, skeletally immature individuals are more likely to sustain an injury to the growth plate (fracture) than a sprain (ligamentous injury). Clinically, patients present with history of trauma, overuse, or both. Pain is produced with active and passive range of motion of the associated joint, in addition to palpation over the affected physis. Depending on the severity of the injury and fracture, various degrees of swelling, bruising, and pain may be present. X-rays vary depending on the type of injury, as described below. However, it is important to note that X-rays often are negative for obvious fracture lucency in the setting of a nondisplaced Salter-Harris I fracture. Thus, clinical exam is important in diagnosis of these injuries. Physeal injuries are commonly described using the Salter-Harris classification. This classification provides a standard method to describe the fracture pattern. In addition, the Salter-Harris classification provides guidance for treatment and some information regarding expected prognosis. (See Figure 22–9.) Treatment varies depending on the fracture and age of the patient. Displaced physeal fractures should be urgently referred to an orthopedist. Nondisplaced fractures can be splinted and referred to a pediatric orthopedic or sports medicine specialist within 7 to 10 days.

> **Helpful Tip**
>
> The health care provider should have a low threshold for fracture in a skeletally immature patient or athlete. Children with open growth plates are more likely to sustain a physeal injury (fracture) than a sprain (ligament injury).

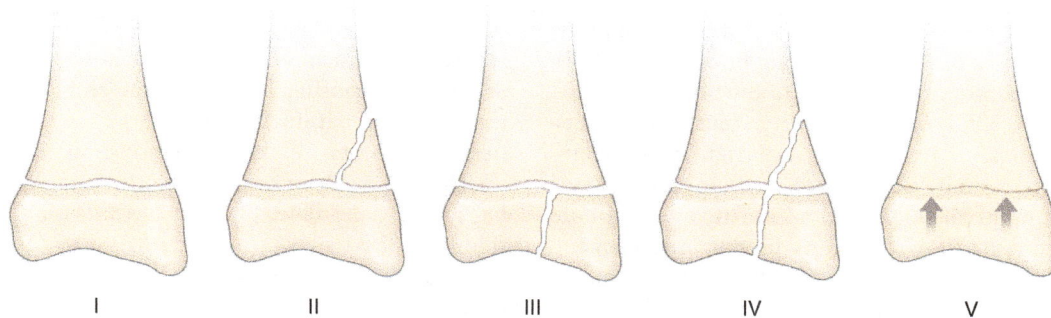

FIGURE 22–9. Salter-Harris classification of physeal fractures: I—fracture extends through the physis; II—fracture extends through the physis and into the metaphysis; III—fracture extends through the physis and into the epiphysis; IV—fracture extends through the physis and into the metaphysis *and* epiphysis; V—crush injury. (Used with permission from Blaise Nemeth, MD, MS.)

▶ CASE 23

An 8-year-old right-hand dominant male patient presents for evaluation of right shoulder pain. While playing in a little league game over the weekend he was hit in the shoulder by a line drive. He had immediate onset of pain over the proximal aspect of his shoulder. There was mild bruising, which his parents thought was the cause of his pain. However, due to persistent pain and refusal to use the arm they decided to seek medical care. The patient denies pain in the elbow and denies any pain in his other extremities, including the left shoulder. On exam, you note tenderness with palpation over the right proximal humerus. You decide to obtain X-rays of his right humerus to evaluate further. On review of the X-rays, you notice a cystic lesion of the right proximal humerus. (See Figure 22–10.) In talking with radiology, this appears most consistent with a unicameral bone cyst.

Question 23-1

What do you discuss with family regarding the natural history of this bone lesion?

A) This lesion requires an emergent referral to oncology and orthopedic surgery for prompt treatment.

B) The lesion remains dormant in childhood and typically expands after skeletal maturity.

C) The lesion starts near the physis, typically migrates away from the physis with growth, and can spontaneously resolve.

D) The lesion is very aggressive, causing significant disruption of the cortex, pain, periosteal reaction, and associated soft tissue swelling.

Discussion 23-1

The correct answer is "C." This child has a unicameral bone cyst or a simple bone cyst. Unicameral bone cysts are typically found in the metaphysis of long bones. The proximal humerus and proximal femur are two common locations where this cyst can occur; the calcaneus is another location. The diagnosis is often made when patients present for care with a pathologic fracture through the cyst, as the isolated cyst generally does not produce symptoms. The diagnosis can be made given the characteristic

FIGURE 22–10. Cystic lesion consistent with unicameral bone cyst. (Reproduced with permission from Doherty GM (Ed). Current Diagnosis & Treatment: Surgery, 14ed. McGraw-Hill Education, Inc., 2015. Fig 40-40.)

appearance on X-ray. Radiographically, the lesion appears as an isolated central, lucent lesion, located within the medullary canal of the metaphysis of the affected long bone. In an active lesion, it often lies immediately adjacent to the physis. Cortical thinning may be present; however, the cortex generally remains intact, unless a pathologic fracture has occurred. The differential diagnosis includes nonossifying fibroma, chondroblastoma, and focal fibrous dysplasia. Observation is a treatment option for asymptomatic cysts. If a fracture is present management includes appropriate treatment of the fracture. Surgical treatment is indicated for large cysts in weight-bearing or dominant limbs or cysts at high risk of fracture. Intralesional corticosteroid injection have been used with some success in treatment of unicameral bone cysts; however, multiple injections may be required. Surgical curettage and bone grafting or intramedullary pinning is occasionally necessary.

> **Helpful Tip**
> Unicameral bone cysts are a common bone lesion in children and may present incidentally, or with indolent onset of pain and stress fracture or acute fracture through the cyst and thin cortex.

▶ CASE 24

A 13-year-old girl presents for evaluation of right leg pain. She denies any injury prior to onset of pain. She states the pain has progressively increased over the past few weeks. It is located over her right shin and is fairly constant. At times it is worse with ambulation. She is accompanied by her mother, and both deny any history of skin changes or swelling. On exam the patient's gait appears symmetric without a limp. The skin over her shin is intact without bruising or erythema. With palpation, she has pain located over the proximal tibia on the right relative to the left. AP and lateral X-rays of her right tibia and fibula demonstrate a rather large, expansive, lucent lesion located in the proximal tibia at the metadiaphyseal junction. There is associated cortical thinning, disruption, and associated periosteal reaction.

Question 24-1

What is the most appropriate next step?
A) Referral to oncology to start chemotherapy.
B) Referral for an incisional biopsy to confirm diagnosis.
C) Reassure family and plan to follow up in 9 to 12 months with repeat X-rays.
D) Intralesional corticosteroid injection.

Discussion 24-1

The correct answer is "B." The patient has any aneurysmal bone cyst—a type of cyst that is typically benign but can be a rather aggressive bone lesion, often mimicking a malignant process. Aneurysmal bone cysts generally occur in adolescents, with the peak incidence in the second decade of life. They can

affect any bone but are most commonly found in the femur, tibia, and spine. Although the natural history of these lesions is often unpredictable, they can demonstrate rapid expansion and growth causing localized pain and swelling. Aggressive lesions found within the spine grow to produce compressive nerve symptoms. X-rays will demonstrate a radiolucent lesion, which is expansile in nature, with the metaphysis often appearing to "balloon" wider than the physis with associated cortical thinning. The lesion can cause cortical disruption and periosteal reaction. The differential diagnosis includes osteosarcoma, chondroblastoma, giant cell tumor, and fibrous dysplasia. Given the aggressive nature and appearance of the lesion, incisional biopsy is recommended to confirm the diagnosis. Treatment often requires curettage and bone grafting or excision. Between 20% and 30% of patients have recurrence, typically within 12 to 24 months.

> **Helpful Tip**
> Unicameral bone cysts are often found immediately adjacent to the physis. They are benign cysts, typically asymptomatic unless a pathologic fracture is present. Aneurysmal bone cysts are benign but potentially aggressive, expansile bone cysts that often mimic a malignant process. An incisional biopsy is required to confirm diagnosis, and surgical curettage versus excision for treatment.

▶ CASE 25

A 12-year-old girl presents for her well-child check. On standing her right shoulder is slightly higher than the left, and the Adams forward bending test demonstrates elevation of the ribs to the right of her spine. Her neurologic examination is normal, including sensation, strength, and reflexes in upper and lower extremities. Skin is clear, including over the lumbar spine. Her height is 130 cm; her right leg measures 68 cm and her left leg measures 68.4 cm. Standing, full-length spine X-rays demonstrate a 25-degree thoracic curve to the right and a 25-degree lumbar curve to the left. (See Figure 22–11.) No vertebral anomalies are noted.

Question 25-1

The most likely cause her curve is:
A) Congenital scoliosis.
B) Leg-length discrepancy.
C) Tethered spinal cord.
D) Marfan syndrome.
E) Unknown.

Discussion 25-1

The correct answer is "E." Scoliosis, defined as a curve of greater than 10 degrees as measured by the Cobb method (see Figure 22–11), occurs in 3% to 5% of adolescents, equally in boys and girls. Girls more commonly present for evaluation

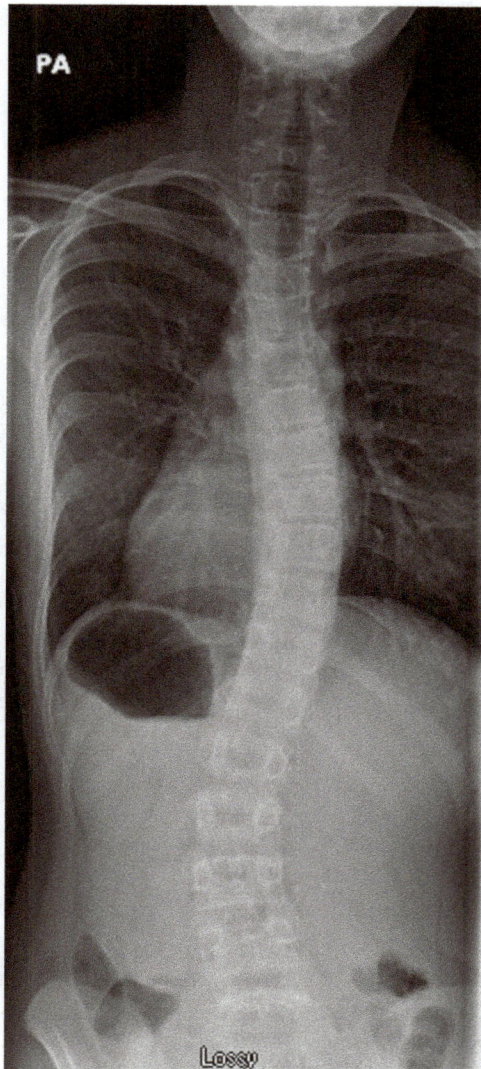

FIGURE 22–11. PA X-ray of the spine, as noted in the upper left. As a result, the patient's right side is to the right, and the cardiac silhouette and gastric air bubble are to the left. (Used with permission from Blaise Nemeth, MD, MS.)

due to more significant curves. Spinal curves can occur due to abnormalities of vertebral body development (in which case the term *congenital scoliosis* is used), tethered cord (often signaled by cutaneous lesions over the lumbar spine or an abnormal neurologic exam with hyperreflexia, spasticity, or foot deformities on one or both sides), and neuromuscular diseases or genetic syndromes, such as Marfan syndrome, neurofibromatosis, or achondroplasia, in which cases other findings of the syndromes should be present. Children younger than 10 years of age are more likely to have scoliosis secondary to one of these causes. Physical exam utilizing the Adams forward-bending test is the primary means of evaluation and detection. Curves related to leg-length discrepancies occur in the lumbar spine and resolve when the leg-length difference is corrected. Typically a leg-length difference of 0.5 to 1 cm is necessary to create a clinically identifiable curve. If no other cause of the curve is identified and the patient is at least 10 years old, the

term *adolescent idiopathic scoliosis* is used. Numerous theories exist, considering the association of scoliosis with neurologic, bone, and connective disorders and the prevalence during puberty, but the exact cause is unknown in most cases.

The patient's mother reveals that there is a cousin with scoliosis who required surgery, and she is concerned that her daughter might need surgery.

Question 25-2
What is the most reliable predictor for curve progression in a female patient with adolescent idiopathic scoliosis?
A) Patient age.
B) Curve magnitude.
C) Sexual maturity rating.
D) Family history.
E) Type of curve.

Discussion 25-2
The correct answer is "C." While age is important in defining adolescent idiopathic scoliosis (ie, older than 10 years), risk of progression is related to both curve magnitude and proximity to skeletal maturity, which is closely related to sexual maturity rating. Larger curves have an increased risk of progression, but skeletal maturity status determines the extent to which progression is likely to occur. Patients who have not yet passed peak height velocity have the greatest risk of progression. For females, menarche occurs shortly after peak height velocity, and skeletal maturity occurs about 2 years later. Boys take longer to reach skeletal maturity. On scoliosis X-rays, the Risser sign is used to estimate remaining growth potential after peak height velocity. The Risser sign utilizes the ossification of the iliac crest apophysis, which starts after peak height velocity. The iliac crest is divided into four quadrants (see Figure 22–12), and as ossification proceeds, the iliac crest apophysis grows posteriorly. Chronologic age and sexual maturity rating may vary greatly at any given age.

The patient is premenarchal.

Question 25-3
What is the most appropriate next step in management?
A) Return in 6 months for repeat evaluation.
B) Referral to physical therapy.
C) Referral to orthopedics for bracing.
D) Referral to orthopedics for surgery.

Discussion 25-3
The correct answer is "C." Adolescent idiopathic scoliosis typically progresses during times of growth, but currently it is not possible predict how quickly and to what degree. There is greater risk of progression in younger individuals and in the presence of higher degree curves. Bracing has been shown to decrease the rate of progression to surgery and is usually indicated for growing individuals with curves exceeding 20 to 25 degrees, so referral to pediatric orthopedics is appropriate. Surgery is usually not indicated unless curves exceed 40 to 50 degrees. Beyond

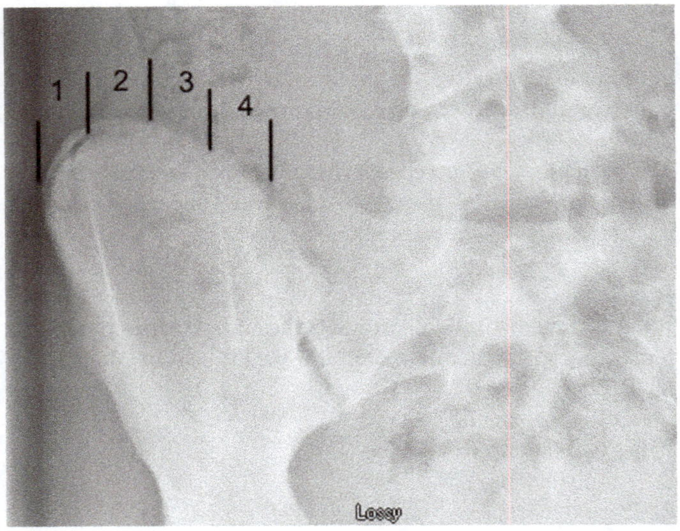

FIGURE 22–12. Ossification of the iliac crest apophysis, as seen on a PA scoliosis X-ray, is used to approximate time following peak height velocity until skeletal maturity. (Image has been cropped to exclude spine and magnify findings of the left iliac crest.) No ossification is graded as Risser 0; 1% to 25% is Risser 1; 26% to 50% is Risser 2; 51% to 75% is Risser 3; and greater than 75% is Risser 4. Closure of the apophysis is Risser 5 and represents skeletal maturity. This patient would be assigned Risser 2 status since the iliac crest apophysis ossification has advanced posteriorly into the second quadrant. (Used with permission from Blaise Nemeth, MD, MS.)

this point curves may progress after skeletal maturity, and patients may develop cardiorespiratory compromise. Physical therapy has not been shown to be effective in preventing significant curve progression. Continued monitoring would not be appropriate in this case given the curve parameters and skeletally immature status of the patient suggesting high risk for curve progression, although for a patient older than 10 years of age with minimal asymmetry on Adams forward-bending test (or radiographic curve < 20 degrees), follow-up evaluation in 6 months is recommended with referral and X-ray if progression is noted.

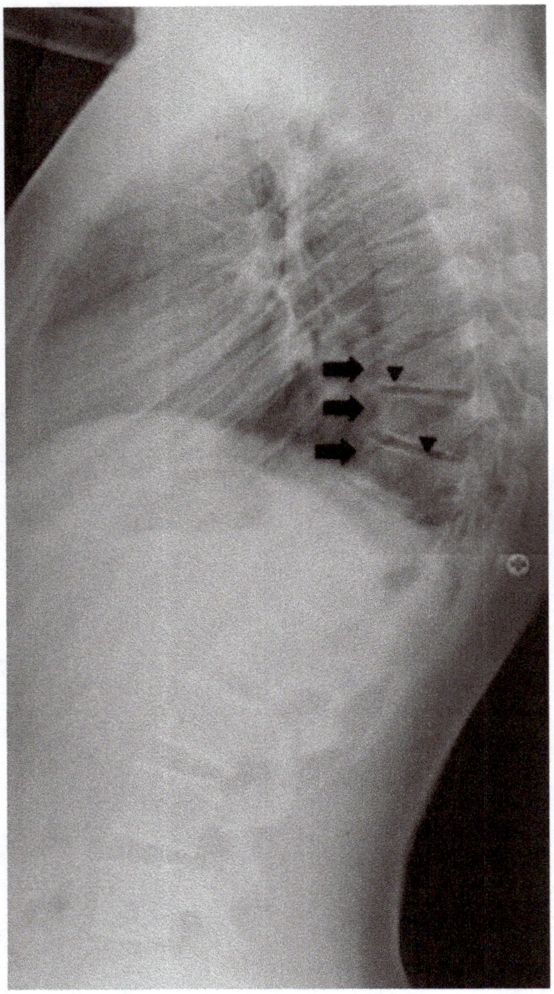

► CASE 26

A 14-year-old boy presents with his mother, who is concerned about his posture. She tells him to sit up straight, but he continues to slouch. She first had concerns 2 years ago and thinks his posture is worsening. He denies pain or neurologic symptoms. On forward bending, there is no asymmetry to his spine or ribs, but he has an abrupt forward angulation to his spine. X-rays are obtained (see Figure 22–13) demonstrating 55 degrees of kyphosis and wedging of multiple vertebral bodies with irregularity of the endplates.

Question 26-1

The most appropriate next step in management is:
A) Referral to physical therapy.
B) Referral to pediatric orthopedics.
C) Referral for chiropractic manipulation.
D) Continued observation.

FIGURE 22–13. Lateral scoliosis X-ray demonstrating wedging of vertebral bodies (*block arrows*) and endplate irregularities (*arrowheads*). (Used with permission from Blaise Nemeth, MD, MS.)

Discussion 26-1

The correct answer is "B." Normal kyphosis of the thoracic spine is 25 to 45 degrees. Scheuermann kyphosis is defined as increased thoracic kyphosis with anterior wedging of at least 5 degrees involving three or more consecutive vertebral bodies. (See Figure 22–13.) The etiology is unknown. Scheuermann kyphosis progresses during adolescence and bracing may slow progression in individuals who are still growing, although referral to pediatric orthopedics for further discussion and shared decision making with the patient and family is most appropriate. Surgery typically is not considered until curves exceed 75 to 85 degrees. Physical therapy and chiropractic manipulation have not been shown to decrease the risk of progression of Scheuermann kyphosis, although physical therapy may be useful for patients with associated muscular back pain. Patients with postural kyphosis have normal X-rays and resolution of their kyphosis with laying down; observation or physical therapy may be appropriate, depending on patient and family preference.

A 4-year-old boy presents with persistent right leg pain. His mother states that for the past 2 weeks he has been "walking funny." He has continued to run and play, but he will stop playing earlier than everyone else secondary to pain. She has noticed he generally points to his right thigh and knee when complaining of pain. She denies any history of injury prior to onset of pain. The patient has been otherwise well and at his baseline health. There is no history of fevers, no other joint swelling or erythema, and no abnormal rashes. His gait exam in the hallway demonstrates asymmetry. You notice his upper body tends to lurch or lean laterally toward the right side through stance phase on his right leg. On examination of his hips, you also note asymmetry in abduction, in the frog-leg position, with about 60 degrees of abduction on the right relative to about 75 degrees of abduction on the left. An AP/frog-leg X-ray of the pelvis demonstrates the findings seen in Figure 22–14.

Question 27-1

All of the following statements regarding the patient's diagnosis are true EXCEPT:

A) Residual deformity and hip joint congruity at skeletal maturity are two of the most important prognostic factors.

B) Age of onset before 8 years of age is associated with a worse prognosis.

C) Long-term studies report most patients do well until the fifth decade.

D) Girls have a worse prognosis than boys.

Discussion 27-1

The correct answer is "B." Legg-Calvé-Perthes (LCP) disease is defined as idiopathic osteonecrosis of the femoral head. The true etiology is unknown, though many theories have been proposed. LCP is more common in males than females, with a peak age of onset between 4 and 8 years. It can affect both hips in about 10%

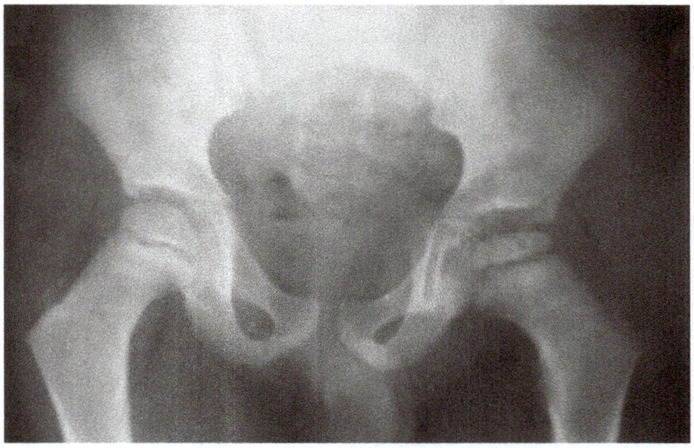

FIGURE 22–14. Legg-Calvé-Perthes disease of the left hip. X-ray demonstrates fragmentation and flattening of the femoral head. (Reproduced with permission from Skinner HB, McMahon PJ: *CURRENT Diagnosis & Treatment in Orthopedics*, 5th ed. New York: McGraw-Hill; 2014.)

to 12% of cases. Patients often present with an insidious onset of limp and pain. Pain can be nonspecific, with patients describing hip, thigh, or knee pain, or a combination of these. Pain is generally worse with activity. On exam, patients with an acute presentation demonstrate an antalgic gait. They also have limited range of motion of the affected hip, most commonly involving hip abduction and internal rotation. Four different radiographic stages are used to describe LCP. The first, appropriately named the initial stage, is characterized by synovitis and early necrosis. On radiographs, there may be subtle widening of the joint space, a subchondral fracture of the femoral epiphysis, or both. During the second stage, fragmentation, the femoral epiphysis begins to collapse. Radiographs demonstrate fragmentation of the femoral epiphysis with areas of increased radiolucency apparent. The degree of deformity depends on the amount of collapse that occurs during this phase. The third stage, reossification, is characterized by new bone formation. The final stage is the healed stage. In this stage the residual deformity of the femoral head and proximal femur is apparent. The true natural history of LCP is unknown; however, various long-term follow-up studies have provided us with what is currently known. Most patients do well without significant pain or limitations until about the fifth decade. Thereafter hip function begins to deteriorate. Most patients develop degenerative joint disease by the sixth and seventh decades of life. Residual femoral head deformity and hip joint congruity at skeletal maturity, age at onset, and sex are all prognostic factors. Age of onset before 6 to 8 years carries a better prognosis due to the remodeling potential. Female patients also appear to have a poorer prognosis relative to their male counterparts. The treatment goals include preserving a round femoral head and joint congruency in addition to maintaining hip range of motion. Treatment is somewhat controversial and varies depending on the age, symptoms, severity of femoral head involvement, and joint congruency. Nonsurgical treatment options include activity limitations, physical therapy, and abduction bracing or casting. Surgical treatment includes both femoral or pelvic surgical options.

> **Helpful Tip**
> Consider hip pathology in a limping child who complains of knee pain.

A 9-year-old female soccer player presents with bilateral heel pain. The pain started about 3 to 4 weeks ago. There was no known injury prior to onset of pain. The pain is located over the bilateral heels and is worse with activity, specifically, worse after soccer activities. Rest and ibuprofen alleviate the pain. The family denies any swelling or redness of the heels. She did have to sit out of part of the last game secondary to pain. On exam, her gait is normal without evidence of antalgia. Bench exam demonstrates mild heel cord contractures with passive dorsiflexion just a few degrees past neutral (legs extended). She has a positive calcaneal squeeze test bilaterally.

Question 28-1

Which of the following is characteristic of this patient's diagnosis?

A) It is a rare cause of heel pain in the preteen age group.
B) Treatment often involves repeated corticosteroid injections or surgery.
C) Maximal pain is elicited with medial and lateral compression along the posterior calcaneus.
D) This condition is more common in females than males.
E) Patients often present with morning stiffness and swelling.

Discussion 28-1

The correct answer is "C." This patient has Severs disease, also known as calcaneal apophysitis, a common cause of heel pain in children between 8 and 13 years of age. It is more common in boys than girls, is bilateral about 60% of the time, and is often seen in children participating in soccer, basketball, running, and gymnastics. Patients present with heel pain that is worse with activity. Clinically, the calcaneal squeeze test (medial and lateral compression of the posterior third of the calcaneus) reproduces the pain. In addition, patients may have associated heel cord tightness and midfoot pronation. Severs disease is a clinical diagnosis. X-rays (AP calcaneal view and lateral view) are generally not necessary but should be considered to rule out other causes of heel pain if history and exam are not classic. Calcaneal apophysitis does not present after skeletal maturity. Treatment includes a combination of activity modifications, anti-inflammatories, and addressing any biomechanical issues with the use of orthotics, gel heel cups, or both. Occasionally, a short leg walking cast or walking boot may be used in patients with more significant pain or activity limitations. Symptoms resolve, on average, after about 2 months with a range between 1 and 6 months.

Discussion 29-1

The correct answer is "B." This patient has Osgood-Schlatter disease (OSD), a common cause of anterior knee pain in patients between 10 and 15 years of age. OSD is a traction apophysitis that occurs at the insertion of the patellar tendon at the tibial tubercle. Sinding-Larsen-Johannsen (SLJ) disease, another apophysitis responsible for anterior knee pain, occurs at the inferior pole of the patella. Both OSD and SLJ are thought to occur secondary to overuse of the extensor mechanism and thus are common in athletes participating in jumping sports. OSD is more common in males and is typically diagnosed with history and clinical exam. Patients present with anterior knee pain that localizes to the tibial tubercle. Pain is worse with activity, and improved with rest and anti-inflammatories. Some patients may develop mild swelling or a prominence over the tibial tubercle. X-rays (AP and lateral knee) should be considered in atypical clinical cases to evaluate for other pathology (eg, tumor, fracture, infection). They commonly demonstrate fragmentation of the tibial tubercle, but this finding may also be seen in asymptomatic patients so is not diagnostic. (See Figure 22–15.) As with other apophysitis conditions, OSD, is an age-limited process and generally improves with skeletal maturity; however, some patients continue to report pain with kneeling after skeletal maturity. Treatment includes activity modifications, ice, and anti-inflammatories. Physical therapy can be used as an adjunct to focus on quadriceps and hamstring stretching and strengthening exercises. More recently, an injection of hyperosmolar dextrose has been used with some success in recalcitrant cases of OSD.

► CASE 29

A 13-year-old previously healthy boy presents for evaluation of bilateral knee pain, left greater than right. He states pain was gradual in onset and denies any significant knee injury prior to onset of pain. The pain is located over the anterior, inferior aspect of his knee and is worse with running and jumping. It has increased since he started basketball season a month ago. On exam, he has symmetric range of motion of the knees bilaterally, and no appreciable swelling. His exam is negative for a ligamentous injury. The point of maximal tenderness is along the tibial tubercle bilaterally. X-rays demonstrate fragmentation of the tibial tuberosity.

Question 29-1

Of the following, the most likely cause of the patient's symptoms is:

A) Physeal fracture of the proximal femur.
B) Traction apophysitis at the insertion of the patellar tendon on the tibia.
C) Avascular necrosis of the femoral head.
D) Acute fracture of the tibial tubercle.

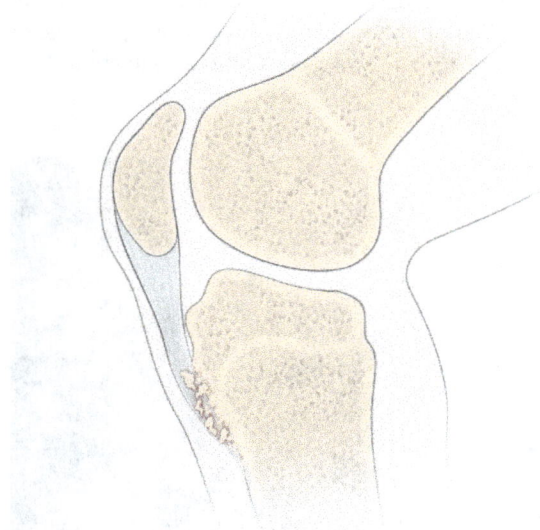

FIGURE 22–15. Osgood-Schlatter disease. It is common, but not necessary, to see fragmentation of the tibial tubercle apophysis, similar to the diagram. (Reproduced with permission from Skinner HB, McMahon PJ, eds. *Current Diagnosis & Treatment in Orthopedics.* 5th ed. New York, NY: McGraw-Hill Education; 2014, Fig. 10-29.)

▶ **CASE 30**

Your first patient of the afternoon is a 12-year-old boy who recently transferred to your clinic for care. He presents for evaluation of right knee pain that began about 2 months ago when he twisted his knee as he was pushed into the pool. He states his whole leg hurt at that time and he had difficulty bearing weight. He was seen in a local emergency department and X-rays of his knee were negative (the family did not bring a copy today). He was diagnosed with a knee sprain and discharged home with crutches. He was seen by a physician a few weeks after the injury and instructed to wean off the crutches as tolerated. He continued to use the crutches for another month and discontinued use about 1 week ago because school started, despite continued pain. On exam, you notice asymmetry in his gait. He demonstrates antalgia and appears to lean to the right with stance phase. On bench exam he has vague knee pain when flexing the right hip and knee relative to the left. He has no pain with palpation around the knee, and the exam is negative for any ligamentous injury. In addition, you note about 40 to 50 degrees of abduction on the right and about 70 to 75 degrees of abduction on the left. He also has limited internal rotation at about 10 degrees on the right and about 30 degrees of internal rotation on the left.

Question 30-1

What is the most appropriate next step?
A) AP and lateral X-rays of femur.
B) AP, lateral, Merchant, and tunnel X-rays of knee.
C) Referral for MRI of right knee.
D) AP and frog-leg X-rays of pelvis.
E) Referral to orthopedics.

Discussion 30-1

The correct answer is "D." Slipped capital femoral epiphysis (SCFE) is a physeal fracture involving the proximal femoral physis that results in anterior displacement of the proximal femoral neck and shaft. It is an orthopedic emergency. Obesity is the most common risk factor. SCFE occurs more commonly in males, and up to 60% of cases may have bilateral involvement (either at presentation or later). Endocrinopathies (thyroid disease, hypopituitarism, and renal osteodystrophy) are another common risk factor and should be considered in the workup of patients with an atypical presentation. Clinically, patients present with a variety of symptoms, including pain located over the anterior groin, thigh, knee, or a combination of these. When a child presents with knee pain, it is important to also examine the gait and hips to assess for possible hip pathology referring pain distally to the knee. Pain can be acute or insidious in onset. Other associated findings include limp (antalgic or Trendelenburg gait, out-toed gait) and decreased range of motion (most commonly involving flexion, abduction, and internal rotation). Diagnosis is based on history, clinical exam, and radiographic studies. Many

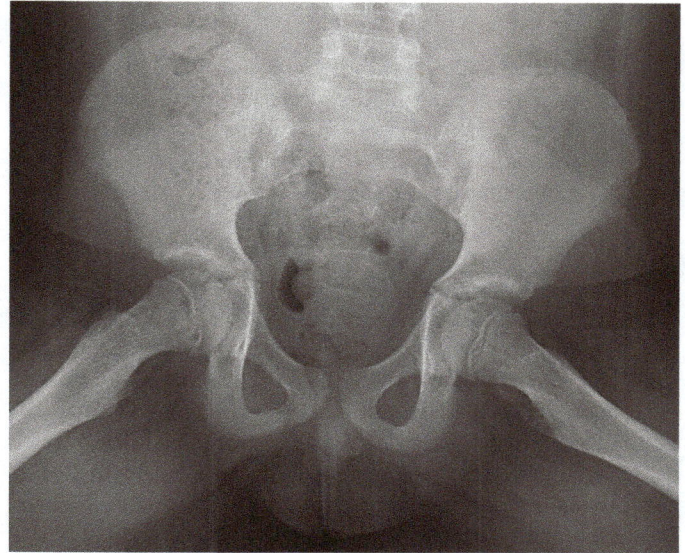

FIGURE 22–16. Slipped capital femoral epiphysis. Note the step-off between the metaphysis and epiphysis on this frogleg-lateral view of the right hip. (Used with permission from Natalie Stork, MD.)

cases of SCFE are diagnosed by AP and lateral films of the pelvis. Up to 50% of patients can have bilateral involvement on presentation. Thus, it is important to obtain radiographs of the bilateral hips and pelvis at the time of presentation. The AP view may show irregularity along the physis and or widening of the physis. The lateral hip film is important, as it is more sensitive in detecting mild slips. On the lateral film the posterior translation of the head relative to the femoral neck and shaft becomes more apparent. (See Figure 22–16.) MRI is an important tool when there is a high clinical suspicion for SCFE but X-rays are normal. This presentation has been referred to as a pre-slip SCFE. Increased signal on both sides of the physis seen on MRI is consistent with a pre-slip SCFE. Various classification systems are used to describe the fracture. One approach focuses on the time frame, classifying fractures as acute (symptom onset < 3 weeks) versus chronic (prodrome of symptoms > 3 weeks), and acute on chronic. The classification of SCFE as stable (the patient can bear weight either with or without crutches) versus unstable (patient unable to bear weight with or without crutches) can be helpful in making treatment decisions. Classification systems also are available for assessing severity based on the degree of slip measured radiographically. Patients diagnosed with SCFE should be made non—weight bearing immediately upon diagnosis despite ambulatory status prior to diagnosis, duration of symptoms, or degree of slip. In addition, upon diagnosis, the patient should be urgently or emergently (in the case of unstable slips) referred to an orthopedist. Treatment generally requires surgical fixation of the fracture. Complications associated with missed diagnosis or untreated SCFE include further progression and subsequent osteonecrosis of the femoral head leading to various other complications.

> **Helpful Tip**
>
> An obese adolescent with a painful limp and anterior thigh pain, groin pain, or unspecified knee pain should raise concern for SCFE. Patients demonstrate an antalgic and Trendelenburg gait with limited range of motion (flexion, abduction, and internal rotation).

▶ CASE 31

A 4-year-old boy presents with a complaint of back pain for the last 3 days. Today he awoke and refused to get out of bed. He is laying down when you enter the exam room and has difficulty rising to a sitting position, pointing to his lower back as the area of discomfort. His mother denies vomiting, diarrhea, urinary frequency, or complaints of nausea or dysuria. His temperature is 38°C (100.4°F). His abdomen is soft and he has negative obturator but positive psoas signs bilaterally. He is tender over the spine in the lumbar region, and his paraspinous muscles are tense and also tender. Neurologic examination of the lower extremities is normal, other than decreased strength with hip flexion due to back discomfort.

Question 31-1

The most likely diagnosis is:

A) Histiocytosis.
B) Urinary tract infection.
C) Discitis.
D) Spondylolysis.
E) Appendicitis.

Discussion 31-1

The correct answer is "C." Back pain in children should always raise concern for a pathologic etiology. In younger children, spine-associated abnormalities may manifest with back pain, abdominal pain, or refusal to walk, stand, or even sit. Discitis is the most likely cause of back pain in a young child, especially if fever is present, although fever is not always present. Often patients present with ill-defined symptoms and normal lab values, leading to delayed diagnosis. The psoas sign may be positive due to irritation from the psoas at its origin at the level of the spine. Discitis can be differentiated from pyelonephritis with associated costovertebral angle tenderness by the absence of urinary symptoms, although urinalysis may be helpful to rule out urinary tract infection. X-rays may reveal narrowing of the disc space at the level of involvement. MRI demonstrates edema within the disc and the adjacent vertebral bodies and is the diagnostic modality of choice. (See Figure 22–17.) Antibiotics typically yield resolution of symptoms, and bracing may provide comfort; *Staphylococcus aureus* is the most common infectious organism. Histiocytosis (previously termed *eosinophilic granuloma*) may occur in the spine and is the most common spinal tumor in children. The clinical presentation may be very similar to discitis, but X-rays will demonstrate vertebra plana (flattening of the vertebral body). (See Figure 22–18.) Patients may have other lesions, and biopsy evaluation confirms the diagnosis.

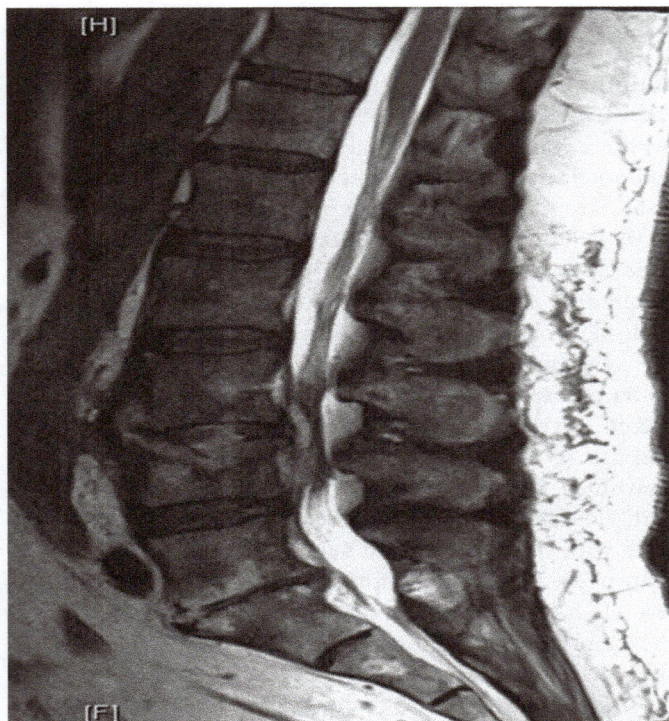

FIGURE 22–17. Sagittal MRI scan of the lumbar spine shows increased signal in the disc space and soft tissue posterior to the vertebral bodies suggestive of discitis. This patient had blood cultures positive for *Staphylococcus aureus*, confirming the diagnosis. (Reproduced with permission from McKean SC, Ross JJ, Dressler DD, Brotman DJ, Ginsberg JS, eds. *Principles and Practice of Hospital Medicine.* New York, NY: McGraw-Hill Education; 2012, Fig. 200-1.)

Treatment usually proceeds with chemotherapy. Most intraspinal soft tissue tumors do not cause back pain but instead present with abnormalities in neurologic exam or radicular pain, or both. Spondylolysis, a stress fracture of the vertebra, is a rare cause of back pain in younger children unless there is an episode of acute trauma with immediate onset of back pain.

▶ CASE 32

A 13-year-old girl presents with complaints of low back pain. Her pain started 1 month ago, about 2 weeks after starting gymnastics. She does not recall any traumatic episode that occurred at the time of pain onset. Initially the pain occurred only during activity, but it has progressively worsened in severity and is now present all the time. She points to the right side of her low back as the area of maximum discomfort. She denies any radiation of pain down her leg, and has no encopresis or enuresis. Heat and ibuprofen help her pain. Examination demonstrates pain with back extension, but minimal limitation or discomfort with forward flexion. Neurologic examination is normal.

Question 32-1

What is the most likely diagnosis?

A) Spondylolysis.
B) Herniated disc.

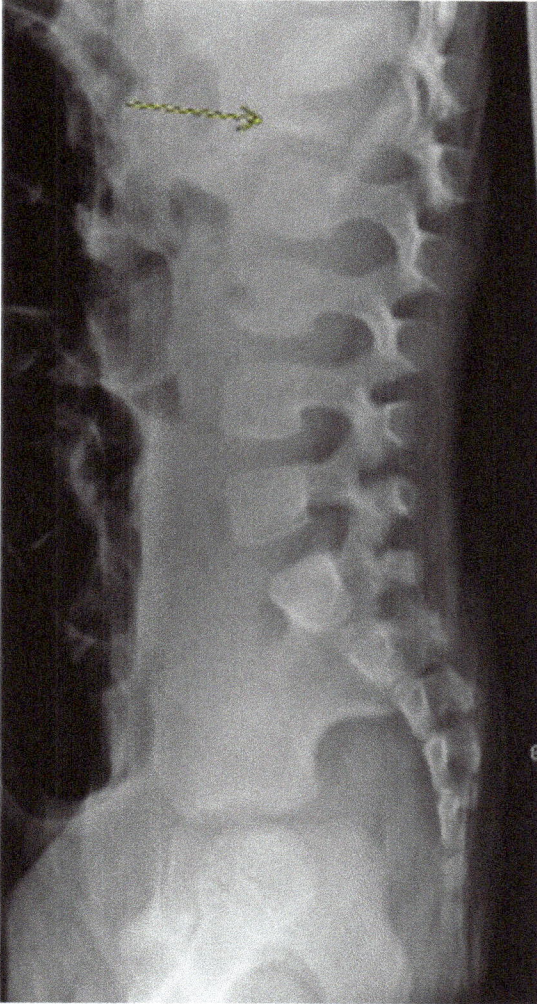

FIGURE 22–18. Lateral lumbar X-ray demonstrating vertebra plana (flattening) of L1 (*arrow*) secondary to infiltration from histiocytosis. This patient presented with refusal to walk secondary to back pain. Note that the disc spaces above and below are preserved, unlike in discitis (Figure 22–20). (Used with permission from Blaise Nemeth, MD, MS.)

C) Mechanical low back pain.
D) Endometriosis.

Discussion 32-1

The correct answer is "A." The most common pathologic cause of acute-onset, atraumatic back pain in adolescents is isthmic spondylolysis, a stress fracture within the pars interarticularis, a narrow part of the posterior ring of the vertebra, as a result of repetitive overuse. (See Figure 22–19.) The most common location is at L5, although other lumbar vertebrae may be involved. Spondylolysis typically develops in school-aged children, and athletes in sports that involve spinal extension, such as gymnastics and football linemen, are at greatest risk for development. Physical examination typically demonstrates pain with back extension. AP and lateral X-rays of the lumbar spine may demonstrate the fracture, especially if both sides are involved. Oblique X-rays may help improve diagnostic accuracy but may

not be necessary if there is clinical suspicion and advanced imaging will be performed regardless. Bone scan is the most sensitive modality for identification (see Figure 22–20) but does not help in determining the acuity of the fracture, or differentiating other potential causes (eg, osteoid osteoma), and involves relatively high radiation exposure. CT scan is the most specific modality, providing good bony detail, but utilizes high radiation doses and does not detect stress reactions ("pre-fractures"). MRI avoids ionizing radiation and is useful if there is concern regarding other abnormalities (eg, discitis in a younger patient); false negatives, when compared with bone and CT scans, may occur due to lack of edema in the dense pars interarticularis and use of disc-specific, rather than pars-specific, imaging protocols. Patients with spondylolysis should be referred to a sports medicine or orthopedics specialist for management. Treatment protocols vary from relative rest to bracing, followed by physical therapy to correct biomechanical issues contributing to stress at the pars interarticularis (such as tight hamstrings) and gradual return to play. Herniated discs are rare in children, although disc bulging and desiccation is commonly found incidentally on MRI; disc herniation presents in a manner similar to that in adults: sudden onset of low back pain that is worse with flexion and often produces radicular symptoms. Treatment involves acute pain management, typically for 1 to 2 weeks, and physical therapy for long-term "back health." Mechanical low back pain also occurs commonly in adolescents but should be a diagnosis of exclusion, considering the other etiologies in the differential diagnosis. Onset is usually insidious, and the pain may limit activity but is often worse with sitting or standing and better with movement. Radicular symptoms are absent, and advanced imaging may not be necessary if the pain is of long duration without change in symptoms. Physical therapy is the mainstay of treatment, addressing biomechanical issues contributing to altered spinal mechanics.

▶ CASE 33

You are meeting a family who is establishing care prior to the birth of their infant in a few months' time. The mother-to-be reports she recently had a good friend with a daughter who was diagnosed with hip dysplasia. Both parents would like to know more about hip dysplasia and the risk factors associated with this condition.

Question 33-1

All of the following combinations of history and exam would raise your suspicion for developmental dysplasia of the hip EXCEPT:

A) A male infant born to a G_2P_2 mother with an intermittent high-pitched hip click at the termination of abduction.
B) A female infant born to a G_1P_1 mother with asymmetry noted in the height of her knees when flexed at 90 degrees.
C) A male infant born by cesarean section due to breech presentation with limited abduction.
D) A female infant with torticollis on exam, born to a G_1P_1 mother with a maternal history positive for hip dysplasia.

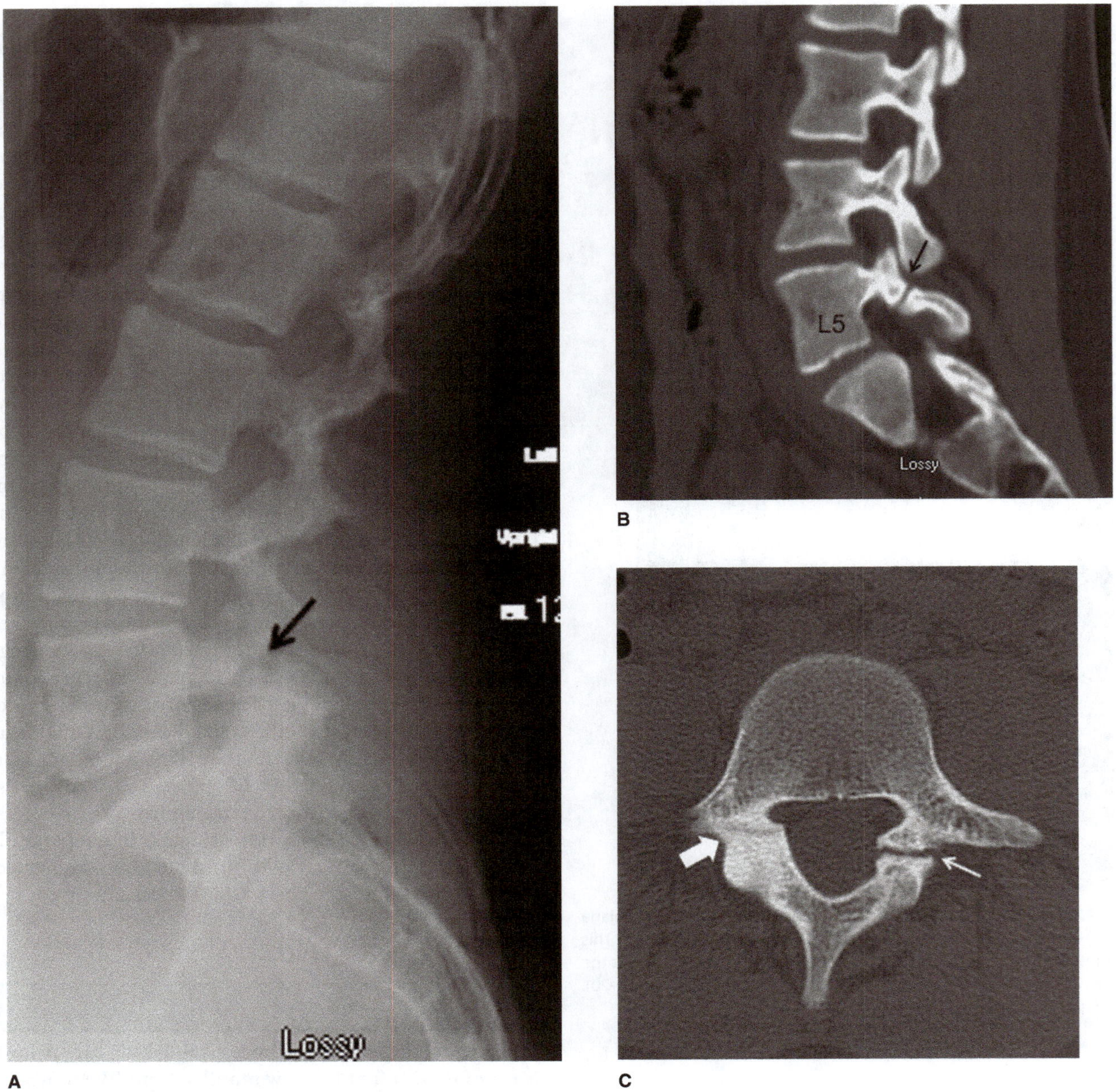

FIGURE 22–19. (A) Lateral lumbar X-ray demonstrating lucency within the pars interarticularis of L5 (*arrow*) in an adolescent soccer player with low back pain for 2 months. (B) The lucency is more easily seen on this sagittal CT scan through the left L5 pars interarticularis (*arrow*) of the same patient. (C) An axial image from the same CT scan also demonstrates the fracture through the left pars interarticularis (*arrow*), as well as hypertrophic healing of an early spondylolytic lesion on the right side (*block arrow*). (Used with permission from Blaise Nemeth, MD, MS.)

Discussion 33-1

The correct answer is "A." Developmental dysplasia of the hip (DDH) is a general diagnosis of abnormal hip development that encompasses a variety of pathologic findings relating to the relationship between the femoral head and acetabulum. The true etiology of DDH is unknown, although it is thought to be multifactorial, including both genetic and environmental influences. Risk factors include a positive family history, female sex, breech presentation, and a restricted intrauterine environment (first born, multiple gestation, oligohydramnios, large for gestational age). Often diagnosis is made on exam, shortly after birth; however, DDH may be detected at any age.

> ▶ **CASE 34**

A 10-week-old female infant presents for her well-child check. She was recently placed in foster care, and her foster mother states they are still working on gathering her medical records.

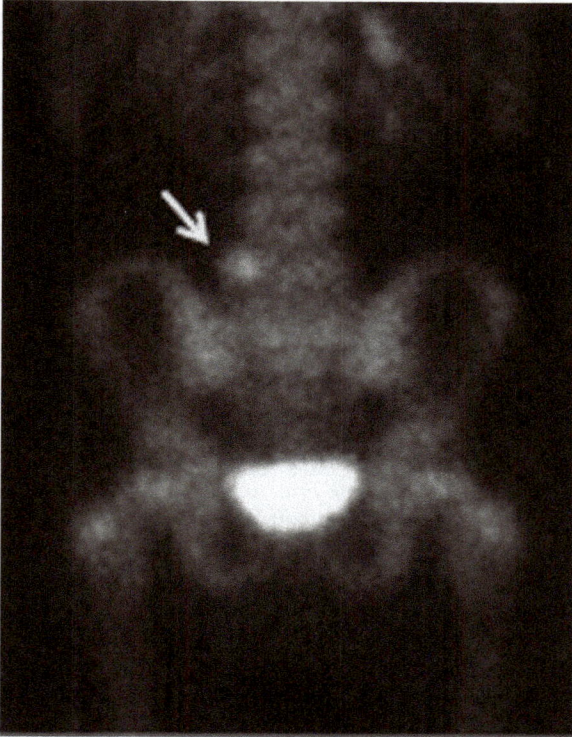

FIGURE 22–20. Bone scan in a different patient demonstrating increased uptake of technetium-99m in the right pars interarticularis of L5 in this pediatric patient with acute onset of low back pain. The finding of spondylolysis was confirmed by CT scan. (Used with permission from Blaise Nemeth, MD, MS.)

The foster mother knows the infant was born at term by cesarean section secondary to breech presentation. Her biological mother is 15 years old, and the foster mother believes this was her first child. On exam, the infant is well appearing, her head is round, and she demonstrates full range of motion of her neck. Knees are symmetric in height when flexed at 90 degrees. With abduction you notice mild asymmetry, with 75 degrees of abduction on the right and 65 to 70 degrees on the left. No overt clunk is noted when performing Ortolani and Barlow tests during your exam today. Given her risk factors—female, breech presentation, first born—and exam findings you are concerned for hip dysplasia (DDH).

Question 34-1
What is the most appropriate next step?
A) Make an urgent referral to orthopedics.
B) Obtain an AP and frogleg film of her pelvis.
C) Reassure the foster mother and follow up at her 4-month checkup.
D) Obtain an ultrasound of her hips bilaterally.

Discussion 34-1
The correct answer is "D." Clinically, patients with DDH can present with a variety of different signs and symptoms, depending on age and the pathology involved. The exam may be normal in patients with mild dysplasia. When present, certain exam

findings will raise the concern and may also provide diagnosis of DDH. In neonates and young infants the Ortolani and Barlow tests have been used to assess for stability (ie, evidence of a dislocated or dislocatable hip). The Ortolani test assesses for reduction of a potentially dislocated hip. With this test the hip is flexed and gently abducted. A positive test occurs if there is a palpable clunk when the hip is brought into this position, indicating reduction of the femoral head into the acetabulum. The Barlow test assesses whether a reduced hip can be subluxed or dislocated. This test is performed by gently bringing the hip into flexion and adduction while palpating for an associated clunk indicating movement of the femoral head out of the acetabulum. The Ortolani and Barlow tests are more useful in the neonatal period. After 2 to 3 months of age these tests become less reliable. In older infants or children the physical exam may demonstrate limited abduction or a painless limp, or both. Asymmetric thigh folds or a leg-length discrepancy may be present in the context of a dislocated hip. Proper physical exam remains the most important aspect in the diagnosis of DDH. Imaging can provide further information to help support the diagnosis. The choice of imaging modality depends on the age of the patient. In infants younger than 4 to 6 months, the femoral head is not yet ossified and cannot be visualized on plain X-rays. This limits the use of plain X-rays in the young infant population. In these young infants, ultrasound is helpful for assessing anatomy and allows for a static and dynamic assessment of the hip anatomy. In infants younger than 6 weeks of age, screening ultrasounds may be overly sensitive and may result in overtreatment. Universal ultrasound screening in infants is generally not practiced in the United States for a number of reasons, including but not limited to low disease prevalence, cost, lack of trained personnel to assure quality imaging and interpretation, subjectivity, and a high false-positive rate.

BIBLIOGRAPHY

Arkader A, Gebhardt MC, Dormans JP. Bone and soft tissue tumors. In: Weinstein SL, Flynn JM, eds. *Lovell and Winter's Pediatric Orthopaedics*. Vol 1. 7th ed. Philadelphia, PA: Wolters Kluwer Health/Lippincott Williams and Wilkins; 2014.

Arndt CAS. Neoplasms of the bone. In: Kleigman RM, Stanton BF, St Geme JW, Schor NF, Behrman RE, eds. *Nelson Textbook of Pediatrics*. 19th ed. Philadelphia, PA: Elsevier/Saunders; 2011.

Baxter WR, Kocher M, Ganley T. Sports medicine in the growing child. In: Weinstein SL, Flynn JM, eds. *Lovell and Winter's Pediatric Orthopaedics*. Vol 2. 7th ed. Philadelphia, PA: Wolters Kluwer Health/Lippincott Williams and Wilkins; 2014.

Brooks W, Gross R. Genu varum in children: Diagnosis and treatment. *J Am Acad Orthop Surg*. 1995;3(6):326–335.

Caird MS, Flynn JM, Leung YL, Millman JE, D'Italia JG, Dormans JP. Factors distinguishing septic arthritis from transient synovitis of the hip in children. A prospective study. *J Bone Joint Surg Am*. 2006;88(6):1251–1257. doi:10.2106/JBJS.E.00216.

Dubnov-Raz G, Ephros M, Garty B-Z, et al. Invasive pediatric *Kingella kingae* infections: A nationwide collaborative study. *Pediatr Infect Dis J.* 2010;29(7):639–643. doi:10.1097/INF.0b013e3181d57a6c.

Dunbar JS, Owen HF, Nogrady MB, Mcleese R. Obscure tibial fracture of infants—the toddler's fracture. *J Can Assoc Radiol.* 1964;15:136–144.

Engström P, Tedroff K. The prevalence and course of idiopathic toe-walking in 5-year-old children. *Pediatrics.* 2012;130(2):279–284. doi:10.1542/peds.2012-0225.

Farsetti P, Weinstein SL, Ponseti IV. The long-term functional and radiographic outcomes of untreated and nonoperatively treated metatarsus adductus. *J Bone Joint Surg Am.* 1994;76(2):257–265.

Flaherty EG, Perez-Rossello JM, Levine MA, et al. Evaluating children with fractures for child physical abuse. *Pediatrics.* 2014;133(2):e477–e489. doi:10.1542/peds.2013-3793.

Flynn JM, Skaggs DL. Supracondylar fractures of the distal humerus. In: Flynn JM, Skaggs DL, Waters PM, eds. *Rockwood and Wilkins' Fractures in Children.* 8th ed. Philadelphia, PA: Lippincott Williams and Wilkins; 2015.

Friedman JE, Richard S. Davidson. Leg-length discrepancy. In: Kleigman RM, Stanton BF, St Geme JW, Schor NF, Behrman RE, eds. *Nelson Textbook of Pediatrics.* 19th ed. Philadelphia, PA: Elsevier/Saunders; 2011.

Halanski MA, Noonan KJ. Limb-length discrepancy. In: Weinstein SL, Flynn JM, eds. *Lovell and Winter's Pediatric Orthopaedics.* Vol 2. 7th ed. Philadelphia, PA: Wolters Kluwer Health/Lippincott Williams and Wilkins; 2014.

Heath CH, Staheli LT. Normal limits of knee angle in white children—genu varum and genu valgum. *J Pediatr Orthop.* 1993;13(2):259–262.

Hecht AC, Gebhardt MC. Diagnosis and treatment of unicameral and aneurysmal bone cysts in children. *Curr Opin Pediatr.* 1998;10(1):87–94.

Herman MJ, James J. McCarthy. The principles of pediatric fracture and trauma care. In: Weinstein SL, Flynn JM, eds. *Lovell and Winter's Pediatric Orthopaedics.* Vol 2. 7th ed. Philadelphia, PA: Wolters Kluwer Health/Lippincott Williams and Wilkins; 2014.

Hosalkar HS, Spiegel DA, Davidson RS. The foot and toes. In: Kleigman RM, Stanton BF, St Geme JW, Schor NF, Behrman RE, eds. *Nelson Textbook of Pediatrics.* 19th ed. Philadelphia, PA: Elsevier/Saunders; 2011.

Kay RM, Kim YJ. Slipped capital femoral epiphysis. In: Weinstein SL, Flynn JM, eds. *Lovell and Winter's Pediatric Orthopaedics.* Vol 2. 7th ed. Philadelphia, PA: Wolters Kluwer Health/Lippincott Williams and Wilkins; 2014.

Kocher MS, Mandiga R, Zurakowski D, Barnewolt C, Kasser JR. Validation of a clinical prediction rule for the differentiation between septic arthritis and transient synovitis of the hip in children. *J Bone Joint Surg Am.* 2004;86-A(8):1629–1635.

Krause BL, Williams JP, Catterall A. Natural history of Osgood-Schlatter disease. *J Pediatr Orthop.* 1990;10(1):65–68.

Lincoln TL, Suen PW. Common rotational variations in children. *J Am Acad Orthop Surg.* 2003;11(5):312–320.

Micheli LJ, Ireland ML. Prevention and management of calcaneal apophysitis in children: An overuse syndrome. *J Pediatr Orthop.* 1987;7(1):34–38.

Mosca VS. The foot. In: Weinstein SL, Flynn JM, eds. *Lovell and Winter's Pediatric Orthopaedics.* Vol 2. 7th ed. Philadelphia, PA: Wolters Kluwer Health/Lippincott Williams and Wilkins; 2014.

Mubarak SJ, Owen CA, Hargens AR, Garetto LP, Akeson WH. Acute compartment syndromes: Diagnosis and treatment with the aid of the wick catheter. *J Bone Joint Surg Am.* 1978;60(8):1091–1095.

Oetgen ME, Peden S. Idiopathic toe walking. *J Am Acad Orthop Surg.* 2012;20(5):292–300. doi:10.5435/JAAOS-20-05-292.

Rathjen KE, Kim HKW. Physeal injuries and growth disturbances. In: Flynn JM, Skaggs DL, Waters PM, eds. *Rockwood and Wilkins' Fractures in Children.* 8th ed. Philadelphia, PA: Lippincott Williams and Wilkins; 2014.

Rosman NP, Douglass LM, Sharif UM, Paolini J. The neurology of benign paroxysmal torticollis of infancy: Report of 10 new cases and review of the literature. *J Child Neurol.* 2009;24(2):155–160. doi:10.1177/0883073808322338.

Sankar WB, Horn BD, Wells L, Dormans JP. The Hip. In: Kleigman RM, Stanton BF, St Geme JW, Schor NF, Behrman RE, eds. *Nelson Textbook of Pediatrics.* 19th ed. Philadelphia, PA: Elsevier/Saunders; 2011.

Schoenecker PL, Rich MR. The lower extremity. In: Weinstein SL, Flynn JM, eds. *Lovell and Winter's Pediatric Orthopaedics.* Vol 2. 7th ed. Philadelphia, PA: Wolters Kluwer Health/Lippincott Williams and Wilkins; 2014.

Schwend RM, Shaw BA, Segal LS. Evaluation and treatment of developmental hip dysplasia in the newborn and infant. *Pediatr Clin.* 2014;61(6):1095–1107. doi:10.1016/j.pcl.2014.08.008.

Sharrard WJ. Knock knees and bow legs. *Br Med J.* 1976;1(6013):826–827.

Skaggs DL, Flynn JM, Grill, F, Moseley CF. Leg length inequality. In: Skaggs DL, Flynn JM, eds. *Staying out of Trouble in Pediatric Orthopaedics.* Philadelphia, PA: Lippincott Williams and Wilkins; 2006.

Staheli LT. Rotational problems in children. *Instr Course Lect.* 1994;43:199–209.

Tiwari A, Haq AI, Myint F, Hamilton G. Acute compartment syndromes. *Br J Surg.* 2002;89(4):397–412. doi:10.1046/j.0007-1323.2002.02063.x.

Topol GA, Podesta LA, Reeves KD, Raya MF, Fullerton BD, Yeh H. Hyperosmolar dextrose injection for recalcitrant Osgood-Schlatter disease. *Pediatrics.* 2011;128(5):e1121 –e1128. doi:10.1542/peds.2010-1931.

Warman ML, Cormier-Daire V, Hall C, et al. Nosology and classification of genetic skeletal disorders: 2010 revision. *Am J Med Genet A.* 2011;155A(5):943–968. doi:10.1002/ajmg.a.33909.

Weinstein SL. Developmental hip dysplasia and dislocation. In: Weinstein SL, Flynn JM, eds. *Lovell and Winter's Pediatric Orthopaedics.* Vol 2. 7th ed. Philadelphia, PA: Wolters Kluwer Health/Lippincott Williams and Wilkins; 2014.

Weinstein SL. Legg-Calve-Perthes syndrome. In: Weinstein SL, Flynn JM, eds. *Lovell and Winter's Pediatric Orthopaedics.*

Vol 2. 7th ed. Philadelphia, PA: Wolters Kluwer Health/ Lippincott Williams and Wilkins; 2014.

Weinstein SL, Dolan LA, Wright JG, Dobbs MB. Effects of bracing in adolescents with idiopathic scoliosis. *N Engl J Med*. 2013;369(16):1512–1521. doi:10.1056/ NEJMoa1307337.

Wells L, Sehgal K. The knee. In: Kleigman RM, Stanton BF, St Geme JW, Schor NF, Behrman RE, eds. *Nelson Textbook of Pediatrics*. 19th ed. Philadelphia, PA: Elsevier/Saunders; 2011.

Wells L, Sehgal K. Torsional and angular deformities. In: Kleigman RM, Stanton BF, St Geme JW, Schor NF, Behrman RE, eds. *Nelson Textbook of Pediatrics*. 19th ed. Philadelphia, PA: Elsevier/Saunders; 2011.

White GR, Mencio GA. Genu valgum in children: Diagnostic and therapeutic alternatives. *J Am Acad Orthop Surg*. 1995;3(5):275–283.

Neurologic Disorders

Satsuki Matsumoto and Leah Zhorne

23

► CASE 1

A 15-year-old obese adolescent girl presents to the clinic with a 1-month history of near-daily, throbbing, early morning headaches and nausea. She is being bullied at school because of her weight and acne. Her medications include a combined oral contraceptive pill (OCP) and retinoic acid cream. Her mother thinks she is faking symptoms to stay home from school. Her vital signs and general, and neurologic exams are normal except for blurred optic disc margins.

Question 1-1
What is the most likely diagnosis?
A) Tension headache due to social stressors.
B) Chronic migraine.
C) Idiopathic intracranial hypertension.
D) Acute hydrocephalus.
E) None of the above.

Discussion 1-1
The correct answer is "C." The early morning headache with nausea and papilledema on exam should clue you in to increased intracranial pressure as the underlying cause of the patient's symptoms. Although option "D," acute hydrocephalus, could also cause these symptoms, the patient would likely present in a more emergent manner with vomiting, altered level of consciousness, and possibly focal neurologic findings. Idiopathic intracranial hypertension (IIH), also known as pseudotumor cerebri syndrome, can be truly "idiopathic"; however, it is also associated with obesity, pregnancy, endocrinopathies, medications (tetracyclines, retinoic acid), vitamin A toxicity, and anemia. Although the neurologic exam in affected children should otherwise be normal, cranial nerve (CN) VI palsy is allowed as it is a "false localizing sign" of increased intracranial pressure.

Question 1-2
What is the next appropriate step in her evaluation?
A) Lumbar puncture with opening pressure.
B) Magnetic resonance imaging (MRI) of the brain with magnetic resonance venography (MRV) of the head.
C) Treatment with a carbonic anhydrase inhibitor.
D) Intravenous opiates.
E) Nutrition consultation.

Discussion 1-2
The correct answer is "B." You first need to assess for secondary causes of increased intracranial pressure with an MRI scan of the brain (looking for tumor and hydrocephalus) and an MRV (looking for venous sinus thrombosis) prior to performing a lumbar puncture with opening pressure (option "A") in the left lateral decubitus position. If her MRI and MRV are normal (venous sinus narrowing is allowed) and the opening pressure is elevated (> 25 cm H_2O in most cases) with normal cerebrospinal fluid (CSF) cell count, she may be treated with a carbonic anhydrase inhibitor (option "C") to lower her CSF pressure. IIH is typically co-managed by ophthalmology and neurology specialists. The risk in untreated IIH is permanent vision loss. Patients who are refractory to medications may require optic nerve sheath fenestration or ventriculoperitoneal shunt placement.

> **Helpful Tip**
> Symptoms of increased intracranial pressure include headaches that wake a patient up in the middle of the night or occur first thing in the morning, especially those with accompanying vomiting. Other warning signs include Valsalva- or exertion-induced headaches. Physical exam findings include papilledema and focal neurologic signs (CN VI palsy).

> **Helpful Tip**
>
> Neuroimaging is indicated in children with headaches who have signs of increased intracranial pressure, seizures, an abnormal neurologic exam, or focal neurologic symptoms (weakness, numbness). It should also be considered in children with new-onset severe headaches (< 1 month duration) or worsening headaches, and in children younger than 6 years of age.

▶ CASE 2

You are seeing, a 10-year-old boy with asthma and attention deficit hyperactivity disorder (ADHD), for his well-child check. On review of systems he complains of frequent headaches during which he stops playing, is irritable with others, and demands that the television (TV) and lights be turned off. He is also uncharacteristically still and prefers to lie on the couch. He describes the headache as being "like a hammer hitting his head." He sees spots and then feels numbness and tingling in his left arm for 15 minutes before the headache begins, but these go away once the headache starts. He is obese, but his examination is otherwise normal.

Question 2-1

What is the most likely diagnosis?
A) Tension-type headache.
B) Migraine with aura.
C) Hemiplegic migraine.
D) Basilar-type migraine.
E) Cluster headache.

Discussion 2-1

The correct answer is "B." A migraine is a long (4- to 72-hour) headache characterized by two of more of the following characteristics: unilateral, pulsating quality, moderate-to-severe intensity, and worsening that causes the sufferer to avoid physical activity; *and* associated with one or more of the following: nausea, vomiting, or photophobia *and* phonophobia. Some of these symptoms can be inferred by this child's behavior (light and noise avoidance). A typical aura includes sensory or visual phenomena (weakness is excluded) that are fully reversible, last 5 to 60 minutes, and are followed shortly by a migraine. Hemiplegic migraine (option "C") includes an aura of fully reversible weakness (must first rule out intracranial pathology), and cluster headache (option "D") includes an aura of several symptoms referable to the brainstem (ataxia, aphasia, vertigo, tinnitus, etc). Tension-type headache (option "A") is essentially the opposite of a migraine and defined as a headache with two or more of the following characteristics: bilateral, mild-to-moderate severity, nonthrobbing (pressing, tight), not aggravated by physical activity, and without nausea or vomiting. The patient may have photophobia *or* phonophobia, but not both. Cluster headaches (option "E") and other trigeminal autonomic cephalgias are uncommon in children and by definition must include autonomic features such as *unilateral* conjunctival injection, tearing, rhinorrhea, or eyelid edema. It can be a bear to remember all of the headache subtypes, so put the International Headache Society's website (http://ihs-classification.org/en/) on your favorites list. It contains a handy index of diagnostic criteria. (Bet you have a headache from reading all of this!)

Question 2-2

What treatment will you recommend?
A) Lifestyle management with adequate sleep, regular meals, improved hydration, avoidance of caffeine, stress management, and regular physical activity.
B) Acetaminophen or ibuprofen as needed, no more than 10 times per month.
C) Headache diary.
D) Prophylactic medication if headaches are disabling or occur more than once a week.
E) All of the above.

Discussion 2-2

Of course the correct answer is "E"! Most pediatric headaches can be managed through simple lifestyle changes and the judicious use of over-the-counter analgesics. If your patient uses any as-needed (PRN) meds more than 10 times per month, he may develop a medication overuse headache. Although select triptans have been approved for use in children by the Food and Drug Administration (FDA), nonsteroidal anti-inflammatory drugs (NSAIDs) typically work just as well if utilized at a proper dose at the onset of the headache.

⧗ QUICK QUIZ

Which should NOT be used for management of headaches in the clinic?
A) NSAIDs.
B) Acetaminophen.
C) Opiates.
D) Meditation (stress reduction).
E) Sleep.

Discussion

The correct answer is "C." Opiates are *not* an appropriate choice for outpatient headache management.

When you see the patient in follow up 2 months later, his headaches are worse. Despite your expert counseling on proper lifestyle management, his mother cannot seem to get him to stop drinking soda, and he will not go to bed before 10:00 PM because he watches TV for hours after dinner. His mother is frustrated because he is now having daily headaches and she does not know what to do. They have adhered to your order of using ibuprofen less than 10 times per month.

Question 2-3

Which prophylactic medication would be the best choice for this child?

A) Cyproheptadine.
B) Propranolol.
C) Topiramate.
D) Valproic acid.
E) None of the above.

Discussion 2-3

The correct answer is "C." When planning a prophylactic medication, you must think about the patient's comorbidities. Topiramate may cause weight loss and thus would be the preferred choice for an obese patient. At higher doses, such as when it is used for seizure medication, it can also cause word-finding difficulties and brain fog. Another potential side effect is kidney stones. Option "B" is incorrect because beta-blockers should be avoided in patients with asthma. Options "A" and "D" are not the best choices for an obese patient as their side effects include weight gain.

▶ CASE 3

A 2-year-old girl is brought to the emergency department by her family because she has been acting strangely ever since she was awakened from her afternoon nap. Her mother says the girl was at her baseline when she and her 4-year-old brother were put down for their naps 3 hours ago. When the mother went to wake her up, the girl was difficult to arouse and seemed confused. On examination, the patient's vital signs are heart rate 70 beats per minute, respiratory rate 12 breaths per minute, and blood pressure 75/50 mm Hg; she has a Glasgow Coma Scale score of 10: she opens her eyes briefly only to voice or tactile stimulation; and she cries and pulls away when you pinch her arm. She does not speak. Her general examination is unremarkable except for miotic pupils.

Question 3-1

Define her mental status.

A) Alert.
B) Lethargic.
C) Obtunded.
D) Stuporous.
E) Comatose.

Discussion 3-1

The correct answer is "C." It is exceedingly important to correctly document the patient's mental status in this situation. If you cannot recall what the words listed in options "A" through "E" mean, then you should document what you see on exam (the patient opens eyes only to voice/pain, etc). From most alert to least, the options choices for this question are defined as follows: option "A," Alert = fully awake (duh); option "B," lethargic = difficulty staying awake (but it connotes a clearly

abnormal state, so please do not document lethargy when you really mean tired); option "C," obtunded = opens eyes only to tactile or verbal stimulation; option "D," stupor = opens eyes only to pain; and option "E," coma = a state of unresponsiveness or unconsciousness without eye opening that is due to brain dysfunction. The differential diagnosis for pediatric altered mental status or encephalopathy is enormous but can be broken down into three main categories: toxic/metabolic, infectious, and structural. It is important to remember that major organ system dysfunction (liver, kidneys, heart, lungs) can lead to encephalopathy as well.

> **Helpful Tip**
> Metabolic etiologies should be very high on your differential diagnosis in an encephalopathic neonate, and metabolic tests (eg, urine organic acids and ammonia) should be included in your first line of testing.

Your initial lab work comes back normal, including full electrolytes (sodium, potassium, chloride, bicarbonate, glucose), renal function (creatinine, blood urea nitrogen), liver function tests (alanine aminotransferase, aspartate aminotransferase), ammonia, and blood gases. A noncontrast computed tomography (CT) scan of the head is also normal. When you go back to the family to gather more information for the history, the little brother proudly volunteers that he found some "candy" and gave it to his sister while they were supposed to be sleeping. You ask mother what medications are accessible in the house. She notes that her husband recently had back surgery and was prescribed hydrocodone for postoperative pain. You quickly administer naloxone to the child, and she returns to her baseline mental status.

Question 3-2

Which of the following acute ingestions would NOT be expected to cause a depressed mental status?

A) Amitriptyline.
B) Aspirin.
C) Cyanide.
D) Lead.
E) All of the above would cause a depressed mental state.

Discussion 3-2

The correct answer is "D." Although lead can cause permanent neurologic sequelae, it would be unusual for a child to be exposed to enough lead to cause an acute poisoning with coma. Lead is more likely to build up over time with repeated exposures. The substances classically known to induce coma include central nervous system (CNS) depressants such as sedatives, narcotics, alcohol, and barbiturates, as well as tricyclic antidepressants, cholinergics, cyanide, and carbon monoxide.

⧖ QUICK QUIZ

What is a potential cause of altered mental status in a pediatric patient?
A) Intracranial hemorrhage.
B) Acute disseminated encephalomyelitis.
C) Hyperinsulinemia.
D) Acute respiratory failure.
E) All of the above.

Discussion

The correct answer is "E." Option "B" actually has the base term encephalitis as part of its disease name! Hyperinsulinemia may cause hypoglycemia, leading to altered mental status. Hypercapnia or hypoxia, or both, may also cause altered mental status. Remember the mnemonic AEIOU-TIPS when evaluating a patient for altered mental status:

A – Ammonia

E – Electrolytes (sodium, glucose, calcium)

I – Infection

O – Overdose

U – Uremia

T – Trauma

I – Intussusception

P – Psychiatric

S – Stroke or Seizure

▶ CASE 4

You are seeing a 4-month-old boy for his well-child check. He was a former 38-week average gestational age (AGA) infant born to a 23-year-old G_1P_0 (now 1) mother by normal spontaneous vaginal delivery after an uncomplicated neonatal course. His Apgar scores at birth were normal. His parents are concerned because he still cannot hold his head up, but note that he has no problems eating. On exam he is alert and reactive with normal general exam findings. His neurologic exam is notable for proximal greater than distal weakness, hypotonia with significant head lag, tongue fasciculations, absent Moro reflex, and absent biceps and patellar reflexes (you even used a real reflex hammer!). There is no family history of neuromuscular disorder. You are worried about the cause of his hypotonia, areflexia, and weakness.

Question 4-1

What is the next appropriate diagnostic step?
A) Obtain a creatine kinase (CK) level.
B) Order an MRI of the brain.
C) Order an electromyogram (EMG) and a nerve conduction velocity (NCV) test.
D) Provide reassurance and close follow-up.
E) Refer for early access and intervention.

Discussion 4-1

The correct answer is "A." The evaluation of a floppy infant is based on the clues found in the history and physical exam that help you determine if the hypotonia is central or peripheral in origin. (See Table 23–1.) This infant most likely has a peripheral cause of his hypotonia; therefore, you should check the CK level to help narrow your differential. In muscular dystrophies the CK level is significantly elevated, but this is not the case in congenital myopathies and spinal muscular atrophy (SMA). This infant's presentation (with profound hypotonia, absent reflexes, and *tongue fasciculations*) is strongly suggestive of SMA type 1, which involves progressive loss of the anterior horn cells. You confirm the diagnosis by sending a sample for molecular testing of the *SMN1* gene. Treatment is supportive. An MRI of the brain (option "B") would be more appropriate if you were worried about a central cause of hypotonia. EMG/NCV (option "C") can be useful in differentiating whether peripheral hypotonia or weakness is related to nerve (anterior horn cell or motor nerve/axon disorders), neuromuscular junction (acquired or congenital myasthenic disorders, or botulism), or muscle disorders but would not be an appropriate first step. If you have a high suspicion for SMA from the start, you should send that specific gene test early in the workup. "D" isn't appropriate as this infant has significant gross motor developmental delay. Referral for services is important in neuromuscular disorders but the first step in this case is a diagnostic work-up. Spinal muscular atrophy (SMA) is classified 1 through 4 depending on the severity of features

TABLE 23–1 CHARACTERISTICS OF CENTRAL VERSUS PERIPHERAL HYPOTONIA

	Central	Peripheral
Mental status	Impaired, lethargic	Intact, alert
Reflexes	Normal to brisk	Diminished or absent
Strength	Movement through postural reflexes, axial hypotonia, mild to no weakness	More profound weakness, no movement through postural reflexes
Other organ system dysfunction	May have multiple congenital malformations, dysmorphic features, brain malformations, seizures, abnormal breathing	Poor feeding, respiratory compromise
Exam clues	Scissoring on vertical suspension, fisted hands with cortical thumbs	Muscle fasciculations, tongue fasciculations, muscle atrophy, weak/soft cry, weak cough

and age of onset. SMA type 1 (Werdnig-Hoffmann disease) is the most common and severe with onset in early infancy. Decreased fetal movement may be noted by the mother in late pregnancy. SMA type 2 and type 3 are milder and present in late infancy or early in toddlerhood. SMA type 4 onsets in adulthood.

► CASE 5

A 10-day-old male infant is admitted to the pediatric intensive care unit (PICU) for fever, seizures, and somnolence. His anterior fontanelle is full. A CT scan of the head did not show acute abnormalities. CSF showed elevated white blood cells with mostly neutrophils, elevated protein, and low glucose. You suspect meningitis and start antibiotics.

Question 5-1

What are the most likely organisms in a patient of this age?
A) *Streptococcus pneumoniae, Neisseria meningitidis, Haemophilus influenzae* type b.
B) *N. meningitidis, S. pneumoniae.*
C) Group B *Streptococcus, Escherichia coli, Listeria monocytogenes.*
D) *S. pneumoniae, N. meningitidis, L. monocytogenes.*

Discussion 5-1

The correct answer is "C." It is important to know the common organisms causing acute bacterial meningitis in each age group. (See Table 23–2.) The most common causes of meningitis in a newborn are group B *Streptococcus*, *E. coli*, and *Listeria*. The typical empiric antibiotic regimen for neonatal meningitis is ampicillin and cefotaxime or gentamycin. *Listeria* is resistant to cephalosporins, which is why you need to include ampicillin. Group B *Streptococcus* is sensitive to penicillins. *E. coli* is a gram-negative rod, and is covered by cefotaxime and gentamycin.

TABLE 23–2 CAUSES OF ACUTE BACTERIAL MENINGITIS BY AGE

Age Group	Common Organisms
Newborn to infant (3 months)	Group B *Streptococcus*, *Escherichia coli*, *Listeria monocytogenes*
Infant (> 3 months) to child	*Streptococcus pneumoniae*, *Neisseria meningitidis*, *Haemophilus influenzae* type b
Adolescent to young adult	*N. meningitidis, S. pneumoniae*
Older adult	*S. pneumoniae, N. meningitidis, Listeria monocytogenes*

► CASE 6

An 18-year-old college freshman is brought to the emergency department (ED) for altered mental status. His roommate reports that the patient was well this morning but when the roommate returned tonight, he found the patient on the floor, barely responsive. The roommate does not suspect drug or alcohol exposure. In the ED, the patient looks toxic. He is febrile, hypotensive, and obtunded, with diffuse petechiae. The head CT scan was unremarkable, and a drug screen was negative. You suspect meningitis.

Question 6-1

What is the most likely organism causing his meningitis?
A) *Streptococcus pneumoniae.*
B) *Escherichia coli.*
C) *Listeria monocytogenes.*
D) *Neisseria meningitidis.*
E) Enterovirus.

Discussion 6-1

The correct answer is "D." *N. meningitidis* is one of the common organisms causing meningitis among adolescents and young adults (college students, military personnel). The doubling time of this organism is very short, leading to the rapid clinical progression. *N. meningitidis* can cause disseminated intravascular coagulation (DIC), with resulting petechiae, purpura, and adrenal insufficiency (Friderichsen-Waterhouse syndrome). A third-generation cephalosporin, such as ceftriaxone is the therapeutic choice.

> **Helpful Tip**
> Petechia and purpura in meningitis should prompt you to think meningococcus; however, these findings are also seen in *Streptococcus pneumoniae* and *Haemophilus influenzae* meningitis.

► CASE 7

You are the senior resident in the emergency department in July when a 3-year-old boy who was sick with fever, cough, and congestion for 4 days presents with irritability, headaches, and a persistent fever. His exam is notable for photophobia and pain with neck flexion. There are no focal neurologic findings, altered mental status, or papilledema. You suspect meningitis and plan to perform a lumbar puncture (LP).

Question 7-1

With what symptoms should you first do neuroimaging prior to LP?
A) Imaging is required before any LP when you suspect meningitis.
B) Any focal neurologic symptoms or altered mental status.
C) Papilledema.
D) Seizures.
E) Options B, C, and D.

Discussion 7-1

The correct answer is "E." Routine neuroimaging is not needed unless the patient has seizures, you are suspicious for a mass lesion (eg, brain abscess), or there are abnormalities on neurologic examination. You should also consider imaging for neonates with meningitis.

Initial CSF results show no organisms on Gram stain, but a high white blood cell count with lymphocytic predominance, mildly elevated protein, and normal CSF glucose.

Question 7-2

What is the most likely etiology?
A) Enterovirus.
B) *Streptococcus pneumoniae*.
C) *Neisseria meningitides*.
D) Partially treated bacterial meningitis (mother forgot to mention the antibiotics he was on last week).
E) None of the above.

Discussion 7-2

The correct answer is "A." Enteroviral meningitis is the most likely pathogen given the time of year (summer) and the patient's CSF results, which are suggestive of a viral aseptic meningitis. While pretreated bacterial meningitis is possible, the initial CSF studies would be expected to show a neutrophilic predominance and a low glucose level. Other etiologies of aseptic meningitis include other viruses and bacterial pathogens such as tuberculous, spirochete, or rickettsial infections. Noninfectious etiologies are also possible and include disorders such as lupus, malignancy, and Kawasaki disease, as well as medications (eg, NSAIDs, intravenous immunoglobulin [IVIG]). (See Table 23–3.)

Over the course of the next day, your patient becomes progressively more lethargic and has a focal seizure.

TABLE 23-3   CEREBROSPINAL FLUID COMPOSITION IN MENINGITIS

Etiology	WBC Count	Protein	Glucose
Bacterial	↑↑ Neutrophil predominance	↑	↓
Viral	↑[a] Lymphocyte predominance	Normal to mildly ↑	Normal
Mycobacterial	↑[a] Monocyte predominance	↑	↓
Fungal	↑[a] Lymphocyte predominance	↑	↓

[a] Mildly elevated to high.

Question 7-3

What acute complications of meningitis could account for these new symptoms?
A) Cerebral edema.
B) Syndrome of inappropriate antidiuretic hormone secretion (SIADH).
C) Subdural effusion.
D) Dural venous sinus thrombosis.
E) All of the above.

Discussion 7-3

The correct answer is "E." All of the listed options are potential complications of meningitis. Careful fluid management is key in meningitis treatment. Acute management of cerebral edema can include steroids, mannitol, diuretics, brief hyperventilation if intubated, and hypertonic saline solution. Subdural effusion may require surgical intervention if there is suspicion for empyema or if it causes increased intracranial pressure. Intracranial thrombosis may require anticoagulation therapy. Long-term complications of meningitis can include permanent neurologic deficits such as intellectual impairment, hydrocephalus, spasticity, and seizures. Hearing loss is also a noted complication of bacterial meningitis and warrants testing in this population.

⧗ QUICK QUIZ

Which is NOT a characteristic of the CSF in acute bacterial meningitis?
A) Elevated protein.
B) Elevated white blood cell count.
C) Elevated glucose.
D) Positive Gram stain.
E) Neutrophilic predominance.

Discussion

The correct answer is "C." In acute bacterial meningitis, the white blood cell count is typically elevated (> 1000 cells/mm³) and comprises primarily neutrophils. The protein content is elevated, and the Gram stain may be positive for bacteria. Hypoglycorrhachia (low CSF glucose) strongly suggests a bacterial infection. Be sure to obtain concurrent serum glucose to calculate the CSF-to-serum glucose ratio (normally ~60%). The normal number of white blood cells in the CSF varies slightly by age, with 0 to 12 for neonates, 0 to 6 for infants 1 to 2 months old, and 0 to 7 for infants and children older than 2 months of age. (See Table 23–3, earlier.)

> **Helpful Tip**
> *Aseptic meningitis* is a catch-all term for CSF inflammation (leukocytosis) with negative bacterial cultures. The most common cause is viral meningitis.

► CASE 8

A 7-year-old girl presents to the emergency department with a 4-day history of fever to 38.9°C (102°F), headache, photophobia, and irritability. Her parents brought her in because she "has not been acting right" for the past 24 hours. They note that she is sleepier, is slow to respond, and seems "out of it." The parents also mention that she developed a "cold sore" on her lip last week. You are testing her for nuchal rigidity (absent) when she has a focal seizure. An electroencephalogram (EEG) shows a temporal lobe seizure focus. A CT scan does not show any contraindication to lumbar puncture (LP). CSF studies show a mononuclear pleocytosis, elevated protein, and normal glucose.

Question 8-1

What diagnosis and organism do you suspect?
A) Meningitis; enterovirus.
B) Encephalitis; enterovirus.
C) Encephalitis; herpes simplex virus type 1.
D) Encephalitis; West Nile virus.
E) Meningitis; chikungunya virus.

Discussion 8-1

The correct answer is "C." Encephalitis caused by herpes simplex virus (HSV) type 1 infection should be high on your differential diagnosis given the clinical picture consistent with encephalitis (brain inflammation manifesting as altered level of consciousness, fever, headache, and possibly focal neurologic features such as seizure) in a child with a history of a recent herpes lesion (cold sore). An overlap syndrome of meningoencephalitis may also develop, in which both the meninges (nuchal rigidity) and brain are affected. HSV is a common cause of encephalitis, second only to enterovirus in children. Other infectious causes include viral agents such as arboviruses and influenza, as well as a myriad bacterial, amoebic, and parasitic agents. If you are suspicious of HSV encephalitis and the first CSF HSV PCR is negative, repeat the test because false negatives have been known to occur in early infection. Always start your patient on empiric acyclovir while awaiting the test results, as morbidity and mortality are high without therapy. Treatment of herpes encephalitis includes 21 days of intravenous (IV) acyclovir followed by an end-of-therapy LP for repeat CSF HSV PCR testing. The repeat testing ensures infection resolution prior to stopping IV acyclovir.[13]

You start empiric treatment for HSV and monitor the patient closely. You start mentally reviewing the differential diagnosis of encephalitis in a child.

Question 8-2

Which is NOT a cause of encephalitis?
A) Intoxication.
B) Arbovirus infection.
C) Cat-scratch disease.
D) Malignancy.
E) Autoimmune disorders.

Discussion 8-2

The correct answer is "A." Intoxication causes CNS depression (encephalopathy) not inflammation (encephalitis). Viruses are the most common cause of encephalitis. Anti-NMDA (N-methyl-D-aspartate) receptor encephalitis is an autoimmune process that manifests with behavior and personality changes, then progresses to autonomic instability, seizures, coma, and even death. It is commonly a paraneoplastic process in adults (associated with ovarian teratoma). It is one of several antibody-mediated encephalitis conditions that are all rare in children. (See Table 23–4.)

> **Helpful Tip**
> Encephalitis and encephalopathy both cause cerebral dysfunction. The difference is that encephalitis results from inflammation of the brain; encephalopathy is a noninflammatory manifestation of a systemic illness.

TABLE 23–4 CAUSES OF ENCEPHALITIS

Cause	Example
Infectious	Enterovirus
	Parechovirus
	HSV 1 and 2
	Adenovirus
	Epstein-Barr virus
	HIV
	West Nile virus
	St. Louis virus
	California encephalitis virus
	LaCrosse encephalitis virus
	Eastern equine encephalitis virus
	Western equine encephalitis virus
	Rickettsia rickettsii (Rocky Mountain spotted fever)
	Borrelia burgdorferi (Lyme disease)
	Bartonella henselae (cat-scratch disease)
	Mycoplasma pneumoniae
	Parasites
	Fungus
Autoimmune	Anti-NMDA receptor encephalitis
Postinfectious	Acute disseminated encephalomyelitis
Vasculitis	
Metabolic	
Malignancy	

HIV, human immunodeficiency virus; HSV, herpes simplex virus; NMDA, N-methyl-D-aspartate.

▶ CASE 9

Apparently it is seizure day in the emergency department. The third chart you open is a 9-year-old boy who has been transferred from outside the hospital. He has a history of chronic otitis media, was diagnosed with another ear infection last week, and was placed on amoxicillin. He presented to the emergency department with persistent fevers and new-onset seizure characterized by unresponsive staring, lip smacking, and then generalized jerking. The outside CT scan was "abnormal" so he was sent to you for further evaluation. On examination, the child is back to baseline mental status, and the parents deny any alteration of consciousness before or after the seizure. You see a hypodense lesion in the left temporal lobe. (See Figures 23–1 and 23–2.)

Question 9-1

What is the lesion, and what will be your next diagnostic step?

A) Acute stroke; brain MRI without contrast.
B) Acute stroke; brain MRI and MRV with and without contrast.
C) Brain tumor; brain MRI with and without contrast.
D) Brain abscess; brain MRI with and without contrast.
E) Brain arteriovenous malformation (AVM); MRV with and without contrast.

FIGURE 23–1. Temporal lobe brain abscess on CT scan. (Used with permission from Nathan Price, MD.)

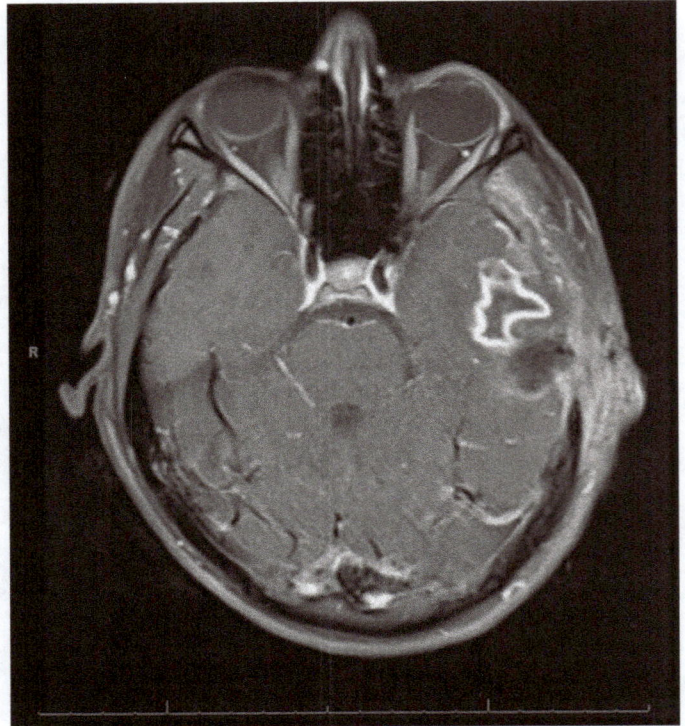

FIGURE 23–2. Temporal lobe brain abscess on MRI. (Used with permission from Nathan Price, MD.)

Discussion 9-1

The correct answer is "D." Although stroke, tumor, and AVM are included in the differential diagnosis for new-onset seizure in the setting of a brain lesion, this is more likely to be an abscess given the infectious history. Infection of the middle ear or sinuses can rarely lead to more invasive infection of nearby areas such as the meninges and brain. Brain abscess secondary to otitis media tends to affect the temporal lobe, whereas sinusitis can lead more often to frontal lobe abscess. This complication should be suspected if the patient has altered mental status, meningeal signs, seizures, or focal neurologic abnormalities. An MRI with and without contrast will better define the lesion and assist with medical and surgical management. Abscesses are characteristically ring-enhancing with contrast studies.

> **Helpful Tip**
> Ear and sinus infections can extend intracranially, causing meningitis, encephalitis, epidural abscess, subdural empyema, brain abscess, dural venous thrombosis, cavernous sinus thrombosis, stroke, and osteomyelitis of the skull.

⏳ QUICK QUIZ

Which is NOT a common risk factor for a brain abscess?
A) Congenital heart disease.
B) Chronic otitis media.

C) Endocarditis.
D) Viral meningitis.
E) Craniotomy.

Discussion

The correct answer is "D." Pathogenesis of brain abscess involves hematogenous seeding (endocarditis), direct spread from contiguous structures such as sinuses and middle ear (untreated otitis media), and direct inoculation in head trauma (open skull fracture, oral trauma) and neurosurgical cases. Congenital heart disease, especially with right-to-left shunting, may cause a brain abscess in the setting of bacteremia. The causative organism reflects the mechanism of infection. For example, brain abscess that formed due to complication of sinusitis reflects the common sinusitis organisms (*Streptococcus pneumoniae*, *Haemophilus influenzae*, anaerobes). Organisms from the lungs (*Aspergillus, Cryptococcus, Nocardia*) can seed the brain through the bloodstream; this most often occurs in immunocompromised hosts. Hematogenous spread from endocarditis is often caused by *Staphylococcus aureus* and Streptococcus viridans. A positive blood culture for *S. viridans* is not always a skin contaminant!

MRI with and without contrast is performed in your 9-year-old patient, revealing a solitary 2.5 mm ring-enhancing lesion consistent with abscess, and no signs of cerebral edema or mass effect. You perform a lumbar puncture and initial studies are pending.

Question 9-2

What factors will lead you to consider *antibiotic therapy alone* over medical and surgical management (aspiration, drainage, excision)?
A) Isolation of a causative organism in the CSF with concomitant meningitis.
B) Abscess location that is very deep or in a high-risk area.
C) An unstable, poor surgical candidate.
D) All of the above.

Discussion 9-2

The correct answer is "D." Multiple factors will weigh into this treatment decision, including the need to isolate an organism for proper treatment. Given that your patient was pretreated with antibiotics, it may not be possible to identify the organism without surgical intervention. Likewise, he is an excellent surgical candidate given that he is otherwise healthy and has a small, solitary abscess without significant mass effect. Antibiotic regimens to treat a parenchymal abscess are prolonged and typically range from 3 to 6 weeks, with repeat imaging often used to assist in determining length of therapy.

▶ CASE 10

A 15-year-old boy presents to the emergency department with a 5-day history of progressive leg weakness and numbness. He has not been able to walk for the past 2 days and has not urinated all day today despite drinking plenty of fluids. He has no preexisting health problems and no prior episodes of weakness, but did have a mild upper respiratory infection 10 days ago. On exam, his mental status, cranial nerves, and upper extremity function are intact. He has decreased sensation below the level of the umbilicus, with diminished reflexes and flaccid asymmetric leg weakness (affecting the right more than the left). He is catheterized and a large amount of urine is drained from the bladder. MRI of the spine reveals a contrast-enhancing, demyelinating lesion in the lower thoracic spine. CSF is notable for elevated protein with a normal WBC count.

Question 10-1

What is the most likely diagnosis?
A) Guillain-Barré syndrome.
B) Multiple sclerosis.
C) Transverse myelitis.
D) Spinal cord tumor.
E) None of the above.

Discussion 10-1

The correct answer is "C." Transverse myelitis (TM) is an acute to subacute, often postinfectious inflammation of the spinal cord that can lead to significant flaccid weakness and depressed or absent reflexes below the level of the lesion. There is often a *sensory level* and, depending on the site of the lesion, bowel and bladder dysfunction. It is treated with high-dose IV steroids or plasma exchange, or both. TM can be distinguished from Guillain-Barré syndrome (option "A"), another common postinfectious neurologic syndrome, by the presence of the spinal level and the focal lesion in the spinal cord. Guillain-Barré syndrome is classified as a polyradiculoneuropathy (typically demyelinating) and affects the peripheral nervous system (PNS; nerves and nerve roots), whereas TM affects the CNS (spinal cord). Although TM may be the initial sign of a future demyelinating disease, you cannot diagnose multiple sclerosis (option "B") at this time without evidence of previous clinical attacks of weakness or old lesions on MRI. Option "D," a spinal cord tumor, is most definitely on your differential diagnosis and is the reason you obtained emergent neuroimaging in the emergency department.

▶ CASE 11

A 15-month-old girl is brought to the clinic for language regression. You do a brief chart review before going in to see her. She was born at term, has no significant past medical history, and has met all developmental milestones on time. Notably, her head circumference has dropped from the 25th to the 2nd percentile in her last few well-child checks. Her mother reports that she has been fussier, is not sleeping well, has lost interest in her surroundings, and is no longer feeding herself. In addition, she has stopped saying several of the words she previously knew. On examination, you note a small child with no dysmorphic features. There is no hepatospleno-megaly and her funduscopic exam is normal. She has poor eye contact. She appears mildly anxious and has an irregular breathing pattern with periods of breath-holding. She is wringing her hands together in the midline in a nonpurpose-ful fashion. Her gait is clumsier than expected for her age. During the exam, she has a brief complex partial seizure. There is no family history of neurologic conditions.

Question 11-1

What is the most likely diagnosis?

A) Tay-Sachs disease.
B) Krabbe disease.
C) Rett syndrome.
D) Autism.
E) None of the above.

Discussion 11-1

The correct answer is "C." Neurodegenerative disorders present with developmental regression or arrest and include numerous hereditary and metabolic causes. Rett syndrome is a neurode-generative disorder characterized by an initial period of normal development followed by a period of rapid developmental regres-sion that typically occurs around 12 months of age (range, 5 to 18 months). This is accompanied by postnatal deceleration of head growth, complete or partial loss of purposeful hand use and language, stereotypical hand movements (midline wringing, clapping, tapping), and gait ataxia. Patients then have a period of relative stability following the regression, unlike other neurode-generative diseases that continually worsen. However, they even-tually have motor regression. Girls are almost exclusively affected. While awake many children with Rett syndrome cycle between hyperventilation and hypoventilation/apnea. Management is supportive, and survival is usually into adulthood. Children with Krabbe disease (option "B"), a lysosomal storage disorder, may initially present with irritability; however, the disorder usually manifests earlier in infancy, around 4 months of age. It is a rap-idly progressive demyelinating disorder characterized by progres-sively increased muscle tone, psychomotor regression, blindness, and seizures. Tay-Sachs disease (option "A") likewise manifests with psychomotor regression around 6 months of age and is accompanied by a cherry red spot on funduscopic exam and hepatosplenomegaly. Autism (option "D") should not be accom-panied by marked developmental regression or microcephaly.

> **Helpful Tip**
> Any child with loss of developmental milestones (regression) warrants a neurologic consultation and MRI of the brain. These should be completed urgently.

▶ CASE 12

You are rotating in the emergency department (ED) and pick up the chart of a previously healthy 5-year-old girl who was brought in by emergency medical services (EMS) with

a first-time generalized seizure that lasted less than 2 min-utes and self-resolved 20 minutes ago. She is afebrile and has no history of recent head trauma or illness. She is sleepy on exam, but follows commands and has a completely nor-mal neurologic exam. Results of a full electrolyte panel with renal and liver function tests and a urine drug screen are all normal.

Question 12-1

What is the next appropriate management step?

A) Obtain a head CT scan stat.
B) Obtain an EEG before discharge from the ED.
C) Counsel the family about epilepsy and provide a prescrip-tion for levetiracetam.
D) Order an outpatient EEG.
E) Admit the patient overnight for hospital observation.

Discussion 12-1

The correct answer is "D." Outpatient EEG is recommended based on the American Academy of Neurology practice param-eter for a first-time afebrile (unprovoked) seizure of a child aged 6 months or older. The only reason to get an urgent EEG in the ED (option "B") is if there are concerns for ongoing subclini-cal status epilepticus. This patient is sleepy because she is still postictal, but she readily follows commands and has a normal neurologic exam, making subclinical status unlikely. Laboratory studies are recommended if clinically appropriate to evaluate for toxic or metabolic etiologies (hyponatremia, hypoglycemia, ingestions). Neuroimaging recommendations are also clinically based. An emergent head CT (option "A") is indicated only to rule out an acute intracranial process that may require immedi-ate intervention. There is no need to obtain a CT scan for every child with a seizure who walks through the door! MRI is always the preferred imaging choice for seizures, but this can be done on an outpatient basis. In most cases, these children should all receive an outpatient EEG, MRI, and neurologic consultation. Option "C" is incorrect, as there is no benefit in treating a child with a first-time seizure rather than waiting to see if he or she develops epilepsy. Patients are more likely to develop epilepsy if they have an abnormality on EEG, prior febrile seizures, a prior insult known to cause seizures (encephalitis), nocturnal seizures, or a postictal Todd paralysis.

⏳ QUICK QUIZ

In which of the following situations would patients require emergent neuroimaging?

A) Seizure after high-speed collision with a tree in a skiing accident.
B) Seizure accompanied by early morning headache, vomiting, and papilledema.
C) Seizure followed by prolonged postictal period (more than several hours).
D) Seizure with postictal weakness of the right arm and leg.
E) All of the above.

Discussion

The correct answer is "E." Emergent neuroimaging is required to rule out acute intracranial processes in all of these scenarios. Option "A" is worrisome for an epidural hematoma; option "B" is suggestive of acute hydrocephalus; option "C" suggests an underlying toxic, metabolic, or infectious etiology; and although option "D" may simply be a postictal Todd paralysis, you must rule out an acute stroke or other intracranial pathology in anyone with a focal neurologic deficit.

> **Helpful Tip**
> Epilepsy is defined as two or more unprovoked seizures occurring at least 24 hours apart. Once the diagnosis is made, children are placed on an antiepileptic medication based on their seizure type. The majority of children can be completely controlled with medications (60–70%). Attempts to wean off of medications are typically made if the patient remains seizure-free for 2 years on medications.

Question 12-2

Would your initial evaluation and differential diagnosis change if the child was a 5-day-old infant with a first afebrile seizure?

A) No, a seizure is a seizure, and workup is independent of age.
B) Yes, I would be more worried about serious underlying pathology.

Discussion 12-2

The correct answer is "B." Neonatal seizures are a whole different beast. First of all, their appearance is different than typical childhood seizures because neonatal brains are immature and not well myelinated. As a result, neonates cannot have a classic generalized tonic-clonic seizure. Typical neonatal seizure manifestations include apnea and stiffening, rhythmic jerking of one limb or side of the body, jerking of multiple limbs but at different times, or even bicycling movements of the legs. Neonatal seizures require emergent workup looking for underlying metabolic or toxic etiology, structural brain defects, and serious bacterial infection. Some examples include hypocalcemia, drug withdrawal, meningitis, sepsis, hypoxic ischemic encephalopathy, urea cycle disorders, intracranial hemorrhage, and glycine encephalopathy.

▶ CASE 13

A 6-year-old girl presents to the clinic with her mother for evaluation of a possible learning disability or attention deficit disorder (ADD). She is having a hard time learning in kindergarten and is often caught "daydreaming." Last night at dinner she suddenly stopped eating, stared for 15 seconds, and then resumed as if nothing was wrong. This event scared the parents so they brought her in today. She is a normal, healthy child with an intact neurologic examination. When you have her blow repeatedly on a tissue, she suddenly stops blowing, stares straight ahead with eyelid fluttering, and does not respond to touch or voice. About 15 seconds later she resumes blowing on the tissue. When you ask her about it she has no idea that she stopped blowing. Her parents note that this was exactly what happened at dinner.

Question 13-1

What is the most likely diagnosis and recommended treatment?

A) Complex partial epilepsy; oxcarbazepine or carbamazepine.
B) Childhood absence epilepsy; ethosuximide.
C) ADHD; stimulant medication.
D) Behavioral staring spells; no treatment necessary.

Discussion 13-1

The correct answer is "B." Childhood absence epilepsy is an epilepsy syndrome characterized by brief seizures (5–15 seconds) consisting of behavioral arrest, staring, and occasional repetitive, nonpurposeful facial movements (blinking, chewing) called *automatisms*. The seizures can occur upwards of 100 times per day and can significantly impact learning abilities. The characteristic EEG finding is a 3-Hz generalized spike-and-wave pattern. The seizures can usually be provoked in the office by hyperventilation (tissue blowing). Interestingly, children with absence epilepsy also have coexisting learning issues and ADHD, so careful screening will still be necessary once seizures are controlled. Ethosuximide is the first-line treatment. The vast majority of children outgrow the seizures. A minority also have generalized tonic-clonic seizures. Although it can be difficult to distinguish a complex partial seizure (option "A") from an absence seizure, typically complex partial seizures last longer (> 1 minute) and are preceded by an aura and followed by a postictal period of fatigue. They are not induced by hyperventilation. Behavioral staring or daydreaming (options "C" and "D") can be distinguished from seizures by the fact that they are interruptible by voice or touch. (Children may ignore being called, but have a hard time ignoring a tickle or pinch!)

> **Helpful Tip**
> Seizure mimics include breath-holding spells, Sandifer syndrome (reflux-related opisthotonic posturing), tics, syncope, and self-stimulation or gratification behavior. These mimics can be differentiated from seizure by a careful history of event timing, triggers, and the ability to distract a child out of an episode.

⌛ QUICK QUIZ

Which of the following is true regarding seizures?
A) Partial seizures may or may not impair consciousness.
B) Generalized seizures always involve changes in motor activity or tone.
C) Absence seizures are focal seizures.
D) Simple partial seizures may be preceded by an aura.
E) Complex partial seizures always involve lip smacking.

TABLE 23–5 SEIZURE CHARACTERISTICS

Seizure Type	Simple Partial (aura)	Complex Partial	Absence	Generalized	Infantile Spasms
Level of consciousness	Preserved	Impaired	Impaired	Impaired	Impaired
Appearance	Focal jerking, stiffness, or sensory symptom	Focal stiffness or jerking	Behavior arrest, facial automatisms (blinking, chewing)	Generalized stiffness, jerking, or both	Brief flexion or extension of arms/abdomen, looks like a "crunch"
Typical duration	< 2 min	< 2 min	5–20 sec	< 2 min	Clusters upon awakening
Postictal period	N	Y	N	Y	N
AED	Oxcarbazepine, levetiracetam, lamotrigine		Ethosuximide, valproic acid, lamotrigine	Levetiracetam, topiramate, valproic acid	ACTH or vigabatrin (if child has tuberous sclerosis)
EEG	Focal discharges/abnormalities		3-Hz generalized spike-and-wave pattern	Generalized discharges	Hypsarrhythmia

ACTH, adrenocorticotropic hormone; AED, antiepileptic drug; EEG, electroencephalogram.

Discussion

The correct answer is "A." Seizures are classified as partial or generalized. Consciousness is not impaired with simple partial seizures. Complex partial seizures may be preceded by an aura, cause impaired consciousness, and may or may not be associated with automatisms (lip smacking, drooling). Partial seizures can evolve into generalized seizures. Generalized seizures include absence, myoclonic, tonic, clonic, tonic-clonic, and atonic. (See Table 23–5.)

► CASE 14

A 13-year-old postmenarchal girl comes to the clinic with concerns of early morning clumsiness after several episodes of breaking dishes and glasses at breakfast. She describes an uncontrollable brief jerk of her shoulders and arms that causes them to fling out, resulting in the broken dishes. On further questioning, she admits to having had a few episodes where she woke up having wet the bed at night and with blood in her mouth from biting his tongue. Her exam is normal. You suspect seizures and order an MRI, which is normal, and an EEG, which shows a 4- to 6-Hz generalized polyspike-and-wave pattern.

Question 14-1

What is the most likely diagnosis?
A) Juvenile myoclonic epilepsy.
B) Benign rolandic epilepsy.
C) Complex partial epilepsy.
D) Childhood absence epilepsy.
E) None of the above.

Discussion 14-1

The correct answer is "A." Myoclonic seizures are brief, involuntary (usually single), asymmetric jerks typically involving the arms. They characteristically occur in the morning hours, leading to dropped toothbrushes, curling irons (and burns!), and broken dishes. Children are often accused of being clumsy until they have their first generalized tonic-clonic seizure. A minority of children also have absence seizures. Benign rolandic epilepsy (option "B") is a form of autosomal dominant epilepsy that is typically "benign" because the majority of children only have a handful of seizures over their lifetime. It typically manifests around 8 years of age and remits by age 14. The typical seizure occurs at night and consists of one-sided facial tingling followed by twitching, drooling, and difficulty speaking. The child is fully aware of what is going on. The seizure can spread to involve the arm or even go on to a generalized tonic-clonic seizure. Treatment is not needed unless seizures are frequent or disruptive, in which case oxcarbazepine or carbamazepine is preferred. The seizures described in this patient are all generalized (myoclonic and presumed generalized tonic-clonic) and would not be part of complex partial or absence epilepsy.

Question 14-2

What is the proper treatment?
(Bonus question: What are the most common side effects of the following drugs?)
A) Oxcarbazepine.
B) Valproic acid.
C) Levetiracetam.
D) Ethosuximide.
E) Any of the above.

Discussion 14-2

The correct answer is "C." Levetiracetam is a well-tolerated medication. Typical side effects include behavioral issues (irritability, moodiness). Although valproic acid (option "B") is also used, it is preferentially avoided in women of childbearing age due to the potential for birth defects (neural tube defects). It can also cause pancreatitis, liver failure, and thrombocytopenia and requires careful blood monitoring. Ethosuximide (option "D") is used in childhood absence epilepsy (but note that it does not treat generalized tonic-clonic seizures). Side effects include gastrointestinal upset and risk of Stevens-Johnson syndrome (which also can occur with lamotrigine). Oxcarbazepine (option "A") is an excellent choice for partial seizures but may actually worsen generalized seizures. Side effects include hyponatremia and ataxia. Carbamazepine has a similar side effect profile to oxcarbazepine, with the added concern for bone marrow suppression and DRESS (drug reaction with eosinophilia and systemic symptoms). All seizure medications have the potential to cause cognitive issues and sleepiness at higher doses. For intractable seizures, the child may be placed on a ketogenic diet.

► CASE 15

During another busy day in clinic, a 5-month-old boy is referred to you for evaluation of atypical movements. The infant was born at term and had been healthy with normal development. A few weeks ago, he started having attacks during which his body crunches up repeatedly then stops. The clusters frequently occur right after he wakes up. The mother shows you a video on her phone. During the episode, the infant's head thrusts forward while his entire body repeatedly flexes together and then extends.

Question 15-1

What is the most likely cause of these events?
A) Infantile spasms.
B) Lennox-Gastaut syndrome.
C) Dravet syndrome.
D) Sleep myoclonus.
E) Tremors.

Discussion 15-1

The correct answer is "A." Infantile spasms (also known as West syndrome) begin in the first year of life with peak onset between 4 and 6 months of age. Seizures occur in clusters and consist of head bobbing with flexion and extension of the trunk and extremities (like opening and closing a jackknife). The infant may cry out before seizing. The EEG shows hypsarrhythmia. (If a test question mentions hypsarrhythmia, stop reading and look for infantile spasms in the answer choices.) Approximately 70% of children have an underlying CNS disorder or malformation. Lennox-Gastaut syndrome is characterized by multiple seizure types, difficult to control seizures, cognitive impairment, and a slow spike-and-wave pattern on EEG. Severe myoclonic epilepsy of infancy (Dravet syndrome) is associated with intractable seizures beginning in the first year of life.

> **Helpful Tip**
>
> When evaluating a child who may be seizing, put your hand on the shaking body part to see if you can extinguish the movement. If you can, the child is not having a seizure.

► CASE 16

There is a full moon and the emergency department is full of seizing children. EMS brings in another seizing patient; this time it is a 9-month-old girl who has been having rhythmic twitching of her left side for 25 minutes. The paramedics gave a dose of IV lorazepam 5 minutes ago. She is febrile to 38.8°C (102°F) and her airway and breathing are stable. She has no past medical history, is up-to-date with immunizations, and has never had a seizure before.

Question 16-1

What is the next treatment step for status epilepticus?
A) Fosphenytoin 20 mg/kg IV.
B) CT of the head stat.
C) Repeat dose of IV lorazepam.
D) Phenobarbital 20 mg/kg IV.
E) Neuromuscular blocking medication.

Discussion 16-1

As with any critically ill patient, first complete a primary survey, the ABCs, and stabilize the patient's cardiorespiratory status. Also think about calling a code blue. Regarding the seizing, the correct answer is option "C": repeat the dose of IV lorazepam if the seizure does not stop 5 minutes after the first dose. If the infant continues to seize 5 minutes after the second dose, your next step in the treatment of status epilepticus will be an IV bolus of an antiepileptic drug such as fosphenytoin or phenobarbital. It is helpful to obtain a drug level 2 to 4 hours after the antiepileptic load in case further medications are needed. Iatrogenic paralysis (option "E") will stop the infant's body from jerking, but it will not stop the seizure. For practical purposes, status epilepticus is defined as a seizure lasting more than 5 minutes, because this is typically when you will intervene. It is more traditionally defined as a seizure lasting more than 30 minutes, or two or more seizures without return to baseline in between. (See Table 23–6.)

You administer the second dose of lorazepam and the seizure stops. You obtain a full electrolyte panel, including calcium, glucose, sodium, and magnesium; urinalysis; urine drug screen; and CBC. All labs come back normal. The patient returns to baseline and looks well, and you go to counsel the parents. She has no signs of meningitis and has not received any antibiotics recently.

Question 16-2

What is her diagnosis?
A) Simple febrile seizure.
B) Complex febrile seizure.

TABLE 23–6 MANAGEMENT OF STATUS EPILEPTICUS

Time in minutes	Action
0–5	Stabilize the patient:
	ABCs: assess airway, breathing, circulation
	Obtain access (IV or intraosseous)
	Administer oxygen
	Obtain stat blood glucose and correct if low
	Obtain blood work
	Identify and treat reversible causes
5–10	Give medications:
	Lorazepam, 0.05–0.1 mg/kg IV, or
	Diazepam, 0.2–0.5 mg/kg IV
10–15	If seizures persists:
	Repeat lorazepam or diazepam
15–25	If seizure persists, load with one of the following:
	Fosphenytoin, 15–20 mg PE/kg IV or IM
	Phenytoin, 15–20 mg/kg IV
	Phenobarbital, 15–20 mg/kg IV
25–40	If seizure persists, give one of the following:
	Levetiracetam, 20–30 mg/kg IV
	Valproate, 20 mg/kg IV
	Phenobarbital (if fosphenytoin or phenytoin given)
	Additional phenytoin or fosphenytoin
40–60	If seizure persists:
	Pentobarbital, lorazepam, or general anesthesia-induced coma
	Avoid paralytics

IM, intramuscular; IV, intravenous; PE, phenytoin equivalents.

Discussion 16-2

The correct answer is "B." A simple febrile seizure occurs between 6 and 60 months of age, is associated with a fever of 38°C (100.4°F) or higher, is generalized, lasts 15 minutes or less, and only occurs once in 24 hours. Febrile seizures are considered complex if they are focal (as in our patient), last longer than 15 minutes (as in our patient), or reoccur in a 24-hour period. Children with simple febrile seizures have only a slightly higher incidence of epilepsy (2% versus 1%) than the general population and typically do very well. Children with complex febrile seizures are slightly more likely to develop epilepsy. Febrile seizures occur in families. Evaluation of simple febrile seizures includes evaluation for the source of fever. Routine lab testing,

EEG, and MRI are not indicated. LP should be considered in (1) a child with clinical signs of meningitis, (2) a 6- to 12-month-old who is not fully immunized, or in whom the immunization status is unknown, or (3) a child who has been pretreated with antibiotics.

> **Helpful Tip**
> Beware of calling everything a febrile seizure. Pay careful attention to the age cutoffs in the definition of febrile seizures. A 5-month-old with fever and seizure has a serious infection until proven otherwise. Likewise, a 7-year-old with a fever and seizure deserves further workup and neurologic evaluation.

> **Helpful Tip**
> Psychogenic nonepileptic events (pseudoseizures) are a conversion disorder best managed through psychological care. Clues to psychogenic events include eye closure, intact awareness during generalized shaking, pelvic thrusting, prolonged or waxing and waning events, and lack of a postictal period. The underlying stressors are not always apparent (or even particularly severe), but patients should *always* be screened for abuse.

► CASE 17

A 2-year-old previously healthy girl presents to the emergency department for unsteady gait. She was in her normal state of health until last night. This morning, she has not been able to walk since she woke up. Otherwise, she is in good spirits and does not appear to be in pain. She is currently afebrile but had a viral illness 2 weeks ago. On exam, she is alert and talks normally. She has no focal neurologic signs, but has truncal ataxia and dysmetria when she reaches for her toy. She is ataxic and unable to walk unassisted. Reflexes are normal throughout.

Question 17-1

What is the most likely diagnosis?
A) Drug ingestion.
B) Posterior fossa tumor.
C) Acute cerebellar ataxia.
D) Acute demyelinating encephalomyelitis (ADEM).
E) Behavioral.

Discussion 17-1

The correct answer is "C." Acute cerebella ataxia is a postinfectious autoimmune process, and is thought to be due to cross-reactivity of antiviral antibodies to cerebellar epitopes. It is most commonly associated with varicella zoster virus and Epstein-Barr virus, but can occur with other infectious processes. A previously healthy child develops ataxia mostly affecting his or her gait over hours to a few days (rapid progression). Mental status is not affected. MRI may be normal or may show enhancement of cerebellum (cerebellitis). CSF usually shows mild pleocytosis. Acute cerebellar ataxia is usually a self-limiting disease, and affected children improve over weeks to a few months. Prognosis for complete recovery is excellent. Only a minority of patients experience persisting ataxia. ADEM is also a postinfectious process, but patients have encephalopathy (mental status change), multifocal deficits on exam, and multifocal lesions on MRI. A child with a posterior fossa tumor does not present with acute ataxia unless there is acute associated hemorrhage or it leads to acute obstructive hydrocephalus. Unlike the child described in the case, such patients do not appear well.

> **Helpful Tip**
> Toxic exposure is the most common cause of acute ataxia in children. In toddlers, accidental ingestion is most common, whereas recreational drug use is often suspected in adolescents. In addition to ataxia, patients also have slurred speech and mental status change. Alcohol, benzodiazepines, antiepileptics, and drugs of abuse all may cause these symptoms.

QUICK QUIZ

Which of the following antiepileptic medications is NOT associated with drug-induced tremors?
A) Phenytoin.
B) Carbamazepine.
C) Sodium valproate.
D) Levetiracetam.

Discussion

The correct answer is "D." Phenytoin, carbamazepine, and sodium valproate can all cause tremors.

▶ CASE 18

A 7-year-old boy presents to your office for evaluation of worsening gait instability and incoordination. His symptoms started shortly after he started walking as an infant and have been progressive. He is experiencing increasing difficulty with walking, and he sometimes trips and falls. His hands are shaky. He has had frequent sinus infections and pneumonias. Physical exam is remarkable for dysarthria, dysmetria on finger to nose, truncal ataxia, and ataxic gait. Dilated blood vessels are noted on the conjunctiva, auricles, and nasal bridge. (See Figure 23–3.)

Question 18-1

The most likely diagnosis in this patient is:
A) Friedreich ataxia.
B) Ataxia telangiectasia.
C) Neuroblastoma.

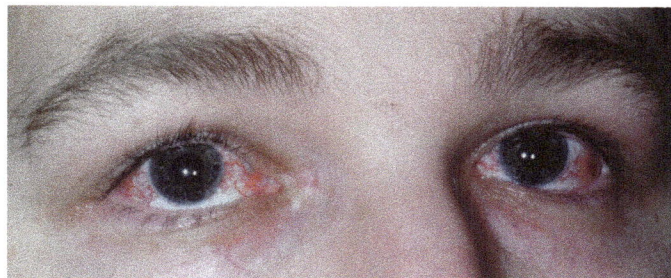

FIGURE 23–3. Conjunctival telangiectasias in a patient with ataxia-telangiectasia. (Reproduced with permission from Goldsmith LA, Katz SI, Gilchrest BA, Paller AS, Leffell DJ, Wolff K, eds. *Fitzpatrick's Dermatology in General Medicine*. 8th ed. New York, NY: McGraw-Hill Education; 2012, Fig. 143-8.)

D) Guillain-Barré syndrome.
E) None of the above.

Discussion 18-1

The correct answer is "B." Ataxia telangiectasia is characterized by progressive childhood onset ataxia, oculocutaneous telangiectasias, sinopulmonary infections, hematologic malignancies (leukemia and lymphoma), and radiosensitivity. Telangiectasias may not be present initially. Patients are immunodeficient and have recurrent sinopulmonary infections requiring aggressive treatment. It is an autosomal recessive disorder, and the causative gene is the *ATM* (ataxia telangiectasia mutated) gene, which is involved in DNA damage response and cell cycle regulation. Alpha-fetoprotein is elevated in the majority of patients. Friedreich ataxia is also an autosomal recessive disorder presenting with gait ataxia. Symptoms typically begin around puberty (later than ataxia telangiectasia). Loss of lower extremity deep tendon reflexes is typical. Other clinical features include diabetes and cardiomyopathy. Opsoclonus-myoclonus syndrome is a rare immune-mediated condition, characterized by irritability, ataxia, opsoclonus, myoclonus, and developmental regression. Opsoclonus consists of chaotic, often conjugate, rapid irregular eye movement in all directions. Myoclonus involves uncoordinated jerking of the limbs and trunk. Neuroblastoma is discovered in about half of cases of opsoclonus-myoclonus syndrome. The course of symptoms for ataxia telangiectasia evolves over days (not years) in Guillain-Barré syndrome.

> **Helpful Tip**
> Children with ataxia telangiectasia are extremely sensitive to radiation. Imaging with ionizing radiation (X-rays, CT scans) should not be ordered casually, given their already increased risk of malignancy.

QUICK QUIZ

Dopamine antagonists such as antipsychotics and some antiemetics can cause acute dystonic reactions (gaze deviation, torticollis, twisting of the trunk).

Choose a drug that can reverse acute dystonia caused by anti-dopaminergic agents.

A) Dantrolene.

B) Bromocriptine.

C) Diphenhydramine.

D) Metoclopramide.

E) All of the above.

Discussion

The correct answer is "C." Diphenhydramine is effective in treating acute drug-induced dystonia. Benztropine is also effective. Dantrolene and bromocriptine are used for treatment of neuroleptic malignant syndrome, which is also caused by dopamine antagonists. Metoclopramide (Reglan) is an antiemetic and a dopamine antagonist; therefore, it can cause dystonia and neuroleptic malignant syndrome.

► CASE 19

A 10-year-old girl is brought to the clinic for evaluation of behavioral changes and abnormal movements. A few weeks ago, she became anxious and emotionally labile, crying for no apparent reason. She has become fidgety. She recently started to have random writhing movements of her arms and legs, and she has not been able to sit still during class. Her handwriting is affected. A few months ago, she had an acute febrile illness with headache and sore throat. The symptoms went away without treatment. On exam, she has good strength and no focal neurologic signs, but she has difficulty maintaining hand grip (repeatedly squeezing and releasing the examiner's fingers). She has facial tics and unpredictable, purposeless flowing movements of her arms and legs.

Question 19-1

What would you do next?

A) Evaluate her for ADHD.

B) Refer her to a psychiatrist.

C) Obtain diagnostic studies, including antistreptolysin O (ASO), and anti-DNase B antibodies, as well as throat culture.

D) Start her on valproate.

Discussion 19-1

The correct answer is "C." Sydenham chorea is the most common cause of chorea in childhood. It occurs several weeks to several months after an untreated group A beta-hemolytic streptococcus (GABHS or *Streptococcus pyogenes*) or "strep throat" infection. Sydenham chorea is one of the major manifestations of acute rheumatic fever, along with migratory arthritis, carditis, erythema marginatum, and subcutaneous nodules. Difficulty with hand grip ("milkmaid's grip") is due to motor impersistence (inability to maintain a posture). Most children with Sydenham chorea have positive serology, although this is not necessary as Sydenham chorea alone is enough to diagnosis acute rheumatic fever. Children should be evaluated for concurrent carditis. Long-term prophylactic antibiotic treatment for the prevention of GABHS infections is required to reduce

the risk of recurrent rheumatic fever. Although most patients with Sydenham chorea do not require symptomatic treatment with medications, when the impairment is considerable, antiepileptic medications such as valproate or carbamazepine can be utilized. In such cases, you will need to confirm the diagnosis before discussing symptomatic treatment.

⧗ QUICK QUIZ

In what percentage of children with Sydenham chorea is serology negative for GABHS?

A) 1%.

B) 5%.

C) 25%.

D) 60%.

Discussion

The correct answer is "C." Most children with Sydenham chorea have positive serology (ASO and anti-DNase B antibodies), but more than 25% have negative serology. Negative serology does not rule out Sydenham chorea (acute rheumatic fever). The anti-DNase B titer remains elevated longer compared with the ASO titer, and may be more helpful as Sydenham chorea develops several weeks to months after a GABHS infection.

► CASE 20

A 7-year-old boy is being evaluated for facial movements. While you are speaking with the father, you hear the boy repeatedly sniffing.

Question 20-1

Which of the following is the most likely cause of the boy's symptoms?

A) Tourette syndrome

B) Habit cough

C) Tardive dyskinesia

D) Chorea

Discussion 20-1

The Best answer is "A" Tourette syndrome is characterized by involuntary motor and vocal tics that have their onset in childhood. The cause is unknown. It is frequently associated with obsessive compulsive disorder (OCD), ADHD, or learning problems. Children can often suppress their tics but then "tic out" in private. Children feel an urge before and sense of relief after a tic. Examples of motor ticks include blinking, grimacing, shrugging, kicking, jumping, and obscene gestures. Examples of vocal tics include swearing/obscenities (coprolalia), repeating words (echolalia), sniffing, barking, and throat clearing. The school should be educated that the tics are not intentional or bad behavior. Medications such as risperidone (antidopaminergic), clonidine, or guanfacine may be prescribed if the tics are severe and interfering with school, work, or social interactions.

► CASE 21

An 8-month-old girl with myelomeningocele is seen in the emergency department for changes in behavior. She has a ventriculoperitoneal (VP) shunt, and her neurogenic bladder is managed by intermittent clean catheterization. She has been fussy for the past few days, has not been eating well, and has vomited a few times. She has been afebrile. She awakes during the exam, but drifts back to sleep. Her anterior fontanelle is bulging. She has limited upward gaze. Her blood pressure is moderately elevated compared with her previous normal measurements.

Question 21-1

What would likely yield the correct diagnosis?
A) Urinalysis and urine culture.
B) Head CT scan.
C) Urine toxicology screen.
D) Tap the VP shunt reservoir and send CSF for analysis, including Gram stain and culture.

Discussion 21-1

The correct answer is "B." Between 60% and 90% of patients with myelomeningocele have hydrocephalus, and it occurs more frequently with higher lesions. VP shunts are often used for treatment of hydrocephalus. A VP shunt can be complicated by shunt failure and infection. In cases of shunt failure, patients present with signs and symptoms of increased intracranial pressure (ICP), such as headache, irritability, lethargy, vomiting, and eye movement abnormality. They may have hypertension with reflex irregular bradycardia. In infants, increasing head circumference, bulging anterior fontanelle, split sutures, and "setting sun" sign (limited upward gaze) may be noted. Some patients with shunt failure present with more subtle symptoms, such as "not acting normal" or moodiness. It is important to consider the possibility of a shunt malfunction when evaluating a patient with a VP shunt presenting with nonspecific complaints. The diagnostic study of choice is a noncontrast head CT scan, which often shows increased ventricle size. Single-shot T2-weighted MRI is becoming the initial imaging study of choice at some institutions. It provides the same information as a head CT scan and avoids radiation. Sedation is usually not required, as the test can be performed quickly. Be aware that programmable shunts may require resetting as the valve-pressure may be changed after exposure to an MRI magnetic field. Neurosurgical consultation is required whenever a shunt malfunction or infection is suspected. Be prepared to hear "It's not the shunt," to which you will reply, "It's the shunt." Urinary tract infections are common in children with bladder dysfunction. However, the patient described has clear signs and symptoms of increased ICP; therefore, urinary tract infection is not at the top of the differential. A patients with toxic ingestion can present with acute mental status change, and it is a reasonable differential diagnosis. However, given signs of increased ICP in a patient with VP shunt, shunt malfunction is more likely. Although shunt infection is possible, imaging is done first before collecting a CSF sample.

Shunt infections most commonly occur within the first few months of placement. The most common organisms are coagulase-negative staphylococci followed by *Staphylococcus aureus*. Patients with shunt infections may be asymptomatic or present with signs of increased ICP, peritonitis (VP shunts), septicemia (ventriculoatrial [VA] shunt), or cellulitis (distal external portion). Treatment includes IV antibiotics, removal of the shunt, and placement of an external ventricular drain.

⧗ QUICK QUIZ

What is NOT a risk factor for hydrocephalus?
A) Intraventricular hemorrhage.
B) Bacterial meningitis.
C) Posterior fossa tumor.
D) Chiari malformation.
E) All of the above.

Discussion

The correct answer is "E." Obstructive hydrocephalus develops whenever the normal flow of CSF is blocked and fluid accumulates within the ventricles or subarachnoid space. It presents with signs and symptoms of increased ICP. CSF is primarily produced by the choroid plexus in the ventricles. CSF flows through the ventricular system (lateral → third → fourth ventricle) into the subarachnoid space, where it is absorbed by the arachnoid granulations into the venous circulation. Remember, CSF flows from the lateral ventricles through the foramen of Monroe into the third ventricle; through the cerebral aqueduct to the fourth ventricle; and through the foramina of Luschka and Magendie into the subarachnoid space. Risk factors for developing hydrocephalus include CNS malformations, CNS infection, intraventricular hemorrhage, trauma, and tumors.

> **Helpful Tip**
> Folic acid supplementation during pregnancy can prevent many cases of neural tube defects. It is recommended that all women of childbearing age take 400 to 800 micrograms (mcg) of folic acid per day. If the woman has a neural tube defect or has given birth to a child with neural tube defect, the recommended dose of folic acid is 4 g (4000 mcg) per day.

⧗ QUICK QUIZ

Patients with myelomeningocele are at risk for which of the following?
A) Constipation.
B) Urinary tract infection.
C) Vesicoureteral reflex.
D) Renal failure.
E) All of the above.

Discussion

The correct answer is "E." Spinal cord pathology can lead to bowel and bladder dysfunction. Clean intermittent catheterization is done to reduce the risk of urinary tract infection and bladder overdistention, which can lead to vesicoureteral reflex, hydronephrosis, and chronic kidney disease. In some cases, a vesicostomy is placed. Ultrasonography and urodynamics are often utilized to assess the morphology and function. Constipation and fecal incontinence are often managed medically (timed toileting, fiber, stool softener, enemas).

> **Helpful Tip**
>
> A Chiari type II malformation (also known as an Arnold-Chiari malformation) is downward displacement of the lower cerebellum and cerebellar tonsils through the foramen magnum, with a concurrent myelomeningocele. Symptoms of Chiari malformation result from compression of the brainstem and cranial nerves and include dysphagia, aspiration, breathing problem (hoarse voice, strider, apnea), and arm weakness. A Chiari I malformation is downward displacement of the cerebellar tonsils only, without a concurrent myelomeningocele. A syrinx (fluid-filled cavity within the spinal cord) can be associated with a Chiari I malformation. (See Figure 23–4.)

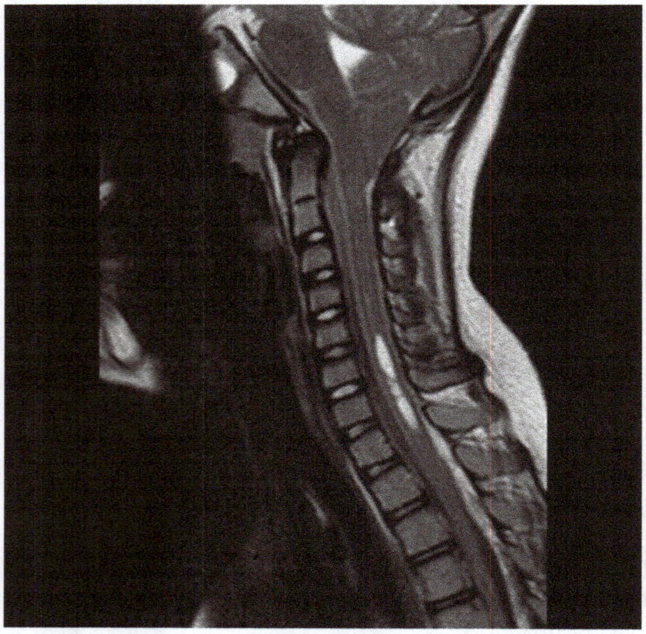

FIGURE 23–4. Sagittal MRI showing downward displacement of the cerebellar tonsils and an associated syrinx in this patient with a Chiari malformation. (Reproduced with permission from Doherty GM, ed. *Current Diagnosis & Treatment: Surgery.* 14th ed. New York, NY: McGraw-Hill Education; 2015, Fig. 36-18.)

▶ CASE 22

A pregnant woman's alpha-fetoprotein, checked as part of screening for neural tube defects, is elevated at 20 weeks' gestation. A prenatal ultrasound reveals signs of a neural tube defect. She and the father-to-be want more information, and they are referred to the neurology clinic for a prenatal consultation visit. You discuss the various types of neural tube defects; anticipated care needs for the newborn, including surgery in the postoperative period; long-term complications; and need for long-term multispecialty care.

Question 22-1

When discussing neural tube defects, what do you tell them?

A) Neural tube defects result from failure of the neural tube to close between the third and fourth week of gestation.

B) Spina bifida occulta may have cutaneous markers.

C) In a meningocele the meninges herniate through a midline defect in the lumbosacral spine.

D) A sacral dimple or cutaneous marking may indicate an underlying tethered cord.

E) All of the above.

Discussion 22-1

The correct answer is "E" *Spinal dysraphism* is a collective term for malformations of the spinal cord. Neural tube defects are included under the term *spinal dysraphism*. Myelomeningocele, also known as spina bifida, is the most common neural tube defect. The proximal or distal portion of the neural tube may be affected. The various types of neural tube defects are summarized in Table 23–7.

TABLE 23–7 TYPES OF NEURAL TUBE DEFECTS

Open spinal defects:
- Meningocele: herniation of the meninges through a lumbosacral defect
- Myelomeningocele: herniation of the meninges and spinal cord through a lumbosacral defect

Closed spinal defects (spina bifida occulta):
- Tethered cord: attachment of the cord to distal structures
- Dermal sinus tract: communication between the skin and the spinal cord
- Caudal regression: incomplete formation of the sacrum

Cranial defects:
- Encephalocele: herniation of the meninges and cerebral cortex, cerebellum, or part of the brainstem through a midline skull defect
- Anencephaly: failure of the part of the brain, brainstem, and skull to develop

Helpful Tip
Encephaloceles may involve the anterior portion of the skull, manifesting with nasal bridge swelling, hypertelorism, proptosis, nasal mass, or CSF rhinorrhea. Add it to your differential diagnosis of nasal obstruction.

⏳ QUICK QUIZ

Which is NOT an overlying cutaneous marker of a closed spinal neural tube defect such as a tethered cord?
A) Sacral dimple.
B) Hair tuft.
C) Lipoma.
D) Hemangioma.
E) None of the above.

Discussion

The correct answer is "E." Trick question! Options "A" through "D" are all correct. Cutaneous markers over the sacrum or coccyx may indicate underlying issues. Order an ultrasound (newborn) or an MRI of the spine.

⏳ QUICK QUIZ

True or false: Most patients with an epidural hematoma have a typical history of initial loss of consciousness, followed by a lucid interval, then clinical deterioration.
A) True.
B) False.

Discussion

The correct answer is "B." In contrast to classic teaching, only about 20% of patients with epidural hematoma experience loss of consciousness. They typically present with mental status changes or focal neurologic findings, or may have more subtle symptoms such as headache and emesis.

▶ CASE 23

A 4-year-old boy is brought in for evaluation of behavior issues. He was born at 27 weeks' gestational age. He was mildly delayed in achieving early developmental milestones even corrected for his prematurity, but he is mostly "caught up" per the mother. However, his preschool teacher has been expressing concerns about his behaviors. He cannot sit still during circle time, and he has difficulty following directions. The child is hyperactive and is exploring the exam room while you talk to his mother. He needs to be redirected multiple times during the exam. You note hyperreflexia at the knees and Achilles in bilateral lower extremities. He has several beats of ankle clonus bilaterally. Toes are upgoing bilaterally. Increased tone is noted at the ankles. He has mild bilateral toe walking. A brain MRI shows increased hyperintensity on T2 images at the frontal and occipital horns of lateral ventricle.

Question 23-1

Which condition would best explain his presentation?
A) Neonatal hyperbilirubinemia.
B) Cerebral palsy.
C) Perinatal stroke.
D) Congenital cytomegalovirus infection.
E) None of the above.

Discussion 23-1

The correct answer is "B." The physical exam finding of lower extremity hyperreflexia, spasticity, ankle clonus, and extensor toe signs (upper motor neuron signs), along with the history of prematurity and the described brain MRI finding (periventricular leukomalacia or white matter injury of prematurity) all point toward the diagnosis of spastic diplegia, one type of cerebral palsy. In addition to spastic diplegia, cognitive deficits and behavioral/attentional deficits are some of the clinical correlates of periventricular leukomalacia. (See Figure 23–5.) Kernicterus is caused by brain damage due to high level of bilirubin in newborn period. Patients develop hearing loss, dystonic cerebral palsy, and abnormal eye movements (limited upward gaze). Perinatal stroke is most common in the left middle cerebral

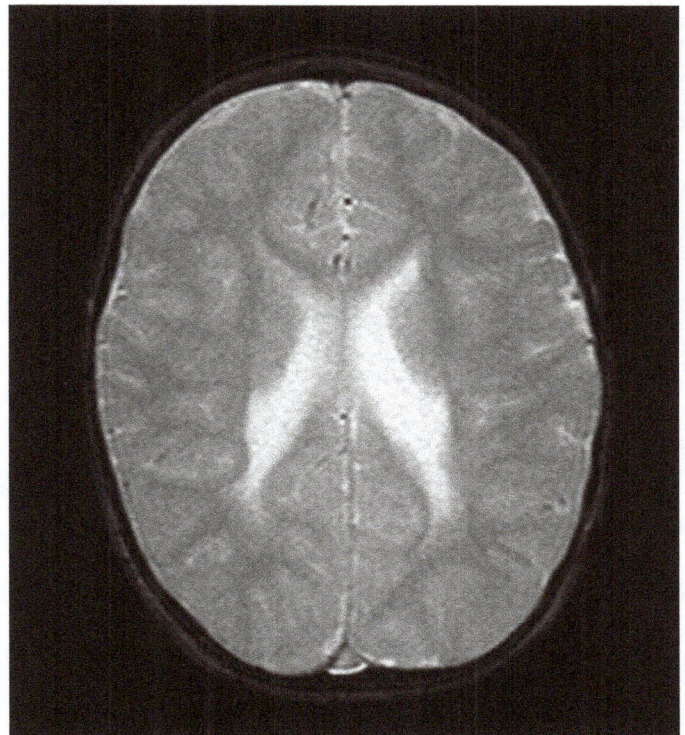

FIGURE 23–5. Axial brain MRI showing periventricular leukomalacia. (Reproduced with permission from Maitin IB, Cruz B, eds. *Current Diagnosis and Treatment: Physical Medicine and Rehabilitation.* New York, NY: McGraw-Hill Education; 2015, Fig. 20-3.)

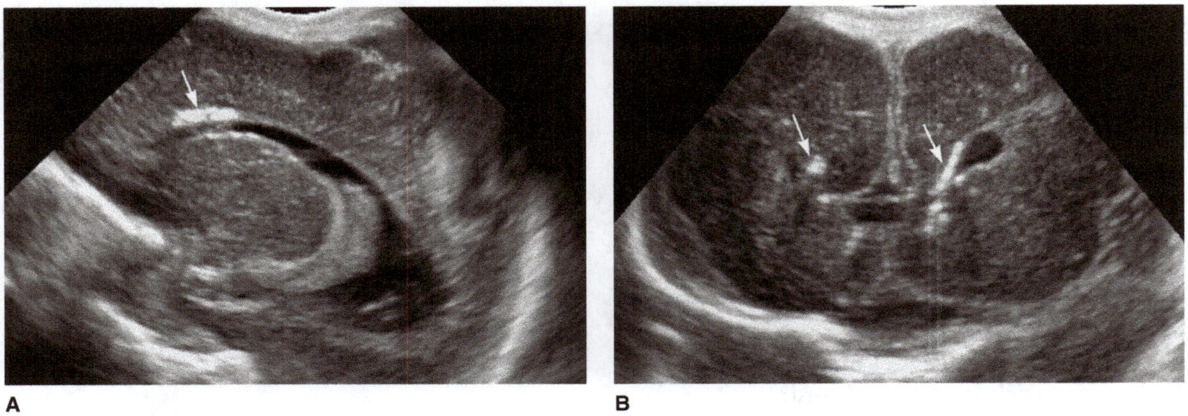

FIGURE 23–6. Ultrasound images of an infant with periventricular calcifications due to congenital cytomegalovirus infection. (Reproduced with permission from Cunningham FG, Leveno KJ, Bloom SL, et al, eds. *Williams Obstetrics*. 24th ed. New York, NY: McGraw-Hill Education; 2014, Fig. 64-3A&B.)

artery distribution, and usually causes focal deficits or seizures. Congenital cytomegalovirus infection is the most common congenital infection in the United States, with prevalence of approximately 1%. Between 10% and 15% of affected patients develop symptoms (intrauterine growth restriction, microcephaly, hepatosplenomegaly, jaundice, thrombocytopenia, and retinitis). Brain imaging shows periventricular calcifications. (See Figure 23–6.)

⧗ QUICK QUIZ

Which is NOT a cause of cerebral palsy?
A) Stroke.
B) Prematurity.
C) Traumatic brain injury.
D) Hypoglycemia.
E) Intracranial hemorrhage.

Discussion

The correct answer is "D." Cerebral palsy is a disorder of movement, muscle tone, or posture that is caused by a nonprogressive disturbance that occurred in the fetal or infant brain. Etiology includes perinatal brain injury (hypoxic ischemic encephalopathy [HIE], stroke), brain injury related to prematurity (periventricular leukomalacia, intraventricular hemorrhage), developmental abnormality (brain malformation, genetic or metabolic abnormality), postnatal brain injury (kernicterus, CNS infection, traumatic brain injury), and prenatal risk factors (congenital TORCH infections, toxin exposure). Obstetric complications are commonly blamed as a cause of cerebral palsy, but in fact perinatal asphyxia only accounts for 6% to 28% of such cases. Cerebral palsy is classified by the predominant motor abnormality and affected body area. Spastic hemiplegia (classically due to perinatal stroke), spastic quadriplegia (classically due to HIE), spastic diplegia (prematurity), and dystonic cerebral palsy (kernicterus, HIE) are some of the examples.

▶ CASE 24

An 8-year-old previously healthy girl presents to the emergency department after a focal seizure with secondary generalization. She is afebrile. She returns to her baseline after brief observation. Her skin exam is normal. A head CT scan shows a contrast-enhancing mass without surrounding edema or mass effect.

Question 24-1

What is the most likely cause of the lesion seen on head imaging?
A) Glioblastoma multiforme.
B) Arteriovenous malformation.
C) Brain abscess.
D) Sturge Weber syndrome.

Discussion 24-1

The correct answer is "B." Arteriovenous malformations (AVMs) are collections of abnormal blood vessels that connect arteries to veins without the intervening capillaries. The imaging shows a typical contrast-enhancing tangled clump of vessels. AVMs can hemorrhage, with clinical presentation of sudden headache, altered mental status, and possible focal neurologic deficits. (See Figure 23–7.) Glioblastoma multiforme is an aggressive tumor, and has a heterogeneous appearance, with surrounding edema and mass effect. A brain abscess has a different appearance at different stages of its evolution, but typically has ring enhancement. (See Figures 23–1 and 23–2, earlier.) A tram-track sign is a reflection of cortical calcifications due to leptomeningeal vascular malformations in Sturge-Weber syndrome. It often is seen in the posterior lobe and has characteristic gyriform parallel lines.

▶ CASE 25

A 5-year-old African American girl with known sickle cell disease presents to the emergency department with drooling and left-sided weakness since yesterday. Yesterday was July

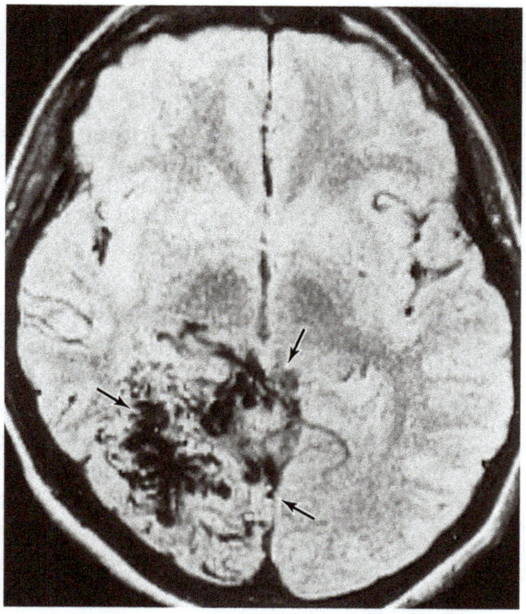

FIGURE 23–7. Axial brain MRI demonstrating a large arteriovenous malformation. (Reproduced with permission from Waxman SG, ed. *Clinical Neuroanatomy.* 27th ed. New York, NY: McGraw-Hill Education; 2013, Fig. 12-23.)

4th, and the patient was having fun blowing and spinning a pinwheel. Her parents noticed that she was not moving the left side of the body well last night. She was drooling as well, which is unusual for her. They decided to bring her in today as her condition is not improving. She has not had fever, cough, diarrhea, or headache. The patient does not have a history of seizures, and her parents have not noticed any seizure-like episodes. There is no family history of seizures, migraines, or early stroke or myocardial infarction. On exam, the patient has left-sided lower facial weakness, as well as decreased strength of the left arm and leg. The sensory exam is difficult to interpret given her age. Deep tendon reflexes are exaggerated on the left arm and leg. A magnetic resonance angiogram (MRA) of the brain shows bilateral stenosis of the intracranial internal carotid arteries with collateral vessels.

Question 25-1

What is the most likely cause of her symptoms?
A) Hemiplegic migraine.
B) Todd paralysis.
C) Brain hemorrhage.
D) Ischemic stroke.
E) None of the above.

Discussion 25-1

The correct answer is "D." The patient likely suffered an ischemic stroke with underlying vascular pathology in the setting of hyperventilation (blowing on a pinwheel), leading to cerebral vasoconstriction. Moyamoya disease is characterized by progressive stenosis of the intracranial internal carotid arteries with formation of collateral vessels. Moyamoya means "puff of smoke" in Japanese, describing the appearance of the fine networks of

TABLE 23–8 **CAUSES OF PEDIATRIC STROKE**

Ischemic

Sickle cell disease

Congenital heart defects (cardiogenic thrombi, right-to-left shunt)

Clotting disorders (antiphospholipid antibodies, factor V Leiden deficiency, protein C or S deficiency, prothrombin mutation)

Hyperhomocystinemia

Arteriopathy (arterial dissection, Moyamoya disease, Infections)

Hemorrhagic

Arteriovenous malformation

the collateral blood vessels. When the condition occurs with a well-known associated disorder, such as sickle cell disease, neurofibromatosis 1, and trisomy 21, it is categorized as Moyamoya syndrome. Typically, both internal arteries are affected, but some cases have unilateral involvement only. The child described in this case had ischemic lesions at the right middle cerebral artery territory on brain MRI. Hemiplegic migraine presents with usually reversible weakness often associated with headache. Todd paralysis is one of the differential diagnoses for new-onset hemiplegia, but the lack of convulsion in this case makes Todd paralysis unlikely. Brain hemorrhage can lead to hemorrhagic stroke, but patients typically also have headache. Furthermore, the vast majority of vascular complications seen in Moyamoya disease in children are ischemic. (See Table 23–8.)

> **Helpful Tip**
> Sickle cell disease is the most common cause of stroke in children. Other etiologies include congenital heart disease, CNS infection, trauma, vascular lesions, thrombophilia, and genetic conditions.

QUICK QUIZ

Which is NOT a presenting sign of stroke in pediatric patients?
A) Seizure.
B) Hemiparesis.
C) Altered mental status.
D) Tremor.
E) Aphasia.

Discussion

The correct answer is "D." Presentation varies by age. Infants typically have seizures and altered mental status while older children present with hemiparesis, headache, and focal deficits (aphasia, vision changes).

► CASE 26

A 10-year-old girl is admitted to the general pediatrics floor for progressive weakness. She started to have weakness in her legs several days ago, and the weakness has progressed to involve her arms and face. She has not been able to walk since yesterday. She denies back pain and bladder or bowel dysfunction. Until her leg weakness started, she had been healthy except for a diarrheal illness 3 weeks ago. Deep tendon reflexes are not present in the legs and are diminished in the arms. CSF and electrophysiologic study results are consistent with Guillain-Barré syndrome.

Question 26-1

Regarding the management of this patient, which statement is NOT correct?
A) Her forced vital capacity (FVC) should be monitored.
B) Her blood pressure should be monitored closely.
C) IVIG or plasma exchange should be considered.
D) Oral steroid should be given.

Discussion 26-1

The correct answer is "D." The pathophysiology of Guillain-Barré syndrome is thought to be an autoimmune phenomenon in the setting of recent infection or immunization. Various pathogens have been implicated, including cytomegalovirus, Epstein-Barr virus, varicella zoster virus, *Campylobacter jejuni* (this child's probable diarrheal illness), *Mycoplasma pneumoniae,* and *Haemophilus influenzae.* Patients present with ascending weakness, usually occurring 1 to 4 weeks after the infection or immunization. Weakness can involve respiratory muscles leading to respiratory compromise, and this can occur rapidly. Therefore, FVC needs to be monitored intermittently to identify patients at risk. Patients whose FVC is 20 mL/kg or less, as well as those with rapidly progressing weakness, bulbar palsy, quadriparesis, and cardiovascular autonomic dysfunction need to be monitored in the PICU. More than 10% of patients require intubation and mechanical ventilation during the course of the illness. Autonomic dysfunction such as cardiac dysrhythmias, hypotension, hypertension, paralytic ileus, and bladder dysfunction are common, occurring in about 50% of patients at the peak of the illness. Cranial nerve involvement can occur in up to 50% of patients, with involvement of the facial nerve being the most common. IVIG or plasma exchange hastens recovery. Steroids, either intravenous or oral, are not indicated. Oral corticosteroids may actually hinder improvement based on adult studies.

Helpful Tip

CSF analysis in Guillain-Barré syndrome typically shows an elevated protein level without pleocytosis (albuminocytologic dissociation). CSF results may not match the expected pattern, especially when the CSF is obtained early in the course of illness. CSF protein begins to rise toward the end of the first week of illness, and peaks in 4 to 6 weeks. Table 23–9 summarizes the differential diagnosis in Guillain-Barré syndrome.

TABLE 23–9 DIFFERENTIAL DIAGNOSIS OF GUILLAIN-BARRÉ SYNDROME

	Presentations and Distinguishing Features
Tick paralysis	Presents with acute ataxia, ascending flaccid paralysis, or both. Removal of tick is the treatment.
Botulism	Descending (*not* ascending) weakness, pupillary abnormalities, and bulbar symptoms. Infant botulism is caused by colonization of the immature bowel by botulinum spores and occurs in patients younger than 1 year of age. In older patients, botulism is caused by botulinum toxin in food or wounds.
Myasthenia gravis	Fatigable weakness. Ptosis, diplopia.
Viral myositis	Muscle pain, tenderness, and weakness after a viral infection. Elevated creatine kinase.
Spinal cord pathology (transverse myelitis, spinal cord compression)	Back pain, bowel or bladder dysfunction, sensory level

► CASE 27

A 15-year-old boy presents to your office with a 1-day history of unilateral facial weakness. On exam, he is unable to fully close his right eye. He also cannot raise his right eyebrow. The nasolabial fold on the right side is less prominent compared with the left side. His extraocular movement is full bilaterally, and he has normal pupillary responses. Strength in the arms and legs is full bilaterally.

Question 27-1

Where do you localize the lesion?
A) Motor cortex.
B) Facial nerve.
C) Neuromuscular junction.
D) Facial muscles.

Discussion 27-1

The correct answer is "B." Due to bi-hemispheric innervation of facial nerve nuclei, a lesion above the facial nerve nucleus (as in stroke) produces facial weakness below the forehead. In the case of facial nerve palsy, the entire face is weak on the affected side, including the forehead. It is therefore very important to assess the presence or absence of forehead weakness when evaluating a patient with facial weakness. (See Figures 23–8 and 23–9.)

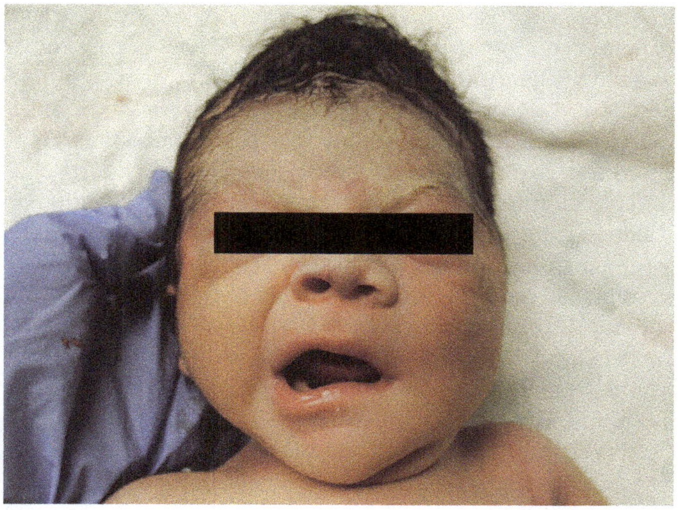

FIGURE 23–8. Left facial nerve injury in a 2-day-old infant. (Reproduced with permission from Cunningham FG, Leveno KJ, Bloom SL, et al, eds. *Williams Obstetrics.* 24th ed. New York, NY: McGraw-Hill Education; 2014, Fig. 33-3.)

When you diagnose facial nerve palsy or Bell palsy in Lyme-endemic regions, testing for Lyme disease is indicated if season is right, as Lyme disease can cause facial nerve palsy (unilateral or bilateral). Idiopathic facial nerve palsy or Bell palsy generally has a good prognosis with minimal residual deficits. However, eye care needs to be discussed to prevent corneal injury. Eye ointment, eye drops, and occasionally an eye patch are recommended. Oral steroids are often prescribed.

▶ CASE 28

A 13-year-old girl presents with an abnormal gait. She has always been a bit clumsy, often twisting her ankles, and she never learned how to ride a scooter. She quit basketball a few

years ago as she was no longer able to keep up with her peers. When she walks, her feet drop, forcing her to lift her legs higher to avoid stumbling. Her father has a similar condition and was diagnosed with hereditary motor and sensory neuropathy (Charcot-Marie-Tooth disease).

Question 28-1
Which finding do you NOT expect on her physical exam?
A) High-arched feet.
B) Decreased position and vibration sense in feet.
C) Calf hypertrophy.
D) Difficulty with heel walking.
E) Absent or depressed deep tendon reflex at Achilles.

Discussion 28-1
The correct answer is "C." Charcot-Marie-Tooth (CMT) disease is a demyelinating disorder of the peripheral nerves. Patients present with foot weakness and often have foot drop, leading to steppage gait (raising legs higher to compensate for the foot drop). Affected children are unable to walk on their heels, owing to weakness of foot dorsiflexion. High-arched feet (pes cavus) are common. Hammer toe deformity develops later. A characteristic inverted "champagne bottle" or "stork leg" appearance of legs is caused by atrophy of the muscles. There is length-dependent position and vibration sense loss beginning in the feet. Hand muscles may become weaker later in the course of the disease, leading to difficulty with fine motor skills. Option "C," calf hypertrophy, is associated with Duchenne muscular dystrophy.

▶ CASE 29

You are evaluating a term newborn boy just after delivery. The pregnancy was complicated by gestational diabetes and excessive maternal weight gain. The newborn was delivered

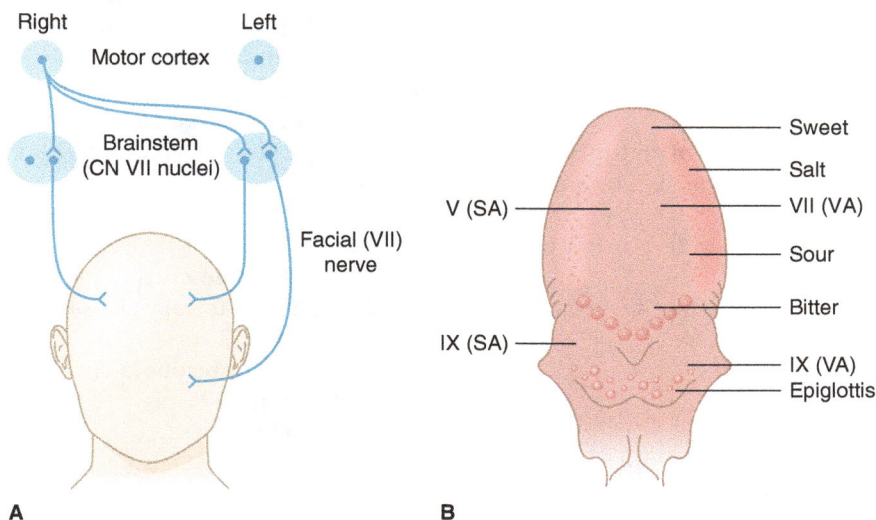

FIGURE 23–9. Facial nerve (CN VII). (A) Central and peripheral motor innervation of the face. The forehead receives motor projections from both hemispheres and the lower face (eyes and below) from the contralateral hemisphere only. (B) Somatic afferent (SA, touch) and visceral afferent (VA, taste) innervation of the tongue. (Reproduced with permission from Aminoff MJ, Greenberg DA, & Simon RP (Eds). *Clinical Neurology*, 9th ed. McGraw-Hill Education, Inc., 2015. Figure 1-17)

vaginally with vacuum assistance. His birth weight is 3900 g. On exam, he has decreased movement of his right arm. He is holding the right arm internally rotated with elbow extension and forearm pronation. Tone in the right arm is decreased. Tone in the rest of the extremities is normal. He is moving his left arm and both legs well. You also note that the right eyelid is droopy and the left pupil is larger than the right. The difference in pupil size is more apparent in the dark.

Question 29-1

Are the eye findings related to the arm weakness?

A) Yes, the eye findings are related to the arm weakness.
B) No, the eye findings are not related to the arm weakness.
C) Unsure. (You haven't a clue but you have a 50-50 shot of guessing correctly.)

Discussion 29-1

The correct answer is "A." The patient has Erb palsy, which is a type of brachial plexus injury. The brachial plexus is formed by nerve roots arising from C5 through T1. Superior trunk or C5 and C6 nerve roots are involved in Erb palsy, which is the most common type of obstetric brachial plexus injury. When the oculosympathetic pathway, which travels through the spinal cord, is also damaged, it causes ipsilateral Horner syndrome (ptosis, miosis, and anhidrosis). (See Figure 23–10.) A physical therapist, neurologist, orthopedic surgeon, or neurosurgeon may be involved in the care. Most patients with Erb palsy have a good prognosis. However, if no or minimal improvement is noted during the first 3 months or so, surgical intervention may be considered.

▶ CASE 30

An 11-year-old girl has experienced ptosis and diplopia for the past 3 weeks. Her symptoms worsen during the course of the day, and ptosis worsens with sustained upward gaze. The acetylcholine receptor antibody is positive, and you make a diagnosis of myasthenia gravis.

Question 30-1

What is the pathophysiologic mechanism of myasthenia gravis?

A) Acetylcholine release into the neuromuscular junction is blocked.
B) Autoantibodies bind to acetylcholine receptors, leading to lysis of the acetylcholine receptors.
C) Mutations occur in acetylcholine receptor subunits.
D) Acetylcholinesterase activity is decreased.
E) None of the above.

Discussion 30-1

The correct answer is "B." Myasthenia gravis is the most common disorder of neuromuscular transmission. It is an autoimmune process in which antibodies binding to acetylcholine receptors lead to lysis of the acetylcholine receptors. Most patients present with ocular symptoms such as ptosis and diplopia (ocular

myasthenia gravis). Other muscles can also be involved, and patients can progress to generalized myasthenia gravis. Bulbar weakness (dysarthria, dysphasia), masticatory weakness (jaw fatigue, jaw closure weakness), respiratory weakness, and axial/limb weakness need to be monitored. The edrophonium (Tensilon) test, electrophysiologic studies, and a positive acetylcholine receptor antibody test aid the diagnosis. Edrophonium is a short-acting acetylcholinesterase inhibitor and improves the symptoms transiently. The classic electrophysiologic finding is decremental response of the compound muscle action potential with repetitive stimulation of a motor nerve. Treatment involves pyridostigmine (Mestinon), which is an anticholinesterase. Immunosuppressive agents such as prednisone, cyclosporine, azathioprine, and mycophenolate mofetil are also used. Plasmapheresis and IVIG are usually reserved for myasthenic crisis or acute worsening. The mechanism listed in option "A" occurs in botulism, as the toxin blocks the calcium-dependent release of acetylcholine. Children with infantile botulism present with constipation, hypotonia, poor feeding, and weak cry. The paralysis in botulism is descending, whereas that in Guillain-Barré syndrome is ascending. Congenital myasthenic syndromes are a group of disorders caused by genetic defects of the neuromuscular junction (presynaptic defects, synaptic defects, postsynaptic defects). Acetylcholine receptor subunit mutation (option "C") is one of the examples of congenital myasthenia syndrome due to postsynaptic defect. Decreased acetylcholinesterase activity (option "D") is the goal of treatment, not the underlying pathophysiology, of myasthenia.

▶ CASE 31

A 4-year-old boy is brought for evaluation because of gait concerns. Gestational and birth histories were unremarkable, and he started walking at 18 months. However, recently he began having difficulty going up the stairs, and now he has to pull himself up holding onto the hand-rails. He is slightly behind his peers in terms of learning. He has not had any recent illnesses. There is no pertinent family history. On exam, you note hypotonia and enlarged calf muscles. When he runs, a waddling gait is apparent. When he stands up from the floor, he places his hands on his knees and then his thighs to stand up.

Question 31-1

What would you do next?

A) Start physical therapy and see how he improves. Follow up in 6 months.
B) Check serum creatine kinase (CK).
C) Order a muscle biopsy.
D) Obtain a brain MRI.
E) Order genetic testing.

Discussion 31-1

The correct answer is "B." Muscular dystrophies are a group of progressive myopathies characterized by muscle weakness. The

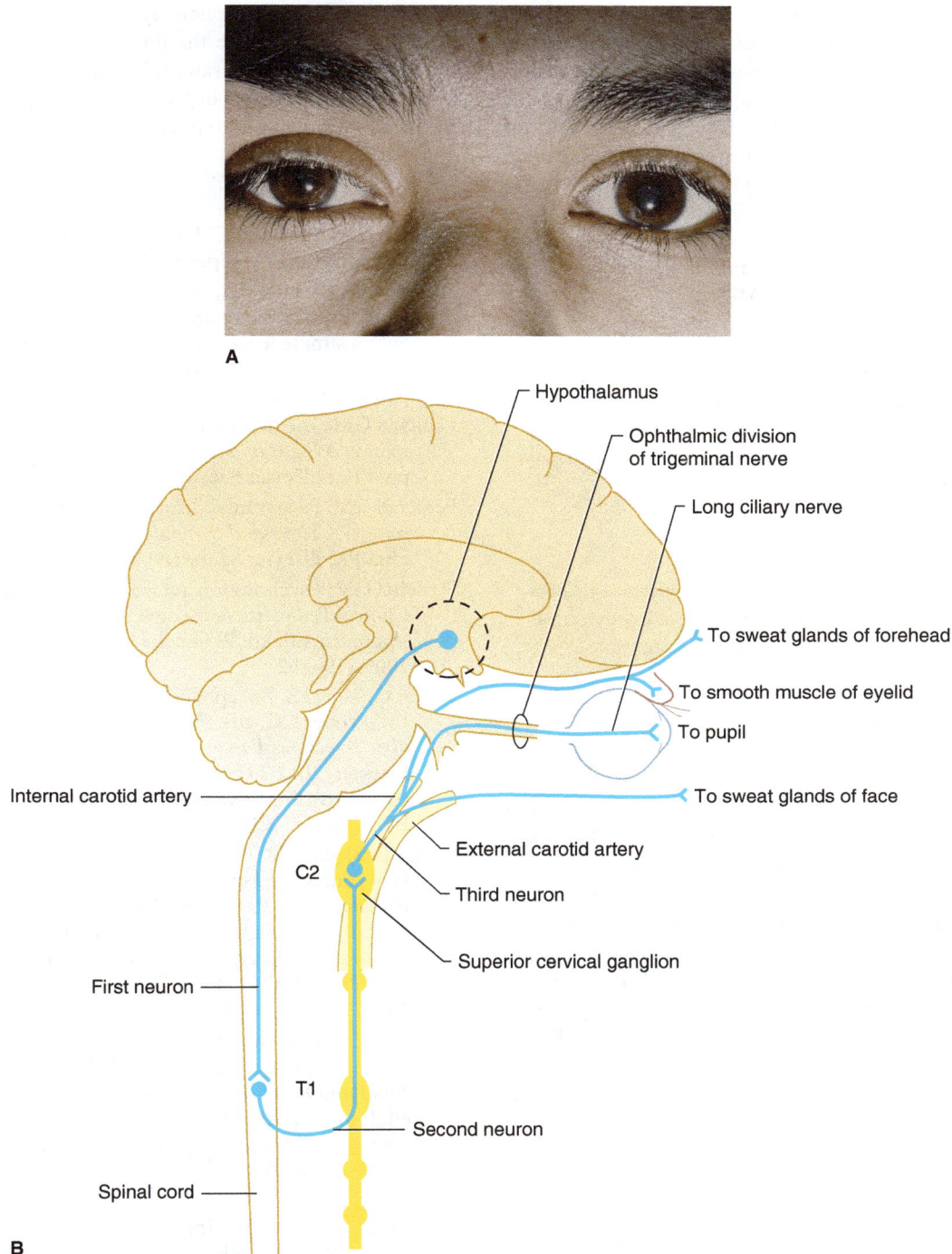

FIGURE 23–10. Oculosympathetic pathway affected in Horner syndrome. Injury to these pathways causes ptosis, miosis, and anhydrosis to the ipsilateral face. (Reproduced with permission from Aminoff MJ, Greenberg DA, Simon RP, eds. *Clinical Neurology.* 9th ed. New York, NY: McGraw-Hill Education; 2015, Fig. 7-10.)

boy's presentation is typical of Duchenne muscular dystrophy (DMD). Patients may have mild developmental delays in the first few years of life. Delayed walking is often seen. Proximal leg weakness usually becomes apparent by 3 years of age. Typically the child has difficulty rising from the floor and negotiating stairs. Additional features such as waddling gait, Gower sign (walking the hands up the legs when standing up from

the floor), calf pseudohypertrophy, and lumber lordosis also appear. Patients often become wheelchair bound in early teenage years. Kyphoscoliosis and cardiomyopathy are later problems. DMD is an X-linked recessive disorder, affecting about 1 in 3500 live male births. It is caused by a mutation in the dystrophin gene on chromosome Xp21. Dystrophin is a critical protein in muscle. Serum CK is very elevated in patients with

DMD due to muscle fiber degeneration. When a mother is a carrier, there is 50% chance of transmitting the dystrophin mutation in each pregnancy. Sons who inherit the abnormal gene will be affected, and daughters who inherit the abnormal gene will be carriers. Therefore, it is important for the parents to be counseled about future pregnancies. Becker muscular dystrophy (BMD) is caused by the same mutation as DMD and is also inherited as an X-linked recessive disorder. Compared to DMD, BMD has a later age of onset and milder symptoms including being able to ambulate for longer. Cardiac involvement is present, as in DMD.

> **Helpful Tip**
> Creatine kinase (CK) is a relatively inexpensive test, and you should consider checking CK when evaluating a boy with developmental delay, weakness, or gait abnormalities to screen for DMD.

> **Helpful Tip**
> Muscle pathology causes proximal muscle weakness (struggle going down stairs). Nerve pathology causes distal muscle weakness (struggle going up stairs).

► CASE 32

A 13-year-old boy is urgently referred to your clinic. He is always sleepy and has a hard time getting up in the morning. If his parents allowed, he would easily sleep all day. He still will take naps after school and on weekends. He sometimes yells out just as he is falling asleep. When his mother checks on him, he is fast asleep. Recently at school, his friend made a sarcastic comment about a teacher. The adolescent started laughing then abruptly fell to the floor. He felt that his legs "gave out." He did not lose consciousness. Shortly after, he was able to stand up and was fine. This has happened two more times, prompting a referral. His exam is entirely normal.

Question 32-1
Which is NOT a symptom of his condition?
A) Daytime sleepiness.
B) Insomnia.
C) Hallucinations.
D) Drop attacks.
E) Sleep paralysis.

Discussion 32-1
The correct answer is "B." Narcolepsy is a chronic disorder. Excessive daytime sleepiness (sleeping for prolonged periods, difficulty waking up, daytime naps in older children) must be present and is typically the first sign. Hallucinations occur as the child is starting to wake (hypnopompic) or fall asleep (hypnagogic). Cataplexy (drop attacks) is an abrupt loss of bilateral

muscle tone, often triggered by strong emotion, which may cause the child to fall to the floor. The other cardinal feature of narcolepsy is sleep paralysis. Treatment includes good sleep hygiene, avoiding CNS depressants, taking power naps, and medication (modafinil) to treat daytime sleepiness.

BIBLIOGRAPHY

Barkovich AJ, Raybaud C. *Pediatric Neuroimaging*. Philadelphia, PA: Lippincott Williams and Willkins; 2012.

Duffner PK, Berman PH, Baumann RJ, et al. Febrile seizures: Guideline for the neurodiagnostic evaluation of the child with a simple febrile seizure. Subcommittee on Febrile Seizures. *Pediatrics*. 2011;127(2):389–394. doi: 10.1542/peds.2010-3318.

Fenichel GM. The hypotonic infant. In: *Clinical Pediatric Neurology: A Signs and Symptoms Approach*. 6th ed. Philadelphia PA: Elsevier Saunders; 2009:153–176.

Fenichel GM. Paroxysmal disorders. In: *Clinical Pediatric Neurology: A Signs and Symptoms Approach*. 6th ed. Philadelphia PA: Elsevier Saunders; 2009:1–48.

Fenichel GM. Psychomotor retardation and regression. In: *Clinical Pediatric Neurology: A Signs and Symptoms Approach*. 6th ed. Philadelphia PA: Elsevier Saunders; 2009:119–152.

Glaser C, Long SS. Encephalitis. In: Long, SS, Pickering LK, Prober CG, eds. *Principles and Practice of Pediatric Infectious Diseases*. 4th ed. Philadelphia, PA: Elsevier; 2012:297–314. https://www-clinicalkey-com.proxy.lib.uiowa.edu/#!/content/book/3-s2.0-B9781437727029000441. Accessed April 28, 2015.

Glaser C, Strober JB. Para- and postinfectious neurologic syndromes. In: Long SS, Pickering LK, Prober CG, eds. *Principles and Practice of Pediatric Infectious Diseases*. 4th ed. Philadelphia, PA: Elsevier; 2012:314–319. https://www-clinicalkey-com.proxy.lib.uiowa.edu/#!/content/book/3-s2.0-B9781437727029000453. Accessed April 28, 2015.

Harrison CJ. Focal suppurative infections of the nervous system. In: Long SS, Pickering LK, Prober CG, eds. *Principles and Practice of Pediatric Infectious Diseases*. 4th ed. Philadelphia, PA: Elsevier; 2012:319–330. https://www-clinicalkey-com.proxy.lib.uiowa.edu/#!/content/book/3-s2.0-B9781437727029000465. Accessed April 28, 2015.

Hershey AD. Headaches. In: Kliegman RM, Stanton BF, St Geme JW, Schor NF, Behrman RE, eds. *Nelson Textbook of Pediatrics*. 19th ed. Philadelphia, PA: Saunders; 2011:2039–2046. https://www.clinicalkey.com/#!/content/book/3-s2.0-B9781437707557005881. Accessed January 24, 2015.

Hirtz D, Ashwal S, Berg A, et al Practice parameter: Evaluating a first nonfebrile seizure in children: Report of the quality standards subcommittee of the American Academy of Neurology, the Child Neurology Society, and the American Epilepsy Society. *Neurology*. 2000;55:616–623.

IHS Classification: International Classification of Headache Disorders (ICHD)–2. International Headache Society website. http://ihs-classification.org/en/. Accessed January 24, 2015.

Lewis, DW. Headaches in infants and children. In: Swaiman K, Ashwal S, Ferriero DM, Schor NF, eds. *Swaiman's Pediatric Neurology: Principles and Practice.* 5th ed. Edinburgh, Scotland: Elsevier Saunders; 2012:880–899. https://www.clinicalkey.com/#!/content/book/3-s2.0-B9781437704358000639. Accessed January 24, 2015.

Liptak GS, Dosa NP: Myelomeningocele. *Pediatr Rev.* 2010;31(11):443–450.

Mann K, Jackson MA: Meningitis. *Pediatr Rev.* 2008;29(12):417–430.

Marcdante KJ, Kliegman RM. Altered mental status. In: Marcdante KJ, Kliegman RM, eds. *Nelson Essentials of Pediatrics.* 7th ed. Philadelphia, PA: Elsevier Saunders; 2015:634–642. https://www.clinicalkey.com/#!/content/book/3-s2.0-B9781455759804001843. Accessed May 30, 2015.

Mink JW, Zinner SH: Movement disorders II: Chorea, dystonia, myoclonus, and tremor. *Pediatr Rev.* 2010;31(7):287–295.

Mix AC, Romero JR. Central nervous system infections. In: Zaoutis LB, Chiang VW, eds. *Comprehensive Pediatric Hospital Medicine.* Philadelphia, PA: Elsevier; 2007:340–351.

O'Donnell KA, Ewald, MB. Poisoning. In: Kliegman RM, Stanton BF, St Geme JW, Schor NF, Berman RE, eds. *Nelson Textbook of Pediatrics.* 19th ed. Philadelphia, PA: Elsevier; 2011:250–270. Accessed May 30, 2015. https://www.clinicalkey.com/#!/content/book/3-s2.0-B9781437707557000580

Ogle JW, Anderson MS. Infections: Bacterial & spirochetal. In: Hay WW Jr, Levin MJ, Deterding RR, Abzug MJ, eds. *Current Diagnosis & Treatment: Pediatrics.* 22nd ed. New York, NY: McGraw-Hill; 2013. http://accessmedicine.

mhmedical.com/content.aspx?bookid=1016&Sectionid=61607535. Accessed May 30, 2015.

Peredo DE, Hannibal MC. The floppy infant: Evaluation of hypotonia. *Pediatr Rev.* 2009;30;e66. doi: 10.1542/pir.30-9-e66.

Plosa EJ, Esbenshade JC, Fuller MP, Weitkamp JH: Cytomegalovirus infection. *Pediatr Rev.* 2012;33(4):156–163.

Roos KL, Brosch JR. Meningitis and encephalitis. In: McKean SC, Ross JJ, Dressler DD, Brotman DJ, Ginsberg JS, eds. *Principles and Practice of Hospital Medicine.* New York, NY: McGraw-Hill; 2012. http://accessmedicine.mhmedical.com/content.aspx?bookid=496&Sectionid=41304186. Accessed May 30, 2015.

Rosen BA: Guillain-Barré syndrome. *Pediatr Rev.* 2012;33(4):164–171.

Schunk JE, Schutzman SA: Pediatric head injury. *Pediatr Rev.* 2012;33(9):398–411.

Shinnar S, Berg AT, Moshe SL, et al. The risk of seizure recurrence after a first unprovoked afebrile seizure in childhood: An extended follow-up. *Pediatrics.* 1996;98(2 pt 1):216–225.

Singer HS, Mink JW, Gilbert DL, Jankovic J. *Movement Disorders in Childhood.* Philadelphia, PA: Saunders Elsevier; 2010.

Stephan M, Carter C, Ashfaq S. Pediatric emergencies. In: Stone C, Humphries RL, eds. *Current Diagnosis & Treatment Emergency Medicine.* 7th ed. New York, NY: McGraw-Hill; 2011. http://accessmedicine.mhmedical.com/content.aspx?bookid=385&Sectionid=40357266. Accessed April 16, 2015.

Swaiman KF, Ashwal S, Ferriero DM, Schor NF, eds. *Swaiman's Pediatric Neurology.* Philadelphia, PA: Elsevier Saunders; 2012.

Tsao CY: Muscle disease. *Pediatr Rev.* 2014;35(2):49–61.

Nutrition

24

Kelly E. Wood

▶ CASE 1

While eating a snack you start reading the nutritional label. You note the total calories listed and start thinking about daily nutritional needs.

Question 1-1
Which factor is NOT used to calculate daily energy needs?
A) Health conditions.
B) Age.
C) Activity level.
D) Height.
E) Gender.

Discussion 1-1
The correct answer is "A." The estimated energy requirement is the estimated daily calorie needs for both baseline metabolism and growth. The complicated equation is based on age, gender, height, weight, and physical activity of healthy children. It will not account for the increased needs seen with acute and chronic illnesses. Calorie and nutrition needs relative to body size are greatest in infancy when rapid growth and brain development are occurring. Birth weight triples during the first year of life. After infancy, the stages of childhood followed by puberty have the next highest energy needs per body size.

You look at the fat content. You wonder what this means for different age groups.

Question 1-2
Which of the following statements is true?
A) Dietary fat requirements are greatest in adolescence.
B) Total fat intake should not exceed 25% of daily calories.
C) Fat is not needed for absorption of vitamin D.
D) Fat is the main energy source for infants.
E) Trans fats decrease the risk of heart disease.

Discussion 1-2
The correct answer is "D." Fat (lipid) is broken down by lipase (pancreatic enzyme), combined with bile and fat-soluble vitamins, absorbed in the jejunum, and enters the lymphatic system for transport to the blood. Any disruption of this process will cause malabsorption with steatorrhea. Newborns have decreased ability to absorb fat due to low pancreatic lipase and bile acid activity. Fat is the most calorie dense nutrient. The majority of dietary fat is triglycerides. The high calorie requirements of infants to support growth and brain development are met by having a diet high in fat; 50% of infant calories come from fat. Vitamin D is a fat-soluble vitamin. Saturated and trans fatty acids increase low-density lipoprotein (LDL) cholesterol and the risk of coronary heart disease.

The label lists the total grams of carbohydrates and protein. The front wrapper boldly proclaims "no added sugars."

Question 1-3
Which of the following is false?
A) Added sugars should be less than 25% of daily calories.
B) Glucose is the primary energy source for the brain.
C) Fiber is a digestible protein.
D) Protein should make up 10% to 35% of daily calories.
E) Protein intake is limited in some inborn errors of metabolism.

Discussion 1-3
The correct answer is "C." Carbohydrates supply the body with glucose especially the central nervous system, which is the largest utilizer of glucose for energy. Digestive enzymes (amylase and disaccharidases) break down carbohydrates into monosaccharides for absorption in the small intestine. Amylase is produced in the saliva and pancreas. Disaccharidases, such as lactase, are brush border enzymes found in the small intestine villi epithelium. Newborns are born with decreased amylase and lactase, which can cause asymptomatic lactose malabsorption. Carbohydrates are the main energy source of children

and adolescents. Carbohydrates should constitute 45% to 65% of daily caloric intake. Sugars, such as fructose in high-fructose corn syrup, are frequently added to beverages to improve the taste. Intake of added sugars is linked to obesity, diabetes, and cavities. Fiber is a nondigestible carbohydrate important to prevent constipation and overeating. Protein is needed for every cell in the body, and intake must meet amino acid needs. If intake is inadequate, muscle is broken down to meet the body's needs. In certain hypermetabolic states, such as burns, protein intake should be increased but in general increased intake is not needed. Intake of protein or specific amino acids may need to be limited in gout, renal disease, and certain inborn errors of metabolism.

▶ CASE 2

You are caring for a premature infant in the neonatal intensive care unit. She is "feeding and growing." With her current feedings, her weight gain and growth velocity are on target. The mother asks why you are adding fortifier to her breast milk.

Question 2-1

Which of the following is true?
A) Premature infants have increased nutritional needs.
B) Iron stores are built up during the second trimester.
C) Unfortified breast milk provides adequate protein.
D) Fortification increases the risk of necrotizing enterocolitis.
E) Fortifier is added to thicken the milk.

Discussion 2-1

The correct answer is "A." Nutrition is important for brain development in premature infants. The third trimester is important for building fat, glycogen, protein, vitamin, and mineral stores. To build up missing stores and grow, premature infants have high nutrient needs especially protein, iron, calcium, and phosphorus. Breast milk is fortified to meet the preterm infant's nutritional needs especially protein. Adding human milk fortifier increases the calories, protein, vitamin, iron, calcium, and phosphorus content. Fortification meets the infant's nutritional needs while providing the benefits of human milk (decrease necrotizing enterocolitis, late-onset sepsis).

▶ CASE 3

While visiting a developing country, you meet a young toddler. His face is full and he has a pot belly. His hair is brittle with depigmented areas. A reddish weeping rash is present on his legs and groin. Pitting edema of his feet, legs, and periorbital areas is present.

Question 3-1

He is at risk of which of the following?
A) Death.
B) Sepsis.

C) Dehydration.
D) Zinc deficiency.
E) All of the above.

Discussion 3-1

The correct answer is "E." This toddler has kwashiorkor. Marasmus and kwashiorkor are two types of severe protein energy malnutrition. Features of both may be present in the same child. Marasmus is associated with total calorie deficiency with loss of fat stores and muscle wasting. Affected infants and children appear emaciated, tired, and apathetic. Their skin and hair is thin. Bradycardia, hypotension, and hypothermia may be present. The buttocks and extremities are shrunken with minimal muscle mass. The skin hangs due to loss of subcutaneous fat. (See Figures 24–1 through 24–3.) Kwashiorkor is associated with energy and protein deficiency but the full pathophysiology is not understood. Edema (anasarca) is the defining characteristic. In contrast to marasmus, fat stores are relatively preserved and height and weight are normal or near normal for age. A weeping, scaly, reddish-brown rash; brittle hypopigmented hair; and irritability may be present. Children with severe malnutrition are at increased risk for infection including sepsis, pneumonia, and diarrhea. Death is frequently due to an overwhelming infection. Dehydration may result from acute or chronic diarrhea. Nutrient deficiencies including zinc are very common.

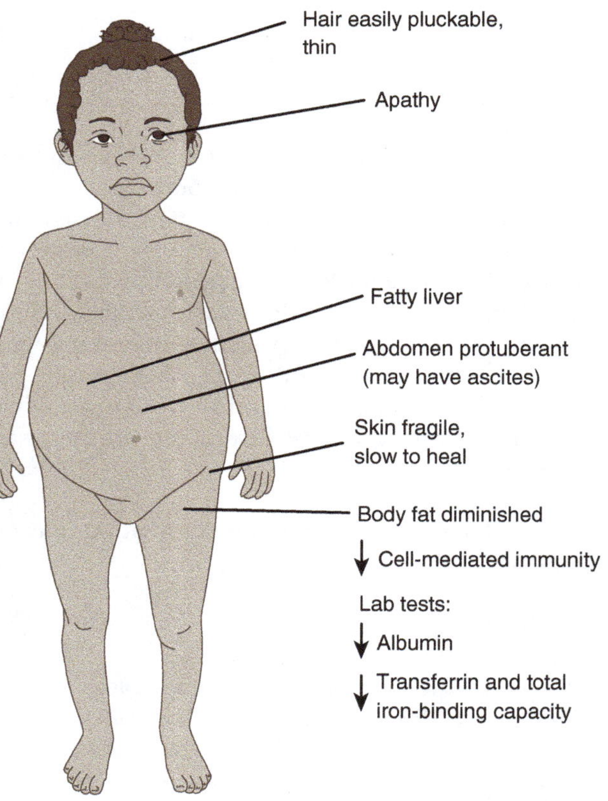

Hair easily pluckable, thin

Apathy

Fatty liver

Abdomen protuberant (may have ascites)

Skin fragile, slow to heal

Body fat diminished

↓ Cell-mediated immunity

Lab tests:

↓ Albumin

↓ Transferrin and total iron-binding capacity

FIGURE 24–1. Kwashiorkor. Manifestations of kwashiorkor. (Reproduced with permission from Murray RK, Bender DA, Botham KM, Kennelly PJ, Rodwell VW, Weil PA, eds. *Harper's Illustrated Biochemistry.* 29th ed. New York, NY: McGraw-Hill Education; 2012, Fig. 57-17.)

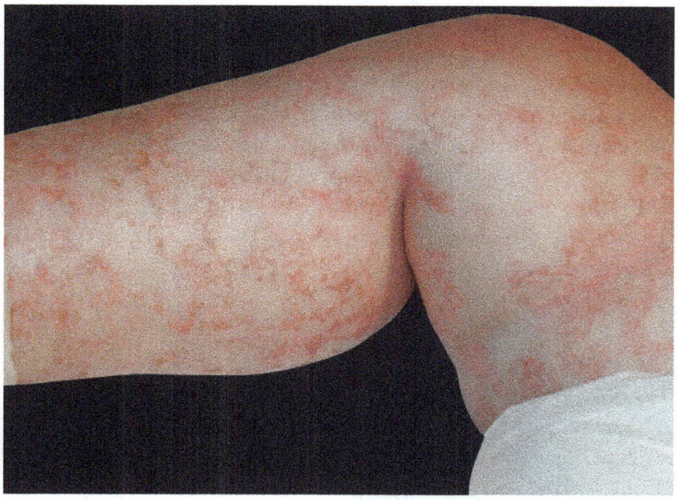

FIGURE 24–2. Kwashiorkor Dermatitis. A "flaky paint" or "crazy pavement" dermatitis is seen in children with kwashiorkor. (Reproduced with permission from Goldsmith LA, Katz SI, Gilchrest BA, Paller AS, Leffell DJ, Wolff K, eds. *Fitzpatrick's Dermatology in General Medicine.* 8th ed. New York, NY: McGraw-Hill Education; 2012, Fig. 130-3.)

⧗ QUICK QUIZ

The defining characteristic of kwashiorkor is:

A) Hanging skin.
B) Edema.
C) Diarrhea.

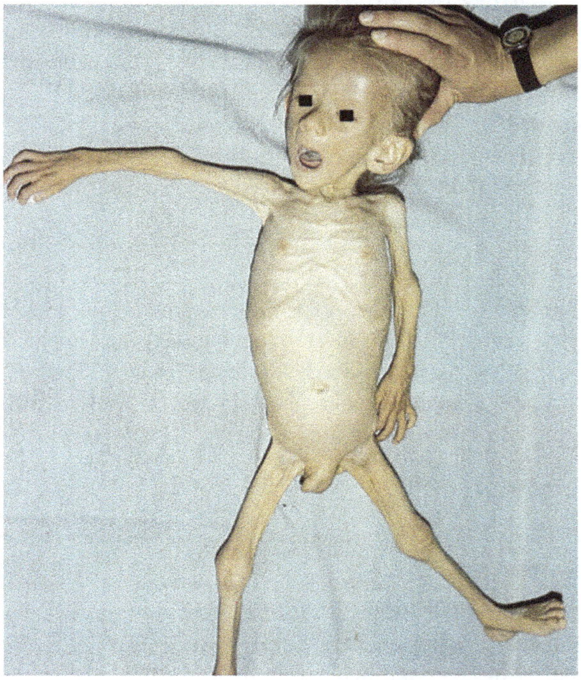

FIGURE 24–3. Marasmus. A child with extreme marasmus with atrophied arms, loose skin, and no subcutaneous fat. (Reproduced with permission from Goldsmith LA, Katz SI, Gilchrest BA, Paller AS, Leffell DJ, Wolff K, eds. *Fitzpatrick's Dermatology in General Medicine.* 8th ed. New York, NY: McGraw-Hill Education; 2012, Fig. 130-1.)

D) Hair loss.
E) None of the above.

Discussion
The correct answer is "B."

► CASE 4

While in the newborn nursery, you talk with a new mother who is breastfeeding. She is exhausted and considering changing to formula feeding for her newborn. She asks if formula is the same as human milk.

Question 4-1
Which of the following statements is true?
A) Human milk contains more casein than whey protein.
B) Cow's milk formula is lactose free.
C) Both provide 100% of daily vitamin D requirements.
D) Gastric emptying is faster for newborns fed human milk.
E) Carbohydrates make up the majority of calories.

Discussion 4-1
The correct answer is "D." The American Academy of Pediatrics (AAP) recommends exclusive breastfeeding for the first 6 months of life with continuation for 1 year or longer. Formula has 50% more protein than human milk. The primary protein in human milk is whey (70%) whereas casein (80%) predominates in cow's milk formulas. Whey protein is easier to digest and promotes faster gastric emptying. The majority of calories in both come from fat. Human milk contains lipase, which increases fat absorption. Lactose is the primary carbohydrate found in human and cow's milk formula. Human milk is deficient in vitamin D, and sun exposure is limited in infants; therefore, breast-fed infants should be supplemented with 400 IU of vitamin D daily to prevent rickets. The vitamin K content of human milk is low. All newborns, especially those who are breastfed, should receive a single intramuscular injection of vitamin K after birth. The iron content of human milk is low but better absorbed and should be adequate for the first 6 months of life.

Question 4-2
Which is an absolute contraindication to breastfeeding?
A) Galactosemia.
B) Active maternal tuberculosis infection.
C) Herpes simplex virus breast lesions.
D) Maternal substance abuse.
E) All of the above.

Discussion 4-2
The correct answer is "E." Galactosemia is a congenital disorder of impaired metabolism of galactose. Galactose and glucose make up the disaccharide lactose. Human and bovine milk naturally contain lactose. Infants with galactosemia require soy formula and lifelong avoidance of lactose. Tuberculosis is transmitted by respiratory droplets to those in close contact.

Breastfeeding should be avoided to minimize close contact between the mother and infant. Herpes simplex virus infections can be deadly in young infants, especially newborns. Direct contact with the lesions may transmit the infection from the mother to the infant. Mothers infected with human immunodeficiency virus (HIV) or human T-cell lymphotropic virus should not breastfeed. Both viruses are transmitted through breast milk. Some medications, drugs, and alcohol are transmitted in breast milk. Before starting any medication, it is important to ensure it is safe to take while breastfeeding. Mothers who abuse drugs should not breastfeed. Amphetamines, cocaine, tetrahydrocannabinol (THC), and phencyclidine (PCP) are passed through breast milk and can adversely affect the infant.

> **Helpful Tip**
>
> Breast milk contains immunologic proteins, including secretory IgA and lactoferrin. IgA is important for mucosal immunity, helping to protect against diarrheal and respiratory illnesses. (See Table 24–1.)

TABLE 24–1 BREASTFEEDING PROTECTS AGAINST THESE CONDITIONS

Infections

Otitis media

Respiratory infections

Diarrhea and gastrointestinal infections

Chronic Conditions

Inflammatory bowel disease

Diabetes mellitus type 1

Asthma

Eczema

Malignancy

Leukemia

Lymphoma

Prematurity

Necrotizing enterocolitis

Sepsis

Nutrition and Gastrointestinal Conditions

Obesity

Other

Sudden infant death syndrome (SIDS)

Data from Kleinman RE, Committee on Nutrition, eds. *Pediatric Nutrition Handbook*. 6th ed. Elk Grove Village, IL: American Academy of Pediatrics; 2009; and Section on Breastfeeding. Breastfeeding and the use of human milk. *Pediatrics*. 2012;129(3):e827–841.

▶ CASE 5

You are seeing an infant girl for her 4-month well-child check. She was recently switched from breast milk to formula. Her father is worried she is constipated. Her stools are soft, non-bloody, and brown but she does not poop every day. She does not strain or act in pain when passing a bowel movement. As a newborn, she passed meconium on the first day of life. She is having 8 wet diapers per day. She is growing well. On exam, she is happy and healthy. He is very worried.

Question 5-1

What do you tell him?

A) She is constipated. Use glycerin suppositories.

B) She has cow's milk protein intolerance. Switch to a protein hydrolyzed formula.

C) She is dehydrated. Give her two ounces of water every day.

D) She may have Hirschsprung disease. You will refer her to a gastroenterologist.

E) She is normal. Now let's talk about vaccines.

Discussion 5-1

The correct answer is "E." Constipation is more common in formula-fed infants, but she is not constipated. Her stools are soft and effortless to pass. Formula-fed infants stool less frequently than breastfed infants. Formula-fed infants have formed, brown stools in contrast to the semiliquid, seedy, yellow stools of breastfed infants. Glycerin suppositories are safe to use in this age group but she does not need medical treatment. Cow's milk protein intolerance may present as failure to thrive, bloody stools, diarrhea, or constipation. Your patient is fat, healthy, and growing. Infants do not need water or juice. Formula or human milk will meet their fluid needs. Infants have 8 to 10 wet diapers per day. Fewer than this may suggest dehydration. Other signs of dehydration would be weight loss, tachycardia, sunken fontanelle, dry lips, and poor capillary refill. Hirschsprung disease is unlikely without a history of delayed passage of meconium.

> **Helpful Tip**
>
> Breastfed infants eat 8 to 12 times per day. Formula-fed infants eat less frequently, usually every 3 to 4 hours for 6 to 8 feedings per day. Increased feeding frequency is the result of faster gastric emptying of breast milk than formula and not due to insufficient maternal milk supply.

▶ CASE 6

A 6-week-old male infant is brought to the emergency department for evaluation of bright red blood in his stool. He has no history of fever, vomiting, diarrhea, rash, bruising, or lethargy. He received an intramuscular injection of vitamin K after birth. He is formula fed and has been growing well. The family noticed the bright red blood tonight in his stool when changing his diaper. On exam, he is alert, well-nourished and healthy. His abdomen is soft with good bowel sounds. His anus has no lesions or fissures. An abdominal X-ray is normal.

Question 6-1

What is best first action to take?
A) Check coagulation studies.
B) Obtain a thorough history.
C) Obtain stool cultures.
D) Obtain an abdominal ultrasound.
E) Consult surgery.

Discussion 6-1

The correct answer is "B." The infant in this case likely has allergic proctocolitis due to cow's milk protein intolerance, which can occur in formula and exclusively breastfed infants. Cow's milk is the most common food allergy of infants and toddlers, with the highest incidence in infancy. Gastrointestinal symptoms are most common but other organ systems may be involved. (See Table 24–2.) Adverse reactions may be IgE mediated (allergy), non–IgE mediated (intolerance), or mixed. Differentiation

TABLE 24–2 COW'S MILK PROTEIN ALLERGY AND INTOLERANCE SYMPTOMS IN INFANTS AND CHILDREN

Gastrointestinal	Failure to thrive
	Gastroesophageal reflux
	Bloody stools (gross and occult)
	Diarrhea
	Constipation
	Protein-losing enteropathy
	Abdominal pain
	Food impaction
	Iron deficiency anemia
	Oral aversion or refusal to eat Vomiting
	Anorexia
Respiratory	Rhinorrhea
	Wheezing or stridor
	Chronic cough
Skin	Urticaria
	Atopic dermatitis
	Angioedema
Systemic	Anaphylaxis
	Shock-like symptoms with severe vomiting, diarrhea, and metabolic acidosis (food protein–induced enterocolitis, [FPIES])

Adapted with permission from Koletzko S, Niggemann B, Arato A, et al: Diagnostic approach and management of cow's-milk protein allergy in infants and children: ESPGHAN GI Committee practical guidelines, *J Pediatr Gastroenterol Nutr.* 2012 Aug;55(2):221–229.

and diagnosis is difficult. Improvement on an elimination diet with subsequent return of symptoms when cow's milk protein is reintroduced confirms the diagnosis. Negative cow's milk protein IgE and skin prick testing does not rule out the diagnosis. Bloody stools can occur with a coagulopathy. The infant received vitamin K prophylaxis after birth and is formula fed. Bacterial infections can cause bloody diarrhea and would be detected by stool cultures. Infection is unlikely as the infant is well and is not having diarrhea. Intussusception can present with bloody stools but typically in an older infant or toddler. Classically infants have colicky abdominal pain, vomiting, and bloody stools described as "currant jelly."

> **Helpful Tip**
> An oral challenge of cow's milk to confirm the diagnosis of cow's milk protein intolerance may be skipped in situations that would be too risky, such as anaphylaxis, hives, wheezing, or stridor. These patients should be managed by a specialist.

You suspect cow's milk protein intolerance in this 6-week-old infant.

Question 6-2

How should the infant be managed?
A) Instruct the parents to switch to an extensively hydrolyzed formula.
B) Instruct the parents to switch to a soy formula.
C) Instruct the parents to switch to a partially hydrolyzed formula.
D) Prescribe diphenhydramine.
E) No management or treatment is necessary.

Discussion 6-2

The correct answer is "A." He should be started on an extensively hydrolyzed formula, which contains only whey or casein peptides. For severe disease or failure to improve, an amino acid–based formula is indicated. Beware—both types of formula taste bad and are costly. A soy formula is not preferable as 10% to 15% of infants with cow's milk intolerance have soy sensitivity as well. Breastfeeding mothers will need to adopt a diary-free diet. After 1 year of age, most infants can have cow's milk reintroduced into their diet. Differentiating from lactose intolerance may be difficult as most hydrolyzed and amino acid formulas are lactose free. Lactose intolerance, other than congenital lactase deficiency, typically presents at an older age and does not produce respiratory, cutaneous, or severe gastrointestinal symptoms.

> **Helpful Tip**
> Congenital lactase deficiency (primary lactase deficiency) is rare. Symptoms begin at birth with watery diarrhea after the first feeding. Infants should be changed to soy formula (lactose free).

The infant is lost to follow-up. He presents 2 months later with diarrhea. He has gained weight. On exam, he has generalized pitting edema, a full abdomen, and respiratory distress. On chest X-ray he has bilateral pleural effusions. His serum albumin level is 2 g/dL, with normal urinalysis, and coagulation studies.

Question 6-3

Which is NOT a cause of his condition?
A) Nephrotic syndrome.
B) Celiac disease.
C) Intestinal lymphangiectasia.
D) Fontan procedure.
E) Cirrhosis with portal vein thrombosis.

Discussion 6-3

The correct answer is "A." Protein-losing enteropathy (PLE) results in gastrointestinal protein loss, hypoalbuminemia, diarrhea, and anasarca. PLE is caused by intestinal mucosal damage or lymphatic system abnormalities. Severe cow's milk protein intolerance is one of many different causes. (See Table 24–3.) Other causes of hypoalbuminemia must be excluded. In PLE, stool is positive for alpha-1 antitrypsin. Hypogammaglobulinemia may be present. Lymphopenia may occur with lymphatic pathology. Functional imaging can localize the site of protein loss. Nephrotic syndrome causes hypoalbuminemia and edema due to loss of protein in the urine. Proteinuria will be present on urinalysis.

⧖ QUICK QUIZ

Which is NOT a cause of hypogammaglobulinemia?
A) Protein-losing enteropathy.
B) Malnutrition.
C) Liver failure.
D) Nephrotic syndrome.
E) Angioedema.

Discussion

The correct answer is "E."

⧖ QUICK QUIZ

Which is an indication for soy formula use?
A) Families wanting a vegetarian diet.
B) Acute gastroenteritis.
C) Prevention of atopic disease.
D) Colic.
E) Premature infant.

Discussion

The correct answer is "A." Soy formula is indicated in galactosemia, congenital lactase deficiency, and when a vegetarian diet is

TABLE 24–3 CAUSES OF PROTEIN-LOSING ENTEROPATHY (PLE)

Mucosal Injury	
Inflammation and ulcerative diseases	Crohn disease
	Ulcerative colitis
	Infections
	Malignancies
	Graft-versus-host disease
	Necrotizing enterocolitis
Nonulcerative diseases	Celiac disease
	Food induced enteropathy
	Eosinophilic gastroenteritis
	Vasculitis (SLE, HSP)
Lymphatic Abnormalities	
Congenital disease	Primary intestinal lymphangiectasia
Acquired diseases	
• Obstruction	Sarcoidosis
	Crohn disease
	Lymphoma
• Elevated lymphatic pressure *from elevated venous pressure*	Congestive heart failure
	Constrictive pericarditis
Syndromes	Noonan
	Turner
	Klippel-Trenaunay
Other	Post–Fontan procedure for congenital heart disease

HSP, Henoch-Schönlein purpura; SLE, systemic lupus erythematosus.

Adapted with permission from Braamskamp MJ, Dolman KM, Tabbers MM: Clinical practice. Protein-losing enteropathy in children, *Eur J Pediatr*. 2010 Oct;169(10):1179–1185.

preferred. Premature infants have increased osteopenia when fed soy formula. There is no proven value in the use of soy formula for the management and/or prevention of colic or atopic disease.

▶ CASE 7

A medical student is shadowing in your clinic. She asks when solid foods may be introduced into the diet of infants.

Question 7-1

Which of the following should you tell her?
A) Pureed meats are good first foods to introduce.
B) Cow's milk can be introduced before 1 year of age.
C) Exclusive breastfeeding should continue until 9 months of age.

D) Egg should not be introduced until 2 years of age to prevent development of a food allergy.

E) None of the above.

Discussion 7-1

The correct answer is "A." Complimentary feeding includes the introduction of foods or liquids other than breast milk. Timing of introduction of solid foods is a common question from caregivers. The AAP recommends exclusive breastfeeding for the first 6 months with continuation until 12 months of age. Solid foods can be introduced at 4 to 6 months of age. The infant must be developmentally ready, including good head control, and loss of the tongue-thrust reflex. One single-ingredient food should be introduced at a time, waiting 3 to 5 days to introduce another new food. Should the infant have an allergic reaction it will be easier to identify the responsible food. The AAP recommends iron-fortified infant cereals and pureed meats as good first foods as they contain ample protein, iron, and zinc. Pureed fruits or vegetables can be added next. It may take repeated exposure before a new food is accepted. Introduction of cow's milk before 1 year of age increases the risk of developing iron deficiency anemia as cow's milk is low in iron and may cause gastrointestinal blood loss in infants. Some authorities recommend delaying the introduction of certain foods (eg, egg, peanuts, soy) to prevent the development of food allergies. Data are currently lacking or conflicting to delay the introduction of such potentially allergenic foods.

> **Helpful Tip**
> Cow's milk does not meet the growing infant's nutritional needs and should not be introduced in the first year of life. Iron, zinc, vitamin E, and essential fatty acid deficiencies as well as excessive renal solute load from protein and sodium are associated with early introduction. Breastfeeding or formula feeding should continue for the first year of life.

> **Helpful Tip**
> Infants should not drink fruit juices in the first 6 months of life. For children up to age 6 years, 100% juices should be offered and limited to 4 to 6 ounces of juice per day. Children 7 to 18 years old may have 8 to 12 ounces of juice per day. Fruit drinks, sport drinks, soda, or other sugar-sweetened beverages should be discouraged.

⏳ QUICK QUIZ

Which is NOT a fat-soluble vitamin?
A) Vitamin E.
B) Vitamin K.
C) Vitamin B_1.
D) Vitamin A.
E) Vitamin D.

Discussion

The correct answer is "C." Vitamin B_1 (thiamine) is a water-soluble vitamin. Water-soluble vitamins are easily absorbed but not stored in the body, requiring ongoing intake to prevent deficiencies. With the excess excreted, the risk of toxicity is low. (See Table 24–4 and Figure 24–4.) Fat-soluble vitamins are stored in the body and need pancreatic enzymes and bile acids for absorption. (See Table 24–5.)

▶ CASE 8

A 12-year-old girl presents with diarrhea that is worse with eating. Stool fecal fat is elevated. Her growth is poor. She has clubbing and a chronic cough. She complains that her eyes burn and are dry. On exam, she has foamy, triangle-shaped infiltrates on her conjunctiva. Her funduscopic exam is normal.

Question 8-1

You suspect a vitamin deficiency, but which one?
A) Vitamin D.
B) Vitamin K.
C) Vitamin A.
D) Vitamin E.
E) Vitamin C.

Discussion 8-1

The correct answer is "C." The girl described has cystic fibrosis with fat malabsorption due to pancreatic insufficiency. Conditions associated with fat malabsorption, such as celiac disease, cystic fibrosis, biliary tract disease, and pancreatic insufficiency, result in fat-soluble vitamin (A, D, E, K) deficiencies. She has xerophthalmia (dry eyes) and Bitot spots (keratin accumulation in the conjunctiva) on exam, which is consistent with vitamin A deficiency. Vitamin A is important for proper vision and eye health. Deficiency may increase morbidity and mortality from measles. Supplementation for those deficient or living in vitamin A–deficient areas during active measles infection has been shown to decrease morbidity and mortality. Routine prophylaxis is not indicated for healthy infants and children who are well fed.

▶ CASE 9

A 3-year-old African American girl is brought to the clinic. She does not like milk and gets minimal sun exposure as the family lives on a busy street requiring adult supervision to play outside. You are worried about vitamin D deficiency.

Question 9-1

Which of the following is NOT a risk factor for vitamin D deficiency?
A) Prematurity.
B) Sunscreen (sun protection factor 30 or greater).
C) Dark pigmented skin.
D) Vegan diet.
E) Unlimited sun exposure.

TABLE 24–4 WATER-SOLUBLE VITAMINS

	Source	Deficiency	Toxicity
Vitamin B_1 (Thiamine)	Legumes Yeast Brown rice Whole grain cereal Pork	Wet beriberi: cardiomyopathy, congestive heart failure, edema Dry beriberi: peripheral neuropathy Infantile beriberi: hoarse cry, aphonia, vomiting, shock Wernicke encephalopathy: ataxia, confusion, nystagmus, ophthalmoplegia	None known
Vitamin B_2 (Riboflavin)	Meat Dairy Eggs Green vegetables Fortified cereals	Angular stomatitis (see Figure 24–4) Glossitis Seborrheic dermatitis: genital area, nose	None known
Vitamin B_3 (Niacin)	Meat Dairy Eggs Beans Fortified cereals	Pellagra: dermatitis of sun-exposed skin (dry, cracked, thickened skin), diarrhea, and dementia Cheilosis	Flushing Pruritus Hives Vomiting Elevated liver enzymes
Vitamin B_5 (Pantothenate)	Egg yolk Liver Milk Broccoli	Burning feet syndrome: distal paresthesia	None known
Vitamin B_6 (Pyridoxine)	Meats Grains Vegetables Nuts	Cheilosis Angular stomatitis Glossitis Seizures in infants Irritability Anemia	Neuropathy Photosensitivity
Vitamin B_7 (Biotin)	Egg yolks Milk Meat Vegetables	Hypotonia Dermatitis Alopecia	None known
Vitamin B_9 (folate)	Green vegetables Liver Yeast Fortified cereal/bread	Megaloblastic anemia (macrocytic) Hypersegmented neutrophils Neural tube defects	Masks vitamin B_{12} deficiency in pernicious anemia
Vitamin B_{12} (Cobalamin)	Meat Fish Dairy Eggs	Megaloblastic anemia (macrocytic) Cheilosis Peripheral neuropathy Neuropsychiatric symptoms Hypersegmented neutrophils	None known Elevated levels may be associated with malignancy, autoimmune conditions, renal failure, and liver disease

(Continued)

TABLE 24–4 WATER-SOLUBLE VITAMINS (*CONTINUED*)

	Source	Deficiency	Toxicity
Vitamin C (Ascorbic acid)	Citrus fruits	Scurvy: ecchymoses, bleeding gums, perifollicular hemorrhage	False-negative stool guaiac
	Strawberries		
	Tomatoes	Coiled "corkscrew" hairs	Diarrhea
	Potatoes	Impaired wound healing	Abdominal bloating
	Brussel sprouts	Hysteria	
	Spinach	Painful extremities	
		Diarrhea	

Data from Kleinman RE, Committee on Nutrition, eds. *Pediatric Nutrition Handbook*. 6th ed. Elk Grove Village, IL: American Academy of Pediatrics; 2009.

Discussion 9-1

The correct answer is "E." Sunlight exposure is the major source of vitamin D for children. Fortified foods such as milk or breakfast cereals are good sources of dietary vitamin D_2. Vitamin D_3 is synthesized in the skin by exposure to sunlight. Both are converted to 25-hydroxyvitamin D (25-OH-D, calcidiol) in the liver then transported to the kidney to form 1,25-dihydroxyvitamin D (1,25-OH$_2$-D, calcitriol). Calcitriol, the active form of vitamin D, increases intestinal absorption of calcium and phosphorus and renal reabsorption of calcium. Risk factors for vitamin D deficiency include prematurity, dark skin pigmentation (interferes with sunlight absorption), inadequate sun exposure, certain medications, fat malabsorption, obesity, liver and kidney disease, and inadequate dietary intake. Medications associated with vitamin D deficiency include certain anticonvulsants and antiretrovirals, glucocorticoids, and antifungals (ketoconazole). Using a sunscreen with a sun protection factor of 30 or greater decreases vitamin D production in the skin. All infants and children younger than 18 years of age should receive supplemental vitamin D per current recommendations. Supplementation should begin in the first few days of life for breastfed infants. Formula-fed term infants who consume at least 33 ounces per day do not need additional supplementation. (See Table 24–5.)

Helpful Tip
Vitamin D deficiency causes decreased bone mineralization, hypocalcemia, and hypophosphatemia, which may result in seizures, tetany, muscle weakness, rickets, or osteomalacia and increased susceptibility to infections.

When examining the toddler, you note bilateral genu varum, widening of her wrists, and frontal bossing. The mother states she noticed her child's bowlegs when the child started walking and it has been getting worse with time.

Question 9-2

What additional possible clinical features would you expect in this patient?
A) Delayed anterior fontanelle closure.
B) Rachitic rosary.
C) Craniotabes.
D) Harrison grove.
E) All of the above.

Discussion 9-2

The correct answer is "E." This toddler has nutritional rickets from inadequate vitamin D intake. Rickets results from inadequate mineralization of growing bone at the growth plate (physis). This results in pathologic enlargement of the physis and metaphysis which leads to bowing of the affected bone. Impaired mineralization in skeletally mature individuals (growth plates closed) affects the bone matrix, resulting in osteomalacia. Rickets is classified as calcipenic or

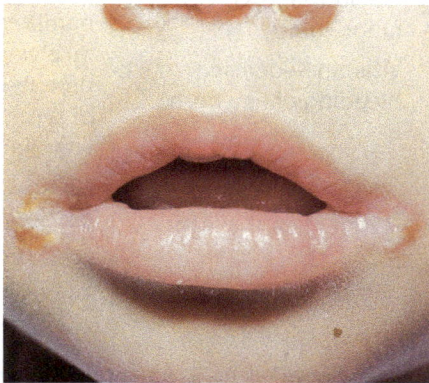

FIGURE 24–4. Angular Stomatitis. Erosions that macerate and bleed at the corners of the mouth are seen in B-complex vitamin (riboflavin and pyridoxine) deficiencies, protein energy malnutrition, and zinc deficiency. (Reproduced with permission from Goldsmith LA, Katz SI, Gilchrest BA, Paller AS, Leffell DJ, Wolff K, eds. *Fitzpatrick's Dermatology in General Medicine*. 8th ed. New York, NY: McGraw-Hill Education; 2012, Fig. 130-7.)

TABLE 24–5 FAT-SOLUBLE VITAMINS

	Source	Dietary Reference Intake	Function/ Target	Deficiency	Toxicity
Vitamin A (Retinol, retinal, retinoic acid, retinyl esters)	Animal sources: dairy, fish, liver, eggs Green/yellow vegetables (carotene): carrots, broccoli, sweet potatoes	Varies by age: 1000–3000 IU	Eye Epithelial cells	Night blindness Xerophthalmia (dryness) Bitot spots Keratomalacia Cornea damage Retinopathy Severe measles infection	Anorexia Increased intracranial pressure Liver damage Peeling skin rash Painful bone lesions Teratogen
Vitamin D (Cholecalciferol $[D_2]$, ergocalciferol $[D_3]$)	Sunlight Fatty fish Vitamin D–fortified foods, including milk	400 IU/day (infants) 600 IU/day (1–18 years of age) Goal 25-OH-D levels > 20 ng/mL	Bone Calcium regulation	Rickets (skeletally immature): craniotabes, rachitic rosary, genu varus (bow legs), splaying of wrists Osteomalacia (skeletally mature): pathologic fractures, hypocalcemia with or without tetany, hypophosphatemia	Hypercalcemia Nephrolithiasis Nephrocalcinosis Ectopic calcification Constipation Depression
Vitamin E (Tocopherols)	Oils Grains Meat Vegetables	Varies by age: 4–15 mg	Antioxidant CNS Eye Skeletal muscle	Motor and sensory neuropathy Ataxia Hemolytic anemia in premature infants Retinal degeneration	Impaired response to iron in anemia Impaired neutrophil function Sepsis in premature infants
Vitamin K (Phylloquinone $[K_1]$, menaquinone $[K_2]$, menadione $[K_3]$)	Green vegetables Oil Fruits Seeds Cow's milk Intestinal bacteria Chemical synthesis	AI: 2–2.5 mcg/day (infants) Varies by age: 30–75 mcg/day (1–18 years of age)	Coagulation: factors II, VII, IX, X, C, and S Bone mineralization	Hypoprothrombinemia Hemorrhage: GI, GU, lungs, joints, CNS Vitamin K–deficient bleeding of newborn	Hemolysis Hyperbilirubinemia in infants receiving large parenteral dose of synthetic vitamin No toxicity from oral intake

AI, adequate intake; CNS, central nervous system; GI, gastrointestinal; GU, genitourinary; IU international units.

Data from Kleinman RE, Committee on Nutrition, eds. *Pediatric Nutrition Handbook*. 6th ed. Elk Grove Village, IL: American Academy of Pediatrics; 2009.

TABLE 24–6 CLINICAL MANIFESTATIONS OF RICKETS

Skeletal	Nonskeletal
Delayed anterior fontanelle closure	Bone pain
Frontal and parietal bossing	Poor growth
Craniotabes (soft skull bones)	Hypocalcemic seizures or tetany
Widening of the wrist or ankles	Dental abnormalities
Genu varum (bowlegs): tibia bowing	Muscle weakness
Genu valgus (knock knees): femur bowing	Motor delays
Cox vera: distal radius/ulna bowing	Ambulation difficulties
Rachitic rosary: enlargement of costochondral junctions	Lethargy
Harrison sulcus groove: flaring of ribs at diaphragm level	Irritability
Pigeon breast deformity	Visceroptosis: sinking or sagging of abdominal viscera (pot belly)
Kyphoscoliosis	

Data from Nield LS, Mahajan P, Joshi A, Kamat D. Rickets: Not a disease of the past. *Am Fam Physician*. 2006;74(4):619–626.

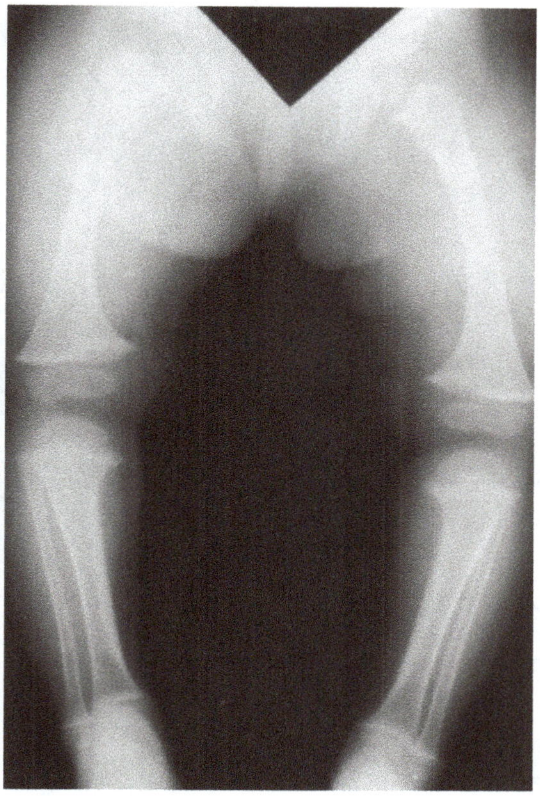

FIGURE 24–5. Genu Varum. X-rays showing bowing of the long bones (genu varum) and flared, irregular physes in a child with rickets. (Reproduced with permission from Skinner HB, McMahon PJ, eds. *Current Diagnosis & Treatment in Orthopedics*. 5th ed. New York, NY: McGraw-Hill Education; 2014, Fig. 10-3.)

phosphopenic. Phosphopenic rickets usually results from renal phosphorus wasting. Calcipenic rickets is most commonly due to insufficient intake, absorption, or metabolism of vitamin D. Initial skeletal manifestations occur at sites of rapid bone growth, including the distal forearm, knee, and costochondral junctions and are influenced by the child's age and weight-bearing patterns of limbs. Forearm changes are commonly seen in infants. Walking toddlers classically have exaggerated bowing of the legs (genu varum). (See Table 24–6 and Figure 24–5.) An anteroposterior X-ray of the knee or wrist is can be helpful to diagnosis rickets. Changes seen include widening of the distal physis, metaphyseal fraying, flaring or cupping, decreased bone density, angular deformities of the arm and leg bones, and pathologic fractures. (See Figure 24–6.)

Discussion

The correct answer is "C." In vitamin D–deficient rickets, serum vitamin D (calcidiol and calcitriol), calcium, phosphorus, and urine calcium are low. Alkaline phosphatase, parathyroid hormone, and urine phosphorus levels are increased. Alkaline phosphatase levels are a useful marker of disease activity with levels frequently exceeding 1500 IU/L.

Helpful Tip
Vitamin K exists in two natural forms: K_1 comes from dietary sources; K_2 is synthesized by gram-negative bacteria in our intestines. Broad-spectrum antibiotics may cause vitamin K deficiency from decreased synthesis of vitamin K_2.

Helpful Tip
Intramuscular vitamin K prevents life-threatening hemorrhage in newborns. Prior reports have associated intramuscular vitamin K with an increased risk of leukemia. This association has not been proven, and vitamin K prophylaxis is recommended for all newborns.

QUICK QUIZ

Which laboratory value is elevated in vitamin D–deficient rickets?
A) Vitamin D.
B) Phosphorus.
C) Alkaline phosphatase
D) Calcium.
E) Urine calcium.

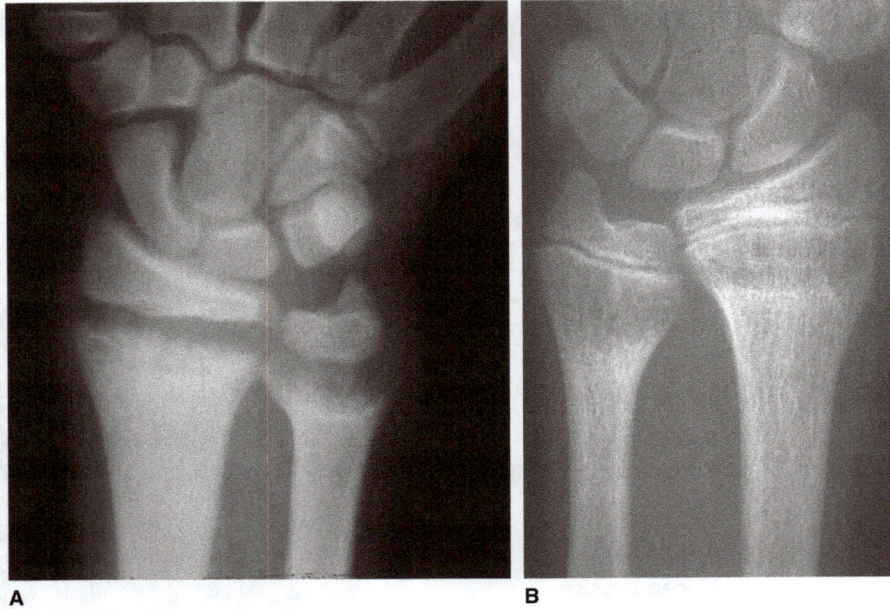

FIGURE 24–6. Metaphyseal Changes in Rickets. Widening, fraying, and cupping of the distal metaphysis of the radius and ulna in a child with rickets. (Reproduced with permission from Feldman D, Pike JW, Adams JS: *Vitamin D*. 3rd edition. London: Academic Press/Elsevier; 2011)

Helpful Tip

Remember "bones, stones, abdominal groans, and psychiatric moans" for the symptoms of hypercalcemia from vitamin D toxicity.

Bones: pain, fractures

Stones: kidney stones, polyuria

Groans: constipation, anorexia, peptic ulcers, pancreatitis

Moans: confusion, depression, dementia

QUICK QUIZ

Which water-soluble vitamin is found only in animal products (meat, dairy, eggs)?
A) Vitamin B_3 (niacin).
B) Vitamin B_{12} (cobalamin).
C) Vitamin B_9 (folate).
D) Vitamin B_1 (thiamine).
E) Vitamin B_7 (biotin).

Discussion

The correct answer is "B." Water-soluble vitamins (B complex and C) are obtained from dietary sources mostly fruits and vegetables except vitamin B_{12} (cobalamin), which is found exclusively in animal products.

► CASE 10

A 16-year-old girl presents with burning and tingling in her legs for the past few months that is getting progressively worse. She is having trouble remembering things at school. At home, she is fighting more with her parents. On exam, she is ataxic, her tongue is smooth, and she has impaired vibratory sensation. Her blood work is notable for hemoglobin of 10 g/dL, mean corpuscular volume (MCV) of 110 fL, and hypersegmented neutrophils.

Question 10-1

Which of the following is NOT a potential cause of her vitamin deficiency?
A) Vegan diet.
B) Ileum resection.
C) Ulcerative colitis.
D) Treatment with a proton pump inhibitor medication.
E) Gastritis.

Discussion 10-1

The correct answer is "C." She has vitamin B_{12} deficiency. Vitamin B_{12}, cobalamin, is a water-soluble vitamin that is important for red blood cells and the central nervous system. Animal products such as meat and eggs are the only dietary source. Dietary deficiency is rare but may occur in those following a strict vegan diet, including breastfed infants of vegan mothers. Vitamin B_{12} requires intrinsic factor (produced in the stomach) for absorption in the ileum. Gastric resection or bypass, ileum resection, Crohn disease, HIV infection, or acid-suppressing medications may impair absorption leading to deficiency. Pernicious anemia, an autoimmune condition, causes vitamin B_{12} deficiency due to a lack of intrinsic factor. Vitamin B_{12} and folate deficiency may result in a macrocytic (MCV > 100 fL) megaloblastic anemia with hypersegmented neutrophils, but only vitamin B_{12} deficiency produces neurologic symptoms. Neurologic manifestations may be irreversible even with treatment. Classically a symmetric peripheral neuropathy affecting the legs with ataxia, altered sensation, and weakness develops. Neuropsychiatric manifestations include memory loss, irritability and personality changes. Treatment consists of oral, intramuscular, or intranasal cobalamin. Ulcerative colitis is not associated with vitamin B_{12} as neither the ileum nor stomach is involved.

Question 10-2

Which of the following may be associated with folate deficiency?
A) Trimethoprim antibiotic.
B) Chronic hemolytic anemia.
C) Goat's milk.
D) Alcohol.
E) All of the above.

Discussion 10-2

The correct answer is "E." Folate and vitamin B_{12} are needed for red blood cell DNA synthesis. Deficiency of either leads to impaired erythropoiesis and megaloblastic anemia. Folate is found in animal products and leafy vegetables. Deficiency is most commonly nutritional from inadequate intake. In the United States, fortification of flour with folic acid has decreased the prevalence of folate deficiency. Goat's milk is deficient in folate. Infants should not be fed goat's milk without other dietary sources of folate. Certain conditions, such as chronic hemolytic anemia and pregnancy, have increased folate needs which if not met result in deficiency. Alcohol inhibits folate absorption and deficiency is seen in those who abuse alcohol, especially when concurrent malnutrition is present. Trimethoprim, methotrexate, and phenytoin all interfere with folate metabolism and have been associated with folate deficiency. Folate deficiency is treated with oral folic acid.

> **Helpful Tip**
> Folate deficiency during pregnancy is associated with neural tube defects. All pregnant women should receive supplemental folic acid.

▶ CASE 11

A 10-year-old boy presents with bruising that has been getting worse over the past few weeks. His bruises occur with minimal trauma. More recently his gums have been bleeding. His legs ache and he does not want to walk. He has not had fever, weight loss, or abdominal pain. On exam, he appears tired. He has swollen bleeding gingiva, multiple large ecchymosis, and a petechial rash around the hair follicles of his legs. The anterior costochondral junctions are prominent. You notice a cut on his leg that is not healing. He has no lymphadenopathy, hepatosplenomegaly, arthritis, or jaundice.

Question 11-1

Which is the most likely cause of his symptoms?
A) Malignancy.
B) Disseminated intravascular coagulation (DIC).
C) Liver failure.
D) Henoch-Schönlein purpura (HSP).
E) None of the above.

Discussion 11-1

The correct answer is "E." The boy in this vignette has scurvy from vitamin C (ascorbic acid) deficiency. On dietary history, he is picky eater. Humans do not make vitamin C but rather obtain it by eating fruits (citrus) and vegetables. In vitamin C deficiency, synthesis of the collagen walls of blood vessels is disrupted, resulting in hemorrhagic signs and symptoms (ecchymosis, purpura, gingival hemorrhage, petechiae). Bone pain from subperiosteal hemorrhage may present as pseudoparalysis. His physical exam is consistent with scurvy with perifollicular hemorrhages, signs of poor wound healing, and costochondral beading known as scorbutic rosary. (See Table 24–4 and Figures 24–7 and 24–8.) Vitamin C deficiency is treated with oral ascorbic acid. Patients with malignancy may present with thrombocytopenic bruising and bleeding as well as bone pain. The lack of fever, weight loss, lymphadenopathy, and hepatosplenomegaly is reassuring. Coagulation studies would be normal, ruling out DIC and liver failure, which may also manifest with jaundice. HSP is an IgA vasculitis that produces palpable purpura, but this boy lacks arthritis and abdominal pain. Scurvy is often mistaken for vasculitis if cutaneous findings are misinterpreted as purpura. However,

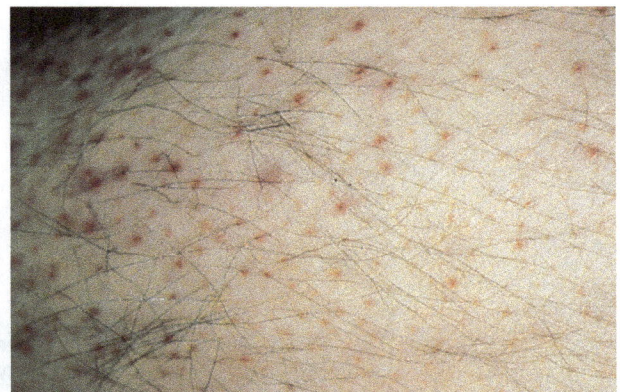

FIGURE 24–7. Scurvy. Perifollicular hemorrhage and follicular hyperkeratosis, which if prominent may be mistaken as palpable purpura associated with vasculitis. (Reproduced with permission from Kaushansky K, Lichtman MA, Prchal JT, eta al: *Williams Hematology*, 9ed. New York: McGraw-Hill Education, Inc; 2016. Figure 122-25.)

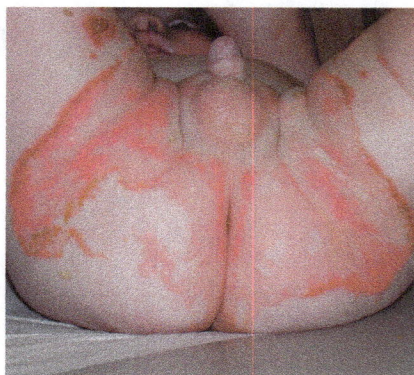

FIGURE 24–8. Corkscrew Hairs. Plugged hair follicles cause hair shafts to coil and are referred to as "corkscrew hairs." (Reproduced with permission from McKean SC, Ross JJ, Dressler DD, Brotman DJ, Ginsberg JS, eds. *Principles and Practice of Hospital Medicine*. New York, NY: McGraw-Hill Education; 2012, Fig 147-16A.)

this patient's rash, gum bleeding, and costochondral changes are not characteristic of the conditions listed.

► CASE 12

An 8-week-old male infant is brought to the clinic to evaluate a diaper rash. His growth has been poor and he has had prolonged diarrhea. His mother has tried zinc oxide cream and a topic antifungal medication without improvement. On exam, he is thin and has erythematous, well-defined, scaly plaques with bullae and erosions. The rash is on his cheeks, around his mouth, and in his diaper area.

Question 12-1

He has a deficiency of what trace mineral?
A) Fluoride.
B) Iodine.
C) Zinc.
D) Chromium.
E) Copper.

Discussion 12-1

The correct answer is "C." This infant has acrodermatitis enteropathica from zinc deficiency. Trace elements or minerals are present in low concentrations in the body but necessary for many enzymatic pathways. Zinc is needed to grow, taste and smell, heal wounds, and fight infections. Zinc is given in developing countries to prevent and treat infections such as diarrhea and pneumonia. Acrodermatitis enteropathica, a hereditary defect in zinc absorption, causes diarrhea, dermatitis, and alopecia. The eczema-like rash has red, scaling plaques that develop bullae, crusting, and erosions in a U-shaped distribution on the face, perioral, acral, and diaper areas. (See Figure 24–9.) Fluoride prevents dental caries but in excess can stain the tooth enamel (fluorosis). Iodine deficiency results in goiter and hypothyroidism. Concurrent selenium, iron, or vitamin A deficiency worsens the effects of iodine deficiency. To prevent deficiency, table salt has added iodine. Chromium is a cofactor for insulin action; deficiency causes impaired glucose tolerance. Skin and hair depigmentation, microcytic hypochromic anemia (unresponsive to iron), neutropenia, and osteoporosis occur with copper deficiency. Menkes (kinky hair) syndrome and Wilson disease are hereditary defects in copper metabolism. Deficiencies of other trace minerals can also cause significant systemic effects. Selenium deficiency causes cardiomyopathy and myositis. Tremor, seizures, arrhythmias including torsades de pointes, and hypocalcemia are seen with magnesium deficiency.

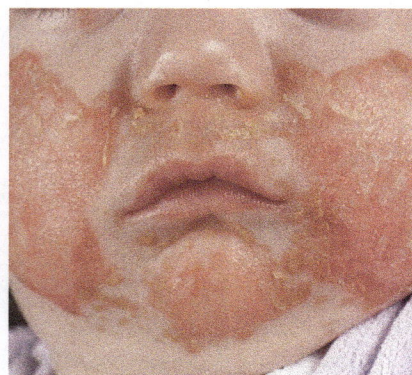

A   B

FIGURE 24–9. Acrodermatitis Enteropathica. Erythematous, well-demarcated lesions with crusting, scale, and erosions involving the anogenital and perioral areas. (Reproduced with permission from Goldsmith LA, Katz SI, Gilchrest BA, Paller AS, Leffell DJ, Wolff K, eds. *Fitzpatrick's Dermatology in General Medicine*. 8th ed. New York, NY: McGraw-Hill Education; 2012, Fig. 130-10A, B.)

A 15-month-old boy is referred for evaluation of anemia (hemoglobin 10 mg/dL). You learn the infant has been receiving cow's milk since 9 months of age.

Question 13-1

What is the best next course of action in the care of this 15-month-old?
A) Switch him to formula.
B) Start empiric treatment with iron.
C) Refer for developmental screening.
D) Dietary modification alone.
E) Repeat his blood work in 3 months.

Discussion 13-1

The correct answer is "B." Early introduction of cow's milk before 1 year of age is associated with iron deficiency. Cow's milk is deficient in iron and may cause gastrointestinal blood loss in infants. In the presence of risk factors, a presumptive diagnosis of iron deficiency anemia can be made and empiric treatment with iron without additional testing may be trialed. If the hemoglobin level has not improved within 1 month, iron studies should be obtained. Alternatively the AAP recommends obtaining confirmatory iron studies as only 40% of 1-year-olds with anemia have iron deficiency and follow-up testing is poor. Dietary modifications, including limiting cow's milk intake to 24 ounces per day and eating iron-rich foods, should be made in addition to iron supplementation.

Question 13-2

Which patient group is NOT associated with an increased risk of iron deficiency and iron deficiency anemia?
A) Premature infants.
B) Menstruating girls.
C) Breastfed infants.
D) Toddlers.
E) Postpubertal boys.

Discussion 13-2

The correct answer is "E." Iron deficiency is the most common nutritional deficiency in the United States. Premature infants are born with low iron stores as are infants with intrauterine growth restriction and those born to mothers with diabetes or anemia. Adolescent girls are at increased risk from menstrual blood loss. After 4 months of age, breastfed infants need iron supplementation to meet their growing needs. Infants who are formula fed should receive only iron-fortified formula. Toddlers who drink excessive cow's milk or are picky eaters will have insufficient iron intake. Boys are at risk during their pubertal growth spurt as demands may exceed stores.

Question 13-3

What has NOT been associated with iron deficiency?
A) Improved test scores.
B) Anemia.
C) Restless leg syndrome.
D) Lead poisoning.
E) Developmental delays.

Discussion 13-3

The correct answer is "A." Consequences of iron deficiency include anemia and possible adverse neurodevelopmental outcomes, including decreased cognition, lower test scores, and motor delays. The neurologic effects may occur before the child becomes anemic. Intestinal absorption of lead is increased, which may result in lead poisoning. Restless leg syndrome, breath-holding spells, febrile seizures, fatigue, and pica have been associated with iron deficiency.

Question 13-4

Which laboratory result is seen with iron deficiency anemia but NOT iron deficiency?
A) Decreased serum ferritin.
B) Elevated serum transferrin receptor 1 concentration.
C) Decreased reticulocyte hemoglobin concentration.
D) Decreased mean corpuscular volume.
E) Elevated red blood cell distribution width.

Discussion 13-4

The correct answer is "D." Universal hemoglobin screening is recommended at 12 month of age and for older children with iron deficiency risk factors. Hemoglobin screening detects anemia but not iron deficiency. Capillary samples should be confirmed by venous measurements to avoid false positive results. Recommended confirmatory iron testing includes serum ferritin and C-reactive protein (CRP) levels or reticulocyte hemoglobin concentration (CHr). A low serum ferritin is a sensitive marker for iron deficiency but it is an acute phase reactant with false elevation in the setting of inflammation as measured by elevation in the CRP. Reticulocyte hemoglobin (CHr) and serum transferrin receptor 1 (TfR1) concentrations are not affected by inflammation. A low CHr has been shown to be the strongest predictor of iron deficiency in children. Currently, TfR1 standards have not been developed for children. An elevated red cell distribution width (RDW) is an early marker of deficiency. (See Table 24–7.)

An 8-month-old boy is hospitalized with vomiting and diarrhea. He is rotavirus-positive. He has been rehydrated with intravenous fluids, and his vomiting has resolved. However, he continues to have diarrhea. He is drinking well and acting hungry. On rounds you are told that he is on a clear liquid diet due to ongoing diarrhea.

TABLE 24–7 LABORATORY TEST RESULTS IN IRON DEFICIENCY VERSUS IRON DEFICIENCY ANEMIA

	Iron Deficiency	Iron Deficiency Anemia
Hemoglobin	Normal	Decreased
Mean corpuscular volume (MCV)	Normal	Decreased
Mean corpuscular hemoglobin concentration (MCHC)	Normal	Decreased
Red cell distribution width (RDW)	Increased	Increased
Serum iron	Decreased	Decreased
Total iron-binding capacity (TIBC)	Increased	Increased
Ferritin	Decreased	Decreased
Transferrin saturation	Decreased	Decreased
Transferrin receptor 1 concentration (TfR1)	Increased	Increased
Reticulocyte hemoglobin concentration (CHr)	Decreased	Decreased

Data from Zimmermann MB, Hurrell RF: Nutritiona iron deficiency, *Lancet* 2007;370(9586):511–520.

Question 14-1

What do you say in response?

A) Oral intake should be delayed for 72 hours in a child with diarrhea.

B) Oral intake should be limited to clear liquids for the first 72 hours of the acute illness.

C) Oral intake should be advanced to a full liquid diet but solid foods should be delayed until the diarrhea resolves.

D) Dairy products should be avoided during an acute diarrheal illness.

E) Oral intake should be started as soon as possible with any illness.

Discussion 14-1

The correct answer is "E." Oral intake should be started as soon as the child is able. Solids should be restarted as tolerated by the child not based on an arbitrary time period. There is no medical reason to withhold food simply because this patient is still having diarrhea. The BRAT (bread, rice, applesauce, toast) diet is no longer recommended as a gateway to reintroducing solid foods after an acute gastrointestinal illness. Absorption of nutrients is decreased with acute diarrhea but not nonexistent. Prolonged periods without enteral nutrition may cause small bowel villi atrophy with subsequent diarrhea. Feeding the gut when able is always a good thing.

The boy is discharged home. Two weeks later he is brought to the clinic for evaluation as he continues to have diarrhea. He is happy, afebrile, and eating well. He is not vomiting. His diarrhea is watery without blood. He takes standard infant formula. On exam, he is a fat, afebrile, healthy infant with plenty of drool. He has regained the weight he lost from his acute illness.

Question 14-2

What is the cause of his prolonged diarrhea?

A) Secondary lactose intolerance.

B) Cow's milk protein intolerance.

C) Osmotic diarrhea from excessive juice intake.

D) *Clostridium difficile* infection.

E) Fat malabsorption.

Discussion 14-2

The correct answer is "A." Before the vaccine, rotavirus was the "winter buddy" of respiratory syncytial virus (RSV). It kept hospital beds full of infants with protracted diarrhea. This child is doing well, eating, and gaining weight. He is hydrated. Protracted diarrhea after an acute gastrointestinal illness may be due to transient lactase deficiency from injury to small bowel villi. Lactase, the enzyme that breaks down lactose, is located in the distal tips of the intestinal microvilli. This period of transient deficiency will resolve with time. Feeding the infant through it or imposing a brief period of a nonlactose formula (soy) feeding may be reasonable though unnecessary.

Question 14-3

What is NOT a cause of secondary lactose intolerance?

A) Bacterial overgrowth.

B) Celiac disease.

C) Crohn disease.

D) Giardiasis.

E) Ethnic lactose malabsorption.

Discussion 14-3

The correct answer is "E." Secondary means it is an acquired condition. You cannot acquire a new ethnicity. Lactose malabsorption is common in Asian and African Americans. They are born with decreased lactase activity. Options "B," "C," and "D" are conditions that damage the small intestinal villi in a manner similar to rotavirus. Treatment is aimed at the underlying cause while awaiting repair of the villi. Symptomatic treatments may include decreasing diary intake or substituting nondairy products (soy, almond milk).

▶ CASE 15

A 9-year-old girl with chronic kidney disease is admitted to the hospital. She is on the renal transplant list and has been admitted for insertion of a dialysis catheter. The child is thin and pale. You enter a general diet order for her. The next morning, your attending is not happy with your choice.

Question 15-1

Which is true regarding dietary restrictions and needs with renal disease?
A) Total fluid intake is never restricted.
B) Potassium requirements are increased.
C) Phosphorus requirements are increased.
D) Sodium intake may be restricted.
E) Nutrition is a minor detail.

Discussion 15-1

The correct answer is "D." Dietary restrictions, needs, and deficiencies depend on the stage of kidney disease. A child with acute renal failure is very different from one with dialysis-dependent disease. Total fluid intake may be restricted depending on glomerular function. If a patient is taking a diuretic agent, unlimited fluid intake is typically counterintuitive. Caloric and protein needs are greater in a child with kidney disease. Protein intake should not be restricted, especially for those on dialysis (associated with protein loss). Those with chronic disease are at risk for malnutrition, especially if the child has associated nausea, vomiting, or lack of appetite. Renal disease may cause hyperkalemia and hyperphosphatemia so giving extra potassium would not be a good idea. Sodium goes hand in hand with fluid retention and hypertension.

···

You begin thinking about nutritional supplements. Vitamins and minerals are good things, but which need to be supplemented in this patient? Unfortunately, a dietician is not on call at 3 AM in your hospital. You decide to try and find the answer by yourself.

Question 15-2

Which is NOT true regarding nutritional deficiencies associated with chronic renal disease?
A) Metabolism of the fat-soluble vitamins A, E, and K is impaired.
B) Bone disease (renal osteodystrophy) is common with progressive chronic kidney disease.
C) Hypovitaminosis D includes deficiencies of both 25-hydroxyvitamin D and 1,25-dihydroxyvitamin D.
D) Potassium intake may need to be restricted.
E) Phosphorus intake must be restricted.

Discussion 15-2

The correct answer is "A." Bone metabolism and mineralization is disrupted in chronic kidney disease. Secondary hyperparathyroidism develops as a result of hyperphosphatemia from renal phosphorus retention. Management includes dietary restriction or phosphate binders. Vitamin D is supplemented, with dosing dependent on the degree of deficiency. Calcium supplementation is not always needed to maintain a normal calcium level.

The kidney is the potassium-wasting machine of the body. Depending on the degree of failure, potassium may need to be restricted. Nutritional supplementation (oral, feeding tube) may be needed if a child cannot meet his or her needs. Vitamins (except vitamin D) and minerals should be supplemented if the child is not meeting 100% of the daily recommended intake (DRI). Hypervitaminosis A may develop in those with advanced kidney disease from decreased renal excretion of metabolites.

▶ CASE 16

An adolescent boy with cystic fibrosis is admitted because of an acute decline in pulmonary function. His weight is down 2 kg from 3 months ago. He has not filled any prescriptions for 2 months.

Question 16-1

Which nutritional problem is he unlikely to have related to his cystic fibrosis?
A) Vitamin D deficiency.
B) Hyponatremia.
C) Vitamin C deficiency.
D) Protein calorie deficiency.
E) Hyperglycemia.

Discussion 16-1

The correct answer is "C." Children with cystic fibrosis have increased calorie and protein needs. The exact amount depends on the severity of their lung disease. Those with pancreatic insufficiency need replacement enzyme therapy in order to absorb fat and fat-soluble vitamins. Fat-soluble vitamins (A, D, E, K) are supplemented in addition to pancreatic enzymes. Excess sodium is lost in the sweat of children with cystic fibrosis. This patient is at risk for hyponatremia if he is sweating significantly. If he has cystic fibrosis–related diabetes, he may develop hyperglycemia. Surgical feeding tubes may be needed for children unable to gain weight or who have persistent malnutrition.

▶ CASE 17

A 2-year-old girl is admitted for routine chemotherapy. She has neuroblastoma. Following procedures, you order a nutrition consult.

Question 17-1

What should you list as the reason for your consult?
A) The child does not like the patient cafeteria menu. She needs food vouchers for the visitor cafeteria.
B) All children on chemotherapy require parenteral nutrition, and you need help ordering it.
C) The child needs iron supplementation, but you are not sure if it should be given via enteral or parenteral route.
D) The child needs to have her growth measurements plotted.
E) The child is receiving high–dose chemotherapy and is at high risk for developing malnutrition. You would like to know her DRI of calories and protein.

Discussion 17-1

The correct answer is "E." The most common characteristic of cancer-associated malnutrition is anorexia. Energy needs are increased due to the metabolic demand of the cancer. Treatment may cause symptoms of anorexia, nausea, vomiting, constipation, diarrhea, altered taste, and mouth sores. Digestion and absorption may be impaired. Children may be unable to eat due to scheduled procedures and surgeries. All contribute to malnutrition in cancer patients. Children receiving high-dose or combination chemotherapy are at high risk for malnutrition and may need nutritional support. If oral intake is inadequate, enteral tube feeding or parenteral nutrition should be started. Tube feedings are the first choice. As the patient's intake improves, it is important to avoid excessive weight gain. If she is receiving frequent blood transfusions, she does not need additional iron.

▶ CASE 18

A 15-year-old boy was involved in a rollover car crash. The car ignited and he was badly burned. He is being admitted to the burn unit in critical condition.

Question 18-1

What nutritional derangements do you anticipate?
A) Lipid catabolism.
B) Protein catabolism.
C) Insensible fluid losses.
D) Electrolyte disturbances.
E) All of the above.

Discussion 18-1

The correct answer is "E." Nutritional support is important to prevent malnutrition, help heal wounds, and handle the increased energy expenditure due to the hypermetabolic state. Burns cause a hypermetabolic response characterized by increased protein catabolism, lipid catabolism, and oxygen consumption with loss of muscle mass. Burn victims may lose huge amounts of fluid from evaporative losses. Enteral support is best, preferred, and maintains the gut integrity. Enteral tube feedings may be needed. Vitamin A and C supplementation help with wound healing.

> **Helpful Tip**
> The most important nutritional intervention in an ill child is adequate protein intake. Protein needs may be 50% greater than baseline during acute illness or stress.

▶ CASE 19

A 5-year-old child with congenital heart disease and chronic heart failure presents with acute worsening of his heart failure. He is on a fluid-restricted diet and takes diuretics daily.

His mother struggles to keep him out of the refrigerator. He is constantly trying to sneak drinks. He went to a birthday party earlier in the day. When no one was watching, he drank 10 juice boxes. He is admitted and placed back on strict fluid restriction.

Question 19-1

What are common nutritional issues encountered in children with congenital heart disease?
A) Total daily caloric needs are increased in the setting of heart failure.
B) Formula may be fortified to meet calorie needs in an infant on a fluid-restricted diet.
C) Potassium supplementation may be required.
D) Fluid restriction can be challenging for children.
E) All of the above.

Discussion 19-1

The correct answer is "E." Congenital heart disease is frequently associated with chronic heart failure and increased calorie needs. In young infants, fluid intake is typically not restricted and diuretics are used to maintain a euvolemic state. Fortification of formula is frequently still needed to meet caloric needs. Children receiving diuretics that cause renal potassium wasting may need oral potassium supplementation. As evident by our young friend, not being able to drink when you want is challenging and may be difficult for a child to understand.

▶ CASE 20

A 17-year-old girl comes to the adolescent clinic to discuss birth control. To be thorough, you ask about her diet and whether she has any weight concerns. Six months ago she watched a documentary on slaughterhouses. From that point on she has been following a strict vegan diet.

Question 20-1

Which nutritional deficiency are you least worried about in this girl?
A) Iron deficiency.
B) Vitamin B_{12} deficiency.
C) Protein deficiency.
D) Vitamin D deficiency.
E) Calcium deficiency.

Discussion 20-1

The correct answer is "C." Vegetarians come in every flavor of the rainbow. It is important to ask specifically what the person will not eat: red meat, fish, fowl, eggs, dairy products, or any combination of these; what he or she is eating (alternative protein sources); and what supplements (vitamin and minerals) he or she is taking. Vegetarians should find alternative protein sources such as legumes, tree nuts, or tofu. Calcium- and vitamin D–fortified foods can ensure adequate intake in someone who "doesn't do dairy." Vegans run the risk of becoming deficient in vitamin B_{12}. Regular consumption of vitamin B_{12}–fortified foods or allowing dairy products in the diet should be encouraged for both vegetarians and vegans. The RDI of iron is greater for herbivores than for carnivores because the iron in a vegetarian diet has lower bioavailability.

Helpful Tip

Iron deficiency is the most common micronutrient deficiency in children and infants who eat a vegetarian diet.

QUICK QUIZ

Which of the following statements regarding nutritional needs in neurologically impaired children is true?
A) Children with neurologic disorders always have increased caloric needs.
B) All children with neurologic disorders require enteral tube feedings.
C) Vitamin D deficiency is not an adverse effect of some anti-seizure medications.
D) Obesity does not occur in children with neurologic impairment.
E) Oral-motor dysfunction contributes to malnutrition in children with neurologic impairments.

Discussion

The correct answer is "E." Children with neurologic impairment have special nutritional needs. If swallowing or sucking is impaired or the child cannot meet nutritional goals, enteral tube feedings typically through a surgical feeding tube are necessary. Calorie needs vary greatly. Children with spasticity (cerebral palsy) have increased energy requirements and have decreased feeding efficiency owing to impaired oral-motor skills (eg, it takes longer to swallow and chew). Those with neuromuscular disorders such as spinal muscular atrophy have lower daily caloric needs. Children with a low resting energy expenditure rate may become obese despite eating very little. Vitamin D deficiency is common with certain antiseizure medications. A ketogenic diet may be prescribed for those with intractable seizures. Adverse effects of the diet include hypoglycemia, dehydration, vomiting, loss of appetite, constipation, hypertriglyceridemia, kidney stones, and pancreatitis. Osteoporosis is very common in this population and pathologic fractures may occur. Factors contributing to poor bone health include lack of sun exposure, antiseizure medications, lack of weight-bearing activity, and inadequate intake of calcium, phosphorus, and vitamin D.

▶ CASE 21

A 5-month-old male infant is brought into clinic because his father has questions about starting solid foods. The infant is exclusively breastfed. His sibling has a peanut allergy, the father has hay fever, and the mother has asthma. To minimize allergen exposure from her breastmilk, the mother has eliminated dairy, eggs, wheat, soy, peanuts, shellfish, and nuts from her diet. The mother does not want the child to start solid foods until he is at least a year old, at which time he will follow a soy-, dairy-, egg-, peanut-, and nut-free diet until age 5. The father does not agree. He wants your opinion as a medical professional.

Question 21-1

What do you tell him?
A) The infant's risk of food allergy is increased as his sibling has a peanut allergy.
B) Breastmilk is more likely than formula to trigger an allergic reaction.
C) A restrictive maternal diet during pregnancy and while breastfeeding protects against the development of food allergies
D) The safest time to introduce solid foods is at 12 months of age.
E) Introducing more than one food at a time is recommended.

Discussion 21-1

The correct answer is "A." Cow's milk, soy, egg, fish, shellfish, peanuts, and tree nuts are common causes of food allergies. An infant is at risk if his or her mother, father, or sibling has asthma, eczema, allergic rhinitis, or food allergy. Though it sounds like a good idea, restricting a mother's diet has not been shown to be protective. (Hooray for mom; she can eat again!) Breast milk is the best option in this case as it builds the immune system and is least allergenic. Exclusive breastfeeding for 4 to 6 months is recommended. When the infant is 4 to 6 months old, single ingredient foods should be introduced one at a time. This approach helps to identify whether or not a food caused a reaction. If more than one food is introduced concurrently and the infant has a reaction, it will be difficult to know which food caused the reaction. Feeding the infant solids should not be delayed beyond 6 months. Families do not need to wait to introduce certain foods. Delayed introduction of potential allergenic foods has not been clearly shown to be beneficial, even in at-risk infants.

▶ CASE 22

A 5-year-old girl has chronic liver cholestasis with diarrhea and poor weight gain. She is receiving medium-chain triglyceride (MCT) oil supplementation. You order laboratory tests to assess her nutritional status.

Question 22-1

Which is NOT associated with cholestatic liver disease?
A) Coagulopathy.
B) Hypercalcemia.
C) Vitamin A deficiency.
D) Hyperparathyroidism.
E) Vitamin D deficiency.

Discussion 22-1

The correct answer is "B." Children with impaired bile acid secretion have impaired absorption of fat and fat-soluble vitamins. Therefore, vitamins A, D, E, and K should be supplemented. Intravenous or intramuscular vitamin K may be needed. A low-fat diet supplemented with MCT oil can decrease steatorrhea as MCT does not require bile salts for intestinal absorption and boosts calorie intake. Children with chronic liver disease may develop hepatic osteodystrophy (a form of rickets). Vitamin D deficiency and hypocalcemia cause secondary hyperparathyroidism, resulting in bone reabsorption. Vitamin D deficiency is only partially to blame as osteopenia may persist even after vitamin D stores have been restored.

▶ CASE 23

A 16-year-old boy is the starting center on his football team. He comes to the office for follow-up care of his acne. You ask about this year's team and how the season is going. During the conversation, he mentions that his coach is encouraging him and his teammates to take protein supplements.

Question 23-1

How do you respond?
A) Adding nonfat powdered milk to foods is an alternative to commercial protein powders.
B) Amino acid supplementation in a healthy athlete is not necessary.
C) "Weight gainers" may result in excessive fat gain.
D) Dietary supplements may vary in quality.
E) All of the above.

Discussion 23-1

The correct answer is "E." A well-balanced diet is the key to athletic success. Diet supplements are not regulated like prescription drugs. Product quality and purity vary even from reliable sources. A healthy athlete who is eating a well-balanced diet does not need protein or amino acid supplements. These supplements have not been shown to significantly improve performance in younger athletes and may decrease performance in endurance sports. "Weight gainers" are high-calorie protein supplements with up to 2000 kilocalories (kcal) per serving. If used as recommended, they add bulk but it will be fat not muscle. If an athlete cannot meet his or her protein needs, adding powdered milk to foods is a reasonable and cheap alternative to over-the-counter supplements.

> **Helpful Tip**
> For athletes looking to increase muscle mass, resistance training is key and should be done on nonconsecutive days (per individual muscle group).

You ask about other dietary supplements he is taking. He found a new energy drink called "Sleep No More." After drinking it, he is really able to focus.

Question 23-2

How do you counsel him about energy and sports drinks?
A) They may contain caffeine.
B) They increase the risk of dehydration.
C) They may cause tremors.
D) They will help you focus but only for a short time.
E) All of the above.

Discussion 23-2

The correct answer is "E." Energy drinks, including those with caffeine, ginseng, and other stimulants, will boost an athlete's performance but only for a short time. An athlete who drinks energy drinks is at increased risk for dehydration and heat-related illness. Muscle tremors and incoordination may occur, so our young athlete will need to hang on to the ball.

> **Helpful Tip**
> A family's culture influences feeding practices, foods and beverages consumed, and how the food is prepared or served. A provider must consider cultural beliefs and practices when making nutrition recommendations.

▶ CASE 24

A 10-week-old male infant is admitted to the hospital with failure to thrive. He is only 30 g above his birthweight. He has profuse, watery, yellow-colored diarrhea. The family cannot differentiate between stool and water. He is on standard cow's milk formula and eats well, taking in 110 kcal/kg body weight per day. His local physician has tried fortifying his formula to 27 kcal per ounce, but the infant has not gained weight. He does not sweat with feedings, vomit, or spit-up. His suck and swallow is normal, and it takes 10 minutes to eat a 4-ounce bottle. He is admitted for nutritional support and diagnostic evaluation. You are concerned he has cow's milk protein intolerance.

Question 24-1

What type of formula should you order for your patient?
A) Intact cow's milk protein formula.
B) Soy formula.
C) Extensively hydrolyzed protein formula.
D) Amino acid–based formula.
E) Both C and D are options.

Discussion 24-1

The correct answer is "E." This child has malabsorptive diarrhea due to severe cow's milk protein–induced enteritis. Extensively hydrolyzed protein formula contains peptides and amino acids. It is first-line treatment for infants with cow's milk or soy protein intolerance and may be used for other causes of malabsorption (prolonged diarrhea, short gut syndrome). If the infant does not improve on a hydrolyzed formula or has severe protein hypersensitivity, an amino acid formula is indicated. Both hydrolyzed and amino acid formulas taste bad and are expensive. Infants are more likely to drink these formulas if introduced early in life before their sense of taste is well developed. The indications for soy formula include galactosemia, parental choice for a vegetarian diet, and lactose intolerance. Infants with severe failure to thrive often require formula fortification to increase the number of kilocalories per ounce. Watch out—concentrated feedings may cause osmotic diarrhea.

You decide to start the infant on an amino acid formula owing to the severity of his symptoms. He does not like the taste and is not meeting his nutritional goals. On a brighter note, his diarrhea has stopped after changing formulas.

Question 24-2
What should you do next to nourish this infant?
A) Add cherry syrup to the formula to improve its palatability.
B) Fortify his formula to 27 kcal per ounce so his total intake goal is less.
C) Switch to intact cow's milk protein formula as you know he will take it.
D) Place an enteral feeding tube and provide supplemental enteral feedings.
E) Place an indwelling venous catheter and start parenteral nutrition.

Discussion 24-2
The correct answer is "D." Infants and children who are unable to meet their caloric intake needs require supplemental nutrition. Enteral feedings through a nasogastric or transpyloric feeding tube are preferred over parenteral nutrition. Enteral feedings stimulate the gut and prevent gut atrophy. Parenteral nutrition is associated with iatrogenic electrolyte imbalances, hypo- and hyperglycemia, complications from an indwelling venous catheter, cholestasis, and liver damage. Situations in which a feeding tube may be needed include prematurity, acute respiratory illness, burns, aspiration, and chronic medical conditions associated with anorexia or increased metabolic needs. If enteral feedings are not tolerated (severe gastroesophageal reflux, delayed gastric emptying, pancreatitis, malabsorption, prolonged diarrhea) or contraindicated (necrotizing enterocolitis, intestinal obstruction or perforation, anatomic abnormality, extreme prematurity), parenteral nutrition is indicated. Parenteral nutrition delivered through a peripheral venous catheter has a dextrose concentration limit of 12.5% or less and it cannot contain calcium. This avoids sclerosis and inflammation of the vein. Electrolytes should be monitored closely when a patient is receiving parenteral nutrition.

You have decided on a formula and enteral supplemental feedings.

Question 24-3
Now which feeding tube should you choose for this infant?
A) Nasojejunal feeding tube.
B) Nasogastric feeding tube.
C) Orogastric feeding tube.
D) Gastrotomy tube.
E) Jejunostomy tube.

Discussion 24-3
The correct answer is "B." An enteral feeding tube inserted through the mouth or nose is not indicated for long-term use. If long-term use is needed, a surgical percutaneous enterostomy tube should be placed. Nasogastric tubes are easy to insert and are the correct choice for most patients. A transpyloric tube (nasojejunal or jejunostomy) may be indicated in cases of severe gastroesophageal reflux or delayed gastric emptying, aspiration, intolerance of gastric feeding, or superior mesenteric artery syndrome, and in patients requiring artificial ventilatory support.

Question 24-4
What is NOT a complication of enteral tube feeding?
A) Tube obstruction.
B) Tube dislodgement.
C) Discomfort with placement.
D) Nasal septum necrosis.
E) All of the above.

Discussion 24-4
The correct answer is "E." Additional complications of nasogastric or transpyloric tubes include misplacement, chronic irritation of the gastrointestinal wall from suctioning, and perforation (trachea, lung, gastrointestinal tract). Surgical tubes are complicated by bleeding, infection, intestinal perforation, tube misplacement, tube problem (clogged, broken, migration), and leakage around the tube.

You decide to place a nasogastric tube. The infant will be allowed to feed orally with the remaining formula given via the feeding tube. The nurse asks whether you would like the feedings given as bolus or continuously.

Question 24-5
Which of the following statements is/are true?
A) Continuous feedings are more likely to cause reflux than bolus feedings.
B) Transpyloric feedings may be given as boluses.
C) Bolus feedings are more physiologic.
D) There is no indication for continuous feedings.
E) All of the above.

Discussion 24-5
The correct answer is "C." Bolus feedings simulate oral feedings—intermittent and given for a similar time period. Minimal supplies are needed (eg, no feeding pump). Bolus feedings are typically used during the day but not at night as the latter are more likely to cause gastroesophageal reflux. Continuous feedings should be used for overnight feedings or intolerance to bolus feedings. Bolus feedings cannot be given through transpyloric feeding tube.

⏳ QUICK QUIZ

What electrolyte abnormality is associated with refeeding syndrome?

A) Hypomagnesemia.
B) Hypophosphatemia.
C) Hypokalemia.
D) All of the above.
E) None of the above.

Discussion

The correct answer is "D." Hypophosphatemia is most common.

> **Helpful Tip**
>
> A child or infant with malnutrition should be monitored for refeeding syndrome and have feedings reintroduced slowly.

BIBLIOGRAPHY

American Academy of Allergy Asthma and Immunology. Prevention of allergies and asthma in children: Tips to remember. http://www.aaaai.org/conditions-and-treatments/library/at-a-glance/prevention-of-allergies-and-asthma-in-children.aspx. Accessed June 2, 2015.

American Academy of Pediatrics. Nutrition and supplement use. http://www.healthychildren.org/English/healthy-living/nutrition/Pages/Nutrition-and-Supplement-Use.aspx. Accessed June 3, 2015.

American Academy of Pediatrics. Performance-enhancing substances. http://www.healthychildren.org/English/healthy-living/sports/Pages/Performance-Enhancing-Substances.aspx. Accessed June 3, 2015.

Baker RD, Greer FR, Committee on Nutrition. Diagnosis and prevention of iron deficiency and iron-deficiency anemia in infants and young children (0–3 years of age). *Pediatrics*. 2010;126(5):1040–1050. doi: 10.1542/peds.2010-2576.

Bhatia J, Greer F, Committee on Nutrition. Use of soy protein-based formulas in infant feeding. *Pediatrics*. 2008;121(5):1062–1068. doi: 10.1542/peds.2008-0564.

Braamskamp MJ, Dolman KM, Tabbers MM. Clinical practice. Protein-losing enteropathy in children. *Eur J Pediatr*. 2010;169(10):1179–1185. doi: 10.1007/s00431-010-1235-2.

Golding J, Paterson M, Kinlen LJ. Factors associated with childhood cancer in a national cohort study. *Br J Cancer*. 1990;62(2):304–308.

Holick MF, Binkley NC, Bischoff-Ferrari HA, et al. Evaluation, treatment, and prevention of vitamin D deficiency: An Endocrine Society clinical practice guideline. *J Clin Endocrinol Metab*. 2011;96(7):1911–1930. doi: 10.1210/jc.2011-0385.

King D, King A. Question 2: Should children who have a febrile seizure be screened for iron deficiency? *Arch of Dis Child*. 2014;99(10):960–964. doi: 10.1136/archdischild-2014-306689.

Kleinman RE, Committee on Nutrition, eds. *Pediatric Nutrition Handbook*. 6th ed. Elk Grove Village, IL: American Academy of Pediatrics; 2009.

Kliegman RM, Stanton BF, St Geme JW, Schor NF, Behrman FR, eds. *Nelson Textbook of Pediatrics*. 19th ed. Philadelphia, PA: Saunders, Elsevier; 2011.

Koletzko S, Niggemann B, Arato A, et al. Diagnostic approach and management of cow's-milk protein allergy in infants and children: ESPGHAN GI Committee practical guidelines. *J Pediatr Gastroenterol Nutr*. 2012;55(2):221–229. doi: 10.1097/MPG.0b013e31825c9482.

Mahant S, Cohen E, Cunningham S, Fine BR. Feeding tubes and enteral nutrition. In: Rausch DA, Gershel JC, eds. *Caring for the Hospitalized Child: A Handbook of Inpatient Pediatrics*. Elk Grove Village, IL: American Academy of Pediatrics; 2013:493–499.

Misra M, Pacaud D, Petryk A, Collett-Solberg PF, Kappy M, Drug and Therapeutics Committee of the Lawson Wilkins Pediatric Endocrine Society. Vitamin D deficiency in children and its management: Review of current knowledge and recommendations. *Pediatrics*. 2008;122(2):398–417. doi: 10.1542/peds.2007-1894.

Nield LS, Mahajan P, Joshi A, Kamat D. Rickets: Not a disease of the past. *Am Fam Physician*. 2006;74(4):619–626.

Oski FA. Iron deficiency in infancy and childhood. *N Engl J Med*. 1993;329(3):190–193. doi:10.1056/NEJM199307153290308.

Prince A, Groh-Wargo S. Nutrition management for the promotion of growth in very low birth weight premature infants. *Nutr Clin Pract*. 2013;28(6):659–668. doi: 10.1177/0884533613506752.

Sahay M, Sahay R. Renal rickets—practical approach. *Indian J Endocrinol Metab*. 2013;17(suppl 1):S35–44. doi: 10.4103/2230-8210.119503.

Schanler RJ, Shulman RJ, Lau C. Feeding strategies for premature infants: Beneficial outcomes of feeding fortified human milk versus preterm formula. *Pediatrics*. 1999;103(6 Pt 1):1150–1157.

Section on Breastfeeding. Breastfeeding and the use of human milk. *Pediatrics*. 2012;129(3):e827–841. doi: 10.1542/peds.2011-3552.

Yan AC, Jen MV. Skin signs of pediatric nutritional disorders. *Curr Probl Pediatr Adolesc Health Care*. 2012;42(8):212–217. doi: 10.1016/j.cppeds.2012.02.003.

Zehetner AA, Orr N, Buckmaster A, Williams K, Wheeler DM. Iron supplementation for breath-holding attacks in children. *Cochrane Database Syst Rev*. 2010;(5):CD008132. doi: 10.1002/14651858.CD008132.pub2.

Zimmermann MB, Hurrell RF. Nutritional iron deficiency. *Lancet*. 2007;370(9586):511–520.

Patient Safety and Quality Improvement 25

Elizabeth H. Mack

▶ **CASE 1**

A child is undergoing sedation for a lumbar puncture. During the preprocedure time out, it is determined that she has diabetes. The child's mother indicates that her daughter did not have her glucose checked this morning despite taking long-acting insulin last night and not eating or drinking this morning. The mother's concern prompts you to check the child's blood glucose level, which is low. She is given dextrose-containing fluids prior to sedation and no harm is done.

Question 1-1

This event can be described as a(n):
A) Near-miss event.
B) Adverse reaction.
C) Sentinel event.
D) Adverse event.
E) Medication error.

Discussion 1-1

The correct answer is "A." The harm did not reach the patient, and therefore this type of error is identified as a near miss. Investigating the root causes of such events, and the safeguards that prevented them from reaching the patient, are just as important as investigating those errors that reach the patient.

Question 1-2

According to the Institute of Medicine's landmark report *To Err Is Human*, preventable medical errors were estimated to cause how many deaths in hospitalized patients annually in the United States?
A) 400–980.
B) 4000–9800.
C) 44,000–98,000.
D) 444,000–980,000.
E) 4,400,000–9,800,000.

Discussion 1-2

The correct answer is "C." *To Err Is Human* estimated that 44,000 to 98,000 inpatients died annually due to preventable medical error. This statistic is quoted regularly throughout the medical and lay literature. Although the validity of these estimates has been questioned, this report served as a "call to action" for health care providers nationwide.

Question 1-3

To Err Is Human estimated the cost associated with preventable adverse events in U.S. inpatients annually to be:
A) $17,000.
B) $17 million.
C) $17 billion.
D) $17 trillion.
E) Unmeasurable.

Discussion 1-3

The correct answer is "C." *To Err Is Human* estimated that preventable medical errors in the United States cost $17 billion annually. Although the validity of this figure has been questioned, this report served as a "call to action" for health care providers nationwide.

▶ **CASE 2**

A 3-year-old boy is prescribed ampicillin for his pneumonia despite his severe penicillin allergy.

Question 2-1

This event is classified as a(n):
A) Near-miss event.
B) Preventable adverse event.
C) Nonpreventable adverse event.
D) Lapse.
E) Latent error.

Discussion 2-1

The correct answer is "B." Whether or not this allergy was documented, the issue reached the patient and was preventable. A near miss represents an error that does not reach the patient. A latent error, often created by employees as a work-around, is typically a system-based problem relating to poor design or workflow that occurred days, weeks, or months before the event. Alternatively, a latent error may not yet be recognized, and thus is often more difficult to identify. A lapse represents memory failure; for example, a nurse forgets to follow a step in the medication administration policy, resulting in an intravenous medication not being unclamped and therefore delayed.

Question 2-2

Suppose the 3-year-old boy had no known drug allergies but developed hives after receiving ampicillin. This event would then be classified as a(n):

A) Nonpreventable adverse event.
B) Preventable adverse event.
C) Blunt error.
D) Lapse.
E) Latent safety threat.

Discussion 2-2

The correct answer is "A." Though the adverse drug event did cause harm, presumably this reaction could not have been anticipated as the child had no prior history of drug allergy or predisposing condition. *Blunt error* is another term for latent error.

Question 2-3

Children are at particularly high risk for adverse drug events because of:

A) Overbearing parents, especially during medication administration.
B) Weight-based dosing and lack of published dosing recommendations.
C) Renal and hepatic metabolism that is not as mature as in the elderly.
D) The wide variety of child-friendly formulations developed by drug companies.
E) Lack of clinical pharmacists who are trained in pediatrics.

Discussion 2-3

The correct answer is "B." Children are at higher risk for adverse drug events because (1) dosing is often weight based, and practitioners deal with a large range of weights in the pediatric population; (2) doses may vary by indication; (3) there is a lack of available dosage formulations; (4) there is a lack of concentrations appropriate for pediatric patients, requiring compounding and other manipulation; and (5) young or delayed children are often unable to communicate.

▶ Case 3

A 13-year-old girl is admitted to the pediatric intensive care unit (PICU). At the same time, a 9-month-old intubated infant develops a pneumothorax. A critical laboratory value for the 13-year-old was not noted until 3 hours after admission.

Question 3-1

PICUs are known to have higher error rates than other locations in children's hospitals because:

A) They are typically located farthest from emergency resources such as code carts and code teams.
B) Fatigue, distraction, and stress are major issues in the context of a huge number of tasks to be performed daily.
C) Violent threats are frequent due to stressed family members.
D) PICUs are more likely to be staffed by residents and fellows.
E) PICUs are more likely to be staffed by inexperienced nurses and respiratory therapists.

Discussion 3-1

The correct answer is "B." Human factors such as distraction, fatigue, and stress are dangerous in the context of the number of tasks that must be accomplished for a critically ill patient.

▶ CASE 4

A new intravenous (IV) pump is introduced on the unit in your children's hospital. A nurse who was out on maternity leave during the in-service education for the new pump is midway through hanging a new IV fluid bag when her other patient's father asks if she can stop his daughter's feeding pump from beeping. When she returns to finish hanging the IV fluids, she discovers the entire 1 liter bag of D_5 0.45% sodium chloride has infused in 15 minutes.

Question 4-1

Through the root cause analysis, the following should be determined:

A) The nurse has a high degree of culpability in this case.
B) The charge nurse is responsible for the error due to inadequate staffing.
C) The nurse's lack of education is responsible for this error.
D) The other patient's father is responsible for distracting her and causing this error.
E) This error reached the patient due to many system-level issues, not one individual.

Discussion 4-1

The correct answer is "E." This error represents the "Swiss cheese model," as described by James Reason. As with most errors, no one person is to blame. This error resulted from a distraction in addition to a system failure to educate all staff who would be working with the new pumps. Likely many other contributing factors would be identified through the root cause analysis. See Figure 25-6 later in this chapter.

Question 4-2

A hospital-wide initiative is under way to improve quality of care and communication among staff members and reduce the number of sentinel events.

Evidence has demonstrated that one way to facilitate good communication in the inpatient setting among care teams is to:

A) Require detailed computerized progress notes by all members of the care team.
B) Implement rounds led by the patient, family, or both.
C) Ensure that the paper chart with copies of the progress notes accompanies the patient on all transports.
D) Implement multidisciplinary family-centered rounds, including a discussion of daily goals.
E) Enter duplicate paper and computerized orders to ensure the plan is followed.

Discussion 4-2

The correct answer is "D." Multidisciplinary rounds that include a discussion of daily goals have been shown to be an effective way of communicating and achieving improved patient outcomes. Communicating in the chart by means of progress notes is clearly not ideal.

> **Helpful Tip**
> Get out from behind the computer. Patient outcomes are improved by family-centered multidisciplinary rounds, not detailed computerized progress notes.

Question 4-3

The 2006 Joint Commission National Patient Safety Goals addressed the fact that this factor contributed to the majority of sentinel events in the hospital:

A) Incomplete documentation.
B) Poor communication.
C) Lack of proper education for staff.
D) Patient and family dissatisfaction.
E) Inadequate staffing.

Discussion 4-3

The correct answer is "B". Poor communication has been shown to be the most common contributor to medical errors and sentinel events.

Question 4-4

A safety culture where voluntary reporting of events effectively occurs will involve:

A) Employees scheduling appointments with the chief quality officer to report errors.
B) Assigning culpability and punishing accountable employees.
C) Changes resulting from reported events where opportunities are identified.
D) Requiring individuals to give their full name when reporting.
E) Hospital attorneys meeting with "whistleblowers."

Discussion 4-4

The correct answer is "C." Event reporting is a key aspect of patient safety culture as measured by the Agency for Healthcare Research and Quality's culture of safety survey. In the context of a strong safety culture, reporting is easy to do, free of retaliation, and results in meaningful change when opportunities are identified.

> **Helpful Tip**
> Medical errors and sentinel events most often are the result of poor communication. Talk with other staff in person rather than through progress notes.

Question 4-5

The model for improvement is a powerful tool for driving quality improvement utilizing cycles involving:

A) Perform, Declare, Synchronize, Assign.
B) Prioritize, Decide, Sequence, Abandon.
C) Prepare, Delve, Sample, Actualize.
D) Publish, Demand, Structure, Allocate.
E) Plan, Do, Study, Act.

Discussion 4-5

The correct answer is "E." The model for improvement describes a methodology for driving quality improvement. The goal is identified, a measurable aim is stated, the key drivers are developed, and then the Plan, Do, Study, Act cycle is repeated until positive change is sustained (often indefinitely). (See Figure 25-1.)

▶ CASE 5

A 10-year-old boy with osteosarcoma of the left lower leg undergoes amputation of the right lower leg. After disclosing the error to the family, the boy still must undergo amputation of the left lower leg.

Question 5-1

This situation is best classified as a:

A) Nonpreventable adverse event.
B) Slip.
C) Near-miss event.
D) Lapse.
E) Sentinel event.

Discussion 5-1

The correct answer is "E." A sentinel event is an unexpected occurrence involving actual or potential death or serious physical or psychological injury. A slip or lapse is an error due to an unconscious lapse in automatic task performance or memory due to distraction; lapses are failures to execute. A near miss is an error that does not result in an adverse event or a "close call." A preventable adverse event occurs when harm caused by medical error reaches the patient; harm that reaches the patient in the absence of medical error is classified as a nonpreventable adverse event.

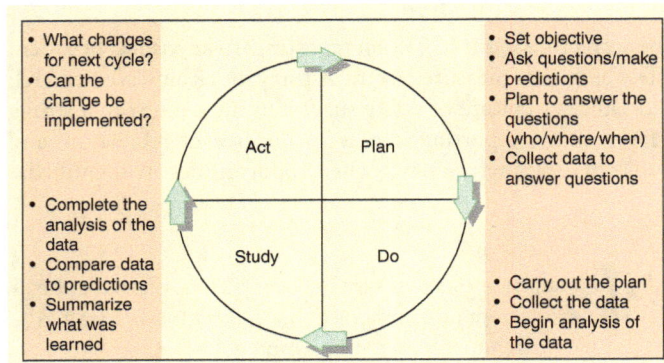

FIGURE 25–1. The PDSA (Plan, Do, Study, Act) cycle is repeated until change is successful in quality improvement projects. (Reproduced with permission from Wachter RM, ed. *Understanding Patient Safety*. 2nd ed. New York, NY: McGraw-Hill Education; 2012, Fig. 3-3.)

▶ CASE 6

A 7 year old male is admitted with hemolytic uremic syndrome (HUS). He has not urinated in over 10 hours and his serum creatinine is 3.5 mg/dL. Ibuprofen is ordered to treat pain as needed despite his acute renal failure.

Question 6-1

Which of the following has been shown to reduce inpatient pediatric medication errors?

A) Hard stops for doses more than 5% outside the recommended range.
B) Involvement of clinical pharmacists trained in pediatric pharmacotherapy.
C) Performance of medication reconciliation by nurses via verbal order.
D) Avoiding conversion of pediatric medication orders to computerized provider order entry.
E) Use of trigger tools to prompt the use of antidotes.

Discussion 6-1

The correct answer is "B." The involvement of clinical pharmacists in inpatient teams has been shown to reduce medication errors. Verbal orders are highly discouraged. Trigger tools are a mechanism for detecting potential errors; for example, ordering naloxone may indicate that a patient received too much narcotic. Hard stops are sparingly used, and pharmacists commonly round medication doses with a wide therapeutic window to reduce cost/waste and increase ease of administration.

Question 6-2

Dose-range checking is extremely useful in preventing pediatric medication errors primarily because:

A) Most pediatric medication errors occur in the ordering phase.
B) Transcription and legibility errors are no longer an issue.
C) Indication or clinical condition will be forced to match the appropriate dose.

D) Dosing will be automatically adjusted for organ dysfunction.
E) Doses can be automatically held if certain laboratory parameters are met.

Discussion 6-2

The correct answer is "A." Seventy-four percent of medication errors and 79% of potential adverse drug events stem from the ordering phase. For a given drug, there is often a wide dosing range due to a wide range of age, weight, and height among our pediatric population. Thus, clinical decision support termed "dose-range checking" recognizes the appropriate dose range for a particular patient's age and size and will prevent a variety of errors in the ordering phase.

Question 6-3

Verbal ordering still occurs in the computerized order-entry era. Errors related to verbal orders can be mitigated by:

A) Limiting use of verbal ordering to computer "downtime."
B) Transcribing these orders onto paper to avoid the pharmacy profiling process.
C) Limiting use of verbal ordering to emergent situations with emphasis on repeat-back technique.
D) Limiting use of verbal ordering by anesthesiologists in the operating room.
E) Requiring nurses to double-check doses with a calculator.

Discussion 6-3

The correct answer is "C." Unfortunately computerized physician order entry (CPOE) does not prevent verbal ordering. Verbal orders should be limited to situations in which the ordering provider cannot possibly enter the order, and the use of repeat-back technique should be employed. During computer downtime, there should be a paper order backup system in place that still involves pharmacy profiling orders.

> **Helpful Tip**
> Verbal orders are a source of potential medical error. If a verbal order is necessary, the person taking the order should repeat back the order to verify it is correct.

Question 6-4

Medication reconciliation is defined as the process whereby:

A) The computerized list of home medications in the electronic health record is continued on admission, transfer, and discharge.
B) The reported home medication list is added to inpatient medications on admission to the hospital.
C) Doses of home medications are checked using dosing calculators on admission to the hospital.
D) An up-to-date medication list is created and compared to the patient's medication orders at times of transition such as admission, transfer, and discharge.
E) A printed list of discharge medications is handed to the patient so he or she can resolve any discrepancies with the pharmacy.

Discussion 6-4

The correct answer is "D." Medication reconciliation involves resolving discrepancies in the medication list at all points of transition as the patient moves through the health care system.

Question 6-5

An effective strategy to prevent inpatient medication errors related to dispensing involves:

A) Storing sound-alike, look-alike drugs in the same area and labeling them with tall-man lettering.
B) Stocking a variety of concentrations, when available, for each medication.
C) Placing the automated dispensing device in a central location in the unit hallway.
D) Having the pharmacy prepare and dispense as many medications as possible.
E) Having nurses compound medications on the inpatient unit.

Discussion 6-5

The correct answer is "D." Having the pharmacy prepare and dispense as many medications as possible reduces the risk of medication errors. Exceptions include emergency medications available in the automated dispensing device. The dispensing area should be free of distraction. Stocking only one concentration of a medication is helpful in avoiding dispensing errors. In addition, sound-alike, look-alike drugs should be stored in separate areas and labeled with tall-man lettering.

> **Helpful Tip**
> Tall-man lettering uses lowercase and uppercase letters to highlight differences among drugs with look-alike names; for example, DOPamine and DOBUTamine.

The Joint Commission requires each institution to create a list of high-alert medications that have a high risk of harm or death if administered improperly.

Question 6-6

Most institutions require the following for high-alert medications:

A) Administration via smart pump.
B) Restricting administration to certain areas.
C) Tall-man lettering.
D) Administration by the attending physician.
E) Independent double-check process.

Discussion 6-6

The correct answer is "E." Most institutions include medications such as chemotherapeutics, anticoagulants, insulin, and neuromuscular blocking agents on the high-alert medication list. Generally, the mechanism in place to handle these high-alert medications involves an independent double-check

process with required co-signatures. The double-check requires verifying the "rights" against the order (medication, dose, patient, route, formulation, time, documentation) before administration and when the dose or medication/administration has changed.

Question 6-7

Trigger tool methodology is used to:

A) Automatically order reversal agents for potentially hazardous medications (eg, narcotic–naloxone).
B) Add corollary orders for medications with common side effects (eg, narcotic–stool softener).
C) Prompt providers to consider laboratory values when ordering relevant medications (eg, creatinine–acyclovir).
D) Screen for potential drug-drug interactions (eg, warfarin–itraconazole).
E) Detect potential adverse drug events by screening for antidote administration (eg, Kayexalate–potassium).

Discussion 6-7

The correct answer is "E." Trigger tool methodology is a quality improvement tool used to detect potential adverse drug events. For example, Kayexalate administration might indicate that an inappropriate amount of potassium was administered (or not discontinued) for the patient's clinical condition. Likewise, administration of naloxone might indicate that too much narcotic was given or that the patient was not monitored appropriately. Administration of these antidotes may also represent the patient's state on admission or an unpreventable adverse event, but it is worth doing a concise chart review to see if there is a lesson that can be learned.

Question 6-8

The gold standard for IV medication delivery involves:

A) Administration by the attending physician after double-checking the "rights" with the nurse.
B) Verification of the "rights," barcode administration, and use of smart pump guardrails.
C) Pharmacist and nurse double-check followed by IV push administration.
D) Use of a basic infusion mode, rather than smart pump guardrails, for children.
E) Avoidance of programming of the smart pump drug library for pediatric patients.

Discussion 6-8

The correct answer is "B." The rights should be verified when administering any medication (medication, dose, patient, route, formulation, time, documentation). Barcode administration involves scanning the patient's identification (ID) bracelet and then verifying the order. Some institutions utilize technology wherein the order will program the pump based on the child's weight and order. However, if a medication or patient is labeled improperly, these technologies are not foolproof. It would be safe to wager that most physicians' working knowledge of an IV pump ends with the alarm silence button.

► CASE 7

You are appointed to your hospital's quality and safety oversight team. The first project is aimed at improving the direct admission process.

Question 7-1

Which of the following describes the best approach for identifying ways in which a process or product can fail, and estimating the associated risk of this failure?

A) Statistical process control charts.
B) Pareto charts.
C) Key driver diagrams.
D) Run charts.
E) Failure mode and effects analysis.

Discussion 7-1

The correct answer is "E." Failure mode and effects analysis involves determining the impact of failure on the patient, the likelihood of failure, and the ability to detect failure. A Pareto chart combines a column and a line graph, relying on the principle that the vast majority of events are caused by a few things. A key driver diagram is structured logic chart with multiple levels depicted as connected boxes. It is a way to look at a problem by breaking it down into parts. A run chart is a line graph of data plotted over time that is used to look at trends—think of patient satisfaction data! (See Figures 25–2 through 25–4.)

Question 7-2

Shewhart, or statistical process control, charts can indicate:

A) Special cause variation by 6 steadily increasing points above a centerline.
B) Common cause variation by 6 steadily decreasing points above a centerline.
C) Random variation by 8 points above a centerline.

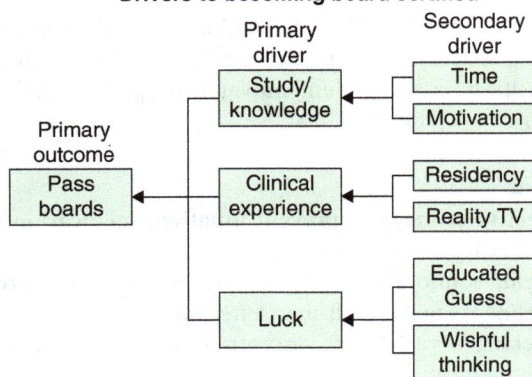

Drivers to becoming board certified

FIGURE 25–3. Key Driver Diagram. This is a structured logic chart that breaks a problem down into its parts.

D) Statistical control by 8 points below a centerline.
E) Single point on the upper or lower control limit.

Discussion 7-2

The correct answer is "A." Common cause, or random, variation is inherent to a system or process. All systems and processes have common cause variation, and systems that only have common cause variation are in statistical control. Special cause variation indicates there is a new factor signal that is not always present in the process. Statistical process control, or Shewhart, charts can help an analyst distinguish between common and special cause variation. Upper and lower control limits generally represent three standard deviations above and below the centerline. Special cause variation is typically represented by a single point outside the upper or lower control limit, 6 steadily increasing points in a row, 2 of 3 points in the outer one-third approaching the upper or lower control limit, or 8 points in a row above or below the centerline. (See Figure 25–5.)

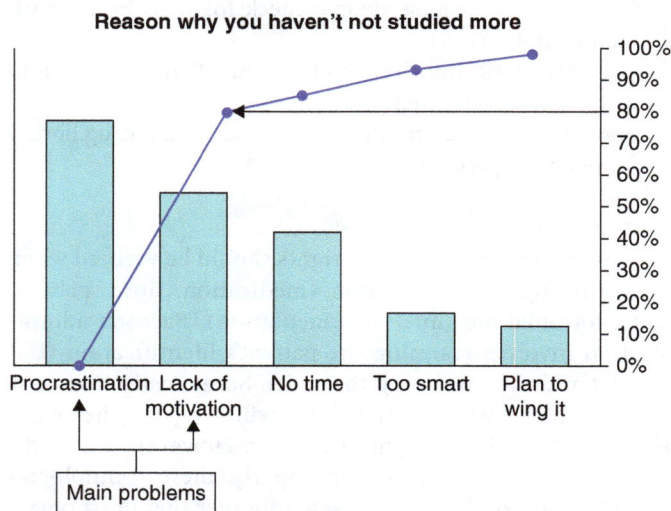

FIGURE 25–2. A Pareto chart combines a column and line graph. It is based on the working theory that 80% of events are attributable to 20% of causes.

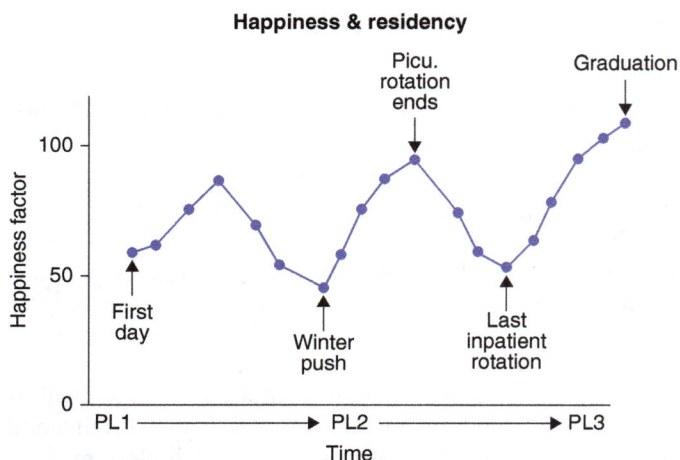

FIGURE 25–4. Run Chart. This is a line graph of data plotted over time that is used to look at trends.

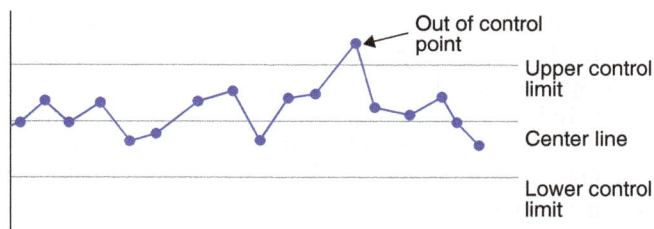

FIGURE 25–5. Statistical process control chart. This type of chart also known as a Shewhart chart helps distinguish between common and special cause variation.

► CASE 8

During a code, a nurse inadvertently administers an improper dose of epinephrine drawn up by another staff member. Unfortunately the infant dies. The nurse administering the dose calls in sick to work for the next 3 days.

Question 8-1

The proper course of action by management includes:

A) Approving a temporary leave of absence until the nurse has taken a medication safety course.
B) Termination.
C) Providing the nurse with counseling resources and institutional support.
D) Requiring the nurse to apologize to the family.
E) Transferring the nurse to another unit within the institution.

Discussion 8-1

The correct answer is "C." "Second victim" syndrome has serious potential consequences, and employees should be supported when human errors occur. This error was clearly a result of multiple systems issues. Additionally, management of the error should not focus on the patient's outcome only, but rather the errors and decisions leading up to the final error. Clearly what happened to the patient and his or her family is awful, but it is important to make sure that such errors do not happen again.

Question 8-2

Disclosure of the details leading up to and involving a medical error should:

A) Consider the risk of lawsuit prior to meeting with the family.
B) Only occur with the hospital attorney present.
C) Not be acknowledged in the medical record.
D) Only be made by the patient's primary care provider.
E) Happen in a timely, thorough fashion with the assistance of risk management personnel.

Discussion 8-2

The correct answer is "E." Failure to communicate is often the trigger for lawsuits. Disclosure of an error does not increase the risk of lawsuits, and in fact often helps the family regain trust and come closer to closure. Disclosure should occur as soon as possible after an event and be documented in the medical

record. Risk management personnel can often help rehearse or guide disclosure.

> **Helpful Tip**
> Disclosure of medical errors does not result in more lawsuits and may help the family find closure and regain trust.

Question 8-3

Patients and their families who experience a medical error should be offered:

A) Compensation for all expenses related to the diagnosis and encounter.
B) Compensation for pain and suffering, but not for related medical bills.
C) Information about how the institution plans to prevent similar future events.
D) Names and credentials of all parties involved in the error.
E) An in-person apology by each of the people involved in the error.

Discussion 8-3

The correct answer is "C." Patients should be offered compensation related to any consequences of the error, but not necessarily the entire encounter or admission, including events preceding the error. Many patients and their families just want to know the results of an investigation or root cause analysis, and how the institution plans to avoid harming patients in a similar situation in the future.

► CASE 9

The nurses on a pediatric ward note a significant amount of variation among the admitting providers caring for infants with bronchiolitis.

Question 9-1

The strategy most likely to improve outcomes and reduce variation would involve:

A) Individual providers writing their own order sets based on their clinical experience.
B) Respiratory therapists writing verbal orders for the treatments that seem to improve each infant.
C) Assigning certain nurses to certain providers' patients so that they learn their ordering patterns.
D) A multidisciplinary group writing evidence-based order sets driving care of this population.
E) Pharmacists making evidence-based recommendations in the chart for each patient.

Discussion 9-1

The correct answer is "D." Reduction in variation is a huge source of cost savings and improved care delivery. Creation of evidence-based order sets or pathways is an efficient way to drive reduction in variation in care. Bronchiolitis guidelines exist, but translating guidelines into practice often takes many years beyond publication of the guideline.

Often different quality improvement methods are used together to bring about improvement.

Question 9-2

One method you might use:

A) Lean methods to reduce variation.
B) The model for improvement to determine common cause variation.
C) Six sigma to reduce waste.
D) Statistical process control, or Shewhart, charts to determine an aim.
E) Key driver diagrams to map out factors likely to affect the desired outcome.

Discussion 9-2

The correct answer is "E." Lean methods, based on the Japanese manufacturing industry and Toyota Production System, refers to a methodology that maximizes value and eliminates waste. The Langley, or Institute for Healthcare Improvement (IHI), model for improvement involves creating an aim statement, then creating, testing, and studying interventions focused on reaching the aim. Six sigma focuses on reducing variation and defects. Statistical process control, or Shewhart, charts are helpful in determining common versus special cause variation. Key driver diagrams facilitate communication of information within a team around factors affecting the desired improvement.

Question 9-3

Quality improvements most likely to succeed include:

A) Education provided to all staff within one discipline.
B) Loosely defined aims.
C) Ownership and buy-in from front-line providers rather than leadership.
D) Limited and defined scope.
E) Feedback and presentation of data at the conclusion of the project.

Discussion 9-3

The correct answer is "D." Common causes of quality improvement project failure include a scope that is too large, lack of involvement of key stakeholders, lack of data feedback, loosely defined aims, and lack of leadership support.

Question 9-4

When special cause variation is demonstrated within a statistical process control chart:

A) Common cause variation is no longer possible.
B) The upper or lower control limit is proven inaccurate.
C) The system is said to be in statistical control.
D) The reason for the special cause can be easily identified.
E) The centerline or mean is recalculated.

Discussion 9-4

The correct answer is "E." Statistical process control, or Shewhart, charts can help an analyst distinguish between common and special cause variation. When special cause is demonstrated, the centerline shifts. The team can speculate as to the reason for the special cause, but within complex systems it may be difficult to isolate one single variable. Systems with only common cause variation are in control: most points are near average, a few points are near the control limits, and no points are beyond the control limits.

Question 9-5

The model for improvement asks the following question:

A) What is the reliability of this intervention? (aim)
B) Is this intervention generalizable? (measure)
C) How will we know if a change is an improvement? (interventions)
D) How many patients should we affect? (scale)
E) How often should we measure? (frequency)

Discussion 9-5

The correct answer is "C." The model for improvement asks three questions: (1) What are we trying to accomplish (aim statement)? (2) How will we know if a change is an improvement (measure)? and, (3) What changes can we make that will result in improvement (interventions)?

Question 9-6

Since human fallibility cannot be avoided, in order to optimize results we must:

Human factors refers to the interaction between humans and other humans, products, equipment, procedures, and their environment.

A) Redesign systems and other exogenous factors to prevent errors from occurring.
B) Use disciplinary action to discourage human error.
C) Focus on the human behavior component as equipment and technology are also fallible.
D) Recognize that endogenous factors such as stress, fatigue, and sleep deprivation are unavoidable.
E) Utilize education repeatedly to ensure human error is minimized.

Discussion 9-6

The correct answer is "A." Human error is unavoidable, but the average error rate is affected by endogenous factors that degrade human capability, such as sleep, stress, and fatigue as well as exogenous factors, such as the systems within which we operate. Redesigning systems to prevent the "Swiss cheese model" from materializing is the optimal approach. (See Figure 25–6.) Imagine a stack of slices of Swiss cheese. If the slices are stacked so that the holes line up an error can easily pass through a hole causing a mistake or accident. If the holes are staggered, an error may pass through one slice but will be caught by the next slice (layer of defense).

▶ CASE 10

A new hospital is being planned to accommodate the needs of a growing community.

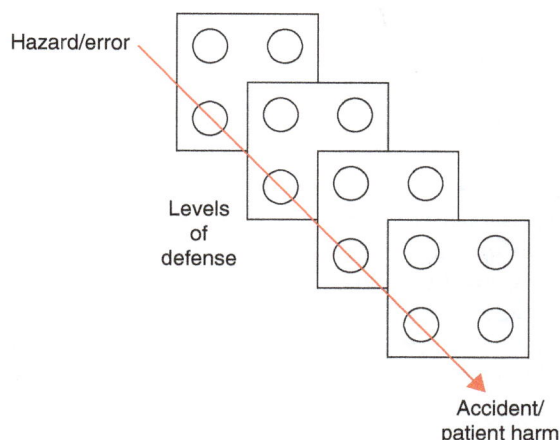

FIGURE 25–6. The "Swiss Cheese Model" of Organizational Accidents. Most accidents occur when an error is not detected repeatedly because failures in a system line up. To detect errors and prevent accidents, the slices of Swiss cheese must be stacked so that the holes don't overlap so that an error that passes through one defense strategy will be detected by the next.

Question 10-1

When building a new children's hospital, increased verticality of the building must be considered as it may have unintended consequences such as:
A) Faster code response.
B) Slower pharmacy turnaround times.
C) Closer-knit relationships between units and floors.
D) Faster transit times from the emergency department.
E) Faster transit times from the operating room.

Discussion 10-1

The correct answer is "B." Increasing verticality can delay pharmacy turnaround times, code response times, and delivery times for specimens or medications that cannot be delivered by tube systems. Verticality may also increase transit times to and from the operating rooms or emergency department. Careful consideration must be given to location of critical services such as pharmacy, and satellite locations may be considered within or near critical units.

Question 10-2

In the process of building a new neonatal intensive care unit, providers and architects decide to transition to all private rooms.

This decision is most likely to have a negative impact on compliance with:
A) Noise regulations.
B) Barcode medication administration.
C) Hand hygiene.
D) Ventilator associated pneumonia bundles.
E) Double-checking breastmilk and high-alert medications.

Discussion 10-2

The correct answer is "E." Moving from a pod arrangement to private rooms will decrease the likelihood that another nurse will be standing close by, and has been observed to decrease compliance with double-checking processes such as for high-alert

medications or breastmilk. (Hospitals without all private rooms could use this to their advantage in a marketing campaign that touts: "Private hospital rooms compromise safe patient care. We care about our patients, so we double-bunk whenever possible.")

Question 10-3

The Consumer Assessment of Healthcare Providers (CAHPS) Child Hospital survey assesses which of the following in relation to other hospitals?
A) Patient and family satisfaction and engagement.
B) Quality metrics such as hospital-acquired infections.
C) Compliance with standard process measures such as venous thromboembolism prophylaxis.
D) Cost-effectiveness of care delivered.
E) Expert opinion of quality of care delivered.

Discussion 10-3

The correct answer is "A." The CAHPS Child Hospital survey is the pediatric version of HCAHPS (Hospital Consumer Assessment of Healthcare Providers and Systems), which assesses patient satisfaction in comparison to other similar institutions.

▶ CASE 11

Recent concerns over unsafe sleep practices on the general pediatric inpatient unit have been brought to the medical director's attention. To improve patient safety, a unit wide educational campaign regarding safe sleep is being planned.

Question 11-1

One might hear the following statement from a staff member in a unit with the most mature learning culture:
A) "Let's do it the way we've always done it; change is too risky."
B) "After that last event happened, we should fix the system so that it doesn't happen again."
C) "If we follow all the rules, we'll avoid causing any harm."
D) "Let's fix this as I think it could cause harm in the future."
E) "Here, nothing is more important than patient and staff safety."

Discussion 11-1

The correct answer is "E." The components of learning and culture are on a spectrum, from least to most mature: unmindful (A), reactive (B), systematic (C), proactive (D), and generative (E).

Question 11-2

The structured communication system SBAR—or situation, background, assessment, recommendation—is a mechanism that:
A) Exposes the transmitter to significant vulnerability.
B) Conveys a message to a provider after verbal orders have been entered.
C) Promotes critical thinking by the transmitter and suggests a solution to the receiver.
D) Is meant only for messages from nurses to physicians.
E) Avoids shared mental models as this can narrow one's thinking.

Discussion 11-2

The correct answer is "C." SBAR is a structured communication system meant to promote analysis of the situation by the messenger and suggest a potential solution to the recipient. This type of tool avoids "read my mind" type of thinking and creates a shared mental model.

▶ CASE 12

A neonatal intensive care nurse may hear thousands of alarms per shift. The staff worry that they may ignore an important alarm, but they cannot possibly treat each alarm with the same degree of concern.

Question 12-1

An effective approach to improving the sensitivity and specificity of the alarms heard in this unit would be to:

A) Silence alarms as soon as they are heard, then evaluate the situation afterward.
B) Lower the low heart rate, oxygen saturation, and blood pressure alarm limits.
C) Turn off the low heart rate, oxygen saturation, and blood pressure alarm limits.
D) Systematically study the trigger, tone, and legitimacy of the alarms heard in this unit.
E) Encourage parents to look for color change, then silence alarms if they are reassured.

Discussion 12-1

The correct answer is "D." Alert fatigue is a very real and dangerous phenomenon. The various alarms should be systematically studied to determine what proportion are legitimate, and whether the issue pertains to limit settings, equipment, or another factor. (Have you ever noticed that an inpatient unit and its alarms can sound like an arcade? Now if only skee-ball was standard equipment on all hospital units, the noise might not be so bad.)

▶ CASE 13

You walk into an operating room and note a scrub nurse trying to perform a "time out," but she is brushed off repeatedly by the surgeon.

Question 13-1

In an attempt to build a culture of safety, in addition to supporting the scrub nurse who tried to be compliant, your actions should include:

A) Disciplining the surgeon.
B) Determining the scope of the problem and implementing widespread safety culture interventions.
C) Disciplining the surgeon's supervisor.

D) Assuming this to be an isolated incident since the scrub nurse was so insistent.
E) Terminating all those involved.

Discussion 13-1

The correct answer is "B." Likely this instance is a symptom of a larger safety culture problem, and the scope of the issue should be investigated. If this is determined to be a widespread issue, there will need to be large-scale safety culture interventions. Leaders will need to be sure there are supportive policies, adequate and appropriately placed champions, user-friendly reporting systems, and lack of retaliation in response to event reporting.

▶ CASE 14

Your staff have come to you as they have repeatedly observed a pediatric gastroenterologist failing to follow proper hand hygiene protocol when he enters patient rooms.

Question 14-1

An effective response to this situation is likely to involve:

A) Taking the situation straight to human resources and recommending termination as compliance with hand hygiene is a hospital policy.
B) Having a "cup of coffee" conversation with the physician, encouraging the staff to speak up, and holding all employees accountable.
C) Explaining to the physician that the standards are higher for gastroenterologists due to the nature of their business.
D) Asking the staff to notify you if they note any further noncompliance.

Discussion 14-1

The correct answer is "B." "Coffee cup" conversations are generally the first step in examining such issues and can help determine the validity of the allegation as well as reasons for noncompliance. However, staff should be encouraged to address situations such as this with the individual. Leaders will be responsible for ensuring that staff can confront such situations without fear of retaliation.

BIBLIOGRAPHY

Argent AC, Montgomery VL. Quality improvement, patient safety, and medical error. In: Nichols DG, ed. *Rogers' Textbook of Pediatric Intensive Care*. 4th ed. Philadelphia, PA: Lippincott; 2008.

Fernandez-Llamazares CM, Calleja-Hernandez MA, Manrique-Rodriquez S, Pérez-Sanz C, Duran-Garcia E, Sanjurjo-Saez M. Impact of pharmacist interventions in reducing paediatric prescribing errors. *Arch Dis Child*. 2012;97:564–568.

Frush KS, Krug SE. *Pediatric Patient Safety and Quality Improvement*. New York, NY: McGraw Hill; 2015.

Hughes RG, Clancy CM. Working conditions that support patient safety. *Nurs Care Qual*. 2005;20:289–292.

Kohn LT, Corrigan JM, Donaldson MS, eds. *To Err Is Human: Building a Safer Healthcare System*. Washington, DC: National Academy Press; 2000.

Langley GJ, Moen RD, Nolan KM, Nolan TW, Norman CL, Provost LP. *The Improvement Guide: A Practical Approach to Enhancing Organizational Performance*. 2nd ed. San Francisco, CA: Jossey-Bass; 2009.

Pronovost P, Berenholtz S, Dorman T, et al. Improving communication in ICU using daily goals. *J Crit Care*. 2003;18:71–75.

Reason J. *Human Error*. Cambridge: Cambridge University Press; 1990.

Pharmacology: Pain Management and Sedation

26

Part 1

Pain Management

Susan S. Vos, Gary Milavetz, Laura Steinauer, and Jeff Van Blarcom

---

▶ CASE 1

A mother calls your office to ask if her child should take a medication with food or on an empty stomach. She does not know the name of the medication. She tells you the pills are small, pink, and diamond shaped and asks, "Isn't that enough information for you to know what medication he is taking?"

Question 1-1

Which of the following are the most important considerations regarding taking medications with food?
A) Decreased gut irritation.
B) Acid degradation.
C) Increased absorption.
D) Decreased absorption.
E) All of the above.

Discussion 1-1

The correct answer is "E." All of the listed options are important considerations when thinking about food and medications. Sometimes medications are taken with food to decrease the likelihood of an upset stomach (eg, ibuprofen). Some drugs can undergo degradation due to changes in gut pH (eg, penicillin V). Food may improve the absorption of some medications (eg, amoxicillin). Food may also bind with a drug, causing decreased absorption (eg, tetracycline). Additionally, food may change the absorption rate and extent of medications. Lastly, some foods can change the metabolism of a medication (eg, grapefruit or grapefruit juice, which interferes with numerous medications).

▶ CASE 2

The father of your 4-year-old patient calls the clinic. His son will not swallow a medication because of the taste. The parents tried holding him down and squirting the medicine in his mouth, but he bit his mother. The father asks if there is anything that can be done to make it taste better.

Question 2-1

Which of the following is the best option?
A) Change to a better-tasting medication.
B) Mask the taste of the medication with flavoring additive.
C) Mix the medication with the child's favorite soft food.
D) All of the above.

Discussion 2-1

The correct answer is "D." One could consider all of these options when the palatability of a medication is decreasing the patient's adherence to the regimen. Knowing the taste of liquid medications is an important consideration when prescribing medications to children. Often, steroids and certain antibiotics are among the worst offenders when it comes to palatability. Changing to a more tolerable-tasting liquid is an option, if one is available. There are some flavoring additives that can be added, but this is not always an option. Some pharmacists are able to extemporaneously compound a medication with a flavoring agent. The parent could mix a medication with a small amount of the child's favorite food (eg, chocolate pudding or applesauce). However, you should be sure to recommend a small amount of food and have the patient consume it right away since there are very little data on the stability of medications when mixed with food. Other options to consider are "chasing" the medication with a strong-flavored drink (eg, chocolate milk, cola, juice).

⧗ QUICK QUIZ

A normal, healthy patient begins taking "Medication A" once daily. "Medication A" has a half-life of 12 hours.

If you start a normal dose of the medication on Monday at 8:00 AM and repeat the dose daily, when will the drug level reach steady state concentration?
A) Tuesday at 8:00 AM.
B) Wednesday at 8:00 AM.
C) Thursday at 8:00 AM.
D) Friday at 8:00 AM.

Discussion
The correct answer is "C." *Half-life* refers to the amount of time it takes for the body to reduce the serum concentration by half. When a medication is taken on a regular basis, an ongoing process occurs in which a continuous amount of the drug is absorbed, metabolized, and eliminated. Eventually, the drug reaches a relatively consistent serum concentration inside the body, called *steady state*. It typically takes between 5 and 6 half-lives for a drug to reach steady state. In this case, it would take about 60 to 72 hours to reach a steady-state concentration. Drug levels should be measured once the drug reaches steady state.

> **Helpful Tip**
> The half-life of a drug is the amount of time it takes the body to reduce the serum drug concentration by half. It takes 5 to 6 half-lives to reach a steady state.

▶ CASE 3

You are seeing an 8-year-old Caucasian girl with a history of generalized tonic-clonic seizures. Owing to poor control on phenytoin, she was switched 3 months ago to carbamazepine, 200 milligrams (mg) by mouth twice daily. Her initial serum level 5 days after starting therapy was 7.1 micrograms/milliliter (mcg/mL). The level was drawn 4 hours after her morning dose, and she reports no missed or extra doses. The goal peak levels of 4 to 12 mcg/mL occur 4 to 5 hours after a dose. On routine recheck of her serum drug concentration today, her level is 4.5 mcg/mL (the level was measured 4 hours after her morning dose, with no missed or extra doses).

Question 3-1
Which of the following factors is most likely influencing the most recent serum level?
A) Laboratory error.
B) Poor adherence to her regimen.

C) Self-induction of metabolism.
D) Drug interaction.

Discussion 3-1
The correct answer is "C." Carbamazepine exhibits self-induction of metabolism. The drug is metabolized more rapidly. Regarding option "A," typically, clinical laboratories do not report a level back if there is any suggestion of error occurring when they include controls or blinded samples. Although option "B" is always possible, it is unlikely in this case because of the history of no missed doses prior to the level being obtained. Since no other medications are being reported in this patient, option "D" is not likely to have occurred. But, it is always a good idea to ask about any new medications, over-the-counter medications, herbal products, and so on.

> **Helpful Tip**
> With carbamazepine, initially check a serum drug concentration after several days of steady-state dosing with no missed or extra doses. The self-induction of metabolism occurs over several weeks to months with maintenance use. Therefore, serum concentrations should be monitored every 3 to 4 months.

▶ CASE 4

A 5-year-old girl is carried into the emergency department by her father. She began seizing approximately 40 minutes ago and the seizure has just stopped following a dose of intramuscular (IM) lorazepam. The father reports that his daughter is currently taking phenytoin (50 mg Infatabs given as 1½ tablets twice daily), and she has not missed any doses in the last week. She weighed 40 pounds at her kindergarten checkup last month.

Question 4-1
What is the patient's daily total dosage of phenytoin in milligrams per kilogram of body weight?
A) 18 mg/kg/day.
B) 8 mg/kg/day.
C) 5.5 mg/kg/day.
D) 4 mg/kg/day.

Discussion 4-1
The correct answer is "B." The patient's weight is 40 pounds, which is equivalent to 18.1 kg. Remember, 2.2 pounds equals 1 kg. The total daily dosage is 150 mg (75 mg twice daily). Therefore, the weight-based dosage per day is 8.2 mg/kg/day. The typical maintenance dosage range for pediatric patients taking phenytoin is 7 to 10 mg/kg/day.

Question 4-2
What should you do next regarding the girl's phenytoin regimen?
A) Give a rapid infusion of phenytoin.
B) Give a partial loading dose of phenytoin.

C) Draw a phenytoin level.

D) Discontinue phenytoin and start a different medication.

E) All of the above.

Discussion 4-2

The correct answer is "C." To be clear, you would first stabilize the patient and administer intravenous lorazepam for status epilepticus. When a patient has a seizure while taking phenytoin, you need to know the drug level at which the patient has seizure activity. Phenytoin is used widely for controlling seizures. Phenytoin has a narrow therapeutic index and dosing and management is often poorly executed. You may decide to give a partial loading dose; however, you must know the patient's current phenytoin level before you can calculate the partial loading dose. Rapid infusion of phenytoin is not recommended due to severe hypotension and cardiac arrhythmias. This warning is considered a "boxed warning" or "black box warning" that is given by the U.S. Food and Drug Administration (FDA). This is the FDA's strongest warning and can require the pharmaceutical company to print the warning on the box of the medication or in literature describing this severe and sometimes life-threatening effect. For phenytoin, the rate of administration should not exceed 50 mg per minute (mg/min) in adults and 1 to 3 mg/kg/min in pediatric patients.

> **Helpful Tip**
> If a black box warning is issued by the U.S. Food and Drug Administration, pharmaceutical companies may be required to print the warning describing the life-threatening effect on the box or on the paper insert.

Upon further questioning of the girl's father, you discover she has recently started enteral nutrition supplementation and has been taking the phenytoin at the same time of day as she is drinking her PediaSure.

Question 4-3

What impact will this have on the bioavailability of phenytoin?

A) Increased phenytoin bioavailability.

B) Decreased phenytoin bioavailability.

C) No effect on phenytoin bioavailability.

Discussion 4-3

The correct answer is "B." Bioavailability is the fraction of an administered dose of unchanged drug that reaches the systemic circulation. In this case, food and enteral feedings will decrease the bioavailability of phenytoin and patients may experience subtherapeutic levels of phenytoin. Patients should be told to take phenytoin on an empty stomach and to take the medication in a consistent manner each day. Phenytoin is a substrate of the enzymes CYP2C19, CYP2C9, and CYP3A4 and therefore has numerous potential drug interactions. It is important to consider drug and nutrient interactions for patients taking phenytoin.

Your 5-year-old patient is stabilized and ready to be discharged from the facility. Her maintenance dose of phenytoin has been increased to 50 mg Infatabs, given as 2 tablets twice daily (11 mg/kg/day).

Question 4-4

When should you check another phenytoin level?

A) Today.

B) Tomorrow.

C) In 1 week.

D) In 1 month.

Discussion 4-4

The correct answer is "C." The serum half-life of phenytoin is variable because it follows Michaelis-Menten pharmacokinetics. This type of nonlinear pharmacokinetics occurs when the drug molecules overwhelm the body's ability to metabolize the drug. This causes the serum drug concentrations to increase in a disproportionate manner. The half-life for phenytoin in adults is about 24 hours; therefore steady-state concentrations are typically reached in 5 to 6 days. Trough concentrations should be measured to ensure that the patient does not experience seizure activity toward the end of the dosing interval as that serum drug concentration decreases.

⏳ QUICK QUIZ

Which of the following statements about linear pharmacokinetics is false?

A) Changes in drug dosing and steady-state drug concentration are proportional.

B) Changes in drug dosing and steady-state drug concentration are disproportional.

C) Clearance is independent of the dose of the drug.

D) The drug's half-life is independent of the drug's plasma concentration.

E) Clearance is independent of dosing schedule.

Discussion

The correct answer is "B." In linear pharmacokinetics, when the dosage of a drug is changed the steady-state plasma drug concentration changes proportionally. For example, if a drug dosage is tripled then the steady-state concentration will also triple. When the drug concentration changes more or less than what would be predicted based on the change in dosage, the pharmacokinetics are said to be nonlinear.

> **Helpful Tip**
> Pharmacokinetics studies what the body does to a drug and includes drug absorption, distribution, metabolism, and elimination. Pharmacodynamics studies what the drug does to the body.

⧗ QUICK QUIZ

Which is NOT an associated laboratory finding with antiseizure medications?

A) Metabolic acidosis.
B) Thrombocytopenia.
C) Elevated liver enzymes.
D) Pancytopenia.
E) All of the above.

Discussion

The correct answer is "E." Valproic acid may cause dose-related thrombocytopenia. Topiramate may cause a metabolic acidosis. Carbamazepine may cause neutropenia and pancytopenia. Oxcarbazepine may cause elevated liver enzymes. This is not an exhaustive list of possible laboratory abnormalities or drugs associated with laboratory derangements.

▶ CASE 5

A 15-month-old girl presents to the emergency department with fever. Her mother reports that "she has slept all day and won't open her eyes." Her weight is 9.6 kg. After lumbar puncture is performed and cerebrospinal and blood cultures are obtained, she is started on the following intravenous (IV) antibiotic therapy:

Vancomycin, 144 mg IV every 6 hours (60 mg/kg/day)

Cefotaxime, 540 mg IV every 6 hours (225 mg/kg/day)

Acyclovir, 190 mg IV every 8 hours (60 mg/kg/day high dose)

On the second day of therapy a trough level reveals the vancomycin serum concentration to be 35 mcg/mL.

Question 5-1

Which of the following actions should be taken to treat this child?

A) Change the interval to every 12 hours.
B) Reduce the dose to 100 mg every 6 hours.
C) Change the interval to every 24 hours.
D) Leave the dose unchanged and recheck the level.

Discussion 5-1

The correct answer is "A." When checking levels, it is important to know the goal trough and peak levels. In meningitis, a high peak level is needed to increase central nervous system penetration. A trough level of 35 mcg/mL is toxic. Save the kidneys! Option "A" is the best answer because it should attain a similar peak but allow the drug to be more fully excreted over the subsequent dosing interval. Option "B" will reduce the peak but maintain a higher serum trough level. Option "C" will likely allow the trough to go sufficiently low as to be ineffective. Option "D" risks keeping the trough to high and permit toxicity to occur.

Helpful Tip

Desired trough serum concentrations of vancomycin to treat a susceptible infection range from 5 to 20 mcg/mL depending on the organism and severity and location of infection. High vancomycin trough levels are associated with renal toxicity. If using vancomycin for an extended period, it is important to monitor trough drug levels!

⧗ QUICK QUIZ

Which of the following statements is false?

A) Dosing of renally excreted medications needs to be adjusted in patients with chronic kidney disease.
B) Pharmacokinetics vary in neonates.
C) Peak drug levels are used to monitor toxicity.
D) It is important to monitor for drug toxicity by checking drug levels.
E) All of the above are true.

Discussion

The correct answer is "C." In general, peak drug levels are followed for therapeutic reasons, and trough levels to monitor for toxicity. Staying with vancomycin as our example, this drug is renally excreted. Therefore, dosing needs to be adjusted based on the patient's glomerular filtration rate to avoid toxicity. In neonates (especially those born prematurely) and infants, pharmacokinetics vary widely as the kidneys are immature. Renal processes gradually mature over the first year of life.

Helpful Tip

Dosage of pediatric medications is weight based. It is important to have an accurate weight to avoid subtherapeutic or excessive dosing of medications.

▶ CASE 6

A 12-year-old boy who weighs 40 kg is taking pimozide, 10 mg/day at bedtime, for the treatment of Tourette syndrome that is unresponsive to other measures. Another caregiver provides him with a prescription for erythromycin to treat acne. Within a few days of starting the erythromycin, he notices an irregular heartbeat. He is subsequently diagnosed with torsades de pointes with a prolonged QTc interval.

Question 6-1

What is the mechanism of the drug interaction between pimozide and erythromycin?

A) Erythromycin stimulates the metabolism of pimozide.
B) Pimozide stimulates the metabolism of erythromycin.
C) Pimozide inhibits the enzyme that metabolizes erythromycin.
D) Erythromycin inhibits the enzyme that metabolizes pimozide.

Discussion 6-1

The correct answer is "D." Medications can be substrates, inhibitors, or inducers of the metabolism of other compounds. Cytochrome P450 enzyme 3A4 (CYP3A4) is responsible for the metabolism of both pimozide and erythromycin and is inhibited by erythromycin, allowing the accumulation of excess pimozide to occur. This is an example of a pharmacokinetic interaction, whereby one drug affects the other's absorption, distribution, metabolism, or excretion. Supratherapeutic serum drug levels of pimozide are associated with torsades de pointes. Cytochrome P450 is a family of enzymes responsible for drug metabolism; these enzymes are primarily found in the liver. At least ten phase 1 cytochrome P450 enzymes are involved in drug metabolism. Some of the metabolites of these phase 1 enzymes may retain pharmacologic activity. Phase 2 enzymes facilitate elimination from the body. Additionally, drug metabolism enzymes mature at different rates from birth to young adulthood.

> **Helpful Tip**
> Erythromycin is commonly associated with drug interactions through inhibition of CYP3A4 (an enzyme that contributes to the drug's metabolism). CYP3A4 is one of the main drug-metabolizing enzymes found in the liver. The metabolism of drugs that are hepatically cleared using this enzyme may be affected.

> **Helpful Tip**
> When prescribing medications, it is important to have an up-to-date list of medications the patient is taking to check for possible drug interactions. Concomitant administration of certain drugs can alter the serum concentrations of other drugs.

▶ CASE 7

A 13-year-old Caucasian boy who weighs 45 kg has a history of motion sickness. He is going on a Caribbean cruise with his parents and siblings. In an attempt to avoid motion sickness while onboard the ship, the parents and child visit a travel clinic for advice and help. A physical exam and review of systems reveals a healthy adolescent who is not on any chronic medications. The provider prescribes a scopolamine patch (1.5 mg) to be placed behind the ear about 4 hours before boarding the cruise ship. This should be left on for 3 days and then discarded. It may be repeated every 3 days for the duration of the cruise. On day 2 of the cruise, the parents have difficulty arousing the boy, and he is confused and cannot remember where he is or why he is there.

Question 7-1

Which of the following pairs are adverse effects of scopolamine?
A) Dry mouth and enuresis.
B) Bradycardia and sweating.
C) Diarrhea and constipation.
D) Drowsiness and confusion.

Discussion 7-1

The correct answer is "D." Scopolamine is an anticholinergic agent. Common central nervous system side effects include drowsiness, dizziness, confusion, hallucinations, and memory disturbances. Other common side effects associated with anticholinergic agents include dry mouth, dry eyes, constipation, tachycardia, and urinary retention. Recall the cholinergic toxicity mnemonic, SLUD (**S**alivation, **L**acrimation, **U**rination, **D**efecation) and think the opposite.

Question 7-2

What type of adverse drug event (ADE) is this patient experiencing?
A) Pharmacokinetic.
B) Pharmacodynamic.
C) Pharmacogenomic.

Discussion 7-2

The correct answer is "B." In a pharmacodynamic-related side effect, the medication dosing and mode of delivery are right but the drug causes an adverse event related to its pharmacologic effect on the body. Had the dosing or mode of delivery been wrong, a pharmacokinetic adverse event would have occurred. In this scenario, the dosing and mode of delivery are correct for a patient 12 years of age or older. An adverse event would have been pharmacogenomic if this drug had been metabolized differently because of his racial or ethnic background.

> **Helpful Tip**
> The U.S. FDA has an online program called MedWatch that is intended to be a mechanism to report ADEs and monitor postmarketing surveillance of medication safety.

⧗ QUICK QUIZ

An idiosyncratic drug reaction:
A) May result from overdosing of a drug.
B) Is a rare and unpredictable event.
C) Is an extension of the drug's pharmacologic effect.
D) None of the above.

Discussion

The correct answer is "B." Idiosyncratic drug reactions are believed to be immune mediated, rare, and unpredictable. The reaction is not dependent on the dose of the drug nor does it involve the known pharmacologic effects of the drug. An adverse drug reaction is an extension of how the drug is supposed to work and may result from giving too much of the drug. For example, diphenhydramine has known anticholinergic effects. Overdosage results in anticholinergic toxicity (excessive symptoms). If syncope occurred this would be an idiosyncratic reaction, as syncope is not a known pharmacologic effect of diphenhydramine.

▶ CASE 8

A 7-week-old girl born at 30 weeks' gestational age is currently receiving caffeine citrate, 5 mg/kg/dose daily, for apnea of prematurity. Following 3 weeks of caffeine therapy in the neonatal intensive care unit, she develops feeding intolerance, which includes gastroesophageal reflux and irritability reported by the parents and nurse during and after feeding.

Question 8-1

Which of the following is the most likely factor causing her feeding intolerance?
A) Caffeine.
B) Gestational age.
C) Postmenstrual age.
D) Feeding technique.

Discussion 8-1

The correct answer is "A." Methylxanthines such as caffeine and theophylline have been the mainstay of treatment for apnea of prematurity for many years. They stimulate the central respiratory drive and decrease the number of apnea episodes. Although caffeine typically is used for apnea due to its ease of administration, wide therapeutic index, and tolerability, sometimes theophylline is used. Methylxanthines are typically safe; however, they can cause adverse drug reactions that include feeding intolerance, diuresis, diaphoresis, and urinary calcium excretion. It is always important to consider adverse drug reactions when new symptoms occur in a patient. In the absence of caffeine administration, the other options could explain the feeding intolerance.

▶ CASE 9

A 12-year-old boy comes to the clinic for an annual physical. Upon examination, you notice he has gray dental staining on his permanent teeth.

Question 9-1

Which drug is the most likely cause of dental staining of permanent teeth?
A) Tetracycline.
B) Levofloxacin.
C) Ceftriaxone.
D) Chloramphenicol.

Discussion 9-1

The correct answer is "A." He may have received a tetracycline medication or his mother may have received this medication while she was pregnant or breastfeeding. Dental staining and darkening of permanent teeth have been reported in patients who received tetracyclines during the time of tooth crown formation. However, recent data have shown that this may not be an issue with doxycycline when used at appropriate doses. Although levofloxacin and other quinolones are often

contraindicated in children owing to the risk of permanent lesions of the cartilage of weight-bearing joints, they may be prescribed if there is no alternative. Ceftriaxone and other drugs in the sulfonamide class are used with caution in jaundiced neonates and infants because of the risk of kernicterus. Kernicterus may be caused by certain drugs that displace bilirubin from protein binding sites, causing hyperbilirubinemia. Chloramphenicol is contraindicated in neonates and infants because of the risk of "gray baby syndrome," which results from their inability to metabolize the drug. The syndrome produces a constellation of symptoms, including vomiting, poor feeding, respiratory distress, and cyanosis, and may lead to death. The takeaway point is that medications safe in adults may pose risks in children given their immature development.

> **Helpful Tip**
> Tetracycline drugs are contraindicated in pregnant women, nursing mothers, and children younger than 8 years (dentition may be permanently stained) unless benefits outweigh the risks.

▶ CASE 10

A 7-month-old infant girl and her mother visit your clinic for the second time this week. The infant's weight today is 16 pounds, unchanged from the visit 4 days ago. Today, the mother reports her daughter has "the worst diaper rash she has ever seen." Four days ago, the infant was diagnosed with acute otitis media and was given a prescription for amoxicillin with clavulanate (Augmentin), 2.5 mL by mouth twice daily for 10 days. The mother reports that they have not missed any doses. The infant's bowel movements have increased in frequency, but they are not described as bloody or watery. Upon physical exam, you notice the skin in the diaper area appears bright red with wet-looking patches. There are no satellite lesions, and the rash is confined to the diaper area.

Question 10-1

Which of the following is the most likely cause of this infant's diaper rash?
A) Her age.
B) Allergic reaction to the antibiotic.
C) Diarrhea associated with antibiotic use.
D) Allergic reaction to the type of wipe used.
E) Allergic reaction to the type of diaper used.

Discussion 10-1

The correct answer is "C." One known and common side effect of amoxicillin with clavulanate is diarrhea, which has an incidence ranging from 3% to 34%. Diarrhea has been shown to be a significant risk factor for diaper dermatitis. Pseudomembranous colitis resulting from *Clostridium difficile* infection can be associated with antibiotic use and is described as watery, bloody stools occurring at a frequency of about 15 stools per day. Treatment for antibiotic-associated pseudomembranous colitis typically includes an oral regimen of metronidazole or vancomycin. It seems ironic that the treatment of an adverse effect of one antibiotic is another antibiotic.

> **Helpful Tip**
> Beta-lactam antibiotics including amoxicillin are bactericidal drugs that inhibit bacterial cell wall synthesis. Bactericidal antibiotics kill bacteria. Bacteriostatic antibiotics inhibit the growth or reproduction of bacteria.

Question 10-2

What is the best treatment option for this patient's diaper dermatitis?
A) Air out the skin.
B) Use barrier cream.
C) Keep the skin clean.
D) All of the above.

Discussion 10-2

The correct answer is "D." The most effective way to treat irritant diaper rash is to reduce skin contact with urine and feces. This can be done by airing out the skin, using a barrier cream, and keeping the skin clean. The goals of diaper dermatitis treatment are typically prevention first, and then cure. Application of a barrier cream is recommended at every diaper change. This can be recommended to prevent and also treat existing diaper dermatitis. Nonprescription topical barrier creams include ingredients such as zinc oxide, petrolatum, or both.

> **Helpful Tip**
> Treatment of diaper rash includes a combination of measures, which are most effective when used together. The letters ABCDE are a useful way to remember all of these measures.

A – Air out the skin by allowing the child to go diaper-free

B – Barrier; apply a generous amount of a diaper paste, cream, or ointment to protect the skin

C – Clean; keep the skin clean using frequent bathing with water and mild cleanser

D – Disposable diapers; consider using disposable rather than cloth diapers during an episode of diaper rash

E – Educate; teach parents and caregivers how to prevent a recurrence of diaper rash

Question 10-3

Since this patient has severe diaper dermatitis and has continued to have symptoms despite treatment with barrier creams, which of the following could be recommended?
A) Topical antifungal cream.
B) Topical steroid cream.
C) Talcum powder.
D) Cornstarch.

Discussion 10-3

The correct answer is "A." Because of the likelihood of fungal infection in this patient secondary to antibiotic use, a topical antifungal (eg, nystatin, clotrimazole) could be recommended for up to 14 days. Talcum powders are not recommended for diaper dermatitis due to the risk of inhalation in the infant. Cornstarch is also not recommended as it can worsen fungal-related diaper dermatitis. Topical steroids could aggravate symptoms and cause adverse systemic effects.

▶ CASE 11

A 12-year-old African-American male has an 8-year history of severe persistent asthma. He uses 2 puffs of an albuterol metered-dose inhaler (MDI) for treatment of acute respiratory symptoms and 2 puffs twice daily of fluticasone, 44 mcg/puff MDI, for maintenance control. Over the past 2 months, he has needed four refills of albuterol while obtaining a monthly refill of his fluticasone. He states he is using his albuterol inhaler five or six times a day with minimal relief of symptoms. He wakes up at night a couple of times a week with coughing. His asthma is poorly controlled and needs additional therapy; therefore, you decide to increase his fluticasone to 220 mcg/puff, in 2 puffs twice a day.

Question 11-1

Which of the following adverse effects is/are associated with long-term inhaled corticosteroid use?
A) Increased heart rate.
B) Longitudinal growth suppression.
C) Skin thinning.
D) Serum electrolyte abnormalities.

Discussion 11-1

The correct answer is "B." Option "A" may be associated with short-acting beta-agonist use (eg, albuterol), option "C" may be associated with topical corticosteroids, and option "D" is unrelated. Adverse effects of long-term inhaled corticosteroids are dose dependent and include hoarseness, oropharyngeal candidiasis, adrenal suppression, cataracts, glaucoma, immunosuppression, short stature, and decreased bone mineralization. Inhaled corticosteroids are used to minimize systemic adverse effects of long-term systemic corticosteroids. Although inhaled corticosteroids have high topical potency in the airways, they have limited—but still some—systemic effects, especially in high doses. Management includes using the lowest dose possible or using alternative (nonsteroidal) medications.

> **Helpful Tip**
> Patients who use inhaled corticosteroids should be monitored for growth, fat redistribution, blood pressure, mood, behavior, and sleep pattern changes as well as cataract formation. When patients exhibit these adverse effects, the dose should be reduced to the lowest effective amount that controls the asthma or an alternative medication should be used.

► CASE 12

A 16-year-old girl weighing 50 kg is being treated for urticaria of unknown origin. She was started on cimetidine, 300 mg at night, after having no response to H_1 antihistamine agents. She is a straight-A student in high school but after a week of cimetidine treatment, she develops confusion, headaches, and right upper quadrant pain. Her provider stops the cimetidine and the adverse events cease after 1 week off therapy.

Question 12-1

Which adverse events are associated with cimetidine?
A) Confusion.
B) Headache.
C) Abdominal discomfort.
D) All of the above.

Discussion 12-1

The correct answer is "D." Cimetidine is a competitive blocker of histamine at the H_2 receptor of the gastric parietal cells. It is important to remember that H_2 receptors are found outside the stomach, including in the brain, lungs, endocrine and exocrine glands, gastrointestinal muscle, genitourinary system, and skin. This answer makes sense if the medication is used to treat a skin condition and toxicity affects multiple organ systems. When prescribing a medication, it is important to think of possible organs that may be affected in addition to the targeted organ.

> **Helpful Tip**
> H_2 receptors are primarily found in the parietal cells of the stomach and inhibit gastric acid secretion. Cimetidine is metabolized by the CYP450 system in the liver and is associated with many drug interactions.

> **Helpful Tip**
> Proton pump inhibitors and H_2 blockers should be judiciously prescribed as use in pediatric patients is associated with increased risk of pneumonia, acute diarrheal illness, and, in premature infants, necrotizing enterocolitis.

> **Helpful Tip**
> Long-term use of H_2 blockers is associated with vitamin B_{12} deficiency, which causes anemia and irreversible peripheral neuropathy.

► CASE 13

A 10-year-old girl is brought to the emergency department by her mother. She is responding inappropriately to questions and displaying combative behavior, vomiting, tachycardia, and hypotension. Ten days earlier, the girl had been seen by her pediatrician but was not prescribed an antibiotic to her mother's disgust. The mother has been giving her daughter acetaminophen, ibuprofen, and occasional aspirin because she had never seen her daughter this uncomfortable with "the flu."

Question 13-1

Which medication is the most likely cause of the patient's current situation?
A) Acetaminophen.
B) Ibuprofen.
C) Aspirin.

Discussion 13-1

The correct answer is "C." There is strong evidence that aspirin therapy following a viral illness (eg, influenza A or B, varicella, adenovirus) may cause Reye syndrome. Reye syndrome is an acute noninflammatory encephalopathy that occurs along with fatty degeneration in the liver. It may cause liver failure, increased intracranial pressure, and death. Signs and symptoms of Reye syndrome include vomiting following a viral illness and confusion that may progress to coma and seizures. Laboratory testing reveals sky-high values for liver function tests, as well as coagulopathy, hyperammonemia, and hypoglycemia. Following the issuances of the Surgeon General's warning as well as package warnings on all products containing aspirin in the 1980s, the incidence of Reye syndrome has decreased.

> **Helpful Tip**
> Aspirin should always be avoided during febrile illnesses in children due to the risk of Reye syndrome, and providers should continue to remind caregivers of this warning. One exception is Kawasaki disease. There is always an exception to the rule!

⧖ QUICK QUIZ

Which is NOT an adverse effect associated with nonsteroidal antiinflammatory drugs (NSAIDs)?
A) Gastritis.
B) Acute kidney injury.
C) Tinnitus.
D) Asthma exacerbation.
E) All of the above.

Discussion

The correct answer is "E." NSAIDs are used for their antiinflammatory, antipyretic, and analgesic properties. Gastrointestinal (GI) symptoms are the most common adverse effects and are generally mild, but serious adverse events, including ulceration, bleeding, and intestinal perforation, may occur. Ibuprofen should be avoided in patients with kidney problems and certain GI conditions.

► CASE 14

An 8-year-old Latino boy has a 5-year history of moderate, persistent asthma. He uses 2 puffs of an albuterol metered-dose inhaler (MDI) for treatment of acute respiratory symptoms and 2 puffs twice daily of a beclomethasone MDI for maintenance control. Over the past 2 months, he has needed six refills of albuterol while obtaining a monthly refill of his beclomethasone. He states he uses his albuterol inhaler six or seven times a day with minimal relief of symptoms. He wakes up at night a couple of times a week with coughing. The assessment is that his asthma is poorly controlled and needs additional therapy. The asthma clinic prescribes salmeterol by dry powder inhaler, 1 puff twice a day.

Question 14-1

How do long-acting beta$_2$-selective sympathomimetic agonists differ pharmacologically from short-acting agents?
A) Longer duration of effect on airways.
B) Exert an additional effect on inflammation.
C) Can be used as oral therapy.
D) Fewer cardiac side effects.

Discussion 14-1

The correct answer is "A." All beta-agonists have a minimal effect on reducing inflammation, so option "B" is not the correct answer to the question. Salmeterol is a long-acting beta-agonist, and albuterol (or levalbuterol) is a short-acting beta-agonist. Since there are no oral formulations of long-acting beta-agonists available, option "C" is incorrect. Owing to B$_1$-receptor stimulation, beta-agonists cause dose-dependent cardiac toxicity, including tachycardia, palpations, and hypertension. A patient must understand which inhaler should be used for relief of symptoms and which inhaler or inhalers should be used daily to prevent symptoms from occurring. The patient must understand that different inhalation techniques are used with the two types of inhalers. Long-acting beta-agonists are not used in the treatment of acute respiratory symptoms because of their slow onset of effect. A long-acting beta-agonist should not be used alone, but only in combination with an inhaled corticosteroid. This is a black box warning by the FDA because of the risk of death from asthma.

Helpful Tip

A long-acting beta-agonist should only be added to inhaled corticosteroid therapy when maximum doses of inhaled corticosteroids have failed to control asthma symptoms. Short-acting beta-agonist inhalers are *always* necessary for the treatment of acute symptoms of asthma because of their rapid onset of action. When using both a long-acting beta-agonist and an inhaled corticosteroid, providers may consider a combination product to improve patient adherence.

Helpful Tip

Beta$_2$-agonists such as albuterol cause hypokalemia because of intracellular shifting of potassium and may be used in the treatment of acute hyperkalemia.

► CASE 15

A 4-week-old girl born at 28 weeks' gestation is being treated for disseminated *Candida albicans*, with known kidney involvement. Conventional amphotericin B has been started. As you are reviewing the morning lab results, you notice her serum creatinine is 2 mg/dL and are concerned about nephrotoxicity.

Question 15-1

Which of the following would be the best choice to treat her infection now that she has developed nephrotoxicity?
A) Discontinue amphotericin B; start fluconazole.
B) Switch to a lipid-based formulation of amphotericin B.
C) Prolong the dosing interval to every 48 hours.
D) Discontinue amphotericin B; start echinocandin (Caspofungin).
E) Both A and D.

Discussion 15-1

The correct answer is "E." Option "A" would be a possible choice because fluconazole has good concentration in the urine and activity against *C. albicans*. However, if this was empiric treatment you would not want to use fluconazole because some non-*albicans* species are resistant to fluconazole. Option "D" is a possible choice because echinocandins have been shown to cover *C. albicans* and are well tolerated in neonates. Conventional amphotericin (amphotericin B) is readily distributed in the kidney; therefore, switching to the lipid formulation may decrease the drug penetration to the site of infection and you may still have kidney damage. A lipid formulation could be used if the infection was outside the kidney, in the central nervous system, for example. Option "C" is not optimal because of the increased serum creatinine. (See Table 26–1.)

► CASE 16

A 12-year-old boy with attention deficit hyperactivity disorder (ADHD) is taking methylphenidate, 20 mg at 8:00 AM and 12:00 noon, followed by 10 mg at 3:00 PM. His symptoms had been under control on methylphenidate in the morning, but he recently added the afternoon dose because of afterschool activities requiring him to be able to focus. He was diagnosed with ADHD at the age of 7 and has no other comorbid disorders. His other medications include acetaminophen as needed for headaches and loratadine as needed for seasonal allergies. Recently, his teacher noticed that he is in a "zombie-like" state and has expressed some concern to the parents.

TABLE 26-1 COMMON TOXICITIES OF ANTIFUNGAL DRUGS

Toxicity	Hepatic	Renal	CNS	Photopsia	Rash	GI[a]	Cardiac	Infusion Reactions	Bone Marrow Suppression
Azoles	Yes	IV voriconazole	Voriconazole	Voriconazole	Yes	Itraconazole, posaconazole	All[b]; itraconazole[c]	No	No
Amphotericin B	Yes	Yes	No	No	Yes	No	No	Yes	Yes[d]
Echinocandins	Yes	No	No	No	Yes	No	No	Yes	No
5-Flucytosine	Yes	No	No	No	Yes	Yes	No	No	Yes

CNS, central nervous system; GI, gastrointestinal.

[a]All medications administered orally have potential to cause GI discomfort.

[b]QTc prolongation.

[c]Myopathy.

[d]Anemia associated with decreased erythropoietin production.

Question 16-1

Which of the following would you recommend at this time?
A) Increase the dose of methylphenidate.
B) Add clonidine.
C) Decrease the dose of methylphenidate.
D) Switch to atomoxetine (Strattera).

Discussion 16-1

The correct answer is "C." Lowering the dose of methylphenidate is the recommended management. Increasing doses of stimulants may worsen symptoms. Adding clonidine (an alpha$_2$-adrenergic agonist) would cause more sedation. Changing to atomoxetine at this point would not be recommended because the patient has not failed to respond to the stimulant; he is likely experiencing a dose-related adverse drug reaction.

> **Helpful Tip**
> Methylphenidate (Ritalin, Concerta) can cause a positive urine drug screen for amphetamines.

► CASE 17

A 12-year-old girl was recently started on dextroamphetamine for treatment of ADHD. Her symptoms have been well controlled since starting treatment and she has shown great improvement in school and social activities. However, she has recently experienced mild weight loss and decreased appetite.

Question 17-1

What should you recommend to address the recent weight loss?
A) Discontinue dextroamphetamine and start atomoxetine.
B) Eat a high-caloric meal at breakfast and bedtime.
C) Discontinue dextroamphetamine and start methylphenidate.
D) Decrease the dose of dextroamphetamine.

Discussion 17-1

The correct answer is "B." Adverse effects are quite common with stimulant therapy, and appetite suppression and weight loss are known adverse effects of stimulants. To manage this adverse reaction, you can recommend a high-caloric meal prior to giving the dose of stimulant, at bedtime, or both. Other adverse effects, such as hypertension, hallucinations, blurred vision, or dysphoria, would be reasons to discontinue the stimulant therapy. Additional side effects of stimulant medications include insomnia, moodiness, and abuse or misuse.

> **Helpful Tip**
> Stimulant medications used to treat ADHD have high potential for abuse and misuse. If a patient requires frequent refills or refuses to take medication holidays, suspect abuse. Remember, you are essentially prescribing "speed."

► CASE 18

A 16-year-old girl was started on fluoxetine, 20 mg daily for depression, 3 months ago. Her mood has improved, but her pants are fitting tighter and she is eating more. She wants to know if this weight gain is related to her medication. You tell her it is complicated.

Question 18-1

What is NOT an adverse effect of selective serotonin reuptake inhibitor (SSRI) use?
A) Decreased libido.
B) Drowsiness.
C) Insomnia.
D) Weight loss.

Discussion 18-1

The correct answer is "D." SSRIs block the uptake of serotonin in the central nervous system, causing increased serotonin activity. SSRIs should be started at the lowest dose possible to avoid adverse reactions, which many are dose dependent. The patient's regimen of 20 mg daily is an appropriate starting dosage for fluoxetine. Dosing is titrated to effect and serum drug levels are not followed. Weight gain is a reported adverse effect of SSRIs but the association is not clear-cut. Once a patient is no longer depressed, his or her appetite may return causing the patient to gain back any weight that was lost. Thus, the weight gain may not be a direct effect of the medication per se. Of the SSRIs, paroxetine has the highest incidence of weight gain. Weight gain with fluoxetine is less likely. Sexual dysfunction includes decreased libido, inability to have an orgasm (anorgasmia), and difficulty achieving an erection. It is a no-win situation. If you are depressed, your libido is likely to be low. If you are treated, your libido may stay low. However, decreasing the dose or dividing the dose during the day may decrease adverse effects.

> **Helpful Tip**
> Antidepressants including SSRIs carry the black box warning that the risk of suicide and suicidal thinking may increase in children and adolescents after starting medication. Every patient started on an antidepressant should be monitored closely for suicidality.

A few months later, the adolescent is admitted to the hospital with confusion, fever, and diarrhea. Her muscles are rigid and stiff. She is tachycardic and hypertensive, and has a fever of 40°C (104°F). She cannot remember her name and is clearly confused. Her reflexes are brisk with clonus, and she has a fine resting tremor. From her records, you see she has been refilling the fluoxetine prescription monthly. She was recently diagnosed with methicillin-resistant *Staphylococcus aureus* (MRSA) cellulitis and started on an oral antibiotic—but she cannot remember its name.

Question 18-2

Which medication may interact with an SSRI to cause serotonin syndrome?

A) Linezolid.
B) Lithium.
C) Tramadol.
D) St John's wart.
E) All of the above.

Discussion 18-2

The correct answer is "E." The patient was prescribed linezolid—an oral antibiotic used to treat MRSA infections. Serotonin syndrome may occur with serotonergic medications (SSRIs, serotonin norepinephrine reuptake inhibitors [SNRIs]), especially when used with other drugs that increase serotonin activity or impair the metabolism of serotonin. Linezolid is a monoamine oxidase inhibitor (MOAI). MOAIs decrease the metabolism of serotonin and may precipitate serotonin syndrome when taken with an SSRI. Other drugs that may cause serotonin syndrome when taken with an SSRI include fentanyl, carbamazepine, valproate, tricyclic antidepressants, triptans, and dextromethorphan. When a patient is taking an SSRI, it is important to check for drug-drug interactions when prescribing a new medication.

> **Helpful Tip**
> Signs and symptoms of serotonin syndrome include altered mental status, autonomic instability, neuromuscular changes, GI symptoms, and seizures.

An ECG is obtained. Her QTc is prolonged at 0.48 seconds.

Question 18-3

True or false: SSRIs can cause QT prolongation.

A) True.
B) False.

Discussion 18-3

The correct answer is "A." SSRIs can cause QT prolongation and ventricular arrhythmias (torsades de pointes). Careful consideration should be given to patients with congenital long QT syndrome, a history of prolonged QT, or a family history of long QT syndrome.

> **Helpful Tip**
> Abrupt discontinuation of SSRIs without a taper can cause discontinuation syndrome, with development of flulike symptoms—dizziness, nausea, chills, and muscle aches.

> **Helpful Tip**
> It is unclear if SSRIs are safe in pregnancy. Fluoxetine is the best choice. Paroxetine increases the risk of congenital heart defects.

▶ CASE 19

A 40-day-old infant was treated successfully with 21 days of IV acyclovir for disseminated neonatal herpes simplex virus (HSV) infection. She is receiving suppressive therapy with oral acyclovir.

Question 19-1

Which is NOT a potential adverse effect of taking acyclovir?

A) Neutrophilia.
B) Neutropenia.
C) Elevated transaminases.
D) Acute kidney injury.
E) Uremia.

Discussion 19-1

The correct answer is "A." Antiviral medications are used to treat serious viral infections. Acyclovir may cause neutropenia, acute kidney injury, or acute liver injury. Oseltamivir (Tamiflu) may cause acute psychosis in pediatric patients. It is impossible to know every side effect of every medication. Just remember to consider a drug reaction when formulating your differential diagnosis, regardless of whether the medication in question is new.

> **Helpful Tip**
> Acute kidney or liver injury and bone marrow suppression are common adverse effects of many different medications.

▶ CASE 20

A 5-year-old Caucasian girl weighing 20 kg has a history of intermittent asthma. Her asthma is controlled with an albuterol MDI with a valved-holding chamber. She uses her inhaler and assist device about once a month, which produces complete resolution of her asthma symptoms. During a school physical exam, her pediatrician diagnoses paroxysmal supraventricular tachycardia and places her on propranolol, 5 mg twice daily. Shortly after she starts the propranolol, her parents notice she is coughing several times a day.

Question 20-1

What is the likely mechanism of her coughing?

A) Adverse drug reaction from propranolol.
B) Drug interaction.
C) Worsening of lung disease.
D) Viral upper respiratory infection.

Discussion 20-1

The correct answer is "B." Propranolol is a non–cardioselective beta-receptor blocking agent (ie, it blocks beta$_1$ and beta$_2$ receptors). Beta$_2$-receptor blockade causes bronchospasm. Some beta-receptor blocking agents (eg, atenolol and metoprolol) at lower doses are less likely to aggravate lung symptoms because they selectively block beta receptors in the heart and not the lungs. Although cough (option "A") is reported in the literature as a side effect of propranolol, given that the patient has a history of asthma, medication-induced bronchospasm is the most likely reason. Option "C" is possible but usually patients with asthma demonstrate more symptoms than just coughing if their asthma is not being controlled. Similarly, option "D" is unlikely without the common additional symptoms associated with a viral upper respiratory infection such as fever, sore throat, or rhinitis.

> **Helpful Tip**
>
> Patients with asthma have airways that are hyperresponsive to triggers that usually do not cause problems to nonasthmatic patients.

⧗ QUICK QUIZ

Which is an adverse effect of beta-blocker drugs?
A) Tachycardia.
B) Hyperglycemia.
C) Fatigue.
D) Hypertension.
E) Hypokalemia.

Discussion

The correct answer is "C." Adverse effects of beta-blockers include bradycardia, hypoglycemia, hypotension, and hyperkalemia.

► CASE 21

An 8-year-old girl (weight, 40 kg; height, 132 cm) presents to your clinic with her mother. She is complaining of increasing frequency and intensity of headaches, fatigue, and blurred vision. She was seen by her primary care provider 6 months ago. The blood pressures recorded at that time were 117/78 mm Hg and 119/79 mm Hg (95th percentile). At that time, she was encouraged to make therapeutic lifestyle changes such as decreasing her sodium intake and increasing her physical activity. She currently has normal renal and hepatic function and is not taking any other medications. Today, she has blood pressure readings of 131/89 mm Hg and 133/90 mm Hg (99th percentile).

Question 21-1

Which of the following is the best initial therapy for her?
A) Losartan, 100 mg once daily.
B) Captopril, 20 mg three times a day.
C) Guanfacine, 2 mg at bedtime.
D) Amlodipine, 10 mg once daily.

Discussion 21-1

The correct answer is "B." Captopril has a short half-life, making it easy to titrate to the desired effect. Its short half-life decreases the chance of angiotensin-converting enzyme (ACE)

inhibitor–induced hypotension. Enalapril and lisinopril are other ACE inhibitors that can be used. They have longer half-lives and only require once- or twice-daily dosing, which may increase adherence and improve quality of life. Losartan, an angiotensin receptor blocker (ARB), and amlodipine, a calcium channel blocker, would both be acceptable as a first-line agent but the dose is too high. Guanfacine, a central alpha-agonist, is not typically used as an initial agent due to the incidence of adverse effects and is usually only used for adjunctive agents in refractory hypertension or in hypertensive emergencies. ACE inhibitors and ARBs interfere with the renin-angiotensin-aldosterone system (RAAS), causing vasodilation and decreased renal sodium and water retention. A brief review of pathophysiology helps clarify the mechanism of action of these drugs. Angiotensinogen is converted to angiotensin I by renin (produced in the kidneys). Angiotensin I is converted to the active form angiotensin II by ACE in the lungs. Angiotensin II causes vasoconstriction and release of aldosterone from the adrenal glands. Aldosterone increases renal sodium and water absorption and potassium excretion. Calcium channel blockers lower blood pressure by peripheral artery vasodilation. Guanfacine blocks sympathetic nervous system activity, resulting in vasodilation and a decreased heart rate.

Question 21-2

Which of the following medications does NOT have direct effect on humoral regulation or RAAS?
A) Lisinopril.
B) Valsartan.
C) Atenolol.
D) Aliskiren.

Discussion 21-2

The correct answer is "C." Atenolol, a cardioselective (at lower doses) beta-blocker, helps regulate blood pressure by acting on parts of the central nervous system. Cardioselective means it antagonizes only $beta_1$ receptors, which results in reduction of cardiac output through negative inotropic and chronotropic effects. Other beta-blockers, such as propranolol and nadolol, block $beta_1$ and $beta_2$ receptors. This additional $beta_2$ blockade can result in pulmonary cross reactivity, but only a minimal number of pediatric patients are affected. Lisinopril (ACE inhibitor), valsartan (ARB), and aliskiren (direct renin inhibitor) all act on different parts of the RAAS, effecting humoral regulation.

At a follow-up visit 1 month later, the girl's blood pressure continues to be uncontrolled and you decide to add a loop diuretic, furosemide.

Question 21-3

Which of the following adverse effects occurs only with loop diuretics and not other classes of diuretics?
A) Dyslipidemia.
B) Hypochloremic metabolic alkalosis.
C) Hyponatremia.
D) Ototoxicity.

Discussion 21-3

The correct answer is "D." Ototoxicity is specific to furosemide. All diuretics may cause a change in blood cholesterol and electrolyte levels. Electrolyte levels are usually monitored in patients taking diuretics. Although the risk of ototoxicity is rare, it is a significant adverse reaction that should be avoided. The exact mechanism is unknown; however, it is likely dose related. Using the lowest effective dose of furosemide and giving divide doses may decrease this risk. Loop diuretics are associated with hypokalemia, hypocalcemia, increased urinary calcium secretion, and nephrocalcinosis (neonates). Thiazide diuretics are potassium sparing and used to treat hypercalciuria (associated with kidney stones) as they decrease urinary calcium excretion.

Part 2

Sedation

Jeff Van Blarcom

▶ CASE 22

An otherwise healthy 9-year-old boy is hospitalized for treatment of encopresis after outpatient treatment has been unsuccessful. Despite having been introduced to the idea of a nasogastric tube prior to admission, he refuses to allow placement of one once in the hospital. In lieu of a struggle, the decision is made to sedate him for the procedure.

Question 22-1

Of the following, what would be the most appropriate medication to sedate a child for a short, likely pain-free procedure?
A) Morphine.
B) Midazolam.
C) Chloral hydrate.
D) Diphenhydramine.
E) Ketamine.

Discussion 22-1

The correct answer is "B." The necessity for sedating children in certain situations can and will continue to be debatable, but sometimes it should be considered to make everyone's life easier, most importantly the child's. Classified as a "short-acting" benzodiazepine, midazolam would be the best of the listed options for the task at hand. Nasogastric tube placement is noxious but in most situations is not painful, making an analgesic such as morphine unnecessary. Anxiolysis, or minimal sedation, is what we seek here. A longer acting agent such as chloral hydrate could also be used, particularly if you are planning on taking several hours to get the tube in. Previously chloral hydrate was commonly used in child younger than 3 years of age, but it is falling out of favor as it can take forever to kick in and once it does it has a prolonged effect. Ketamine, which is an analgesic (pain-killer) and a sedative, could also be used, but this procedure should not be painful and ketamine has no reversal agent. Midazolam is also a good amnestic agent. (If the child cannot remember it, did it really happen?) Diphenhydramine may or may not help, just as in other situations, but is not revered for its use as a sedative per se. (See Table 26–2.)

Question 22-2

Which of the following is properly matched with its definition?
A) Minimal sedation: a drug-induced depression of consciousness during which patients cannot be easily aroused but respond purposefully.
B) Moderate sedation: a drug-induced state during which patients respond normally to verbal commands.
C) Deep sedation: a drug-induced depression of consciousness during which patients respond purposefully to verbal commands.
D) General anesthesia: a drug-induced loss of consciousness during which patients are not arousable, even by painful stimulation.
E) None of the above.

Discussion 22-2

The correct answer is "D." To clarify and simultaneously get all our adverbs straight, minimal sedation implies that a child can respond to commands normally, moderate sedation implies that a child can respond purposefully but not normally, deep sedation implies that a child can respond purposefully but cannot be aroused easily, and general anesthesia implies that a child is not arousable even to painful stimuli. All of these definitions refer to patients who have been drugged, of course. Useful though they are, these definitions imply intended end points, not strictly controlled steady-state conditions. In some children, particularly those who are not communicative, the levels of sedation can be hard to distinguish. It should be noted that use of the term *conscious sedation*, at least according to the American Academy of Pediatrics (AAP), is no longer considered acceptable, given its rather contradictory literal meaning. The different levels of sedation are correlated with differing levels of airway protection and cardiovascular effects: Minimally sedated children are able to maintain their airway

TABLE 26-2 MISCELLANEOUS PEDIATRIC SEDATION DRUGS

Drug	Description	Uses
Ketamine	Dissociative agent that has sedative, analgesic, and amnestic properties	Commonly used in veterinary medicine ("horse tranquilizer") but not often used in adult humans due to risk of hypertension, dysphoria, and agitation
	Preserves airway reflexes and has little effect on respiratory drive	In pediatric patients, rarely causes laryngospasm
	When given IV, peak onset of action occurs within 1 minute and duration of action is about 10–15 minutes	Associated with an emergence reaction characterized by hallucination, confusion, and a dreamlike state
	When given IM, peak onset of action is about 5–10 minutes and duration of action is 15–30 minutes	Causes increased intra-cranial and intra-ocular pressure and should be avoided when either is increased
Propofol	Sedative agent without any anlagesic or amnestic properties	Most frequent use is as an induction agent for general anesthesia
	Functions similarly to barbiturates in the human body	Administered as a continuous IV infusion
		Looks like milk and contains lipids
	Rapid onset of action (within 40 seconds) and short duration of action (1–3 minutes)	Should be avoided in patients who have an egg allergy
Dexmedetomidine	Alpha$_2$-adrenergic receptor (like clonidine) that provides sedation without respiratory depression	Administered as a continuous IV infusion
		Main pediatric use is for prolonged sedation in an intensive care setting
Chloral hydrate	Oral sedative, use of which has persisted despite advent of other sedatives since its first medicinal use in the late 1800s	Continues to be used because of its favorable safety profile and familiarity, although use is decreasing
	Onset of action within about 20 minutes of oral administration	Excessive dosing can cause apnea and hypotension
	Reaches its peak effect at 30–60 minutes	(If you "slipped someone a Mickey," you gave that person a drink laced with chloral hydrate)

IM, intramuscular; IV, intravenous.

without assistance, and their blood pressure and heart rate are not affected by the medication; moderately sedated children are the same; deeply sedated children may require airway or ventilatory support, and their blood pressure and heart rate may be affected; and anesthetized children will likely have a dismal outcome if not properly supported.

. . . .

The child in our scenario is given a dose of nasal midazolam and, once he is dozing, the tube is successfully placed with a minimum of fuss. Later he asks you where the tube came from. Success!

Question 22-3

Which of the following is true?

A) Sedation of children should only occur in a hospital setting.

B) Experience in placing a larygeal mask airway is necessary for a sedation practitioner.

C) A "crash cart" should be available whenever a child is sedated.

D) Nitrous oxide is no longer considered to be an acceptable medication for sedating children.

E) Propofol should only be administered in the operating room under the auspices of an anesthesiologist.

Discussion 22-3

The correct answer is "C." Sedation of children need not occur in a hospital setting, but all of the necessary equipment should be readily available. Advanced airway management skills, such as mastery of placement of a laryngeal mask airway, would be helpful but are not a requirement for a sedation practitioner. Skill in tracheostomy would also be helpful, but those who are adept at that do not frequent sedation areas outside of the operating room, nor should they. An ability to effectively ventilate an overly sedated child is a must, however. Pediatric advanced life support (PALS) training is not an absolute requirement for a practitioner providing minimal sedation (anxiolysis), but it *is* a requirement, per AAP sedation guidelines, for any person providing more than minimal sedation to a child. Anxiolytic medications are frequently given at similar dosages for reasons other than sedation for procedures and generally do not require elaborate monitoring or observation protocols, but any planned sedation of a greater degree mandates the presence of the proper personnel, equipment, and preparation. Although nitrous oxide (N_2O), not to be confused with nitric oxide, has been used for medical purposes for a long time, it is still a perfectly acceptable sedative and analgesic for procedural sedation. And it has also proved useful in drag racing. It cannot be used alone for general anesthesia unless a hazardous degree of hypoxia is acceptable, but it is easy to administer to a child willing to accept a face mask, it is relatively inexpensive, and its effects come and go rapidly. It is, however, rather notorious for causing postanesthesia nausea. Propofol is another handy sedative and does not necessarily need to be administered only by an anesthesiologist. It is powerful enough that painful procedures can be performed on an oblivious patient given an adequate dose, but it is not an analgesic per se. The effects of both nitrous oxide and propofol wear off shortly after the inhalation (nitrous oxide) or the IV infusion (propofol) is stopped. (See Table 26–2.) If whatever you did to the patient when he or she was out was painful, it may well hurt after the sedative wears off, so an analgesic agent (painkiller) should be given as well.

> **Helpful Tip**
> Sedation may cause respiratory and cardiovascular depression. Be prepared to support a child whenever the word *sedation* is uttered. Grab a manikin of choice and practice your bag-and-mask skills.

► CASE 23

A 9-month-old is discovered to have what sounds like a pathologic murmur during a well-child check. He appears healthy, exhibits good growth and development, and has no signs consistent with heart failure. He is sent to get an echocardiogram the following week. For his sedated study, the proper procedures are followed: emergency airway equipment is available, the appropriate personnel are present and properly trained, the child is monitored with continuous pulse oximetry and cardiorespiratory monitoring, the child has been NPO (nil per os) for the recommended amount of time, and the echocardiogram technician has showered and is ready to go.

Question 23-1

Of the following, what would be the most appropriate medication(s) to sedate a child for an echocardiogram?
A) Chloral hydrate, midazolam, and diphenhydramine.
B) Pentobarbital.
C) Propofol.
D) Midazolam.
E) Morphine.

Discussion 23-1

The correct answer is "B." Although echocardiogram technicians might prefer that every child be deeply sedated with a propofol drip so they could get to lunch on time, many would argue that the level of sedation provided by propofol, and the necessity of placing an IV line, would be excessive or even counterproductive. A 9-month-old is unlikely to cooperate enough to ensure an adequate study without sedation, and distraction techniques such as toys, television, pacifiers, and clowns are useful but unlikely to provide the needed tranquility. All of the listed medications can be used to sedate a child for an echocardiogram, but pentobarbital offers the best sedation profile for such an endeavor. Echocardiograms usually take between 15 and 90 minutes, and pentobarbital is an intermediate-acting barbiturate that will cover this time frame adequately. Barbiturates are sedative-hypnotic (ie, anxiolytic and soporific) but not analgesic medications, which when dosed appropriately afford the opportunity for the successful completion of an echocardiogram. Echocardiograms are not painful procedures and only require sedation, so morphine, which is a sedative and an analgesic, would not be necessary although it could also get the job done. Use the right tool for the right job, some say. Midazolam, a benzodiazepine, would also provide appropriate sedation but might not last long enough for a complete study: Grumpy child, grumpy tech. There is of course no prohibition to giving a child repeated doses of an agent for a sedated procedure or study, but administering multiple doses is disruptive, as is whatever behavior necessitated another dose. Using a multidrug regimen offers no significant advantage over a single, appropriately dosed agent and can increase the likelihood of variable or unwanted effects. (See Table 26–3.)

The echocardiogram proceeds without difficulty and is completed in 15 minutes. The child's mother has other things to get done that afternoon and is anxious to get away from all things medical.

Question 23-2

When is it appropriate to discharge the child to home or errands with a caregiver?
A) For narcotics or benzodiazepines, after the reversal agent has been given.
B) 1 hour after completion of the echocardiogram.
C) Once the child is no longer nauseated.

TABLE 26–3 BENZODIAZEPINES COMMONLY USED IN PEDIATRICS

Benzodiazepine	Common Trade Name	Time of Peak Effect	Duration of Action	Commonly Used Dosage Forms
Midazolam	Versed	0.5–1 hour	3 hours	PO, IV, nasal
Lorazepam	Ativan	2–4 hours	10–20 hours	PO, IV
Diazepam	Valium	1–2 hours	36–200 hours	PO, IV, PR
Alprazolam	Xanax	1–2 hours	6–12 hours	PO

IV, intravenous; PO, by mouth; PR, per rectum.

D) Once the child has returned to baseline neurologic status and vital signs are normal.

E) After two half-lives of the sedative agent have passed.

Discussion 23-2

The correct answer is "D." If a child has normal vital signs and has returned to baseline neurologic status after sedation, he or she is likely ready to go. A good test of recovery is the child's demonstration of the ability to drink without difficulty. Recovery from sedation commonly is a nauseating experience and having a child drink without subsequent vomiting is a good sign that he or she is unlikely to arrive at the emergency department later that day or the next dehydrated and unhappy. Vomiting by itself is unpleasant and aspiration events, though uncommon, are best not provoked. Arbitrarily applying a time limit to a child's recovery, as in options "B" and "E," is not a sound practice given the variable effects that a medication can have on a child. On occasion it may take longer than anticipated for a child to return to baseline neurologic status. Most of the effects of a medication, fortunate and unfortunate, can be anticipated and should be known by the practitioner before giving the medication to a patient. Administration of a reversal agent can be an unpleasant experience, which may well be contrary to the sedation goal of minimizing pain and discomfort but probably would be in order if the choice is reversal or intubation. The child would nonetheless need to be monitored thereafter until he or she has returned to baseline neurologic status. Some awareness of what constitutes normal vital signs for children of a particular age is also a necessity. Parental statements such as "She always has a high heart rate" should be accepted diplomatically but should not be unquestioned, in a sedation recovery or otherwise.

Question 23-3

The most common adverse events encountered in the sedation of children by nonanesthesiologists are of what nature?

A) Cardiac (eg, arrhythmia, arrest).

B) Respiratory (eg, hypoxia, hypoventilation).

C) Inadequate sedation.

D) Oversedation.

E) Aspiration.

Discussion 23-3

The correct answer is "C." Inadequate sedation with subsequent failure to complete a study may not be the worst adverse outcome, but it is nonetheless an adverse outcome. In a study by Cote and colleagues from 2000, 13% of sedated children were inadequately sedated. The next most common category of adverse events involved the respiratory system. The events in this category included respiratory depression, most commonly oxygen desaturation (54 of 1140, or 4.7%), and a rare necessity for positive-pressure ventilation (2 of 1140). Thankfully, adverse events that result in long-term morbidity or mortality are uncommon; most of these can be attributed to medication errors, lack of appropriate monitoring or personnel, or sending a child home before appropriate recovery. Vigilance is always in order.

⌛ QUICK QUIZ

Which medication does NOT provide analgesia?

A) Propofol.

B) Ketamine.

C) Morphine.

D) Nitrous oxide.

E) All of the above provide analgesia.

Discussion

The correct answer is "A."

> **Helpful Tip**
> Sedation is not the same as analgesia. Know the indications and effects of the medications that are used. Chemical distraction does not treat pain.

▶ CASE 24

A 4-year-old boy is brought to the emergency department in the early afternoon after falling while trying to learn to ride his new bike. The bike was not significantly damaged but the same cannot be said of the boy's left forearm, which is obviously deformed. The child appears to be in a fair amount of pain. There is no vascular or neural compromise distal to the injury, so you have some time to get some history; notably: He is an otherwise healthy child who has not had anything to eat since a healthy, well-balanced breakfast early that morning. His most recent ingestion was some ginger ale on the way to the hospital. He has never been sedated or been operated upon. The remainder of his physical examination is normal. An IV line is successfully placed and he is given a dose of morphine to good effect. An X-ray confirms a moderately displaced radial fracture, which is not a sustainable position for the bone or the child in general, so preparations are made to reset the fracture.

Question 24-1

For a nonemergent procedure requiring sedation, what is the minimum recommended time between the ingestion of solid food and the administration of a sedative?

A) 1 hour.

B) 2 hours.

C) 6 hours.

D) 8 hours.

E) 12 hours.

Discussion 24-1

The correct answer is "C." NPO status is an element of the child's history that should be taken into account prior to sedation. Most sedating medications can also cause nausea and we do not want any partially digested breakfast items in our patient's right mainstem bronchus, especially if the procedure for which the child is to be sedated is not emergent. Other historical elements

TABLE 26-4 ASA PHYSICAL STATUS CLASSIFICATION

Class	Description
I	A normally healthy patient
II	A patient with mild systemic disease (eg, controlled reactive airway disease)
III	A patient with severe systemic disease (eg, a child who is actively wheezing)
IV	A patient with severe systemic disease that is a constant threat to life (eg, a child with status asthmaticus)
V	A moribund patient who is not expected to survive without the operation (eg, a patient with severe cardiomyopathy)

ASA – American Society of Ansthesiologists

that should be evoked are gathered in a standard history and physical exam, with the addition of any past experiences with sedation or anesthesia and any family history of problems with anesthesia. Although this child is described as a normal, healthy child, an assessment of his neck and his airway should be undertaken such that the sedating provider will be aware of how difficult it will be to ventilate or intubate the child should that be necessary, or if the child is even safe to be sedated without first securing his airway and ventilating him with the help of an anesthesiologist and an anesthesia machine. The overall assessment of the child's health can be used to stratify the risk of an adverse event using the American Society of Anesthesiologists' (ASA) classification system. It is recommended that anesthesiology be consulted for sedations of children in classes III and higher. (See Table 26–4.) A child's Mallampati classification, which is determined by looking into the oropharynx while the child, in a sitting position, sticks out the tongue, is a proxy for determining the difficulty of endotracheal intubation. If you can see the base of the uvula and the tonsillar pillars, and the child is class I, it should be an easy intubation. If all you can see is the palate, the child is class IV (hard intubation) and you may not be able to get a tube in the right spot if need be. If you can successfully bag-mask-valve ventilate and place a nasogastric tube, you still may be on solid ground, however. Ginger ale can be considered a clear liquid, which requires a 2-hour waiting period; solid items such as pancakes and sausage require at least a 6-hour waiting period. Breast milk requires a shorter waiting period than infant formula. Yet another plug for breast feeding. (See Table 26–5.)

TABLE 26-5 ASA 2011 PREOPERATIVE FASTING RECOMMENDATIONS

Clear liquids	2 hours
Breast milk	4 hours
Infant formula	6 hours
Solid food	6 hours

ASA, American Society of Ansthesiologists.

During the time in which all of the appropriate personnel and equipment are gathered for sedating the child and resetting his fracture, his father continues to appear very anxious. He eventually says that his son is in pain again.

Question 24-2

How would the child's pain be best treated now?
A) Give a dose of acetaminophen.
B) Tell his father to wait in another room, given that he seems to be heightening the anxiety level.
C) Give another dose of opioid.
D) Put the boy's favorite movie on.
E) Give a dose of diazepam.

Discussion 24-2

The correct answer is "C." The overriding principle in the administration of opioid medications for the relief of pain is: Titrate to effect. There is no need to let him suffer. Weight-based dosing should be viewed only as a starting point. Dosing of sedatives in general is a guess based on medical experience; the same dose of a particular drug could have different effects on different children. We know the effects of opioids, wanted and unwanted, but those should not deter us from using opioids when they will be helpful. Acetaminophen may not be sufficiently potent and likely will take longer than desired to have an effect, but would not be contraindicated. Giving a dose of another opioid would also be acceptable, assuming it has a reasonably fast onset and short duration of action and assuming that the child's fracture is going to be reset in a timely fashion. Perhaps fentanyl may be used, but not methadone or oxycontin (a sustained-release form of oxycodone). Morphine, in this setting, would be useful because it has a rapid onset of action if given IV and the effect will last for quite some time. The child's arm is likely to cause some pain for a while. A benzodiazepine would be useful in alleviating some of his anxiety, but benzodiazepines do not have analgesic properties and pain is the bulk of his problem at this point. Diazepam has a long duration of action and may well complicate both the child's sedation and recovery from sedation, so would not be a desirable medication here. The euphoric effect of an opioid likely will alleviate most of the child's anxiety, but it may not be unwarranted to add a anxiolytic. Quite possibly option "B" is the only inappropriate answer here. We certainly see a fair amount of secondary gain–influenced behavior in pediatrics, but this is a situation in which a child has an obvious need for pain relief and removing an anxious parent will only exacerbate the child's discomfort. No doubt part of being a pediatrician is the ability to calm an anxious parent. If you coincidentally see that the child has lice, now may not be the best time to mention it. In a medical setting where children can be anticipated to be anxious or in pain, caregivers, stickers, dolls, toys, music, movies, goofy employees, child life, and other such nonpharmocologic modalities should always be available and liberally utilized. Suppose a child with osteogenesis imperfecta comes to medical attention with a new fracture. He takes opioids for pain on a regular basis. Do not start with, or default to, standard weight-based dosing. Talk to his caregivers to find out what works for him; he almost certainly will need more than an opioid-naïve patient.

Question 24-3

Concerning opioids, which of the following is NOT true?

A) Heroin was initially synthesized as an alternative to morphine.
B) Opioids comprise opiates, synthetic compounds, and endogenous compounds such as endorphins.
C) Narcotics and opiates are one and the same.
D) Morphine can be considered to be the prototypical opiate agonist.
E) Opiates are derived from opium alkaloids from the poppy plant.

Discussion 24-3

The correct answer is "C." If we are to discuss sedatives and analgesics, we need to know what we are talking about in specifics. All opiates are narcotics but not all narcotics are opiates. A narcotic, as defined in medicine, is a substance that induces a state of stupor, which includes all legal and illegal "mind-altering" substances—opiates, marijuana, and cocaine, to name a few. Opiates are opium alkaloids derived directly from the poppy plant. Opioids include the substances listed above in option "B." Fentanyl, as an example of a synthetic opioid, is produced through a complicated process that does not include anything from the poppy. (See Table 26–6.)

> **Helpful Tip**
> Opioid medications given should be titrated to effect not solely based on recommended weight-based dosing. No two patients are alike. A patient dependent on opioids will need higher doses so do not start at the same dose as an opioid-naïve patient.

Question 24-4

Which of the following is NOT a known complication of opioid administration?

A) Chest wall rigidity.
B) Respiratory depression.
C) Emergence hallucinations.
D) Hypotension.
E) Anaphylaxis.

Discussion 24-4

The correct answer is "C." Emergence phenomena such as delirium or hallucinations are known adverse effects of ketamine, particularly in older children and adults, but are not known to occur with opioid administration. Chest wall rigidity is a frightening occurrence that is a known side effect of fentanyl, a much more potent and faster acting opioid than morphine. As we have discussed, fentanyl is useful for short, painful procedures such as the resetting of a displaced fracture, though other newer agents such as propofol have gained acceptance for use in emergency departments. Chest wall rigidity can make ventilating a sedated patient very difficult; thankfully we have naloxone to reverse the effects of any opioid. Naloxone should be nearby any time an opioid is given, especially in a controlled environment like an inpatient unit or emergency department. All of these effects should make the necessity of proper monitoring apparent. Constipation, nausea, vomiting, and pruritis are also well-known effects of opioids. Allergic reactions, from urticaria up to anaphylaxis, are possible. Remember the history and physical exam? A discussion of allergies is part of that, but that does not eliminate the possibility of an allergic issue. Morphine causes histamine release and thereby causes itching, but this reaction is not an allergy per se. Synthetic opioids are useful for opiate-allergic patients (notably fentanyl, meperidine, and methadone).

> **Helpful Tip**
> Naloxone is frequntly given to reverse opioid-induced respiratory depression. Full reversal will take away all analgesia leaving you with a patient writhing in pain. Abrupt reversal in a opioid-dependent patient may lead to seizures and withdrawal. Use the smallest dose possible to reverse the unwanted effect while keeping the desired effect.

The boy in question is properly sedated with propofol and his fracture is promptly and properly reset. Perhaps we should discuss what kind of monitoring was used during his procedure.

Question 24-5

Which of the following is NOT considered a necessity when monitoring a moderately or deeply sedated patient?

A) Continuous pulse oximetry.
B) A licensed practitioner whose sole responsibilty is monitoring the patient.
C) Continuous cardiorespiratory monitoring.
D) Blood pressure measurements every 5 minutes.
E) End-tidal carbon dioxide monitoring.

TABLE 26–6 OPIOIDS COMMONLY USED IN PEDIATRICS			
Opioid	**Common Trade Name**	**Duration of Action**	**Commonly Used Dosage Forms**
Morphine	(Many)	4–5 hours	PO, IV, IM
Hydromorphone	Dilaudid	4–5 hours	PO, IV
Oxycodone	OxyContin	3–4 hours	PO, IV
Fentanyl	Duragesic	1–1.5 hours	IV
Methadone	Dolophine	4–6 hours	PO, IV

IM, intramuscular; IV, intravenous; PO, oral.

Discussion 24-5

The correct answer is "E." End-tidal CO_2 monitoring is useful for monitoring sedated patients, particularly if the view of their body is obstructed by something like a magnetic resonance imaging (MRI) scanner, but currently is not seen as a necessity for most sedation situations. The other listed safety measures are seen as mandatory. The most important of these is the sedation provider, who, by paying close attention to the patient, can avert most untoward occurences. All sedation of whatever level is indeed *sedation*, so the practitioner responsible for the child should be prepared for things to go awry. Our accepted terminology regarding the levels of sedation, namely minimal sedation, moderate sedation, deep sedation, and general anesthesia, represents a spectrum of altered mental status and children can certainly go from one state to another without announcing their intentions. Adverse events and outcomes are rare, but there is no excuse not to be ready. A working knowledge of the medications to be used and airway management skills are a necessity. This may sound intimidating, but a calm demeanor and knowledge of the workings of a bag-valve-mask contraption and its intended effects on the human body should keep everyone clean and out of trouble. All obligatory sedation equipment can be summarized by the mnemonic SOAPME:

S – Suction (a suction apparatus and an appropriate suction catheter)

O – Oxygen (a supply of oxygen and a delivery apparatus; eg, nasal cannula)

A – Airway (airway management equipment; eg, nasopharyngeal and oropharyngeal airways, laryngoscope and blades, endotracheal tubes, stylets, face mask, bag-valve-mask or equivalent device)

P – Pharmacy (drugs needed to support life during an emergency, including antagonists such as naloxone and flumazenil)

M – Monitors (pulse oximeter with appropriate probes, sphygmomanometer, end-tidal carbon dioxide monitor, ECG/cardiorespiratory monitor, stethoscope [old-fashioned but useful])

E – Equipment (special equipment for particular cases; eg, defibrillator)

▶ CASE 25

An 11-year-old boy is hospitalized for treatment of meningitis. The infection appears to be viral based on his laboratory studies, but bacterial infection has not been ruled out; therefore he is admitted for IV antibiotics at least for a day or two while the blood and spinal fluid cultures mature. Beyond that, his head pain is probably significant enough to get him admitted. He was given a IV dose of morphine in the emergency department prior to admission and now he is upstairs, obviously uncomfortable. He likes the room dark because "the light hurts his head," he does not want to move his head, and he says that his back hurts at the site of his lumbar puncture. He is stable both from a respiratory standpoint and from a cardiovascular standpoint, although he is somewhat tachycardic with a heart rate of 110 beats per minute, which seems most likely to be due to his pain and the anxiety of being in a unfamiliar environment.

Question 25-1

Of the following, which option would be a good first step in controlling his pain?

A) Ibuprofen on demand.

B) A PCA (patient-controlled analgesia) machine.

C) Acetaminophen on demand.

D) Fentanyl on demand.

E) Regularly scheduled acetaminophen.

Discussion 25-1

The correct answer is "E." It could be reasonably assumed that his pain is going to last for a while, perhaps a day or two, and we should have it within our power to alleviate most of his pain. Regularly scheduled analgesia is likely to be more beneficial than on-demand dosing, so the on-demand options probably are not a good starting point. Appropriately and regularly dosed acetaminophen will be metabolized in due course by a healthy liver, and as such will be safe quite possibly to give for many days, should the need arise or should you be questioned by a parent. Pain from meningitis most often does not rise to the point of necessitating a PCA machine. PCA would not be the first step in controlling the pain of the child in question, although if the child is requiring opioids at a regular interval, it may be appropriate to take that step. A patient in certain situations can be anticipated to benefit from PCA and an acute pain service consult, if the service is available. Pancreatitis or a major operation such as an open reduction and internal fixation of a fractured femur, for instance. Do not, under any circumstances, ask the acute pain service consultant about chronic pain control, yours or anyone else's, without the expectation of redirection.

Question 25-2

What is the pain-killing mechanism of action of acetaminophen?

A) Unknown.

B) Anti-inflammatory property.

C) Inhibition of cyclooxygenase.

D) Endorphin effect.

E) Placebo-like effect.

Discussion 25-2

The correct answer is "A." The mechanism of action of acetaminophen is indeed unknown, but it is effective in reducing fever and controlling pain. NSAIDs (nonsteroidal anti-inflammatory drugs)—notably aspirin, ibuprofen (Motrin, Advil), ketorolac (Toradol), and naproxen (Aleve, Naprosyn)—block the action of cyclooxygenase 1 and 2 in the inflammatory process, thus diminishing pain related to inflammatory conditions, such as injury and infection.

By the way, increasing the amount of ibuprofen or acetaminophen is unlikely to be fruitful unless they were underdosed from the start. There appears to a ceiling for the effectiveness of both of these drugs, unlike the effect of opioids.

> **Helpful Tip**
>
> Patient-controlled analgesia (PCA) is complex and should not be implemented by untrained personnel, although a working knowledge of the subject is useful for any clinician working in an inpatient setting. The PCA device usually requires an awake patient of somewhat sound mind, able to comprehend what it is intended to do. Children younger than perhaps age 5 years are not likely to understand its use, even if diligently instructed. The PCA device allows the patient to receive a programmed amount of opioid at a programmed minimum interval, and if need be, administer a basal (continuous) rate of opioid. That may be common knowledge, but the following are the parameters that must be set for the device to function, for which there is no snappy mnemonic:
>
> - Loading bolus
> - Clinician bolus
> - Number of clinician boluses per hour
> - Lockout (time interval)
> - Basal medication infusion rate
> - Total drug over time
> - Maximum number of patient demand doses per hour
>
> Obviously this is not for the uninitiated. Additionally, terms can vary depending on the manufacturer. More information about PCA devices can be obtained during an anesthesia residency.

The child's mother expresses concern, not about acetaminophen, but about the possibility of addiction if he gets "a lot of narcotics."

Question 25-3

Which of the following is true?

A) Physical dependency can be anticipated after 2 weeks of regular opioid use.

B) Physical dependency can be anticipated after 2 days of continuous use (ie, a drip).

C) Dependency is not common when appropriate dosing of opioids is used for an appropriate indication.

D) Psychological dependency can be reasonably anticipated after three doses of opioid.

E) Withdrawal symptoms are unavoidable after the administration of more than 1.5 mg/kg of fentanyl or an equipotent dose of another opiate.

Discussion 25-3

The correct answer is "C." You reassure his mother that in the anticipated amount of time during which his pain

appropriately necessitates medication, dependency is highly unlikely to occur. Additionally, and more importantly, he is unlikely to experience any symptoms of withdrawal once he no longer needs any pain medication. He may well become constipated, which is a problem that you address with his mother. Although the likelihood of dependency in a particular situation cannot be accurately calculated, it can be predicted, and in some situations has been quantified: After a cumulative dose of greater than 60 mg/kg of midazolam, there is a 17% to 30% incidence of withdrawal symptoms; after a total fentanyl dose of greater than 1.5 mg/kg there is a greater than 50% chance of withdrawal symptoms (not "unavoidable"); and after a continuous infusion of fentanyl for more than 9 days, 100% of infants developed withdrawal symptoms. Now, having embedded those numbers into your fund of knowledge, you should also keep in mind that any time a patient has been given a significant amount of benzodiazepine or opioid, a high index of suspicion for withdrawal is warranted. What constitutes a "significant amount" can be left to the eye of the beholder, but either withdrawal or addiction would be extremely unlikely in the scenario presented here.

BIBLIOGRAPHY

American Academy of Pediatrics Committee on Infectious Diseases. The use of systemic fluoroquinolones, policy statement. *Pediatrics.* 2006;118:1287–1292.

American Academy of Pediatrics, American Academy of Pediatric Dentistry, Coté CJ and the Work Group on Sedation, et al. Guidelines for monitoring and management of pediatric patients during and after sedation for diagnostic and therapeutic procedures: An update. *Pediatrics.* 2006;118:2587–2602.

Bauer LA, eds. *Applied Clinical Pharmacokinetics.* 2nd ed. New York, NY: McGraw-Hill; 2008.

Belay ED, Bresee JS, Holman RC, et al. Reye's syndrome in the United States from 1981 through 1997. *N Engl J Med.* 1999;340:1377–1382.

Benavides S, Nahata M. *Pediatric Pharmacotherapy.* Lenexa, KS: American College of Clinical Pharmacy; 2013:155–178.

Bhutta AT, Savell VH, Schexnayder SM. Reye's syndrome: Down but not out. *South Med J.* 2003;96(1):43–45.

Cote CJ, Karl HW, Notterman DA, Weinberg, JA, McCloskey C. Adverse sedation events in pediatrics: Analysis of medications used for sedation. *Pediatrics.* 2000;106(4):633.

Grossman ER, Walchek A, Freedman H. Tetracyclines and permanent teeth: The relation between dose and tooth color. *Pediatrics.* 1971;47:567–570.

Guerrini R. Epilepsy in children. *Lancet.* 2006;367:499–524.

Gulian JM, Gonard V, Dalmasso C, et al. Bilirubin displacement by ceftriaxone in neonates: Evaluation by determination of free bilirubin and erythrocyte-bound bilirubin. *J Antimicrob Chemother.* 1987;19:823–829.

Hart LS, Berns SD, Houck CS, et al. The value of end-tidal CO2 monitoring when comparing three methods of conscious sedation for children undergoing painful procedures in the emergency department. *Pediatr Emerg Care.* 1997;13:189–193.

Ho CW, Loke KY, Lim YY, Lee YS. Exogenous Cushing syndrome: A lesson of diaper rash cream. *Horm Res Paediatr.* 2014;82(6):415–418.

Hoeger PH, Stark S, Jost G. Efficacy and safety of two different antifungal pastes in infants with diaper dermatitis: A randomized, controlled study. *J Eur Acad Dermatol Venereol.* 2010;24(9):1094–1098.

Lexi-Drugs. Lexicomp. Hudson, OH: Wolters Kluwer Health, Inc. Available at: http://online.lexi.com. Accessed January 16, 2015.

Malviya S, Voepel-Lewis T, Tait AR. Adverse events and risk factors associated with the sedation of children by non-anesthesiologists. *Anesth Analg.* 1997;85:1207–1213.

National Heart Lung, and Blood Institute. Guidelines on asthma. [April 2012.] http://ww.nhlbi.nih.gov/health-pro/guidelines/current/asthma-guidelines/full-report. Accessed on June 1, 2015.

Practice guidelines for preoperative fasting and the use of pharmacologic agents to reduce the risk of pulmonary aspiration: Application to healthy patients undergoing elective procedures: An updated report by the American Society of Anesthesiologists Committee on Standards and Practice Parameters. *Anesthesiology.* 2011;114(3):495–511.

Rybak LP. Pathophysiology of furosemide ototoxicity. *J Otolaryngol.* 1982;11(2):127–133.

Sáez-llorens X, Macias M, Maiya P, et al. Pharmacokinetics and safety of caspofungin in neonates and infants less than 3 months of age. *Antimicrob Agents Chemother.* 2009;53(3):869–875.

Sanborn PA, Michna E, Zurakowski D, et al. Adverse cardiovascular and respiratory events during sedation of pediatric patients for imaging examinations. *Radiology.* 2005;237:288–294.

Stamatas GN, Tierney NK. Diaper dermatitis: Etiology, manifestations, prevention, and management. *Pediatr Dermatol.* 2014;31:1–7.

Subcommittee on Attention-Deficit/Hyperactivity Disorder, Steering Committee on Quality Improvement and Management. ADHD: Clinical practice guidelines for the diagnosis, evaluation, and treatment of attention-deficit/hyperactivity disorder in children and adolescents. *Pediatrics.* 2011;128:1007 and suppl.

Thyagarajan B, Deshpande SS. Cotrimoxazole and neonatal kernicterus: A review. *Drug Chem Toxicol.* 2014;37:121–129.

Tobias JD. Tolerance, withdrawal, and physical dependency after long-term sedation and analgesia of children in the pediatric intensive care unit. *Crit Care Med.* 2000;28(6):2122–2132.

Todd SR, Dahlgren S, Traeger MS, et al. No visible dental staining in children treated with doxycycline for suspected Rocky Mountain spotted fever. *J Pediatr.* 2015;166:1246–1251.

U.S. Food and Drug Administration. MedWatch: The FDA safety information and adverse event reporting system. [June 3, 2015.] http://www.fda.gov/safety/medwatch/default.htm. Accessed on June 5, 2015.

Warden CN, Bernard PK, Kimball TR. The efficacy and safety of oral pentobarbital sedation in pediatric echocardiography. *J Am Soc Echocardiogr.* 2010;23(1):33–37.

Yldzda D, Yapcoglu H, Ylmaz HL. The value of capnography during sedation or sedation/analgesia in pediatric minor procedures. *Pediatr Emerg Care.* 2004;20:162–165.

Poisoning and Environmental Exposure to Hazardous Substances

27

Christopher Hogrefe

▶ CASE 1

A 2-year-old boy is brought into the emergency department with altered mental status, appearing lethargic. The boy was found in his parents' bathroom surrounded by various bottles, including household cleaners, over-the-counter medications, and a couple of unspecified prescription medications. He has otherwise been healthy, and his recent 2-year-old well-child visit was unremarkable. The boy has received all of his vaccinations and has no known sick contacts.

Question 1-1

What information should be gathered next to assist in treating this ill-appearing patient?
A) The specific household cleaners found at the scene.
B) The names of the over-the-counter medications in the bathroom.
C) The types and doses of medications prescribed to the parents.
D) Any interventions that may have been administered prior to arrival.
E) All of the above.

Discussion 1-1

The correct answer is "E." The approach to a patient with an unknown ingestion should start with gathering as much information about the scene as possible. The patient's vital signs and physical examination can help immensely in identifying potential etiologies, but care should be given to understanding the likely causative agents based on exposure. Collecting insight into the facts suggested above will help direct conversations with the Poison Control Center and guide potential interventions.

....

While evaluating the patient you find that he is suffering from epistaxis. Inspection of his diaper reveals a red tinge to the front of his diaper.

Question 1-2

What additional inquiry may further your diagnosis and potential treatment?
A) Has the child been ill recently?
B) Are there any alternative/complimentary medications in the home?
C) Has the child had any traumatic injuries lately?
D) All of the above.
E) None of the above.

Discussion 1-2

The correct answer is "B." Option "A" has previously been addressed, and option "C" is unlikely given the distribution of the patient's symptoms. However, option "B" references an important aspect of the evaluation of patients with suspected ingestions that should not be ignored. Approximately 38% of adults in the United States, and an additional 12% of children, use alternative/complimentary treatments. Such medications include glucosamine, garlic supplements, ginseng, herbal pills, and scores more. In this case, fish oil toxicity can lead to hemorrhagic symptoms, including but not limited to epistaxis and hematuria. There have even been case reports of hemorrhagic stroke. Be sure to inquire about alternative/complimentary medications in poisoning cases.

....

The Poison Control Center can be an extremely valuable resource when treating patients with suspected poisonings.

Question 1-3

What information is not available from the Poison Control Center?
A) Guidance directly to families.
B) Disposition recommendations.
C) Treatment options and dosages.
D) Diagnostic considerations.
E) Additional details regarding the patient's past medical history.

Discussion 1-3

The correct answer is "E." Contacting the Poison Control Center (by dialing 1-800-222-1222 from anywhere in the United States) is an important step in the management of suspected poisonings. In fact, it is a tremendous resource for families as well, given that an estimated 90% of pediatric poisonings can be managed from home when the Poison Control Center is contacted before medical intervention is sought. With that said, the Poison Control Center can provide useful information in the management of poisonings, as listed above. However, they are not a central repository for personalized medical information. That information should be obtained elsewhere (ie, from the patient, family, the hospital's medical record system, etc).

Helpful Tip

In patients with suspected but unknown ingestions, always consider the possibility of multiple ingestions, particularly in cases of potential suicide. Utilizing the Poison Control Center (1-800-222-1222) can be a very valuable resource in diagnosing and treating these patients.

Left, Reproduced with permission from the Children's Hospital of Pittsburgh of UPMC and the Pittsburgh Poison Center; Right, Reproduced with permission from the U.S. Department of Health and Human Services.

The 2-year-old makes a full recovery. Before discharge and during future well-child visits, it is important to counsel families regarding the prevention and treatment of accidental ingestions or poisonings.

Question 1-4

Which of the following is NOT worth including during such a discussion?

A) Using cabinet and drawer locks.
B) Elevating substances out of reach.
C) Keeping ipecac accessible in the house.
D) Using childproof bottles and containers.
E) Counseling children directly on the general dangers of common household substances and medications.

Discussion 1-4

The correct answer is "C." Syrup of ipecac was formally recommended to help induce vomiting following a potential toxic ingestion. Subsequent studies have shown that it is very

effective in producing emesis; however, it has not been shown to be effective at improving outcomes. The American Academy of Pediatrics (AAP) recommends that ipecac not be stored in the home. In fact, the United States Food and Drug Administration (FDA) is considering classifying it as a prescription-only medication. The other answers are all important points to highlight when counseling families on preventing poisonings, including advising children of the risks of exposure to common household products and the medications found in their homes.

QUICK QUIZ

Which of the following regarding ingestions and poisonings is false?

A) Always consider complimentary/alternative medications in your differential for toxic ingestions.
B) Remember to utilize the Poison Control Center as a valuable resource in diagnosing, treating, and dispositioning patients.
C) Counseling parents and children can help in preventing future ingestions.
D) Remember to consider the possibility that multiple substances were ingested.
E) Encourage families to keep syrup of ipecac in the home but to call the Poison Control Center before administering to a child after ingestion.

Discussion

The correct answer is "E."

▶ CASE 2

A 15-year-old girl on the high school track and field team has been suffering from a particularly painful case of bilateral medial tibial stress syndrome (ie, shin splints) over the past week. In order to continue training for the upcoming district track meet she has been taking an over-the-counter oral medication three times a day along with applying an over-the-counter topical cream on her bilateral shins. One morning before school her parents find her lying on her bed complaining of abdominal pain, nausea, mild dizziness, and a ringing in the ears. The patient presents to your clinic secondary to these symptoms.

Question 2-1

To what clinical toxidrome do you attribute her presentation?

A) Acetaminophen.
B) Salicylates.
C) Tricyclic antidepressants.
D) Topical anesthetics (eg, lidocaine).
E) Opioids.

Discussion 2-1

The correct answer is "B." Abdominal pain and nausea are common symptoms that can be associated with numerous medications, including acetaminophen, non-steroidal anti-inflammatory drugs (NSAIDs), and opioids. Even dizziness can result from some of these medications. However, ringing in the ears should raise one's suspicion for salicylate toxicity or NSAIDs, as opposed to the other options. Aspirin (a salicylate) is readily accessible as an over-the-counter medication, and it is also found in numerous over-the-counter analgesic creams. Patients can exhibit systemic symptoms from topical anesthetics such as lidocaine (eg, LMX, Bactine), including dizziness. However, systemic toxicity requires very large amounts and typically results in cardiovascular (bradycardia, arrhythmias, cardiac arrest) or neurologic (altered taste, paresthesias, agitation, seizures) manifestations, or both. Lastly, keep in mind that several other commonly used household products include salicylates, including oil of wintergreen, antiseptic mouthwashes, and bismuth subsalicylate (ie, Pepto-Bismol). Ingesting as little as 5 mL of wintergreen oil can be fatal in a child.

> **Helpful Tip**
> The use of aspirin in children has been associated with Reye syndrome, a potentially lethal condition that can result in numerous symptoms, including fatty liver, hyperreflexia, cerebral edema, and multiorgan failure. The AAP advises against the use of aspirin in febrile illnesses for patients younger than 19 years old. The unintentional ingestion of aspirin by children has also dropped as a result of decreasing the dose of chewable, flavored aspirin tablets to 81 mg, limiting the number of tablets per bottle to 36, and emphasizing child-resistant bottles.

You obtain a salicylate level on the patient. It is 35 mg/dL, within the range of mild to moderate toxicity.

Question 2-2

What should you utilize to guide your management now and moving forward?
A) Clinical symptoms.
B) Arterial blood gases (ABGs).
C) Actual salicylate level and its trend after treatment.
D) Done nomogram.
E) Rumack-Matthew nomogram.

Discussion 2-2

The correct answer is "A." The patient in this case is suffering from chronic salicylate toxicity rather than an acute exposure. This alters the utility of the Done nomogram, which is only useful in acute salicylate ingestions. Additionally, many have argued that this nomogram is of minimal clinical significance at best given that it does not predict the need for therapy. The actual salicylate level is of importance; however, it is less

important in chronic salicylate exposure and should not trump a patient's clinical symptoms. ABGs are beneficial and may be helpful in guiding some aspects of treatment, but this test is not more significant than the clinical presentation. Lastly, the Rumack-Matthew nomogram is germane to a different toxidrome (discussed later).

The results of her laboratory tests begin to return. She is found to have an anion gap metabolic acidosis and a pH of 7.1 on her ABGs.

Question 2-3

Given the patient's presentation, which treatment should you initiate for her salicylate toxicity?
A) Activated charcoal.
B) Intravenous sodium bicarbonate.
C) Acetazolamide.
D) Both A and B.
E) Both B and C.

Discussion 2-3

The correct answer is "D." This question is difficult given the chronic nature of the ingestion. However, it is still recommended that patients who have consumed salicylates be administered activated charcoal. Some authorities have advocated for multidose activated charcoal, but this remains controversial. Indications for urinary alkalization include a rising salicylate level, metabolic acidosis, and serum concentration greater than 30 mg/dL in acute ingestions. Sodium bicarbonate should be used to help enhance the elimination of the salicylate, in the process also alkalinizing the urine. Acetazolamide is contraindicated in salicylate ingestions as it causes the renal elimination of bicarbonate and a subsequent systemic metabolic acidosis. In general, forced diuresis in these patients should be avoided.

> **Helpful Tip**
> Salicylate poisoning causes a mixed metabolic acidosis and respiratory alkalosis.

Activated charcoal and repeated doses of sodium bicarbonate fail to improve the patient's clinical symptoms. In fact, she appears to be more lethargic upon reevaluation. Repeat laboratory analysis shows a worsening metabolic acidosis, an indication for hemodialysis.

Question 2-4

Which of the following is NOT an indication for hemodialysis in salicylate toxicity?
A) Central nervous system depression.
B) Acute heart failure.
C) Salicylate level greater than 40 mg/dL.
D) Coagulopathy.
E) Seizures.

Discussion 2-4

The correct answer is "C." Absolute salicylate levels do not determine the need for hemodialysis in isolation, unless the level is greater than 80 to 100 mg/dL in acute ingestions, greater than 50 to 60 mg/dL in chronic ingestions, or the level continues to rise despite treatment. The patient in this case is the victim of a chronic ingestion, as previously stated. Indications to pursue hemodialysis in salicylate toxicity include acute renal failure (acute kidney injury), congestive heart failure, pulmonary edema, altered mental status, coma, seizures, cerebral edema, and worsening metabolic acidosis or rising salicylate level despite the aforementioned interventions (eg, activated charcoal, sodium bicarbonate).

> **Helpful Tip**
> In salicylate toxicity, activated charcoal and sodium bicarbonate are the treatments of choice; hemodialysis can be considered in patients who do not respond to treatment and for specific indications (eg, seizures, coagulopathy).

> **Helpful Tip**
> Salicylate toxicity can be acute or chronic; consider common over-the-counter medications as potential culprits (eg, aspirin, mouthwashes, topical pain-relieving creams, etc). The Done nomogram is of limited clinical utility.

▶ CASE 3

A 2-year-old girl is brought into the emergency department by her mother after the patient was found playing with an open bottle of naproxen. For the preceding 45 minutes, the child had been playing with her siblings without direct supervision. The bottle had only recently been opened, and while it is not clear how many pills had been taken previously there are more than twelve 200 mg pills missing. You find pill residue in the child's mouth, but she is otherwise asymptomatic at this time.

Question 3-1

What initial intervention should be implemented?
A) Copious oral hydration.
B) Aggressive intravenous hydration.
C) Activated charcoal.
D) Gastric lavage.
E) No intervention is indicated at this time.

Discussion 3-1

The correct answer is "C." Enough evidence exists in this case to warrant prompt intervention. And while the time course and amount of naproxen (an NSAID) consumed is not precisely known, one should assume that it has been up to 45 minutes since the child ingested up to 2400 mg of the medication. Accordingly, activated charcoal is the initial treatment of choice. This intervention is indicated in children who consume more than 100 mg/kg or five adult doses of an NSAID. Presentation should generally be within 1 hour if administering activated charcoal. Gastric lavage has fallen out of favor and is no longer recommended given the associated risks (eg, aspiration) and relative dearth of evidence to support improved outcomes. Hydration (oral or otherwise) may aid in addressing sequelae of NSAID toxicity (ie, renal toxicity), but this is not the primary initial treatment needed.

Question 3-2

How much and how often should the activated charcoal be administered?
A) 1 to 2 g/kg up to 90 g orally, once.
B) 2 to 4 g/kg up to 200 g orally, once.
C) 1 to 2 g/kg up to 90 g orally, twice.
D) 2 to 4 g/kg up to 200 g orally, twice.
E) 3 g/kg up to 150 g orally, once.

Discussion 3-2

The correct answer is "A." The ideal dose of activated charcoal should not exceed 90 g. Given orally, the weight-based dose is 1 to 2 g/kg and it is typically administered as a slurry (sometimes mixed with sorbitol; premixed slurry formulations are commercially available). Multiple-dose activated charcoal (MDAC) may further decrease absorption rates. However, its efficacy has not been extensively studied, and it is not thought to result in significantly improved outcomes. (See Table 27–1.)

You call the Poison Control Center to review the patient's case, including her signs and symptoms of toxicity, laboratory evaluation, and acute management. You report that you have given activated charcoal. The Poison Control Center asks if the child is symptomatic.

TABLE 27–1 INDICATIONS AND CONTRAINDICATIONS FOR ADMINISTERING ACTIVATED CHARCOAL

Indications	Contraindications
Presentation within 1 hour of ingestion	Altered mental status (aspiration risk)
Ingestant absorbed by charcoal	Ingestant not absorbed by charcoal (eg, iron, alcohol, or lithium)
Ingestant is potentially toxic or may cause injury	Bowel obstruction or perforation
	Inability to protect airway (aspiration risk)

Question 3-3

Acute NSAID toxicity does NOT result in which of the following sequelae?
A) Aseptic meningitis.
B) Gastrointestinal hemorrhage.
C) Seizures.
D) Hypertension.
E) Hepatocellular injury.

Discussion 3-3

The correct answer is "D." NSAID toxicity typically results in hypotension rather than hypertension. Gastrointestinal symptoms are most common, including abdominal pain, vomiting, and diarrhea. Aseptic meningitis has been reported in cases secondary to hypersensitivity (along with asthma exacerbations). Gastrointestinal hemorrhage can result and is treated by standard means. Seizures have been associated with specific NSAID use, in particular piroxicam, naproxen, ketoprofen, and mefenamic acid. The treatment for such seizures involves the use of benzodiazepines. Lastly, liver function can be impaired as a result of excessive NSAID ingestion in addition to being associated with cholestasis. Acute kidney injury may occur.

> **Helpful Tip**
> Know your NSAIDs! There can be differences in the presentation among patients who present with specific NSAID ingestions (eg, naproxen can cause seizures.). It is not necessarily important to memorize these subtleties; however, it is important to identify which NSAID was consumed to anticipate potential clinical symptoms and prepare for possible subsequent treatment.

She has thrown up once but is otherwise doing well. You have ordered laboratory testing, and are waiting for the results. The mother asks if the child will have to spend the night in the hospital.

Question 3-4

In the setting of an asymptomatic patient with a normal laboratory evaluation, how long should the patient be observed?
A) No observation is needed.
B) 4 to 6 hours.
C) 8 to 12 hours.
D) 12 to 18 hours.
E) At least 24 hours.

Discussion 3-4

The correct answer is "B." Generally speaking, NSAID toxicity is relatively benign and symptoms typically develop within 4 hours of ingestion. Ingestions of 100 mg/kg or less are usually asymptomatic. Patients with normal laboratory tests—complete blood count (CBC) with differential, basic metabolic panel (including blood urea nitrogen [BUN], creatinine, and glucose), and a urinalysis at minimum—and no further symptoms should be observed for 4 to 6 hours to ensure no further development of symptoms or sequelae. Patients with abnormal laboratory tests should be admitted for further observation and supportive measures (eg, intravenous hydration) as appropriate. A nephrologist should be consulted in the setting of acute kidney injury.

⏳ QUICK QUIZ

Regarding NSAID toxicity, which of the following is true?
A) Generally, NSAIDs ingestions and overdoses are benign.
B) Patients who are otherwise asymptomatic may be safely discharged after 4 to 6 hours of observation.
C) Patients should be assessed for acute kidney injury, and if present a nephrologist should be consulted.
D) Gastrointestinal symptoms are the most common with NSAID toxicity.
E) All of the above.

Discussion

The correct answer is "E."

▶ CASE 4

A 17-year-old girl is brought into the emergency department by ambulance. She was found sleeping sonorously in her bedroom lying next to an empty bottle of acetaminophen. Her best friend contacted the patient's parents after seeing a social media post detailing the patient's breakup with her boyfriend. Upon arrival at the emergency department her vital signs are stable and she is arousable. The patient notes nausea and generalized malaise. She admits to consuming a large quantity of acetaminophen in an attempt to harm herself roughly 4 hours ago, but she is unsure of the number of pills ingested.

Question 4-1

Given the patient's presentation, what other symptoms might you expect to find with further probing or upon physical examination?
A) Right upper quadrant abdominal pain.
B) Emesis.
C) Spontaneous bleeding (eg, from the gums, ecchymosis).
D) Seizures.
E) Hypotension.

Discussion 4-1

The correct answer is "B." The patient is still in the early stages of acetaminophen toxicity, which typically entails nausea, vomiting, and malaise. These nonspecific symptoms mimic many other processes, which can lead to underappreciating the potential severity of illness if the proper historical points are not elicited (or provided for you, as in this case). Right upper quadrant pain and spontaneous bleeding can occur, although these findings develop further along in the course of acetaminophen ingestions. Seizures and hypotension are not typically associated with acetaminophen toxicity.

> **Helpful Tip**
> Remember that co-ingestion with other medications, including opioids and cold medications, is common in acetaminophen toxicity. In fact, there are more than 100 cold medications that contain acetaminophen. Be sure to consider, and treat when appropriate, these co-ingestions.

You remember that timing is important with acetaminophen ingestions and that symptoms depend on time elapsed since ingestion. The Poison Control Center mentioned that the progression of acetaminophen toxicity is generally described in phases.

Question 4-2

Which of the following pairings of phase timing with symptoms and laboratory abnormalities is INCORRECT?

A) Phase 1 (30 minutes to 24 hours postingestion) → nausea, vomiting, malaise.

B) Phase 2 (24 hours to 72 hours postingestion) → right upper quadrant pain, oliguria, elevated liver transaminases, prothrombin time (PT), and international normalized ratio of PT (INR).

C) Phase 3 (72 hours to 96 hours postingestion) → peak liver function testing abnormalities, acute liver and renal failure, jaundice.

D) Phase 4 (96 hours to 10 days postingestion) → hepatic encephalopathy.

E) All of the above are correct.

Discussion 4-2

The correct answer is "D." The phases and associated time courses are all paired correctly. However, hepatic encephalopathy is indicative of phase 3. At this stage if a patient's PT/INR continues to rise or renal insufficiency develops there is a high likelihood that hepatic transplantation may be necessary. Phase 4 brings with it either resolution of hepatic abnormalities or continued progression to complete hepatic failure and death. Here is an abbreviated version that may help keep the phases of acetaminophen toxicity straight.

Phase 1: mild symptoms (≤ 24 hours)

Phase 2: hepatoxicity and nephrotoxicity develop (1–3 days)

Phase 3: acute liver failure and acute kidney injury develop (3–4 days)

Phase 4: recovery or death from liver failure occurs (4–10 days)

Shortly after the patient's arrival you astutely ordered an acetaminophen level. Her 4-hour level returned at 150 mmol/L.

Question 4-3

How should you proceed, given this information?

A) Discharge the patient as her level is not hepatotoxic.

B) Observe the patient for an additional 4 hours.

C) Admit the patient for 24-hour observation.

D) Initiate medical management.

E) Prepare the patient for hemodialysis.

Discussion 4-3

The correct answer is "D." Ingestions of greater than 200 mg/kg or 10 g (whichever is less) are considered potentially toxic. The patient's initial acetaminophen level is in the "possibly hepatotoxic" range according to the Rumack-Matthew nomogram. (See Figure 27–1.) It is important to note that the acetaminophen level in cases of toxicity should be drawn at 4 hours postingestion or at presentation if the suspected ingestion was more than 4 hours prior. Acetaminophen levels before that point in time may warrant treatment if markedly elevated (an ominous sign), but a normal level prior to the 4-hour mark does not rule out acetaminophen overdose or the need for treatment. It is not appropriate to discharge this patient, and medical treatment should be initiated given the relatively high level so acutely. Hemodialysis is not indicated for the treatment of acetaminophen toxicity. (See Table 27–2.)

You astutely decide to initiate medical treatment for this patient. Well-trained, you recall that *N*-acetylcysteine (NAC) is the treatment of choice.

Question 4-4

Which route and loading dose should be utilized to administer this medication initially?

A) Oral; 140 mg/kg.

B) Oral; 70 mg/kg.

C) Intravenous; 140 mg/kg.

D) Nasogastric tube; 140 mg/kg.

E) Nasogastric tube; 70 mg/kg

Discussion 4-4

The correct answer is "A." The preferred initial route of administration of NAC is orally at a loading dose of 140 mg/kg. Often this medication is diluted in juices or soft drinks to facilitate consumption. The utilization of antiemetics (eg, ondansetron)

TABLE 27–2   INDICATIONS FOR TREATMENT OF ACUTE ACETAMINOPHEN TOXICITY

Acetaminophen level above the treatment line on Rumack-Matthew nomogram

Ingestion > 200 mg/kg or 10 g and acetaminophen level results not rapidly available

Unknown time of ingestion with detectable acetaminophen level

Unknown time of ingestion with elevated liver transaminases

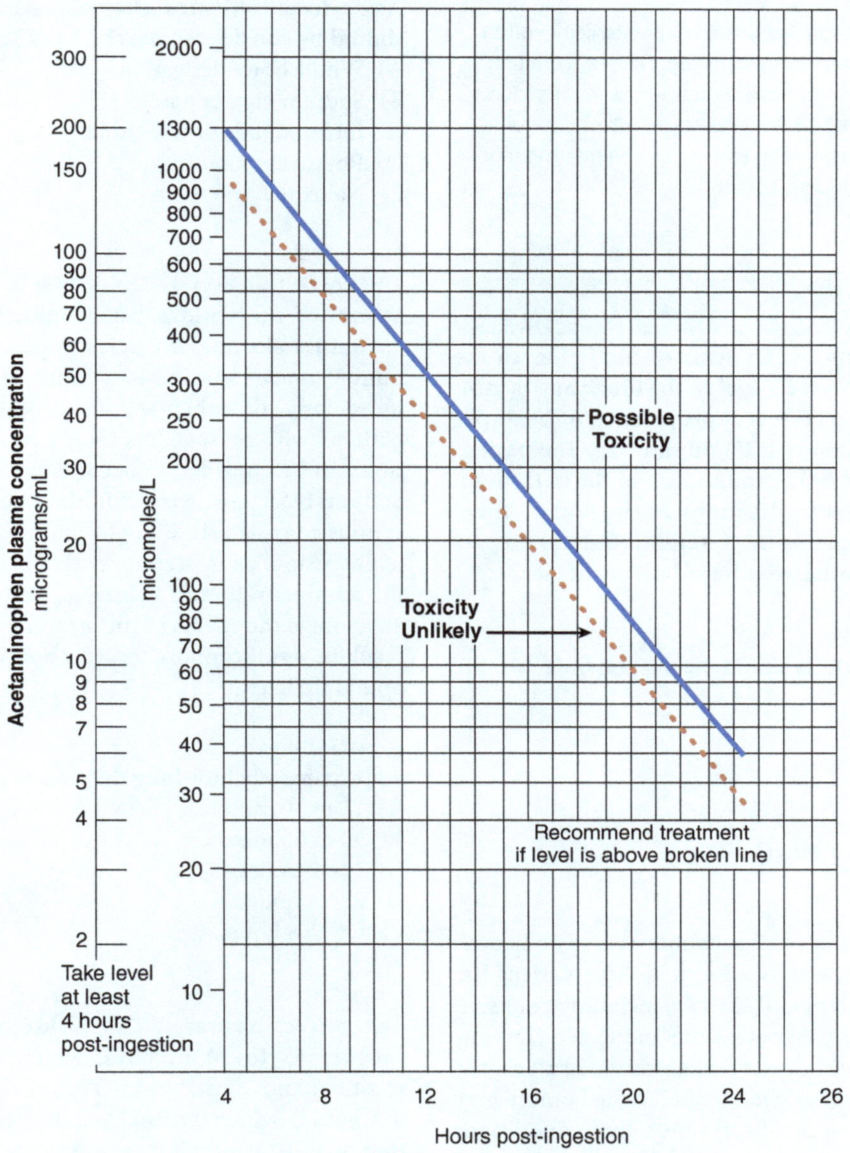

FIGURE 27–1. The Rumack-Matthew nomogram is used for assessing acetaminophen toxicity. Treatment is recommended for acetaminophen levels above the lower nomogram line (*broken line*). Serum levels obtained prior to 4 hours after ingestion are uninterpretable. (Reproduced with permission from Tintinalli JE, Stapczynski JS, Ma OJ, Yealy DM, Cline DM, Meckler GD, eds. *Tintinalli's Emergency Medicine: A Comprehensive Study Guide.* 8th ed. New York, NY: McGraw-Hill Education; 2016, Fig. 190-2.)

should be entertained to facilitate the administration of this medication. Since this patient is not actively vomiting, oral administration is the best answer. If the patient does happen to vomit up the NAC, an attempt to repeat the dose orally after giving an antiemetic should be pursued. Persistent vomiting is an indication to attempt administration by nasogastric tube. For patients who cannot tolerate either enteral routes, intravenous NAC can be given. The dosing of the intravenous medication is dictated by the package insert and can be guided by the Poison Control Center. Of note, once initiated NAC is then given orally every 4 hours at 70 mg/kg for 17 additional doses or until the patient's acetaminophen

level is nontoxic. Overall, when initiated within 8 hours of ingestion, NAC is 100% hepatoprotective. Activated charcoal should also be administered if the patient presents 2 hours or less after ingestion.

> **Helpful Tip**
>
> For acute acetaminophen ingestions, a serum level must be obtained 4 hours after ingestion. Normal levels before this time point do not rule out liver injury nor do they obviate the need for treatment.

Helpful Tip

Patients with acute acetaminophen toxicity often present with minimal symptoms (eg, nausea, vomiting, or malaise). Be sure to have a high index of suspicion. Utilize the Rumack-Matthew nomogram to help guide treatment decisions. *N*-acetylcysteine is the treatment of choice in acetaminophen toxicity.

► **CASE 5**

A 6-year-old boy presents in the arms of his father to the emergency department. He feels cool to the touch and is minimally responsive. His heart rate is appropriate at 65 beats per minute but his blood pressure is 70/30 mm Hg. The patient appears apneic. The boy's father found him in the bathroom. They have no prescription medications in the house. There are no signs of external trauma on the child, who has no past medical history and has otherwise been healthy of late.

Question 5-1

Which of these medications could be responsible for the patient's presentation?
A) Aspirin.
B) Ibuprofen.
C) Lomotil.
D) Acetaminophen.
E) Prenatal vitamins with iron.

Discussion 5-1

The correct answer is "C." Lomotil is a combination of diphenoxylate and atropine, which acts as an opioid. This patient has many signs consistent with opioid toxicity, including cool skin (suggestive of hypothermia), hypotension, and apnea (respiratory depression). One would expect a bradycardic heart rate as well; however, the atropine (anticholinergic) in the Lomotil may result in a normal or low-normal heart rate. Other typical signs of opiate overdose include pinpoint pupils (although this does not occur in this particular ingestion secondary to the effects of atropine), central nervous system depression, and palpitations. Aspirin overdoses should precipitate tachypnea. NSAID toxicity may appear similarly (very rarely), although signs of hypothermia are not present. These patients typically have a benign course and are much less likely to be this critically ill. Acetaminophen and iron ingestions primarily present with gastrointestinal manifestations.

Helpful Tip

Opioid ingestions can also result from narcotic prescriptions such as hydrocodone and oxycodone. Another consideration that should be considered is heroin. The use of heroin has been on the rise since 2007, in part because it has become more readily available and is a cheaper alternative to prescription narcotics.

Question 5-2

Aside from activated charcoal, what medical intervention should be considered next?
A) Whole bowel irrigation.
B) Sodium bicarbonate.
C) Intravenous normal saline.
D) Physostigmine.
E) Naloxone.

Discussion 5-2

The correct answer is "E." While a case could be made for several of the options listed, initially the most appropriate answer is naloxone, which is an opioid-antagonist. Effective in minutes, naloxone can be administered intravenously, intramuscularly, or subcutaneously. Whole bowel irrigation for patients who present less than 1 hour after an opioid ingestion can be considered, but it is not the treatment of choice. Sodium bicarbonate is not initially indicated, and while intravenous normal saline might be appropriate in the setting of hypotension, as is present in this case, it should not precede the administration of naloxone. Lastly, physostigmine would antagonize the effects of the atropine in Lomotil. Yet, this may result in significant bradycardia and would do nothing for the opioid toxicity itself.

Question 5-3

Approximately how long does naloxone have efficacy?
A) 15 to 30 minutes.
B) 30 to 60 minutes.
C) 1 to 2 hours.
D) 2 to 4 hours.
E) Up to 8 hours.

Discussion 5-3

The correct answer is "A." Naloxone remains effective for roughly 15 to 30 minutes, which can be problematic for most opioid ingestions. Typical opioid action can last for hours, which means that the usual dose for naloxone treatment (0.1 mg/kg/dose in infants and young children and 0.01 mg/kg/dose in neonates) may need to be repeated. With ingestions of long-acting opioids such as methadone, patients may require increased doses of naloxone, repeated doses, or even a continuous infusion. Absorption of the diphenoxylate is delayed owing to atropine-induced delayed gastric motility, which may cause prolonged or delayed symptoms (24 hours after ingestion).

Two hours into his evaluation the young boy stabilizes after the administration of several doses of naloxone and a bolus of normal saline. His vital signs return to normal, and his physical examination is unremarkable.

Question 5-4

What is this patient's disposition?
A) Pediatric consultation in the emergency department.
B) Observation for 2 additional hours.
C) Observation for 4 additional hours.

D) Admission for 24 hours.

E) Discharge to home promptly.

Discussion 5-4

The correct answer is "D." Owing to the prolonged half-life of diphenoxylate, particularly compared with the short half-life of naloxone, and prolonged symptoms from atropine-induced delayed gastric motility, 24-hour admission is recommended for all patients who require the administration of naloxone. Discharge before this period of observation leaves the patient vulnerable to a return of the initial symptoms secondary to opioid toxicity (eg, hypotension, central nervous system depression, apnea, etc). For other opioid ingestions, patients can be discharged if asymptomatic 6 hours after ingestion or if asymptomatic 4 hours after the administration of naloxone.

⏳ QUICK QUIZ

Which statement regarding opioid ingestion is false?

A) Naloxone should not be administered to neonates.

B) Symptoms of opioid toxicity commonly include hypotension, bradycardia, respiratory depression, miosis, hypothermia, and seizures.

C) Naloxone is the treatment of choice for opioid toxicity, but remember that the half-life of this medication is often shorter than that of the opioid ingested.

D) It is important to consider concomitant ingestions resulting from combination products (eg, hydrocodone-acetaminophen, etc).

E) Full opioid reversal in patients with opioid dependence may precipitate withdrawal.

Discussion

The correct answer is "A." Naloxone may be given to neonates. Are you NRP (neonatal resuscitation program) certified? The dose is 10 times less than that given to infants and young children.

> **Helpful Tip**
>
> Symptoms of opioid toxicity commonly include hypotension, bradycardia, respiratory depression, miosis, hypothermia, and seizures. Naloxone is the treatment of choice in such patients, but remember that the half-life of this medication is often shorter than that of the opioid ingested. Be sure to consider concomitant ingestions (eg, hydrocodone-acetaminophen, etc).

⏳ QUICK QUIZ

What is NOT a potential ingestant for which whole bowel irrigation should be considered?

A) Iron pills.

B) Lithium pills.

C) Sustained-release drugs.

D) Packages of cocaine.

E) Ibuprofen.

Discussion

The correct answer is "E." Others that should be considered include ingestions of enteric-coated pills, illicit drug packages, and other drugs not bound by charcoal, such as iron and lithium.

▶ CASE 6

An 8-year-old girl is on a camping trip with her mother. She returns from the woods, and her mother notices that she appears to be confused and tachypneic. The mother checks her pulse and it seems accelerated. You happen to be accompanying the group on this outing. After quickly evaluating the patient you suspect anticholinergic effects. Emergency services are called and an ambulance is dispatched to the camp to facilitate transportation for further medical care.

Question 6-1

Which symptom is NOT a part of the classic toxidrome associated with this child's presentation?

A) Dry as a bone.

B) Red as a beet.

C) Blind as a bat.

D) Cool as a cucumber.

E) Mad as a hatter.

Discussion 6-1

The correct answer is "D." The classic presentation of a patient with anticholinergic toxicity is mad as a hatter (altered mental status, hallucinations), hot as a hare (hyperthermia), red as a beet (flushed skin), dry as a bone (dry mucous membranes, skin, or both), blind as a bat (mydriasis-induced blurry vision), and full as a flask (urinary retention). Cool as a cucumber is the opposite physiologic response to an anticholinergic exposure.

> **Helpful Tip**
>
> Hyperthyroidism (eg, thyroid storm) may present clinically in a manner similar to anticholinergic toxicity.

Question 6-2

Which plant is NOT potentially responsible for her presentation?

A) Jimson weed.

B) Nightshade.

C) Mushrooms.

D) Belladonna.

E) Foxglove.

Discussion 6-2

The correct answer is "E." Foxglove is also known as *Digitalis purpurea*, and exposure to this plant can cause cardiac dysrhythmias, shock, cardiovascular collapse, agitation, lethargy, and gastrointestinal symptoms. However, foxglove does not precipitate a typical anticholinergic toxidrome. Each of the other options can precipitate anticholinergic toxicity. Regarding mushrooms, those with anticholinergic properties include *Amanita muscaria* and *Amanita pantherina*. Also, keep in mind that medications can result in an anticholinergic toxidrome as well. These medications include atropine, scopolamine, antihistamines (eg, diphenhydramine), cyclobenzaprine, and antispasmodics (eg, hyoscyamine).

Once the ambulance arrives the patient is placed on the cardiac monitor. Her vital signs show a normal temperature and blood pressure. Peering from the periphery, you observe the monitor closely. You find that she appears to have the most common cardiac monitor/ECG abnormality associated with anticholinergic toxicity.

Question 6-3

What is that finding?
A) Sinus tachycardia.
B) QRS prolongation.
C) Atrioventricular (AV) block.
D) Right bundle branch block.
E) Ventricular bigeminy.

Discussion 6-3

The correct answer is "A." ECG findings associated with anticholinergic exposure are generally nonspecific, in contrast to some other toxicities. Although each of the options listed can result, sinus tachycardia is the most common ECG finding.

Question 6-4

What is the treatment of choice for this patient?
A) Benzodiazepines.
B) Phenobarbital.
C) Aggressive intravenous hydration.
D) Physostigmine.
E) Sodium bicarbonate.

Discussion 6-4

The correct answer is "D." Depending on a patient's presenting symptoms, each of the aforementioned options may be appropriate. However, given this case the patient would benefit most from physostigmine. This medication reverses both the central and peripheral anticholinergic effects. It should be used with caution as it can cause dysrhythmias and cholinergic crises. Its use should be avoided in those with asthma, cardiovascular disease, or concurrent or suspected tricyclic antidepressant overdose. The pediatric dose is 0.02 mg/kg intravenously over 5 minutes. In the case of this patient, she has not had any

seizures, negating the use of benzodiazepines or phenobarbital. Nor is she hypotensive, and while intravenous hydration may be beneficial it will not directly address any active symptoms. Sodium bicarbonate is effective in some cardiac dysrhythmias, but one has not been identified in this case.

⧗ QUICK QUIZ

Which is NOT a symptom of a cholinergic crisis?
A) Diarrhea.
B) Drooling.
C) Urinary retention.
D) Sweating.
E) Pinpoint pupils.

Discussion

The correct answer is "C." The symptoms of cholinergic excess can be remembered using the mnemonic SLUD (**S**alivation, **L**acrimation, **U**rination, **D**iarrhea) or DUMBELS (**D**iarrhea, **U**rination, **M**iosis, **B**ronchospasm, **E**mesis, **L**acrimation, **S**weating).

▶ CASE 7

A group of rebellious teenagers conduct an unsupervised house party one evening. It is billed as a "pharm party" or "pill party" in which the guests bring prescription medications that are then combined into a large bowl. Adventurous party-goers can choose to sample random, unknown pills. Three of the patrons who engage in the festivities become ill. After the local authorities break up the soirée, the three patients needing medical attention are brought to your emergency department by ambulance for further evaluation and treatment. The EMS crew was able to ascertain that a preponderance of the medications collected at the party were antihypertensive medications. The first patient presents with a heart rate of 33 beats per minute and mild hypotension, and his bedside glucose level is 55 mg/dL. You astutely suspect that the patient is suffering from ill-effects related to a beta-blocker overdose.

Question 7-1

Which medication is NOT used in the management of such an ingestion?
A) Atropine.
B) Sodium bicarbonate.
C) Glucagon.
D) Insulin.
E) Inamrinone.

Discussion 7-1

The correct answer is "B." The initial treatment of choice in beta-blocker toxicity, particularly in the setting of bradycardia, hypotension, or both, is atropine (0.02 mg/kg/dose IV in the pediatric population) and intravenous fluids. Although its efficacy is not outstanding, it is recommended as a primary treatment modality. Glucagon (0.03–0.1 mg/kg as a bolus followed by 0.07 mg/kg/h as an infusion) should then be attempted if atropine is unsuccessful. Other medications such as insulin (which promotes improved myocardial metabolism) and inamrinone (a phosphodiesterase inhibitor with positive inotropic effect) can be attempted as well. Sodium bicarbonate may be effective in treating an arrhythmia secondary to beta-blocker toxicity, but it is not a primary treatment. Of note, another treatment option includes calcium gluconate or calcium chloride. These medications improve conduction, inotropy, and blood pressure.

The next party-goer to require your attention has a very similar presentation to the first patient. Although her heart rate is 33 beats per minutes and she is hypotensive, her blood glucose level is 178 mg/dL. The Poison Control Center is contacted, and it is suggested that the patient may have consumed a significant amount of a calcium channel blocker.

Question 7-2
Which strategy should be used to treat this patient?
A) Calcium gluconate bolus.
B) Calcium gluconate continuous infusion.
C) Calcium chloride bolus.
D) Calcium chloride continuous infusion.
E) Norepinephrine.

Discussion 7-2
The correct answer is "A." Calcium salts may be given for the treatment of calcium channel blocker overdose, but not all patients respond. Calcium chloride may cause tissue necrosis from extravasation and should be given through central venous access; therefore, calcium gluconate may be preferred. The ideal dose for the administration of calcium gluconate in the pediatric population is 60 mg/kg/dose, which may be repeated at the same dosage in 10 minutes, if necessary. Keep in mind that calcium channel blockers are notorious for refractory bradycardia and hypotension. If repeated doses of calcium gluconate are administered be sure to follow the patient's serum calcium levels or consider a continuous infusion, or both. Vasopressor infusions (eg, norepinephrine) may be beneficial in hypotensive patients. As with beta-blocker ingestion, glucagon, insulin with glucose, and atropine may be used.

Helpful Tip
Differentiating between beta-blocker overdoses and calcium channel overdoses can be very difficult as both cause bradycardia and hypotension. The patient's glucose level may provide additional insight to help delineate between the two. Beta-blockers cause hypoglycemia and calcium channel blockers cause hyperglycemia.

With treatment for the first two patients underway, you turn your attention toward patient #3. She too is bradycardic, but she is found to be hypertensive. Additionally, her breathing is quite slow, and her pupils are pinpoint. With stimulation her heart rate and breathing improve.

Question 7-3
What is the most likely causative antihypertensive agent for this presentation?
A) Diltiazem.
B) Hydrochlorothiazide.
C) Lisinopril.
D) Clonidine.
E) Metoprolol.

Discussion 7-3
The correct answer is "D." The patient presentation is similar to an opioid overdose with respiratory depression and miosis standing out among her symptoms. Clonidine is a centrally acting alpha$_2$-agonist, which mimics opioid effects. Generally, this medication first causes hypertension before its antihypertensive effects surface, sometimes up to 10 hours later. Children tend to be more affected by this medication than adults. Diltiazem is a calcium channel blocker that results in hypotension, whereas metoprolol is a beta-blocker that likewise leads to hypotension shortly after excessive ingestion. Hydrochlorothiazide is a loop diuretic that causes neither apnea nor miosis. As for lisinopril, this medication does have some activity on opioid receptors, but like loop diuretics it does not result in respiratory depression or miosis. Naloxone should be given if central nervous system or respiratory depression is present, but not all patients will respond.

Helpful Tip
Atropine is a good first treatment for symptomatic bradycardia, administered at 0.02 mg/kg/dose IV. It may buy you time to decide your next step.

▶ CASE 8

A 15-year-old male patient who had been diagnosed with postconcussive syndrome had previously been started on amitriptyline for symptoms associated with his concussion. Unable to participate in football, he developed worsening depression. He presents to the emergency department after admitting to consuming a "handful" of his 10 mg amitriptyline tablets. His vital signs are within normal limits, and he does not appear to be in any distress. You obtain a stat ECG upon the patient's arrival, which is shown below.

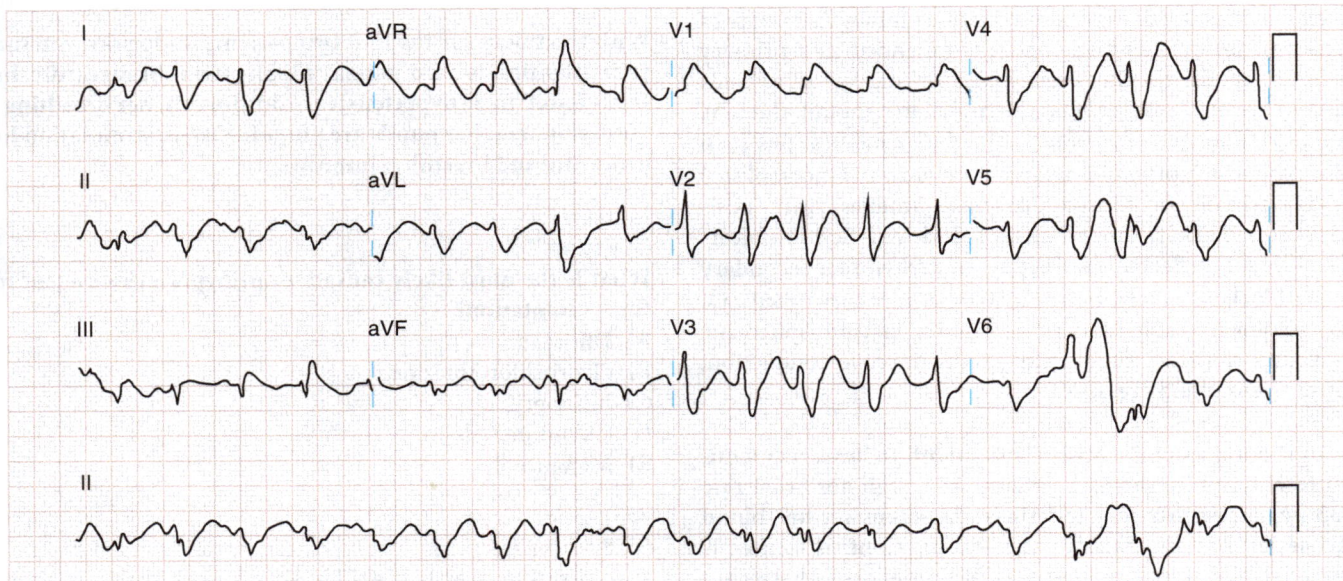

(Reproduced with permission from Life in the Fastlane.com. http://lifeinthefastlane.com/ecg-library/basics/tca-overdose/)

Question 8-1

Which of the following would you expect to find on the ECG of a patient with a tricyclic antidepressant overdose?
A) Sinus tachycardia.
B) QTc prolongation.
C) QRS complex widening.
D) Right bundle branch block.
E) All of the above.

Discussion 8-1

The correct answer is "E." QRS widening (> 100 msec) is a common initial finding associated with tricyclic antidepressant (TCA) overdoses. Due to blockade of sodium channels in the His-Purkinje system and myocardium, this ECG finding usually precedes bundle branch blocks. Tachycardia is almost always present at some point in a patient's course, but QRS widening is more concerning and dictates management moving forward. Prolongation of the PR interval, ST/T-wave changes, heart block, ventricular fibrillation or tachycardia, torsades de pointes, and asystole may occur as well.

Question 8-2

What is the initial treatment that should be initiated for this adolescent in the setting of a TCA overdose with QRS widening?
A) Epinephrine.
B) Procainamide.
C) Calcium chloride/calcium gluconate.
D) Sodium bicarbonate
E) Flumazenil.

Discussion 8-2

The correct answer is "D." Sodium bicarbonate is the most effective and initial treatment of choice for abolishing arrhythmias, shortening the QRS duration, and increasing blood pressure.

Bolus doses of 1 to 2 mEq/kg should be administered intravenously and repeated as needed. Epinephrine is generally not utilized in this context, with dopamine or norepinephrine preferred for cases of significant hypotension. Calcium chloride or calcium gluconate have no role in the management of TCA overdoses. Procainamide (increases myocardial toxicity) and flumazenil (increases risk of seizure) are contraindicated in such cases.

> **Helpful Tip**
>
> - TCAs block sodium and potassium channels, leading to increased cardiovascular toxicity. Other depressants (particularly new antidepressants such as citalopram) block amine reuptake and cause less life-threatening toxicity.
> - Look for QRS widening on ECG and treat with sodium bicarbonate.
> - Patients with symptoms after 6 hours of observation (including tachycardia), co-ingestions, dysrhythmias, or altered mental status warrant admission. Psychiatric evaluation may be necessary if a suicide attempt is suspected.

Once the sodium bicarbonate is ordered you reevaluate the patient. Clinically he appears to be deteriorating.

Question 8-3

Which symptom would you NOT expect relative to his TCA toxicity?
A) Hypotension.
B) Seizures.
C) Agitation.

D) Lethargy.
E) Bradycardia.

Discussion 8-3

The correct answer is "E." Bradycardia develops later in the course of TCA toxicity once a patient's catecholamines are depleted. Initially, patients exhibit tachycardia resulting from a blockade of norepinephrine and concomitant anticholinergic effects. The other options are all potential symptoms that can develop as a result of this poisoning. Hypotension may be refractory to initial treatment and require vasopressor support (norepinephrine). In fact, seizures can be particularly detrimental, as the associated acidemia that develops can worsen subsequent cardiovascular toxicity.

> **Helpful Tip**
> Do not let well-appearing patients with a suspected TCA ingestion fool you. They can deteriorate rapidly, developing significant cardiovascular compromise that necessitates emergent intervention.

The patient's clinical course continues to worsen, and he develops a tachydysrhythmia.

Question 8-4

With sodium bicarbonate already administered, what is the treatment of choice for this cardiac abnormality in the setting of a TCA overdose?
A) Lidocaine.
B) Metoprolol.
C) Procainamide.
D) Physostigmine.
E) Flecainide.

Discussion 8-4

The correct answer is "A." In general, antiarrhythmic drugs should be avoided. Lidocaine is the preferred second-line agent in the treatment of tachydysrhythmias in the setting of TCA toxicity. Metoprolol, a beta-blocker, will not affect sodium channels. Procainamide (a class 1A medication) and flecainide (a class 1C agent) are actually contraindicated, as they can result in a "quinidine-like" effect on the myocardium, increasing the toxicity of the TCA. Lastly, physostigmine is also contraindicated because of the risk of cardiac toxicity potentially deteriorating into asystole.

QUICK QUIZ

What is NOT a sign or symptom of TCA ingestion?
A) Hypertension.
B) Coma.
C) Blurred vision.
D) Seizure.
E) Heart block.

Discussion

The correct answer is "A." Tricyclics cause hypotension. The cardiovascular, central nervous system, and peripheral nervous system (anticholinergic effects) are affected by TCA ingestion. Do you remember mad as a hatter, hot as a hare, and blind as a bat? If not, you did not learn the signs and symptoms of anticholinergic toxicity discussed earlier. Remember, physostigmine should not be used to treat anticholinergic toxicity in the setting of a TCA ingestion.

> **Helpful Tip**
> Antidepressants other than tricyclics have different cardiovascular toxicity. For instance, selective serotonin reuptake inhibitors (SSRIs) have less cardiovascular toxicity in general and a wider margin for safety. Citalopram is the most cardiotoxic SSRI and may have delayed cardiovascular toxicity, generally more than 12 hours after ingestion.

► CASE 9

A 16-year-old boy and his best friend are brought into the emergency department by his mother very late at night. The mother states that the teens had attend an unsupervised party in the woods that night. You interview the son first, who stumbles as he walks from the door to the bed. He reports consuming beer for the first time. His vital signs reveal tachycardia (110 beats per minute) but are otherwise unremarkable. Upon examination his speech is a bit slurred, but he is able to follow commands appropriately.

Question 9-1

Which of the following is the least relevant question when evaluating this patient?
A) How much alcohol did you consume?
B) When did you eat last?
C) Have you fallen or sustained any additional trauma?
D) Did you take any other drugs or medications?
E) Do you have any other medical conditions?

Discussion 9-1

The correct answer is "B." Evaluating patients intoxicated with ethanol may appear mundane, particularly in patients who otherwise appear well. However, there are important questions that should be asked to rule out more significant pathology. For instance, one should take care to investigate whether the amount of alcohol consumed roughly correlates with the clinical presentation. If this patient had only consumed one can of beer but was slurring his speech and was tachycardic, an investigation for other causes of his symptoms should be entertained. A traumatic fall can be the cause of such a presentation or the sequela from alcohol intoxication. Concomitant medical conditions (eg, diabetes mellitus) can also affect the presentation of these patients. Additionally, it is critically important to inquire about the ingestion of other medications or illicit substances. Alcohol intoxication can mask the toxicity of other medications, particularly in severely intoxicated patients. Although it may affect the rate of clearance, the last meal consumed is of far less clinical significance.

The patient admits to consuming four cans of beer in less than an hour. His physical examination reveals no other significant abnormalities, including signs of trauma. You elect to obtain a plasma ethanol level, which registers 150 mg/dL.

Question 9-2

What treatment should be initiated?
A) An intravenous bolus of normal saline.
B) Thiamine, folate, and a multivitamin.
C) Glucose.
D) Activated charcoal.
E) None; observe the patient.

Discussion 9-2

The correct answer is "E." Patients with ethanol intoxication and no co-ingestions warrant observation and supportive measures if needed. They may benefit from antiemetics and hydration, but this is not necessary in all, or even most, patients. If the patient can tolerate oral hydration and it is safe to do so, this intervention should be attempted first. The administration of thiamine, folate, and a multivitamin are typically reserved for malnourished patients who consume the bulk of their daily caloric intake from alcohol. Glucose may be warranted in patients who develop hypoglycemia from severe alcohol intoxication, although this is not evident in this case. Lastly, patients may benefit from gastric decontamination (activated charcoal) with co-ingestions but not as a rule for isolated ethanol ingestions. Remember alcohols (ethanol, methanol, ethylene glycol) are rapidly absorbed and do not bind to charcoal. Knowing the patient's alcohol level can help predict how long it will take for metabolism of the alcohol (serum level of 0). The ethanol level typically decreases by 15 mg/dL/h in a nonalcoholic patient. The level for the adolescent described in this case should be 0 in 10 hours.

While you were treating the first patient your colleague was attending to his friend. He asks for your thoughts on the case. Apparently, this patient did not consume beer; he was handed a bottle of "moonshine" at the party. The patient has no idea how much "moonshine" he consumed, but after his maiden voyage into the world of alcohol consumption he is rethinking his decision to drink it. The patient reports significant nausea with four associated bouts of nonbilious, nonbloody emesis. His abdomen is diffusely painful, and his vision is blurry.

Question 9-3

What do you suspect to be the cause of his presentation?
A) Ethanol.
B) Ethylene glycol.

C) Methanol.
D) Isopropyl alcohol.
E) Glycerol.

Discussion 9-3

The correct answer is "C." The patient's presentation, particularly the blurry vision, should significantly raise your suspicion for methanol toxicity, which can be found in "moonshine." Often there is an 8- to 30-hour latent period that can exist before the onset of symptoms, but this is not always the case. A normal eye examination may be present initially, but as formic acid (a methanol metabolite) accumulates, it can have direct toxic effects on the retina and optic nerve. A funduscopic examination may reveal hyperemia of the disc, papilledema, or optic neuropathy.

Question 9-4

Given the apparent methanol toxicity, which laboratory testing (or associated value) will not be beneficial in managing this patient's presentation?
A) Urinalysis.
B) Serum anion gap.
C) Serum osmolar gap.
D) Ethanol level.
E) Methanol level.

Discussion 9-4

The correct answer is "A." A urinalysis is not likely to add anything to the treatment of this patient. Calculating the anion gap, which is $(Na^+) - (Cl^- + HCO_3^-)$, can help confirm an anion gap metabolic acidosis, which is present in methanol poisonings. The osmolar gap equals the measured osmolarity minus the calculated osmolarity. A normal value is −7 to 10 mOsm. A widened serum osmolar gap, or $(2*Na^+) + (BUN/2.8) + (Glucose/18) + (EtOH/4.6)$, also helps confirm methanol toxicity. However, a low or negative osmolar gap does not completely rule out a methanol ingestion (or another toxic alcohol ingestion). The ethanol level can be useful not only in calculating the osmolar gap but also in guiding treatment. Lastly, methanol concentrations do confirm the presence of methanol. But, if a patient's presentation is late, the methanol concentration may be normal due to the formation of the associated toxic metabolites (ie, formaldehyde and formic acid). Formaldehyde is metabolized to formic acid, which is primarily responsible for toxicity. In these cases a high anion gap metabolic acidosis should be present.

> **Helpful Tip**
> The mnemonic ME DIE A is helpful in recalling the substances that can cause an increased osmolar gap:
>
> **M** – Methanol **D** – Diuretics/Diluents **A** – Acetone,
> **E** – Ethanol (eg, mannitol, sorbitol) ammonia
>   **I** – Isopropyl alcohol
>   **E** – Ethylene glycol

The patient has both an anion and osmolar gap; a methanol level is pending. You decide to initiate treatment for this patient.

Question 9-5

What medication(s) is/are appropriate for methanol ingestions?
A) Fomepizole (4-methylpyrazole [4-MP]).
B) Ethanol.
C) Activated charcoal.
D) Both A and B.
E) Both A and C.

Discussion 9-5

The correct answer is "D." Methanol toxicity results from its metabolites (formic acid) rather than the parent alcohol. Methanol is primarily metabolized by alcohol dehydrogenase. Fomepizole and ethanol are appropriate treatments for methanol overdoses. Fomepizole works by inhibiting alcohol dehydrogenase and is FDA-approved for methanol ingestions. Its indications include an accidental ingestion of methanol (even a sip), intentional methanol ingestion, and altered mental status or visual symptoms with an otherwise unexplained osmolar gap or anion gap metabolic acidosis. This medication should be administered in these contexts even before a methanol level has returned. Ethanol has a higher affinity for alcohol dehydrogenase than methanol, thereby slowing the production of form-aldehyde and formic acid. While not FDA-approved, it is still an appropriate treatment either orally or intravenously. Serum ethanol levels must be followed when administering ethanol, with a target range of 100 to 150 mg/dL. Activated charcoal does not absorb methanol, and it has no role in methanol ingestions. Additionally, since methanol is rapidly absorbed, gastric lavage is not likely to be beneficial. Dialysis rapidly clears methanol and its metabolites and may be needed in cases of severe toxicity.

> **Helpful Tip**
> Enhanced elimination via dialysis may be used to treat methanol, ethylene glycol, lithium, theophylline, and salicylate toxicity.

> **Helpful Tip**
> • Ethanol toxicity is generally treated with supportive measures, but be certain to evaluate for co-ingestions, signs of trauma, or other comorbid medical conditions.
> • Methanol is metabolized to formaldehyde and formic acid, which directly affect the retina and optic nerve. Be sure to perform a funduscopic examination.
> • The anion and osmolar gap calculations in possible methanol ingestions are quite beneficial in confirming the diagnosis and guiding treatment.
> • The use of fomepizole or ethanol, or both, is indicated for methanol ingestions.

▶ CASE 10

A 3-year-old boy is brought into the emergency department after his father found him with a bottle of antifreeze. The liquid had been spilled on the ground surrounding the child. The child's clothes are stained and his breath smells sweet. He has vomited twice and is sleepy. On exam, he is somnolent but arousable. His gait is ataxic.

Question 10-1

Which is expected to be seen on laboratory testing?
A) Anion gap metabolic acidosis.
B) Elevated serum osmolar gap.
C) Hypocalcemia.
D) Elevated creatinine.
E) All of the above.

Discussion 10-1

The correct answer is "E." Ethylene glycol is found in antifreeze. Ethylene glycol and methanol both may be found in de-icing solutions, windshield wiper fluid, and industrial solvents. Often the toxic alcohol is present in high concentrations. Toddlers may ingest ethylene glycol due to its sweet taste. Ethylene glycol is metabolized to glycoaldehyde, glycolic acid, glyoxylic acid (glycolate), and oxalic acid. The latter two are responsible for toxicity. Mild toxicity presents similar to intoxication from ethanol, with central nervous system depression, ataxia, nausea, and vomiting. Severe toxicity may cause acute kidney injury, seizures, coma, and cerebral edema. Similar to methanol, ethylene glycol causes an anion gap metabolic acidosis and elevated osmolar gap, but hypocalcemia and elevated creatinine are unique to ethylene glycol ingestion.

Question 10-2

What organ is targeted by the toxic metabolites of ethylene glycol?
A) Retina.
B) Liver.
C) Heart.
D) Kidney.
E) Muscle.

Discussion 10-2

The correct answer is "D." Oxalic acid combines with calcium, causing hypocalcemia and the formation of calcium oxalate crystals. Glycolate-induced renal tubule damage and precipitation of calcium oxalate crystals cause acute kidney injury. Treatment of ethylene glycol ingestion is the same as that for methanol ingestion: fomepizole, ethanol, dialysis, or a combination of these measures. Dialysis removes the toxic alcohol and its metabolites as well as fomepizole and ethanol; therefore, dosing should be increased for both.

⏳ QUICK QUIZ

Which of the following is true regarding alcohol ingestion?
A) Methanol is metabolized to glycolate.
B) Fomepizole is used in the treatment of methanol and ethylene glycol ingestions.
C) Ethylene glycol metabolites are toxic to the retina and optic nerve, so a funduscopic exam should be performed in cases of ingestion.
D) Methanol and ethylene glycol ingestion causes a nonanion gap metabolic acidosis.
E) Ethylene glycol ingestion always requires dialysis.

Discussion

The correct answer is "B." Ethylene glycol is metabolized to glycolate and is toxic to the kidneys. Methanol is metabolized to formic acid and is toxic to the retina and optic nerve. Fomepizole or ethanol are used as treatment, but dialysis may be required for some ingestions of methanol or ethylene glycol. Ingestion causes an anion gap metabolic acidosis and increased osmolar gap.

▶ CASE 11

A 14-year-old boy is brought into the emergency department after his father caught him hovering over a substance that the family had been using to thin paint as they remodel their home. The patient is clearly euphoric, singing and skipping about the room. A strong aromatic presence is found on the patient (including his breath). His vital signs reveal mild tachycardia. The patient's only physical examination finding is diffuse wheezing.

Question 11-1

Which question is least relevant in evaluating this patient?
A) What was the specific product around which he was found?
B) Have you ever done this in the past?
C) How much of the substance was used or how many times did you use the substance?

D) How did you come into contact with the substance—ingestion, inhalation, or another way?
E) What was the intent behind using the substance?

Discussion 11-1

The correct answer is "B." The patient's past exposure to this substance does not alter his management moving forward, as it does not suggest an increased risk of an adverse outcome. However, the other questions do further the evaluation of this patient. Obtaining as many details as possible about the product in question helps guide your potential intervention and can aid the Poison Control Center in making recommendations. The amount of the exposure to the substance can also suggest the extent of toxicity. Additionally, being aware of the manner in which the substance was consumed can provide insight into the organ systems most likely to be affected. Lastly, being cognizant of whether the patient intended harm to himself has a significant impact on the disposition of the patient.

After further inquiry, you ascertain that the patient had been huffing (inhaling a substance from a soaked rag) xylene, a hydrocarbon substance commonly used for thinning paint. Additionally, he states that he inadvertently swallowed some of the substance during his hijinks. Your further evaluation, particularly in the setting of his wheezing, includes obtaining a chest X-ray.

Question 11-2

All of the following findings can be seen in hydrocarbon inhalation EXCEPT:
A) Bibasilar or perihilar infiltrates, or both.
B) Lobar consolidation.
C) Pneumomediastinum.
D) Pleural effusion.
E) Tension pneumothorax.

Discussion 11-2

The correct answer is "E." Hydrocarbons are commonly found around the home and encompass a range of products (eg, paint thinners, lamp oil, kerosene) that can be inhaled, ingested, or both. (See Table 27–3.) The most common chest X-ray finding

TABLE 27–3 COMMON HOUSEHOLD PRODUCTS THAT CONTAIN HYDROCARBONS				
Aliphatic	**Aromatic**	**Alicyclic**	**Halogenated**	**Essential Oils**
Methane	Benzene	Pine oil (Pine Sol)	Chloroform	Camphor
Butane	Toluene	Turpentine	Methylene chloride	Cinnamon
Gasoline	Xylene		Pine oil (Pine Sol)	Clove oil
Kerosene				Eucalyptus
Mineral seal oil (furniture polish)				Pennyroyal
Paraffin wax				Peppermint
Propane				
Tar				

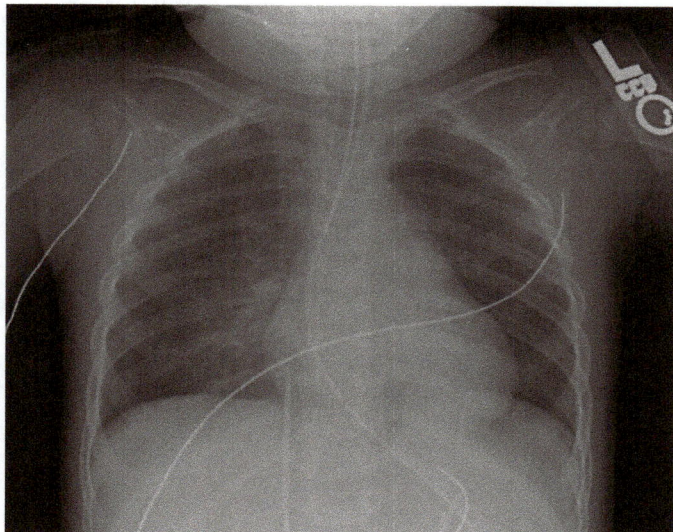

FIGURE 27–2. Hydrocarbon aspiration pneumonitis. A pediatric chest X-ray that reveals perihilar and bibasilar infiltrates, as can be seen in hydrocarbon aspiration pneumonitis. (Reproduced with permission from Tintinalli JE, Stapczynski JS, Ma OJ, Yealy DM, Cline DM, Meckler GD, eds. *Tintinalli's Emergency Medicine: A Comprehensive Study Guide.* 8th ed. New York, NY: McGraw-Hill Education; 2016, Fig. 199-1B.)

associated with hydrocarbon aspiration is increased bronchovascular markings and bibasilar or perihilar infiltrates, or both. (See Figure 27–2.) These abnormalities can actually arise as quickly as 20 minutes postexposure or be delayed by hours. Other chest X-ray abnormalities associated with hydrocarbon inhalation include lobar consolidation (which is uncommon) along with pneumomediastinum and pleural effusions (which are both rare). Tension pneumothorax is not associated with hydrocarbon exposure.

Question 11-3
In an attempt to treat this patient's xylene exposure, which of the following measures should be initiated?
A) Nasogastric aspiration.
B) Activated charcoal.
C) Corticosteroids.
D) Sodium bicarbonate.
E) Epinephrine.

Discussion 11-3
The correct answer is "A." Aromatic hydrocarbons are among those substances that respond to small-bore nasogastric tube aspiration. The CHAMP mnemonic can aid in remembering when nasogastric aspiration is indicated: **C**amphor, **H**alogenated hydrocarbons, **A**romatic hydrocarbons, **M**etals (eg, mercury and lead), and **P**esticides. Before implementing this treatment, be sure to consider the risk of aspiration. Activated charcoal is not likely to be effective in the current setting. Corticosteroids might be considered because of the patient's wheezing, but they do not have an appreciable effect on the hydrocarbon itself. Sodium bicarbonate does not have a role in the management of hydrocarbon toxicity. Lastly, epinephrine (which could otherwise be considered in the setting of bronchospasm) should be

avoided, particularly in aromatic hydrocarbon exposure. This medication sensitizes the myocardium and can lead to potentially lethal dysrhythmias.

This 14-year-old boy will require admission secondary to his pulmonary symptoms and abnormal chest X-ray, among other indications. Not all patients with hydrocarbon exposure require admission.

Question 11-4
Which is NOT an appropriate criterion for discharge?
A) Symptomatic patient who quickly becomes asymptomatic.
B) Asymptomatic patient with an abnormal chest X-ray.
C) Patient observed for 2 hours without symptoms.
D) Patient without evidence of intent to harm self.
E) Asymptomatic patient with a normal chest X-ray and normal pulse oximetry.

Discussion 11-4
The correct answer is "C." Patients should be observed for at least 6 hours following hydrocarbon exposure. If asymptomatic at that time patients can be discharged to home. This even applies in the setting of an asymptomatic patient with an abnormal chest X-ray provided that his or her vital signs are normal. It is imperative, however, that this type of patient have reliable follow-up. Barring other abnormalities during the evaluation, symptomatic patients who quickly become asymptomatic (without intervention) are considered appropriate for discharge, as are patients who have remained asymptomatic with a normal chest X-ray and vital signs. Finally, prior to discharge it is important to ensure that the patient is not a threat to himself or herself.

The patient recovers while hospitalized but no one on the health care team has addressed his "huffing" habit. You talk to the patient about the dangers of hydrocarbon inhalation.

Question 11-5
Which of the following will you tell him?
A) Use may result in irreversible brain damage.
B) He is at risk for sudden death.
C) He may develop an erythematous rash on his face.
D) Both A and B.
E) All of the above.

Discussion 11-5
The correct answer is "E." Hydrocarbons are intentionally inhaled as a means to "get high" and may be a gateway drug to other illicit substances. They are cheap, legal, and readily available. The practice may be called huffing, bagging, or sniffing. Onset of effect is rapid (seconds) but the duration is short (15 to 45 minutes). An eczema-like rash ("glue-sniffers rash") may develop around the mouth and on the face due to the drying effect of hydrocarbons. Sudden cardiovascular collapse and death (sudden sniffing death) are rare but may occur. Long-term use may result in permanent brain damage, including cognitive impairment, neuropathy, and cerebellar dysfunction.

Helpful Tip

- Hydrocarbons are commonly found around the home and encompass a range of products that can be inhaled, ingested, or both.
- Obtain a chest X-ray as a component of the evaluation for hydrocarbon exposure, looking for bibasilar and perihilar infiltrates as the most common findings.
- Supportive care is generally the treatment of choice for hydrocarbon toxicity, although nasogastric aspiration should be considered for certain subclasses (eg, halogenated and aromatic hydrocarbons).

▶ CASE 12

A 9-year-old girl is brought in after picking a handful of purple bell-shaped flowers. She has thrown up twice and states that her vision is blurry, and she feels weak. Her heart rate is 32 beats per minute.

Question 12-1

What is the cause of her presentation?
A) Jimson weed.
B) Poinsettia.
C) Foxglove.
D) Lilac.
E) Petunia.

Discussion 12-1

The correct answer is "C." Foxglove (*Digitalis purpurea*), along with lily-of-the-valley and oleander, contains cardiac glycosides and can produce a digitalis effect. The patient classically presents with weakness, syncope, visual changes, nausea, vomiting, anorexia, confusion, and bradycardia. Toxicity results in multiple different arrhythmias. Hyperkalemia can occur as well. Treatment entails activated charcoal. Digibind (digoxin-specific antibody Fab fragments) is the specific antidote, which is indicated in patients with cardiovascular collapse, a potassium level greater than 5.5 mEq/L, or life-threatening arrhythmias. Toxicity does not always correlate with the serum digitalis level. Jimson weed produces anticholinergic effects, including tachycardia. Poinsettia toxicity is less severe than once thought, with mild gastrointestinal discomfort as the primary symptom. Lilac and petunia plants are nontoxic. It has been speculated that Vincent van Gogh suffered from digitalis toxicity, as his paintings appear to contain haloes and primarily yellow hues similar to those occurring from toxicity-induced glaucoma and xanthopsia (objects appear to have a yellow hue).

▶ CASE 13

An adventurous 2-year-old boy was brought in by a home daycare provider. She reports that the child had been playing in the garden when he developed watery eyes, began drooling, and appeared sweaty. She states that he has been teething, but this amount of drooling seemed excessive. Additionally, the child had a couple of bouts of profusely runny diarrhea. Although a couple of other kids at the daycare recently had a viral gastroenteritis, the acute onset of this symptom appeared abnormal to her. Thus, she brought him into your clinic to have the boy evaluated. Further inquiry reveals there are no unusual plants or vegetables in the garden. However, you learn that it was recently treated with an unspecified insecticide. You immediately suspect organophosphate exposure.

Question 13-1

Other classic symptoms that you might expect in this patient include all of the following EXCEPT:
A) Mydriasis.
B) Bradycardia.
C) Emesis.
D) Bronchospasm.
E) Increased urination.

Discussion 13-1

The correct answer is "A." This is the classic presentation of cholinergic toxicity, which can be seen in organophosphate exposure from insecticides, pesticides, and chemical nerve agents (sarin, VX gas), and is perhaps best remembered with the DUMBELS mnemonic:

D – Diarrhea, diaphoresis

U – Urination

M –Miosis, muscle fasciculations

B – Bradycardia, bronchorrhea, bronchospasm

E – Emesis

L – Lacrimation

S – Salivation

In this case, one might expect the patient to have pinpoint pupils (miosis) as opposed to dilated pupils (mydriasis). It is also important to remember that seizures can occur in up to 25% of cases of pediatric organophosphate toxicity (compared with 3% of adult exposures). Ingestion of wild mushrooms containing muscarine (toxin) can also result in cholinergic toxicity. Organophosphates inhibit acetylcholinesterase, resulting in excess acetylcholine and increased postsynaptic receptor stimulation in the parasympathetic nervous system (muscarinic) and at the neuromuscular junction (nicotinic). Muscarine binds directly to acetylcholine postsynaptic receptors of the parasympathetic nervous system.

Helpful Tip
Symptoms of the cholinergic toxidrome in toddlers can be very difficult to differentiate. For instance, increased urination can be difficult to gauge at times, as can increased salivation. Have a low index of suspicion when the clinical context suggests possible exposure or even access to organophosphates.

Question 13-2

When evaluating this patient, which of the following laboratory testing is essential in guiding the treatment course?
A) Plasma acetylcholinesterase level.
B) ABGs.
C) CBC with differential.
D) Basic metabolic and electrolyte panel.
E) None of the above.

Discussion 13-2

The correct answer is "E." Although the plasma acetylcholinesterase level will help confirm the diagnosis, one should not wait for this result nor is it necessary before initiating treatment. Institute treatment based on the clinical presentation and index of suspicion. The other laboratory tests may assist in evaluating for concomitant end-organ damage and subsequent response to treatment, but they do not provide additional insight into when treatment should be initiated either.

A plasma acetylcholinesterase level is ordered from the laboratory, but it will be quite some time before it returns. You astutely elect to initiate treatment for this young boy.

Question 13-3

What medication is the treatment of choice for organophosphate toxicity?
A) Atropine.
B) Pralidoxime (2-PAM).
C) Epinephrine.
D) Either A or B.
E) Either A or C.

Discussion 13-3

The correct answer is "D." Appropriate treatments for the cholinergic toxidrome include both atropine and pralidoxime. Atropine, at a dose of 0.05 to 0.2 mg/kg, blocks acetylcholine at the muscarinic receptor sites and works within 1 to 4 minutes. Pralidoxime (2-PAM), regenerates cholinesterase by reversing the phosphorylation of the enzyme reversing neuromuscular blockade (nicotinic receptors). It has a synergistic effect with atropine, and symptoms generally start to resolve within 10 to 40 minutes. The dose of 2-PAM is 25 to 50 mg/kg. These medications can be given until muscarinic findings subside, but be wary of using pupillary response as the only indicator of treatment efficacy. Epinephrine does not have a role in such cases. Benzodiazepines may be used to treat seizures.

Question 13-4

In addition to initiating the appropriate antidote therapy, all of the following treatment interventions should be strongly considered in organophosphate toxicity EXCEPT:
A) Decontamination and removal of clothing.
B) Frequent suctioning.
C) Intravenous hydration.
D) Naloxone.
E) Sodium bicarbonate.

Discussion 13-4

The correct answer is "E." One of the most important aspects of managing a patient with an organophosphate exposure is to remove the clothing from the patient and consider a shower if it is possible. Failure to do so can lead to persistent symptoms (cutaneous absorption) even in the face of appropriate therapy. Intravenous hydration should be considered as symptoms necessitate, and naloxone may be warranted in situations when a patient is altered with a question as to the cause. (See Table 27–4.) Frequent suctioning can be very beneficial in significant exposures, particularly until the atropine aids in drying up the secretions. Sodium bicarbonate does not have a significant role in the management of these cases.

> **Helpful Tip**
> In organophosphate poisoning, treatment including atropine and pralidoxime (2-PAM) should be initiated based on the clinical presentation as opposed to waiting for a plasma acetylcholinesterase level.

TABLE 27–4 ANTIDOTES AND INGESTANTS

Ingestant/Toxicant	Antidote
Salicylate	None
Nonsteroid anti-inflammatory drugs (NSAIDs)	None
Acetaminophen	*N*-acetylcysteine (NAC)
Tricyclic antidepressants	None
Iron	Deferoxamine
Lithium	None
Selective serotonin reuptake inhibitors (SSRIs)	None
Diphenhydramine	Physostigmine
Opioids / narcotics	Naloxone
Insulin	Glucagon
	Dextrose
Sulfonylureas	Octreotide
Benzodiazepines	Flumazenil
Organophosphates	Atropine
Heparin	Protamine
	Fresh frozen plasma
Warfarin	Vitamin K
	Fresh frozen plasma
Beta-blocker	Glucagon
Carbon monoxide	Hyperbaric oxygen
Ethylene glycol/Methanol	Fomepizole and Ethanol

► CASE 14

On a very cold winter night a 5-year-old boy is brought into the emergency department by his parents. They report that he woke them up complaining of feeling sick to his stomach and having a significant headache. When they tried to walk him back to his room, he stumbled into a wall. These symptoms concerned the parents enough to seek medical intervention. The boy had otherwise been healthy recently. On arrival, his vital signs reveal tachycardia to 115 beats per minute, tachypnea at 20 respirations per minute, and a normal pulse oximetry reading of 98%.

Question 14-1

Pertinent additional questions related to this patient's presentation include all of the following EXCEPT:

A) Does anyone in the home have similar symptoms or otherwise feel ill?
B) Have you noticed any issues with your furnace recently?
C) Has the child or family recently taken a long trip?
D) Does the child have a space heater or other source of supplemental heat in the room?
E) Do you have any pets?

Discussion 14-1

The correct answer is "C." The presentation of this patient is concerning for carbon monoxide poisoning. Carbon monoxide is an odorless, tasteless gas. Poisoning may result from smoke inhalation (eg, house fire), malfunctioning furnaces, poor ventilation when using a fuel-burning device (eg, heaters, charcoal grills, generators), or running vehicle engines in enclosed spaces. The symptoms of this toxicity can be subtle and nonspecific, including headache, dizziness, ataxia, confusion, nausea, vomiting, and dyspnea. Thus, gathering additional information about possible sources or other affected individuals and pets can be exceptionally valuable. Be sure to ask whether anyone else in the home has symptoms, including pets. Asking about the status of the furnace (eg, "Has your furnace been serviced recently?"; "How old is your home or furnace?") can provide valuable insight. Sources of supplemental heat can result in carbon monoxide toxicity and should be considered. A patient's recent travel history is not germane to the evaluation of possible carbon monoxide poisoning. Cherry red lips and nail beds are useful when present but frequently are absent.

> **Helpful Tip**
> Furnaces, space heaters, fires, and automobile exhaust are all commonly considered as potential causes of carbon monoxide poisoning, but remember that substances containing methylene chloride (eg, paint removers, furniture strippers) can also cause carbon monoxide toxicity.

Upon further questioning you learn that everyone in the home feels well. However, the patient has been using a space heater in his room because of a recent cold snap.

Question 14-2

What laboratory testing should be obtained to help confirm the diagnosis while you initiate treatment?

A) CBC with differential.
B) Basic metabolic panel.
C) ABGs.
D) Carboxyhemoglobin level (COHb).
E) No testing is required; pulse oximetry is all that is needed to guide management of this patient.

Discussion 14-2

The correct answer is "D." The COHb, measured by co-oximetry of a blood sample, is vital in the management of this patient. Although the value of this test may be deceptive at times (eg, not markedly elevated despite the patient being critically ill, or unexpectedly low if a significant amount of time has passed) and may not correlate with the severity of poisoning, it is the first test that should be obtained when carbon monoxide exposure is expected. Normal values tend to be elevated to approximately 3%, although patients who smoke can have a COHb value up to 10%. ABGs would be beneficial in the management of the patient to assess for hypoxemia (and even metabolic acidosis, in severe cases); however, this test would not confirm the diagnosis. A CBC with differential and basic metabolic panel can provide some useful information as well (eg, anion gap), but again they will not confirm the diagnosis. Remember, too, that pulse oximetry readings would likely be normal in carbon monoxide poisoning because this device cannot differentiate between oxyhemoglobin, carboxyhemoglobin, and other abnormal hemoglobins (ie, methemoglobin).

Once the patient's blood work is obtained and sent to the laboratory for analysis you immediately institute treatment.

Question 14-3

What is the first intervention that should be provided to this patient?

A) Intravenous dextrose.
B) Supplemental oxygen.
C) Rapid sequence intubation.
D) Methylene blue.
E) Thiamine.

Discussion 14-3

The correct answer is "B." The most important initial treatment for carbon monoxide poisoning is to provide 100% oxygen by face mask. If the patient is not protecting his or her airway, intubation may be necessary. However, that is not the case in this scenario. High-flow oxygen decreases the half-life of COHb from 300 minutes to approximately 90 minutes. Intravenous dextrose may be necessary as a supportive measure but is not a first-line treatment. Thiamine is reserved for patients with altered mental status of unknown etiology, which is most common in adults. Lastly, methylene blue is the antidote for methemoglobinemia.

He is receiving supplemental oxygen and remains unsteady on his feet. The lab calls. The young boy's COHb level is 22%.

Question 14-4

What intervention should now be considered, given his presentation?
A) Hyperbaric oxygen.
B) Continued high-flow supplemental oxygen.
C) Observation without supplemental oxygen.
D) Rapid sequence intubation.
E) None of the above.

Discussion 14-4

The correct answer is "A." Indications for hyperbaric oxygen therapy in acute carbon monoxide poisoning are unclear and controversial. The goal of hyperbaric therapy is to prevent long-term neurocognitive damage. Possible indications include loss of consciousness, syncope, persistent neurologic symptoms, cardiac ischemia on ECG, elevated COHb level in pregnant patients, and a high COHb level. For many providers this may necessitate a transfer to a facility with the appropriate resources. Treatment with hyperbaric oxygen will further reduce the half-life of COHb to 20 minutes. Additional supplemental oxygen therapy may be beneficial for the patient, but more aggressive intervention is indicated. And, although the patient is ill, he is otherwise stable; thus rapid sequence intubation is not necessary at this time. In this case, the patient has persistent neurologic findings (eg, ataxia) and an elevated COHb level despite high-flow supplemental oxygen, therefore; hyperbaric oxygen therapy is indicated.

⌛ QUICK QUIZ

What is NOT measured by co-oximetry testing of a blood sample?
A) Oxyhemoglobin.
B) Carboxyhemoglobin.
C) Methemoglobin.
D) Reduced hemoglobin.
E) All of the above.

Discussion

The correct answer is "E." A standard pulse oximeter is not useful to screen for carbon monoxide poisoning or methemoglobinemia. It cannot differentiate COHb or other abnormal hemoglobins from oxyhemoglobin, thus giving a falsely elevated normal reading. Do not be falsely reassured by a normal pulse oximetry reading.

► CASE 15

A 16-year-old female patient inadvertently swallowed her imitation tongue piercing, which consisted of two metallic pieces. Plain X-rays of the abdomen (anteroposterior and lateral) suggest that the metallic objects are in the fundus of the stomach.

Question 15-1

What should be your next step in the management of this patient?
A) No interventions are necessary; the patient can be discharged to home.
B) Observe the patient for at least 4 hours to ensure passage of the magnets.
C) Administer a promotility agent to facilitate passage of the magnets.
D) Consult a pediatric surgeon for an exploratory laparotomy.
E) Consult a pediatric gastroenterologist to discuss removing the magnets.

Discussion 15-1

The correct answer is "E." Magnet ingestion by pediatric patients is a growing concern, particularly as magnets are being used increasingly in products. The use of magnets in commercial products includes jewelry as in the aforementioned case. This patient has swallowed two magnets that formed her imitation tongue ring. The number of magnets and their location are the most important concerns in managing these patients. Initially, a provider should obtain anteroposterior and lateral X-rays of the abdomen to assess their location within the abdomen. Single magnet ingestions found in the esophagus or stomach should be considered for endoscopic removal, although some advocate for serial imaging to ensure movement of the magnet in otherwise asymptomatic patients. Multiple magnets or magnetic/metallic objects may attract one another between two loops of bowel causing pressure necrosis, perforation, obstruction, or volvulus. All patients with multiple magnet ingestions should have all magnets that are accessible by endoscopy removed. If the magnets are further along the gastrointestinal tract in an asymptomatic patient, serial abdominal X-rays can be obtained every 4 to 6 hours. However, removal by enteroscopy or colonoscopy is still advised if the magnets can be accessed. Patients who are symptomatic after ingesting multiple magnets located beyond the reach of endoscopy should be evaluated by a pediatric surgeon for consideration of a surgical intervention. Promotility agents are not used to facilitate passage of magnets through the gastrointestinal tract.

► CASE 16

A 7-year-old boy is playing outside his home, an old farmhouse, unsupervised. His father finds him lying on the ground seizing. He is brought directly into the emergency department where you evaluate him. Although his seizures have stopped, physical examination reveals dark linear lines on the gingiva.

Question 16-1

What is the likely cause of the patient's presentation?
A) Iron toxicity.
B) Organophosphate toxicity.
C) Lead toxicity.
D) Anticholinergic toxicity.
E) Ethylene glycol toxicity.

Discussion 16-1

The correct answer is "C." The patient history suggests an older home, possibly one painted with lead-based paint. The occurrence of seizures may not be specific, but it is associated with severe lead toxicity and may be both prolonged and refractory. Burton lines are blueish-black lines on the gingiva seen in lead toxicity, though uncommonly. This constellation of contextual clues and symptoms is not associated with the other options listed. Lead is a neurotoxin, and even at minimally elevated levels is associated with long-term effects on cognition and learning. The primary sources are lead paint, and dust and soil contaminated by flakes of lead paint. Certain folk remedies may contain lead. Symptoms of lead intoxication include irritability, headaches, abdominal pain, constipation, and clumsiness. Severe toxicity may cause seizures, coma, vomiting, and encephalopathy. Intervention is based on the blood lead level of a venous sample. An abnormal capillary value must be confirmed by a venous lead level. A lead level less than 10 mcg/dL is acceptable. Patients with values higher than 10 mcg/dL require repeat testing, monitoring, education, and possible environmental investigation for lead sources or treatment, depending on the exact value. (See Table 27–5.) A diet containing adequate vitamin C, iron, and calcium is recommended. Parents should be educated about lead toxicity, especially as it relates to infants and toddlers, who like to put objects in their mouths.

Suspecting chronic lead toxicity, you order a venous lead level.

Question 16-2

In chronic cases, at which level do most patients become symptomatic?
A) Greater than 10 mcg/dL.
B) Greater than 20 mcg/dL.
C) Greater than 40 mcg/dL.
D) Greater than 60 mcg/dL.
E) Greater than 100 mcg/dL.

Discussion 16-2

The correct answer is "D." A normal lead level is less than 10 mcg/dL, whereas levels greater than 100 mcg/dL can result in severe encephalopathy. Generally, it is thought that acute lead exposures resulting in lead levels greater than 40 mcg/dL can result in symptoms. However, while manifesting acutely, this patient's presentation is more consistent with chronic exposure (suggested by the farmhouse exposure and presence of gingival changes). Clinical examination findings may not become apparent until the lead level surpasses 60 mcg/dL.

> **Helpful Tip**
> There is controversy as to the lead level at which even asymptomatic children should be treated. Regardless, any level greater than 10 mcg/dL should prompt an investigation into possible sources of lead exposure.

The patient's venous lead level returns at 80 mcg/dL. It has been 3 hours since his initial presentation.

TABLE 27–5 TREATMENT OF LEAD TOXICITY

Blood Lead Concentration	Classification	Interventions	Chelation Agent	Route of Administration
10–19 mcg/dL	Mild intoxication	Diet, Education[a]	None	NA
20–44 mcg/dL		Diet, Education[a]	None	NA
		Environmental evaluation		
		± Bowel decontamination		
45–69 mcg/dL	Moderate intoxication	Diet, Education[a]	Dimercaptosuccinic acid (succimer)	PO
		Environmental investigation	*or*	
		± Bowel decontamination	CaNa$_2$ EDTA	IV
≥ 70 mcg/dL	Severe intoxication	Hospitalize	BAL (dimercaprol)	IM
Symptomatic		± Bowel decontamination	*and*	
Intolerant of succimer			CaNa$_2$ EDTA	IV

BAL, British anti-Lewisite; CaNa$_2$ EDTA, calcium disodium ethylenediamine-tetraacetate; CNS, central nervous system; IM, intramuscular; IV, intravenous; NA, not applicable; PO, oral.

[a]Education includes dietary and environmental changes.

Question 16-3

What treatment should you implement?

A) Activated charcoal.
B) Dimercaprol (British antilewisite [BAL]).
C) Calcium disodium ethylenediamine-tetraacetate (CaNa₂ EDTA).
D) Deferoxamine.
E) Both B and C.

Discussion 16-3

The correct answer is "E." The initial treatment in severe lead toxicity is dimercaprol (BAL) and CaNa₂ EDTA. Both medications are chelating agents. CaNa₂ EDTA should be started after the second dose of BAL is administered. Chelation therapy is continued for 5 days. Lead levels should be rechecked after stopping therapy, as repeat courses may be needed. Activated charcoal is not effective in lead toxicity. Deferoxamine is a treatment agent for iron ingestions. The magical number to start chelation therapy is a lead level of 45 mcg/dL or higher. A value of 70 mcg/dL or higher, symptoms of lead poisoning, or inability to tolerate oral succimer requires hospital admission and treatment with intravenous chelation therapy. If lead flecks are present on an abdominal X-ray, whole bowel irrigation should be performed. Consult the Poison Control Center or an experienced toxicologist when managing lead toxicity.

After 5 days of treatment with BAL and CaNa₂ EDTA, the patient appears well and at his baseline. He has had no additional seizures. His lead level is rechecked and found to be 40 mcg/dL. Interestingly, his lead level the day before was 15 mcg/dL.

Question 16-4

How can you explain this result?

A) The child has been exposed to additional lead.
B) There has been a treatment failure.
C) A laboratory error has likely transpired.
D) The child has hematochromatosis.
E) Lead redistributes into the serum after chelation.

Discussion 16-4

The correct answer is "E." Chelation therapy (with either BAL or CaNa₂ EDTA) results in lead redistribution into the serum. Thus, while a patient may be clinically asymptomatic, one might note a rise in the serum lead level. This is not uncommon and does not signify a treatment failure. It is unlikely that a patient would be exposed to additional lead while hospitalized. Although a laboratory error should be considered, it is far less likely to occur. Lastly, hematochromatosis is an inherited condition involving iron accumulation.

> **Helpful Tip**
> A lead level of 45 mcg/dL or higher requires chelation therapy. Make sure the child will take the oral succimer, as it has a "rotten egg" odor.

► CASE 17

A 14-year-old boy was practicing a new magic trick with a nickel. In his attempt to make the coin disappear, and while technically successful, he inadvertently "swallowed" the coin. He presents to the emergency department after this episode. He appears to be in no acute distress. The patient's vital signs are normal. A chest X-ray shows a circular radiopaque object just above carina.

Question 17-1

What is the next step in your management of this patient?

A) Consult pediatric gastroenterology for endoscopy.
B) Consult pediatric pulmonology for bronchoscopy.
C) Secure additional testing.
D) Observe the patient in the emergency department.
E) Discharge the patient; no further evaluation or intervention is necessary.

Discussion 17-1

The correct answer is "C." The information provided by the chest X-ray is not sufficient to determine if the patient has aspirated or swallowed the coin. As such, selecting a disposition for the patient is difficult at this juncture. Obtaining a lateral chest X-ray might provide additional insight. Aspirated coins often become tilted when caught on tracheal rings. Thus, one might see an angulated coin. Another benefit of the lateral view is that one might be able to appreciate the air-filled trachea distinctly from the location of the coin, suggesting that it has been swallowed. (See Figure 27–3.)

Additional imaging determines the coin is in the patient's distal esophagus. He is having no trouble breathing or swallowing.

Question 17-2

What should be done now?

A) Consult pediatric gastroenterology for endoscopy.
B) Consult pediatric pulmonology for bronchoscopy.
C) Secure additional testing.
D) Observe the patient.
E) Discharge the patient; no further evaluation or intervention is necessary.

Discussion 17-2

The correct answer is "D." Asymptomatic patients with esophageal coins may be observed for 24 hours to see if the coin will pass into the stomach. Coins in the proximal esophagus are less likely to pass. An esophageal coin should be removed if the patient is symptomatic (cannot swallow secretions), the time of ingestion is unknown, there is uncertainty about whether object is a disc (button) battery or coin, or the object fails to pass into the stomach after 24 hours of observation. (See Table 27–6.)

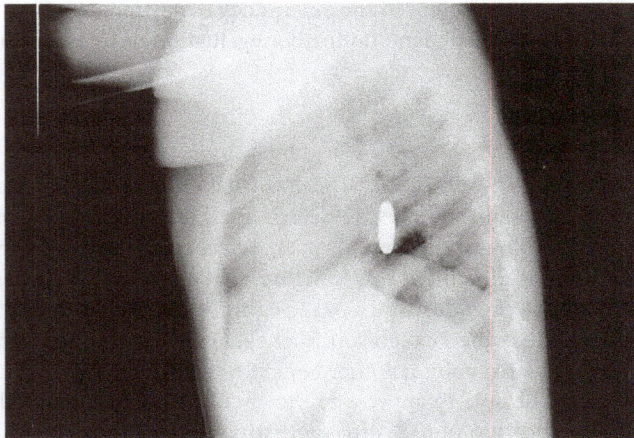

A

B

FIGURE 27–3. Esophageal foreign body. Posteroanterior (A) and lateral (B) chest X-rays show a round radiopaque foreign body in the esophagus consistent with a coin. A lateral chest X-ray may help identify the anatomic location of the coin, as the air-filled trachea can often be delineated from the esophagus. (Reproduced with permission from Stone CK, Humphries RL, eds. *Current Diagnosis and Treatment: Emergency Medicine.* 7th ed. New York, NY: McGraw-Hill Education; 2011, Fig. 50-9A, B.)

TABLE 27–6 SWALLOWED FOREIGN BODIES THAT REQUIRE ENDOSCOPIC REMOVAL

Sharp object

High-powered magnet

Multiple magnets

Long object (> 6 cm)

Lead-containing objects

Coins in the esophagus > 24 hours

Button/disc battery in esophagus

Button/disc battery or cylindrical battery in stomach > 48 hours

Airway obstruction (tracheal compression)

Esophageal obstruction (cannot swallow secretions)

Intestinal obstruction

QUICK QUIZ

Which is NOT an indication for emergent endoscopy with removal of the foreign body?
A) A toddler with a swallowed safety pin located in the esophagus.
B) A 10-year-old who is unable to swallow his secretions and has a swallowed quarter in the proximal esophagus.
C) A 17-year-old with a disc (button) battery in his distal esophagus.
D) A 5-year-old with multiple magnets in the stomach.
E) All of the above are indications for emergent endoscopy.

Discussion

The correct answer is "D." Multiple magnets in the stomach require urgent endoscopic removal but not emergent.

▶ CASE 18

A 3-year-old girl found her way into her mother's medicine cabinet roughly 7 hours prior to presentation at your clinic. The only medication in the cabinet was an iron supplement for iron-deficiency anemia. This bottle was opened when the mother found the young girl playing at the cabinet, but it was not initially clear if the girl had consumed any tablets. Shortly after being found the girl reported some vague "tummy pain," which resolved. After a period of observation at home, the mother thought it best to have her daughter evaluated. Upon arrival the child appears well and has no complaints. Her vital signs are within normal limits.

Question 18-1

What test will provide you with the most efficient means for determining whether the patient consumed any iron tablets?
A) CBC with differential.
B) Liver function tests.
C) Serum iron level.
D) Computerized tomography (CT) scan of the abdomen and pelvis.
E) Abdominal X-ray.

Discussion 18-1

The correct answer is "E." Iron tablets are radio-opaque, and thus they should be apparent on X-ray in the gastrointestinal tract of a patient who has consumed them. However, there are caveats to consider with regard to the utility of abdominal X-rays in iron ingestions. The absence of radio-opaque pills or tablets does not rule out iron ingestion, including a potentially lethal ingestion. It could also be the case that the iron has dissolved. Additionally, liquid preparations and children's chewable tablets and multivitamins are not often visible on X-rays. A CBC with differential may suggest signs of anemia due to gastrointestinal hemorrhage from iron toxicity, while liver function tests may suggest end-organ damage later in a patient's course. However, neither test is likely to help determine if any iron has been consumed.

Serum iron levels should certainly be evaluated, as peak absorption of the iron occurs between 2 and 6 hours after ingestion. In a patient with acute iron toxicity, an anion gap metabolic acidosis, leukocytosis, hyperglycemia, or a combination of these findings may be present. With that said, one can gain more prompt insight into a possible ingestion with X-rays, utilizing the serum iron level as further evidence of an iron ingestion. A CT scan of the abdomen and pelvis would likely reveal iron tablets if they have been consumed. Yet, the significant radiation, financial cost, and delay in securing this imaging negates its utility in the initial assessment of potential iron ingestions. Iron toxicity depends on the quantity of elemental iron ingested. Different formulations (ferrous fumarate > ferrous sulfate > ferrous gluconate) contain different amounts of elemental iron. Ingestions of less than 20 mg/kg of elemental iron typically do not result in symptoms. Toxic levels generally occur with ingestions of greater than 40 mg/kg elemental iron and lethal levels with ingestions of greater than 60 mg/kg elemental iron.

> **Helpful Tip**
> Iron ingestions have historically resulted in the highest ingestion-related mortality in children. With that said, children's chewable iron products have been shown to be safe for use as directed, although they frequently will not show up on plain film imaging.

X-rays of the child's abdomen confirm the presence of radio-opaque tablets in the stomach.

Question 18-2
Given the apparent iron ingestion, in which stage of iron toxicity is this patient?
A) Stage 1.
B) Stage 2.
C) Stage 3.
D) Stage 4.
E) Stage 5.

Discussion 18-2
The correct answer is "B." The stages of iron toxicity are important, particularly the second stage. During stage 1 (30 minutes to 6 hours after ingestion), patients typically experience nonspecific gastrointestinal symptoms such as abdominal pain, nausea, emesis, and diarrhea or gastrointestinal hemorrhage (hematemesis, melena) may occur. Stage 2 can be clinically problematic, as it is referred to as the latent stage. Typically commencing 6 to 12 hours after ingestion, patients are often asymptomatic, with their previous gastrointestinal symptoms having resolved. It is not uncommon for patients to present at this stage. Between 12 hours and 48 hours after ingestion patients can enter stage 3, denoted by hypoperfusion, shock, metabolic acidosis, coma and acute liver failure with hypoglycemia and coagulopathy. This can progress to stage 4 (2 to 6 weeks after ingestion), highlighted by liver failure from hepatic cirrhosis and emesis from gastric outlet or small bowel obstructions from intestinal scarring. This stage usually

manifests 2 to 4 weeks later. It should be noted that patients can skip any of these stages. But if a patient does not experience stage 1 within 6 hours of an ingestion the amount of iron consumed is likely not significant. This "6-hour rule" does not apply if enteric-coated tablets were consumed.

> **Helpful Tip**
> Iron is directly corrosive to the gastrointestinal mucosa and may cause life-threatening hemorrhage, necrosis, or both.

Her iron level returns from the laboratory at 550 mcg/dL.

Question 18-3
What is the first-line therapy that should be initiated for this patient?
A) Activated charcoal.
B) Gastric lavage.
C) Oral deferoxamine.
D) Intravenous deferoxamine.
E) Sodium bicarbonate.

Discussion 18-3
The correct answer is "D." A peak serum iron level should be obtained 4 to 6 hours after ingestion. Deferoxamine is a highly specific iron chelator. It binds with ferric iron, forming a water-soluble compound excreted by the kidneys. Because it results in more constant levels in the bloodstream, intravenous deferoxamine is preferred over other formulations. Indications for the use of deferoxamine include metabolic acidosis, severe symptoms, and serum level greater than 500 mcg/dL or greater than 350 mcg/dL when pill fragments are present on X-ray. The preferred dosing of this medication is an initial continuous infusion rate of 15 mg/kg/h, increasing the dose as needed. Maximum doses up to 45 mg/kg/h have been reported. The infusion rate should be decreased if hypotension occurs. Activated charcoal will not absorb iron, and studies have not shown gastric lavage to improve outcomes in such ingestions. Sodium bicarbonate, without an associated metabolic acidosis, is not a therapy for iron toxicity. Of note, endoscopic removal of the tablets or whole bowel irrigation (eg, polyethylene glycol at 10–15 mL/kg/h) would be appropriate treatment options as well, given the presence of pills in the patient's stomach.

The pharmacist calls you regarding your order for intravenous deferoxamine. There is some question as to whether this medication is actually indicated.

Question 18-4
Which of the following is NOT an indication for implementing deferoxamine treatment in the setting of an iron overdose?
A) Altered mental status.
B) Persistent gastrointestinal symptoms.
C) A serum iron level greater than 500 mcg/dL.
D) Hypotension.
E) Metabolic alkalosis.

Discussion 18-4

The correct answer is "E." The presence of a metabolic acidosis is an indication to initiate deferoxamine therapy, but metabolic alkalosis is not. The other options are all appropriate reasons to commence with treatment. In the case described, the patient had a serum iron level greater than 500 mcg/dL and the presence of pill fragments on plain films. Also consider that patients with late presentations (> 8 hours) may have artificially lower serum iron levels owing to redistribution intracellularly yet still warrant deferoxamine therapy.

⧗ QUICK QUIZ

Regarding iron toxicity, which of the following is false?

A) Iron is often radiolucent, and plain films of the abdomen can be useful in detecting an ingestion.

B) Iron ingestions can involve many different potential sources, including iron tablets, toys, weights, and imported items such as pottery or cooking vessels.

C) The stages of iron toxicity are important, particularly stage 2, when patients may appear asymptomatic. One must have a high index of suspicion at this stage.

D) The treatment of choice for iron toxicity is intravenous deferoxamine, which has several indications, including an iron level greater than 500 mcg/dL or an iron level greater than 350 mcg/dL when pill fragments are seen on plain films.

E) Patients who have accidentally ingested less than 40 mg/kg of elemental iron with only mild gastrointestinal symptoms may be watched at home.

Discussion

The correct answer is "A." Iron is radio-opaque not radiolucent, but iron tablets may not always be seen on X-ray.

► CASE 19

An 18-month-old toddler was cruising through the kitchen one morning when he discovered a bright and shiny dishwasher detergent pod on the floor. The young lad promptly placed this directly into his mouth. Minutes later his mother noticed the presence of detergent granules around his mouth. The patient was immediately brought into your emergency department for further evaluation and treatment.

Question 19-1

What is the immediate concern regarding this ingestion?

A) Coagulation necrosis of the esopagus due to a caustic acid ingestion.

B) Liquefaction necrosis of the esophagus due to a caustic acid ingestion.

C) Coagulation necrosis of the esophagus due to a caustic alkali ingestion.

D) Liquefaction necrosis of the esophagus due to a caustic alkali ingestion.

E) Both coagulation and liquefaction necrosis of the esophagus due to a caustic acid ingestion.

Discussion 19-1

The correct answer is "D." Dishwasher and laundry pods are concentrated forms of cleaning detergents, which have become an increasing hazard for young children. Not only is their concentrated formulation a concern for a more severe esophageal or airway injury if ingested or aspirated, their appearance is often bright and shiny, leading young children to perceive them as candy. Common household agents such as oven and drain cleaners along with traditional laundry detergents can also lead to significant esophageal injury if ingested. Acidic preparations of such substances lead to coagulation necrosis. These types of injuries tend to be less severe because they are self-limiting as the coagulation process prevents deeper penetration of the caustic substance. Alkali ingestions, including those that might result from the ingestion of a dishwasher detergent pod or classically lye, can lead to liquefaction necrosis. This type of injury causes the disintegration of the mucosa and potentially perforation of the esophagus. In treating these ingestions, neutralizing substances, diluting agents (eg, milk), and activated charcoal are not recommended. Patients with symptoms (dysphagia, hematemesis, retrosternal chest pain) or oral burns following an ingestion or those known to have ingested a substance associated with significant esophageal injury (eg, drain cleaner) should undergo endoscopy. Otherwise, asymptomatic patients should be observed for several hours to ensure no further complications develop (so long as the substance ingested is of low causticity). Long-term complications include the formation of esophageal strictures, which may cause obstruction.

> **Helpful Tip**
> After caustic ingestion of an alkali or acidic agent, patients should not be forced to vomit. This may cause repeat esophageal burn as the caustic substance moves back into the esophagus.

► CASE 20

A 6-year-old boy presents to your clinic with his mother, who is concerned that he may have inadvertently swallowed a small, cylindrical battery from his Billy the Bot toy. The child denies any associated symptoms, and he appears well. His vital signs are within normal limits, and his pulmonary and abdominal examinations are unremarkable. You obtain plain films of the chest and abdomen to evaluate for the presence of a battery. A small radio-opaque object seemingly consistent with a battery is noted in the stomach.

Question 20-1

What is your next course of action?

A) Consult a pediatric gastroenterologist to discuss endoscopic removal of the battery.
B) Admit the patient for serial abdominal examinations and repeat imaging.
C) Observe the patient in the clinic with repeat plain films in 6 hours.
D) Discharge the patient to home with follow-up as needed.
E) Discharge the patient to home with follow-up scheduled for 2 days.

Discussion 20-1

The correct answer is "E." The management of battery ingestions is important as they may result in caustic alkaline injuries to the esophagus. Fortunately, there are several guidelines that can help with the management of patients with battery ingestions. When the battery (disc or cylindrical) is found to be in the stomach, any child younger than 5 years old (symptomatic or otherwise) should be seen by a pediatric gastroenterologist at the initial presentation. For asymptomatic children 5 years of age and older, a pediatric gastroenterologist should be consulted if the battery remains in the stomach on follow-up plain films 48 hours after the ingestion. A disc (button) battery located in the esophagus is a different story. This requires emergent removal to prevent necrosis. Thus, in this case the asymptomatic 6-year-old can be discharged to home with a regular diet and normal activity level with instructions to return in 48 hours for repeat imaging. If the battery remains in the stomach at that time it should be removed endoscopically. Follow-up imaging is also indicated if the patient develops symptoms, to prove passage of the battery if it has not been visualized in the stool 1 to 2 weeks after ingestion, and to monitor the weekly progression of the battery if it has not passed and has been previously seen in the intestines on plain films. Batteries that find their way out of the stomach and into the intestines generally pass without complication. Lastly, keep in mind that the larger the battery (> 15–20 mm) the more likely it is that there will be some difficulty with passage.

> **Helpful Tip**
> A disc (button) battery located in the esophagus is an emergency whereas a coin may not be. On X-ray, look for a double-ring or halo appearance, which reflects the battery's biconvex shape. (See Figure 27–4.)

▶ CASE 21

As a civic-minded physician, you agree to speak at the local school to parents, students, and teachers regarding health and the environment for Earth Day. Although the majority of the presentation is left to your discretion, the organizers have asked you to touch on a couple of specific topics aimed at highlighting the interplay between the health of the

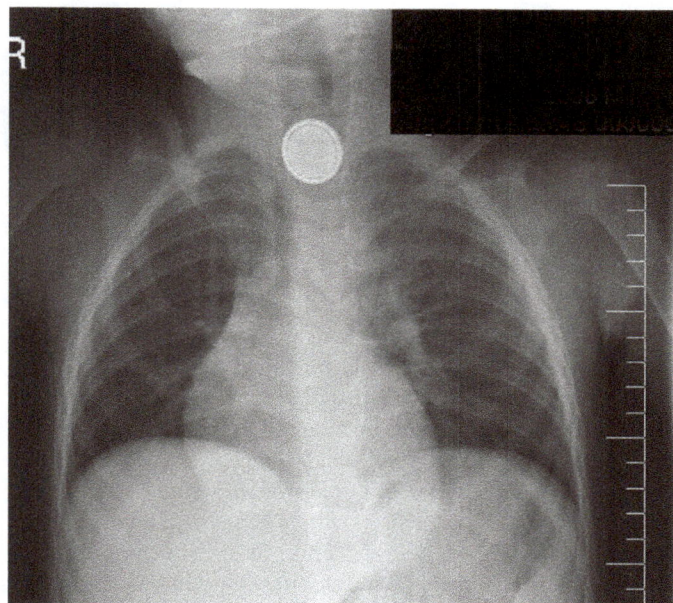

FIGURE 27–4. A disc battery is located in the proximal esophagus. On X-ray, a disc battery has a double-ring or a surrounding halo, which helps differentiate it from a coin. (Reproduced with permission from Knoop KJ, Stack LB, Storrow AB, Thurman RJ (Eds). *The Atlas of Emergency Medicine*, 3ed. McGraw-Hill Education, Inc., 2010. Photo contributor: Scott Manning, MD.)

community and the environment. It is suggested that you spend a portion of your presentation discussing the possible dangerous substances that could find their way into the community's food and water supply if individuals and industries are not vigilant.

Question 21-1

Which of the following is NOT an example you might cite as such a contaminant?

A) Mercury.
B) Fluoride.
C) Arsenic.
D) *Escherichia coli* (*E. coli*).
E) *Cryptosporidium*.

Discussion 21-1

The correct answer is "B." Toxic substances can contaminate food and water supplies, impacting the health of an entire community. Fluorinated water has been shown to reduce cavities in children by up to 40% in children. Fluoride is generally not thought to be a significant hazard to a community's food or water supply. The other remaining options present noteworthy potential harms to public health, particularly to developing children. Heavy metals such as mercury and arsenic or bacteria (eg, *E. coli* and *Cryptosporidium*) can result in both acute illness and chronic sequelae.

One of your talking points will center on the chemical hazards that can exist in the community.

Question 21-2

Which of the following is NOT a common source of contamination that may affect the health of the community?

A) Pesticide runoff.

B) Nuclear power.

C) Electric or magnetic fields (eg, power lines, household appliances).

D) Automobile exhaust.

E) Industrial waste.

Discussion 21-2

The correct answer is "C." It is worthwhile to be aware of the potential chemical hazards that exist around us. The list of these entities is lengthy and includes all the options listed above except electric and magnetic fields. Recent studies have suggested that these fields (which are generated by electrical power lines and household appliances) likely do not result in leukemia, brain tumors, or other types of cancer as previously speculated. To date, the literature on the topic suggests that only extremely high levels of exposure to magnetic fields (affecting < 1% of the child population) may result in an increased risk. However, even this conclusion is not clear.

....

The final area to be emphasized during your noble endeavor relates to possible chemical exposures in the home.

Question 21-3

In contemplating this issue, which question will be least successful in highlighting the various types of chemical hazards in their homes?

A) Do you have any exotic pets?

B) Are you currently remodeling your home?

C) Do you work with chemicals on the job site?

D) Does your job entail working in or around those that are ill?

E) Do you smoke tobacco products?

Discussion 21-3

The correct answer is "A." Substances found within the home and those brought home can all impact the health of the children in a home. While exotic pets may present some health risks they are not likely to be chemical in nature. On the other hand, during a home remodeling there are often numerous cleaning products introduced into the home. These products can emit fumes that can present a health risk, represent a source for a possible cutaneous exposure or burn, and serve as a source for an unintentional ingestion. Similarly, exposure to chemicals on the job site can be transferred to one's family. Sprayed chemicals such as insecticides or pesticides, industrial solvents, and other substances can present a home health hazard. Similarly, illnesses can be transmitted from someone working in or around the health care profession to family members in the home. And lastly, it is well known that exposure to tobacco smoke can have a significant impact on the health of everyone in the home, not just the primary user. For each of these entities, one should also consider the duration of exposure and the age(s) at which the exposure transpired. The physiologic effects of such exposures can be cumulative and result

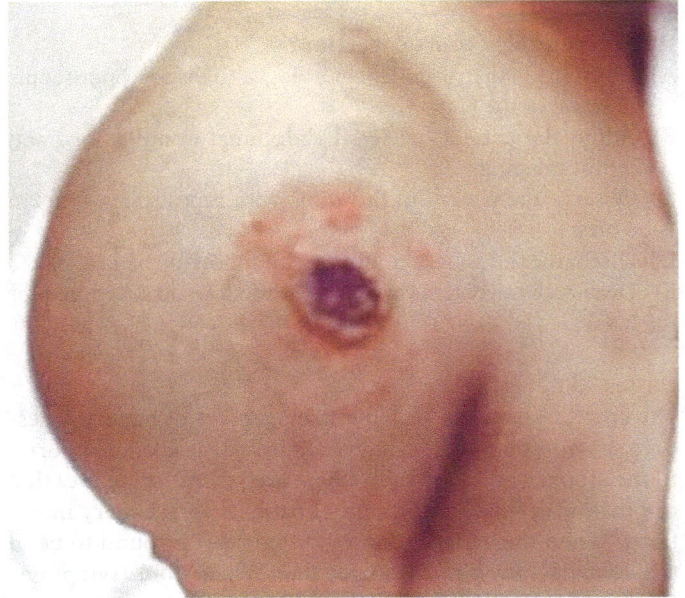

FIGURE 27–5. Anthrax spores from the bacteria *Bacillus anthracis* have been used in biological warfare. Cutaneous anthrax can manifest with small pruritic papules that quickly evolve into a vesicle that necrosis into an ulcer with a black eschar as seen in this photograph. (Reproduced with permission from Tintinalli JE, Stapczynski JS, Ma OJ, Yealy DM, Cline DM, Meckler GD, eds. *Tintinalli's Emergency Medicine: A Comprehensive Study Guide.* 8th ed. New York, NY: McGraw-Hill Education; 2016, Fig. 9-2.)

in more pronounced symptoms. Additionally, younger patients may be more susceptible to certain hazardous materials or more likely to suffer long-term sequelae. Remember, when evaluating patients for potential toxic ingestions, be sure to consider the home setting and parents' activities as well.

> **Helpful Tip**
> The signs and symptoms of a toxic exposure are influenced by both the duration of and age at which the exposure occurs.

BIBLIOGRAPHY

American Academy of Pediatrics Committee on Drugs. Naloxone dosage and route of administration for infants and children: Addendum to emergency drug doses for infants and children. *Pediatrics.* 1990;86:484.

Brent J, McMartin K, Phillips S, et al. Fomepizole for the treatment of methanol poisoning. *N Engl J Med.* 2001;344:424.

Brok J, Buckley N, Gluud C. Interventions for paracetamol (acetaminophen) overdose. *Cochrane Database Syst Rev.* 2006;(2):CD003328.

Chamberlain JM, Klein BL. A comprehensive review of naloxone for the emergency physician. *Am J Emerg Med.* 1994;12:650.

Committee on Environmental Health. Lead exposure in children: Prevention, detection, and management. *Pediatrics.* 2005;116(4):1036–1046. doi: 10.1542/peds.2005-1947.

Greene SL, Dargan PI, Jones AL. Acute poisoning: Understanding 90% of cases in a nutshell. *Postgrad Med J.* 2005;81(954):204–216.

Hampson NB, Piantadosi CA, Thom SR, Weaver LK. Practice recommendations in the diagnosis, management, and prevention of carbon monoxide poisoning. *Am J Resp Crit Care Med.* 2012;186(11):1095–1101. doi: 10.1164/rccm.201207-1284CI.

Hann G, Duncan D, Sudhir G, West P, Sohi D. Antifreeze on a freezing morning: Ethylene glycol poisoning in a 2-year-old. *BMJ Case Rep.* 2012 Mar 27; 2012. doi: 10.1136/bcr.07.2011.4509.

Ikenberry SO, Jue TL, Anderson MA, et al. Management of ingested foreign bodies and food impactions. *Gastrointest Endosc.* 2011;73(6):1085–1091.

Kao LW, Nañagas KA. Carbon monoxide poisoning. *Emerg Med Clin North Am.* 2004;22:985.

Kerr GW, McGuffie AC, Wilkie S. Tricyclic antidepressant overdose: A review. *Emerg Med J.* 2001;18(4):236–241.

Kramer RE, Lerner DG, Lin T, et al. Management of ingested foreign bodies in children: A clinical report of the NASPGHAN Endoscopy Committee. *J Pediatr Gastroenterol Nutr.* 2015;60:562.

Krenzelok EP, Proudfoot AT. Salicylate toxicity. In: Haddad LM, Winchester J, eds. *Clinical Management of Poisoning and Drug Overdose.* Philadelphia, PA: WB Saunders; 1998:675.

Lanthony P. [Van Gogh's xanthopsia]. *Bull Soc Ophtalmol Fr.* 1989;89(10):1133–1134.

Mills KC, Curry SC. Acute iron poisoning. *Emerg Med Clin North Am.* 1994;12:397.

National Capital Poison Center. NBIH button battery ingestion triage and treatment guideline. http://www.poison.org/battery/guideline.asp. Accessed June 28, 2015.

Rumack BH, Matthew H. Acetaminophen poisoning and toxicity. *Pediatrics.* 1975;55:871.

Sidell FR. Clinical effects of organophosphorus cholinesterase inhibitors. *J Appl Toxicol.* 1994;14:111.

Smolinske SC, Hall AH, Vandenberg SA, et al. Toxic effects of nonsteroidal anti-inflammatory drugs in overdose. An overview of recent evidence on clinical effects and dose-response relationships. *Drug Saf.* 1990;5:252.

Thomas TJ, Pauze D, Love JN. Are one or two dangerous? Diphenoxylate-atropine exposure in toddlers. *J Emerg Med.* 2008;34(1):71–75.

Tormoehlen LM, Tekulve KJ, Nañagas KA. Hydrocarbon toxicity: A review. *Clin Toxicol (Phila).* 2014;52:479.

UW Health. Common plants: What's poisonous and what's not? American Family Children's Hospital and Wisconsin Poison Center. https://www.uwhealth.org/files/uwhealth/docs/pdf/poisonous_ plants.pdf. Accessed on June 12, 2015.

Warniment C, Tsang K, Galazka SS. Lead poisoning in children. *Am Fam Physician.* 2010;81(6):751–757.

Preventative Pediatrics

28

Ashley Miller and Rebecca Lozman-Oxman

► CASE 1

A 2-year-old girl presents in mid-October for her yearly routine vaccinations. She is up to date with her primary vaccinations. She has never had the flu shot before, but her parents would like her to have it this year because she had the flu last year. The patient has a history of wheezing at 2 months of age associated with respiratory syncytial virus (RSV) infection and at 6 months of age with a viral upper respiratory tract infection. She also has a history of rash around her mouth after eating scrambled eggs but is able to eat baked products containing eggs without difficulty.

Question 1-1
Which of the following statements correctly describes the influenza vaccine(s) that can be offered to this child, and why?
A) None, due to her history of egg allergy.
B) Inactivated influenza virus (IIV) vaccine only, due to her history of wheezing.
C) Live attenuated influenza virus (LAIV) vaccine only, due to her history of egg allergy.
D) Both vaccines can be offered as there is no contraindication.
E) None of the above.

Discussion 1-1
The correct answer is "E." Influenza vaccination is recommended yearly for all children older than 6 months of age. Children aged 6 months to 8 years require two doses (≥ 4 weeks apart) during the first season they receive the vaccine. The IIV vaccine is given as an injection. The LAIV vaccine is given intranasally as a mist. The LAIV vaccine is contraindicated in (1) children younger than 2 years of age, (2) those who have had a prior allergic reaction to the LAIV, (3) those who are currently taking aspirin or aspirin-containing products, (4) those with egg allergy, (5) pregnant women, (6) immunosuppressed people, (7) those who have taken influenza antiviral medications in the last 48 hours, or (8) children aged 2 to 4 years with asthma or who had wheezed in the past 12 months. For older children with

asthma, the LAIV vaccine should be avoided as it is associated with increased risk of wheezing. Most formulations of influenza vaccines contain a small amount of egg protein as they are produced from chick embryos. All children with an egg allergy may receive the IIV vaccine but should be monitored in the office afterward. Children with egg anaphylaxis should receive their vaccine in an allergy clinic. New research suggests that the LAIV vaccine may be used in children with egg allergy, but the Advisory Committee on Immunization Practices (ACIP) and Centers for Disease Control and Prevention (CDC) currently recommend the IIV. This child should receive the IIV vaccine due to her history of egg allergy. Her wheezing was too long ago to matter. For any immunization questions, consult the CDC's website. (See Figure 28–1.)

> **Helpful Tip**
> The occurrence of Guillain-Barré syndrome within 6 weeks following a previous dose of influenza vaccine is considered a precaution for use of all influenza vaccines.

What if the 2-year-old's favorite food was eggs and she had never wheezed, but she had a history of chronic kidney disease. In fact, she is eating a hardboiled egg in your office right now.

Question 1-2
What vaccine would you recommend for her?
A) IIV vaccine.
B) LAIV vaccine.
C) Either the IIV or LAIV vaccine.
D) Neither; children with chronic health diseases are too fragile to receive vaccinations.

Discussion 1-2
The correct answer is "A." Children with chronic health conditions should be vaccinated with the IIV. They are at high risk for complications from influenza infection. Those around them

Figure 1. Recommended immunization schedule for persons aged 0 through 18 years –United States, 2015.
(FOR THOSE WHO FALL BEHIND OR START LATE, SEE THE CATCH-UP SCHEDULE [FIGURE 2]).
These recommendations must be read with the footnotes that follow. For those who fall behind or start late, provide catch-up vaccination at the earliest opportunity as indicated by the green bars in Figure 1.
To determine minimum intervals between doses, see the catch-up schedule (Figure 2). School entry and adolescent vaccine age groups are shaded.

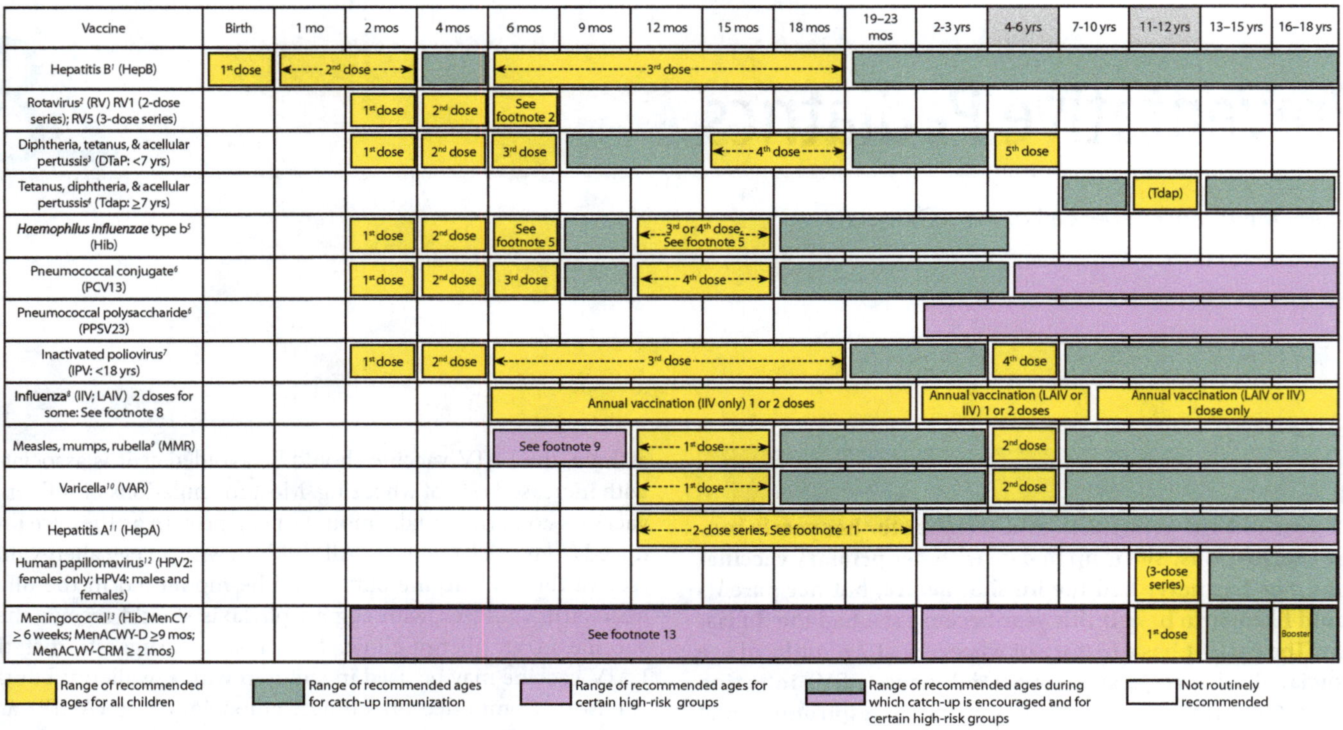

This schedule includes recommendations in effect as of January 1, 2015. Any dose not administered at the recommended age should be administered at a subsequent visit, when indicated and feasible. The use of a combination vaccine generally is preferred over separate injections of its equivalent component vaccines. Vaccination providers should consult the relevant Advisory Committee on Immunization Practices (ACIP) statement for detailed recommendations, available online at http://www.cdc.gov/vaccines/hcp/acip-recs/index.html. Clinically significant adverse events that follow vaccination should be reported to the Vaccine Adverse Event Reporting System (VAERS) online (http://www.vaers.hhs.gov) or by telephone (800-822-7967). Suspected cases of vaccine-preventable diseases should be reported to the state or local health department. Additional information, including precautions and contraindications for vaccination, is available from CDC online (http://www.cdc.gov/vaccines/recs/vac-admin/contraindications.htm) or by telephone (800-CDC-INFO [800-232-4636]).
This schedule is approved by the Advisory Committee on Immunization Practices (http://www.cdc.gov/vaccines/acip), the American Academy of Pediatrics (http://www.aap.org), the American Academy of Family Physicians (http://www.aafp.org), and the American College of Obstetricians and Gynecologists (http://www.acog.org).

NOTE: The above recommendations must be read along with the footnotes of this schedule.

FIGURE 28–1. Recommended immunization for newborns through 18 years of age. *(Footnotes not included.)* (Reproduced with permission from the Centers for Disease Control and Prevention [CDC].)

should be vaccinated to boost herd immunity and "cocoon" the child. A chronic health condition is not a contraindication to the LAIV vaccine but is listed as a precaution along with asthma in a child 5 years of age or older.

The child received two doses of the IIV last year. The father cannot understand why she needs to be vaccinated every year.

Question 1-3

What do you tell him?

A) The vaccine protects against more than one strain of the virus.
B) The vaccine may contain different viral strains from year to year.
C) Immunization is the best way to prevent infection.
D) Immunizing his child contributes to herd immunity.
E) All of the above.

Discussion 1-3

The correct answer is "E." The virus strains included in the vaccine are updated every year to match the circulating strains predicted to cause infection during the upcoming flu season. Both influenza A and B strains are included.

Helpful Tip

Children with egg allergy may receive the influenza virus as long as they can be monitored afterward. If the child only has a history of hives, go for it in the office; if anaphylaxis, send the child to the allergist's office. The only contraindicated vaccine for those allergic to eggs is the yellow fever vaccine.

Your staff have been talking about the influenza vaccine. Some are complaining that last year's vaccine "didn't work" so they do not want to be vaccinated this year. Others are saying they hate shots and wish they did not have to get theirs.

Question 1-4

What do you tell them?

A) It is the virus's fault the vaccine was less effective last year.
B) Staff members who do not like shots can receive the LAIV.
C) Health care providers should be vaccinated yearly.

D) Vaccination is optional for health care providers; the purpose is to protect the provider from getting sick from a patient.

E) The LAIV is not available in the clinic currently, but those who prefer it can wait rather than receive the IIV today.

Discussion 1-4

The correct answer is "C." Each influenza season the CDC samples the influenza virus circulating to evaluate which strains are causing disease. These strains mutate, called antigenic drift, which can happen between seasons or even within a season. Vaccines must be produced many months in advance, so unfortunately because of drift, they may not be exact matches to currently circulating strains; therefore, the vaccine may be more effective some years than others. Health care providers should be immunized both to prevent infection in themselves and transmission to others. If a staff member received the LAIV, he or she would have to wait 7 days before returning to work as to not infect a susceptible patient. You can expect problems with your coworkers if they have to cover your shifts for 7 days because you are scared of a needle. The vaccine should be administered when it is available rather than waiting.

► CASE 2

A 12-month-old girl is in your office for routine vaccination. She has previously received her routine 2-, 4-, and 6-month vaccinations. You noticed that her record states that she was given the measles, mumps, and rubella (MMR) vaccine at 10.5 months of age. Her parents state that she was given the vaccine then because they had traveled out of country to India. The family has another trip to India upcoming in 3 weeks.

Question 2-1

Which vaccines does she need today?
A) None; she is up to date with her routine vaccines.
B) Varicella vaccine only.
C) MMR and varicella vaccines.
D) MMR, varicella, and hepatitis A vaccines.
E) MMR and meningococcal vaccine.

Discussion 2-1

The correct answer is "D." Because rates of seroconversion of MMR are lower if given before 12 months of age, MMR should be given again at 12 months and at 4 years of age. Routine varicella and hepatitis A vaccines should be given. Meningococcal vaccine is a consideration for children traveling to countries where the disease is common. Hepatitis B, *Haemophilus influenzae* type b (Hib), and pneumococcal conjugate (PCV-13) vaccines could be administered today or at her 15-month checkup. (See Figure 28–1.) MMR is a live attenuated vaccine that is given in two doses at ages 12 months and 4 to 6 years. Doses must be administered 4 or more weeks apart. A combination preparation including varicella (MMRV) is also available. Infants 6 to 11 months of age traveling internationally should receive one dose of the MMR vaccine before departure and then resume the

regularly scheduled two-dose series. Children 12 months and older should receive two doses separated by 4 weeks before traveling, to fulfill their vaccine requirement. Recommendations are the same during an outbreak.

You counsel the parents regarding potential adverse effects while handing them a copy of the Vaccine Information Sheet from the CDC.

Question 2-2

What is NOT a possible adverse effect of the MMR vaccine listed on this sheet?
A) Fever.
B) Seizure.
C) Immune thrombocytopenia (ITP).
D) Autism.
E) Arthritis.

Discussion 2-2

The correct answer is "D." Unfortunately, a single bogus study and a female celebrity who shall not be named helped create an antivaccine movement. Autism is a terrible disorder, but it is not caused by vaccines. The benefits of vaccination outweigh the small chance of an adverse effect in most situations. Certain adverse reactions from vaccines should be reported to the U.S. Department of Health and Human Services using the Vaccine Adverse Event Reporting System (VAERS).

The mother pats her apparently pregnant belly and asks if she may receive the MMR vaccine before travel.

Question 2-3

What do you tell her?
A) You have no reason to know anything about vaccines and pregnancy.
B) She should have been vaccinated in the first trimester.
C) She may receive the vaccine but not until the third trimester.
D) She should be vaccinated after the baby is born.
E) Women should only be vaccinated while pregnant.

Discussion 2-3

The correct answer is "D." The MMR vaccine is contraindicated in pregnancy. Mothers needing the vaccine should wait until after delivery. Women should not become pregnant in the 4 weeks after vaccination.

► CASE 3

For Christmas your cousin took her family, including her three children aged 9 months to 3 years, to Disneyland. They were accompanied by another family with a 5-year-old who had finished chemotherapy for acute lymphoblastic leukemia (ALL) 8 months earlier. It is now early January and your cousin calls in a panic because she just heard on the news that a measles outbreak has been linked to Disneyland!

Question 3-1

What do you tell her about each of her own children?

A) She should monitor the children for runny nose, cough, and runny eyes, followed by a rash that starts from the fingers and toes and works toward the trunk, which would suggest they have measles.

B) The 3-year-old is okay because he received his first MMR vaccine at 11 months before the family traveled to Mexico, and his second at his 13-month well-child visit.

C) All of the children should have titers drawn to see if they have immunity.

D) The 9-month-old, who is not showing signs or symptoms, should receive his first MMR vaccine now.

E) All of the children should receive intramuscular immunoglobulin as it has been more than 72 hours since they might have been exposed.

Discussion 3-1

The correct answer is "D." Those who are underimmunized and exposed should receive the MMR vaccine within 72 hours of the exposure (postexposure prophylaxis). Immunoglobulin is recommended for those who are at high risk for measles complications after a direct exposure. It is not used to control an outbreak. In this setting as part of outbreak control, the 9-month-old should be vaccinated now but will still require two doses after age 1 to be considered immune. Doses given before 12 months do not count but are important if traveling internationally. Sorry, 3-year-old sibling, but you are getting vaccinated, too! Vaccination is recommended for those who are unvaccinated or incompletely vaccinated rather than drawn serum antibody titers.

> **Helpful Tip**
> MMR vaccine may be effective if given within the first 3 days (72 hours) after exposure to measles; however, as postexposure prophylaxis with MMR vaccine does not prevent or alter the clinical severity of mumps or rubella, it is not recommended for those who are fully vaccinated.

The 5-year-old with ALL completed his chemotherapy 8 months ago after starting treatment 2 years previously. He was up to date on immunizations before starting treatment. His pediatrician gave him catch-up shots 2 months ago.

Question 3-2

What do you tell your sister regarding this child?

A) He is at higher risk because of his recent immunosuppression and should be watched more closely.

B) He may not mount the same symptoms since he was recently immunosuppressed.

C) He should have received his MMR vaccine at 1 year of age, and again 3 to 6 months after he finished his chemotherapy, so he should be fully immunized and not at higher risk.

D) He should be given immunoglobulin now.

E) All of the above.

Discussion 3-2

The correct answer is "C." He is no longer considered immune suppressed; if he was, the correct answer would be "D."

> **Helpful Tip**
> Measles immunoglobulin may be effective for as long as 6 days after exposure.

Question 3-3

Which of the following children should NOT receive single antigen varicella vaccine?

A) Child with neomycin anaphylaxis.

B) Child with gelatin anaphylaxis.

C) Chid with leukemia.

D) Pregnant teenager with only one varicella vaccination.

E) All of the above.

Discussion 3-3

The correct answer is "E." Varicella is a live attenuated vaccine available as a single antigen varicella vaccine and combination MMRV vaccine. It is given in two doses at 12 months and 4 to 6 years of age. If patient has anaphylaxis to any component of the vaccination (this includes neomycin and gelatin), then the vaccine should be avoided. Because the effects of varicella vaccine on the fetus are not known, varicella vaccination is contraindicated in pregnant individuals. Live viruses are contraindicated in immunosuppressed patients.

⧖ QUICK QUIZ

Who should NOT receive the MMRV vaccine?

A) Child who received intravenous immunoglobulin for Kawasaki disease 18 months ago.

B) Child with benign thyroid nodule.

C) Child with an acute febrile illness last week.

D) Child with a sibling who had a febrile seizure after receiving her vaccines.

E) Child with HIV.

Discussion

The correct answer is "E." Live attenuated virus vaccines include MMR, varicella, rotavirus, oral polio, and influenza (LAIV). You do not want to give a live virus to a host with the potential to develop infection. Is it surprising, then, that immunosuppression is a contraindication to receiving live viral vaccines? This category includes children with leukemia, lymphoma, solid tumors, acquired immunodeficiency syndrome (AIDS), HIV with immunosuppression, congenital immunodeficiencies, and those receiving long-term immunosuppressant medications. MMR and single antigen varicella vaccines can be safely given to HIV-positive children as long as they are not immunosuppressed. The combination MMRV vaccine should not be given to an HIV-positive child.

Pregnant women should not receive live viral vaccines. MMR and varicella vaccination should be delayed if a child has a significant acute febrile illness. A family or personal history of seizures is a precaution but not a contraindication for the MMR vaccine. Children who have received immunoglobulin should not receive their MMR or varicella vaccinations for 3 to 11 months (the time frame depends on the dose of immunoglobulin) as it may block the host's response to the vaccine.

► CASE 4

A 3-year-old has recently come into the care of his grandmother. While with his mother he received two doses of the hepatitis B vaccine and one dose of Hib; PCV-13; rotavirus; diphtheria, tetanus, and acellular pertussis (DTap); and inactivated poliovirus (IPV).

Question 4-1

What vaccines is the patient due for today?

A) Hepatitis B, Hib, PCV-13, DTap, IPV, MMR, varicella, and hepatitis A.
B) Hepatitis B, Hib, PCV-13, DTap, IPV, MMR, varicella, hepatitis A, and rotavirus.
C) Hepatitis B, Hib, DTap, IPV, MMR, varicella, and hepatitis A.
D) Hepatitis B, DTap, IPV, MMR, varicella, and hepatitis A.

Discussion 4-1

The correct answer is "A." After the Boards, pull up the CDC's catch-up schedule rather than going from memory. The catch-up schedule itself is confusing. (See Figure 28–2.) The rotavirus vaccine cannot be given past 8 months of age so option "B" is wrong. Catch-up boosters of hepatitis B, Hib, PCV-13, DTap, and IPV must be given. Initial catch-up of MMR, varicella, and hepatitis A must be given as well. Let's hope your office stocks combination vaccines as you have just ordered eight individual vaccines. Rotavirus is a live oral vaccine given as a two-dose

FIGURE 2. Catch-up immunization schedule for persons aged 4 months through 18 years who start late or who are more than 1 month behind —United States, 2015.
The figure below provides catch-up schedules and minimum intervals between doses for children whose vaccinations have been delayed. A vaccine series does not need to be restarted, regardless of the time that has elapsed between doses. Use the section appropriate for the child's age. Always use this table in conjunction with Figure 1 and the footnotes that follow.

Vaccine	Minimum Age for Dose 1	Minimum Interval Between Doses			
		Dose 1 to Dose 2	Dose 2 to Dose 3	Dose 3 to Dose 4	Dose 4 to Dose 5
Children age 4 months through 6 years					
Hepatitis B[1]	Birth	4 weeks	8 weeks *and at least 16 weeks after first dose.* Minimum age for the final dose is 24 weeks.		
Rotavirus[2]	6 weeks	4 weeks	4 weeks[2]		
Diphtheria, tetanus, and acellular pertussis[3]	6 weeks	4 weeks	4 weeks	6 months	6 month[3]
Haemophilus influenzae type b[4]	6 weeks	4 weeks If first dose was administered before the 1st birthday. 8 weeks (as final dose) If first dose was administered at age 12 through 14 months. No further doses needed if first dose was administered at age 15 months or older.	4 weeks[5] if current age is younger than 12 months **and** first dose was administered at younger than age 7 months, **and** at least 1 previous dose was PRP-T (ActHib, Pentacel) or unknown. 8 weeks *and age 12 through 59 months (as final dose)[5]* • if current age is younger than 12 months **and** first dose was administered at age 7 through 11 months; OR • if current age is 12 through 59 months **and** first dose was administered before the 1st birthday, **and** second dose administered at younger than 15 months; OR • if both doses were PRP-OMP (PedvaxHIB; Comvax) **and** were administered before the 1st birthday. No further doses needed If previous dose was administered at age 15 months or older.	8 weeks (as final dose) This dose only necessary for children age 12 through 59 months who received 3 doses before the 1st birthday.	
Pneumococcal[6]	6 weeks	4 weeks If first dose administered before the 1st birthday. 8 weeks (as final dose for healthy children) If first dose was administered at the 1st birthday or after. No further doses needed for healthy children if first dose administered at age 24 months or older.	4 weeks if current age is younger than 12 months and previous dose given at <7months old. 8 weeks (as final dose for healthy children) If previous dose given between 7-11 months (wait until at least 12 months old); OR If current age is 12 months or older and at least 1 dose was given before age 12 months. No further doses needed for healthy children if previous dose administered at age 24 months or older.	8 weeks (as final dose) This dose only necessary for children aged 12 through 59 months who received 3 doses before age 12 months or for children at high risk who received 3 doses at any age.	
Inactivated poliovirus[7]	6 weeks	4 weeks[7]	4 weeks[7]	6 months[7] (minimum age 4 years for final dose).	
Meningococcal[13]	6 weeks	8 weeks[13]	See footnote 13	See footnote 13	
Measles, mumps, rubella[9]	12 months	4 weeks			
Varicella[10]	12 months	3 months			
Hepatitis A[11]	12 months	6 months			
Children and adolescents age 7 through 18 years					
Tetanus, diphtheria; tetanus, diphtheria, and acellular pertussis[4]	7 years[4]	4 weeks	4 weeks If first dose of DTaP/DT was administered before the 1st birthday. 6 months (as final dose) If first dose of DTaP/DT was administered at or after the 1st birthday.	6 months if first dose of DTaP/DT was administered before the 1st birthday.	
Human papillomavirus[12]	9 years		Routine dosing intervals are recommended.[12]		
Hepatitis A[11]	Not applicable (N/A)	6 months			
Hepatitis B[1]	N/A	4 weeks	8 weeks and at least 16 weeks after first dose.		
Inactivated poliovirus[7]	N/A	4 weeks	4 weeks[7]	6 months[7]	
Meningococcal[13]	N/A	8 weeks[13]			
Measles, mumps, rubella[9]	N/A	4 weeks			
Varicella[10]	N/A	3 months if younger than age 13 years. 4 weeks if age 13 years or older.			

NOTE: The above recommendations must be read along with the footnotes of this schedule.

FIGURE 28–2. Recommended catch-up immunization schedule for children of age 4 months through 18 years of age. *(Footnotes not included.)* (Reproduced with permission from the Centers for Disease Control and Prevention [CDC].)

(2 and 4 months) or three-dose (2, 4, and 6 months) series, depending on the vaccine used. It should also not be initiated after 15 weeks of age due to lack of safety data for older infants. Eight months of age is the latest time point at which the final dose can be given. After the infant swallows the vaccine the virus will be shed in the poop; therefore, caregivers should use good hand hygiene after changing diapers to avoid getting sick. Newer preparations are not associated with intussusception, as was a former version that is no longer available. Infants who are mildly ill may receive the rotavirus vaccine, but if they have severe vomiting or diarrhea, the vaccine should be delayed. Other contraindications include allergic reaction to a previous dose of the rotavirus vaccine and infants with immunodeficiencies such as severe combined immunodeficiency (SCID). The vaccine is *not* contraindicated in infants whose household contacts are immunocompromised as long as hand hygiene is enforced.

Question 4-2

What would be the next set of booster vaccines this patient receives, and when?

A) In 4 weeks, he may receive hepatitis B, IPV, DTap, PCV-13, and hepatitis A.

B) In 4 weeks, he may receive IPV, DTap, PCV-13, and rotavirus.

C) In 6 weeks, he may receive PCV-13, DTap, and IPV.

D) In 8 weeks, he may receive IPV, DTap, and hepatitis A.

E) In 4 weeks, he may receive DTaP and IPV.

Discussion 4-2

The correct answer is "E." This child requires only DTaP and IPV booster vaccines. No rotavirus: He is still too old. No hepatitis B: He completed the third dose of the three-dose series at the last visit. No Hib: He only needs one dose since his previous was after 15 months of age. No PCV-13: He only needs one dose since his previous was after 24 months of age. Other considerations include the following:

- DTap and IPV: The third dose is given 4 weeks after the second.

- Hepatitis A: The second dose may be given 6 months after the first.

- MMR and varicella: The second dose may be given according to the regular schedule at 4 to 6 years of age.

> **Helpful Tip**
> Premature infants should follow the same standard childhood vaccine schedule as full-term infants. The schedule should be based on the premature infant's chronological age not gestational age.

▶ CASE 5

A 2-year-old child comes in for her well-child check. She has sickle cell disease (SCD) and is receiving hydroxyurea. She missed her 18-month checkup but was up to date on vaccines at her 12-month well-child check.

Question 5-1

Which vaccines are very important in a patient with SCD?

A) Hib.

B) PCV-13.

C) Meningococcal.

D) Influenza.

E) All of the above.

Discussion 5-1

The correct answer is "E." Children with SCD are functionally asplenic—an acquired immunodeficiency. Children with asplenia whether functional or anatomic are at risk for infections with encapsulated bacteria such as *Haemophilus influenzae* type b, *Streptococcus pneumoniae,* and *Neisseria meningitidis.* Children with SCD should receive all routine childhood immunizations, especially Hib, PCV-13, and meningococcal vaccines.

....

Reviewing her records, you see she has received three doses of the Hib and PCV-13 vaccines. She has not received the meningococcal vaccine. She is current on all other vaccines.

Question 5-2

Which vaccines should your sickle cell disease patient receive today?

A) Hib and PCV-13.

B) Hib and pneumococcal polysaccharide unconjugated vaccine (PPSV-23).

C) PCV-13 and meningococcal.

D) Hib, PCV-13, and meningococcal.

E) Hib, PPSV-23, and meningococcal.

Discussion 5-2

The correct answer is "D." Pneumococcal vaccines include both a 13-valent pneumococcal conjugate vaccine (PCV-13) and a 23-valent pneumococcal polysaccharide unconjugated vaccine (PPSV-23). PCV-13 is given as a four-dose series (at 2, 4, 6, and 12 to 15 months) to children younger than 2 years of age. The number refers to the number of bacterial serotypes included in the vaccine. Children with asplenia, HIV, congenital immunodeficiency, SCD, cochlear implant, nephrotic syndrome, chronic kidney disease, blood or solid organ tumor, organ transplant, chronic lung disease, and chronic heart disease (especially cyanotic heart disease) should receive the PPSV-23 at 24 months of age and a single booster dose 5 years later. If a child with one of the conditions listed above did not complete the PCV-13 series, he or she should receive catch-up doses before receiving the PPSV-23. Since your patient has received three of four doses of the pneumococcal series, he should receive the PCV-13 today followed 8 weeks later by the PPSV-23. Hib is administered as a three-dose series at 2, 4, and 6 months of age. A booster dose is given between 12 and 15 months. Children aged 12 to 59 months old at a high risk for Hib disease (eg, SCD, HIV) who haven't received a booster dose will need 1 or 2 dose(s) depending on number of doses previously received.

⧖ QUICK QUIZ

Which child should NOT receive the meningococcal vaccine?

A) 12-year-old who has not previously received the meningococcal vaccine.

B) 13-year-old with HIV who received his first dose 1 year ago.

C) 19-year-old who has not previously received the meningococcal vaccine.

D) 2-month-old with asplenia.

E) 12-month-old with complement deficiency.

Discussion

The correct answer is "C." Several different types of meningococcal vaccines are available in the United States. Quadrivalent conjugate vaccines contain serotypes A, C, Y, and W. In 2014, the U.S. Food and Drug Administration (FDA) approved a serogroup B meningococcal vaccine for use in people aged 10 to 25 years and in 2015, the ACIP voted to recommend use of the vaccine in high-risk people within that age group. A single meningococcal vaccine should be administered to all adolescents aged 11 to 12 years, with a booster dose at age 16. If the first dose is given at age 16 or older, a booster is not needed. If the adolescent is 18 years or older, the vaccine should only be administered in specific high-risk situations (eg, travel to an endemic area, or community outbreak). HIV-positive adolescents aged 11 to 18 years should receive a two-dose initial series, with 8 weeks between doses. Children with asplenia, including SCD and complement deficiency, should receive doses at 2, 4, 6, and 12 months of age.

▶ CASE 6

An infant is born at 30 weeks' gestation by vaginal delivery to a hepatitis B surface antigen (HBsAg)–negative mother. The infant weights 2600 g. You are unsure whether to order the hepatitis B vaccine (HBV). The infant is premature and small. You wonder if that makes a difference.

Question 6-1

What is true regarding hepatitis B vaccination and premature infants?

A) Premature infants weighing more than 2 kg should receive the HBV at the same time as a term infant would.

B) Premature infants weighing less than 2 kg should never receive the HBV.

C) Premature infants weighing less than 2 kg should receive the HBV at 60 days of age.

D) Premature infants born before 32 weeks' gestational age should not receive the HBV at birth.

E) All premature infants born to HBsAg-positive mothers should receive the HBV.

Discussion 6-1

The correct answer is "A." All term infants should receive the HBV within 12 hours of birth to prevent vertical transmission of infection from the mother to the infant. Hepatitis B

TABLE 28–1 HEPATITIS B VACCINATION IN PREMATURE INFANTS			
	Maternal Hepatitis B Status and Birthweight		
	HBsAg Negative *and* ≥ 2 kg	**HBsAg Negative *and* < 2 kg**	**HBsAg Positive (any birthweight)**
Hepatitis B vaccine	At birth	At 30 days of age	At birth
Hepatitis B immunoglobulin	N/A	N/A	At birth

kg, kilogram; N/A, not applicable.

immunoglobulin (HBIG) should be given in addition to the vaccine to infants born to HBsAg-positive mothers. Additional doses should be given at 1 to 2 and 6 months. With premature infants, birthweight above or below 2 kg and maternal hepatitis B status drive the decision of timing of vaccination. For an infant of a mother who is HBsAg positive, birthweight does not matter. If the HBV is given at birth to an infant weighing less than 2 kg, the infant will need to complete a four- rather than three-dose series. (See Table 28–1.) As long as we are talking about hepatitis, do not forget that the hepatitis A vaccine series is two doses, starting at 12 months of age.

▶ CASE 7

You are rounding in the neonatal intensive care unit (NICU). The mother of an infant girl who was born prematurely at 26 weeks' gestational age, now corrected to a gestational age of 35 weeks, asks you when her daughter may be vaccinated.

Question 7-1

What do you tell her?

A) Great question! We should give your baby her 2-month vaccines now, including DTap, Hib, HBV, IPV, and PCV-13.

B) Great question! As long as your baby is in the NICU she can't receive her vaccines, as she would put the other babies at risk while she is shedding the virus. Once she is discharged we should start her scheduled vaccines immediately.

C) Great question! Even though she weighed less than 2 kg at birth, your baby can get all of her immunizations on time.

D) Great question! She is at increased risk of adverse effects from the vaccines.

Discussion 7-1

The correct answer is "A." Premature infants should receive all routine childhood immunizations based on their chronological age. This infant is 63 days old; therefore, she should receive her 2-month vaccines. The vaccines given typically at 2, 4, and 6 months are all killed viruses, except for the rotavirus, which should not be given in the NICU setting. Not all premature infants weighing less than 2 kg at birth receive the HBV. You already learned this! Otherwise they should receive their vaccines consistent with their chronological age. Preterm and low birth weight infants are not at increased risk for adverse reactions to vaccines.

> **Helpful Tip**
> Preterm infants are at increased risk of vaccine-preventable diseases and their complications; however, they are less likely to receive their immunizations on time.

> **Helpful Tip**
> The CDC publishes vaccine information for people who travel internationally. Remember, your passport and vaccine record go hand in hand.

▶ CASE 8

The parents of one of your patients would like to discuss the pros and cons of the human papillomavirus vaccine (HPV) for their 11-year-old son.

Question 8-1

Which of the following statements is true?
A) It will help prevent cervical cancer for his female partners but does not protect against any other cancers.
B) There are no adverse effects to the HPV vaccine.
C) The vaccine may cause premature ovarian failure.
D) The HPV vaccine is a three-part series given over a 6-month period; it is important to complete the whole series.
E) Fainting may occur after vaccine administration, but having the patient sit or lay down for 5 to 10 minutes afterward reduces the occurrence.
F) Boys may not receive the HPV vaccine before age 11.

Discussion 8-1

The correct answer is "D." HPV is a sexually transmitted infection. It can cause genital warts and cancer. Acquisition of the virus occurs in more ways than just intercourse (penetration). The vaccine is most effective if given to those who have not yet been infected. The vaccine protects against anal, vaginal, and vulvar cancers as well as anogenital warts. Syncope is a common adverse effect of the HPV vaccine and can be prevented with 15 minutes of sitting or lying down following vaccination. Pain is also a side effect commonly complained of after vaccination. There is no evidence that ovarian failure is an adverse effect of the HPV vaccine. The three-dose series should be administered to all adolescents aged 11 to 12 years but it may be started as young as 9 years old.

⧗ QUICK QUIZ

Regarding vaccination for diphtheria, tetanus, and pertussis, which of the following statements is true?
A) Pregnant women should receive the tetanus, diphtheria, and acellular pertussis (Tdap) vaccine in the third trimester of each pregnancy.
B) Children younger than 7 years of age should receive the tetanus, diphtheria, and acellular pertussis (Tdap) vaccine.
C) Children older than 7 years of age should receive the DTap vaccine.
D) DTap and Tdap contain the whole-cell pertussis vaccine.
E) Only adults working in the health care or child care industry need a booster dose.

Discussion

The correct answer is "A." Children younger than 7 years of age should receive the DTap vaccine. It is a five-dose series given at 2, 4, 6, and 15 to 18 months, and at 4 to 6 years. Tdap is administered to children 7 years of age and older and adults. All adolescents (ages 11 to 12) and adults should receive a one-time booster dose due to the waning immunity of the acellular pertussis component. Booster is indicated even for those recently infected as natural infection does not produce lifelong immunity. Pertussis ("whooping cough") causes a prolonged respiratory illness and can be severe in young infants. A booster dose is very important for adults caring for young infants to "cocoon" the infant who is too young to be vaccinated. Currently the vaccine available in the United States is acellular pertussis; whole-cell pertussis vaccines are no longer available. The whole-cell vaccine provided better immunity but had more adverse side effects. Children younger than age 7 years with a contraindication to pertussis should receive DT instead of DTap. DT should be substituted for those aged 7 years and older. Aside from anaphylaxis, there are few contraindications for the DTap or Tdap vaccine; the most common side effects include fever, tenderness/redness at site of the injection, and prolonged crying or fussiness.

> **Helpful Tip**
> Common adverse side effects of all vaccines include fever, tenderness or redness at the injection site, and fussiness. Other side effects are minor. In the risk-benefit ratio of this situation, vaccines will always win. Children should continue to receive their vaccines.

▶ CASE 9

A 5-year-old child is brought for his kindergarten checkup. His parents have his school immunization request form for you to fill out. He is undergoing chemotherapy for ALL and is currently doing well, with good blood counts.

Question 9-1

Which is false regarding immunizations in children receiving chemotherapy?

A) There are limited data regarding immunizations in children undergoing chemotherapy.

B) Only live viral vaccines should be administered.

C) The response to vaccination may be reduced as a result of immunosuppression.

D) Only inactive immunizations should be administered.

E) After completion of chemotherapy, children should receive catch-up doses of any vaccines they missed.

Discussion 9-1

The correct answer is "B." If you have not learned that live vaccines are contraindicated in immunosuppressed patients, you need to start this chapter over. Vaccines provide immunity by stimulating an immune response in the host. If your *immune* system is shut down, it makes sense that your *immune* response may be decreased. A little protection is better than no protection and not all children will respond the same, so give the vaccines but check vaccine titers 3 to 6 months postchemotherapy. If titers are low, revaccinate.

> **Helpful Tip**
> Vaccines received prior to chemotherapy and radiation are valid unless the patient undergoes a hematopoietic cell transplant.

▶ CASE 10

You are living in Iowa and visit the Amish community, providing door-to-door care as in the old days. The people of this community do not vaccinate. You recently diagnosed and treated a young boy in the community for polio. His mother is pregnant with her seventh child.

Question 10-1

Which of the following is applicable to your efforts to protect the unvaccinated mother, fetus, and six other children?

A) Unvaccinated adults living in a community with a case of wild-type polio should complete a three-dose primary vaccine series.

B) Vaccinated adults living in a community with a case of wild-type polis should receive a single booster dose of the vaccine.

C) The injectable polio virus vaccine is used in the United States.

D) Vaccination is typically not recommended during pregnancy.

E) All of the above.

Discussion 10-1

The correct answer is "E." Wild-type polio infection was a horrible disease but is nonexistent in the United States thanks to vaccination. Vaccines work and are great! The live oral polio virus vaccine (OPV) has been replaced by the inactivated polio vaccine (IPV) administered in a four-dose series at 2, 4, and 6 to 18 months and 4 to 6 years. OPV should not be counted in the four needed doses. The IPV is safe, with no serious reactions, including vaccine-associated paralytic polio. The pregnant mother, children, and father as well as other community members exposed should be vaccinated. As all are unvaccinated, they should complete the primary series (four doses for children and three doses for those 4 years of age and older). Vaccination is typically not recommended in pregnancy but in this case the mother is at risk and requires immediate protection. A one-time booster is indicated for a vaccinated adult in exposure situations (community case, international travel, exposed health care workers).

> **Helpful Tip**
> The dosing schedule for infants is somewhat easy to remember but the rules for catch-up immunizations vary by recommended interval between doses, number of doses required, and who to vaccinate. Consult the CDC's catch-up schedule for help.

▶ CASE 11

A mother of a 6-month-old brings her infant in for a well-baby check. As part of your routine questioning, you ask about water sources. The family has well water but the fluoride level has not been checked. The mother asks, "Does my baby need fluoride at this age?" On exam the infant is fat and happy, and his bottom two incisors have erupted.

Question 11-1

Which of the following statements is/are true regarding fluoride?

A) Fluoride should be started at 2 months of age.

B) Fluoride varnish application should start once the secondary teeth have erupted.

C) Fluoride supplementation should be considered for children who exclusively drink bottled water.

D) Fluoride toothpaste should be avoided until 2 years of age.

E) If a well has fluoride, supplementation is not needed.

F) Both A and B.

G) Both B and C.

H) Options B, D, and E.

Discussion 11-1

The correct answer is "C." Fluoride supplementation prevents cavities. Drinking fluorinated water and brushing twice daily with a fluoride-containing toothpaste is adequate exposure. Bottled water contains very little to no fluoride, and well water may contain insufficient fluoride. Fluoride supplementation should not be started until 6 months of age. The concentration of fluoride in a well determines the amount of supplementation needed. If greater than 0.6 parts per million (ppm), supplementation is not needed. If the concentration is less than 0.3 ppm, supplementation should be started at 6 months of age. If the concentration is between 0.3 and 0.6 ppm, supplementation should begin at 3 years of age. Fluoride toothpaste can be used as soon as teeth have erupted. The key is to use a very small amount (size of a grain of rice) until 3 years old (size of a pea). The American Academy of Pediatrics (AAP) recommends universal application of fluoride varnish to all infants and children starting when the first tooth appears. Varnish should be repeated every 3 to 6 months. Remember too much fluoride is not good and may cause fluorosis (staining of the teeth).

....

The mother asks what she should be doing to take care of her baby's teeth.

Question 11-2
Which of the following regarding oral hygiene is true?
A) The leading cause of chronic disease in children is dental caries.
B) Children should begin dental cleanings at 2 years of age.
C) Dental pain has not been shown to affect focus and learning.
D) Dental health care is easily accessible to children under the age of 5.
E) None of the above are true.

Discussion 11-2
The correct answer is "A." Dental caries are more prevalent than asthma and allergies. Children should begin dental cleanings at 1 year of age. Dental pain has been associated with educational disruption. Many families have a difficult time accessing dental care.

⏳ **QUICK QUIZ**

Younger drivers are more likely to be distracted while driving. Which of the following statements is false regarding distracted driving?
A) Over 70% of teens have admitted to composing or sending text messages while driving.
B) Over 65% of teens have admitted to reading a text message while driving.
C) 10% of all drivers under the age of 20 involved in fatal crashes were reported as distracted at the time of the crash.
D) 25% of teens respond to one or more text messages every time they drive.
E) Headset use while driving is considerably safer.

Discussion
The correct answer is "E." Using hands-free headsets has not been proven safer and is still considered distracted driving. Motor vehicle crashes are the leading cause of death in adolescents. Crashes are associated with (1) other teenagers in the car, (2) night driving, and (3) using electronic devices while driving (distractions).

▶ **CASE 12**

You are the attending physician in the newborn nursery. You have standard discharge teaching for parents that includes fever, feeding, pooping, peeing, safe sleep, and car seats. The parents of a newborn also have a 6-year-old daughter. They ask if they need to listen, noting that as parents of a 6-year-old they are well aware of the importance of car seats.

Question 12-1
What do you tell them?
A) Infants should remain in a rear-facing car seat in the back seat until 2 years of age.
B) Children should not ride in the front seat before age 13.
C) A five-point harness should be used until the child is age 4.
D) School-aged children should ride in a booster seat to ensure the seatbelt is properly positioned until age 8 or the seat belt fits correctly.
E) All of the above.

Discussion 12-1
The correct answer is "E." The AAP undated its car seat recommendations in 2011. The options listed above reflect current recommendations.

....

Moving along in your discharge teaching monologue, you discuss safe sleeping to prevent sudden infant death syndrome (SIDS).

Question 12-2
Which is a safe sleep environment?
A) Infant sleeping in a sleep sack with a pacifier, lying flat on his back in the crib without bumpers, toys, or blankets. The crib is located in the parents' bedroom.
B) Infant sleeping in a co-sleeper in the parents' bed.
C) Infant sleeping in a sleep sack, lying flat on his back in the crib with a teddy bear. The crib is located in the parent's bedroom.
D) Infant sleeping prone in a crib on an alarm mat. The crib is in the parents' bedroom.
E) Infant sleeping in a car seat.

Discussion 12-2
The correct answer is "A." This is one no pediatrician should get wrong. Have you heard of the Back to Sleep campaign? Evidence supports the contention that room sharing without bed sharing decreases the risk of SIDS by up to 50%. The crib or bassinet should have a firm, flat mattress covered with a fitted sheet. Crib slates should be no more than 2 inches apart—a soda can should not fit through the space. Throw the bumpers, toys, blankets, and anything else in the crib on the floor. You do not want to suffocate or overheat the infant. Sleep sacks work well. The arms are swaddled while the hips are free (key). SIDS alarms have not been shown to decrease the risk. Devices that place an infant in a sitting position, such as a car seat, stroller, or swing, increase the risk of SIDS, especially in infants younger than 4 months of age, likely related to the ability of the infant's head to assume a position that closes off the airway.

Helpful Tip
Pacifier use at the beginning of sleep has been shown to decrease the risk of SIDS. Although the mechanism is unknown, the protective effect continues even after the pacifier falls out, so it does not need to be reinserted.

► CASE 13

A 13-month-old boy is brought to the clinic after a fall. He recently started walking and is still unsteady. The child was playing on the couch and rolled off onto the carpet, bonking his head. He cried immediately but is now acting fine. He has a small hematoma on his forehead. You reassure the mother that he is okay and take the time to go over important safety points for early walkers.

Question 13-1

Which of the following statements regarding injury prevention for newly mobile toddlers is false?

A) All infants and children should wear sunscreen when outside.
B) Early walkers are unsteady, and stair gates are important to prevent falls down the stairs.
C) Siblings should not supervise younger siblings in the bathtub.
D) Childproofing the home is important, especially as children become mobile, develop better fine motor skills, and become curious.
E) Heavy objects and hot liquids should not be left on the edge of tables or counters to prevent children from pulling the objects or liquids onto themselves.

Discussion 13-1

The correct answer is "A." Once a toddler becomes mobile he or she can get into anything. Childproofing the home includes (1) locking up medications and cleaning products, (2) keeping small toys out of reach, (3) making sure cords are not dangling, (4) using outlet safety covers, (5) not having young children take care of their baby siblings, (6) keeping sharp objects out of reach, and (7) making sure hot and heavy overhead items are secured and not reachable by children. (See Table 28–2.)

⧗ QUICK QUIZ

Which of the following regarding sun safety is false?

A) Children and infants should stay in the shade.
B) Sunscreen is generally recommended for use in infants younger than 6 months of age.
C) Sun exposure should be limited during peak hours.
D) Infants and children should wear brimmed hats when in the sun.
E) Sunscreen should be SPF 15 or higher, with protection against UVA and UVB rays.

Discussion

The correct answer is "B." Infants younger than 6 months of age should stay in the shade and wear adequate clothing (eg, long-sleeved shirt, lightweight long pants, hat) to prevent sunburn. When neither is adequately available, a small amount of sunscreen may be applied. All children 6 months of age and older should use sunscreen, making sure to put enough on and reapply every 2 hours or after swimming or sweating. Peak sun hours are from 10 AM to 4 PM. Sunglasses and tightly woven clothes are recommended as well.

► CASE 14

You join a practice in the very northern parts of New Hampshire, near the Canadian border, and after meeting several of your patients and their families have several safety concerns relating to their activities. You meet a 13-year-old boy, who excitedly tells you about his four-wheeler and how much fun he is having tearing around the fields and trails after his dad. He assures you he always wears his helmet!

Question 14-1

How do you respond?

A) You praise him for always wearing his helmet and leave it at that.
B) You ask if his four-wheeler has an "adult engine" (> 90 mL), and recommend his father drive if it does, as these are not recommended for children or teens younger than 16 years of age.
C) You ask if he is wearing a motorcycle helmet with eye protection and not just a bicycle helmet.
D) You suggest that riding the all-terrain vehicle (ATV) on the road would be safer, especially if he is going to go fast.
E) Both B and C.

Discussion 14-1

The correct answer is "E." ATVs with adult engines can reach speeds of 50 miles per hour (mph). Teenagers younger than 16 years of age should not be the operator as their reaction times and ability to concentrate (immature motor and judgment skills) are not sufficiently developed. (For the same reason car licenses are not given out before age 16, and many states now have graduated license programs.) Riding with a passenger is not recommended. An appropriate helmet (motorcycle), eye protection, and reflective clothing should be worn. Street use of off-road vehicles is a no-no.

> **Helpful Tip**
> Children younger than 12 years of age represent 15% of the deaths related to ATV crashes.

► CASE 15

Your brother is looking for a house with a pool. He has two young children, 2 and 4 years old, and asks your advice to keep them safe.

Question 15-1

What do you tell him regarding safety around a pool?

A) The pool should be surrounded on all four sides by a fence.
B) The pool should have a gate that latches.
C) Children should always be supervised when swimming.
D) Children should begin swimming lessons at 4 years of age.
E) All of the above.

TABLE 28-2 INJURY PREVENTION AND SAFETY RECOMMENDATIONS

Age	Recommendation	Age	Recommendation
Infants (0–12 months)	Rear-facing car seat	All ages	Stay away from drugs, alcohol, and tobacco
	Safe sleeping • Back to sleep • No co-sleeping • No excess bedding, stuffed animals, crib bumpers • Firm mattress • Crib slats < 2 inches apart • Do not overdress • Pacifier is okay		Discuss bullying and fighting
			Tobacco-free environment • Home and car
			Pet safety • Supervise near pets • Do not leave infant or young child alone with a pet
	SIDS prevention • No tobacco smoke exposure • Safe sleep		Gun safety • No gun is safest • Store locked, unloaded, with ammunition locked in a separate place
	Choking hazards • Keep small toys out of reach • Feed age-appropriate finger foods cut into appropriate-sized bites		Water safety • Pools should be surrounded by a 4-sided fence with childproof gate • Never allow children to swim unattended • Supervise around water
Toddlers (1–4 years)	Remove all dangling cords		Bathtub safety • Turn hot water heater to < 48.8°C (120°F) • Never leave an infant or young child unattended
	Keep overhead objects secured and out of reach		
	Keep overhead hot liquids out of reach and turn pot handles to back of stove		Supervision • Younger children should not supervise their young siblings • Never leave a child alone in a car or home
	Childproof stairs, windows, and electrical outlets		
	Lock up medications and cleaning products		Use appropriate car restraints and car seats
	Choking hazards • Only age-appropriate toys • Cut hotdogs and grapes into quarters • Cut food into small bite-sized pieces		Sun safety • Limit sun • Avoid midafternoon sun exposure • Use sunscreen • Wear hats
	Put away sharp objects		Insect safety • Use DEET
	Do not use baby walkers		Test and use smoke alarms and carbon monoxide detectors
Children (5–10 years)	Street safety • Look both ways before crossing • Use crosswalk		Wear a bicycle helmet • Anytime on a moving object or animal
	Teach child to swim		Wear proper safety equipment for activities (roller blading, skiing, etc)
Adolescents (11–21 years)	No ATV if younger than 16 years of age		Teach stranger safety
	Safe driving • No distractions • Never ride with a friend who is under the influence of drugs or alcohol		Wear a life jacket on a boat

ATV, all-terrain vehicle; DEET, *N,N*-diethyl-meta-toluamide (insect repellent); SIDS, sudden infant death syndrome.

Discussion 15-1

The correct answer is "E." Swimming pools, including inflatable and portable pools, should be enclosed by a four-sided fence with a latching gate. A fence is important for pool safety, but it only works if it keeps the pool completely blocked off from children and the gait remains closed with a childproof lock. Avoid chain-link fences, because children are resourceful and may climb over. Even with a good fence, a child still needs to be supervised. Other methods to prevent drowning include swimming lessons starting at age 4 years if the child is developmentally ready (starting at an earlier age does not offer an advantage), ensuring that parents are trained in cardiopulmonary resuscitation, and using appropriate personal floatation devices.

▶ CASE 16

At a 3-year-old well-child check, the mother mentions that the family will be spending time at the lake this summer. She is concerned about water safety and asks you for advice.

Question 16-1

What do you recommend?
A) She always be close enough to hear him.
B) She always be close enough to see him.
C) She always be close enough to touch him.
D) As long as he knows not to go near the water without her, he'll be safe.

Discussion 16-1

The correct answer is "C." Toddlers are unlikely to thrash, splash, or call out if they fall into a body of water. They are more likely to sink silently below the surface and drown. Toddlers, infants, or other weak swimmers should be within an arm's length of an adult ("touch supervision"). Parents can be advised to think of water like the street; you always hold their hand crossing the street, you should do the same around water.

Now the 3-year-old's mother is worried. She asks, "Isn't he old enough to be alone in the bathtub? He likes to play in there for hours!"

Question 16-2

You respond:
A) As long as you don't fill the tub up too much, and you can hear him, he's fine by himself.
B) Children shouldn't be left alone in the tub until age 6.
C) As long as his 8-year-old sister is watching him he should be fine.
D) Children are fine in the bathtub as young as age 2 if they have a special bath seat.
E) Children should only take showers.

Discussion 16-2

The correct answer is "B." Children can drown in minimal amounts of water. Not only should tubs and pools be supervised, but 5-gallon buckets should be emptied when toddlers are around and toilets or bathrooms should have locks. Supervisors of bath time should be at least a teenager or adult, as older siblings can be distracted easily. Bath rings and seats can fall over, leading to drowning. They offer a false sense of security.

The mother suddenly looks up as if she had a bright idea. "What about arm floaties when swimming. Won't that make up for his missing swimming skills?"

Question 16-3

What is an appropriate personal flotation device (PFD) for a weak swimmer?
A) Swim wings.
B) Swim bubble.
C) Vest-style PFD.
D) Horseshoe-style PFD.
E) Both C and D.

Discussion 16-3

The correct answer is "E." "Swim wings" or other inflatable flotation devices are meant to help children learn to swim. They do not hold their face out of the water to help prevent drowning. They also might pop and allow the child to sink. The "bubble" is also a learning-to-swim tool; it actually positions the child face down in the water, which could be very dangerous in a panicked, weak swimmer.

▶ CASE 17

The mother of a child in your practice is concerned about tick-borne diseases and asks you whether treatment is always necessary if a child is bitten by a tick.

Question 17-1

Who should receive prophylactic treatment for a tick bite?
A) A 10-year-old who had a deer tick bite 5 days ago while on a Boy Scout camping trip in New Hampshire. The boy reports the tick was on for 2 days before he told anyone about it. He is asymptomatic currently.
B) A 7-year-old who had a deer tick bite. The tick was attached for more than 36 hours ago, and the local Lyme rates are greater than 20%.
C) A 9-year-old who had a deer tick removed 3 hours ago from rural Maine. The tick was on for more than 36 hours.
D) A pregnant 16-year-old who had a deer tick attached for more than 36 hours and is in your office for removal.
E) Both A and B.
F) Both A and D.
G) Options A, B, and C.
H) All of the above.

Discussion 17-1

The correct answer is "C." Lyme prophylaxis is given if (1) the bite is from a deer tick, (2) the tick is attached for more than 36 hours, (3) it has been less than 72 hours since tick removal, (4) local Lyme rates are greater than 20%, and (5) doxycycline is not contraindicated (eg, younger than 8 years of age; pregnant or breastfeeding patient).

Question 17-2

Which of the following sequences describes the correct method of removing a tick?

A) Paint tick with nail polish or petroleum jelly; once it stops moving use tweezers to grasp tick as close to skin surface as possible and, with steady pressure, pull out tick; clean area with soap and water; dispose of tick by flushing down toilet.

B) Using fine-tipped tweezers, grasp tick as close to skin surface as possible; pull upward with steady even pressure; clean area after removing tick with soap and water or rubbing alcohol; dispose of tick by submerging in alcohol, flushing down toilet, or placing in sealed bag or container.

C) Using fine-tipped tweezers, grasp tick as close to skin surface as possible; pull upward with steady pressure and twist gently to ensure head is removed fully; clean area with soap and water; dispose of tick by submerging in alcohol, flushing down toilet, or placing in sealed bag or container.

D) Heat tick with flame cautiously so not to burn the skin; once it stops moving use tweezers to grasp tick as close to skin surface as possible and, with steady pressure, pull out tick; clean area with soap and water; dispose of tick by flushing down toilet.

Discussion 17-2

The correct answer is "B." Children should be searched for ticks when coming indoors after playing in or near wooded areas. The tick should be removed as quickly as possible.

QUICK QUIZ

Which of the following statements regarding firearms is true?

A) The leading cause of firearm deaths in individuals aged 0 to 19 years is homicide.

B) The leading cause of firearm deaths in individuals aged 0 to 19 years is suicide.

C) The leading cause of firearm deaths in all ages is homicide.

D) The leading cause of firearm deaths in all ages is suicide.

E) Firearms are the most lethal method for suicide in individuals aged 15 to 19 years.

F) Prevention of firearm related deaths should be discussed as part of a well-child exam starting as a young toddler.

G) Both B and E.

H) Options A, C, and F.

I) Options A, D, E, and F.

J) All of the above.

Discussion

The correct answer is "I." In 2009, among individuals from birth to 19 years of age, 66% of firearm-related deaths were homicide, 28% were suicide, 4% were unintentional, 1% were undetermined, and 1% were police related. Among all age groups, 60% were suicide, 36% were homicide, 2% were unintentional, 1%

were undetermined, and 1% were police related. Firearms are the most lethal cause of suicide attempts in 15- to 19-year-old individuals, having a 90% fatality rate. The AAP recommends that pediatricians discuss prevention of firearm-related deaths and injuries, including the dangers of access to guns both inside and outside the home. It is recommended that pediatricians incorporate questions regarding access and safety of storage, as well as counsel on the increased risk of suicidal acts when a gun is present in the home. The safest home is one without a gun. Guns should be stored unloaded and locked, with ammunition stored in a separate locked location.

QUICK QUIZ

Which of the following statements regarding trampolines is false?

A) 10% or more of trampoline injuries involve the head and neck.

B) Younger children are at risk for proximal tibial fractures.

C) Approximately three quarters of trampoline injuries occur when there is more than one occupant on a trampoline.

D) Trampoline falls account for over 25% of all trampoline-related injuries.

E) The APP states that consumer use of trampolines is only safe if the trampoline meets the safety guidelines, there is appropriate supervision, and there is only one child on the trampoline at a time.

Discussion

The correct answer is "E." The AAP does not recommend consumer use of trampolines, regardless of safety measures taken. The other statements are all true.

▶ CASE 18

You are teaching a resident in your clinic about well-child care and recommended screenings at 12 months. She asks how to decide who to screen for lead exposure.

Question 18-1

Which of the following is the best response?

A) All children receiving Medicaid should be screened.

B) A child who lives in a home built in 2000 that is undergoing extensive renovation should be screened.

C) All children who attend daycare should be screened.

D) All children who play outside in the dirt should be screened.

Discussion 18-1

The correct answer is "A." Environmental lead exposure can result in lead toxicity, with subsequent cognitive impairment. In the past all children were screened. Today screening targets those at risk for lead toxicity, with lead testing at 1 and 2 years of age. Among children eligible for Medicaid, 80% were found to have increased blood levels. Others at increased risk include

(1) siblings or playmates who have had elevated blood lead levels; (2) children who visit houses built before 1970, including private in-home daycares; and (3) children exposed to structures with damaged or recently remodeled lead-painted surfaces.

> **Helpful Tip**
> When considering environmental lead sources, think about soil and leaded gasoline that may have leaked into the soil before the area became a neighborhood. Consider airborne lead from combustion, which was a common cause of elevated lead levels before 1980. Use of lead paint on interior surfaces ceased in the 1970s; however, dust and surrounding soil may still be contaminated.

Question 18-2

Which of the following statements describes the risks of elevated lead levels?
A) Children with lead levels higher than 10 mcg/dL are at risk for delinquent behaviors in adolescence.
B) Children with lead levels lower than 10 mcg/dL are at no increased risk for adverse effects.
C) Chelation of children with moderately elevated lead levels will remove all risk for changes in neuropsychology or cognitive testing.
D) All of the above.
E) None of the above.

Discussion 18-2

The correct answer is "A." A lead level of 10 mg/dL or greater has been shown to affect a child's cognitive ability. Lead level, even below 10 mcg/dL, is inversely related to IQ points. It is estimated that there is an IQ loss of 2 to 3 points for lead levels higher than 20 mcg/dL. Chelation therapy has not proven effective at removing all risk, but it does lower the blood lead level so damage is not ongoing.

A child is found to have elevated lead levels.

Question 18-3

In addition to the causes already discussed, what else should be considered as an environmental source of lead exposure?
A) The family has been burning painted and unusual wood and other materials to heat the home.
B) The older sibling likes to make ceramic pots, and food is often stored in them.
C) The mother makes stained glass windows.
D) The father is an active hunter and fisher.
E) All of the above.

Discussion 18-3

The correct answer is "E." This child needs to be removed from these exposures. In addition, the child and family should be instructed to wash hands often and consistently as frequent hand washing, especially before eating, can decrease environmental lead exposure and ingestion. Remember that an elevated capillary lead level should be confirmed by venous sample.

> **Helpful Tip**
> Peak lead concentration in children is usually reached at age 2 years, even if the lead exposure in the environment has not abated, since this is when hand-to-mouth activity decreases.

▶ CASE 19

You are talking at dinner with a friend, and the topic of eye exams comes up. Your friend wants to know when her children should have the first eye exam.

Question 19-1

What do you tell her?
A) At 6 months of age.
B) At 1 year of age.
C) At 3 years of age.
D) At 5 years of age before beginning school.
E) None of the above.

Discussion 19-1

The correct answer is "E." The first eye exam should occur at birth, to check for cataracts, retinoblastoma, and ptosis—all problems which, if not caught early, can have a significant effect on lifelong vision. Eye exams should be continued at every well visit, with visual acuity testing being done as early as possible, usually ages 3 to 4 years. Well-child eye exams should include assessment of ability to track objects, extraocular movements, simultaneous red reflex, pupillary response, inspection (lid, cornea, iris), corneal light reflex, and cover-uncover test. Early detection and treatment of strabismus in infants and children can prevent vision loss (amblyopia).

Question 19-2

When should a child be referred to a pediatric ophthalmologist?
A) When he or she has failed vision testing or is unable to be tested in the office.
B) When he or she has an anatomic abnormality on exam.
C) When he or she is 3 years old.
D) When he or she is 6 months old.
E) Both A and B.

Discussion 19-2

The correct answer is "E." An abnormal exam, failed visual acuity test, and positive history warrant referral to a specialist. Important history details include family history of eye problems (congenital cataracts, retinoblastoma), developmental delay, systemic disease with associated eye issues, parental concerns (head tilt, squinting, tearing, or lazy eye, inability to recognize or look at objects, etc).

▶ CASE 20

A new mother comes to your office. During the health screening she admits to smoking and expresses the desire to quit. She asks you about the risks of secondhand smoke for her infant.

Question 20-1

You emphasize which of the following in your response?

A) Recurrent respiratory illnesses and wheezing.
B) Ear infections.
C) Dental decay.
D) Increased risk of SIDs.
E) All of the above.

Discussion 20-1

The correct answer is "E." Infants and children should not be exposed to secondhand smoke, which increases the risk of SIDS, ear infections, viral respiratory illnesses, and wheezing. It takes longer for children who live in households with secondhand smoke to get over colds. Asthmatics may have increased attacks that are more severe and require hospitalization. In addition, children who grow up with parents who smoke are more likely to smoke. Clearly it adversely affects their health. Encouraging and counseling parents to quit smoking to improve the health of their children can sometimes be more effective than making the same argument on behalf of their own health.

> **Helpful Tip**
> Children of smokers miss more days of school than those of nonsmokers.

⏳ QUICK QUIZ

Which of the following statements regarding health screening is false?

A) All children should have a nonfasting lipid profile checked at 10 years of age.
B) All infants should have a hemoglobin or hematocrit checked at 12 months of age.
C) Blood pressure should be checked yearly starting at 6 months of age.

Discussion

The correct answer is "C." Blood pressure should be measured yearly starting at 3 years of age. Hypertension is defined as a blood pressure greater than the 95% for age, sex, and height on three different occasions. A blood pressure cuff that is too small falsely elevates the measurement. Children should have their risk factors for dyslipidemia checked biannually from age 2 through 10 years, then yearly afterward. If a risk is identified, a nonfasting lipid panel should be obtained. All children should have a nonfasting lipid panel at ages 9 to 11 years and 17 to 21 years. Keep your patients' hearts healthy to prevent early onset of cardiac and coronary artery disease! Screening for iron deficiency should be done at all well-child checks starting at 4 months. Any child at risk, as well as all infants at 12 months of age, should have hemoglobin or hematocrit measured. Save your patients' brains as iron deficiency adversely affects cognition!

> **Helpful Tip**
> A blood pressure cuff is the correct size if the bladder length encircles 80% to 100% of the arm and the bladder width encircles 50% of the arm.

▶ CASE 21

A 7-year-old boy is brought to the office because he fell off the couch and hurt his arm. His arm turns out to be fine. The child had not been to a health care provider in 2 years, so the father completed the history form while waiting to be seen. As you read through it, you notice the child has a history of being overweight, and the family history indicates several members who were hypertensive or had heart attacks at young ages.

Question 21-1

Which of the following is a risk factor for dyslipidemia?

A) Child's BMI at 80th percentile.
B) Maternal aunt with history of myocardial infarction at age 60 years.
C) Maternal uncle with history of myocardial infarction at age 60 years.
D) Mother with history of gestational diabetes.
E) None of the above.

Discussion 21-1

The correct answer is "B" Here is the bad news: atherosclerosis can begin in young people with dyslipidemia, and the presence of risk factors in a child increase the likelihood of heart disease as an adult. Early identification and management decreases the risk of heart disease. The first step in management focuses on diet and physical activity. You just learned to when to perform lipid testing. This 8-year-old should be screened due to his risk factors. (See Tables 28–3 and 28–4.) Children and

TABLE 28–3 RISK FACTORS FOR DYSLIPIDEMIA

Myocardial infarction, angina, stroke, surgery for coronary artery disease, or sudden unexplained cardiac death in parent, grandparent, aunt or uncle.
- Male younger than 55 years old
- Female younger than 65 years old

Parent with high cholesterol or dyslipidemia

Diabetes

Hypertension

Obesity

Cigarette smoker

Moderate or high-risk medical condition (see Table 28–4)

TABLE 28–4 RISK CONDITIONS ASSOCIATED WITH DYSLIPIDEMIA

High Risk	Moderate Risk
Diabetes, types 1 and 2	Kawasaki disease with regressed coronary aneurysms
Chronic kidney disease	Chronic autoimmune diseases (lupus, JIA)
Kidney transplant	HIV
Kawasaki disease with current aneurysms	Nephrotic syndrome
Heart transplant	

HIV, human immunodeficiency virus; JIA, juvenile idiopathic arthritis.

adolescents are initially screened with a nonfasting lipid profile. If the results are abnormal, a fasting lipid panel is needed. The risk of heart disease increases as the number of personal risk factors (obesity, hypertension) increases.

► CASE 22

A new mother brings her 18-month-old son for his well-child check. She tells you that he is very smart and can use her electronic tablet by himself. He even knows how to move from one app to the next. You wonder if anyone has had the "screen time" discussion with the mother.

Question 22-1

What do you tell her?
A) Screen time should be limited to 3 hours per day for children aged 2 to 5 years.
B) Screen time should be limited to 30 minutes per day for children younger than 2 years of age.
C) Children may have a television in their bedroom if time limits are followed.
D) Screen time includes time spent watching television, only.
E) Children younger than 2 years of age should avoid television and other forms of entertainment media.

Discussion 22-1

The correct answer is "E." Screen time includes time on any electronic device, including computers, video games, phones, tablets, and television. Children younger than 2 years of age should have no screen time. Children aged 2 and older should be limited to 2 hours per day. Televisions should not be in bedrooms. (This may be less common now in the age of electronic devices, but the same prohibition applies to use of smartphones and tablets before bedtime.)

Question 22-2

Which of the following statements is false regarding entertainment media and children?
A) Excessive screen time is associated with being overweight.
B) Screen-free zones should include children's bedrooms and the dinner table.

C) The average child spends 7 hours per day on entertainment media.
D) Children and teens are at risk for cyberbullying, online solicitation, and access to inappropriate materials.
E) Young toddlers and children who are exposed to a small amount of educational electronic media show fewer language delays.

Discussion 22-2

The correct answer is "E." No studies have shown benefits of early television and video-viewing before 2 years of age. Studies have shown that language *delays* have been associated with viewing in children younger than 18 months of age.

► CASE 23

A father arrives at your office with his twins for a quick checkup. As he takes off his bicycle helmet upon entering, he tells you they biked to the office today. The 2-year-old twins ride in a trailer towed behind the bicycle. The children are strapped in with 5-point harnesses.

Question 23-1

Bicycle safety includes all of the following EXCEPT:
A) Parents and children should wear bicycle helmets every time they ride a bike.
B) Infants may ride on a rear-mounted bicycle seat as long as it has a 5-point harness.
C) Children aged 1 to 4 years may ride in a bicycle-mounted seat or tow-behind trailer.
D) Children over 4 years of age or whose weight can shift the bike should not ride in mounted bicycle seats.
E) Children should ride appropriately sized bicycles.

Discussion 23-1

The correct answer is "B." Infants younger than 1 year of age should not ride as passengers on bicycles. Remember to emphasize the importance of wearing the helmet correctly: low (covers forehead), snug, and level. Two fingers should fit under the fastened chin strap.

BIBLIOGRAPHY

American Academy of Pediatrics. Bright futures. https://brightfutures.aap.org. Accessed June 1, 2015.

American Academy of Pediatrics. Sun and water safety tips. http://www.aap.org/en-us/about-the-aap/aap-press-room/news-features-and-safety-tips/pages/Sun-and-Water-Safety-Tips.aspx. Accessed June 1, 2015.

American Academy of Pediatrics, Committee on Injury and Poison Prevention. All-terrain vehicle injury prevention: Two-, three-, and four-wheeled unlicensed motor vehicles. *Pediatrics*. 2000;105(6):1352–1354.

American Academy of Pediatrics, Committee on Injury and Poison Prevention. Policy statement—Prevention of drowning. *Pediatrics*. 2010; doi: 10.1542/peds.2010-126.

American Academy of Pediatrics, Committee on Practice and Ambulatory Medicine; Bright Futures Periodicity Schedule Workgroup. 2014 recommendations for pediatric preventive health care. *Pediatrics.* 2014;133(3):568–570. doi: 10.1542/peds.2013-4096.

American Academy of Pediatrics, Council on Communications and Media. Media education. *Pediatrics.* 2010;126(5):1012–1017. doi: 10.1542/peds.2010-1636.

American Academy of Pediatrics, Council on Sports Medicine and Fitness. Trampoline safety in childhood and adolescence. *Pediatrics.* 2012;130(4):774–779. doi: 10.1542/peds.2012-2082.

American Academy of Pediatrics, Task Force on Sudden Infant Death Syndrome. SIDS and other sleep-related infant deaths: Expansion of recommendations for a safe infant sleeping environment. *Pediatrics.* doi: 10.1542/peds.2011-2284.

Centers for Disease Control and Prevention. Catch-up immunization schedule. http://www.cdc.gov/vaccines/schedules/hcp/imz/catchup.html. Accessed June 1, 2015.

Centers for Disease Control and Prevention. Frequently asked questions about HPV vaccine safety. http://www.cdc.gov/vaccinesafety/Vaccines/HPV/hpv_faqs.html#one; http://www.cdc.gov/hpv/prevention.html. Accessed June 1, 2015.

Centers for Disease Control and Prevention. Measles (rubeola). http://www.cdc.gov/measles. Accessed June 1, 2015.

Centers for Disease Control and Prevention. Prevention of varicella—Recommendations of the Advisory Committee on Immunization Practices (ACIP). *MMWR Morb Mortal Wkly Rep.* 2007;56. http://www.cdc.gov/mmwr/pdf/rr/rr5604.pdf. Accessed June 1, 2016.

Centers for Disease Control and Prevention. Recommended immunization schedule for persons age 0 through 18 years. http://www.cdc.gov/vaccines/schedules/hcp/imz/child-adolescent.html. Accessed June 1, 2015.

Centers for Disease Control and Prevention. Ticks. http://www.cdc.gov/ticks/removing_a_tick.html. Accessed November 26, 2015.

Committee on Practice and Ambulatory Medicine Section on Ophthalmology; American Association of Certified Orthoptists; American Association for Pediatric Ophthalmology and Strabismus; American Academy of Ophthalmology. Eye examination in infants, children, and young adults by pediatricians. *Pediatrics.* 2003;111(4):902–907. doi: 10.1542/peds.111.4.90.

Dowd MD, Serge RD; Council on Injury, Violence, and Poison Prevention Executive Committee; American Academy of Pediatrics. Committee on Injury and Poison Prevention. Firearm-related injuries affecting the pediatric population. *Pediatrics.* 2012;130(5):e1416–e1423. doi: 10.1542/peds.2012-2481

Monk HM, Motsney AJ, Wade KC. Safety of rotavirus vaccine in the NICU. *Pediatrics.* 2014;133(6):e1555–e1560. doi: 10.1542/peds.2013-3504.

National Heart, Lung and Blood Institute. Expert Panel on Integrated Guidelines for Cardiovascular Health and Risk Reduction in Children and Adolescents: Summary report. http://www.nhlbi.nih.gov/health-pro/guidelines/current/cardiovascular-health-pediatric-guidelines/summary. Accessed June 1, 2015.

Saari TN. Immunization of preterm and low birth weight infants. American Academy of Pediatrics Committee on Infectious Diseases. *Pediatrics.* 2003;112(1 Pt 1):193–198.

Tanski SE, Wilson KM. Children and secondhand smoke: Clear evidence for action. *Pediatrics.* 2012;129(1):170–171. doi: 10.1542/peds.2011-3190.

Wyckoff AS. From prenatal visit to anticipatory guidance up to age 21 Academy's new Periodicity Schedule is now online, providing up-to-date reference. *AAP News.* 2014;35(3):10. doi: 10.1542/aapnews.2014353-10.

Psychosocial Issues and Child Abuse 29

Cassandra Collins, James Burkhalter, and Kelly E. Wood

Part 1
Psychosocial Issues

► CASE 1

A 9-year-old boy is brought to the clinic for an appointment by his mother. The mother reports that she and the boy's father have recently gotten divorced and she is concerned about the effect that the divorce has had on the boy.

Question 1-1
Which of the following problems can children experience as a result of parental divorce?
A) Behavioral problems.
B) Social withdrawal.
C) Depression and anxiety.
D) Decline in academic achievement.
E) All of the above.

Discussion 1-1
The correct answer is "E." Divorce can affect children of all ages in various ways. Children may feel a sense of loss, confusion, guilt, and disruption to their routine as a result of parental divorce. Children have not yet developed a concrete set of coping skills to deal with the emotions brought on by divorce. Boys have a higher likelihood of demonstrating behavioral problems or outbursts as a result of the emotions they may be experiencing. In addition to behavioral problems, social withdrawal, depression, anxiety, and decline in academic achievement are all ways in which divorce can be associated with diminished psychosocial well-being in children. (See Table 29–1.)

Helpful Tip
Approximately 60% of marriages in the United States end in divorce, and more than 1 million children under the age of 18 are involved in divorce each year.

Helpful Tip
Recommending individual and family therapy to help the child and family develop positive coping and communication skills is one of the most important recommendations a physician can make during and after a family is experiencing divorce.

► CASE 2

A kindergartner and his mother present to your office for a school physical. The mother informs you that her son, who is 5 years old, suddenly started sucking his thumb again and occasionally has been soiling his underwear. She mentions that her father, who suffered from Alzheimer disease, passed

TABLE 29–1 EFFECTS OF DIVORCE BY AGE-GROUP

Infancy/Toddlerhood (1–3 years)	Childhood (4–12 years)
• Developmental milestones can be affected • Attachment patterns can be affected	• Behavioral problems • Lower self-esteem, self-efficacy • Academic difficulties • Emotional distress • Difficulty in interpersonal relationships
Adolescence (13–17 years)	**Young Adulthood (18–24 years)**
• Depression • Altered attitudes toward marriage • Early sexual activity • Academic difficulty • Higher dropout rate • Antisocial behavior	• Greater number of sexual partners • Reluctance to commit to long-term relationships • Negative perceptions of family and interpersonal relationships

away nearly 2 weeks ago. Her son has been struggling with sleep, admits to a decreased appetite, and has been isolating from his siblings. According to the mother, he believes his grandfather will return at some point. She does not think he is experiencing difficulties with the loss.

Question 2-1

What, if any, symptoms in this scenario suggest the kindergartner is struggling with the loss of his maternal grandfather?
A) Thumb sucking.
B) Belief that death is reversible.
C) Decreased appetite.
D) Social isolation.
E) All of the above.

Discussion 2-1

The correct answer is "E." Death is an emotionally charged issue for most patients, and this is especially true for children. Sadness, anxiety, guilt, and fear over the separation that comes with the loss of life are typical emotional responses by children. Younger children may demonstrate regressive behaviors and suddenly show signs of thumb sucking and bed wetting. They struggle with understanding death as a biologic event, which is important for practitioners to acknowledge. It is also important for adults to avoid assumptions about what children understand and instead inquire about their perceptions. Concrete explanations of death and visual reminders, such as tombstones, help with the grief process. Children younger than 5 years of age do not understand the finality of death. They may believe it is reversible and find it difficult to grasp the

universality of death. Those 5 to 10 years old begin to realize death is irreversible but resist the idea that dying is a possibility for children as well. Older children are able to understand the biologic, social, and psychological changes that occur during the death process.

> **Helpful Tip**
> Shock, disbelief, confusion, numbness, anger, loneliness, and helplessness, along with sleeping difficulties, appetite problems, social isolation, and minor illnesses, are additional responses to death frequently seen in children.

Question 2-2

What factors influence a child's response to death?
A) Relationship to deceased.
B) Significance of relationship.
C) Way the death occurred.
D) Previous death experiences.
E) All of the above.

Discussion 2-2

The correct answer is "E." All four of these factors, along with personality, chronological age, and developmental level, influence a child's response to death. With regard to terminal illness, it is important to understand that family members will likely experience anticipatory grief in preparation for their loved one's death. Children and their families will also go through the stages of mourning and grief. These stages do not necessarily occur in a specific order, and all people grieve differently.

> **Helpful Tip**
> Elisabeth Kübler-Ross's five stages of loss and grief are:
> 1. Denial and isolation: We deny the reality of the situation, block out words, and hide from the facts.
> 2. Anger: Reality and pain reemerge as denial and isolation subside.
> 3. Bargaining: We try to regain control and protect ourselves from the painful reality.
> 4. Depression: A reaction relating to the loss.
> 5. Acceptance: Withdrawal and calmness.

▶ CASE 3

A 15-year-old boy is referred to your office by a counselor at the local high school. The counselor has noticed the sophomore is lethargic at school, seems sleep deprived, has increased irritability, and his grades are starting to slip. She has also witnessed him act more aggressively toward some of his classmates, which is not his usual behavior.

Question 3-1

What is the most likely reason behind his behavioral changes?

A) Developmental stage of adolescence.
B) Increase in electronic screen time.
C) Start of a new relationship with a significant other.
D) All of the above.
E) None of the above.

Discussion 3-1

The correct answer is "B." Youth spend an average of at least 7 hours per day using electronic screen media. Most have access to a home television, video-game console, computer, the Internet, and a cell phone. Exposure to mass media can influence a child's behavior negatively, leading to increased aggression, sexual behavior, substance use, unhealthy eating patterns, and academic difficulties. It can also be beneficial by increasing empathy, highlighting acceptance of diversity, and assisting with early literacy skills. Sleeping is the only activity in which children spend more time than connecting with electronic screen media. Heavy mass media exposure has been associated with depression, psychological distress, mood disorders, sleep disorders, and increased prevalence of asthma, hypertension, and high cholesterol. The American Academy of Pediatrics recommends that parents avoid electronic screen time for children younger than 2 years, limit screen time for children older than 2 years to no more than 1 to 2 hours per day, keep children's bedrooms free of screen media, and co-view and openly discuss the content of media with their children.

> **Helpful Tip**
> Two important questions practitioners can ask parents are: How much time per day does your child spend with entertainment media? Is there a television or Internet connection in your child's bedroom? It is then helpful to provide education about limiting electronic screen time and recommend moving the television and Internet access to an area that can be monitored by adults.

▶ CASE 4

A 16-year-old girl is referred to her primary care physician for evaluation of depression by the school nurse, who is concerned because she has missed several classes each day. The patient has been in her current school for approximately 2 months. She has had to change schools frequently in response to eviction, crime in her neighborhood, and employment opportunities for her mother, and is currently enrolled an academic grade below her age group. After reviewing the patient's records, the physician notes that she has a history of fighting, little adult supervision, and difficulty concentrating. The mother holds three part-time jobs, and it can be difficult to reach her to discuss the girl's care.

Question 4-1

The most likely cause of the patient's difficulties is related to:

A) Child abuse.
B) Socioeconomic stressors.
C) Substance abuse.
D) Depression.
E) Denial of critical care.

Discussion 4-1

The correct answer is "B." Socioeconomic and poverty-related stressors are directly linked to symptoms of depression, social problems, attention problems, and delinquency in children and adolescents. Frequent moves and transitions are accompanied by difficulty in developing and maintaining positive relationships and environmental stability. Children who live in families with socioeconomic stress often experience chronic and uncontrollable life events that affect their psychological health. They witness higher rates of violence in their neighborhoods and experience more conflict and instability in their families. For teenagers, parental employment may mean less adult supervision, and this decreased parental presence can lead to an increase in difficulties for the teen.

> **Helpful Tip**
> Assisting families in finding and utilizing neighborhood and family resources can help them cope with the stressors brought on by socioeconomic difficulties. Learn what resources are available!

▶ CASE 5

A couple presents to their pediatrician's office with their son, who was adopted as an infant. The adoptive parents and son are of different races, and their son is now asking why he looks different from his family. The couple is unsure how to handle these questions. They ask why their son is asking these questions at this age, and how they should respond to these questions.

Question 5-1

The most likely age group of this child is:

A) 1 to 3 years.
B) 3 to 6 years.
C) 6 to 12 years.
D) 12 to 18 years.

Discussion 5-1

The correct answer is "B." At age 3 years, children's self-concept and thinking begin to change. Until this age, children do not recognize that there is a difference between themselves and their adoptive families. Additionally, at this age as children are entering school, peers may begin to ask questions about a child's physical differences from his or her adoptive parents, and inquire about the child's biologic and cultural heritage.

Question 5-2

Adoptive parents should do all of the following EXCEPT:

A) Tell their child the story of his or her adoption and how the family came to be.

B) Openly acknowledge the racial or physical differences that exist between themselves and their child.

C) Discourage the child from learning more about his or her heritage or ethnic group.

D) Give the child permission to talk about and ask questions about adoption.

E) Help guide the child in what information he or she will share with others and how it will be shared.

Discussion 5-2

The correct answer is "C." If parents discourage the child from learning more about his or her biologic heritage or avoid discussions about the child's heritage or ethnic identity, they may convey the perception that the child's biologic heritage or ethnicity is "bad" or that adoption is "bad." Families need to openly acknowledge racial differences that exist between themselves and their children. Open conversations using positive adoption language should be a natural part of a family's conversation. (See Table 29–2.)

> **Helpful Tip**
> Pediatricians should be aware of the complex developmental, medical, behavioral, psychological, and educational challenges that adoptive children may face. Pediatricians may be asked to review medical and mental health records to help families understand the issues that may affect their adoptive child currently and in the future. Pediatricians should help families access needed developmental and mental health services, be available to provide support, and model positive adoptive language and vocabulary.

► CASE 6

The foster parents of a 4-year-old girl present to a pediatrician's office and inquire about appropriate medical care for their new daughter, who was placed with them less than 2 weeks ago. They have not received a great deal of guidance from the foster care system and are curious about the next steps. The American Academy of Pediatrics issued guidelines on meeting the developmental and health care needs of children in foster care.

Question 6-1

These recommendations state that children should:

A) Receive a health evaluation shortly after entering foster care to identify any immediate medical needs.

B) Receive a thorough pediatric assessment within 30 days of entering the foster care system.

C) Be assigned a consistent source of medical care to ensure continuity of care.

TABLE 29–2	DEVELOPMENTAL UNDERSTANDING OF ADOPTION
Age	**Conceptual Understanding**
3–6 Years	• Thinking and self-concept change • Recognize differences between themselves and adoptive family • Can be self-absorbed and think they can magically cause things to happen • May have more separation issues than peers • May feel responsible for loss of their birth family • May fear adoptive parents will abandon them
6–12 Years	• Will realize they have lost a biologic family • Fantasize about what life may have been like with their birth family • May be upset with differences they notice between their families and those of peers • May experience denial of differences between themselves and their adoptive families • May experience denial of their adoption • Self-esteem issues may complicate their emotions • Peer and school problems may be related to underlying adoption issues • Some may be diagnosed with PTSD or RAD
12–16 Years	• Develop identity • Begin task of separation and individuation • Can become angry over differences between their life experiences and society's norm • May idealize their "perfect" biologic family • May engage in risk-taking behaviors • May "try on" other identities

PTSD, posttraumatic stress disorder; RAD, reactive attachment disorder.

D) Receive ongoing developmental, educational, and emotional assessments.

E) All of the above.

Discussion 6-1

The correct answer is "E." Many children in foster care have been exposed to extreme poverty and maltreatment, and this could lead to compromised brain development, emotional problems, and behavior difficulties. Children in foster care tend to suffer from more health problems than the general population. This is especially true for mental health issues, developmental delays, and the diagnosis of intellectual disability. Many foster children feel depressed, anxious, uncertain, rejected, and guilty owing to their foster placement. They also have higher levels of hearing and vision impairment, asthma, lead toxicity, and tuberculosis. Foster care children have less access to adequate care, but utilize it more frequently and require more specialized services compared with children not in the foster care system. Both foster parents and teachers report more problematic behavior by a foster child at home than at school. Fewer externalizing behaviors are exhibited at school, and this is likely due to the structure, consistent routine, controlled setting, and defined limits of the academic setting.

> **Helpful Tip**
> In the United States, approximately 750,000 children are in foster care. Each year, 20,000 to 25,000 children "age out" of the foster care system.

> **Helpful Tip**
> Approximately 70% of foster children are placed with a foster family because of child abuse or denial of critical care.

Question 6-2

Child welfare and foster care include which systems?
A) Courts.
B) Mental health services.
C) Government agencies.
D) Private providers.
E) All of the above.

Discussion 6-1

The correct answer is "E." We told you "all of the above" is usually a sure bet. The child welfare system consists of state and local agencies, legal system, private service providers, public assistance, mental health services, Medicaid, and any other services available to children and their families. Foster families provide daily care of the foster child, but the biologic parents usually remain the child's legal guardians and make legal decisions on his or her behalf. Birth families tend to have many psychosocial stressors and few resources. Some of these stressors include substantial poverty, limited education, substance abuse, chronic mental illness, and domestic violence. Foster families assume an extremely challenging task when attempting to raise a foster child as these children frequently require a high level of care. The families receive very low financial reimbursement rates and limited support from the child welfare system. The transition from adolescence to adulthood may be one of the more challenging developmental stages, and aging out of the foster care system only adds to the difficulty. Foster children tend to have limited family support, often lack a high school education, may

have an unplanned child, and have difficulties obtaining health care. Supportive adult relationships with foster children who are aging out of the system may influence the outcome by helping these adolescents maintain positive future expectations.

> **Helpful Tip**
> *Positive future expectations* refer to the degree which a child in foster care has optimism about his or her future. This includes believing a positive outcome may come one's way and that one has control over one's future.

▶ CASE 7

You meet a Hispanic couple and their 8-year-old son during the child's appointment to establish care in your clinic. Although English is the parents' second language they are able to communicate fairly well regarding their son's health. Your interaction with the family makes you wonder how you can help your organization become more welcoming to patients of various cultures.

Question 7-1

"Cultural competence" in health care entails:
A) Understanding the importance of social and cultural influences on patients' health beliefs and behaviors.
B) Considering how these social and cultural factors interact at multiple levels of the health care delivery system.
C) Devising interventions that take social and cultural issues into account to ensure quality health care delivery to diverse patient populations.
D) Including a framework for organizational, structural, and clinical interventions that encompass social and cultural factors.
E) All of the above.

Discussion 7-1

The correct answer is "E." Option "E" strikes again. A health care system that is culturally competent is defined as one that acknowledges and incorporates the importance of culture, assessment of cross-cultural relations, vigilance toward the dynamics that result from cultural differences, expansion of cultural knowledge, and adaption of services to meet culturally unique needs. (You may be thinking, how many times can some variation of the word *culture* be used in one sentence?) Evidence clearly highlights racial and ethnic disparities in physical health conditions, and data show that minorities suffer disproportionately from cancer, diabetes, asthma, cardiovascular disease, and other medical conditions. These disparities are multifactorial. Compared with the majority population, members of minority communities are typically more socioeconomically disadvantaged, have less education, have more hazardous occupations, and live in areas with greater environmental hazards. A patient's lack of insurance leads to inadequate access to preventative care, higher rates of emergency department visits and avoidable inpatient admissions, later stage diagnosis of cancer and other medical conditions, and barriers to obtaining affordable prescription medications.

> **Helpful Tip**
> A culturally competent health care system is also built on an awareness of the integration and interaction of health beliefs and behaviors, disease prevalence and incidence, and treatment outcomes for different patient populations. No two groups of people are alike.

► CASE 8

A 2-year-old girl is brought to your clinic by her mother. The child has been coughing since she awoke, and the mother is concerned she may have bronchitis or pneumonia. The mother would like her child to be seen right away, stating "she may need to be hospitalized." This mother frequently brings her daughter to the clinic with excessive concerns about her child's health. In the child's chart, it is documented that her life was at risk in utero and she was born prematurely at 27 weeks' gestation, followed by a long hospitalization in the neonatal intensive care unit after birth.

Question 8-1
Which of the following is likely affecting the patient's mother?
A) Vulnerable child syndrome.
B) Munchausen syndrome.
C) Munchausen syndrome by proxy.
D) Generalized anxiety disorder.
E) "No fevers in daycare" predicament.

Discussion 8-1
The correct answer is "A." Vulnerable child syndrome (VCS) is used to describe children who are perceived by their parents as being vulnerable and at greater risk for physical, developmental, or behavioral disturbances or problems. This causes parents to have unfounded anxiety about the health of their child. These excessive parental concerns, and related high frequency of health care use, are often precipitated by an event or situation that has exacerbated the parent's perception of the child's vulnerability. (See Table 29–3.)

> **Helpful Tip**
> The best management of vulnerable child syndrome is prevention. Be aware of the risk factors that may affect parents. Recognize these families and begin communicating and educating them about their child's health. Pediatricians may need to uncover the parent's underlying anxiety about the child's health and make a referral for therapy.

TABLE 29–3 RISK FACTORS FOR VULNERABLE CHILD SYNDROME

- Child's life was at risk during pregnancy, delivery, or both
- Child was born prematurely
- Physician predicted child might die
- Mother's life was at risk during pregnancy, delivery, or both
- Child has a history of serious illness or injury
- Parent has previously experienced unexpected death of a child or infant
- Mother has a history of multiple spontaneous abortions or stillbirths
- Parents have fertility issues
- Mother has had postpartum depression

► CASE 9

A teenage girl has been seeing a therapist for approximately 3 months to address concerns about social withdrawal, decline in grades, and possible depression. At her most recent appointment, she told the therapist she often finds herself lost in thought, repetitively and passively focusing on her distress and its possible causes. She cannot seem to stop going over the details in her head.

Question 9-1
The patient is likely experiencing:
A) A psychotic break.
B) Panic attacks.
C) Daydreams.
D) Rumination.
E) Hallucinations.

Discussion 9-1
The correct answer is "D." Rumination is a way of responding to distress that involves passively and repetitively focusing on symptoms of its possible causes and consequences. Rumination is typically associated with a maladaptive response that is linked with depressed mood. Rumination demonstrates a cognitive vulnerability factor for both adolescent and adult depression. Adolescents who are experiencing social anxiety may be more likely to experience rumination, especially when coping with ambiguous or socially distressing situations.

> **Helpful Tip**
> Female adolescents report higher levels of rumination than their male counterparts.

► CASE 10

A 14-year-old girl presents with her mother in the emergency department for a severe migraine. The physician on call talks with the patient's mother to obtain a thorough medical history and learns that the girl has had daily migraines for nearly 2 years. Magnetic resonance imaging (MRI) scans, computed tomography (CT) scans, and various other medical tests have been performed. The girl has also seen several specialists, including traditional and naturopathic doctors, and psychological professionals. None of these tests or specialists has been helpful in her diagnosis or pain management.

Question 10-1

Which of the following conditions is affecting the patient?
A) Chronic pain syndrome.
B) Munchausen syndrome.
C) Ear infection.
D) Encephalitis.
E) Insomnia.

Discussion 10-1

The correct answer is "A." The unknown etiology and poor response to treatment noted in this case make chronic pain syndrome the best fit for the condition currently affecting the patient and the presenting problem for her emergency department visit. Chronic pain is characterized by its ongoing, persistent nature. A diagnosis of chronic pain typically requires that the pain has lasted 3 months or longer. It is a diagnosis of exclusion. Chronic pain is a complex diagnosis associated with many factors, such as the child's development, as well as biologic, psychological, and social factors. These factors can also affect the child's understanding of his or her pain, ability to communicate about pain, and ability to cope with pain. The syndrome is best managed by a multidisciplinary team with knowledge of different organ systems and psychological needs. Exhaustive diagnostic workup and treatment does not help in managing the condition.

Question 10-2

Chronic pain could be affecting what area(s) of functioning for the patient?
A) Communication.
B) Social.
C) Emotional.
D) Behavioral.
E) Physical.
F) All of the above.

Discussion 10-2

The correct answer is "F." (This one was sneaky. "All of the above" is still the safe bet, but did you notice it was option "F," not "E"?) It can be very difficult for children and adolescents to cope with chronic pain. Children may struggle to communicate about their pain, their needs, and their wants to others, including family members, teachers, and friends. Children can struggle to interact in an age-appropriate manner with their peers and others in social situations, or lack regular interaction with others due to their pain. Children can also be affected by depression, anxiety, and behavioral outbursts as a result of their inability to cope with their pain and the effects on their mood.

Helpful Tip
It is estimated that 15% to 20% of children experience chronic pain.

▶ CASE 11

A 13-year-old girl lives with both of her parents, along with a 7-year-old brother and 10-year-old sister. The teen has been in the gifted children program at school since age 7, when she first scored three grades ahead of her age group. She participates in several extracurricular learning groups and competitive knowledge-based groups at her school. Her parents are very active in attending these events and are supportive of their daughter's perfectionistic tendencies, often allowing her to dictate the family's schedule so that she can complete homework and projects.

Question 11-1

What is the most likely way the teenager's siblings are affected?
A) They are proud of her achievements.
B) They are jealous of the attention she receives from their parents.
C) They are happy about having less focus on them and their schoolwork.
D) They feel pressure to achieve as highly as their sister.
E) Both B and D.

Discussion 11-1

The correct answer is "E." Siblings of gifted children can feel jealous of the attention that their gifted sibling receives. This can occur for various reasons, including the gifted sibling having more one-on-one time with parents, participating in more activities, and receiving more recognition from others, such as teachers and peers. Siblings of gifted children tend to feel pressure to achieve and perform at the same level of their sibling. When this does not occur, siblings can feel inadequate. The pressure that siblings feel can be actual pressure from parents but it can also be perceived pressure that they feel to perform at the same level as their sibling.

Question 11-2

When should professionals assist parents in management of their gifted child?
A) Immediately upon identification of the child as gifted.
B) When the gifted child begins school.
C) When the gifted child's siblings begin school.
D) Only if problems arise with the gifted child.
E) Only if problems arise within the family.

Discussion 11-2

The correct answer is "A." Professionals should provide anticipatory guidance to parents and families to assist them in the management of their gifted child. Professionals can include physicians, teachers, therapists, and other professionals who may come in contact with the family. Professionals should help the parents to understand ways in which to help their gifted child while also helping them to understand how having a gifted child may affect family dynamics. Parents should be encouraged to model appropriate behaviors and a mindset that encourages growth in all areas for the gifted child, rather than one focused solely on achievement. It should be emphasized that gifted children are children first and foremost. Helping the child understand social cues and respond appropriately to them will be important, especially if the child has skipped a grade due to his or her abilities. Continued communication among parents, teachers, and counselors will be important to ensure that all the child's needs are met. Gifted children should be encouraged to enjoy nonacademic achievements, have down time, and have hobbies that are not achievement related. Individual counseling may be suggested to help the gifted child develop and utilize appropriate coping skills. Family counseling may be suggested to help the family communicate and develop positive relationships with one another.

▶ CASE 12

A 3-month-old girl has multiple heart problems and is in need of an eventual heart transplant. Her parents are understandably upset, frustrated, and confused about the situation. They regularly speak to the medical team and inquire about next steps. They have to take their daughter to numerous medical appointments, and their lives have been turned upside down.

Question 12-1

Coping in families of children with chronic illness may be improved by which of these variables?
A) Openness in communication.
B) Emotional support.
C) Positivity.
D) Spirituality.
E) All of the above.

Discussion 12-1

The correct answer is "E." Socioeconomic status, marital satisfaction, and satisfaction with health care the child receives are other factors that may be associated with positive coping. Chronic illness refers to an incurable illness that lasts for 3 months or more. The severity of symptoms, the child's personality, traits of the family, and the child's social environment influences how well he or she can cope with a chronic illness. Chronically ill children go through the same developmental stages as healthy kids, but they may struggle at mastering and coping with typical childhood stressors. Physical symptoms of the illness, continual treatment, medications, hospitalizations, interruptions in daily life, and heightened family stress may also interfere with normal child development. It is imperative for a practitioner to understand the development stage of any child who is receiving care, but especially children who suffer from chronic illness and handicapping conditions. Children with chronic illness will likely develop in different ways than the general population owing to their condition.

> **Helpful Tip**
> Between 10% and 20% of children suffer from chronic illnesses; the most common of these are asthma, congenital heart disease, and chronic kidney disease.

Question 12-2

What services can a pediatric medical home provide to children with chronic illnesses and their families?
A) Specialty care.
B) Educational services.
C) Out-of-home care.
D) Family support.
E) All of the above.

Discussion 12-2

The correct answer is "E." Families are assuming a greater role in care of their chronically ill children at home owing to shorter inpatient hospitalizations. Quality care can be provided in the community, but it is quite costly. A family-centered medical home is an approach to providing comprehensive primary care to children with chronic or handicapping conditions. The pediatric care team partners with the family to meet all of their medical and nonmedical needs. Medical homes can also provide services to families involved with a child who has received an organ transplant. Families with children who undergo transplantation experience similar psychosocial and family issues as those with a child that has a chronic illness or handicapping condition. In traditional families, mothers tend to bear the burden of caring for their chronically ill child more so than fathers. Opportunities for these mothers to work outside the home are often limited because of their child's illness, and their mental health is more likely to be worse than that of fathers or mothers of healthy children. Marital satisfaction and social interactions also can be negatively affected by the increased caretaking needs of a child with chronic illness.

▶ CASE 13

A preschool-aged boy has been brought into the school nurse's office several times following aggressive outbursts in the classroom. His teacher reports that the boy struggles to interact with peers, plays aggressively with toys, struggles to show empathy toward others, and has exceptionally low self-esteem for his age. While "playing house" with peers, he often demonstrates aggression toward the mother figure of the home. He is also prone to temper tantrums and frequently resists comfort from others.

Question 13-1

The cause of this boy's behavior is most likely:
A) Learning disability.
B) Attention deficit hyperactivity disorder.
C) Depression.
D) Intimate partner violence in the home.
E) Autism spectrum disorder.

Discussion 13-1

The correct answer is "D." This preschooler is most likely acting out in school because he has witnessed intimate partner violence at home. Children who witness violence at home often display their distress behaviorally. They struggle to develop secure attachments and accept comfort from adults. Their extreme fear can also manifest in psychosomatic complains such as stomachaches, headaches, enuresis, and insomnia. These children are more aggressive, display behavioral problems, demonstrate anxiety symptoms, and have posttraumatic stress symptoms. (See Table 29–4.)

Question 13-2

What are precipitants of intimate partner violence?
A) Substance use.
B) Socioeconomic stress.
C) Mental health issues.
D) Experiencing violence in childhood.
E) All of the above.

Discussion 13-2

The correct answer is "E." Substance use has been linked to higher rates of intimate partner violence. Socioeconomic stress, such as extreme poverty, is identified as a factor that is linked to intimate partner violence. Mental health issues, especially when left untreated, can affect individual's ability to cope with stress and it may lead to intimate partner violence. Experiencing violence in childhood is a large precipitant of intimate partner violence. Without intervention or therapy in childhood, children can grow up to utilize and demonstrate the same methods of interaction and violence that they experienced as children. When children experience societal violence, it can also be linked to higher rates of demonstrating these same violent and aggressive behaviors as adults.

> **Helpful Tip**
> Children can witness domestic violence in ways other than by direct observation. Examples include overhearing violence, seeing the aftermath of broken property, or seeing evidence of injuries on their parent.

TABLE 29–4 EFFECTS OF FAMILY AND SOCIETAL VIOLENCE BY AGE GROUP

Infancy/Toddlerhood	Early Childhood
• Excessive irritability • Regressed behavior around language and toilet training • Sleep disturbances • Fear of being alone • Difficulty separating from parents	• Behavioral problems • Social problems • PTSD symptoms • Difficulty developing empathy • Poor self-esteem • Aggression and temper tantrums • Despondency and anxiety • Psychosomatic complaints
School-Aged Children	**Adolescence**
• May blame themselves for the abuse • May try to rationalize the violence • At risk of developing antisocial rationales for their own behaviors • Sadness, depression, or vulnerability • Poor social skills and peer differences • Difficulty adhering to rules • Learning difficulties • Poorly developed verbal skills	• Difficulty forming healthy, intimate relationships • Higher likelihood of avoidant attachment style • May continue abusive patterns in their own intimate relationships • May adopt caretaking roles for their parents or siblings • Social isolation • Involvement in crime

PTSD, posttraumatic stress disorder.

Part 2
Child Abuse

▶ CASE 14

A 5-week-old girl is brought to the emergency department for evaluation of fussiness. The infant was born at term. Nothing remarkable occurred during the delivery or pregnancy. She is being bottle fed and gaining weight well. The only symptom is fussiness. On exam, she is awake and appears healthy. Her frenulum is torn and there is bruising of her gums. Her family cannot explain what happened.

Question 14-1

Which of following is the best next course of action?
A) Prescribe gas drops.
B) Discharge the infant home.
C) Recommend changing infant formulas.
D) File a report with child protective services (CPS).
E) Perform a lumbar puncture.

Discussion 14-1

The correct answer is "D." The differential for a "fussy baby" is broad. This infant has physical findings concerning for child abuse. A torn frenulum and oral bruising occurs when a bottle or other object is forcefully shoved in the mouth, usually to silence a crying infant. (See Figure 29–1.) Red flags for abuse include the following:

- Changing history
- Inconsistent histories
- History not consistent or plausible with injury or the child's development
- No or vague history of trauma
- Delayed seeking of medical care for injuries
- Multiple injuries present
- Injuries classically seen with child abuse

Health care workers are mandatory reporters. Any concern, suspicion, or documented abuse (physical, sexual, neglect) must be reported to CPS.

Question 14-2

Which is NOT a risk factor for child abuse?
A) Alcohol abuse.
B) Teenage caregiver.
C) Married caregiver.
D) Child with chronic medical conditions.
E) History of abuse.

Discussion 14-2

The correct answer is "C." For everything except sexual abuse, the parents are usually to blame—especially fathers in abusive head trauma. Caretaker risk factors include young age, single,

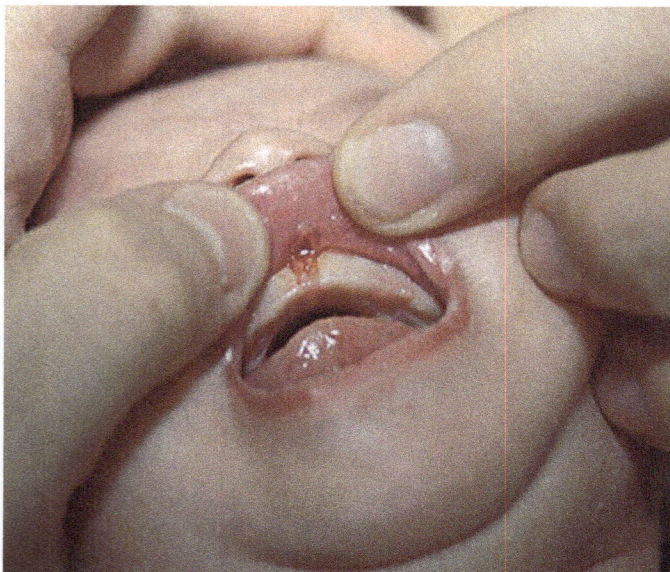

FIGURE 29–1. Torn Frenulum. Frenulum tears occur from trauma, such as when an object is forcefully shoved in the mouth. (Used with permission from Paul Bellino, MD.)

isolation, stress, lower level of education, lower income, unstable home life, domestic violence, substance abuse, and mental illness. Abusive caretakers were frequently abused or neglected themselves as children. Abusive parents may have unrealistic expectations that are beyond the age or development of the child. Young children and those with chronic medical conditions are at increased risk. Abuse that is undetected at previous medical encounters puts the child at risk for repeated episodes of abuse, including fatal injury.

Question 14-3

What is NOT part of a diagnostic workup for suspected physical child abuse?
A) Skeletal survey.
B) Dilated eye exam.
C) Noncontrast head CT scan.
D) Coagulation studies.
E) All of the above are part of the diagnostic evaluation of suspected child abuse.

Discussion 14-3

The correct answer is "E." A full skeletal survey is mandatory for all children younger than 2 years of age with suspected physical abuse. Head imaging (CT, MRI, or both) and dilated eye exam by an ophthalmologist looking for retinal hemorrhages are obtained when intracranial injury is suspected. A noncontrast head CT scan is a good first test as it can be perform rapidly and identifies hemorrhage and injuries requiring immediate surgical intervention. Additional testing will depend on the case and may include abdominal imaging and drug testing. When extensive bruising or hemorrhage is present a coagulopathy, such as hemophilia or von Willebrand disease, or thrombocytopenia should be ruled out.

You order a skeletal survey and blood work, and call an ophthalmologist.

Question 14-4

Which of the following is NOT a radiographic finding of physical child abuse?
A) Rib fractures.
B) Metaphyseal bucket-handle or corner fracture.
C) Multiple fractures of various ages.
D) Femur or humerus fracture.
E) All of the above are radiographic findings of physical child abuse.

Discussion 14-4

The correct answer is "E." Inflicted fractures of almost any bone have been described. The majority of cases involve children younger than 2 years of age. (See Table 29–5.) Fractures in a child who is walking are very suspicious. Rib fractures result from squeezing or hitting the child's chest. Classic metaphyseal (bucket-handle or corner) and spiral fractures of the long bones result from forceful twisting or pulling of an extremity. (See Figures 29–2 and 29–3.) Accidental injuries and fractures may occur in healthy children, especially those who are ambulatory

TABLE 29–5 FRACTURES SUGGESTIVE OF INFLICTED INJURY

Multiple fractures

Rib fractures at any location

Femur fracture, especially if child is not walking

Humerus fracture especially midshaft

Skull fractures, including simple and complex

Classic metaphyseal lesions
- Bucket-handle fracture
- Corner fracture

Sternum, scapula, or spinous process fractures

Hand or foot fractures, especially if child is not walking

Bilateral long bone fractures

Vertebral body fractures

Finger or toe fractures in infants and toddlers

FIGURE 29–3. Rib Fractures. Four-month-old with right-sided posterior rib fractures. Rib fractures associated with abuse can occur at any location. (Reproduced with permission from van Rijn RR: How should we image skeletal injuries in child abuse? *Pediatr Radiol*. 2009 Apr;39 Suppl 2:S226-S229.)

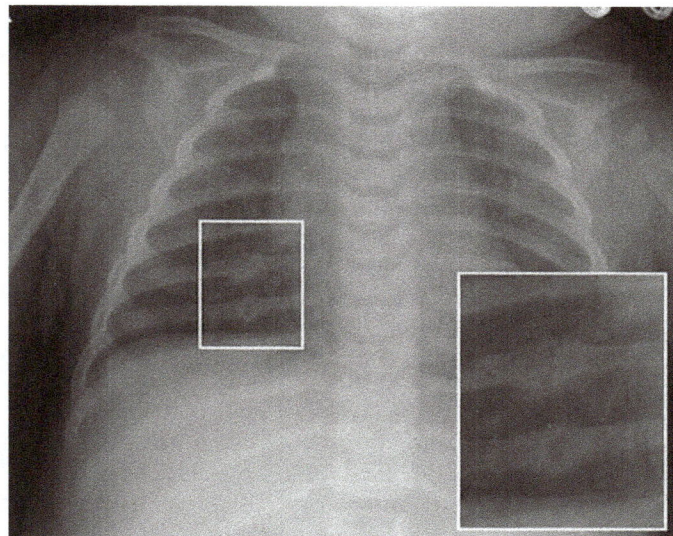

and older in age. With accidental injuries, the story should make sense and be consistent with the developmental age of the child, multiple injuries are usually not present, and medical care is not delayed. If in doubt, a CPS report should be filed.

Question 14-5

Which is NOT associated with an alternative medical explanation for fractures?
A) Blue sclera.
B) Metaphyseal cupping.
C) Osteopenia.
D) Prematurity.
E) All of the above can increase risk of fracture and may explain fractures seen in the course of a child abuse investigation.

Discussion 14-5

The correct answer is "E." Differentiating medical causes of fractures from abuse may be difficult. The differential diagnosis of child abuse includes accidental injury, normal variants, birth trauma, congenital insensitivity to pain, drug toxicity, infection, skeletal dysplasia, and metabolic bone disease. Osteogenesis imperfecta ("brittle bone disease") is a rare genetic condition of weakened bones that fracture with minimal trauma. Most commonly fractures involve the long bones. Associated blue sclera, osteopenia or osteoporosis, wormian bones, abnormal teeth (dentinogenesis imperfecta), short stature, and family history (if present) help differentiate it from abuse. Genetic testing and culture of skin fibroblasts confirm the diagnosis. Fractures caused by rickets usually produce associated radiographic changes (metaphyseal cupping or widening, osteopenia) and abnormal results on laboratory testing. Prematurity may be associated with osteopenia, resulting in pathologic fractures.

FIGURE 29–2. Classic Metaphyseal Fractures. One-month-old asymptomatic infant with bilateral metaphyseal corner fractures of the distal femur. Imaging was performed because the infant's twin brother presented with multiple bruises suspicious for abuse. Evidence supports imaging of both twins if one presents with injuries as the other twin is at risk. (Reproduced with permission from van Rijn RR: How should we image skeletal injuries in child abuse? *Pediatr Radiol*. 2009 Apr;39 Suppl 2:S226-S229.)

▶ CASE 15

An ambulance arrives at a house after a 9-1-1 call reporting a 4-month old infant who is not breathing. The mother tells responders that the infant has not been sick. He was laid on his back in his crib last night. When she went to check on him this morning, he was not breathing. She blew in his face and called 9-1-1. On exam, the infant does not move or open his eyes. His breathing is shallow. He is stabilized and transferred to the pediatric intensive care unit. A CT scan of his head shows an acute subdural hemorrhage, bilateral skull fractures, and brain swelling. **Bilateral retinal hemorrhages are seen on dilated eye exam.**

Question 15-1

Which of the following is true about this case?

A) Shaking is always involved.

B) Delayed diagnosis never occurs.

C) Blindness is not a possible long-term sequela.

D) Subdural hemorrhages may occur from birth trauma.

E) Short falls may cause extensive retinal hemorrhages.

Discussion 15-1

The correct answer is "D." Abusive head trauma, including "shaken baby syndrome," involves shaking, blunt impact to the head, or a combination of both. It is the leading cause of death from child abuse. Infants typically present with subtle signs and symptoms and without a history of trauma, resulting in misdiagnosis or delayed diagnosis. Most victims are younger than 1 year of age, male, and have a history of prior abuse. The most common injuries are subdural and retinal hemorrhages. Epidural, subarachnoid, and parenchymal hemorrhage may also occur. Associated skeletal and skull fractures may be present, but external signs of trauma may be minimal or absent. (See Figures 29–4 and 29–5.) Short falls (from less than 5 feet) usually result in no injury or scalp hematomas. Asymptomatic subdural and retinal hemorrhages from birth trauma should resolve by 3 months and 1 month of age, respectively, and usually are not associated with other injuries. Nearly one third of severely shaken infants die

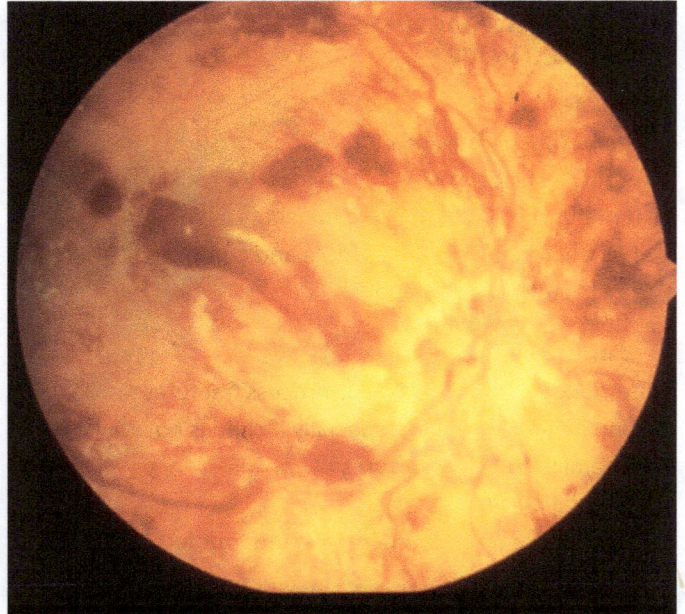

FIGURE 29–5. Retinal hemorrhages are strongly associated with abusive head trauma, can occur with normal head imaging, and most often are numerous, extensive (extend to periphery), multilayer, and bilateral. (Reproduced with permission from Knoop K, Stack L, Storrow A. *Atlas of Emergency Medicine*. 2nd ed. New York, NY: McGraw-Hill; 2002, Fig. 15-33.)

and many suffer long-term consequences such as seizures, blindness, spasticity (cerebral palsy), developmental delay, and cognitive impairment.

FIGURE 29–4. Acute Subdural Hematoma. Head CT scan with an acute subdural hematoma (SDH) appearing as a crescent-shaped, hyperdense collection over the right cerebral hemisphere with mass effect. Multiple SDHs located over the convexities or interhemispheric fissure are associated with abusive head trauma. (Reproduced with permission from Knoop KJ, Stack LB, Storrow AB, Thurman RJ, eds. *The Atlas of Emergency Medicine*, 3d ed. McGraw-Hill Education, Inc., 2010. Photo contributor: Cincinnati Children's Hospital Medical Center. Fig 15-30.)

► CASE 16

An 18-month-old girl has fever. She recently started walking and has a waddling wide-based gait when you see her walking around the room. She has different-colored bruises on her legs and one on her forehead.

Question 16-1

Which is NOT a characteristic of physical abuse?

A) Bruises on bilateral shins.

B) Loop-shaped bruises.

C) Nasal septum perforation.

D) Tympanic membrane perforation.

E) Small circular burn of uniform depth.

Discussion 16-1

The correct answer is "A." Bruises are the most common finding in physical abuse. This toddler's bruising pattern is consistent with accidental falls in an early walker. Unintentional bruises occur over boney prominences such as the shins and forehead. Bruising of atypical areas and patterns of bruising should raise concern for physical abuse. (See Table 29–6 and Figures 29–6 through 29–8.) The tongue, gingiva, frenulum, or teeth may be injured. The nasal septum may be dislocated, bruised, or perforated. Tympanic membrane perforation and pinna bruising

TABLE 29-6 BRUISING PATTERNS

Concerning for Abuse	Not Concerning for Abuse
Buttocks and back	Knees
Ear	Shins
Neck	Forehead
Genitalia	Elbows
Abdomen	Forearms
Chest	Hips
Patterned	
• Loop marks	
• Belt marks (possibly with buckle mark)	
• Hand or finger prints	
• Spanking (parallel to intergluteal cleft)	
Symmetric	
Multiple	
Bruising in an infant who is not walking	

result from direct impact. (See Figure 29–9.) The burn described in option "E" is from a cigarette. Burns in the shape of an object with uniform depth are consistent with an inflicted injury. (See Figures 29–10 and 29–11.) Unintentional burns are usually shallow, with a partial object outline, as the natural reflex is to pull away. Burns of uniform depth on the buttocks or underside of the legs without splash marks occur with immersion in a hot liquid. A sharp line separates normal from burned skin. (See Figure 29–12.) Children flex and lift their legs, sparing the skin folds of the knee and hip. A glove-and-sock (hand or foot immersion) pattern may also be seen.

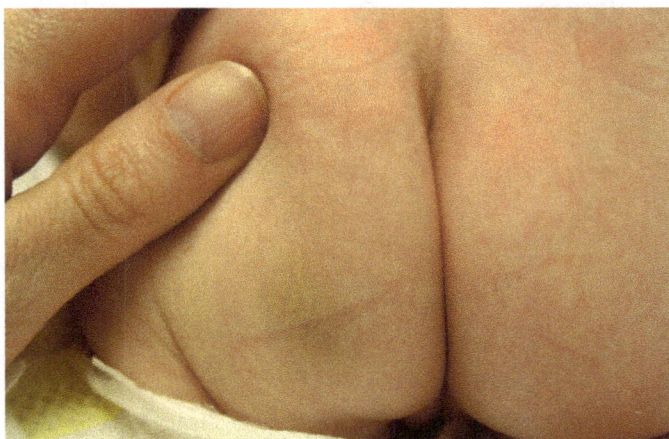

FIGURE 29–7. Pattern Bruising. Loop and linear bruises on the thigh and buttock from being struck with an extension cord, belt, or similar object. (Reproduced with permission from Knoop KJ, Stack LB, Storrow AB, Thurman RJ, eds. *The Atlas of Emergency Medicine*, 3d ed. McGraw-Hill Education, Inc., 2010. Photo contributor: Cincinnati Children's Hospital Medical Center. Fig 15-10.)

> **Helpful Tip**
> Certain cultural practices may be confused with physical abuse. In cupping, a heated cup is suctioned to the skin (usually on the back), causing circular burns with central bruising. In coining, a coin is forcibly rubbed on oiled skin; a similar practice, spooning, causes linear red streaks and bruising. (See Figure 29–13.)

FIGURE 29–6. Buttock bruising on a 1-year-old infant. In the absence of a bleeding disorder, bruising in an immobile child is highly suspicious for physical abuse. (Used with permission from James Anderst, MD, MS.)

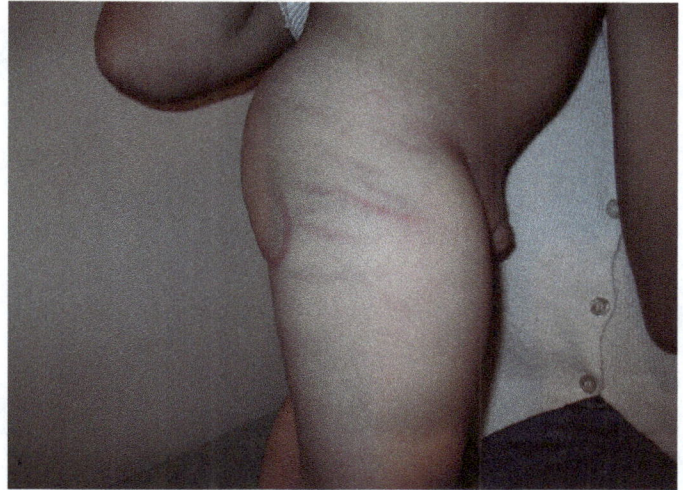

FIGURE 29–8. Spanking Bruises. Linear, parallel bruises near the gluteal folds from spanking. (Reproduced with permission from Knoop KJ, Stack LB, Storrow AB, Thurman RJ, eds. *The Atlas of Emergency Medicine*, 3d ed. McGraw-Hill Education, Inc., 2010. Photo contributor: Charles Schubert & Robert A. Shapiro, MD. Fig 15-8.)

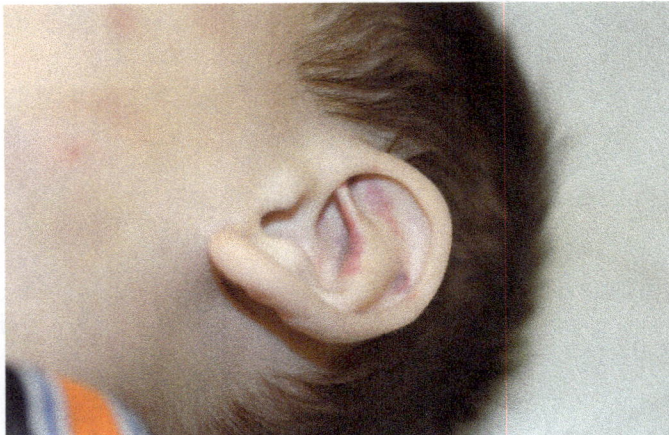

FIGURE 29–9. Ear Bruising. Inflicted ear and cheek bruising, with a pattern on the cheek suggestive of an object or hand print. Bruising of the helix occurs with pinching the outer ear. (Used with permission from James Anderst, MD, MS.)

⧗ QUICK QUIZ

Which is NOT a form of neglect?
A) Educational.
B) Physical.
C) Transportation.
D) Emotional.
E) Medical.

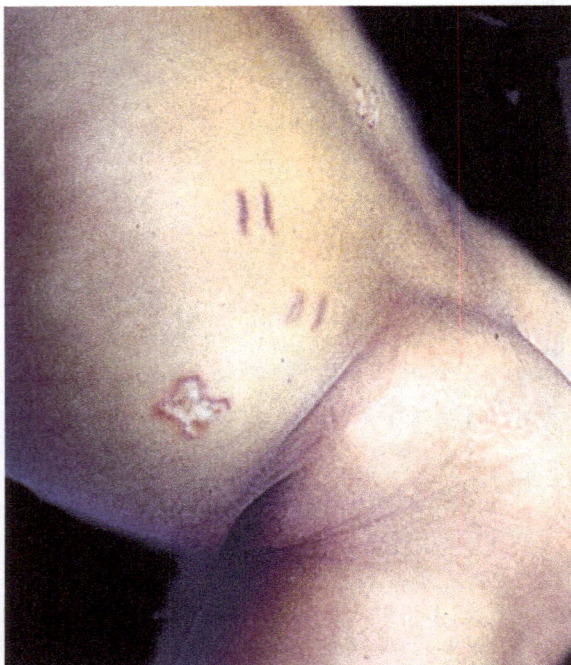

FIGURE 29–10. Pattern Burns. Burn from a cigarette lighter. (Used with permission from Frank A. Maffei, MD.)

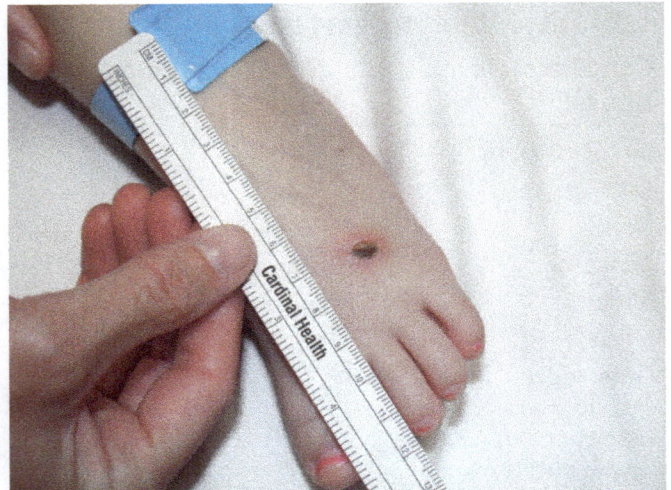

FIGURE 29–11. Cigarette Burn. Circular burn with a diameter of less than 1 centimeter, characteristic of an inflicted cigarette burn. These burns have distinct margins and are of uniform depth. In contrast, accidental burns from running into a lit cigarette usually occur on the face or distal extremities and are superficial, not fully outlined, and have an uneven depth. (Reproduced with permission from Knoop KJ, Stack LB, Storrow AB, Thurman RJ, eds. *The Atlas of Emergency Medicine*, 3d ed. McGraw-Hill Education, Inc., 2010. Photo contributor: Kathi L. Makoroff, MD. Fig 15-5.)

Discussion

The correct answer is "C." Neglect is the most common form of abuse. Four types are commonly differentiated:

- Physical—failure to provide basic needs and supervision
- Medical—failure to seek or provide care to maintain a child's health
- Educational—failure to provide appropriate education, including ensuring school attendance
- Emotional—failure to meet the child's emotional needs, such as withholding affection and allowing the child to witness domestic violence

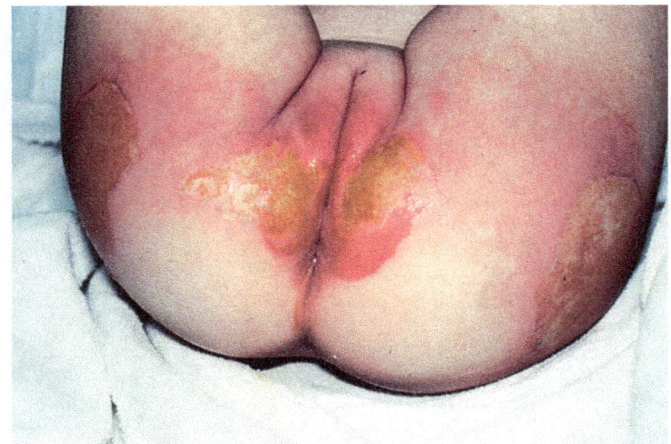

FIGURE 29–12. Scald burn of upper arm, back, and buttock. Pink areas are superficial partial-thickness burn, whereas whiter areas are deeper burns in the dermis. (Reproduced with permission from Brunicardi FC, Andersen DK, Billiar TR, et al, eds. *Schwartz's Principles of Surgery*, 10th ed. McGraw-Hill Education, Inc., 2015. Fig 16-6, pg 482.)

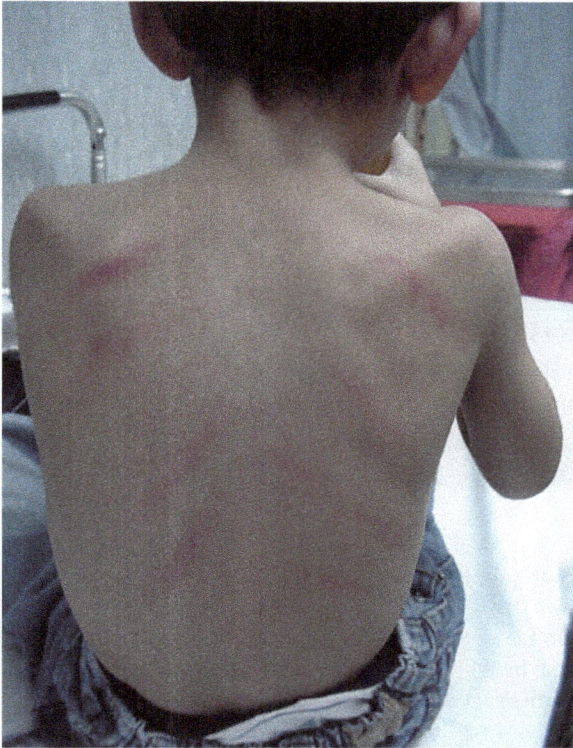

FIGURE 29–13. Coining. A young boy with coining marks from rubbing a coin across his back to heal his acute illness. Coining is a common culture practice in Asia. It can be confused with child abuse. (Used with permission from Maria McColgan, MD.)

► CASE 17

A 3-year-old girl is brought to the clinic. She has been demonstrating sexual acts with her dolls for the past few months. She describes in detail what is going on and uses adult language. Her exam including genitalia is normal.

Question 17-1

What should you do next?
A) Reassure the mother.
B) Perform vaginal swabs for evidence collection.
C) Refer the child to a behavioral specialist.
D) Refer the child to the emergency department.
E) File a child protective services (CPS) report.

Discussion 17-1

The correct answer is "E." This toddler is acting out sexually which is the most specific sign of sexual abuse. Victims of sexual abuse may present with behavioral problems, including sexual acting out, depression, aggression, school problems, and regression (eg, return to thumb sucking). Medical complaints include encopresis, enuresis, dysuria, anogenital trauma, bleeding or discharge, chronic abdominal pain, pregnancy, and sexually transmitted infection (STI). As there is a suspicion for sexual abuse in this child's history, it is mandatory that a report be filed with CPS. As this event is not acute and no findings are present on exam, evidence collection is not necessary.

⧗ QUICK QUIZ

Which statement regarding sexual abuse is false?
A) Sexual abuse is underreported.
B) Boys are more likely than girls to report sexual abuse.
C) Perpetrators are typically male and a trusted acquaintance.
D) Victims may have lifelong mental illness and low self-esteem.
E) Perpetrators are not usually parents or caregivers.

Discussion

The correct answer is "B." Girls are more frequently abused than boys, but boys are less likely to report abuse.

► CASE 18

A 10-year-old boy is brought to the emergency department. He reports someone hurting him "down there." When asked for more information, he tells you someone put something in his bottom.

Question 18-1

Which is part of the evaluation of acute sexual abuse?
A) Limited genitalia exam.
B) Brief history.
C) Collection of evidence only if acute injuries are present.
D) Sexually transmitted infection (STI) testing.
E) None of the above.

Discussion 18-1

The correct answer is "E." This child needs urgent evaluation. The interview is crucial as physical findings are usually absent. (See Table 29–7.) A complete physical exam, including mouth, anus, and genitalia, should be performed in a well-lighted area. A normal physical exam does not rule out abuse. Diagnostic findings of penetrating trauma include hymen injury (lacerations, bruising, absent posterior tissue, healed transection or cleft) and deep anal laceration. Genitalia exam in young girls before puberty is best performed in the frog-leg (supine legs apart) or knee-chest (prone with knees, chest, and head touching table) position. Boys can be examined standing, sitting, or lying down. Evidence should be collected if the abuse with exchange of bodily fluids occurred less than 72 hours earlier to try to recover bodily fluid from the perpetrator. Testing for STIs is recommended for postpubertal children and prepubertal

TABLE 29–7 STEPS IN INTERVIEWING CHILDREN ABOUT POSSIBLE SEXUAL ABUSE

- Use open-ended questions
- Interview child alone
- Have a trained interviewer
- Make sure documentation is complete
- Record answers in child's own words

children with risk factors (penetration, high prevalence of STIs in community). When indicated, postexposure prophylaxis for pregnancy and STIs should be given.

▶ CASE 19

A 3-month-old infant is admitted for workup of apnea. This is his third admission for the same problem in so many months. He was born at term, and the results of his newborn metabolic screen were normal. Likewise results of his exam today are normal; he appears healthy with no symptoms. During his past hospitalizations, he underwent evaluation for sepsis, including a lumbar puncture, viral testing, electroencephalography (EEG), brain MRI, upper gastrointestinal series (UGI) and metabolic disorder testing. All results were normal. Apnea was reported by the mother but never witnessed by a health care provider. At discharge, the mother remains upset and worried that something has been missed despite staff attempts to reassure her.

Question 19-1

Which is NOT a characteristic associated with this disorder?
A) Reported symptoms do not match a particular diagnosis.
B) Repeated diagnostic testing and medical interventions are common.
C) Mortality has not been reported.
D) Mothers are the usual caregivers involved.
E) It is a form of child abuse.

Discussion 19-1

The correct answer is "C." Fabricated or induced childhood illness (Munchausen syndrome by proxy) occurs when a caregiver causes or makes up an illness in a child. Symptoms resolve or improve when the child is removed from the caregiver. It may take months to years before the diagnosis is made. Unnecessary medical testing and interventions are common. No typical presentation exists. Thirty percent of children may have a concurrent real medical problem for which the symptoms are exaggerated. (See Table 29–8.) Perpetrators are most commonly an

TABLE 29-8 FABRICATED CHILDHOOD ILLNESS: COMMON PRESENTATIONS

Exaggerated symptoms of real medical problem

Apnea

Feeding problems

Fever

Diarrhea

Bleeding

Seizures or central nervous system depression

Vomiting

Bizarre symptoms

Treatment refractory symptoms

TABLE 29-9 FABRICATED CHILDHOOD ILLNESS: PERPETRATOR CHARACTERISTICS

Mother

Overly attentive to child

Attention seeking

Involved in the medical profession

Knowledgeable about medicine

Psychiatric illness

Likes to play the sick role

Insists on invasive procedures and hospitalizations

Unhappy when child improves or diagnosis is ruled out

History of death of a child

Hospital hopping; care at multiple facilities

overly attentive mother. (See Table 29–9.) Mortality is reported at 9% to 10%. Long-term outcomes include disability, permanent injury, behavioral or emotional illness, and the victim's eventual belief the symptoms are real, with development of factitious disorder as an adult. The diagnosis may be made by video surveillance or a trial of removing the child from the caregiver to monitor the child's condition.

BIBLIOGRAPHY

Bass S, Shields M, Behrman R. Children, families, and foster care: Analysis and recommendations. *Future Child.* 2004;14(1):4–29.

Betancourt J, Green A, Carrilo J, Ananeh-Firempong O. Defining cultural competence: A practical framework for addressing racial/ethnic disparities in health and healthcare. *Public Health Rep.* 2003;118(4):293–302.

Bilaver L, Kienberger Jaudes P, Koepke D, Goerge R. The health of children in foster care. *Social Service Rev.* 1999;73(3):401–417.

Borchers D, American Academy of Pediatrics Committee on Early Childhood, Adoption, and Dependent Care. Families and adoption: The pediatrician's role in supporting communication. *Pediatrics.* 2003;112:1437–1441.

Cantos A, Gries L. Therapy outcome with children in foster care: A longitudinal study. *Child Adolesc Social Work J.* 2010;27(2):133–149.

Carter B. Chronic pain in childhood and the medical encounter: Professional ventriloquism and hidden voices. *Qual Health Res.* 2002;12(1):28–41.

Charkow W. Inviting children to grieve. *Professional School Counseling.* 1998;2(2):117.

Chen J, Li X. Genetic and environmental influences on adolescent rumination and its association with depressive symptoms. *J Abnorm Child Psychol.* 2013;41:1289–1298.

Cross T. *On the Social and Emotional Lives of Gifted Children.* Waco, TX: Prufrock Press; 2011.

Davies J, Gentile D. Responses to children's media use in families with and without siblings: A family development perspective. *Fam Relations.* 2012;61(3):410–425.

Davis HW, Carrasco MW. In: Zitelli BJ, McIntire S, Nowalk AJ, eds. *Zitelli and Davis' Atlas of Pediatric Physical Diagnosis.* 6th ed. Philadelphia, PA: Saunders; 2012:181–257.

Dell'Api M, Rennick JE, Rosmus C. Childhood chronic pain and health care professional interactions: Shaping the chronic pain experiences of children. *J Child Health Care.* 2007;11(4):269–286.

Duncan AF, Caughy MO. Parenting style and the vulnerable child syndrome. *J Child Adolesc Nurs.* 2009;22(4):228–234.

Flaherty EG, MacMillan HL; Committee on Child Abuse and Neglect. Caregiver-fabricated illness in a child: A manifestation of child maltreatment. *Pediatrics.* 2013;132(3):590–597. doi: 10.1542/peds.2013-2045.

Greeson J, Thompson A. Aging out of foster care. In: Arnett JJ, ed. *The Oxford Handbook of Emerging Adulthood.* New York, NY: Oxford University Press; 2014;1–21.

Hymel KP, Jenny C. Child sexual abuse. *Pediatr Rev,* 1996;17(7):236–249. doi: 10.1542/pir.17-7-236.

Holt S, Buckley H, Whelan S. The impact of exposure to domestic violence on children and young people: A review of the literature. *Child Abuse Negl.* 2008;32(8):797–810.

Jackson J, Miller M, Moffatt M, Carpenter S, Sherman A, Anderst, J. Bruising in children: Practice patterns of pediatric hematologists and child abuse pediatricians. *Clin Pediatr (Phila).* 2015;54(6):563–569. doi: 10.1177/0009922814558249.

Jenny C, Crawford-Jakubiak JE; Committee on Child Abuse and Neglect. The evaluation of children in the primary care setting when sexual abuse is suspected. *Pediatrics.* 2013;132(2):e558–e567. doi: 10.1542/peds.2013-1741.

Jose PE, Wilkins H, Spendlow JS. Does social anxiety predict rumination and co-rumination among adolescents? *J Clin Child Adolesc Psychol.* 2012;41(1):86–91.

Kemp AM, Dunstan F, Harrison S, et al. Patterns of skeletal fractures in child abuse: Systematic review. *BMJ.* 2008;337:a1518.

Kirkorian H, Wartella E, Anderson D. Media and young children's learning. *Future Child.* 2008;18(1):39–61.

Kivlin JD, Simons KB, Lazoritz S, Ruttum MS. Shaken baby syndrome. *Ophthalmology.* 2000;107(7):1246–1254. doi: http://dx.doi.org/10.1016/S0161-6420(00)00161-5.

Kleinman PK. Diagnostic imaging in infant abuse. *Am J Roentgenol.* 1990;155(4):703–712. doi: 10.2214/ajr.155.4.2119097.

Kokotos F. The vulnerable child syndrome. *Pediatr Rev.* 2009;30(5):193.

Kot L, Shoemaker H. Children of divorce. *J Divorce Remarriage.* 1999;31:161–178.

Krug EG, Dahlberg LL, Mercy JA, Zwi AB, Lozano R. Child abuse and neglect by parents and other caregivers. In: *World Report on Violence and Health.* Geneva, Switzerland: WHO; 2002:59–86 (chap 3).

Lahoti SL, McClain N, Girardet R, McNeese M, Cheung K. Evaluating the child for sexual abuse. *Am Fam Physician.* 2001;63(5):883–892.

Midence K. The effects of chronic illness on children and their families: An overview. *Genet Social Gen Psychol Monographs.* 1994;120(3):311.

Morad Y, Kim YM, Armstrong DC, Huyer D, Mian M, Levin AV. Correlation between retinal abnormalities and intracranial abnormalities in the shaken baby syndrome. *Am J Ophthalmol.* 2002;134(3):354–359. doi: 10.1016/S0002-9394(02)01628-8.

Narang S, Clarke J. Abusive head trauma: Past, present, and future. *J Child Neurol.* 2014;29(12):1747–1756. doi: 10.1177/0883073814549995.

Nimkin K, Kleinman PK. Imaging of Child Abuse. *Radiol Clin North Am.* 2001;39(4):843–864. doi: 10.1016/S0033-8389(05)70314-6.

Pettle S, Britten C. Talking with children about death and dying. *Child Care Health Dev.* 1995;21(6):395–404.

Potter D. Psychosocial well-being and the relationship between divorce and children's academic achievement. *J Marriage Fam.* 2010;72:933–946.

Ruh Linder J, Werner N. Relationally aggressive media exposure and children's normative beliefs: Does parental mediation matter? *Fam Relations.* 2012;61(3):488–500.

Samide L, Stockton, R. Letting go of grief. *J Specialists Group Work.* 2002;27(2):192–204.

Santiago CD, Wadsworth ME, Stump J. Socioeconomic status, neighborhood disadvantage, and poverty-related stress: Prospective effects on psychological syndromes among diverse low-income families. *J Econ Psychol.* 2001;32:218–230.

Sawyer M, Spurrier N. Families, parents and chronic childhood illness. *Fam Matters.* 1996;44:12–15.

Section on Radiology. Diagnostic imaging of child abuse. *Pediatrics.* 2009;123(5):1430–1435. doi: 10.1542/peds.2009-0558.

Sedlak AJ, Mettenburg J, Basena M, Peta I, McPherson K, Greene A. *Fourth National Incidence Study of Child Abuse and Neglect (NIS-4).* Washington, DC: U.S. Department of Health and Human Services; 2010.

Slaughter V. Young children's understanding of death. *Austral Psychol.* 2005;40(3):179–186.

Strasburger V, Jordan A, Donnerstein, E. Health effects of media on children and adolescents. *Pediatrics.* 2010;125(4):756–767.

Squires JE, Squires RH Jr. Munchausen syndrome by proxy: Ongoing clinical challenges. *J Pediatr Gastroenterol Nutr.* 2010;51(3):248–253. doi: 10.1097/MPG.0b013e3181e33b15.

Starling SP, Holden JR, Jenny C. Abusive head trauma: the relationship of perpetrators to their victims. *Pediatrics.* 1995;95(2):259–262.

Research and Statistics

30

Andrew R. Peterson

Question 1

List the following types of study design from most valid to least valid (hierarchy of study design).

- Randomized controlled trial
- Case control study
- Case series/case report
- Animal research
- Systematic review
- Prospective cohort
- Ideas/opinions/editorials/anecdote
- Meta-analysis
- Controlled, nonrandomized study
- Cross-sectional/observational study

Discussion 1

The correct answer sequence is: (1) meta-analysis, (2) systematic review, (3) randomized controlled trial, (4) controlled, nonrandomized study, (5) prospective cohort, (6) case control study, (7) cross-sectional/observational study, (8) case series/case report, (9) animal research, and (10) ideas/opinions/editorials/anecdote.

Question 2

Which is a true statement regarding a randomized controlled trial?
A) Subjects pick which treatment to receive.
B) All subjects receive the same treatment.
C) The person giving the treatment chooses who receives what treatment.
D) Subjects do not get to choose a treatment arm.
E) None of the above.

Discussion 2

The correct answer is "D." Subjects are randomized to receive one or another specific treatment or intervention. They are followed prospectively to evaluate the effects of the intervention. The process of randomization limits the amount of confounding that might affect the results. If all potential confounders are distributed evenly by randomization. The only variable that might explain the outcome is the treatment being studied. Often randomized controlled trials are blinded (the subject does not know what treatment is being received) or double-blinded (the subject and the person administering the treatment do not know what treatment is being received). This is meant to limit the amount of unintentional confounding that might occur from the subject or investigator knowing too much about the interventions. Randomized controlled trials are considered the gold standard clinical study. (See Figure 30–1.) However, they are not always practical. While it might be relatively easy to do a randomized controlled trial of a new pain medication versus a placebo pill, it is not easy to do such a study on the effectiveness of parachutes for preventing death when jumping from an airplane.

> **Helpful Tip**
> Randomized controlled trials are considered the gold standard for clinical study.

Question 3

Which is a true statement regarding a controlled clinical trial?
A) Subjects are blinded to the intervention.
B) All subjects receive the same intervention.
C) The person administering the intervention is blinded.
D) The study is without confounding variables.
E) None of the above.

Discussion 3

The correct answer is "B." This is similar to a randomized controlled trial, except the intervention is not randomized. For this reason, the potential confounding variables are not equally distributed and might influence the validity of the study. For

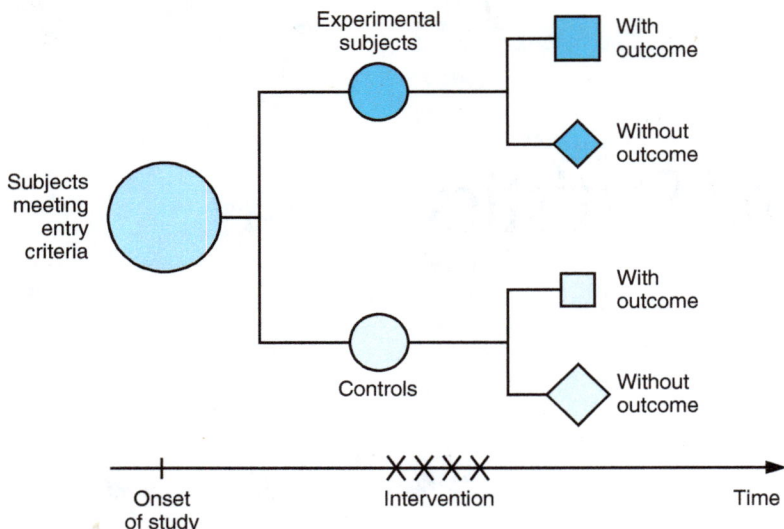

FIGURE 30–1. Randomized controlled trial. Schematic diagram of a randomized controlled trial in which (1) dark-shaded areas = subjects assigned to treatment, (2) light-shaded areas = subjects assigned to control, (3) squares = subjects with outcome of interest, and (4) diamonds = subjects without outcome of interest. (Reproduced with permission from Dawson B, Trapp RG, eds. *Basic and Clinical Biostatics.* 4th ed. New York, NY: McGraw-Hill Education; 2004, Fig. 2-6.)

example, one might do a controlled clinical trial of two types of knee surgery by comparing the surgical outcomes of one surgeon who uses one technique with those of another surgeon who uses a different technique. While any difference in outcome might be due to the differences in surgical technique, they might also be due to patient selection issues, referral bias, differences in insurance status (a common marker of differences in socioeconomic status), or differences in the skill of the surgeon.

Question 4

Which is a true statement regarding a prospective cohort study?
A) It is a retrospective analysis.
B) It does not have a control subject group.
C) It involves an intervention.
D) It follows subjects prospectively.
E) All of the above.

Discussion 4

The correct answer is "D." This study design takes a population and follows it over time to compare patients with a specific condition or treatment with another group that has not been affected by the treatment or condition being studied. (See Figure 30–2.) Cohort studies are observational and no additional variables are controlled for. It is entirely possible that the two groups are different in ways other than the variable being tested. However, a cohort study is often the best method of studying a problem in the real world. For example, my colleagues and I are currently studying injuries in youth football players. It is not practical to randomize children to playing tackle or flag football, so instead we are following children who play tackle football and children who play flag football and comparing the number and types of injuries each sustains.

Question 5

Which is a true statement regarding a case-control study?
A) It controls for all variables.
B) It is a prospective study.
C) It is retrospective study.
D) It does not involve a control group.
E) All of the above.

Discussion 5

The correct answer is "C." A case control study is a retrospective study design that compares patients who already have a specific condition with people who do not. (See Figure 30–3.) The risk of confounding is high in case-control studies because there is no method of controlling for any other variables that might influence

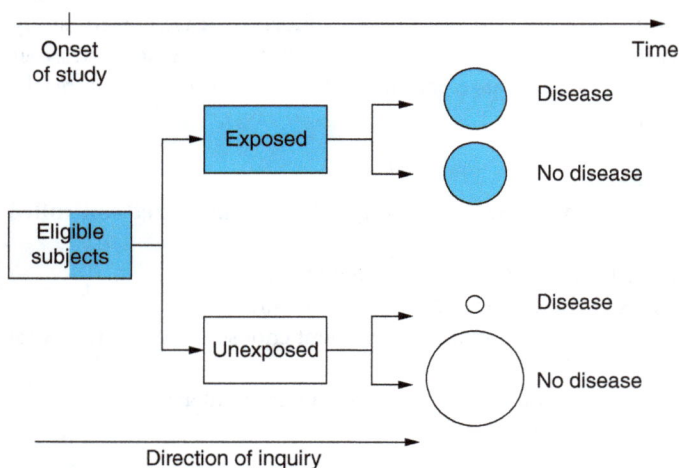

FIGURE 30–2. Cohort study. Schematic diagram of a cohort study in which (1) shaded areas = subjects exposed, (2) unshaded areas = subjects not exposed, (3) big circles = subjects with outcome of interest, and (4) small circles = subjects without outcome of interest. (Reproduced with permission from Greenberg RS, Daniels SR, Flanders WD, Eley JW, Boring JR, eds. *Medical Epidemiology.* 4th ed. New York, NY: McGraw-Hill Education; 2005, Fig. 8-2.)

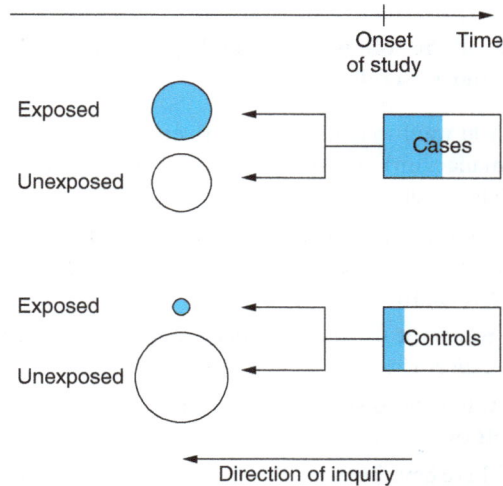

FIGURE 30–3. Case-control study. Schematic diagram of a case-control study in which shaded areas = subjects exposed to risk factor of interest. (Reproduced with permission from Greenberg RS, Daniels SR, Flanders WD, Eley JW, Boring JR, eds. *Medical Epidemiology*. 4th ed. New York, NY: McGraw-Hill Education; 2005, Fig. 9-1.)

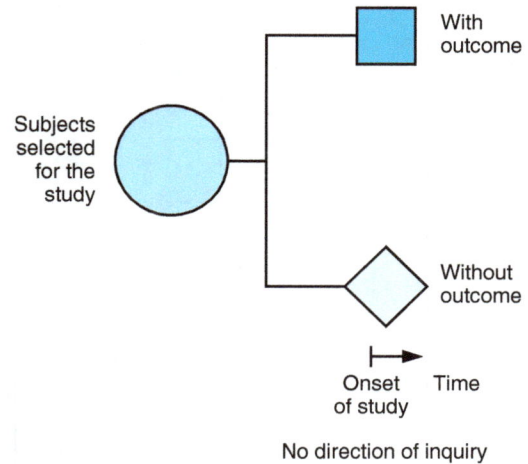

Question: "What is happening?"

FIGURE 30–4. Cross-sectional study. Schematic diagram of a cross-sectional study in which (1) squares = subjects with outcome of interest, and (2) diamonds = subjects without outcome of interest. (Reproduced with permission from Dawson B, Trapp RG, eds. *Basic and Clinical Biostatics*. 4th ed. New York, NY: McGraw-Hill Education; 2004, Fig. 2-2.)

who gets the condition and who does not. However, it is often the only method of identifying what exposure might have caused a disease. For example, suppose you were doing a study of fourth-year medical students with depression and you were trying to figure out what caused their depression. You could use a group of case subjects (students with depression) and compare any historical information you could find with the historical information of a group of control subjects (students without depression) to try to determine what might be the cause of the depression. Let's say you found that all the depressed students had Dr. Wood as their pediatric clerkship mentor and all the not-depressed students had Dr. Peterson. You might conclude that it was something about Dr. Wood that made these students depressed. In this case you would be right, but it could also be any number of other variables that affected where and when the student did their pediatric rotation (these are true confounders) or variables completely unrelated to their time on the pediatrics wards.

Question 6

Which is NOT a true statement regarding a cross-sectional study?
A) It measures a variable continuously over time.
B) It measures a variable at one point in time.
C) It does not determine causality.
D) It does not involve an intervention.
E) It does not compare two populations of subjects.

Discussion 6

The correct answer is "A." A cross-sectional study measures a population or variable at one point in time. (See Figure 30–4.) It does not say anything about causality. For example, you might do a survey of pediatric residents to see how many are depressed. You would be able to say that, at the time of the survey, X% were exhibiting signs of depression. But you would not be able to say why or whether that percentage had changed over time.

Question 7

What is a meta-analysis?
A) An editorial piece.
B) A type of systematic review.
C) A haiku.
D) A study involving three treatment or intervention arms.
E) None of the above.

Discussion 7

The correct answer is "B." A meta-analysis is a type of systematic review that evaluates the results of multiple studies on a single topic and combines them using specific statistical methods as if they were from one study. (See Figure 30–5.) A systematic review is a type of study that reviews all of the literature on a particular topic in a systematic way and evaluates the validity of each study.

Question 8

You cared for patient with a very rare disease that is not well described in the literature. Your consultants have cared for a handful of similar patients. You write a manuscript and are in the process of submitting it for publication when you are asked to indicate the type of study. What do you choose?
A) Case report.
B) Cohort study.
C) Case-controlled study.
D) Case series.
E) All of the above; the journal can decide which is correct.

Discussion 8

The correct answer is "D." A case report is a description of a single patient, and a case series is a description of several similar patients. These reports do not necessarily tell you anything about what causes a disease or what might be useful for treating

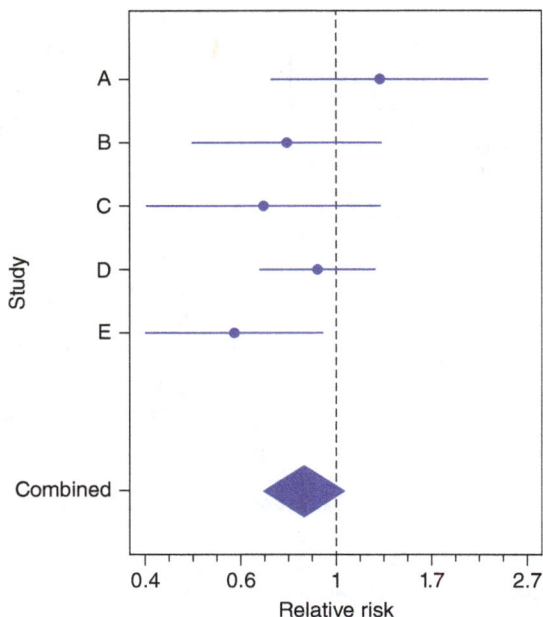

FIGURE 30–5. Meta-analysis. Meta-analysis of five hypothetical epidemiologic studies (A–E) of the relationship between decreased dietary fat intake and risk of developing breast cancer. The results from all five studies are combined and statistically analyzed as if they were from one study. (Reproduced with permission from Greenberg RS, Daniels SR, Flanders WD, Eley JW, Boring JR, eds. *Medical Epidemiology*. 4th ed. New York, NY: McGraw-Hill Education; 2005, Fig. 13-5.)

it, but they are very useful for generating hypotheses. It is common for a clinician-researcher with an idea for a new treatment to first create a case series of patients who undergo the treatment. This allows the clinician-researcher to gain familiarity with the treatment and potential pitfalls. If all goes well, the clinician-scientist then expands his or her inquiry to prove whether or not the treatment works, using a prospective cohort study or controlled trial.

Question 9
All else being equal, which of the following is the more powerful study?
A) Low sample size.
B) High sample size.
C) Both may have limitations.

Discussion 9
The correct answer is "C." This might seem like a silly question, but it is an important tenet of clinical research. Studies of small patient populations are more likely to yield erroneous results than studies on large patient populations. However, when the study becomes too large, it is possible to find statistically significant differences that are not clinically significant (ie, the study is over-powered). There is one area where a larger sample size is always beneficial: in the detection of adverse events. If a treatment has a rare, but bad, side effect, having a larger sample size increases the chance that the researcher finds the side effect.

Question 10
For each of the following research questions, which study design is most useful?

10-1: You want to study the effectiveness of a new antibiotic (Killemallacillin) for treating staphylococcal infections in otherwise healthy patients.

10-2: You want to study the utility of a new diagnostic test for diagnosing anterior cruciate ligament (ACL) tears in athletes with knee injuries.

10-3: You want to study the benefits of regular exercise on breast cancer risk.

10-4: You want to study what happens to depressed medical students over time.

10-5: There have been a lot of studies done on whether or not Killemallacillin is effective for treating staphylococcal infections, but they are contradictory. You want to see if the data from the existing studies might be combined in a way that make them more useful.

10-6: You have 12 patients with recent ACL tears. You want to know if the sport they played caused their injury.

10-7: Against the advice of the Food and Drug Administration (FDA), you have treated 12 patients with staphylococcal infections using Killemallacillin. You want to share your results.

Select from the following list:
A) Meta-analysis.
B) Systematic review.
C) Randomized controlled trial.
D) Controlled, nonrandomized study.
E) Prospective cohort.
F) Case-control study.
G) Cross-sectional/observational study.
H) Case series/case report.
I) Animal research.
J) Ideas/opinions/editorials/anecdote.

Discussion 10
The correct answers follow.

10-1: The correct answer is "C." The randomized controlled trial is the gold standard for treatment studies. There are a lot of potential confounders in this study and they can be minimized by randomizing treatment allocation.

10-2: This is a trick question. Send a complaint to the question writer as this research question does not fit neatly into one of the described study designs. But you want to compare the results you get with the new diagnostic test to some gold standard reference. For ACL tears, you could compare the test to magnetic resonance imaging (MRI) or to the appearance of the ACL at the time of arthroscopy.

10-3: The best answer is "C," but in reality option "E" and in the worst-case scenario option "F" are used. It would be great if you could randomize women into exercising or nonexercising groups, follow them longitudinally, and see which ones developed breast cancer. But that study probably would not get past the Institutional Review Board (IRB), and you would have a hard time recruiting and retaining subjects. So, often these types of questions are answered with the prospective cohort study. You follow two groups of women longitudinally, one group that exercises and one that does not, and see who develops breast cancer. Obviously, these two groups might be different in other ways, confounding the results. Finally, if you did not have time for all that, you might look at one group of women who have breast cancer and one group that does not and have them recall how much exercise they have gotten throughout their lives. Again, these groups may be quite different in ways other than their exercise exposure, but they might also be different in how they recall their exercise history, adding an additional confounder.

10-4: The correct answer is "E." The prospective cohort study is commonly used to determine how an exposure affects people over time. In this case there may be differences between the students other than whether or not they are depressed, but it will be very difficult to control for those differences. Sometimes, researchers use matching to try to control for some of those unmeasured variables. They try to make the control subjects as much like the case subjects as possible. So for example, if a depressed medical student is male, tall, blonde and going into pediatric cardiology, they will try to find a nondepressed medical student who is also male, tall, blonde and going into pediatric cardiology. Obviously, not all of the unmeasured confounders can be accounted for this way, but it is better than nothing.

10-5: The correct answer is "A." That is the description of a meta-analysis. You would evaluate the quality of the studies that have been done and use statistical wizardry to combine their results as though they were one study.

10-6: The correct answer is "F." Hopefully this question illustrates the pitfalls of case-control studies. In this example, you would take the 12 injured patients and compare them with 12 uninjured patients to see if they played different sports. Obviously a lot of other variables might explain the reason why they tore their ACLs. But sometimes all you have is the condition. Imagine you are working with the Environmental Protection Agency (EPA) and you identify a group of people in the same community who all have lymphoma. There is no better way to find the cause of their cancer than to compare them to others in the community who do not have the disease.

10-7: The correct answer is "H." This is a case series. It is not an experiment. The pleural of "anecdote" is not "data." However, if you are the first person to try such a thing, a case series like this might be useful for developing experiments to answer the question of whether or not Killemallacillin is useful for treating *Staphylococcus*.

Question 11
Match the following terms with their definitions:

Term:

A) Validity.
B) Reliability.
C) Bias.
D) Confounding.
E) Generalizability.
F) Intention to treat analysis.
G) Type I error.
H) Type II error.
I) Null hypothesis.

Definition:

11-1: A study is done under specific conditions. This term refers to how well the construct holds up outside of those specific conditions. How valid is the result in the real world?

11-2: The extent to which a conclusion corresponds accurately to the real world. All other errors in study design affect this.

11-3: A statement that there is no difference between two phenomena. This statement is rejected if there is sufficient evidence to the contrary.

11-4: Repeatability. Consistency.

11-5: Incorrect rejection of the null hypothesis. Detecting an effect when none is present.

11-6: Failure to reject a false null hypothesis. Failing to detect an effect that is present.

11-7: In prospective studies, this technique ensures that subjects are measured in the arm of the study that they started in. Ignoring this technique, limits the power of the study.

11-8: An inclination towards a specific outcome or belief. It may affect the results of a study in unmeasured or unintentional ways.

11-9: An extraneous variable that correlates with both the dependent and independent variable. These types of errors affect the interpretation (but not the results) of studies that do not account for them.

Discussion 11
The correct answers follow:

11-1: Option "E," generalizability.

11-2: Option "A," validity.

11-3: Option "I," null hypothesis.

11-4: Option "B," reliability.

11-5: Option "G," type I error.

11-6: Option "H," type II error.

11-7: Option "F," intention to treat analysis.

11-8: Option "C," bias.

11-9: Option "D," confounding.

Question 12

Pull out a piece of paper and draw two 2 × 2 tables (one for diagnostic tests and one for treatments) that explain the following concepts:

- Relative risk reduction
- Absolute risk reduction
- Number needed to treat
- Sensitivity
- Specificity
- Positive predictive value
- Negative predictive value

2 × 2 table for treatment

	Treatment group	Control group	
Events	A	B	A+B= total number of events
Non-events	C	D	C+D= total number of non-events
	A+C= total number in treatment group	B+D= total number in control group	

Experimental event rate (EER) = $\frac{A}{A+C}$

Control event rate (CER) = $\frac{B}{B+D}$

Absolute risk reduction = EER–CER

Relative risk reduction = $\frac{EER-CER}{CER}$

Number needed to treat = 1/(EER–CER)

2 × 2 table for diagnosis

	Condition present	Condition absent	
Test outcome positive	True positive	False positive (type 1 error)	Total number with positive test
Test outcome negative	False negative (type 2 error)	True negative	Total number with negative test
	Total number with condition	Total number without condition	

Sensitivity = $\frac{\text{True positives}}{\text{Total number with condition}}$

Specificity = $\frac{\text{True negatives}}{\text{Total number without condition}}$

Positive predictive value = $\frac{\text{True positive}}{\text{Total number with positive test}}$

Negative predictive value = $\frac{\text{True negative}}{\text{Total number with negative test}}$

Question 13

Match the following terms with their definitions:

Term:

A) Prevalence.
B) Incidence.
C) Pretest probability.
D) Posttest probability.
E) Standard deviation.
F) Confidence interval.
G) Likelihood ratio.
H) Relative risk.
I) Odds ratio.

Definition:

13-1: An estimate of a population parameter from a single sample. If an experiment were repeated over and over, there would be an $X\%$ chance that each of the sampling intervals contained the true value.

13-2: The probability of an event occurring in an exposed group divided by the probability of an event occurring in an unexposed group.

13-3: The probability of having an event occur in an exposed group divided by the probability of an event not occurring in an unexposed group.

13-4: The number of new cases in a population over a given time period.

13-5: The chance that a person has a disease before a diagnostic test is done.

13-6: The chance that a person has a disease after a test is done (takes into account the chance that the person has the disease and the accuracy of the test).

13-7: A measure of the amount of variation around a sample mean. The larger this value is, the larger the margin of error or confidence interval around a result. This value increases with smaller sample sizes (n) and increased intrinsic variance around the true population mean and decreases with larger n and smaller intrinsic variance around the true population mean.

13-8: The proportion of a population that has a condition.

13-9: Probability of an individual with the condition having a positive test divided by the probability of an individual without the condition having a positive test. When doing a test, you have a certain pretest probability. If the test is positive, you use this value to determine what your posttest probability should be.

Discussion 13

The correct answers follow.

13-1: Option "F," confidence interval.

13-2: Option "H," relative risk.

13-3: Option "I," odds ratio.

13-4: Option "B," incidence.

13-5: Option "C," pretest probability.

13-6: Option "D," posttest probability.

13-7: Option "E," standard deviation.

13-8: Option "A," prevalence.

13-9: Option "G," likelihood ratio.

Question 14

What is the difference between statistical significance and clinical significance?

A) Clinical but not statistical significance is determined by the *P* value.
B) A result can be clinically significant but not statistically significant.
C) A result must be statistically significant to be clinically significant.
D) A statistically significant result is always clinically significant.
E) None of the above.

Discussion 14

The correct answer is "C." A result that is statistically significant is likely true. A result that is clinically significant is relevant to clinical practice. A result cannot be clinically significant if it is not statistically significant. That is, a result should not influence clinical care if it is not likely to be true. Imagine you tested a new drug to treat staphylococcal infections that was effective in treating the infections 6 of 12 times whereas a placebo was effective 4 of 12 times, with a $P = 0.40$. This is well above the commonly accepted *P*-value of $P = 0.05$ that signifies statistical significance. You should not interpret this study to say that the new drug is more effective than placebo. If it were, that would be clinically important, but since it is not statistically significant, it cannot be clinically significant. A result may be statistically significant but not clinically significant. Imagine you had investigated a new drug that increased the rate of fingernail growth by 0.001 inches per year and, because you studied the drug in more than a million people, you were able to demonstrate that it was more effective than placebo at increasing fingernail growth rate with a $P = 0.00001$ certainty. This is highly statistically significant, but most readers would agree that it is not clinically significant at all.

Question 15

Which of the following is an example of a "PICO" question?

A) Is pneumonia more likely to lead to death than pancreatitis?
B) Among adolescents with Chlamydia urethritis, what is the rate of Gonnococcal urethritis?
C) Among 3- to 6-month-old infants with RSV bronchiolitis, is nebulized hypertonic saline or nebulized albuterol better for decreasing hospital length of stay?
D) Among children with acute otitis media who are treated with amoxicillin, how long does it take ear pain to resolve?

Discussion 15

The correct answer is "C" In evidence-based medicine, most questions are phrased as PICO questions (whether we realize it or not). The acronym stands for:

P – Patient or population

I – Intervention or indicator

C – Comparator or control

O – Outcome

Here are two more examples: (1) "In patients treated with Killemallacillin compared to patients treated with placebo, which group clears their infection more rapidly?" (2) "In a group of coal miners over 6 feet tall compared to coal miners less than 5 feet tall, who bumps their head more often?"

BIBLIOGRAPHY

Motulsky H. *Intuitive Biostatistics: A Nonmathematical Guide to Statistical Thinking.* 2nd ed. New York, NY: Oxford University Press; 2010.

Silver N. *The Signal and the Noise: Why Most Predictions Fail—But Some Don't.* New York, NY: Penguin Press; 2012.

Wheelan CJ. *Naked Statistics: Stripping the Dread from the Data.* New York, NY: WW Norton; 2014.

Renal and Urologic Disorders

31

Jen Jetton and Kathy Lee-Son

The medical students rotating with you report being generally baffled by the mysterious entity known as the kidney and, in fact, report having near–posttraumatic stress responses to their renal module exam. They ask you to explain to them once more what it is the kidneys do and why there is so much fuss about them.

Which one of the following is NOT produced by the kidney?
A) Renin.
B) Aldosterone.
C) 1, 25-dihydroxyvitamin D (calcitriol).
D) Erythropoietin.
E) All of the above are made by the kidney.

Discussion

The correct answer is "B." Aldosterone is produced by the adrenal glands under the stimulation of the renin-angiotensin-aldosterone system. The kidneys play multiple roles in body homeostasis. These include:

- Disposal of waste products of daily metabolism and medications
- Maintenance of water and fluid balance
- Regulation of blood pressure through the production of renin
- Regulation of body salt homeostasis (sodium, chloride, potassium)
- Regulation of bone mineral homeostasis (calcium, magnesium, phosphorus)
- Production of the active form of vitamin D
- Regulation of growth and the growth hormone axis
- Production of erythropoietin (stimulates bone marrow to produce red blood cells)

Depending on the nature and severity of the particular kidney disease or disorder, you may see dysregulation in one, many, or all of these functions.

▶ **CASE 1**

A 2-day-old newborn boy was born at term by normal vaginal delivery weighing 3.5 kg. The pregnancy was the product of in vitro fertilization. The mother had multiple ultrasounds throughout pregnancy and all were normal per her report. The newborn has been a perfect baby—peeing, eating, sleeping and crying. For a reason unknown to your resident, the newborn had serum electrolytes, blood urea nitrogen (BUN), and creatinine measured. The results flag red, and you see the creatinine is 0.9 mg/dL.

Question 1-1

What do you do next?
A) Order a stat renal ultrasound.
B) Place an indwelling urinary catheter.
C) Transfer the newborn to the neonatal intensive care unit.
D) Consult your nephrology friends.
E) Look up the mother's creatinine value.

Discussion 1-1

The correct answer is "E." Creatinine and BUN levels are used to monitor kidney status. Creatinine varies by age, gender, muscle mass, and hydration. To be useful, the creatinine must be interpreted in the context of the clinical situation. A boy with muscular dystrophy is expected to have a low creatinine due to lack of muscle. In children with chronic disease, knowing the patient's baseline is helpful. A creatinine of 0.6 mg/dL may be normal for the patient's age but not normal if the patient's baseline is 0.3 mg/dL. Trends are also useful to monitor. In neonates, creatinine reflects the maternal value during the first days of life and then declines over the course of a week or so to typical values. Glomerular filtration rate (GFR) is different. It is a measurement of kidney function and is useful for staging chronic kidney disease (CKD; eg, chronic kidney disease 2 = GFR 60–89 mL/min/1.73 m^2). We want to make sure the GFR (usually estimated based on the serum creatinine) is stable for at least 3 months before assigning a CKD stage. (See Table 31–1.)

TABLE 31–1 KIDNEY FUNCTION MEASUREMENTS

Measures of Kidney Function	What Is It?	Factors That Affect Interpretation
Serum creatinine	• Muscle breakdown product. • Easy to measure through a simple blood test.	• See Discussion 1-1. • Level varies depending on age, gender, diet, and hydration status. Expect an infant to have a level 0.2–0.3 mg/dL, a school-aged child 0.4–0.6 mg/dL, and an adolescent male 0.8–1 mg/dL. • Different lab methods may produce values that vary as much as 0.2–0.3 mg/dL. • Impacted by gestational age and degree of nephrogenesis in preterm infants (will trend down more slowly from maternal values in preterm infants than term infants). • Does not differentiate nature, type, or timing of renal insult in patient with acute kidney injury (AKI). • May rise as much as 48 hours after an AKI event.
Glomerular filtration rate (GFR)	• Measure of the filtration function of the kidney. • Normal is > 90 mL/min/1.73 m². • GFR < 15 mL/min/1.73 m² suggests need for dialysis or kidney transplant. • Whether or not GFR is stable or changing is important for assessing chronic kidney disease (CKD) progression. • May be estimated using mathematical equations that take into account serum creatinine or may be measured using a 24-hour urine collection or nuclear medicine test.	• Fall in GFR will cause a rise in serum creatinine (though remember this may happen 24–48 hours after the injury). Serum creatinine may not rise even if there is progression of CKD if there is also compensatory hypertrophy in the remaining nephrons. • Estimating equations are not always accurate, especially in children with GFR >75, and rely on accuracy of the serum creatinine. • 24-hour urine collections require the patient to follow directions carefully and collect *all* of the urine in a 24-hour period and not more. Obviously a child who is not potty trained or who wets the bed at night will have a hard time with this. • Nuclear medicine GFRs require two peripheral IV placements and serial blood draws over several hours, which may not be acceptable to the child.

Helpful Tip

Nephrogenesis begins at the fifth week of gestation and continues until 34 to 36 weeks' gestation.

Helpful Tip

The GFR in a term infant is 10 to 20 mL/min/1.73 m² during the first days of life. GFR doubles within the first 2 weeks of life, then rises steadily until reaching adult levels (>90 mL/min/1.73 m²) by age 2 years.

▶ CASE 2

A usually healthy 17-year-old boy comes to the office after school for a sports physical. He is well appearing and well grown. Blood pressure is 117/76 mm Hg. He is afebrile. He has no abnormalities on physical exam. He provides a urine sample that shows 2+ protein on urine dipstick with specific gravity 1.030. The rest of the urinalysis is normal.

Question 2-1

What is the next step in the diagnosis?
A) Obtain a stat kidney biopsy.
B) Admit for further evaluation.
C) Obtain a first morning urine specimen for urinalysis.
D) Order a renal ultrasound.

Discussion 2-1

The correct answer is "C." (See Discussion 2-2.)

Question 2-2

What is the most likely cause of proteinuria in this scenario?
A) Benign orthostatic proteinuria.
B) Focal segmental glomerulosclerosis.
C) Atypical hemolytic uremic syndrome.
D) Undiagnosed posterior urethral valves.

Discussion 2-2

The correct answer is "A." Low level proteinuria may have benign causes such as exercise, fever, or dehydration. Benign orthostatic proteinuria is the finding of proteinuria in a specimen obtained later in the day with a negative urine protein on a first morning sample. For this adolescent boy who is otherwise healthy, the next step in the evaluation would be to have him bring in a first morning urine sample for urinalysis. The most likely cause is benign orthostatic proteinuria (key features of the case are afternoon sample and high specific gravity that may reflect mild dehydration after sports practice). Normal growth, normal blood pressure, and absence of edema or other abnormalities on physical exam are reassuring findings. With persistent or more severe proteinuria, the risk of glomerular disease or renal scarring increases, and renal biopsy may be indicated. Microscopic hematuria with or without proteinuria, ill appearance, and hypertension would be expected with atypical (non–diarrhea-associated) hemolytic uremic syndrome. Posterior urethral valves obstruct the bladder and typically present in the newborn period. Delayed presentation is associated with poor urinary stream, hypertension, urinary tract infections, poor growth, and enuresis; proteinuria may be seen in these cases if scarring is severe or chronic kidney disease is advanced. If this patient was a girl, you would be laughed at if you included that on the differential. Focal segmental glomerulosclerosis is not a good disease. Affected patients typically present with nephrotic syndrome—massive proteinuria and edema. If proteinuria is still present on first morning sample (typically, a urine protein/creatinine greater than 0.5 mg/dL on several samples is a good measure), then additional workup should include serum creatinine, BUN, electrolytes, glucose, and serum albumin. Consider a renal ultrasound. A voiding cystourethrogram or renal scan to evaluate for scarring may be indicated if there is a history of frequent urinary tract infections that started early. See Case 22 on nephrotic syndrome, later in this chapter, for additional workup if proteinuria is severe. Early consultation with a nephrologist is indicated for high-grade proteinuria.

▶ CASE 3

A 6-year-old girl provides a urine sample during evaluation for urinary frequency. She is well grown and well appearing. Blood pressure is 91/52 mm Hg. Urinalysis shows 3+ blood with 8 to 10 red blood cells per high power field (RBCs/HPF), no proteinuria, and urine specific gravity of 1.020.

Question 3-1

What is the next step in her diagnosis?
A) Renal biopsy.
B) Urine culture.
C) Urine calcium and urine creatinine.
D) Renal ultrasound.
E) Options A, B, and C.
F) Options B, C, and D.
G) All of the above.

Discussion 3-1

The correct answer is "F." (See Discussion 3-2.)

Question 3-2

What is the most likely diagnosis?
A) Urinary tract infection.
B) Hypercalciuria.
C) Thin basement membrane disease.
D) Alport syndrome.

Discussion 3-2

The correct answer is "B." Microscopic hematuria is defined as the presence of greater than 4 to 5 RBCs/HPF in a fresh specimen (note: RBCs may lyse if a urine sample is left to sit for a long time). The differential diagnosis is very broad, including both benign and more serious conditions such as idiopathic microscopic hematuria, hypercalciuria, crystalluria, thin basement membrane disease, kidney stones, cystitis/urinary tract infection (UTI), trauma, exercise-induced hematuria, tumor or mass anywhere in the urinary tract, and glomerular disease (eg, Alport syndrome, IgA nephropathy). Look for historical clues to help narrow the differential: dysuria, abdominal or flank pain, family history of hematuria, or kidney disease. Key findings that suggest a more serious diagnosis include presence of proteinuria, hypertension, abnormal serum creatinine, systemic signs (eg, arthritis, rashes, respiratory distress). Workup includes urinalysis, urine microscopy, urine calcium, urine creatinine, serum creatinine, urine culture, and renal and bladder ultrasound. You could also consider antistreptolysin O (ASO), antinuclear antibody (ANA), and complement proteins (C3, C4), depending on the presentation. RBC casts or dysmorphic RBCs on microscopy suggest glomerular disease. In this case, normal blood pressure, absence of pyuria, and lack of proteinuria are good signs and reassuring. Hypercalciuria is a common cause of isolated microscopic hematuria and may be associated with dysuria or urinary frequency. A random urine calcium and creatinine level is a good screen, although you will need a 24-hour urine collection to confirm the diagnosis. Thin basement membrane disease, formerly called familial benign hematuria, is common, *usually* benign, and may be inherited from the child's mother or father (obtain a good family history to be sure there is no hidden renal failure in the past). It is an autosomal dominant disease. Ask the parents if they have ever had their urine checked (in this case no family history was mentioned). Alport syndrome is in the same spectrum of collagen abnormalities but classically is associated with a family history, more severe renal disease, and in some cases hearing loss and unusual eye malformations. Again, be sure to get a good family history! A UTI can cause microscopic hematuria, but you would expect concurrent pyuria as well as some dysuria and maybe a fever. Nonetheless it is important to rule it out. You should get a renal ultrasound to make sure she does not have a mass or stone or other concerning condition. Remain alert to changes in growth or blood pressure in these children over time as their condition may evolve.

▶ CASE 4

A 15-year-old healthy adolescent boy presents to your office for his annual sports physical examination. He was noted to have mildly elevated blood pressure in triage, 134/85 mm Hg, but 120/81 mm Hg and 124/78 mm Hg on repeat manual assessments. Repeated urinalyses show 30 to 50 RBCs/HPF and 2+ protein. He has no complaints of pain, gross hematuria, recent illnesses, or travel. Family history is positive for a maternal grandfather who was told he had blood in the urine, but he does not go to the doctor. Mother also has microscopic hematuria. Lab results are as follows: CBC normal, Na 139 mEq/L, K 3.9 mEq/L, Cl 107 mEq/L, CO_2 25 mEq/L, BUN 20 mg/dL, and creatinine 0.9 mg/dL. You suspect Alport syndrome given the family history.

Question 4-1

The following would be expected findings on subsequent evaluation EXCEPT:

A) Bilateral normal kidneys on renal ultrasound.
B) Proteinuria noted on first morning urine specimen.
C) Hypercalciuria on random urine sample.
D) Dysmorphic RBCs on urine microscopy.
E) Thin glomerular basement membrane on renal biopsy.

Discussion 4-1

The correct answer is "C." Alport syndrome is an inherited glomerular basement membrane defect of type IV collagen in its formation of the collagen trimer. There are three forms. The X-linked (80%) form is a defect of the *COL4A5* gene; the autosomal recessive (15%) and autosomal dominant (5%) forms both have defects in *COL4A3* or *4A4* genes. Patients generally have persistent microscopic hematuria, possibly associated with intermittent episodes of gross hematuria. In addition, true proteinuria is suggestive of worsening glomerular disease. Because this is a glomerular basement membrane defect, dysmorphic RBCs will most likely be seen on microscopy. Alport syndrome is not typically associated with hypercalciuria. Finally, renal ultrasound of patients with AS is generally normal. Please note extrarenal findings of Alport syndrome that include sensorineural hearing loss, anterior lenticonus, or retinopathy.

▶ CASE 5

A 12-year-old boy is brought to his pediatrician's office by his mother because he had bright red blood in his urine. He had no pain with voiding; his urine just looked red in the toilet. He has recently had runny nose and congestion. On further questioning, he thinks he might have had similar episodes in the past but did not want to tell anyone about them.

Question 5-1

Which of the following is the most likely diagnosis?

A) Kidney stones.
B) Urinary tract infection.
C) IgA nephropathy.
D) Hemolytic uremic syndrome.
E) Minimal change disease.

Discussion 5-1

The correct answer is "C." Recurrent episodes of painless gross hematuria associated with an upper respiratory infection are typical of a patient with IgA nephropathy, although only 40% to

50% of patients present in this way. Other patients may present with microscopic hematuria with or without proteinuria or, in the most severe cases, with nephrotic syndrome and rapid progression to end-stage renal disease. Severe colicky flank pain would suggest kidney stones. Sometimes the child may report seeing a stone as it passes. Fever, dysuria, and flank pain would be typical of a urinary tract infection. Hemolytic uremic syndrome usually has a more severe presentation, with symptoms that include persistent gross hematuria (often brown or tea colored), oliguria, ill appearance, vomiting, and hypertension. Minimal change disease is not typically associated with gross hematuria unless the patient has developed a renal vein thrombosis. In this case, you would expect some other clues to nephrotic syndrome (eg, edema, oliguria) long before the gross hematuria.

Question 5-2

What other clinical findings may be seen with this disease entity?

A) Rash.
B) Joint pain or arthritis.
C) Crampy abdominal pain.
D) All of the above.
E) None of the above.

Discussion 5-2

The correct answer is "E." IgA nephropathy is typically limited to the kidney, although patients may develop IgA nephropathy secondary to another systemic illness such as cirrhosis, celiac disease, or HIV infection.

Helpful Tip

Gross hematuria key points:

- Urine may look red, brown, or pink.
- Red cell casts on microscopy suggest glomerulonephritis.
- Similar differential diagnosis as for microscopic hematuria (see earlier discussion): brown or cola-colored urine suggests acute glomerulonephritis. Also consider sickle cell nephropathy (especially with papillary necrosis).
- Clues to diagnosis and key findings are the same as described earlier. Ask about recent sore throat, skin infections (eg, impetigo), or upper respiratory infection (URI) symptoms. Ask about family history. Ask about and look closely for systemic findings such as arthritis, joint pains, anemia or cytopenias, respiratory distress, edema, and hypertension. Ask about recent exposures to animals, petting zoos, or unpasteurized or undercooked food products if there is concern for hemolytic uremic syndrome.
- Workup consists of urinalysis, urine microscopy, serum creatinine, serum electrolytes, BUN, calcium, and renal and bladder ultrasound to look for urinary tract abnormalities, tumors or masses, cysts, or stones. If systemic signs are present check C3, C4, ASO, and ANA.

> **Helpful Tip**
>
> Not all red urine suggests hematuria. Consider myoglobinuria (especially with vigorous exercise in the heat) or hemoglobinuria (such as with hemolysis). Urine will be red or brown with positive blood on dipstick but no or very few RBCs on microscopy. Remember, the urine sample should be fresh as RBCs lyse when sitting for a long time.

▶ CASE 6

A mother comes to your clinic with her 4-year-old daughter, who was sent home from daycare after wetting her pants three times today. The girl was potty-trained without difficulty and has had only occasional accidents, but she has not been pooping every day (only every third day, and her poops are so big they almost clog the toilet). The mother says her daughter feels warm to the touch, but she has not taken her temperature. The girl has been spending a lot of time at the water fountain recently. She has also recently been refusing to stop playing with her new favorite toy for long enough to go to the bathroom.

Question 6-1

What are possible causes of enuresis in this situation?
A) Urinary tract infection.
B) Constipation.
C) New-onset diabetes mellitus.
D) Behavioral/normal response.
E) All of the above.
F) None of the above.

Discussion 6-1

The correct answer is "E." Occasional episodes of enuresis, or wetting (*diurnal enuresis* is wetting in the daytime) can be normal, especially in busy 4-year-olds who do not want to stop what they are doing. Constipation is an important contributor to enuresis and urinary tract infections and should always be addressed if present (parents may seem confused when you ask about poop *and* pee, but it is important). Urinary tract infection is of course on the differential, especially given the sudden onset. Finally, if the child seems to be drinking a lot more than usual, consider diabetes mellitus. Ask about voiding patterns: does the child do the pee-pee dance, barely make it to the bathroom on time, or rush in and out of the bathroom without emptying his or her bladder all the way? For boys, ask about a strong urinary stream (dribbling can be a sign of a urinary tract obstruction such as posterior urethral valves). Physical exam should include examination genital rashes, urethral abnormalities (boys) and labial fusion (girls). Examine the lower back for a hair tuft or abnormal gluteal crease that might suggest a spinal cord or neurologic problem. Workup is guided by the historical clues and should include a urinalysis and urine culture. Treat constipation. Consider a renal ultrasound if symptoms recur often.

Consider having the parents keep a voiding diary. Encourage the child to go to the bathroom every couple of hours even if he or she does not feel the urge.

▶ CASE 7

The next patient is a 12-year-old boy who has been wetting the bed since he was young. In fact he has never been dry. You look at the growth chart and notice that he has not grown much either in the past 6 years. His height is now at the third percentile whereas based on midparental predicted height he should be at the 80th percentile. His blood pressure is also greater than the 95th percentile for age.

Question 7-1

Your workup should include:
A) Renal ultrasound.
B) Urinalysis.
C) Serum electrolytes.
D) BUN and creatinine.
E) All of the above.

Discussion 7-1

The correct answer is "E." Nocturnal enuresis (nighttime wetting) occurs in a small percentage of children aged 12 years and older who have no other medical issues. In the absence of any other concerning findings on history and physical, workup can be limited to a first morning urinalysis. This will indicate if the kidneys are able to concentrate urine appropriately, and you can evaluate for glucosuria that would suggest diabetes. In this case (and since this is a *renal* chapter), the child has some signs of chronic kidney disease, including short stature and high blood pressure, so your evaluation should be more extensive. Renal conditions that might present as nocturnal enuresis include renal dysplasia, undiagnosed posterior urethral valves, and diabetes insipidus. If the child appeared otherwise well without any concerning signs or symptoms, then management could include reassurance, treatment of constipation if it is present, good bladder emptying during the day, reward systems, bell and pad alarms, and desmopressin (DDAVP) if all else fails.

▶ CASE 8

A family comes to your practice for the first time to establish care. The mother introduces you to her two boys. One boy is 4 years old and the other is a 5-month-old infant. Both appear to be on the small side. You plot the infant's length, weight, and head circumference on the growth chart and are shocked to see that he is below the fifth percentile for all three measures. He also seems sleepy. His mother says that he stopped feeding well about 2 months ago when she switched from breastfeeding to formula in order to go back to work. The older boy is on the growth chart, but just barely. You notice that he has to leave the room three times during your half-hour visit to go to the bathroom. His mother has five water bottles in her purse. The older boy asks her for water as soon as he comes back from the bathroom. You are beginning to wonder if something is wrong.

Question 8-1

Your *initial* workup for the older boy should include all of the following EXCEPT:
A) Urinalysis.
B) Serum electrolytes.
C) Brain MRI.
D) Urine osmolality.
E) Serum osmolality.

Discussion 8-1

The correct answer is "C."

Question 8-2

Which findings would be most consistent with the diagnosis you suspect?
A) Hypernatremia and urine specific gravity of 1.030 or higher.
B) Hypernatremia and urine osmolality of 35 mOsm/kg (low).
C) Hyponatremia and urine specific gravity less than 1.005.
D) Hyponatremia and urine osmolality of 450 mOsm/kg (high).

Discussion 8-2

The correct answer is "B." Diabetes insipidus (DI) is a condition characterized by polydipsia, polyuria, and very dilute urine even when the serum sodium is high or the patient is dehydrated. Think of the child who cannot sit through a car ride without needing to stop every 30 minutes to go to the bathroom and who also never stops drinking water. *Congenital nephrogenic DI* is a rare, inherited condition (most often X-linked but can also be autosomal dominant or recessive) that often presents as failure to thrive in an infant or with episodes of recurrent dehydration, vomiting, or seizures. Breastfed infants may present later because breast milk has a much higher water and much lower salt and protein content relative to cow's milk–based formulas (having plenty of water at all times is critical for these patients!). You later find out the older boy was breastfed until he was 1 year old and since then has always been a heavy water drinker. Based on this information you will also want to consider nephrogenic DI in the infant (in addition to other failure-to-thrive workup measures that you will be doing). Remember that DI may be *nephrogenic* (kidney does not respond to antidiuretic hormone and therefore cannot hold onto water) or central (pituitary does not make enough antidiuretic hormone). Nephrogenic DI may be *inherited* or *acquired* (from certain medications such as lithium or longstanding urinary tract obstruction). If the thirst and the frequent bathroom breaks only recently started (eg, in an older child), think about central causes such as a brain tumor. Similarly, recent neurosurgery or head injury may be a clue to central DI. The first step is to confirm the diagnosis. Start by ordering a serum sodium level, urinalysis, and urine and serum osmolality. You are looking for dilute urine (eg, *low* urine specific gravity < 1.005 and *low* urine osmolality) in a patient with

high serum sodium greater than 145 mg/dL, high serum osmolality, dehydration, or a combination of these. If the patient has been drinking plenty of water and your initial screen is not helpful, consult your friendly endocrinologist or nephrologist about a water deprivation test and desmopressin challenge. Option "A" suggests appropriately *very* concentrated urine for a patient who may have hypernatremic dehydration. Option "C" suggests primary polydipsia; that is, someone who drinks *lots* of water but does not have a concentrating defect. The dilute urine (in a patient with low serum sodium) suggests the kidneys are appropriately trying to get rid of all the water the person is drinking. Option "D" suggests the syndrome of inappropriate diuretic hormone in which the kidneys hold onto water even though the serum sodium is low (how inappropriate!).

In the previous question (8-1), you should have been able to think through these scenarios and about what your first line of diagnostic tests would have been. Brain MRI (option "C") may turn out to be an important test if your first line of testing indicates that the underlying problem is central DI. But is not necessary for diagnosing the underlying cause of polyuria and polydipsia.

▶ CASE 9

The next patient is also here to establish care. The family is a young couple who bring their 4-month-old infant boy to see you. While very happy about the birth of their first child, they are a bit worried. They tell you that their son looks smaller than his same-age cousin, who outweighs him by 4 pounds. He throws up a lot, and they are not sure if this is normal. Even though he throws up, he still makes plenty of wet diapers each day. You confirm that he is below the fifth percentile for both length and weight. You wonder if something in the water is causing kidney problems in every infant in your clinic today, but decide that you should obtain some basic lab studies first. The serum chemistry looks something like this: Na 142 mEq/L, K 3.2 mEq/L, Cl 115 mEq/L, and CO_2 10 mEq/L.

Question 9-1

To make a diagnosis of renal tubular acidosis, you should see all of the following EXCEPT:
A) Low serum bicarbonate (CO_2).
B) High serum chloride.
C) Normal serum anion gap.
D) High urine pH.
E) Normal to low serum chloride.

Discussion 9-1

The correct answer is "E." Renal tubular acidosis is a clinical condition in which the kidneys either waste too much base (bicarbonate) or cannot get rid of enough acid in the urine in order to maintain a normal pH. The key point is that it produces a metabolic acidosis with a *normal* anion gap (which comes with a *high* serum chloride). A normal anion gap is 8 to 16. If you see a positive anion gap, then you are dealing with something else. In this case, the anion gap is 14, which is normal: $(142 + 3.2) - (115 + 10)$. The other thing you may see is a high urine pH relative to the low serum CO_2, again highlighting that the kidneys are not able to maintain acid-base balance appropriately. Distal renal tubular acidosis is a rare condition that may present as failure to thrive. The other much more common cause of hyperchloremic *normal* anion gap metabolic acidosis is diarrhea. Ask about diarrhea in a well-grown older child in whom you see this pattern of electrolyte abnormalities. If you find an increased anion gap metabolic acidosis, think about ingestions (especially salicylates, methanol/propylene glycol), diabetic ketoacidosis, and lactic acidosis.

► CASE 10

It is a hot summer day in the great Midwest. A 15-year-old boy is being treated with intravenous (IV) vancomycin at home for osteomyelitis of his distal tibia. During his initial hospitalization, his BUN was 15 mg/dL and his creatinine was 0.8 mg/dL. His vancomycin trough at discharge was 15 mcg/mL. He has missed his last two follow-up appointments but comes to clinic today. His blood pressure is 140/90 mm Hg, and he complains of a headache and generalized malaise. He has been taking ibuprofen multiple times per day for the past few weeks. On repeat laboratory testing, his creatinine is 2.5 mg/dL, BUN 35 mg/dL, and vancomycin level 60 mcg/mL.

Question 10-1
Which factor is likely contributing to his acute kidney injury?
A) Vancomycin toxicity.
B) Use of multiple nephrotoxic medications.
C) Dehydration.
D) Failure to receive proper clinical monitoring.
E) All of the above.

Discussion 10-1
The correct answer is "E." Drug nephrotoxicity is a common cause of acute kidney injury, especially in hospitalized pediatric patients. Risk of nephrotoxicity is increased with concurrent use of multiple nephrotoxic medications, dehydration, preexisting chronic kidney disease or acute kidney injury, long-term use of nephrotoxic medications, and inadequate laboratory and clinical monitoring for signs of toxicity.

Question 10-2
Which is NOT a potential nephrotoxic medication?
A) Acyclovir.
B) Diphenhydramine.
C) Amikacin.
D) Cyclosporine.
E) Indomethacin.

Discussion 10-2
The correct answer is "B." When using or administering nephrotoxic medications, take precautions to avoid hurting the kidneys. Maintain hydration. Monitor for toxicity (drug levels). Avoid use of multiple medications that may hurt the kidney. Minimize long-term use or substitute an alternative medication if possible. (See Table 31–2.)

► CASE 11

A 15-year-old previously healthy boy was hit hard in the back during a basketball game. Later that evening he noticed that his urine was bloody (red). His parents took him to the local emergency department, where he underwent a CT scan that showed many cysts in both kidneys.

Question 11-1
What is his likely diagnosis?
A) Autosomal recessive polycystic kidney disease.
B) Autosomal dominant polycystic kidney disease.
C) Multicystic dysplastic kidney.

Discussion 11-1
The correct answer is "B." (For explanation, see the discussion that follows Case 13 and Table 31–3.)

► CASE 12

A pregnant woman undergoes fetal ultrasound at 22 weeks' gestation. It shows an abnormal-appearing right kidney. The other kidney appears healthy. There is normal amniotic fluid, and no other apparent congenital abnormalities are noted.

Question 12-1
What is the likely diagnosis?
A) Autosomal recessive polycystic kidney disease.
B) Autosomal dominant polycystic kidney disease.
C) Multicystic dysplastic kidney.

Discussion 12-1
The correct answer is "C." (For explanation, see the discussion that follows Case 13 and Table 31–3.)

► CASE 13

An infant is born at 36 weeks' gestation. Oligohydramnios has been noted during the latter part of the pregnancy. Immediately after birth the infant has respiratory distress and requires intubation. In addition, his abdomen is noted to be markedly distended with bilateral palpable masses.

Question 13-1
What is the likely diagnosis?
A) Autosomal recessive polycystic kidney disease.
B) Autosomal dominant polycystic kidney disease.
C) Multicystic dysplastic kidney.

TABLE 31-2 NEPHROTOXIC MEDICATIONS USED IN PEDIATRIC PATIENTS

Medications by Class	Mechanism of Injury	Clinical and Laboratory Findings
Antimicrobials		
Acyclovir	Precipitation of crystals in renal tubules	Oliguria, serum creatinine rise, hyperkalemia
Aminoglycosides (eg, gentamicin, amikacin, tobramycin)	Proximal tubular toxicity	Serum creatinine rise, often no change in urine output (eg, nonoliguric acute kidney injury). Electrolyte, mineral wasting (eg, hypokalemia, hypomagnesemia)
Amphotericin B	Distal tubular toxicity, renal vasoconstriction	Distal renal tubular acidosis, hypokalemia, increased serum creatinine, impaired urine concentrating ability (polyuria)
Cidofovir	Proximal tubular toxicity	Electrolyte and mineral wasting
Cephalosporins Penicillins	May cause acute interstitial nephritis	Pyuria (urine eosinophils)
Vancomycin	Exact mechanism unclear	Elevated serum creatinine, elevated vancomycin level
Nonsteroidal anti-inflammatory drugs		
Ibuprofen Indomethacin Ketorolac Naproxen	Renal vasoconstriction and reduced GFR; may also see acute interstitial nephritis	Serum creatinine, potassium and BUN rise; decreased urine output
Angiotensin-converting enzyme (ACE) inhibitors and angiotensin receptor blockers (ARBs)		
ACE inhibitors (eg, captopril, enalapril, lisinopril) ARBs (eg, losartan)	Decreased renal perfusion	Serum creatinine and potassium rise, especially when used in dehydration or bilateral renal artery stenosis
Immunosuppressives		
Calcineurin inhibitors (eg, tacrolimus, cyclosporine)	Renal vasoconstriction; may trigger thrombotic microangiopathy, especially in bone marrow transplant patients	Oliguria, serum creatinine rise, hyperkalemia; if thrombotic microangiopathy develops, may see severe acute kidney injury; long-term use may result in fibrosis and progressive chronic kidney disease
Radiocontrast agents	Toxicity to the renal tubules related to reactive oxygen species	Serum creatinine rise, mild proteinuria

Discussion 13-1

The correct answer is "A." Kidney cysts may be found incidentally and be of no clinical consequence or may represent renal pathology. Although several names of cystic kidney diseases sound similar, the terms (eg, polycystic and multicystic) are *not* interchangeable and should be used accurately to refer to specific disease processes. Briefly, autosomal recessive polycystic kidney disease (ARPKD) affects the kidneys (bilateral) and liver. Hepatobiliary involvement includes congenital hepatitic fibrosis with portal hypertension and biliary duct dilation. Symptoms depend on the severity and age at presentation. Severe renal disease may cause pulmonary hypoplasia from oligohydramnios and present with respiratory distress in the newborn period. Older children may present with liver disease and signs of portal hypertension. Autosomal dominant polycystic kidney disease is bilateral and outside of a family history is often diagnosed incidentally on imaging. Multicystic dysplastic kidney (MCKD) is typically *unilateral*, and the affected kidney may shrink and disappear (involute). (See Table 31-3.)

▶ CASE 14

You attend an urgent cesarean section of a mother who presented with decreasing fetal movements and worsening oligohydramnios at 34-2/7 weeks' gestation. You are frantically trying to remember the neonatal resuscitation protocol when the infant is delivered and do not hear him cry. He is brought to the resuscitation table where, after stimulating and drying him off, you notice he has retractions but very shallow breaths. His heart rate is 90 bpm. You begin providing continuous positive airway pressure (CPAP) and he slowly improves. You

TABLE 31–3 CYSTIC KIDNEY DISEASES

Entity	Associated Findings	Clinical Significance and Other Considerations
Multicystic dysplastic kidney (MCDK) Unilateral (usually) kidney characterized by multiple cysts of different sizes and no functional or normally formed renal tissue (may contain nonrenal tissue such as cartilage)	• Often detected on fetal ultrasound or incidentally during imaging study for another purpose • Typically involutes over time (patients detected later in life with a "solitary kidney" may have had an MCDK that involuted)	• Usually asymptomatic. About one third of contralateral kidneys have an abnormality such as vesicoureteral reflux, so VCUG is a recommended part of early evaluation • Expect compensatory hypertrophy of contralateral kidney • Usually no associated extrarenal findings
Autosomal dominant polycystic kidney disease (ADPKD) Inherited form of renal cystic disease characterized by bilateral macrocysts Genes involved are *PKD1* (chromosome 16) and *PKD2* (chromosome 4)	• Diagnosis made by combination of ultrasound findings and positive family history • Children are often diagnosed incidentally through imaging studies done for another purpose • Cyst burden increases progressively over time • Progressive CKD and ESRD usually occur later in life (50s–60s) in about half of patients	• Clinical symptoms may include hypertension, pain from cyst enlargement or stretching of renal capsule, hemorrhage or infection in individual cysts, and proteinuria • Extrarenal manifestations include cysts in other organs (liver, pancreas, lungs, spleen), cardiac valve abnormalities, and cerebral aneurysms
Autosomal recessive polycystic kidney disease Inherited form of renal cystic disease characterized by microcysts and cystic dilation of collecting tubules Gene involved is *PKHD1* (chromosome 6)	• Diagnosis based on clinical findings • May manifest as an infant with massively enlarged and echogenic kidneys; kidneys grow rapidly during first days to months to first year of life • Varying degrees of pulmonary hypoplasia may be seen depending on severity of oligohydramnios and underlying kidney disease • Potter sequence (flattened facies, club feet, small chest wall, pulmonary hypoplasia) may be seen in most severe cases; other patients may have minimal lung disease and a more normal infant course • Some patients may have relatively silent kidney disease and present later in childhood with liver disease	• Associated with hepatic disease and fibrosis (Caroli disease—dilated intrahepatic bile ducts) • Hypertension is common and may be difficult to treat • May have rapid progression to ESRD and need for dialysis • Mortality in infancy often related to severity of pulmonary hypoplasia • Many patients progress to ESRD, though with variable timing (childhood to age 40–50 years) • May require liver transplant, although again course is variable between and even within families

CKD, chronic kidney disease; ESRD, end-stage renal disease; VCUG, voiding cystourethrogram.

---

breathe a sigh of relief now that his Apgar scores are improving. As you proceed with a detailed physical exam, you notice that he has a bilateral floppy abdominal wall and undescended testicles. He also has bilateral clubbed feet.

Question 14-1

You may find all of the following in detailed investigations EXCEPT:

A) Undescended testicles that are physiologic based on his prematurity.

B) Pulmonary hypoplasia that will require close monitoring.

C) Renal ultrasound that shows an enlarged bladder and dilated and tortuous ureters.

D) Dilated prostatic urethra on voiding cystourethrogram (VCUG), raising suspicion for posterior urethral valves.

E) Possible alterations in urine output, requiring close monitoring; you are not sure if he will make any urine, or make too much.

Discussion 14-1

The correct answer is "A." The findings of floppy abdominal wall and undescended testicles with oligohydramnios are suggestive

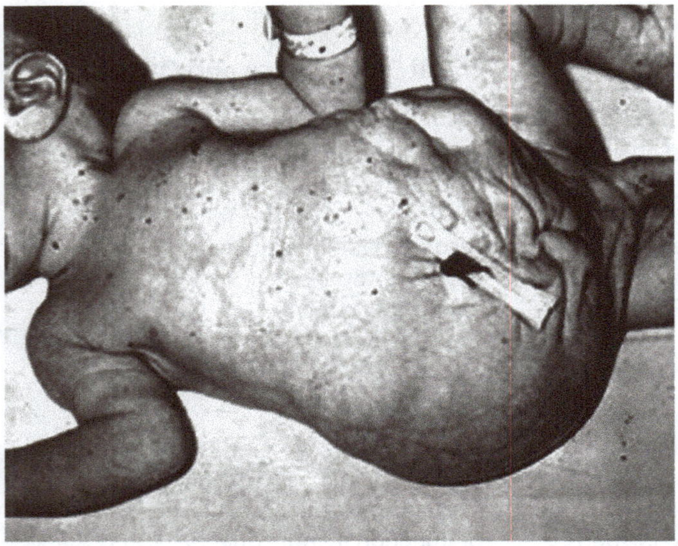

FIGURE 31–1. Prune belly syndrome. This male infant has prune belly (Eagle-Barrett) syndrome with floppy abdominal wall muscles. An abnormally formed urinary tract and bilateral cryptorchidism are also characteristic. (Reproduced with permission from Brunicardi FC, Andersen DK, Billiar TR, et al, eds. *Schwartz's Principles of Surgery*. 10th ed. New York, NY: McGraw-Hill Education; 2015, Fig. 39-34.)

of prune belly syndrome (PBS). (See Figure 31–1.) PBS primarily affects boys. It results from a mesenchymal defect in the neural crest during embryologic development, causing subsequent abnormal development of testes, abdominal muscle wall, and smooth muscle development of the urinary tract. Dilation of the urinary tract results in poor peristalsis and drainage. Renal ultrasound and VCUG are required in this newborn to determine the extent of hydroureteronephrosis and whether there is severe reflux. Because of prostatic hypoplasia, the prostatic urethra may appear dilated, but there is no membrane fold obstructing the urethra as in posterior urethral valves. As a result of this secondary obstructive nephropathy, little urine may be made initially. After an indwelling urinary catheter is placed, however, the infant may have a postobstructive diuresis and then make urine like there is no end. Careful monitoring is required! If oligohydramnios is present, neonates may have lung hypoplasia and respiratory distress after birth.

> **Helpful Tip**
> Prune belly (Eagle-Barrett) syndrome is characterized by floppy abdominal wall muscles, abnormally formed urinary tract, and bilateral cryptorchidism in boys.

▶ CASE 15

Young teenage parents bring their 2-month-old boy to the emergency department with a 2-day history of fever (Tmax 39.4°C [102.9°F]). He does not have any upper respiratory tract symptoms. He just received his 2-month immunizations last week. The parents state that he did not wake up for his usual overnight feed last night. This morning, he had emesis twice and has been inconsolable, crying nonstop for the past 3 hours. Vital signs are weight 5 kg, heart rate 165 bpm, respirations 40 breaths per minute, and blood pressure 89/40 mm Hg. He is fussy on your examination.

Question 15-1

Your infection workup will include the following EXCEPT:
A) Peripheral blood culture.
B) Midstream urine culture.
C) Urine bag culture.
D) Catheter urine culture.
E) Lumbar puncture for cerebrospinal fluid culture.

Discussion 15-1

The correct answer is "C." Since the infant is younger than 3 months of age, neonatal sepsis workup protocols should include peripheral blood to rule out bacteremia, clean urine culture specimen, and possible lumbar puncture (LP) to rule out meningitis (LP varies depending on the scenario). Of the three urine collection choices, urine bag is the least ideal. It carries the highest risk of skin and fecal contamination and therefore should be avoided. If you happen to catch a midstream urine for culture, congratulations! If not, we would recommend sticking with a sterile catheter urine specimen.

Question 15-2

What therapeutic management options should you provide for this infant while awaiting the results?
A) IV ceftriaxone and ampicillin for 48 hours, then switch to oral antibiotics.
B) IV ceftriaxone and ampicillin pending culture results.
C) Ibuprofen for fever and pain.
D) Acetaminophen for fever and pain.
E) Both A and C.
F) Both A and D.
G) Both B and C.
H) Both B and D.

Discussion 15-2

The correct answer is "H." Broad-spectrum antibiotics appropriate for infants younger than 3 months of age should be applied in this case, until culture results can identify the presence or absence of serious bacterial infection. The decision to switch to oral antibiotics should be guided by the specific infection and resolution of fever. In the setting of pyelonephritis, where there is a high likelihood of acute kidney injury, ibuprofen should be avoided as a generic analgesic/antipyretic in children, and ibuprofen is a no-no in infants younger than 6 months of age. Acetaminophen would be the better option as first-line therapy.

The nurses have a difficult time catheterizing the infant, but the urinalysis comes back within 24 hours showing 10×6 colony-forming units (CFUs) of *Escherichia coli*.

Question 15-3

What follow-up investigations would you like to pursue at this time?

A) Dimercaptosuccinic acid (DMSA).
B) Renal ultrasound.
C) VCUG.
D) Mercaptoacetyltriglycine (MAG3) renal scan with furosemide.
E) Options A, B, and C.
F) Both B and C.
G) Options B, C, and D.
H) Both C and D.

Discussion 15-3

The correct answer is "B." This is a male infant who presents with a first episode of pyelonephritis. There is no evident prenatal history to suggest preexisting urogenital anomalies. However, a renal ultrasound will help confirm the presence or absence of hydronephrosis, hydroureter, enlarged bladder, and other potential congenital anomalies of the kidney and urinary tract (CAKUT). VCUG diagnoses vesicoureteral reflux (VUR). According to the most recent American Academy of Pediatrics guidelines (2011), a VCUG is no longer routine after the first UTI or pyelonephritis. If the renal ultrasound is abnormal or this is a repeat infection, then a VCUG should be obtained. DMSA is a radiotracer imaging test used to identify cortical uptake in the kidneys. In the setting of acute pyelonephritis, there may be a region of hypoperfusion defect. However, this test has minimal utility in acute pyelonephritis. There is no evidence to suggest that acute hypoperfusion defect will result in chronic scarring. DMSA is most useful in the setting of chronic pyelonephritis, which is associated with renal scaring. MAG3 renal scan is generally used to compare the differential function of bilateral kidneys. It also aids in distinguishing tracer delay in excretion from the renal pelvis to help diagnose ureteropelvic junction obstruction.

For the same patient, renal ultrasound shows bilateral hydroureteronephrosis. You proceed to order a VCUG. The parents become very anxious about any further testing. They do not want the infant to go through another catheter procedure. He is feeling better now after antibiotics and they want to go home. You are the attending pediatrician and have to address the importance of all these tests. Recalling your nephrology rotation, you explain why it is important to diagnose urinary tract obstruction.

Question 15-4

You emphasize that:

A) VCUG is the definitive diagnostic test for posterior urethral valves (PUV).
B) Bladder anomalies such as ureterocele or ectopic ureter can cause obstruction at the ureterovesicular junction (UVJ).
C) Bilateral hydroureteronephrosis suggests that obstruction at the level of the ureteropelvic junction (UPJ) is unlikely.
D) Given the ultrasound findings, the pretest likelihood that the VCUG will confirm VUR just increased.
E) All of the above.

Discussion 15-4

The correct answer is "E." In the case of a male infant with pyelonephritis and bilateral hydroureteronephrosis, it is important to proceed further and identify urinary tract obstruction and VUR. Urinary obstruction can occur at multiple levels, including PUV, UVJ, and UPJ. In this case the latter is less likely because there is also dilation in the ureters and it is bilateral. VCUG is the definitive diagnosis for PUV, identifying a dilated prostatic urethra, with membranous folds that are causing obstruction. Having a positive renal ultrasound for anomalies in this case does increase the likelihood of diagnosing VUR. Obstructive nephropathy such as PUV is associated with chronic kidney disease and end-stage renal disease. Congenital anomalies of the kidney and urinary tract (CAKUT) make up of 40% of pediatric end-stage renal disease patients who require dialysis or transplantation. Do not miss this!

The infant has now been diagnosed with PUV and you follow him in your outpatient clinic. Following valve ablation, he has been eating and voiding well. You do not have to worry about him not drinking enough. His mother says he never refuses a bottle—unlike some of your other patients. He has been free of UTIs since he has been on antibiotic prophylaxis. He is now 1 year old. He comes to your office with a 1-day history of vomiting and diarrhea. There are other sick children at daycare. His mother is concerned because he seems very tired and his lips are dry. He continues to void clear urine. He has stopped vomiting now, so you ask the mother to give him Pedialyte for rehydration. In the meantime, you ordered some labs. The results are as follows: Na 157 mEq/L, K 5.0 mEq/L, Cl 117 mEq/L, CO_2 20 mEq/L, BUN 24 mg/dL, and creatinine 0.7 mg/dL. His CBC is normal. Urinalysis shows specific gravity of 1.005 and no pyuria, blood, or protein. You plan to admit him to the hospital for fluid management.

Question 15-5

The rationale for your fluid goals is that:

A) He has acute kidney injury secondary to dehydration and therefore can be managed with D_5 ½ NS at maintenance rate.
B) He has hypernatremia and hyperchloremia because of diarrheal water losses and will need D_5 ½ NS at 1.5 times the maintenance rate.
C) He has hypernatremia and hyperchloremia because of total water deficit from diarrhea losses and underlying urine concentrating defect. He will need D_5 ¼ NS at 1.5 times the maintenance rate.
D) He has total water deficit from his underlying urine concentrating defect with additional water loss from diarrhea. You do not have enough information right now to determine what IV fluid to prescribe.

Discussion 15-5

The correct answer is "D." Patients with obstructive nephropathy often have a distal collecting duct dysplasia, resulting in a urine concentrating defect. This infant has been self-regulating his net excess water loss in his urine by drinking all the time.

These children are water seekers, like others with nephrogenic diabetes insipidus. Notice that when he is hypernatremic and clinically volume depleted, his urine is still dilute. When intake decompensates at times of illness or preoperative fasting, access to free water is compromised and rapid hypernatremia can develop. In this case, acute diarrheal losses exacerbated the infant's free water deficit. You will need to be careful when correcting his hypernatremia (no more than 12 mEq in a 24-hour period); therefore, you should calculate his water deficit to aim for a sodium level of 145 mEq/L. You need his current dry weight to complete your fluid order. Do not forget to also factor in what you think he needs for maintenance fluids and ongoing insensible losses. (Maybe it's time to call the nephrology service for help with this mad math!)

> **Helpful Tip**
> Free water deficit (liters) = 0.6 × Weight (kg) × (Actual Na – Goal Na)/Goal Na.

> **Helpful Tip**
> One liter of D_5 0.45% sodium chloride gives you 500 mL of free water.

► CASE 16

A 5-year-old girl presents to your office with complaints of abdominal pain and foul-smelling urine. She does not have fever and is in no distress. Her mother states this is likely another episode of UTI. She had two other episodes last year for which she received antibiotics. The mother does not remember if urine cultures were obtained then. The mother also notes that her daughter has daytime accidents on most days of the week at kindergarten. She is also constipated. You decide to wait for the formal urinalysis and culture before prescribing antibiotics. Urinalysis shows specific gravity greater than 1.030, 50 WBCs/HPF, 5 RBCs/HPF, 1+ protein, and many bacteria.

Question 16-1
What investigations would you like to pursue at this time?
A) Renal ultrasound.
B) VCUG.
C) DMSA.
D) Both A and B.
E) Both A and C.
F) Both B and C.

Discussion 16-1
The correct answer is "A." In the setting of an otherwise well child who presents with childhood-onset recurrent UTIs, a thorough history should first be obtained to identify the risk factors associated with urinary tract infection. Congenital anomalies of the kidney and urinary tract (CAKUT) may be present, and therefore

a renal ultrasound is appropriate. However, having CAKUT associated with VUR is highly unlikely as this would most likely present in infancy. Unless the renal ultrasound suggests any abnormal findings, VCUG is generally not a first-line diagnostic test in this age group. Although this is her third episode of UTI, DMSA should be pursued only if she had any evidence of chronic kidney disease, such as elevated blood pressure, persistent hematuria or proteinuria, or elevated serum creatinine. She has clinical features suggestive of dysfunctional voiding, based on ongoing daytime enuresis and constipation. Counseling management of dysfunctional voiding includes increasing fluid intake, increasing frequency of voiding to every 2 to 3 hours during the day, double voiding, and eliminating constipation.

⧖ QUICK QUIZ

All of the following statements about signs and symptoms of UTI are true EXCEPT:
A) Abdominal pain may be a sign of a UTI in older children.
B) UTIs frequently present with diarrhea.
C) UTIs may present as enuresis.
D) UTIs may present as sepsis.
E) Newborns may present with jaundice as a sign of a UTI.

Discussion
The correct answer is "B." The presentation of UTI in pediatric patients varies by age. (See Figure 31–2.)

► CASE 17

A 4-year-old girl presents to your office with bright red blood in her urine. It is at the end of her urinary stream. She has some discomfort with voiding. She is not febrile. She recently had a runny nose and cough. She is well otherwise, is on no medications, and has no allergies. You remember that urine microscopy can be very helpful in such cases.

Question 17-1
What might you find?
A) RBC casts.
B) WBCs.
C) RBCs that are not dysmorphic.

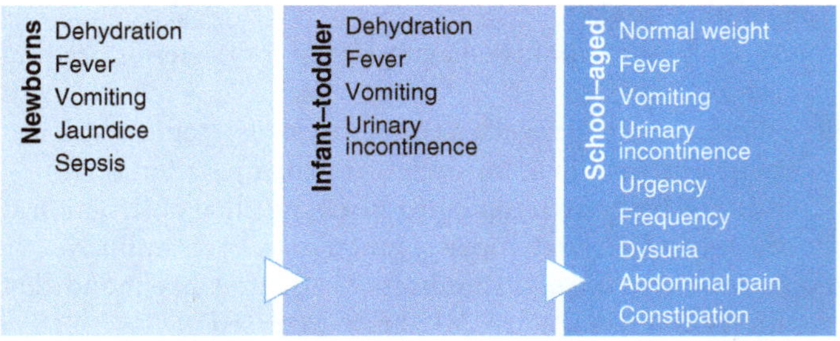

Newborns	Infant-toddler	School-aged
Dehydration	Dehydration	Normal weight
Fever	Fever	Fever
Vomiting	Vomiting	Vomiting
Jaundice	Urinary incontinence	Urinary incontinence
Sepsis		Urgency
		Frequency
		Dysuria
		Abdominal pain
		Constipation

FIGURE 31–2. Signs and symptoms of urinary tract infection by age group.

D) Eosinophils.
E) Both A and B.
F) Both B and C.
G) Both C and D.

Discussion 17-1

The correct answer is "F." This patient has dysuria, with bright red blood at the end of her urinary stream and a recent upper respiratory tract infection. Most likely a viral cystitis is contributing to her symptoms. Cystitis with a viral infection can be associated with a sterile pyuria. Nondysmorphic RBCs arise from lower urinary tract, as in cystitis. RBC casts are suggestive of glomerulonephritis, which does not present with terminal hematuria. Eosinophils in the urine would suggest an interstitial nephritis, most commonly secondary to medications.

▶ CASE 18

The midwife requests your consultation for a newborn girl who has a single umbilical artery. You find a term newborn establishing breastfeeding with normal voiding and stooling. However, physical examination shows a right preauricular tag and a slightly smaller right ear. She also has an asymmetric face, with normal palate and suck.

Question 18-1

You proceed with the following steps and explain to the mother that:
A) Her daughter has established a normal newborn routine and so can be discharged for follow up in your office.
B) Before discharge, the newborn will need a renal ultrasound and hearing screen because you suspect that these findings may be secondary to an oto-renal genetic syndrome.
C) The preauricular tag is cosmetic and not clinically significant.
D) There is no clinical significance to a two-vessel cord.

Discussion 18-1

The correct answer is "B." A two vessel-cord, especially with a single umbilical artery, historically was reportedly associated with increased findings of congenital anomalies. In recent studies, a single umbilical artery was most commonly associated with prematurity and being small for gestational age, and therefore remains a significant clinical finding. The incidence of identifying significant renal anomalies based on single umbilical artery is approximately 0.5%. However, this newborn also has a preauricular tag and an asymmetric facies. This combination of findings should trigger additional consideration of oto-renal syndromes and consequent evaluation of renal anomalies that are readily screened for.

▶ CASE 19

A 7-year-old boy with a history of myelomeningocele presents to the emergency department with a 2-day history of fever and worsening abdominal pain that is most noticeable

with catheterization of the appendicovesicostomy. He has a history of recurrent UTIs and was diagnosed with grade III bilateral VUR at age 2 years. He has flank tenderness, complains of headache, and has photosensitivity in the bright room. His mother notes that he appears to have sunken eyes. Vital signs are temperature 39.5°C (103.1°F), heart rate 125 bpm, respirations 35 breaths per minute, and blood pressure 143/90 mm Hg. Labs show WBCs 13 × 10³/µL, hemoglobin 9.5 g/dL, platelets 235 × 10³/µL. Na 146 mEq/L, K 5.4 mEq/L, Cl 108 mEq/L, CO_2 13 mEq/L, BUN 25 mg/dL, and creatinine 1.5 mg/dL. You notice his baseline creatinine from 6 months ago was 0.8 mg/dL. While collecting urine for culture 400 mL of urine was drained.

Question 19-1

What is the most likely explanation for this hypertensive emergency?
A) Acute abdominal pain that warrants surgical evaluation.
B) Acute kidney injury with intravascular volume overload.
C) Acute pyelonephritis with reflux nephropathy.
D) Pheochromocytoma.

Discussion 19-1

The correct answer is "C." Acute pain can be associated with elevated blood pressure readings but is not typically associated with signs of end organ involvement with headache and photosensitivity. Intravascular volume overload in the context of acute kidney injury with creatinine of 1.5 mg/dL is an appropriate consideration. However, the patient has sunken eyes and there is no evidence of oligoanuria. His longstanding history of VUR in the context of myelomeningocele and appendicovesicostomy is consistent with an underlying neurogenic bladder. Therefore, reflux nephropathy with acute pyelonephritis is the most likely explanation. Longstanding reflux nephropathy can lead to chronic kidney disease and end-stage renal disease. Pheochromocytoma can manifest as an acute hypertensive crisis. However, it is unlikely to present with acute rise in serum creatinine.

▶ CASE 20

A 9-year-old usually healthy boy is brought to his pediatrician because he has not been feeling well for the last week. This morning he started vomiting. He has not been voiding as often, and when he does his urine looks very dark. On further questioning, his mother reports that he was treated 2 weeks ago for a sore throat. He has had no diarrhea or bloody stools, nor has he had unusual rashes. On physical exam his blood pressure is 142/85 mm Hg (confirmed with manual reading). He is mildly tachypneic. His face looks more full than usual—his mother shows you a photo to help you see the difference. Urinalysis results are 3+ protein, 3+ blood, and RBC casts. Visible inspection shows the urine is brown. His serum creatinine is 0.9 mg/dL.

Question 20-1

What is the most likely diagnosis?
A) Childhood nephrotic syndrome.
B) Acute UTI.
C) Acute renal vein thrombosis.
D) Postinfectious glomerulonephritis.
E) Lupus nephritis.

Discussion 20-1

The correct answer is "D." The boy is hypertensive with a blood pressure value greater than the 95% for his age, height, and gender. The combination of hypertension, brown or dark red–colored urine, proteinuria, and hematuria with RBC casts screams glomerulonephritis. His recent strep throat infection strongly suggests this is postinfectious glomerulonephritis. Gross hematuria should not be present in nephrotic syndrome. An acute UTI may produce gross hematuria but not RBC casts, and you would expect dysuria, pyuria, and a positive leukocyte esterase test. Renal vein thrombosis may cause gross hematuria but not signs of glomerular injury (RBC casts), and he has no risk factors. Lupus nephritis is a real possibility but less likely in an otherwise healthy child with no family history of autoimmune disorders and a recent episode of pharyngitis.

> **Helpful Tip**
> Brown-, cola-, or tea-colored urine with hematuria, proteinuria, and RBC casts or fragments is seen with kidney inflammation (ie, glomerulonephritis). Urine with bright red blood and hematuria is more typical of lower urinary tract pathology (eg, UTI, kidney stone).

You have diagnosed the patient with glomerulonephritis and think it is postinfectious.

Question 20-2

What is the best next diagnostic test to help you narrow the differential?
A) Complement protein levels.
B) Urine culture.
C) Renal biopsy.
D) Renal ultrasound.
E) Antinuclear antibody.

Discussion 20-2

The correct answer is "A." *Glomerulonephritis* is a term that describes inflammation of the glomeruli. There are many different etiologies; it is your job to determine the underlying cause. This typically requires laboratory testing, imaging, and specialist consultation. Serum complement proteins, C3 and C4, help narrow the differential based on whether the values are low or normal. The other tests are reasonable and may be needed after you know the serum complement values. Typically in postinfectious glomerulonephritis, C3 is low and C4 is normal or mildly decreased. In lupus nephritis, C3 and C4 are both low (and often very low). *Poststreptococcal glomerulonephritis* is a sequela of

group A strep infection (of either throat or skin, such as impetigo) with a nephritogenic bacterial strain. Key findings include recent sore throat (or maybe just a nonspecific "illness" about 2 weeks before the onset of kidney findings), hypertension, mild edema, mild respiratory distress (may represent pulmonary edema), and brown urine, with both proteinuria and hematuria on urinalysis. Serum creatinine is likely elevated for age as well. Differential diagnosis includes other acute glomerulonephritides such as membranoproliferative glomerulonephritis and lupus nephritis (both associated with low serum complements), as well as normal complement glomerulonephritis such as IgA nephropathy, Alport syndrome, and sickle cell nephropathy. Workup includes urinalysis, urine microscopy, electrolytes, BUN, creatinine, albumin, C3, C4, ASO, and ANA. Complications of poststreptococcal glomerulonephritis may be serious and include hypertension (may be severe), pulmonary edema, heart failure, and acute kidney injury (may see rapidly progressive glomerulonephritis [RPGN]). Initial management includes blood pressure control using fluid and sodium restrictions, diuretics, and antihypertensive medications if needed. Serum creatinine, daily weights, and daily intake and output should be monitored closely. No additional treatment is needed unless the child appears to have an RPGN.

After 6 months the patient's serum C3 remains low. His urinalysis remains positive for both microscopic hematuria and 3+ proteinuria.

Question 20-3

What is the appropriate action at this point?
A) See the patient again in 6 months.
B) Tell the child to eat more salt as this will help to flush out the protein.
C) Restrict the child's physical activity as this is likely exercise-induced rhabdomyolysis.
D) Refer the child to a nephrologist for a kidney biopsy.

Discussion 20-3

The correct answer is "D." Serum C3 should normalize by 8 weeks. Proteinuria should resolve by 6 months. Hematuria may last for up to a year. Based on the persistent proteinuria and low C3 in this patient, a kidney biopsy is likely indicated as the risk of more severe glomerular disease that requires treatment with immunosuppression is high.

Question 20-4

What other diagnoses should be considered at this time?
A) Membranoproliferative glomerulonephritis.
B) Lupus nephritis.
C) Alport syndrome.
D) IgA nephropathy.
E) Both A and B.

Discussion 20-4

The correct answer is "E." Two other causes of hypocomplementemic (ie, low C3 and C4) acute glomerulonephritis are membranoproliferative glomerulonephritis and systemic lupus nephritis. Alport syndrome and IgA nephropathy are not characterized by low serum complement levels. If the patient was an adolescent Hispanic or African-American girl, then look hard for systemic findings such as rash, joint pains or arthritis, respiratory symptoms, and cytopenias that would be consistent with lupus nephritis. Look for low C3 *and* C4 and positive ANA test.

▶ CASE 21

Suppose instead of a sore throat this same 9-year-old boy developed a strange rash on his legs and arms just before he noticed that his urine was dark. He complains of belly cramps and refuses to eat. He also refuses to go to school because he does not feel good and his legs hurt. His mother is wondering whether he might have allergies because his eyes look puffy in the morning. On physical exam he appears uncomfortable. Blood pressure is 122/80 mm Hg. A purple rash appears all over his legs, arms, and buttocks. The spots, or varying sizes, do not blanch. You suspect Henoch-Schönlein purpura.

Question 21-1

Which clinical or laboratory finding would suggest more severe kidney involvement and worse prognosis?
A) Microscopic hematuria.
B) Pyuria.
C) Hypoalbuminemia.
D) Scrotal swelling.

Discussion 21-1

The correct answer is "C." Nephrotic range proteinuria with hypoalbuminemia is associated with a worse outcome. The renal manifestations of Henoch-Schönlein purpura (HSP) range from none, to microscopic hematuria, to gross hematuria with or without proteinuria, to nephrotic range proteinuria and rapidly progressive glomerulonephritis. The renal prognosis is more guarded when nephrotic range proteinuria is present. Kidney biopsy may be indicated. Scrotal pain and swelling are associated with HSP.

Instead of a rash, this same 9-year-old boy tells his mother that his poop looks red. She is alarmed because he appears very sick, and increasingly pale. He does not want to eat or drink. He says he has not needed to pee since yesterday. Three days ago he went apple picking at an orchard where they were serving unpasteurized cider.

Question 21-2

What is the most likely diagnosis now?
A) Alport syndrome.
B) Henoch-Schönlein purpura.
C) Poststreptococcal acute glomerulonephritis.
D) Hemolytic uremic syndrome.

Discussion 21-2

The correct answer is "D." The history of bloody diarrhea, dark urine, and ill appearance should raise concern for D+ (diarrhea) hemolytic uremic syndrome (HUS). This disease can be very serious, with potential for severe acute kidney injury (up to 50% of these children need dialysis—the "U" stands for *uremia*). If you are lucky, the history will suggest a potential exposure such as unpasteurized cider associated with *Escherichia coli* O157:H7 infection. Sometimes these patients come in crops (ie, outbreaks). Shiga toxin is the offending agent that causes endothelial cell damage and leads to shearing of red cells and platelets (*hemolysis*, the "H"—look for schistocytes on the blood smear) that gum up the small blood vessels in the kidneys and other organs. Hemolysis of the cells leads to anemia and thrombocytopenia. All these things together (as in *syndrome*, the "S")—the kidney injury and the hemolytic anemia and thrombocytopenia—give you the diagnosis of **h**emolytic **u**remic **s**yndrome (HUS).

Question 21-3

Which extrarenal manifestations should you watch for?
A) Pancreatitis.
B) Colitis.
C) Seizures.
D) Bowel necrosis.
E) All of the above.
F) None of the above.

Discussion 21-3

The correct answer is "E." HUS can be a horrible disease (even leading to death in some cases). All of these things are possible due to extensive microvascular thrombosis. Patients need very close monitoring and careful management of fluids and electrolytes. Hypertension may be seen in some patients long after they leave the hospital.

> **Helpful Tip**
> A rapidly rising serum creatinine in the context of acute glomerulonephritis symptoms is a renal emergency (likely rapidly progressive glomerulonephritis) and requires immediate nephrology evaluation, including kidney biopsy and pulse steroids.

▶ CASE 22

A 5-year-old boy comes for evaluation of eye swelling. Two weeks earlier he had a cold with runny nose, cough, and congestion. Swelling was first noticeable in his face and both eyes upon waking in the morning. By the end of the day the swelling would go away. Over the next several weeks the swelling progressed to involve his abdomen, extremities, and scrotum. He was treated with oral hydroxyzine 10 milligrams (mg) by mouth 3 times a day with no response. He gained 6 pounds in 9 days, and he was no longer needing to go to the bathroom as often. His urine is neither red nor brown. On exam, he has ascites with a positive fluid wave, an enlarged painless scrotum with palpable testes, and pitting edema over his

lumbosacral spine and shins. He has no rash, swollen joints, hepatosplenomegaly, or lymphadenopathy. He is tachycardic but his heart is regular without murmur or gallop. You suspect nephrotic syndrome.

Question 22-1

What is NOT a typical finding in nephrotic syndrome?
A) Urine protein-to-creatinine ratio greater than 1.
B) RBC casts on urine microscopic examination.
C) Serum albumin less than 3 g/dL.
D) Hyperlipidemia.
E) Normal C3 and C4.

Discussion 22-1

The correct answer is "B." Nephrotic syndrome is characterized by massive proteinuria, edema, and hypoalbuminemia. The most common kind of nephrotic syndrome in children is minimal change disease, which typically presents between the ages of 1 and 10 years (and usually before 6 years of age). Ask about preceding colds or viral illnesses. The swelling may come on slowly. The description of waking up with puffy eyes that improve as the day goes on (thanks to gravity pulling that fluid down to the feet) is classic. Periorbital edema is often mistaken for an allergy, and sometimes these children are treated for "allergies" for some time before someone checks a urinalysis (hence the hydroxyzine our patient was prescribed). Hematuria and RBC casts are characteristic of glomerulonephritis; however, you can see some mild microscopic hematuria with nephrotic syndrome. Low serum complement levels are not associated with nephrotic syndrome. First-line treatment of nephrotic syndrome is steroids as well as fluid and salt restrictions to prevent worsening of the edema.

Question 22-2

Which of the following are potential complications of nephrotic syndrome?
A) Acute kidney injury.
B) Spontaneous bacterial peritonitis.
C) Blood clots and strokes.
D) Stretch marks.
E) All of the above.

Discussion 22-2

The correct answer is "E." All of the listed options are potential complications of nephrotic syndrome. Acute kidney injury can occur because of intravascular volume depletion related to the low oncotic pressure (even though the patient has gallons of extra water onboard!). These patients are at high risk for developing spontaneous bacterial peritonitis when they have severe ascites and have lost all their immunologic proteins (IgG) in their urine. They are also in a hypercoagulable state because of urinary losses of antithrombin III and protein S. The intravascular volume depletion only makes this worse. Diuresis needs to be done *very* carefully as rapid fluid removal puts the patient at great risk for clotting (including sinus venous thromboses). Unfortunately some of our patients have frequent relapses and episodes of anasarca, leading to stretch marks over time.

▶ CASE 23

A 15-year-old girl is admitted to the pediatric intensive care unit with fever and hypotension. Her skin is red as if sunburnt. Her blood pressure is 75/50 mm Hg. She has been vomiting and had diarrhea this morning. She has not peed for about 6 hours. On exam, she is tachycardic with brisk capillary refill. Her skin is diffusely red and her eyes are injected. There is no hepatosplenomegaly. Her BUN is 29 mg/dL and creatinine is 1.9 mg/dL. Her urinalysis has a specific gravity greater than 1.030. She received fluid resuscitation, requiring multiple normal saline boluses, and has been started on a vasopressor continuous infusion. You suspect toxic shock syndrome with acute kidney injury.

Question 23-1

How would you classify her acute kidney injury?
A) Stage 1.
B) Stage 2.
C) Stage 3.
D) Stage 4.

Discussion 23-1

The correct answer is "B." Acute kidney injury (AKI) is an abrupt decrease in GFR and renal function that is reversible in the majority of cases. It is highly prevalent in the pediatric population, occurring in one of three hospital admissions for children. AKI is an independent risk factor for intensive care unit admissions with prolonged length of stay and ventilation days, and increased mortality. AKI can be oliguric or nonoliguric, and the presence of urine output does not exclude the presence of AKI. There are also only three stages of acute kidney injury. Standardized definitions of AKI are based on changes in serum creatinine and presence of oliguria. This patient's creatinine is elevated approximately two times her expected baseline, and she has been oliguric for not more than 12 hours, which fits the criteria for stage 2 AKI. (See Table 31–4.)

TABLE 31–4 ACUTE KIDNEY INJURY CRITERIA

	Serum Creatinine	Urine Output
Stage 1	1.5× increase of baseline SCr or > 0.3 mg/dL	< 0.5 mL/kg/h × 6 h
Stage 2	2.0× increase of baseline SCr	< 0.5 mL/kg/h × 12 h
Stage 3	3.0× increase of baseline SCr or require renal replacement therapy	< 0.3 mL/kg/h × 24 h or anuric × 12 h

SCr, serum creatinine.

TABLE 31–5 COMMON ETIOLOGIES OF ACUTE KIDNEY INJURY

- Decreased effective circulating volume with decreased renal perfusion: dehydration, poor cardiac output, hepatorenal syndrome, capillary leak, active nephrotic syndrome
- Nephrotoxins: NSAIDs (ibuprofen, naproxen, ketorolac, indomethacin), vancomycin, gentamicin, acyclovir, cidofovir, or diuretic use
- Hypoxic ischemic encephalopathy
- Acute tubular necrosis
- Tumor lysis syndrome
- Acute tubulointerstitial nephritis
- Acute glomerulonephritis
- Obstruction
- Vascular thrombosis (umbilical vein and artery catheterization)

NSAIDs, nonsteroidal anti-inflammatory drugs.

Question 23-2

What is the etiology of her AKI?
A) Nephrotoxic medication.
B) Renal vein thrombosis.
C) Hypoperfusion.
D) Acute glomerulonephritis.

Discussion 23-2

The correct answer is "C." Her AKI has resulted from hypoperfusion due to decompensated toxic shock syndrome. Initial diagnostic tests for AKI should include electrolytes, BUN, creatinine, and urinalysis. (See Table 31–5.)

> **Helpful Tip**
> The urinalysis can help identify the cause of AKI. On microscopic exam, look for abnormal urine sediments.
> - Granular casts: acute tubular necrosis, vasculitis, glomerulonephritis
> - RBC casts: vasculitis, glomerulonephritis
> - WBC casts: pyelonephritis, interstitial nephritis, vasculitis, glomerulonephritis
> - Eosinophils: interstitial nephritis (most labs require a specific request for this)
> - Hyaline casts: proteinuria

You suspect the etiology of her AKI is prerenal but you want to be sure you are not missing intrinsic kidney disease, such as acute tubular necrosis (ATN).

Question 23-3

Which finding will help confirm a prerenal etiology?
A) Fractional excretion of sodium greater than 1%.
B) Urinalysis specific gravity 1.005.
C) Urine osmolarity less than 350 mOsm/kg.
D) Fractional excretion of sodium less than 1%.

TABLE 31–6 INVESTIGATIONS TO DISTINGUISH PRERENAL AZOTEMIA FROM ATN

1. Fractional excretion of sodium (FENa):

$$FENa = \frac{UNa \times PCr}{PNa \times UCr} \times 100\%$$

FENa: Child	FENa: Infant	Interpretation
< 1%	< 3%	Prerenal azotemia
1–2%	2–3%	Indeterminate
> 2%	> 3%	ATN

- FENa is used when the creatinine is abnormal.
- FENa is difficult to interpret after diuretic use and aggressive fluid resuscitation

2. Urine osmolarity:
- Elevated > 500 mOsm/kg suggests preserved urine concentrating ability, typical of prerenal azotemia.
- Decreased < 350 mOsm/kg suggests improper urine concentrating ability, typical of ATN.

3. Urine specific gravity:
- Elevated > 1.020 suggests prerenal azotemia.
- Decreased < 1.010 suggests ATN.

4. BUN-to-creatinine ratio (less reliable):
- Elevated BUN/creatinine ratio > 20 = prerenal azotemia.
- Normal BUN/creatinine ratio 10–15 = ATN.

ATN, acute tubular necrosis; BUN, blood urea nitrogen; PCr, plasma creatinine; PNa, plasma sodium; UCr, urine creatinine; UNa, urine sodium.

Discussion 23-3

The correct answer is "D." AKI can be prerenal (poor perfusion), intrinsic (ATN), or postrenal (urinary tract obstruction) in etiology. Prerenal injury indicates inadequate perfusion of the kidney. Etiologies include decreased intravascular volume (dehydration, diuretics, hemorrhage), peripheral vasodilation (sepsis), and inadequate perfusion (heart failure). ATN is due to intrinsic kidney injury. Etiologies include prolonged prerenal state, ischemia, nephrotoxic medications, rhabdomyolysis, and contrast dye. Urine concentrating ability is the key distinguishing feature. In ATN, concentrating ability is lost. Table 31–6 summarizes key tests and findings used in differentiating prerenal azotemia from ATN.

> **Helpful Tip**
> When distinguishing prerenal AKI from ATN (intrinsic kidney injury), think about concentrating ability. If the injury is prerenal (hypoperfusion), the kidney wants to hold onto fluid (FENa is low, urine is concentrated). In ATN, the kidney is damaged and cannot concentrate the urine (FENa is high).

▶ CASE 24

A 6-year-old girl presents to your inpatient service for further evaluation. She has had fatigue, fever, and poor oral intake for the past week. She received two doses of ibuprofen each of the last 3 days for fever. Vital signs on admission are temperature 38.5°C (101.3°F), heart rate 136 bpm, respirations 25 breaths per minute, and blood pressure 85/51 mm Hg. Lab results include:

- CBC, glucose, C-reactive protein (CRP) normal
- Sodium (Na) 148 mEq/L
- Potassium (K) 3.6 mEq/L
- Chloride (Cl) 108 mEq/L
- CO_2 29 mEq/L
- BUN 25 mg/dL
- Creatinine 0.7 mg/dL
- Phosphorus 3.8 mg/dL
- Calcium (Ca) 8.2 mg/dL

Following administration of a 10 mL/kg normal saline (NS) bolus, and 6 hours of D_5 ½ NS maintenance IV fluids, the medical student reports to you that the patient's urine output has been 0.5 mL/kg/h since admission. Repeat vital signs show heart rate 120 bpm, respirations 25 breaths per minute, and blood pressure 90/56 mm Hg.

Question 24-1

What is NOT an appropriate next step in your management?
A) Obtain a urinalysis.
B) Measure fractional excretion of sodium.
C) Give IV furosemide.
D) Order a renal ultrasound.
E) Give a second 10 mL/kg NS bolus.

Discussion 24-1

The correct answer is "C." This patient has a multifactorial AKI presenting with oliguria, as diagnosed with urine output less than 0.5 mL/kg/h for 6 hours, along with elevated creatinine at 0.7 mg/dL. There is a strong history of prerenal dehydration prior to hospital admission, given her persistent fever and poor oral intake for the past week. She also received ibuprofen, which in the setting of dehydration could contribute to nephrotoxic AKI. Obtaining a urinalysis is helpful in many ways. Urine specific gravity greater than 1.020 would suggest intravascular depletion. Hematuria and proteinuria may identify an active glomerular disease. Fractional excretion of sodium (FENa) less than 1% can also confirm intravascular depletion. Giving IV furosemide will likely increase her urine output. However, when she is persistently tachycardic with borderline hypotension, this medication may worsen her AKI. Ordering a renal ultrasound can identify bilateral echogenic kidneys in the setting of AKI and potentially rule out any ureteric obstruction (postrenal injury).

▶ CASE 25

You are staffing the day shift in the emergency department when a 5-year-old boy presents with worsening radiating abdominal pain rated as 8/10, associated with an episode of gross hematuria yesterday evening at around suppertime. His mother states that he has not voided since. He now has persistent emesis. IV morphine was given, providing some relief. Vital signs are temperature 36.4°C (97.5°F), heart rate 125 bpm, respirations 30 breaths per minute, and blood pressure 110/70 mm Hg. He lies still in bed and identifies right-sided flank pain. Lab results are as follows: hemoglobin 10.2 g/dL, WBCs $3.0 \times 10^3/\mu L$, platelets $210 \times 10^3/\mu L$, INR 1.1, PT 11 sec, PTT 29 sec, Na 140 mEq/L, K 4.0 mEq/L, Cl 109 mEq/L, CO_2 24 mEq/L, BUN 20 mg/dL, creatinine 0.8 mg/dL, and CRP less than 0.5 mg/dL.

Question 25-1

Investigations and management should NOT include which of the following?
A) IV NS bolus × 10 mL/kg.
B) IV ceftriaxone.
C) Abdominal X-ray.
D) Renal ultrasound.
E) Obtain urinalysis.

Discussion 25-1

The correct answer is "B." This patient most likely has an obstructive kidney stone presenting with oliguric AKI, as evidenced by oliguria and elevated creatinine of 0.8. There are no clinical signs suggestive of an infective process; therefore, IV antibiotic use is not warranted at this time. He may be clinically dehydrated as indicated by his history, and a fluid bolus challenge given his tachycardia is appropriate. Abdominal X-ray (flat plate) and renal ultrasound are both useful studies that can identify radiopaque kidney stones and evidence of obstruction by examining for hydronephrosis and or hydroureter. Urinalysis is helpful to look for persistent hematuria, or to collect for a kidney stone analysis.

▶ CASE 26

A 3-year-old girl who was previously healthy presents with a history of fever and cough for the past week. Over the past 24 hours, she has had worsening respiratory distress and fatigue. She has only voided once in the past day. On examination, vital signs show temperature 36.5°C (97.7°F), heart rate 130 bpm, respirations 35 breaths per minute, SaO_2 88% on room air, and blood pressure 118/71 mm Hg. Lab results are Na 135 mEq/L, K 4.9 mEq/L, Cl 108 mEq/L, CO_2 20 mEq/L, BUN 25 mg/dL, and creatinine 0.9 mg/dL. She has mild facial edema, is tachypneic with shallow breaths, has soft diffuse crackles on auscultation and a systolic murmur grade II/VI over left sternal border, but is otherwise warm and well perfused. She has mild abdominal distension that is nontender. There is no pitting edema to extremities.

Question 26-1

What is an appropriate management option to consider?
A) IV NS bolus × 10 mL/kg.
B) IV furosemide.
C) IV maintenance fluids D_5 ½ NS + 20 mEq/L KCl.
D) IV maintenance fluids D_5 NS.
E) IV hydralazine.

Discussion 26-1

The correct answer is "B." This patient is presenting with oliguric AKI and a preceding history of an upper respiratory illness within the past 7 to 10 days, suggestive of postinfectious glomerulonephritis. She is fluid overloaded as evidenced by tachycardia, cardiac murmur, elevated blood pressure, pulmonary edema (tachypnea, hypoxia, crackles on auscultation), and facial edema. This is in the setting of abnormal creatinine and BUN. IV furosemide is the drug of choice to stimulate natriuresis and diuresis, which can alleviate her current fluid overload status. Although she is oliguric, providing a normal saline bolus at this time may worsen her fluid overload status, with the potential complication of precipitating or worsening acute congestive heart failure and pulmonary edema. IV maintenance fluids at this time, with or without potassium, would also be inappropriate fluid management given her oliguric state. Potassium should never be included in IV fluids in a patient with an evolving AKI. IV hydralazine would be effective as an acute antihypertensive medication, acting as a vasodilator. However, it would not be a preferred agent over IV furosemide.

> **Helpful Tip**
> Learn the verbiage. Acute kidney injury (AKI) is the en vogue term replacing acute renal failure (ARF).

► CASE 27

You are seeing a 13-year-old adolescent boy who was admitted to the local community hospital for chronic fatigue and significant iron deficiency anemia with hemoglobin of 5.8 g/dL. The history reveals that he has had no recent illnesses, fever, or travel history. He has decreased appetite and nausea without abdominal pain. He is fatigued after sleeping 10 hours at night, and has trouble staying awake at school. He wakes to void several times at night. He complains of generalized weakness, having withdrawn from his soccer team this past month. Growth parameters are significant for weight at the 10th percentile and height at the 50th percentile. Vital signs are temperature 36.7°C, heart rate 100 bpm, respirations 24 breaths per minute, and blood pressure 137/82 mm Hg. Upon admission, lab results are Na 135 mEq/L, K 5.2 mEq/L, Cl 101 mEq/L,

CO_2 16 mEq/L, glucose 102 mg/dL, albumin 3.2 g/dL, calcium 6.8 mg/dL, phosphate 8.2 mg/dL, BUN 85 mg/dL, and creatinine 5.2 mg/dL. Urinalysis is negative for blood, but positive for 1+ protein. You recognize that this patient has renal failure and consider the next steps in his treatment.

Question 27-1

Which of the following should NOT be part of your management plans for him?
A) Renal ultrasound.
B) IV maintenance fluids D_5 ½ NS.
C) IV calcium chloride to correct for hypocalcemia.
D) Low-phosphate and low-potassium diet.
E) Pediatric nephrology consult at a tertiary care hospital for transfer of care to determine modality of renal replacement therapy.

Discussion 27-1

The correct answer is "C." Hypocalcemia in the setting of end-stage renal disease (ESRD) is most commonly associated with hyperphosphatemia and vitamin D deficiency. Control of hyperphosphatemia will generally normalize hypocalcemia by use of phosphate binders, low-phosphate diet, renal replacement therapy (dialysis), or a combination of these. Unless there is symptomatic hypocalcemia, acute calcium repletion is not warranted. Renal ultrasound will be instrumental in diagnosing the etiology of his renal failure. In this setting with a well-grown adolescent, chronic kidney disease (CKD) with a history of polyuria and bland urine may be consistent with a diagnosis of juvenile nephronophthisis, with typical features of normal but diffusely echogenic kidneys. The choice of maintenance IV fluids without potassium is optimal given mild to moderate hyperkalemia, and he is not oliguric with signs of hypervolemia. Similarly, a low-phosphate diet and potassium dietary restrictions would be optimal until renal replacement therapy is provided. As the patient is clinically stable with signs of ESRD, consulting pediatric nephrology and transferring him to begin renal replacement therapy is appropriate.

Question 27-2

Regarding CKD, which of the following is false?
A) CKD has five stages.
B) Most CKD in infants is acquired.
C) Congenital anomalies are a common cause of CKD.
D) Staging of CKD is based on GFR.
E) GFR is reduced starting at stage 2.

Discussion 27-2

The correct answer is "B." CKD is staged 1 through 5 based on GFR. CKD stage 5 is the same as ESRD. Children with CKD stage 5 typically require transplant or dialysis. (See Table 31–7.) Congenital anomalies of the kidney and urinary tract (CAKUT) make up about 40% of all pediatric ESRD. CAKUT is also the most common cause of CKD in children and infants younger than age 10 years. After age 10, most cases of CKD are acquired (eg, glomerulonephritis).

TABLE 31–7 STAGES OF CHRONIC KIDNEY DISEASE

Stage	Glomerular Filtration Rate (GFR) (mL/min/1.73 m²)
1	> 90 (normal)
2	60–89
3	30–59
4	15–29
5	< 15 or dialysis

Question 27-3

Which is NOT a laboratory finding of oliguric AKI or CKD, or both?

A) Hyperkalemia.
B) Hypocalcemia.
C) Hypophosphatemia.
D) Azotemia.
E) Metabolic acidosis.

Discussion 27-3

The correct answer is "C." AKI and CKD presenting with oliguria are generally associated with hyperphosphatemia. Additional findings include elevated creatinine, anemia, low vitamin D level and elevated parathyroid hormone. Hypophosphatemia may occur in cases of CKD with high urine output failure. This is common in CKD due to CAKUT.

> **Helpful Tip**
>
> CKD in children can be *oliguric* or *nonoliguric* (high urine output). Those with an obstructive nephropathy (ie, posterior urethral valves or reflux nephropathy) are typically polyuric and consequently may also have hypokalemia and hypophosphatemia even though they have severe renal failure. In contrast, oliguric renal failure is typical of the glomerulonephritides (ie, hemolytic uremic syndrome, postinfectious glomerulonephritis).

The same patient has been started on peritoneal dialysis, and you are now his primary pediatrician. You review his medical records and learn that his immunizations are incomplete. His most recent vaccines were received at 18 months of age.

Question 27-4

Recognizing that he is now on dialysis and would most likely move forward for kidney transplantation at some point, which is the vaccine that you would like him to catch up on as soon as possible?

A) Diphtheria, tetanus, and acellular pertussis (DTaP).
B) Hepatitis B.
C) Meningococcal.
D) Human papillomavirus (HPV).
E) Measles, mumps, and rubella (MMR).

Discussion 27-4

The correct answer is "E." Due to the lapse of prekindergarten vaccination schedules, he would have missed the second dose of MMR vaccine. This is extremely important for pretransplantation candidates, as he will remain on chronic immunosuppression and will not be able to receive any live vaccines thereafter. He may be incomplete in the DTaP series; however, this vaccine may be received at any point. He should have received the full hepatitis B series by 18 months. HPV vaccine is not a live viral vaccine and does not have the absolute contraindication as does MMR.

⧗ QUICK QUIZ

What is NOT a goal of chronic renal replacement therapy (dialysis)?

A) Correct hyperparathyroidism.
B) Prevent kidney transplantation.
C) Maintain fluid status with fluid restriction.
D) Normalize electrolytes.
E) Treat hypertension.

Discussion

The correct answer is "B." Chronic renal replacement therapy or dialysis is utilized as a bridge towards kidney transplantation in pediatrics. The overall CKD status is generally optimized during the dialysis period. This generally includes normalization of electrolytes and acid-base derangements, control of anemia, control of hypertension, correction or stabilization of secondary hyperparathyroidism in metabolic bone disease, establishment of good nutrition with appropriate growth and development of the child, and determination of psychosocial readiness to receive a kidney transplant, which will require lifelong immunosuppressive treatment.

▶ CASE 28

A 5-year-old girl is on chronic dialysis from *Escherichia coli* shiga toxin–positive hemolytic uremic syndrome (HUS)–induced ESRD. She is doing well on dialysis and is awaiting transplant. You discuss transplant options with the family; specifically, living versus deceased donor transplants.

Question 28-1

Which of the following regarding living donor transplantation is false?

A) Increased long-term survival.
B) Lower risk of delayed graft function.
C) Health of donor cannot be guaranteed.
D) More control over planning time of transplant.
E) May avoid need for a dialysis "bridge."

Discussion 28-1

The correct answer is "C." Transplant is the best choice for pediatric patients with ESRD (CKD stage 5). Overall, living donor

TABLE 31–8 DECEASED VERSUS LIVING DONOR KIDNEY TRANSPLANT

	Living	Deceased
Ischemia time	Shorter	Longer
Immediate function	Better	May result in delayed graft function
Delayed graft function	Lower risk	Higher risk
Donor health	Thorough assessments of donors ensure excellent health and renal function	Donors may have suboptimal health
HLA mismatches	Better ability to find a donor with few or zero HLA mismatches if donor is related	Increased risk of HLA mismatches
Long-term survival	Better	Variables listed above can decrease overall graft survival
Planning	Can identify an appropriate time that is most compatible with school and work schedules	Uncertainty; can be on waiting list for many years
Dialysis needs	There is a movement toward more preemptive transplantation if renal progression is slow; therefore, child may not need bridging period with dialysis	Child will most likely be on dialysis while waiting on deceased donor list
Preference	First choice for pediatrics	—

transplants are superior to deceased donor transplants. (See Table 31–8.)

The parents ask what they can do to make sure the transplant is successful. They want to be proactive.

Question 28-2

What do you tell them about measures that increase long-term transplant survival?

A) Be sure child always takes the prescribed immunosuppression medications.

B) Prevent urinary tract infections.

C) Attend follow-up visits.

D) Seek immediate medical care for fever.

E) All of the above.

Discussion 28-2

The correct answer is "E." Survival, growth, and quality of life are better with transplant than dialysis so it is important to take care of the graft. Preventing acute and chronic rejection of the donor kidney is very important. Some factors that affect transplant survival are within the patient's control, but many are not. (See Table 31–9.)

Your 5-year-old patient received a living donor transplant and has been thriving in the years since. Now a 15-year-old adolescent, she presents to your office with fever and acute abdominal pain. She complains of dysuria, has had decreased intake for the past 2 days, and last voided 6 hours ago. She has no diarrhea or vomiting. She was on a band trip this past week and may have missed a few doses of her immunosuppressive medications. On focused abdominal physical exam, there is no guarding or rebound tenderness. However, there is focal tenderness on deep palpation over her transplant graft. Lab results show the following: Na 138 mEq/L, K 5.9 mEq/L, Cl 109 mEq/L, CO_2 15 mEq/L, BUN 53 mg/dL, and creatinine 2.1 mg/dL (her baseline creatinine is between 1.3 and 1.5 mg/dL). Trough tacrolimus level is pending.

TABLE 31–9 FACTORS THAT AFFECT LONG-TERM SURVIVAL IN TRANSPLANT PATIENTS

- Acute rejection (cellular and antibody mediated)
- Chronic rejection (cellular and antibody mediated)
- Poor adherence to immunosuppression
- Recurrent urinary tract infections
- Ongoing obstructive uropathy especially in congenital neurogenic bladder (eg, posterior urethral valves)
- Recurrence of primary disease
  - Immune mediated (membranoproliferative glomerulonephritis [MPGN], focal segmental glomerulosclerosis [FSGS], IgA nephropathy, membranous nephropathy)
  - Vasculitis (systemic lupus erythematosus, Henoch-Schönlein purpura, granulomatosis with polyangiitis, microscopic polyangiitis)
  - Atypical hemolytic uremic syndrome (complement dysregulation)
  - Sickle cell nephropathy
  - Anti–glomerular basement membrane (Anti-GBM) disease
  - Metabolic disorder with persistent abnormality of a substance (eg, primary hyperoxaluria)
  - Recurrent episodes of acute kidney injury
  - Other health comorbidities (hypertension, diabetes, hyperlipidemia, obesity)

Question 28-3

Your differential diagnosis of this acute kidney injury includes all of the following EXCEPT:

A) Dehydration, which will require provision of IV fluid bolus.
B) Pyelonephritis, which will require urine culture and start of IV antibiotics.
C) Acute transplant rejection, which will require a transplant graft biopsy.
D) Urinary obstruction, which will require ultrasound of transplant graft.
E) Recurrence of primary disease, which will require a transplant graft biopsy.

Discussion 28-3

The correct answer is "E." There always needs to be a broad differential diagnosis for acute kidney injury of the transplanted kidney. In this case there is sufficient history of decreased oral intake to suspect that intravascular repletion is warranted. The patient has fever and complaints of dysuria that warrant workup and IV antibiotic therapy until proven otherwise. Given her report of missed doses of immunosuppressive therapy and exam findings of transplant graft tenderness with fever, acute transplant rejection should remain high on the differential. The gold standard diagnosis for transplant rejection is a renal biopsy. Urinary obstruction also warrants investigation as she is developing oliguria. A renal ultrasound should be ordered to identify any hydronephrosis or hydroureter to suggest an acute obstructive process. Disease recurrence should be considered in most patients who have undergone kidney transplant; therefore, understanding the underlying primary disease is important. However, *E. coli* shiga toxin–positive HUS does not recur whereas atypical (non–diarrhea-associated) HUS can recur.

► CASE 29

The medical student who started this chapter has decided that the kidney is quite interesting though complex. He is given a learning assignment about hypertension in children and adolescents. His presentation is going well, and he starts to discuss risk factors.

Question 29-1

Which statement describes a risk factor for hypertension?

A) Having a Y chromosome.
B) Fast food addiction.
C) Video game fanatic.
D) "He's just 'husky'."
E) All of the above.

Discussion 29-1

The correct answer is "E." Hypertension is a major long-term health condition and a leading cause of premature death among adults. Owing to its hereditary nature, primary hypertension is detectable in children and adolescents. The estimated prevalence

in children aged 3 to 18 years is 3% to 5%. Risk factors such as age, male gender, obesity, physical activity, and dietary salt intake are major contributors to the risk of hypertension.

> **Helpful Tip**
> Childhood obesity is associated with higher rates of hypertension. The likelihood of being diagnosed with prehypertension is two times greater and hypertension is four times greater in overweight adolescents than in those of normal weight.

The student is pleased to see that you, the attending, are still awake. He nervously smiles at you. You give him the thumbs up and say to forge ahead. His next PowerPoint slide defines a normal blood pressure for "kids" as systolic blood pressure of 120 mm Hg or lower and diastolic blood pressure 80 mm Hg or lower.

Question 29-2

On his evaluation, you will be sure to note that:

A) Blood pressure 75% or greater is the magical number to define hypertension.
B) Blood pressure in pediatric patients must account for age.
C) Blood pressure in pediatric patients must account for sex.
D) Blood pressure in pediatric patients must account for height.
E) Options B, C, and D.

Discussion 29-2

The correct answer is "E." Diagnosis of hypertension in a child or adolescent requires three separate visits for blood pressure measurements, with an average blood pressure at or above the 95th percentile for age, sex, and height. Hypertension can be diagnosed in a single visit if the child has symptomatic hypertension (headache, nausea, blurry vision, shortness of breath) or has stage 2 hypertension (blood pressure > 99%). (See Figure 31–3.)

Your blood pressure is rising thinking about the audacity of defining hypertension as a single value. You will need to make an educational handout. Your mind starts to wander as you sip your third cup of coffee. You cannot remember if you have peed today.

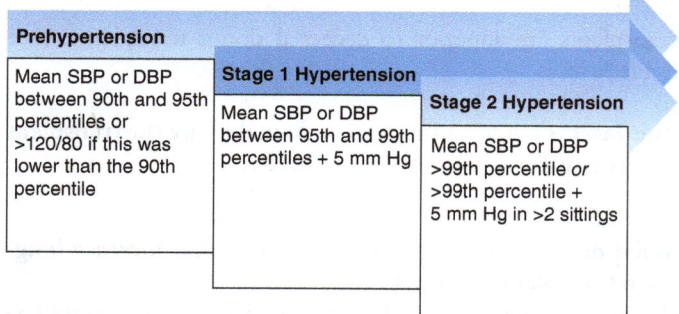

Prehypertension	Stage 1 Hypertension	Stage 2 Hypertension
Mean SBP or DBP between 90th and 95th percentiles or >120/80 if this was lower than the 90th percentile	Mean SBP or DBP between 95th and 99th percentiles + 5 mm Hg	Mean SBP or DBP >99th percentile or >99th percentile + 5 mm Hg in >2 sittings

FIGURE 31–3. Classification of hypertension in children and adolescents. DBP, diastolic blood pressure; SBP, systolic blood pressure.

Question 29-3

Which is true regarding your hormones currently?

A) Renin is elevated.
B) Angiotensin I is low.
C) Aldosterone is low.
D) Angiotensin II is low.
E) Both A and C.

Discussion 29-3

The correct answer is "A." You are dehydrated from excess caffeine ingestion. The renin-angiotensin system is the major hormonal system that affects blood pressure regulation. Renin is produced in the juxtaglomerular cells of the afferent renal arteriole and is stimulated by decreased glomerular perfusion, reduced sodium intake, or activity of the sympathetic nervous system. Renin cleaves angiotensinogen to form angiotensin I. Angiotensin-converting enzyme in the lungs converts angiotensin I to angiotensin II (major active component). Angiotensin II is a potent vasoconstrictor and increases blood pressure. It also stimulates aldosterone release from the adrenal gland, resulting in aldosterone-mediated salt and water retention with further increase in blood pressure.

> **Helpful Tip**
> Angiotensin-converting enzyme inhibitors and angiotensin II receptor antagonists are key medications in hypertension treatment.

▶ CASE 30

An 11-year-old boy is currently hospitalized after surgery to repair a broken arm. He crashed his bike while wearing a helmet. There were no complications with surgery. He is otherwise healthy. You are paged for a pediatric consult in the middle of the night. The boy's blood pressure has been "high." His latest measurement is 125/81 mm Hg using one of those machines the hospital has. The nurse reports it was measured on his left leg while he was calm in bed. He is 150 cm (4 feet, 11 inches) tall. You give him a quick glance and notice he has a cast on his arm and is overweight. He otherwise looks fine. He is peeing well and the rest of his vital signs are normal. He has no complaints.

Question 30-1

What should you do next?

A) Obtain a manual blood pressure.
B) Ask for blood pressure measurements to be obtained in the arm.
C) Ensure the cuff size is correct.
D) Ensure the cuff is placed correctly.
E) All of the above.

Discussion 30-1

The correct answer is "E." Doesn't it sometimes seem that it is impossible to get an accurate blood pressure measurement?

TABLE 31–10 LIMITATIONS OF BLOOD PRESSURE MEASUREMENTS

All methods	• Machine calibration error • Wrong cuff size • Cuff placement incorrect (arm always preferred) • Not true rested blood pressure (moving, arm elevated)
Auscultation	• Soft Korotkoff sounds • Poor hearing • Deflating cuff too quickly • Terminal digit preference (rounding numbers to 0, 5)
Oscillometric	• Machine measures mean oscillations of arterial wall and calculates systolic blood pressure (SBP) and diastolic blood pressure (DBP) with formula unique to the machine • Initial cuff pressure reaches 160–180 mm Hg; can be uncomfortable for young children • Need for separate neonatal and child pressure cuff cables
Home blood pressure monitor	• Not calibrated • Lack of cuff sizes appropriate for children
Palpation	• Only measures SBP • Low accuracy
Ambulatory blood pressure monitor (ABPM)	• Requires ABPMs that are calibrated for use in children • Not available for younger children • High cost

The blood pressure recorded for this child is 125/81 mm Hg (95%). Before ordering tests, it is important to make sure the reading is accurate. Lots of things can go awry when taking a child's blood pressure. (See Table 31–10.) Think about the infant happily kicking his leg as the cuff inflates. What about the toddler being held down to get a measurement, or the adolescent whose pressure is measured using a child-sized cuff? Another glance at the bed confirms your hunch: the cuff being used is appropriate for a small child, not an overweight 11-year-old. Remember that a blood pressure cuff is the correct size if the bladder length encircles 80% to 100% of the arm and the bladder width encircles 50% of the arm. You find a small adult cuff and retake the pressure. The manual reading is 105/60 mm Hg (45%). Good night.

Let's suppose that same 11-year-old has a blood pressure of 136/95 mm Hg (> 99%). You confirm the reading with a manual measurement on both arms using proper technique and an appropriately sized cuff. He is still asymptomatic and peeing clear urine at a rate of 1 mL/kg/h.

Question 30-2

Do you go back to bed?

A) Yes, he has prehypertension.

B) Yes, he needs two more measurements to meet the definition of hypertension.

C) Yes, he needs a BP at or above 95% and symptoms to meet the definition of hypertension.

D) No, he has stage 2 hypertension which requires a diagnostic evaluation and treatment.

E) No, he has stage 2 hypertension and you need to do some reading.

Discussion 30-2

The correct answer is "D" but also "E." He meets the definition of hypertension. If you didn't pick up on this, go back and reread the previous case discussions.

Question 30-3

What is the next step in diagnosis?

A) Renal ultrasound.

B) BUN and creatinine.

C) Urinalysis with microscopy.

D) Review his medications.

E) All of the above.

Discussion 30-3

The correct answer is "E." Always start with a thorough history, including lifestyle habits (physical activity and diet), substance exposure, risk factors, family history, and sleep history. This should help focus the evaluation on necessary areas of investigation. Initial testing should include four-point blood pressures; renal ultrasound to identify anomalies, dysplastic, or atrophic kidneys; echocardiogram to investigate for left ventricular hypertrophy, a sign of end-organ damage; laboratory studies, including electrolytes, BUN, creatinine, and urinalysis to estimate baseline kidney function and electrolyte derangements; urine culture to rule out chronic pyelonephritis; and CBC to screen for anemia consistent with chronic kidney disease. Other tests that may be indicated include fasting lipids and glucose, drug screen to identify abuse of substances that may cause hypertension, and a sleep study to identify obstructive sleep apnea as a potential association with hypertension.

You order all of these tests and arrange for a nephrology consult. You will call the specialist as soon as you get 2 more hours of sleep.

Question 30-4

Will the specialist be happy with your initial workup?

A) Yes.

B) No.

C) Maybe.

D) It depends what time of day you call for a consult.

E) Both C and D.

Discussion 30-4

The correct answer is "E." Young children with stage 1 hypertension or adolescents with stage 2 hypertension should also have the following studies performed:

- Renin, aldosterone levels, to identify mineralocorticoid-related disease
- Plasma metanephrines, to screen for pheochromocytoma
- Renovascular imaging; this includes DMSA, Doppler ultrasound of the kidneys, magnetic resonance angiography (MRA), and arteriography

You gather more details of the history and find the patient loves energy drinks. In fact, several empty cans of "Sleep No More" juice are at his bedside. A look at the label shows that one can has the same amount of caffeine as 3 cups of coffee, with only 10 calories. You need to try one of these. A red flag indicating new tests results flashes across the patient's electronic medical record. His urine drug screen is positive for amphetamines. Did you remember to ask about drug use? Could that be why he is hypertensive?

Question 30-5

All of the drugs listed can cause hypertension EXCEPT:

A) Prednisone.

B) Caffeine.

C) Lorazepam.

D) Ibuprofen.

E) Methylphenidate.

Discussion 30-5

The correct answer is "C." Lorazepam and other benzodiazepines cause hypotension and central nervous system depression. He may need a dose to fall asleep tonight. Methylphenidate, which is commonly prescribed for attention deficit hyperactivity disorder (ADHD), can cause hypertension and a positive urine drug screen for amphetamines. (See Table 31–11.)

The boy tells you that he has been taking "medicine" for ADHD for the past year. Although caffeine and methylphenidate can cause hypertension, you decide to take a full history and perform a physical exam to be sure no other key details have been overlooked. Previously, you did a "drive-by" peak. On exam, his skin is moist, he is tachycardic, and something is palpable at the midline of his neck. He seems to be staring at you with wide-open bug eyes.

Question 30-6

What is the next step in his diagnostic workup?

A) Thyroid studies.

B) Hemoglobin A_{1c}.

C) Four-point blood pressures.

D) Serum caffeine level.

E) Cortisol level.

TABLE 31–11 COMMON CAUSES OF DRUG-INDUCED HYPERTENSION

Drug	Potential Mechanisms
Stimulants caffeine, cocaine	Vasoconstriction with increased sympathetic nervous system activity, and decreased baroreceptor sensitivity
Methylphenidate	Unclear but likely secondary to increased dopamine agonist activity
Oral contraceptives (estrogen, progesterone)	Alterations in sodium retention secondary to renin-angiotensin-aldosterone system stimulation
Glucocorticoids	Stimulation of renin-angiotensin system, enhanced pressor sensitivity to endogenous vasoconstrictors, inhibition of phospholipase A_2, reduced activity of kallikrein-kinin system Blood pressure rise is dose dependent
Mineralocorticoid (licorice, ketoconazole)	Inhibits catabolism of aldosterone; results in sustained effect of aldosterone effect, increasing sodium retention and potassium loss
Tobacco	Increased sympathetic nervous system activity, decreased endothelium-dependent vasodilation, increased arterial wall stiffness
Ephedrine (herbal products)	Stimulation of catecholamine release, increased alpha-, $beta_1$, $beta_2$ receptors
NSAIDs	Inhibition of prostaglandin, decrease in glomerular filtration rate; results in salt and water retention

Discussion 30-6

The correct answer is "A." Aside from primary hypertension, which is a diagnosis of exclusion, it is important to consider secondary causes of hypertension. Etiologies include cardiac, endocrine, and renovascular disease. In this case, the child has symptoms that suggest an endocrine cause of hypertension; specifically, hyperthyroidism due to Graves disease. Hyperthyroidism causes isolated systolic blood pressure elevation. A recheck of his blood pressure shows it is 136/70 mm Hg. (See Table 31–12.)

TABLE 31–12 ENDOCRINE CAUSES OF SECONDARY HYPERTENSION

Hormone Dysregulation	Mechanisms
Primary hyperaldosteronism	Mineralocorticoid excess results in excess aldosterone without stimulation from renin
Cushing syndrome	Glucocorticoid excess produces aldosterone effect and increases sensitivity to endogenous vasoconstrictors (epinephrine and angiotensin II)
Pheochromocytoma	Catecholamine-secreting tumor cells that may arise from neural crest, adrenal glands, or in extra-adrenal sites have a direct effect on blood pressure, through circulating levels of catecholamines (noradrenaline, adrenaline, dopamine); associated with neurofibromatosis type 1, multiple endocrine neoplasia, and von Hippel-Lindau disease
Acromegaly (growth hormone excess)	Growth hormone causes sodium retention with volume expansion
Primary hyperparathyroidism	Parathyroid hormone causes elevated intracellular calcium, hypomagnesemia, and raised plasma renin activity
Hypothyroidism	Reduces renal blood flow and glomerular filtration rate and decreases cardiac output; compensation is by increased peripheral resistance, which increases diastolic blood pressure
Hyperthyroidism	Thyroid hormone stimulates renin-angiotensin-aldosterone axis and increases sodium reabsorption, resulting in isolated systolic hypertension
Reninoma	Juxtaglomerular cell tumors of the kidney or ectopic tumors secrete renin, resulting in subsequent increase of aldosterone; hypertension is often severe and presents acutely
Diabetes mellitus	Type 1 diabetes mellitus: hypertension is secondary to progression of diabetic nephropathy Type 2 diabetes mellitus: hypertension is multifactorial, related to hyperinsulinism, sodium retention, volume expansion, and increased arterial stiffness

QUICK QUIZ

What diagnosis is associated with upper extremity blood pressure greater than lower extremity blood pressure on four-limb measurement?
A) Aortic valve stenosis.
B) Coarctation of the aorta.
C) Renal vein thrombosis.
D) Acute tubular necrosis.
E) None; this is normal.

Discussion

The correct answer is "B." Lower extremity blood pressures should be higher than the upper extremities. In coarctation, the reverse is true. Four-point (limb) blood pressure measurements are a cheap screening test in the workup of hypertension. You can get away with three points—both arms (in case an aberrant right subclavian artery is present) and one leg. Diminished or delayed femoral pulses (brachial-femoral delay) may be present with coarctation.

> **Helpful Tip**
> Coarctation of the aorta contributes to hypertension in three clinical settings:
> 1. Presurgical: Prerenal hypoperfusion results in activation of renin-angiotensin system.
> 2. Immediate postoperative period (after repair): Paradoxical hypertension occurs from increased activity of the renin-angiotensin and sympathetic nervous system.
> 3. Years after repair: Chronic hypertension is recognized in postoperative patients. Delayed diagnosis and repair is associated with more severe chronic hypertension.

▶ CASE 31

A 4-year-old girl with a history of reactive airway disease presents with worsening headache over the past 2 days that is unresponsive to acetaminophen. She has intermittent facial flushing, diaphoresis, and palpitations. On physical exam, her heart rate is 110 bpm, blood pressure is 150/100 mm Hg, and funduscopic exam reveals blurred optic discs. She is admitted for acute management of hypertension.

Question 31-1

The choice of drug for management for the next 24 hours would be:
A) Isradipine PO q6h.
B) Captopril PO q6h.
C) Hydralazine IV q4h prn.
D) Labetalol continuous IV infusion.
E) Nicardipine continuous IV infusion.

Discussion 31-1

The correct answer is "E." For acute hypertensive emergency with suspected end-organ damage, early management in the intensive care unit with continuous infusion of antihypertensive medication is essential. First-line management may include a bolus dose of IV hydralazine or labetalol. Labetalol should be used judiciously in a child with reactive airway disease as this could precipitate bronchospasm. Therefore, nicardipine (calcium channel blocker) would be the treatment of choice. This child has symptoms of severe hypertension, which could include congestive cardiac failure, palpitations, murmur, headache, vomiting, lethargy, acute hypertensive encephalopathy, seizure, or cerebrovascular accident (hemorrhagic stroke). Causes of severe hypertension in pediatric patients include renal disease (glomerulonephritis, reflux nephropathy, obstructive uropathy, acute kidney injury, polycystic kidney disease, end-stage renal disease at presentation), malignancy (pheochromocytoma, Wilms tumor, neuroblastoma), vascular abnormality (aortic coarctation, renal artery stenosis, hemolytic uremic syndrome), or medications (illicit substances, eg, MDMA; rapid withdrawal of clonidine or beta-blockers). Given the presentation of flushing and diaphoresis, this patient should receive a full workup to rule out pheochromocytoma or neuroblastoma.

> **Helpful Tip**
> A hypertensive *urgency* is an elevation of blood pressure with symptoms but no end-organ damage. A hypertensive *emergency* is an elevation of blood pressure with end-organ damage.

▶ CASE 32

A 15-year-old overweight, adolescent boy who is at the 75th percentile for height presents from school physical examination with blood pressure of 135/85 mm Hg. He is asymptomatic, without headache, chest pain, or palpitations. He has mild shortness of breath on exertion.

Question 32-1

Initial investigations should include all of the following EXCEPT:
A) Plasma renin.
B) Echocardiogram.
C) Renal ultrasound.
D) BUN and creatinine.
E) Repeat blood pressure measurements.

Discussion 32-1

The correct answer is "A." This is an adolescent patient with asymptomatic elevated blood pressure readings that fall within the stage 1 hypertensive range (we plotted it for you). He is overweight and is otherwise well. The first-line investigations for adolescent hypertension include four-point blood pressure; renal ultrasound to investigate for dysplasia, atrophic kidneys, or other anomalies; renal function to determine whether there is underlying chronic kidney disease; and echocardiogram to evaluate for chronicity of hypertension and to detect left ventricular hypertrophy as a sign of end-organ damage. Repeat blood pressure measurements at multiple clinic visits, and school or home blood pressure readings over a 3-month period, are required to confirm the presence of true hypertension. Plasma renin is optimally used when investigating a child or adolescent with stage 2 hypertension, and potentially with systemic conditions associated with hypertension.

► CASE 33

Parents bring in their 3-year-old otherwise healthy son to your office with concerns of developmental delay. He has yet to speak in 2-word phrases. The mother has noticed that he prefers to play by himself and is very active all the time. He follows 1-step commands well, but struggles with multistep commands. On physical exam, he is at the 10th percentile for height and weight, and the 40th percentile for head circumference. Vital signs are normal except for manual blood pressure of 115/65 to 120/69 mm Hg on his arms, and 120/70 to 125/72 mm Hg on his legs. He has palpable soft nodules on his upper back, brown patches on his trunk, and freckling in the axillary region.

Question 33-1

You order a renal ultrasound, with specific attention to look for:
A) Angiomyolipoma.
B) Renal dysplasia.
C) Renal artery stenosis.
D) Middle aortic stenosis.
E) Adrenal mass.

Discussion 33-1

The correct answer is "C." This child has developmental delay, macrocephaly, neurofibromas, café-au-lait spots, and axillary freckling, which strongly suggest neurofibromatosis type 1 (NF1). NF1 is associated with hypertension, with renal artery stenosis being the predominant etiology. A Doppler renal ultrasound would be most appropriate. Angiomyolipoma is associated with tuberous sclerosis. Although tuberous sclerosis is associated with developmental delay and produces skin findings such as facial angiofibromas or hypomelanotic macules (ash-leaf spots), affected children do not have axillary freckling or café-au-lait spots. Renal dysplasia can result in hypertension, but the primary genetic syndromes of neurocutaneous findings and hypertension should be ruled out first. There is also no significant past medical history in this case. Supravalvular aortic stenosis is typically a concern in Williams-Beuren syndrome, and this is best investigated with CT angiogram or angiography. An adrenal mass should also be investigated with CT but is unlikely to be associated with developmental delay.

Helpful Tip
Doppler ultrasound has low specificity for renal artery stenosis. If there is strong suspicion of renal artery stenosis, angiographic imaging modalities (CT angiogram, angiography) are definitive diagnostic tests.

Question 33-2

Which of the following disorders is/are associated with abnormal blood vessels that result in findings of renovascular hypertension secondary to either renal artery stenosis or middle aortic syndrome?
A) Fibromuscular dysplasia.
B) Takayasu arteritis.
C) Tuberous sclerosis.
D) Neurofibromatosis.
E) Retroperitoneal fibrosis following abdominal irradiation.
F) All of the above.

Question 33-2

The correct answer is "F." Middle aortic syndrome is characterized by segmental narrowing along the abdominal or distal descending aorta. Narrowing may involve the ostia of the renal artery. Hypertension is noted above the stenosis, with a blood pressure gradient distal to the stenosis. These disorders typically are associated with severe and difficult-to-control hypertension, resulting in use of numerous antihypertensive agents. Surgical intervention, including angioplasty, may be required but has variable success.

Helpful Tip
Do not prescribe an ACE inhibitor if there is bilateral renal artery stenosis. This could result in serious renal failure!

⧗ QUICK QUIZ

What is NOT a sequela of childhood hypertension?
A) Atherosclerosis.
B) Left ventricular hypertrophy.
C) Liver disease.
D) Retinal arteriopathy.
E) Stroke.

Discussion

The correct answer is "C." Elevated blood pressure is associated with the development of end organ damage affecting the kidney, heart and blood vessels. End organ damage is typically seen after longer time periods of elevated blood pressures but if pressures are very high (hypertensive emergency) complications may develop over a short time period.

BIBLIOGRAPHY

Hypertension

Falkner B. Hypertension in children and adolescents: Natural history and epidemiology. *Pediatr Nephrol.* 2010;25:1219–1224.

Flynn JT, Tullus K. Severe hypertension in children and adolescents: Pathophysiology and treatment. *Pediatr Nephrol.* 2009;24(6):1101–1112.

Hansen ML, Gunn PW, Kaelber DC. Underdiagnosis of hypertension in children and adolescents. *JAMA.* 2007;298:874–879.

National High Blood Pressure Education Program Working Group on High Blood Pressure in Children and Adolescents. The fourth report on the diagnosis, evaluation, and treatment of high blood pressure in children and adolescents. *Pediatrics.* 2004;114(suppl 2):555–576.

Tullus K, Brennan E, Hamilton G, et al. Renovascular hypertension in children. *Lancet.* 2008;371(9622):1453–1463.

Viera AJ, Neutze DM. Diagnosis of secondary hypertension: An age-based approach. *Am Fam Physician.* 2010;82(12):1471–1478.

Chronic Kidney Disease

Atkinson MA, Furth SL. Anemia in children with chronic kidney disease. *Nat Rev Nephrol.* 2011;7:635–641.

Dharnidharka VR, Fiorina P, Harmon WE. Kidney transplantation in children. *N Engl J Med.* 2014;371(6):549–558.

Müller D, Goldstein SL. Hemodialysis in children with end-stage renal disease. *Nat Rev Nephrol.* 2011;7:650–658.

Rees L, Mak RH. Nutrition and growth in children with chronic kidney disease. *Nat Rev Nephrol.* 2011;7:615–623.

Schaefer F, Warady BA. Peritoneal dialysis in children with end-stage renal disease. *Nat Rev Nephrol.* 2011;7:659–668.

Schmitt CP, Mehls O. Mineral and bone disorders in children with chronic kidney disease. *Nat Rev Nephrol.* 2011;7:624–634.

Shroff R, Weaver DJ, Mitsnefes MM. Cardiovascular complications in children with chronic kidney disease. *Nat Rev Nephrol.* 2011;7:642–649.

Urologic Disorders

Ingraham SE, McHugh KM. Current perspectives on congenital obstructive nephropathy. *Pediatr Nephrol.* 2011;26(9):1453–1461.

Strand WR. Initial management of complex pediatric disorders: Prunebelly syndrome, posterior urethral valves. *Urol Clin North Am.* 2004;31(3):399–415, vii.

Glomerular Diseases

Cramer MT, Guay-Woodford LM. Cystic kidney disease: A primer. *Adv Chronic Kidney Dis.* 2015;22(4):297–305.

Gipson DS, Massengill SF, Yao L, et al. Management of childhood onset nephrotic syndrome. *Pediatrics.* 2009;124(2):747–757.

Harris PC, Torres VE. Polycystic kidney disease, autosomal dominant. In: Pagon RA, Adam MP, Ardinger HH, et al, eds. *GeneReviews* [Internet]. Seattle, WA: University of Washington, Seattle; 1993–2015.

Acute Kidney Injury

Chan JCM, Williams DM, Roth KS. Kidney failure in infants and children. *Pediatr Rev.* 2002;23(2):47–60.

Moffett BS, Goldstein SL. Acute kidney injury and increasing nephrotoxic-medication exposure in noncritically ill children. *Clin J Am Soc Nephrol.* 2011;6(4):856–863.

Van De Voorde RG 3rd. Acute post-streptococcal glomerulonephritis: The most common acute glomerulonephritis. *Pediatr Rev.* 2015;36(1):3–12.

Respiratory Disorders

Anthony Fischer

32

> ▶ CASE 1

A 2-year-old fully immunized boy is brought to the emergency department for sudden onset of barking cough associated with inspiratory stridor. He has had a runny nose and hoarse voice for the last day. Temperature is 37.6°C (99.7°F), heart rate is 150 beats per minute (bpm), respirations 40 breaths per minute, and oxygen saturation (SpO_2) by pulse oximeter is 98%. He has moderate suprasternal retractions and stridor. Lung fields are clear to auscultation.

Question 1-1
Your treatment plan includes:
A) Albuterol and prednisolone.
B) Aerosolized 3% hypertonic saline.
C) Ceftriaxone.
D) Aerosolized epinephrine and dexamethasone.
E) Amoxicillin.
F) Further diagnostic testing.

Discussion 1-1
The correct answer is "D." The history and physical exam are consistent with viral laryngotracheobronchitis (croup), which is caused by an infection with mucosal edema of the larynx, trachea, and bronchi. Nasal congestion and cough appear first. Over 12 to 48 hours, the cough worsens, becomes barky, and stridor develops. Typically, children 6 months to 3 years of age are affected. If a child is older than age 6 years, it is not croup. Fall is the season of choice, and symptoms are worse at night. Parainfluenza viruses are usually to blame. Swelling makes the airway narrower, increasing airflow resistance and resulting in the classic barky cough with stridor. If a child barks like a seal, chances are he or she has croup. Diagnostic studies are not needed. Croup is a clinical diagnosis that even medical students can make. The edema improves with dexamethasone (typical dose 0.6 mg/kg). For patients with respiratory distress and stridor *at rest*, aerosolized epinephrine should also be given. Symptoms can return 2 to 3 hours later when the medication wears off. Children should be monitored for 3 to 4 hours after treatment with aerosolized epinephrine to ensure that stridor at rest does not return. The key is stridor at rest. Stridor will still be present if the child is crying. Albuterol or prednisolone would be appropriate treatments for an asthma exacerbation, which is characterized by inflammation and bronchoconstriction in the intrathoracic airways (inside the chest). Symptoms include wheezing (not stridor). Three percent hypertonic saline has been proposed as a treatment for bronchiolitis but has not been tested in croup. Ceftriaxone and amoxicillin could be used to treat bacterial pneumonia, but the normal oximetry and lack of fever or localized crackles makes this possibility unlikely. Immunization status is always a relevant question in pediatrics. Epiglottis caused by *Haemophilus influenzae* infection presents with stridor, respiratory distress, and drooling. Lying down makes everything worse so the child sits in a tripod position (upright, leaning forward, hands on knees). This is a life-threatening emergency that could be mostly prevented with Hib vaccination. The airway may become obstructed by the big swollen epiglottis. Do everything in your power to not tick off a child with epiglottis.

> **Helpful Tip**
> Forget the cool mist and steam therapies for croup. These therapies have not been shown to work (sorry!) but are not harmful, so when someone insists they help just smile.

> **Helpful Tip**
> Racemic epinephrine is a 1:1 mixture of D- and L-isomers. It was felt to have fewer side effects and preferred over L-epinephrine. It is now known that both are effective and rates of tachycardia and hypertension are the same.

An anteroposterior (AP) X-ray was ordered just in case the child swallowed a quarter when his dad was not watching.

Question 1-2

What is the classic radiographic finding with croup? (See Figure 32–1.)

A) Thumb sign.

B) Widened retropharyngeal space.

C) Radiopaque circle.

D) Steeple sign.

E) Subcutaneous emphysema.

Discussion 1-2

The correct answer is "D." In a child with croup an AP film of the neck shows narrowing of the subglottic air column, which

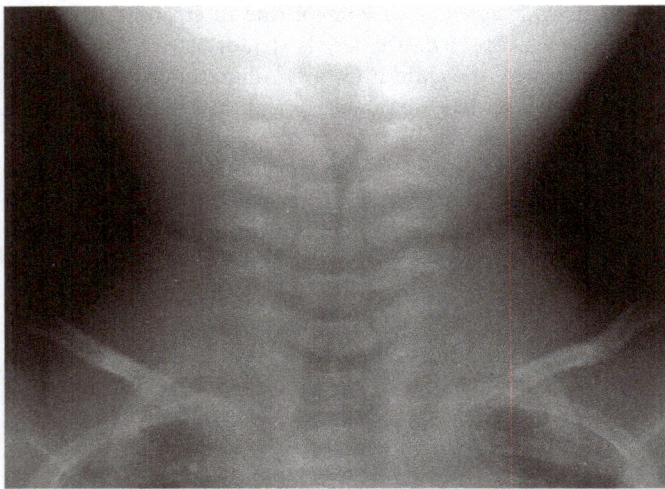

A

B

FIGURE 32–1A, Steeple sign in a 1-year-old with croup. **B,** Steeple sign in a 12-year-old. (Reproduced with permission from Stone CK, Humphries RL, eds. *Current Diagnosis and Treatment: Emergency Medicine.* 7th ed. New York, NY: McGraw-Hill Education; 2011, Fig. 32-10.)

resembles a church steeple. Epiglottitis may show a thumbprint sign on lateral neck film. Remember what you just read—do not aggravate a child with epiglottitis. A widened retropharyngeal space on lateral film may be seen with retropharyngeal abscess. A radiopaque circle would suggest a foreign body. Subcutaneous emphysema is seen when air from a pneumomediastinum extends to the soft tissue.

▶ CASE 2

A mother brings to the clinic a 6-week-old girl who has a high-pitched inspiratory noise that worsens with excitement. The girl has no respiratory distress or hoarseness. She has never turned blue or stopped breathing. She breastfeeds well and is growing normally.

Question 2-1

What is the most likely cause of the inspiratory noise?

A) Foreign body.

B) Vocal cord paresis.

C) Laryngomalacia.

D) Tracheomalacia.

E) Aberrant right subclavian artery.

Discussion 2-1

The correct answer is "C." The most common cause of stridor in newborns is laryngomalacia. Laryngomalacia causes intermittent collapse of the supraglottic structures with inspiration. Infants are squeaky and musical sounding. It is noticed soon after birth, progressively worsens until 4 months of age, and then typically resolves by 1 year. The *inspiratory* stridor is (1) worse with crying, feeding, or excitement; (2) worse with viral upper respiratory tract infections; and (3) positional in nature (worse when supine). Flip the infant prone either on the bed or over your forearm; the stridor should lessen. (People will think you are a diagnostic genius.) The differential diagnosis for stridor is long but all candidate conditions cause airway obstruction typically outside of the chest (extrathoracic). (See Table 32–1.) Unilateral vocal cord paresis may be recognized by a weak cry, hoarseness, or aspiration with feeds. Bilateral disease causes stridor. Laryngomalacia does not cause hoarseness. Tracheomalacia is less common (approximately 1:2000). Tracheomalacia can cause stridor depending on the location, but more frequently is associated with cough and wheezing. Vascular rings are congenital anomalies of the aortic arch that compress the trachea or esophagus, or both, causing stridor. Complete rings fully encircle the trachea and esophagus (ie, double aortic arch). Incomplete rings (ie, pulmonary sling) do not. An aberrant right subclavian artery (incomplete ring) courses posterior to the esophagus and can cause difficulty with swallowing (dysphagia lusoria). Let's hope this child's older sibling did not feed her a peanut that she aspirated.

TABLE 32–1 CAUSES OF STRIDOR BASED ON TIMING DURING RESPIRATORY CYCLE AND LOCATION OF OBSTRUCTION

Inspiratory stridor	Laryngomalacia
• Supraglottis	Croup
	Epiglottitis
	Peritonsillar abscess
	Retropharyngeal abscess
	Foreign body
	Lingual thyroid
	Retro/micrognathia
	Tonsil hypertrophy
	Laryngospasm
	Anaphylaxis
• Biphasic stridor	Vocal cord paralysis
• Glottis	Subglottic hemangioma
• Usually a fixed obstruction	Foreign body
	Laryngeal web
	Laryngeal cyst
	Recurrent respiratory papillomatosis
	Tracheal stenosis
	Complete or near-complete tracheal rings or tracheal stenosis
Expiratory stridor	Subglottic stenosis
• Subglottis	Tracheomalacia
	Bacterial tracheitis
	Vascular ring
	Foreign body

Helpful Tip

Stridor from a subglottic hemangioma is often misdiagnosed as croup, and both improve with steroids. Like hemangiomas on the skin, these subglottic lesions grow rapidly during the early months of life, worsening the airway obstruction. Diagnosis requires a high index of suspicion and endoscopy. Look for recurrent episodes, biphasic stridor, facial hemangiomas in a beard distribution, apnea, and lack of viral prodrome.

Question 2-2

How should this infant girl's problem be managed?

A) Supraglottoplasty.
B) Tracheostomy.
C) Therapeutic trial of lansoprazole.
D) Racemic epinephrine by nebulizer.
E) Close outpatient monitoring of growth and respiratory symptoms.

Discussion 2-2

The correct answer is "E." Laryngomalacia usually has a benign course. For mild symptoms, as in this infant, no intervention is necessary. Severe symptoms warranting intervention and referral to otolaryngology include problems with feeding, poor growth, apneic spells, or persistent respiratory symptoms. Pharyngolaryngeal reflux is frequently associated with laryngomalacia; therefore, antireflux medications (proton pump inhibitor or H_2 histamine antagonist) are recommended by some experts. If needed, a supraglottoplasty may be performed surgically to remove excess tissue. Tracheostomy is not necessary in this patient. Racemic epinephrine is a treatment for croup, which is a cause of acute stridor.

► CASE 3

A 5-year-old immunized girl develops biphasic stridor and high fever. She has a brassy-sounding cough and has severe respiratory distress. She is toxic appearing but not drooling and able to lie flat.

Question 3-1

What diagnosis do you suspect?

A) Croup.
B) Peritonsillar abscess.
C) Pneumonia.
D) Tracheitis.
E) Diphtheria.

Discussion 3-1

The correct answer is "D." The child has symptoms of bacterial tracheitis. This is a life-threatening infection that may require intubation to keep the airway open. Usually it occurs after a viral illness. Affected children want to lie flat, which is the opposite of epiglottitis. Pneumonia does not cause wheezing. Croup produces a barky cough. A peritonsillar abscess gives a muffled "hot potato" voice. Diphtheria can cause pseudomembranous pharyngitis, but this child is immunized.

The child is admitted to the PICU.

Question 3-2

Antibiotic coverage should include all of the following organisms EXCEPT:

A) *Haemophilus influenzae.*
B) *Staphylococcus aureus.*
C) *Pseudomonas aeruginosa.*
D) *Streptococcus pyogenes.*
E) *Mycoplasma pneumoniae.*

Discussion 3-2

The correct answer is "E." Bacterial tracheitis can be polymicrobial and has been reported with all of these organisms except *Mycoplasma*.

▶ CASE 4

An infant has biphasic stridor, poor feeding, and respiratory distress. You suspect vascular compression of the trachea.

Question 4-1

Which of the following tests would be best to address this question?
A) Chest X-ray.
B) Noncontrast chest CT.
C) Barium esophagram.
D) Chest CT angiography.
E) Echocardiography.
F) Bronchoscopy.

Discussion 4-1

The correct answer is "D." CT angiography would give the greatest sensitivity and specificity for identifying vascular compression.

▶ CASE 5

A 7-year-old previously healthy girl was hospitalized for pneumonia requiring emergency intubation in the emergency department of a community hospital. One month after discharge, she developed progressive dyspnea and biphasic stridor. She performs spirometry in your office.

Question 5-1

Which flow-volume loop is most likely? (See Figure 32–2.)
A) Normal.
B) Expiratory small airway obstruction, bronchodilator responsive.
C) Normal expiratory loop, inspiratory obstruction.
D) Inspiratory and expiratory large airway obstruction.
E) Expiratory obstruction, bronchodilator nonresponsive.

Discussion 5-1

The correct answer is "D." This child has developed subglottic stenosis as a complication of traumatic intubation resulting in near complete central airway obstruction, which can be recognized by flow limitation on expiration and inspiration. Subglottic stenosis can be congenital or acquired. Acquired cases are usually associated with endotracheal intubation—traumatic, prolonged (think preemies), or use of an oversized endotracheal tube (most common). Tracheostomies may also cause stenosis. Listen for biphasic stridor. Flow-volume loops or curves plot inspiratory and expiratory airflow (y-axis) against lung volume (x-axis). (See Figure 32–3.) Looking at the flow-volume loops is helpful when assessing central airway obstruction. (See Figure 32–4.) A fixed central airway obstruction decreases inspiratory and expiratory airflow. When obstruction affects expiration or inspiration but not both, it is dynamic and determined by pressure changes in and out of the airways as well as location in or out of the chest. For example, an airway obstruction that is variable and extrathoracic reduces inspiratory flow with resultant stridor. The obstruction resolves with expiration. Think of drinking a milkshake through a flexible straw. When you apply suction, negative inspiratory pressure is generated, the straw collapses and nothing comes up the straw to your mouth. When you release or blow air down the straw (creating positive pressure), it opens again. Subglottic stenosis is a fixed obstruction so this child's loop would look like panel C in Figure 32–3.

> **Helpful Tip**
> Recurrent or persistent croup may signal underlying subglottic stenosis. The airway is already narrowed. Edema from infection or laryngopharyngeal reflux makes it worse.

Question 5-2

What is the next step in evaluation and management?
A) Referral to otolaryngology for direct laryngoscopy and bronchoscopy.
B) Tracheostomy.
C) Therapeutic trial of lansoprazole.

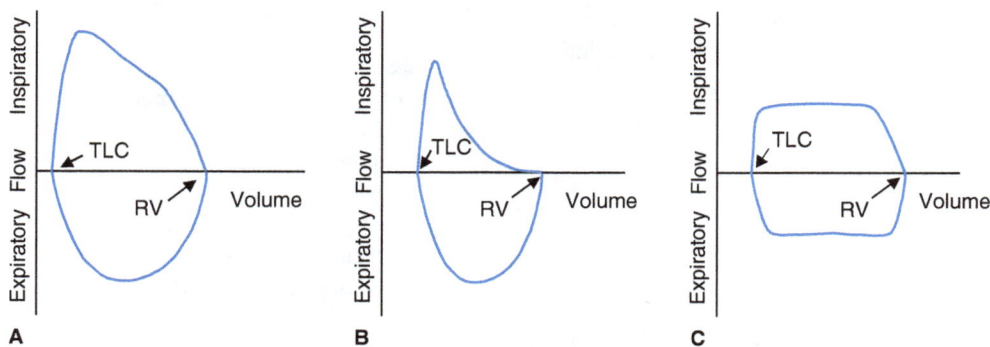

FIGURE 32–2. Flow-volume loops. The y-axis measures airflow in liters per second. The x-axis measures lung volume in liters. The expiratory curve is above the x-axis and inspiratory curve below. (A) Normal: the expiratory flow rate rapidly rises to its peak then falls in linear fashion; the inspiratory curve is symmetric and saddle shaped. (B) Airflow obstruction: the slope of the expiratory curve is scooped out and the peak flow is reduced. (C) Fixed central airway obstruction: flow is limited in both inspiration and expiration with flattening of both curves. RV, residual volume; TLC, total lung capacity. (Reproduced with permission from Kasper DL, Fauci AS, Hauser SL et al: *Harrison's Principles of Internal Medicine*, 19th ed. McGraw-Hill Education, Inc., 2015. Fig 306-4.)

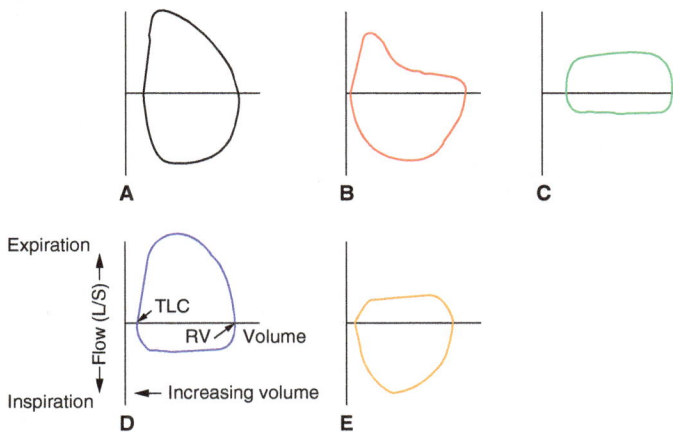

RV-residual volume, TLC-total lung capacity

A Normal
B Lower airways obstruction
C Fixed central airway obstruction
D Valuable central extrathoracic obstruction
E Valuable central intrathoracic obstruction

FIGURE 32–3. The y-axis measures airflow in liters per seconds. The x-axis measures lung volume in liters. The expiratory curve is above the x-axis and inspiratory curve below. (A) Normal: the expiratory flow rate rapidly rises to its peak then falls in linear fashion; the inspiratory curve is symmetric and saddle shaped. (B) Airflow obstruction: the slope of the expiratory curve is scooped out and the peak flow is reduced. (C) Fixed central airway obstruction: flow is limited in both inspiration and expiration with flattening of both curves. (D) Variable or dynamic extrathoracic obstruction: inspiratory flow is limited with flattening of the inspiratory curve. (E) Variable intrathoracic obstruction: expiratory flow is limited with flattening of the expiratory curve.

D) Racemic epinephrine by nebulizer.
E) Close outpatient monitoring of growth and respiratory symptoms.

Discussion 5-2

The correct answer is "A." The patient should be referred to otolaryngology to assess surgical options. Treatment depends on severity and location of the stenosis. This patient already manifests severe respiratory symptoms and outpatient observation without referral is not appropriate. Surgical options include open reconstruction and endoscopic dilation/laser. Tracheostomy is avoided if possible. Acid-suppressive medications will not reverse the degree of airway obstruction. They may have a role in preventing subsequent insult, but this is not proven.

▶ CASE 6

A newborn child was diagnosed with C-type esophageal atresia and tracheoesophageal fistula (EA-TEF) (diagram below) and undergoes surgical repair.

Question 6-1

Which other airway abnormality is most likely to coexist with this defect?

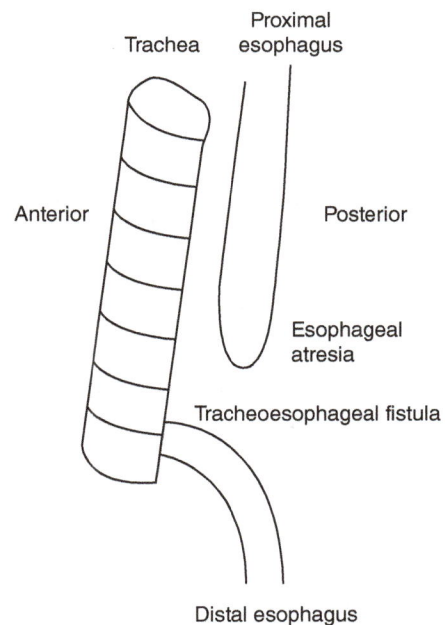

A) Left bronchial stenosis.
B) Complete tracheal rings.
C) Tracheomalacia.
D) Posterior laryngeal cleft.
E) Tracheal compression by anomalous left pulmonary artery.

Discussion 6-1

The correct answer is "C." A tracheoesophageal fistula (TEF) generally results in a wider posterior tracheal membrane at the site of the defect as well as tracheal rings that are less complete. This causes the trachea to collapse with increased air flow. Left bronchial stenosis can be acquired as a complication of some thoracic surgeries, especially cardiac surgeries. However, this complication would be rare. Posterior laryngeal cleft is a disorder that results in communication between the airway and the esophagus at the level of the larynx, causing recurrent aspiration and difficulty handling secretions. It is a rare occurrence compared with tracheomalacia. An anomalous left pulmonary artery (pulmonary sling) results in division of the trachea and esophagus and would be most unlikely in a patient with TEF.

⧗ QUICK QUIZ

What is the most common type of TEF?
A) Type A.
B) Type B.
C) Type C.
D) Type D.
E) Type E.

Discussion

The correct answer is "C." You would think the most common variant would be called type A, but not in this defect. In type C TEF, the upper esophagus ends in a blind pouch and the TEF is connected to the distal esophagus; this variant is present in

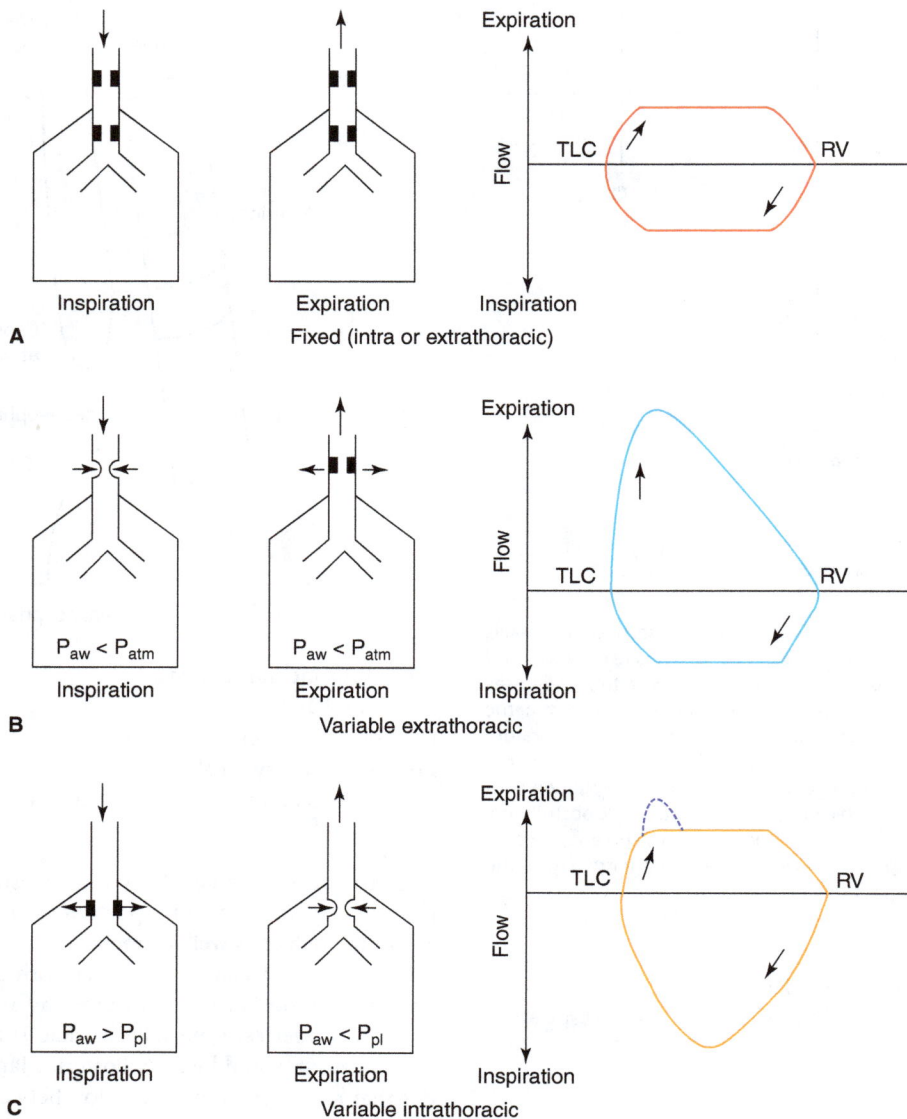

FIGURE 32–4. Flow-volume loops—central airway obstructions. (A) Fixed obstruction: flow is limited in both inspiration and expiration with flattening of both curves. (B) Variable or dynamic extrathoracic obstruction: inspiratory flow is limited with flattening of the inspiratory curve. (C) Variable intrathoracic obstruction: expiratory flow is limited with flattening of the expiratory curve. (Reproduced with permission from Burrows B, Knudson RJ, Quan SF, et al: *Respiratory Disorders: A Pathophysiologic Approach.* 2d ed. Chicago: Year Book Medical Publishers; 1983.)

87% of cases. In proximal TEF, the upper esophagus connects with the trachea allowing aspiration of oral secretions and feeds. In distal TEF, the lower esophagus connects with the trachea allowing aspiration of gastric contents. (See Figure 32–5.)

Wanting to learn more about EA-TEF, you ask the father what symptoms the newborn had that led to the diagnosis.

Question 6-2
Which is NOT a symptom of EA-TEF?
A) Drooling.
B) Coughing immediately after feeds.
C) Respiratory distress.
D) Polyhydramnios in utero.
E) All of the above.

Discussion 6-2
The correct answer is "E." Esophageal atresia (EA) is the most common congenital anomaly of the esophagus. Over 90% of cases have a concurrent tracheoesophageal fistula (TEF). The clinical presentation of TEF depends on the presence or absence of EA. Neonates with EA develop symptoms immediately after birth from excess secretions. Think of a bubbling fountains; affected infants have frothy saliva coming from their mouth and nose in a similar fashion. They will drool, cough, choke, possibly turn blue, and have respiratory distress. Feeding will make everything worse as oral content is aspirated through the proximal fistula. Gastric contents can reflux through a distal fistula, causing chemical pneumonitis. Crying introduces air into the stomach through a distal fistula, just as in a balloon that is being inflated.

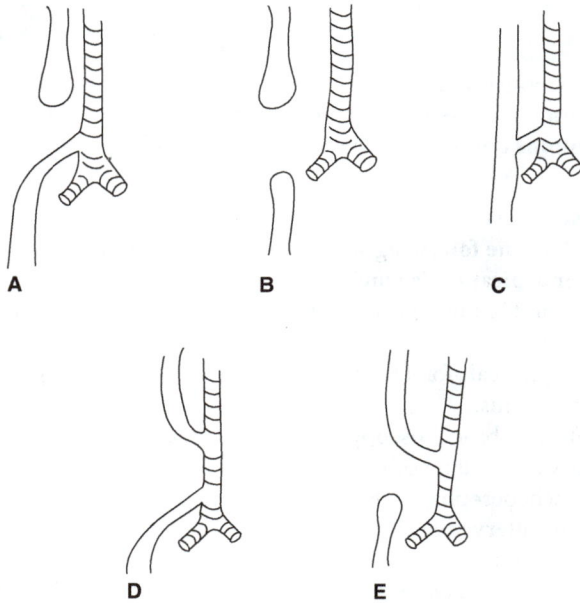

FIGURE 32–5. Types of esophageal atresia and tracheoesophageal fistula. (A) Type C: esophageal atresia with distal tracheoesophageal fistula (87% of cases). (B) Type A: esophageal atresia without tracheoesophageal fistula (8% of cases). (C) Type E: H-type fistula, tracheoesophageal fistula without esophageal atresia (4% of cases). (D) Type D: esophageal atresia with proximal and distal tracheoesophageal fistula (< 1% of cases). (E) Type B: esophageal atresia with proximal tracheoesophageal fistula (1% of cases). (Reproduced with permission from Lalwani A K, ed. *Current Diagnosis and Treatment in Otolaryngology: Head and Neck Surgery.* 3rd ed. New York, NY: McGraw-Hill Education; 2011, Fig. 35-1 A-E.)

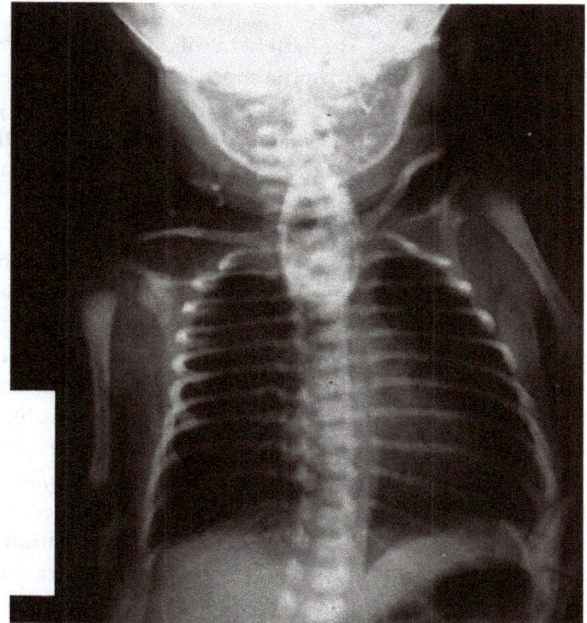

FIGURE 32–6. This is a newborn with esophageal atresia and tracheoesophageal fistula. The feeding tube is coiled in the upper pouch of the esophagus. A tracheoesophageal fistula is present as there is air below the diaphragm. (Reproduced with permission from Brunicardi FC, Andersen DK, Billiar TR, et al, eds. *Schwartz's Principles of Surgery.* 10th ed. New York, NY: McGraw-Hill Education; 2015, Fig. 39-10.)

Helpful Tip

Infants with an isolated TEF without EA (H-type fistula) may present later in infancy with recurrent wheezing or aspiration pneumonias, or both.

Question 6-3

Which is NOT a true statement about EA-TEF?

A) It is associated with CHARGE syndrome.
B) It may cause prenatal oligohydramnios.
C) A nasogastric or orogastric tube will not pass into the stomach.
D) An esophagogram is helpful to diagnosis H-type fistulas (type E).
E) Vertebral defects and anal atresia are associated conditions.

Discussion 6-3

The correct answer is "B." Remember, the fetus swallows amniotic fluid then pees it out. An intestinal obstruction such as EA will cause buildup of unswallowed fluid (polyhydramnios). Concurrent congenital anomalies are present 50% of the time. CHARGE is a mnemonic for **C**oloboma, **H**eart defects, choanal **A**tresia, **R**etarded growth and development, **G**enital defects, and **E**ar defects. Do not be confused; there is no "T" but TEF is associated nonetheless. VACTERL stands for **V**ertebral defects, **A**nal atresia, **C**ardiac defects, **T**racheo**E**sophageal fistula, **R**enal

anomalies, and **L**imb abnormalities. If you find a TEF, look closely for deformities, call a geneticist, and order some imaging. A quick test for EA is to try to pass a nasogastric or orogastric tube. It won't work. On chest X-ray it may be coiled in the esophageal pouch. (See Figure 32–6.) Notice this is for EA that likely has a TEF. Type E TEF (H-type) does not have an EA. (See Figure 32–5.) An esophagogram isn't a perfect test. Endoscopy with bronchoscopy or CT imaging may be needed to clarify findings. For EA and TEF, call a surgeon right away. These defects are treated surgically.

▶ CASE 7

A 2-year-old child acutely developed severe respiratory distress, and stridor. He is unable to swallow secretions. Vital signs are temperature 40°C (104°F), heart rate 190 bpm, respirations 50 breaths per minute, and blood pressure (BP) 80/40 mm Hg. On exam he is toxic appearing, leaning forward, drooling, and in distress.

Question 7-1

Which of the following should be performed first?

A) Endotracheal intubation by a skilled provider.
B) IV placement for fluid administration.
C) Neck CT scan.
D) Intramuscular ceftriaxone.
E) Throat examination and pharyngeal culture.

Discussion 7-1

The correct answer is "A." The patient in this vignette has airway compromise from epiglottitis. The most important first step is to secure the airway (remember those ABCs)—preferably in an operating room setting. IV placement, fluid resuscitation, antibiotic treatment, and diagnostic studies should be delayed until after an artificial airway is established. Epiglottitis is a life-threatening emergency that rapidly progresses to upper airway obstruction from edema of the epiglottis and aryepiglottic folds. A child presents with the abrupt onset of fever, dysphagia, drooling, dysphonia, and distress (the 4 Ds). The illness progresses rapidly over 12 to 24 hours. Children look toxic and sit in a tripod position (mouth open, neck hyperextended, sitting up, leaning forward) to make the airway as wide as possible. As a result of widespread vaccination against Hib, cases of epiglottitis now commonly involve bacteria other than *H. influenzae* and affect older children rather than toddlers. Immunocompromised individuals and those with incomplete vaccination are at risk. Have you caught on that epiglottitis, although rare now with immunizations, is a big deal?

► CASE 8

A 3-year-old boy has fever, stridor, respiratory distress, and torticollis. He has decreased range of motion of his neck, especially lateral rotation and extension. You suspect that the child has a retropharyngeal abscess.

Question 8-1

Which of the following statements about retropharyngeal abscess is true?

A) Lateral neck X-ray has greater sensitivity for retropharyngeal abscess than neck CT with contrast.
B) Anaerobic organism coverage is not necessary for patients with retropharyngeal abscesses.
C) Lateral neck X-ray should be performed with the neck slightly flexed.
D) Direct spreading of the infection can result in mediastinitis or meningitis.
E) Culture of a drained abscess usually reveals a single organism.

Discussion 8-1

The correct answer is "D." Deep neck space infections include retropharyngeal and parapharyngeal abscess. The retropharyngeal nodes that become infected involute by age 5 years, making infection in older children uncommon. Direct spreading of retropharyngeal abscess can result in a variety of complications such as mediastinitis, meningitis, and venous thrombosis. Computed tomography (CT) scan with contrast has greater sensitivity than lateral neck X-ray for diagnosing retropharyngeal abscess. If lateral neck X-ray is obtained, the neck should be slightly extended. Flexion of the neck makes the retropharyngeal space appear widened. Because retropharyngeal abscesses are often polymicrobial and can harbor anaerobic organisms, treatment with ampicillin-sulbactam or clindamycin is recommended.

► CASE 9

An 18-month-old boy presents with acute cough, stridor, and drooling. He was playing with his older brother when these symptoms developed. He was previously well.

Question 9-1

Which of the following statements about foreign body ingestion or aspiration is true?

A) A chest X-ray may rule out the presence of an airway foreign body.
B) Esophageal foreign bodies do not produce respiratory symptoms.
C) Flexible bronchoscopy is the safest procedure for removing airway foreign bodies.
D) Tracheoesophageal fistula is a potential complication of button battery ingestion.
E) On chest X-rays, coins in the trachea usually appear more round on anteroposterior (AP) view compared with lateral view.

Discussion 9-1

The correct answer is "D." This child aspirated a foreign body and it is obstructing his upper airway. Eighteen-month-olds like to put things in their mouths. Older siblings have fun toys with little parts; think Legos and Barbie shoes. The child is usually fine, then suddenly becomes blue and cannot breathe. A history of choking is not always present as the event was likely unwitnessed. Foreign bodies can land in any part of the airway but most commonly end up in the bronchi, especially on the right side. Symptoms vary and may be subtle as well as subacute (eg, persistent wheezing unresponsive to treatment). Button battery ingestion is an emergency because it can cause esophageal necrosis resulting in mediastinitis or tracheoesophageal fistula. Do not mistake a button battery for a coin on a radiograph. Button batteries have a double ring or rounded edge appearance. Coins have a sharp edge. Chest X-ray can locate a radiodense foreign body but will miss many life-threatening foreign bodies such as plastic toys or peanuts. Flexible bronchoscopy is not recommended to remove foreign bodies because there is not a sufficient working channel to grab foreign material. Instead, rigid bronchoscopy should be performed to safely remove an airway foreign body. Coins in the esophagus generally appear more round on AP projection, but coins in the trachea are more round on a lateral view. This is because the posterior membrane of the trachea is more elastic than the cartilaginous anterior and lateral portions of the trachea.

> **Helpful Tip**
> Most foreign bodies (peanuts, plastic objects) are radiolucent and will not be seen on radiograph. Do not be falsely reassured. If your suspicion remains high, the child should undergo rigid bronchoscopy not only to make the diagnosis but to remove the object.

QUICK QUIZ

A friend's teenage son is eating peanuts when he starts laughing. He subsequently starts to cough and choke. He appears anxious and makes a hand gesture toward his throat. At this point, he is no longer coughing.
What should be done next?
A) Administer intramuscular epinephrine.
B) Perform the Heimlich maneuver.
C) Perform back blows and chest compressions.
D) Do not intervene unless he loses consciousness.
E) Sign up for a cardiopulmonary resuscitation (CPR) course.

Discussion

The correct answer is "B." He is choking to death. This is a classic example of complete airway obstruction (cannot cough or speak) from aspiration of a little peanut. Remember to follow the American Heart Association guidelines. The Heimlich maneuver should be performed until the peanut is dislodged or the victim loses consciousness, at which time standard CPR should be performed and 9-1-1 called. Back blows and chest compressions are used to dislodge foreign bodies in infants. Blind finger sweeping is not recommended. Peanuts are a frequent cause of anaphylaxis, for which epinephrine should be administered. However, this scenario does not have features of anaphylaxis as there is no involvement of a second organ system (eg, hives, angioedema, vomiting).

Helpful Tip
In cases of vocal cord paralysis–induced stridor, do not settle after discovering why the child has stridor; look for the underlying etiology of the paralysis. For example, resulting dysphagia and failure to thrive are symptoms of a Chiari malformation (brainstem compression) in infants.

QUICK QUIZ

Which is NOT a typical cause of biphasic stridor?
A) Subglottic stenosis.
B) Vocal cord paralysis.
C) Subglottic stenosis.
D) Croup.
E) Foreign body.

Discussion

The correct answer is "D." Croup typically causes inspiratory stridor; however, if the swelling and inflammation became severe, the stridor could become biphasic.

▶ CASE 10

A 16-year-old patient has a 6-month history of progressive hoarseness.

Question 10-1

What is the next step in evaluation?
A) Reassurance.
B) Trial of omeprazole.
C) Laryngoscopy.
D) Burst of prednisone.
E) Trial of albuterol.

Discussion 10-1

The correct answer is "C." Chronic hoarseness may be related to damage to the vocal cords or abnormal vocal cord movement. It is unlikely that hoarseness lasting 6 months will spontaneously resolve. Hoarseness could be a consequence of reflux or chronic cough, but before making such assumptions, the structure and function of the vocal cords must be examined.

Question 10-2

Which of the following is the most likely risk factor for this disorder?
A) Smoking.
B) Human papillomavirus infection.
C) History of intubation for a surgical procedure.
D) Singing or prolonged vocalization.
E) Gastroesophageal reflux.

Discussion 10-2

The correct answer is "D." Although each of the listed risk factors can contribute to hoarseness, the most common cause of chronic hoarseness in children and adolescents is singing or prolonged vocalization. Think about your voice after an intense sporting event where your team won in overtime or concert. Voice trauma can happen to anyone.

Question 10-3

Vocal cord paresis or paralysis can be a complication of all the following EXCEPT:
A) C2 spinal cord transection.
B) Tracheal reconstruction.
C) Patent ductus arteriosus (PDA) ligation.
D) Chiari II malformation.
E) Thyroid surgery.

Discussion 10-3

The correct answer is "A." Vocal cord movement is controlled by the vagus nerve, which originates in the brainstem; specifically, the superior and recurrent laryngeal branches of the vagus nerve. Central nervous system lesions that increase pressure on the brainstem (eg, Chiari II malformation) may result in cranial neuropathies, including vocal cord paresis. An isolated transection of the spinal cord would not affect vocal cord movement. The left recurrent laryngeal nerve courses below the arch of the aorta. This increases its risk of damage during PDA ligation and other cardiac surgeries. Recurrent laryngeal nerves also pass along the trachea and thyroid tissues.

► CASE 11

A previously healthy 18-year-old college freshman was found unresponsive by his roommate. He recently broke up with his girlfriend. On examination, he was apneic, bradycardic, and pupils were pinpoint. SpO_2 was 90%.

Question 11-1

Which of the following venous blood gas values (pH, PCO_2, HCO_3^-, base excess) is most likely?

A) 7.54, 22, 22, 0.
B) 7.1, 80, 24, 0.
C) 7.1, 18, 12, –12.
D) 7.35, 76, 35, +10.

Discussion 11-1

The correct answer is "B." This patient has an opioid toxidrome with acute respiratory depression. This presentation could also be consistent with alcohol poisoning from binge drinking. Both cause central nervous system depression. The pinpoint pupils (miosis) are suggestive of opioid ingestion. Either way the first step would be stabilization of his cardiorespiratory status. Acute hypoventilation results in a respiratory acidosis with hypercarbia (elevated partial pressure of carbon dioxide [PCO_2]). Option "A" is respiratory alkalosis (seen with hyperventilation), option "C" is an anion gap metabolic acidosis, and option "D" is a compensated chronic respiratory acidosis (HCO_3^- and PCO_2 are elevated). (See Table 32–2.) When interpreting blood gases take a two-step approach. First, determine the primary problem. For example, respiratory acidosis causes a low pH and high PCO_2. (See Table 32–2.) Second, look for compensation. The body tries to keep a neutral status. In respiratory disorders, the kidney will change the bicarbonate (HCO_3^-) level to follow carbon dioxide (PCO_2)—both will increase or decrease. In metabolic disorders, the lungs change the PCO_2 opposite to the HCO_3^-. Mixed disorders are tough.

Helpful Tip
Oxygenation is not the same as ventilation. Ventilation controls carbon dioxide (CO_2). A pulse oximetry measurement of a normal hemoglobin oxygen saturation does not mean the CO_2 level is normal. Check the blood gases.

TABLE 32–2 PRIMARY ACID–BASE DISORDERS

	pH	PCO_2	HCO_3^-
Respiratory acidosis	↓	↑	
Metabolic acidosis	↓		↓
Respiratory alkalosis	↑	↓	
Metabolic alkalosis	↑		↑

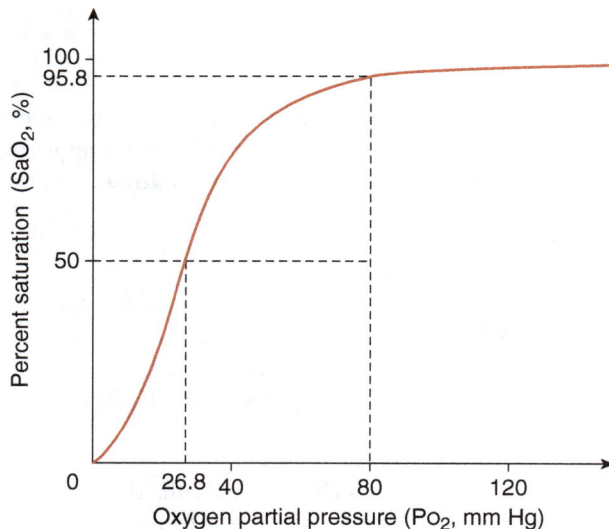

FIGURE 32–7. Oxygen hemoglobin dissociation curve. (Reproduced with permission from McKean SC, Ross JJ, Dressler DD, Brotman DJ, Ginsberg JS, eds. *Principles and Practice of Hospital Medicine.* New York, NY: McGraw-Hill Education; 2012, Fig. 83-2.)

⌛ QUICK QUIZ

Which of the following is false regarding pulse oximetry?

A) Continuous and noninvasive measurement of arterial oxygen saturation.
B) Normal and abnormal values are well defined.
C) Oxygenated hemoglobin and deoxygenated hemoglobin absorb light at different wavelengths.
D) Differences between upper and lower extremity oxygen saturation in a newborn may suggest congenital heart disease.
E) Does not detect changes in PCO_2.

Discussion

The correct answer is "B." Pulse oximetry is an easy way to detect hypoxemia. This "fifth vital sign" estimates arterial hemoglobin saturation (oxygen saturation [SpO_2]) using a probe placed on the finger. In infants, probes can be placed on palms, feet, penis, and other sites. The ratio of deoxyhemoglobin and oxyhemoglobin, each measured by the amount of light absorbed at different wavelengths, is used to estimate saturation. Nothing is perfect. The exact oxygen saturation at which tissue hypoxia occurs is unclear, so absolute normal and abnormal values do not exist. Pulse oximetry does not detect hypoventilation or hyperoxia. The hemoglobin dissociation curve is not linear; therefore, large changes in arterial partial pressure of oxygen (PaO_2) may not change in the SpO_2 if it is already near 100%. For example, the PaO_2 would have to decrease from 145 to 65 mm Hg before the SpO_2 would decrease significantly. (See Figure 32–7.)

► CASE 12

A 10-year-boy with spinal muscular atrophy type 1 is brought by his parents to the emergency department. He has had a runny nose, low-grade fever, and cough for 3 days. His parents have performed suctioning and cough assistance at home. In the emergency department, oxygen saturation (Spo_2) is 80% on room air with coarse crackles bilaterally on lung exam. A capillary blood gas analysis shows Pco_2 of 50 mm Hg.

Question 12-1

Which is the most important factor explaining the patient's hypoxemia?
A) Hypoventilation.
B) Shunting through an atrial or ventricular septal defect.
C) Ventilation-perfusion mismatch.
D) Increased physiologic dead space.
E) Hemoglobin dissociation curve shifted to the left due to acidosis.

Discussion 12-1

The correct answer is "C." The question implies that there is some degree of lung disease (pneumonia) causing ventilation-perfusion (V/Q) mismatch as well as hypoventilation (elevated Pco_2) from muscle weakness. Distinguishing the relative contributions of each process requires knowledge of both the hemoglobin dissociation curve and the alveolar gas equation. At Spo_2 of 80%, the Pao_2 (arterial oxygen level) is estimated to be 50 mm Hg based on the hemoglobin dissociation curve. In hypoxemia, the dissolved oxygen in the blood decreases. To compensate, oxygen is released from hemoglobin, resulting in decreased hemoglobin oxygen saturations. (See Figure 32–7, earlier.) At standard atmospheric pressure with no supplemental oxygen, the alveolar gas equation can be simplified to:

$$PAo_2 = 150 - Pco_2/0.8$$
$$= 150 - 50/0.8$$
$$= 150 - 62.5$$
$$= 87.5 \text{ mm Hg}$$

Estimated Pao_2	per Spo_2	50 mm Hg
Normal Pao_2	(no hypoventilation, no V/Q mismatch)	100 mm Hg
Predicted Pao_2	(hypoventilation only)	87.5 mm Hg

The alveolar gas equation estimates the oxygen level at the alveoli. In the above example, hypoventilation alone cannot explain the hypoxemia because the actual is lower than that predicted value, meaning something else is contributing. The PAo_2 (alveolar partial pressure of oxygen) is used to calculate the alveolar-arterial gradient (A-a gradient = $PAo_2 - Pao_2$). This gradient helps figure out the cause of hypoxemia. When oxygen is not transferred effectively from the alveoli to the blood the A-a gradient is elevated, such as in cases of V/Q mismatch.

> **Helpful Tip**
> Quick reference estimates from the hemoglobin dissociation curve (see Figure 32–7, earlier)

Spo_2	Pao_2
50% =	27 mm Hg
80% =	50 mm Hg

> **Helpful Tip**
> The alveolar gas equation simplifies to $PAo_2 = 150 - Pco_2/0.8$.

> **Helpful Tip**
> Normal PAo_2 is approximately 100 mm Hg.

Question 12-2

Assuming that there was no V/Q mismatch, what is the highest that the Pco_2 could be in this patient ($PAo_2 = Pao_2 = 50$ mm Hg)?
A) 50 mm Hg.
B) 65 mm Hg.
C) 80 mm Hg.
D) 100 mm Hg.
E) 120 mm Hg.

Discussion 12-2

The correct answer is "C." This can be calculated as follows:

$$PAo_2 = 150 - Pco_2/0.8$$
$$Pco_2 = 0.8 \times (150 - PAo_2) = 80 \text{ mm Hg}$$

Online calculators and smartphone apps are make it so much easier to check these values.

The patient is admitted to the intensive care unit and prescribed intravenous antibiotics.

Question 12-3

Supportive cares for the patient should include:
A) Cough assist.
B) Suctioning.
C) Bilevel positive airway pressure (BiPAP).
D) Enteral nutrition to prevent muscle catabolism.
E) All of the above.

Discussion 12-3

The correct answer is "E." Cough assist and suctioning are essential aids for airway clearance to prevent atelectasis. This patient's muscle weakness will make his cough weak and less effective. BiPAP will help maintain normal ventilation. Enteral nutrition is needed to prevent worsening weakness during prolonged periods of fasting and to meet the increased calorie needs during acute illness.

> **Helpful Tip**
> Continuous positive airway pressure (CPAP) and bilevel positive airway pressure (BiPAP) are both forms of noninvasive ventilation. BiPAP gives positive inspiratory and expiratory pressure and has a backup rate. It helps with ventilation and central apnea. CPAP gives positive expiratory pressure, helping keep the alveoli open for oxygenation and obstructive apnea.

> **Helpful Tip**
>
> Ventilation controls the carbon dioxide level in the blood. It is equal to the respiratory rate multiplied by the tidal volume (RR × VT) of each breath. Children with weakness or restrictive lung disease are rate dependent because of low VT.

► CASE 13

An 18-year-old girl with cystic fibrosis presents to an emergency department in summer with vomiting, cough, and dehydration. Her best FEV$_1$ (forced expiratory volume in 1 second) value in the last year was 60% of predicted. She was competing in a softball tournament when symptoms worsened. Vital signs are as follows: heart rate 128 bpm, respirations 28 breaths per minute, BP 115/70 mm Hg, and Spo$_2$ 90% on room air. Examination reveals bilateral inspiratory crackles, mild respiratory distress, and delayed capillary refill. The metabolic panel shows Na$^+$ 130 mEq/L, K$^+$ 3.3 mEq/L, Cl$^-$ 88, total HCO$_3^-$ 32, BUN 29, Cr 0.9, and glucose 200.

Question 13-1

What is her primary acid-base disturbance?
A) Non-anion gap metabolic acidosis.
B) Diabetic ketoacidosis.
C) Metabolic alkalosis.
D) Chronic respiratory acidosis.
E) More diagnostic information is required.

Discussion 13-1

The correct answer is "E." Her cystic fibrosis is poorly controlled. She has severe airway obstruction as evident by her low FEV$_1$. The primary acid-base disturbance cannot be defined because respiratory acidosis with compensation and metabolic alkalosis are both possible with increased total HCO$_3^-$. Children and adolescents with cystic fibrosis are at risk of developing hyponatremic, hypochloremic, metabolic alkalosis as a result of chloride loss, especially after significant perspiration (option "C"). Additionally, this patient has evidence of progressing pulmonary disease (low FEV$_1$) and is at risk of developing respiratory acidosis (option "D"). The laboratory data obtained are not consistent with metabolic acidosis (options "A" and "B") because the total HCO$_3^-$ is increased. Remember:

	pH <7.35	pH >7.45
CO$_2$ ↑	Respiratory acidosis	Metabolic alkalosis
CO$_2$ ↓	Metabolic acidosis	Respiratory alkalosis

► CASE 14

An 18-year-old boy with Duchenne muscular dystrophy comes to your clinic for regular follow-up. He is a college freshman majoring in pre-law. He has no distress on examination and lung fields are clear bilaterally. He has a forced vital capacity (FVC) of 45% of predicted and Spo$_2$ of 97% on room air. Capillary blood gas analysis shows pH 7.35, Pco$_2$ 50, HCO$_3^-$ 28, and base excess of 4. Chest X-ray shows osteopenia and restrictive changes, but no significant atelectasis.

Question 14-1

What is the next step in management?
A) Oxygen at night.
B) CPAP at night.
C) BiPAP at night.
D) Acetazolamide.
E) Tracheostomy and mechanical ventilation.

Discussion 14-1

The correct answer is "C." Duchene muscular dystrophy is a progressive disease that results in restrictive lung disease (low FVC) because of decreased ability to open up the lungs resulting from a combination of weak respiratory muscles and acquired scoliosis. The patient described has chronic respiratory failure due to neuromuscular weakness. His Pco$_2$ is elevated with metabolic compensation (elevated HCO$_3^-$). Nighttime BiPAP will improve tidal volume and ventilation related to neuromuscular weakness. CPAP can help overcome upper airway obstruction but it will not improve hypoventilation related to muscle weakness. Acetazolamide is a carbonic anhydrase inhibitor that can reduce bicarbonate levels but does not help the underlying problem of hypoventilation. Tracheostomy is not necessary and has the potential to interfere with the ability to speak. His oxygenation status is fine, with a normal Spo$_2$.

► CASE 15

An 18-year-old boy has acute shortness of breath and left-sided chest pain with inspiration after being involved in a motor vehicle collision. He is tachypneic, lightheaded, and unable to take deep breaths. Vital signs are temperature 36.5°C (97.7°F), heart rate 140 bpm, respirations 45 breaths per minute, BP 90/50 mm Hg, and Spo$_2$ 90%. Chest auscultation reveals absent breath sound on the left side and tympanic sounds on percussion.

Question 15-1

What is the next step in management?
A) Needle thoracostomy.
B) Chest X-ray.
C) Subcutaneous enoxaparin.
D) Intravenous heparin.
E) Albuterol by continuous nebulizer.

Discussion 15-1

The correct answer is "A." By clinical examination, the patient has a tension pneumothorax, which is causing respiratory failure and obstructive shock. The patient should be immediately stabilized by needle thoracostomy, without awaiting further diagnostic studies. Options "C" and "D" allude to the possibility of pulmonary embolism, but there is clear evidence of pneumothorax on examination. (See Figure 32–8.)

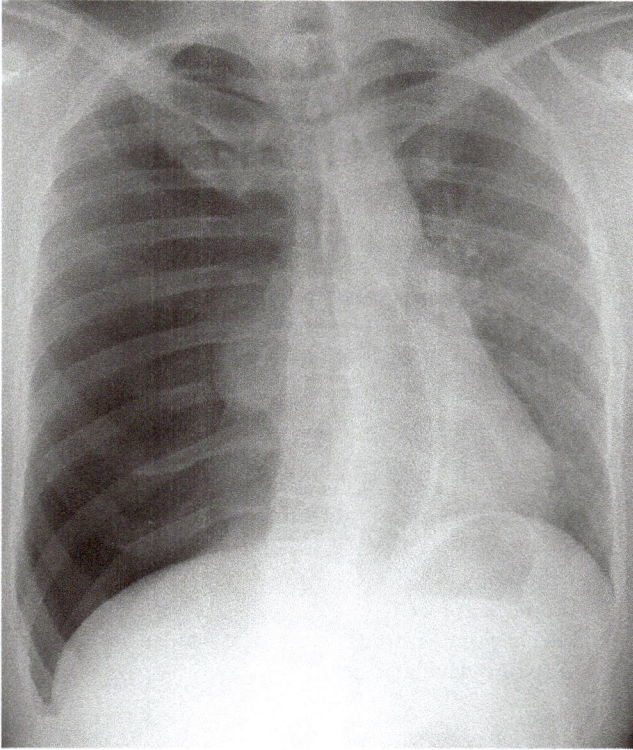

FIGURE 32–8. Tension pneumothorax. On the right side, there is free air outside the lung with flattening of the diaphragm. The mediastinum is shifted to the left. (Reproduced with permission from McKean SC, Ross JJ, Dressler DD, Brotman DJ, Ginsberg JS, eds. *Principles and Practice of Hospital Medicine*. New York, NY: McGraw-Hill Education; 2012, Fig. 107-7.)

⏳ QUICK QUIZ

Which of the following is true regarding tachypnea?
A) Equals a respiratory rate greater than 20 for children 5 to 10 years of age.
B) Definition varies by age.
C) Equals a respiratory rate greater than 50 for newborns.
D) Respiratory rate should be counted for a full 30 seconds.
E) Just look at the child (who needs to count?).

Discussion

The correct answer is "A." Tachypnea varies by age. (See Table 32–3.) Respiratory rate should be counted over a full minute. Determining the actual respiratory rate is important.

TABLE 32-3 NORMAL RESPIRATORY RATES BY AGE	
Age	Normal Respiratory Rate (breaths per minute)
Infant	30–60
Toddler	25–40
Child	20–30
Adolescent	12–16

▶ CASE 16

A 4-year-old girl has had a chronic dry cough lasting 3 months that occurs both in the day and at night. She has had two prior acute care visits for the cough and was diagnosed with an upper respiratory infection. She also has had two prior hospitalizations for wheezing illnesses and has atopic dermatitis.

Question 16-1

What do you recommend for the cough?
A) Montelukast.
B) Bronchoscopy.
C) Albuterol as needed.
D) Inhaled beclomethasone, albuterol as needed.
E) Amoxicillin-clavulanic acid.

Discussion 16-1

The correct answer is "D." Asthma is a *chronic* inflammatory disease of the lungs with reversible bronchospasm. Inflammation means steroids will help. The patient described has persistent or chronic asthma, likely with an allergic basis. Instead of wheezing, cough is her predominant symptom, often referred to as "cough variant" asthma. Albuterol alone would not alter the inflammatory component of the child's asthma, so addition of an inhaled corticosteroid is necessary. Leukotriene receptor antagonists such as montelukast are generally less effective than inhaled corticosteroids. Bronchoscopy may be necessary if there is not an adequate response to a trial of asthma therapy. Amoxicillin-clavulanic helps resolve cough due to protracted bacterial bronchitis, which is usually a wet or productive cough.

Question 16-2

Which is NOT consistent with persistent asthma?
A) Wheezing 3 days or more during the week.
B) Waking up at night weekly.
C) Never needing albuterol.
D) Cannot play tag with friends.
E) Decreased FEV_1 on lung function tests.

Discussion 16-2

The correct answer is "C." Asthma management has two parts: (1) making the diagnosis and (2) long-term control. Symptoms must be recurrent—wheezing, cough, shortness of breath, or a combination of these. Symptoms occur at night or worsen with exposure to triggers (viral infections, exercise, irritant exposure, allergen exposure). Once diagnosed, the next step is to determine the severity—intermittent or persistent. If asthma is persistent a daily preventive medication is needed. Remember the rule of 2s to decide if asthma is intermittent or persistent. Asthma is persistent if any of the following are present: (1) daytime symptoms occur 2 or more days per week, (2) nighttime symptoms occur 2 or more times per month, (3) albuterol is needed 2 or more days per week, and (4) normal activity is impaired in some way. Lung function tests (FEV_1) may also be used. At follow-up visits, asthma control becomes the focus. Finally, do not forget the asthma action plan; ensure that the girl and her family understand the details of the plan, including medication use and when to seek medical care for worsening symptoms.

► CASE 17

The girl returns to your office in January. She has had a runny nose, cough, and fever. Over the past 24 hours, breathing has become increasingly difficult. Albuterol helps but only for a short time period and does not completely relieve the symptoms. On exam, her vital signs are heart rate 160 bpm, respirations 45 breaths per minute, and SpO_2 of 88%. On exam she has retractions, nasal flaring, abdominal breathing, decreased breath sounds, and faint expiratory wheezes.

Question 17-1

What should you do next?
A) Administer albuterol.
B) Administer oxygen if SpO_2 remains low after albuterol.
C) Give systemic steroids.
D) Consider hospital admission.
E) All of the above.

Discussion 17-1

The correct answer is "E." She is having an acute asthma exacerbation. Common triggers include viral respiratory tract infections, exercise, allergen exposure, and smoke exposure. Symptoms that do not respond to bronchodilators are called status asthmaticus. In this child, wheezing is minimal as her air movement is poor. This is a bad sign. With improved air flow, her wheezing may get louder. Albuterol is a beta$_2$-receptor agonist that causes bronchodilation by relaxing the bronchial smooth muscle. It is used for acute symptom relief and improving air flow. The true game changer is systemic steroids. Remember, this is also an inflammatory process. Steroids take time to work, so give them early.

> **Helpful Tip**
> A normal PCO_2 on blood gas analysis in a patient with an acute asthma exacerbation is a sign of impending failure. The CO_2 should be low from hyperventilation. Normalizing may be a sign of impending respiratory failure or "wearing out."

Question 17-2

What would be expected on chest X-ray during an asthma exacerbation?
A) Widened mediastinum.
B) Pleural effusion.
C) Underinflated lungs.
D) Peribronchial thickening.
E) Getting a radiograph is silly.

Discussion 17-2

The correct answer is "D." Asthma is an obstructive pulmonary process. The air gets trapped in the lungs leading to

hyperinflation. Radiographs show flattened diaphragm, retrocardiac air, and a narrow mediastinum as the lungs are overinflated like balloons. Option "E" is also correct as a chest X-ray is not typically needed. Radiographs may be indicated in patients with suspected asthma complications like pneumothorax.

► CASE 18

A 2-year-old boy has a chronic wet-sounding cough lasting 3 months that occurs both in the day and at night. Systemic steroids and inhaled albuterol have not improved the cough. Last year, he had a longstanding cough that fully resolved when he was being treated for a concurrent ear infection.

Question 18-1

What do you recommend for his cough?
A) Montelukast.
B) Bronchoscopy.
C) Albuterol as needed.
D) Inhaled beclomethasone, albuterol as needed.
E) Amoxicillin-clavulanic acid.

Discussion 18-1

The correct answer is "E." The boy has a chronic cough as it has been present for over 1 month. This vignette describes features of protracted bacterial bronchitis, which results from chronic lower airway inflammation and infection by *Streptococcus pneumonia*, *Haemophilus influenzae*, or *Moraxella catarrhalis*. Protracted bacterial bronchitis often occurs in association with tracheomalacia or bronchomalacia. Typically children younger than 5 years of age are affected and have a chronic wet cough but are otherwise well. Symptoms resolved with antibiotic treatment. It is important to rule out other causes of chronic cough, such as cystic fibrosis. (See Table 32–4.) The patient has not responded to albuterol or steroids in the past, so asthma is unlikely. A bronchoscopy may be necessary if response to treatment with amoxicillin-clavulanic acid is not adequate. Consider immunodeficiency evaluation as recurrent sinopulmonary infections is a sign of an underlying immunodeficiency.

► CASE 19

An 18-year-old boy who plays soccer feels short of breath during both practices and competitions. He has no chest pain, palpitations, wheezing, cough, or stridor. Spirometry and baseline electrocardiogram (ECG) are within normal limits. On treadmill testing, he reaches a maximum heart rate of 200 bpm and his oxygen consumption (VO_2) at maximal effort is 130% of predicted. Oxygen saturations are normal, and dead space ventilation is decreased with exercise. There is no airflow obstruction during or after exercise. An anaerobic threshold is detected at 65% of his maximum VO_2. His shortness of breath is reproduced during the later portions of the study.

TABLE 32–4 CAUSES OF CHRONIC COUGH

Asthma	• Most common • Personal or family history of atopy • Recurrent episodes triggered by viral URIs • Exercise intolerance • Nocturnal symptoms • Resolves with albuterol and steroids
Foreign body	• History of choking episode (not always) • Asymmetric breath sounds on exam (not always) • Atelectasis or hyperinflation in one area on chest X-ray
Protracted bacterial bronchitis	• Wet cough • Child looks well • Young children • Resolves with antibiotics
Psychogenic "habit"	• Brassy sounding • May follow a viral URI • Possible associated throat clearing • Annoying to others • Key: not present once asleep
Pertussis (whooping cough)	• Paroxysms of dry cough • Known as the 100-day cough • Classic inspiratory whoop (not always) • Posttussive emesis • Deficient immunizations • Improves over time • Antibiotics do not make cough go away
Prolonged infection	• *Mycoplasma pneumoniae* • *Chlamydia pneumoniae* • Influenza
Cystic fibrosis	• Poor growth • Productive cough • Diagnosed by sweat chloride test • Can be detected on newborn metabolic screening
Immunodeficiency	• Recurrent sinopulmonary infections • Atypical or severe infections • Poor growth
Tracheomalacia	• Symptoms may be worse supine • Hypoxemia and obstructive apnea may occur • Monophonic wheeze on exam

URI, upper respiratory tract infection.

Question 19-1

Which of the following explains his shortness of breath?
A) Metabolic acidosis.
B) Pulmonary vascular disease.
C) Interstitial lung disease.
D) Vocal cord dysfunction.
E) Exercise-induced asthma.
F) Mitral insufficiency.

Discussion 19-1

The correct answer is "A." The athlete described in this vignette has above-average performance on exercise testing and reached his physiologic limitation. Exercise above the anaerobic threshold causes a lactic acidosis, which intensifies the feeling of shortness of breath. Pulmonary vascular disease and interstitial lung diseases should cause hypoxemia. Dead space normally decreases during exercise due to larger tidal volumes (deep breaths). Exercise-induced asthma and vocal cord dysfunction are ruled out by the lack of airway obstruction on inspiration and exhalation. Physiologically significant mitral insufficiency would decrease VO_2 relative to the heart rate and may reduce oxygen saturation. Basically, he is in great shape but must accept he may not be professional athlete material.

▶ CASE 20

A 16-year-old female runner feels short of breath during competitions. A loud inspiratory noise has caused her to miss several track meets. She has no chest pain, palpitations, or wheezing. Spirometry and baseline electrocardiogram (ECG) are within normal limits. On treadmill testing, she reaches a maximum heart rate of 187 bpm and her VO_2 at maximal effort is 100% of predicted. Inspiratory flow limitation and stridor occur near maximal effort.

Question 20-1

What is the most likely diagnosis?
A) Pulmonary hypertension.
B) Interstitial lung disease.
C) Vocal cord dysfunction.
D) Exercise-induced asthma.
E) Cardiomyopathy.

Discussion 20-1

The correct answer is "C." This athlete most likely suffers from vocal cord dysfunction triggered by exercise (a well-known trigger). The vocal cords adduct with inspiration when they should not, causing chest or throat tightness, cough, dyspnea, and stridor. The condition is often misdiagnosed as asthma. Girls are predominately affected, and academic, social, or athletic stressors are typically present. The presentation may be dramatic, resulting in unnecessary invasive procedures such as emergency tracheostomy. Laryngoscopy can confirm the diagnosis. Speech therapy and patient education are the mainstays of treatment. (Did you know this condition was first called "hysteric croup," reflecting the thought that a woman in a fit of hysteria could cause the dysfunction?)

► CASE 21

A 18-year-old boy is undergoing treatment for Hodgkin lymphoma. He is an avid tennis player but has diminished exercise tolerance. He informs you that he has a higher than normal resting heart rate and that he reaches a maximum heart rate of 200 bpm during vigorous exercise.

Question 21-1

Which of the following is NOT consistent with his heart response during exercise?
A) Large airway obstruction related to mediastinal lymphadenopathy.
B) Valvular heart disease.
C) Anemia.
D) Deconditioning.
E) Peripheral myopathy related to chemotherapy.

Discussion 21-1

The correct answer is "A." Patients with a pulmonary limitation to exercise become short of breath before they can achieve a high heart rate. The maximum heart rate expected is approximately 220 bpm minus age in years. The other causes listed would not be expected to impair heart rate response to exercise. Anemia, valvular heart disease, and deconditioning cause less oxygen to be delivered per heartbeat. Peripheral myopathy may decrease the efficiency of work, but should not affect the heart rate response.

⏳ QUICK QUIZ

Which of the following disorders is more strongly associated with obstructive sleep apnea compared with central sleep apnea?
A) Prematurity.
B) Opioid mediations.
C) *PHOX2B* mutations.
D) Heart failure.
E) Congenital hypothyroidism.
F) Pierre Robin sequence.

Discussion

The correct answer is "F." Pierre Robin sequence (small jaw, posteriorly displaced tongue, cleft palate) results in airway obstruction. When the brain does not tell the body to breath central apnea occurs. Prematurity, central nervous system depressants, heart failure, *PHOX2B* mutations, and congenital hypothyroidism are all associated with central sleep apnea. *PHOX2B* mutations cause congenital central hypoventilation syndrome (the so-called Ondine curse).

► CASE 22

The waveforms below represent a 20-second interval obtained during monitoring of a hospitalized patient.

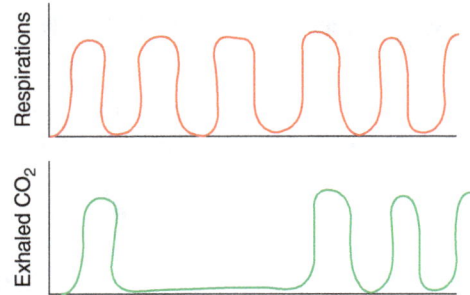

Question 22-1

Which of the following is present?
A) Obstructive apnea.
B) Central apnea.
C) Sighing respiration.
D) Desaturation.
E) None of the above; the waveforms are normal.

Discussion 22-1

The correct answer is "A." No CO_2 is exhaled on the second and third breaths, despite evidence of respiratory effort. This implies obstructive apnea. Central apnea would be characterized by concurrent lack of respiratory effort. Ask if the chest is moving when the child or infant is not breathing. In patients with obstruction, the brain is telling the body to breath, so the chest is moving but the air does not flow.

► CASE 23

A full-term neonate has recurrent apneic spells without noisy breathing or other symptoms of obstruction.

Question 23-1

Which of the following tests should you obtain first?
A) EEG.
B) Bronchoscopy.
C) Capillary blood gas analysis.
D) Polysomnogram.
E) Esophageal pH study.

Discussion 23-1

The correct answer is "C." A basic laboratory evaluation should begin prior to ordering expensive tests. Possible reasons for apnea could include infection, metabolic disorders, or impaired control of breathing. A capillary blood gas analysis can be obtained more quickly than the other studies and may indicate whether there is an acid-base disorder or impaired regulation of ventilation. Bronchoscopy would be useful in the evaluation of suspected airway obstruction, but this infant's history suggests central apnea. Polysomnography would allow for definitive diagnosis of either central or obstructive sleep apnea.

► CASE 24

A 6-year-old boy has obstructive sleep apnea (OSA) with an apnea-hypopnea index (AHI) of 10. His parents are concerned that his classroom performance may be affected by his sleep apnea.

Question 24-1

You advise:

A) Adenotonsillectomy is likely to lower his AHI.
B) Adenotonsillectomy will improve his neurocognitive performance.
C) His sleep apnea will not improve spontaneously with watchful waiting.
D) CPAP will improve neurocognitive performance.
E) None of the above.

Discussion 24-1

The correct answer is "A." In OSA, the upper airway becomes obstructed during sleep. Sleep is disrupted, which may lead to behavioral problems. Signs and symptoms of OSA are listed in Table 32–5. A randomized controlled trial of adenotonsillectomy versus watchful waiting showed that adenotonsillectomy does decrease AHI on average, but this was not associated with an improvement in performance on a neurocognitive testing. In many children, there was spontaneous improvement in sleep apnea.

> **Helpful Tip**
> The apnea-hypopnea index (AHI) is determined during a sleep study. It is calculated as the total number of episodes of apnea and hypopnea divided by the hours of sleep. An AHI of greater than 1 episode per hour of sleep is consistent with OSA.

⧗ QUICK QUIZ

How is OSA diagnosed?

A) History alone.
B) History and tonsillar hypertrophy on exam.
C) Polysomnography.
D) Body mass index.
E) Family members need ear plugs to sleep in the child's vicinity.

TABLE 32–5 SIGNS AND SYMPTOMS OF OBSTRUCTIVE SLEEP APNEA

Symptoms	Signs
Frequent snoring (≥ 3 nights/week)	Enlarged tonsils
Gasping breaths	Facial deformities such as micrognathia
Sleep enuresis	Failure to thrive
Daytime sleepiness	Underweight
Headaches	Overweight or obese
Learning difficulties	Pulmonary hypertension
Hyperactivity/attention problems	

Discussion

The correct answer is "C." History and physical exam are good screening tools. Snoring especially with viral respiratory infections is normal and common. The key is frequent (≥ 3 nights/week) snoring and other signs and symptoms. The exam may be normal. When it comes to the tonsils, size does not matter! If OSA is suspected, the gold standard test is a sleep study (polysomnography), which will decide if OSA is present and if so how severe it is.

Question 24-2

Which of the following ventilator settings is most appropriate for a child who has central sleep apnea? (CPAP is continuous positive airway pressure, IPAP is inspiratory positive airway pressure, EPAP is expiratory positive airway pressure, rate refers to respiratory rate, and V_T is tidal volume. CPAP, IPAP, and EPAP are measured as cm H_2O.)

A) CPAP 6.
B) IPAP 14, EPAP 5.
C) IPAP 14, EPAP 5, with 2 L/min of oxygen (O_2).
D) IPAP 14, EPAP 5, rate 20.
E) Volume control, V_T 10 mL/kg of body weight, high pressure limit 20 cm H_2O.

Discussion 24-2

The correct answer is "D." This is the only selection that has a mandatory rate. In central apnea, a rate is needed to guarantee the child takes the needed number of breaths. The machine has to take over for the brain's dysfunctional respiratory drive. CPAP will not supply a rate, and BiPAP alone (options "B" and "C") relies on the patient's respiratory effort (ie, self-generated respiratory rate) to trigger the ventilator. Option "E" uses volume control, which would be more affected by leaks or disconnection. Moreover, there is also no rate given for choice E.

▶ CASE 25

An 18-year-old girl with cystic fibrosis (FEV_1 50% of predicted value) has bronchiectasis involving the right and left upper lobes.

Question 25-1

Which of the following organisms is the most likely to be chronically colonizing her airways?

A) *Staphylococcus aureus.*
B) *Pseudomonas aeruginosa.*
C) *Burkholderia cepacia.*
D) *Achromobacter xylosoxidans.*
E) *Stenotrophomonas maltophilia.*

Discussion 25-1

The correct answer is "B." Cystic fibrosis (CF) is an autosomal recessive genetic condition resulting in dysfunction of the cystic fibrosis transmembrane regulator (CFTR) protein. The CFTR protein controls the chloride channels in the lungs, pancreas, intestine, and skin. Secretions become thick and are difficult to clear. In the lungs, this leads to chronic infection, inflammation, and progressive airway obstruction (low FEV_1). In CF, the lungs are colonized with weird bacteria (all the listed options) that are specific to CF. By age 18 years, the most common CF airway pathogen is *P. aeruginosa*. In early childhood, *S. aureus* is more common.

Question 25-2

Which of the following pathogens is NOT commonly identified in sputum from patients with bronchiectasis due to cystic fibrosis?

A) *Staphylococcus aureus.*
B) *Pseudomonas aeruginosa.*
C) *Burkholderia cenocepacia.*
D) *Neisseria meningitidis.*
E) *Stenotrophomonas maltophilia.*
F) *Aspergillus fumigatus.*
G) *Mycobacterium abscessus.*

Discussion 25-2

The correct answer is "D." It probably is unfair to list seven instead of five choices. Consider it a test to see if you are paying attention. *N. meningitidis* would not routinely be isolated from CF sputum. The other species listed are regularly seen in CF sputum samples. *Red flag alert:* Finding these bacteria in the lungs is not normal. It means that some underlying disease process is present. Think CF, ventilator-associated pneumonia, or immunodeficiency. Utilize those health care dollars and order diagnostic tests!

Question 25-3

CF lung disease is characterized by all of the following radiologic abnormalities EXCEPT:

A) Bronchial wall thickening.
B) Air trapping.
C) Atelectasis.
D) Bronchiectasis.
E) Pleural effusion.

Discussion 25-3

The correct answer is "E." CF is a progressive disease. Eventually the airways and lungs are damaged and respiratory failure occurs. Early CF disease primarily affects conducting airways. Mucus plugging may result in focal areas of atelectasis and air trapping (hyperinflation). Inflammation can lead to bronchial wall thickening and bronchiectasis. Pneumothorax and pneumomediastinum can occur.

▶ CASE 26

A 17-year-old boy with CF (FEV_1 30% of predicted value) is hospitalized for pulmonary exacerbation. He produces over 200 mL of bright red blood after coughing.

Question 26-1

What is the most likely source of the blood?

A) Alveolar hemorrhage.
B) Branch pulmonary artery.
C) Bronchial artery.
D) Submucosal vessels.
E) Esophageal varices.

Discussion 26-1

The correct answer is "C." CF patients with bronchiectasis are at risk of hemoptysis from hemorrhage of dilated bronchial arteries. This can be life threatening because (1) the bleeding is rapid, owing to the bronchial arteries being under systemic pressure, and (2) there is the possibility for airway compromise. Blood pouring into your airways is not good. Alveolar hemorrhage would be more characteristic of idiopathic pulmonary hemosiderosis. Esophageal variceal bleeding presenting as hematemesis can also occur in patients with CF as a result of portal hypertension secondary to CF-associated liver disease.

Question 26-2

Management of this patient's hemoptysis should include:

A) Correction of vitamin K deficit.
B) Discontinuation of ibuprofen.
C) Consultation of interventional radiology.
D) Temporarily ceasing chest physiotherapy.
E) All of the above.

Discussion 26-2

The correct answer is "E." Correcting any underlying coagulopathy is essential. Bronchial artery embolization by interventional radiology may be required if there is life-threatening hemoptysis. Obviously giving a medication (NSAID) that interferes with platelet function is not a good idea when a patient is hemorrhaging, nor is shaking and pounding on the chest.

▶ CASE 27

A 14-year-old girl with CF (FEV_1 70% of predicted value) is hospitalized for pulmonary exacerbation with methicillin-resistant *Staphylococcus aureus* (MRSA) and mucoid *Pseudomonas aeruginosa*. She is receiving vancomycin, tobramycin, trimethoprim-sulfamethoxazole, and ceftazidime. During treatment, she develops severe abdominal pain, distension, and fever. Examination reveals tachycardia and a diffusely firm and tender abdomen with rebound tenderness.

Question 27-1

Which of the following complications is most likely?

A) *Clostridium difficile* colitis.
B) Distal intestinal obstruction syndrome.
C) Fibrosing colonopathy.
D) Appendicitis.
E) Nephrolithiasis.

Discussion 27-1

The correct answer is "A." Patients with CF commonly receive broad-spectrum antibiotics and run a higher than ordinary risk of *C. difficile* colitis. In CF, pulmonary exacerbations characterized by worsening symptoms and decrease in pulmonary function on testing occur. Patients may be hospitalized depending on the severity. Treatment includes aggressive therapies such as chest physiotherapy to increase mucociliary clearance and systemic antibiotics.

QUICK QUIZ

Which of the following is a manifestation of CF?
A) Rectal prolapse.
B) Nasal polyps.
C) Diabetes.
D) Intestinal obstruction.
E) All of the above.

Discussion

The correct answer is "E." The hallmarks of CF are chronic obstructive lung disease, pancreatic insufficiency, and salty sweat, but there are a multitude of other manifestations. Options "A" and "B" should make you wonder about CF. In CF, the pancreatic duct is plugged, resulting in fat malabsorption, diarrhea, and vitamin deficiencies (ADEK). Endocrine function can be impaired, resulting in CF-related diabetes mellitus. Intestinal obstruction may occur in newborns as meconium ileus or in older children as distal intestinal obstructive syndrome. Sodium and chloride are lost through sweat, which may cause hyponatremic, hypochloremic metabolic alkalosis. Clinical manifestations, especially if pancreatic function is normal, may not present until adulthood. (See Table 32–6.)

▶ CASE 28

A patient of yours recently became pregnant. Her older brother has CF. The father of the child is Caucasian.

Question 28-1

What is the probability that her child will carry at least one *CFTR* mutation?
A) 1 in 3.
B) 1 in 4.
C) 1 in 25.
D) 1 in 75.
E) 1 in 2500.

Discussion 28-1

The correct answer is "A." Because your patient does not have CF, the only remaining possibilities are wild-type (normal CFTR protein present) or carrier. Therefore, there is a 2 in 3 chance she is a carrier (see the Punnett square below). Of the children without CF, two will be carriers and one will not. There is a 50% chance this mutation will be passed to her child. Thus, the chance that her child will be a carrier is $^2/_3 \times ^1/_2 = ^1/_3$.

TABLE 32–6 CLINICAL FEATURES OF CYSTIC FIBROSIS

Respiratory
- Chronic cough (productive)
- Chronic respiratory infections
- Nasal polyps
- Chronic pansinusitis
- Clubbing
- Pneumothorax
- Pneumomediastinum
- Pulmonary hemorrhage

Intestinal
- Meconium ileus
- Distal intestinal obstruction syndrome (DIOS)
- Rectal prolapse
- Biliary cirrhosis
- Cirrhosis with portal hypertension
- Malabsorption
- Greasy, foul-smelling stools
- Fat-soluble vitamin deficiency
- Pancreatitis

Other
- Diabetes or hyperglycemia
- Failure to thrive
- Hyponatremic, hypochloremic metabolic alkalosis
- Male infertility (absent vas deferens, normal sperm production)

	Father	
	CFTR+	CFTR–
Mother CFTR+	Wild-type (normal)	Carrier
CFTR–	Carrier	CF

Question 28-2

What is the probability that the child will have CF?
A) 1 in 3.
B) 1 in 4.
C) 1 in 75.
D) 1 in 150.
E) 1 in 2500.

Discussion 28-2

The correct answer is "D." The allele frequency of *CFTR* mutations in the Caucasian population is approximately 1 in 25. There is a 1 in 3 chance the child will inherit a mutation from the mother (see Question 28-1). There is a 1 in 25 chance the father is a carrier. There is a 1 in 2 chance a paternal mutation would be transmitted to the child. Therefore, the probability the child will have CF is $P = \frac{1}{3} \times \frac{1}{25} \times \frac{1}{2} = \frac{1}{150}$.

▶ CASE 29

A newborn child is identified by newborn screen as having an elevated immunoreactive trypsinogen level of 70 nanogram (ng)/mL and a single copy of *CFTR*-ΔF508 mutation.

Question 29-1

What is the next step?
A) Prescribe pancreatic enzymes.
B) Order full sequencing of *CFTR*.
C) Start fat-soluble vitamin supplementation.
D) Perform diagnostic sweat chloride testing.
E) Reassure the family that a false-positive newborn screen is common.

Discussion 29-1

The correct answer is "D." Infants with CF will typically have elevated blood levels of immunoreactive trypsinogen (IRT). If elevated, the next step is to test for CF gene mutations. If IRT is elevated and mutations are present, sweat chloride testing is done. If sweat chloride is 60 mEq/L or greater on two samples, the diagnosis is confirmed. Pancreatic enzymes and fat-soluble vitamins may not be necessary even in a patient with CF if there is enough residual CFTR function to permit pancreatic sufficiency. Although there are false-positive results of newborn screening, it is not appropriate to reassure the parents until more information is known.

▶ CASE 30

An asymptomatic newborn child is identified as having two deleterious *CFTR* mutations, ΔF508 and Q890X. However, sweat chloride values are not diagnostic for CF (28 and 32 mEq/L).

Question 30-1

Which of the following tests may explain this apparent discrepancy?
A) Repeat sweat testing.
B) Repeat genotype of the child.
C) Genotype parents of the child for these mutations.
D) Perform nasal potential difference testing.
E) None of the above.

Discussion 30-1

The correct answer is "C." Many different mutations of the *CFTR* genes exist. The two *CFTR* mutations are either *cis* (on the same chromosome) or *trans* (on opposite chromosomes). If the mutations are in *trans*, then the patient would likely have CF. To distinguish between these possibilities, genotyping of the parents should be done. If one parent possesses both mutations and does not have CF, then the two mutations exist on the same

chromosome. To have CF, the mutations must be on different chromosomes (*trans*). If both mutations are on the same chromosome (*cis*), the patient is essentially a CF carrier. Clear as mud?

Question 30-2

Which of the following gastrointestinal complications of CF is least likely to occur in infancy?
A) Direct hyperbilirubinemia.
B) Fibrosing colonopathy.
C) Malabsorption.
D) Growth failure.
E) Intestinal obstruction.

Discussion 30-2

The correct answer is "B." Fibrosing colonopathy can occur if pancreatic enzyme therapy is dosed at inappropriately high levels. This would not be expected in the infantile period. All of the other disorders are complications that can be attributed to loss of CFTR protein in hepatobiliary, pancreatic duct, or intestinal epithelial cells.

Question 30-3

Which of the following adulthood complications of CF does NOT occur as a consequence of antibiotic therapy?
A) Male infertility.
B) Hearing loss.
C) Chronic renal failure.
D) Drug-resistant microorganisms.
E) All of the above.

Discussion 30-3

The correct answer is "A." Male infertility is secondary to bilateral obstruction and obliteration of the vas deferens during fetal development. Spermatogenesis is normal. Hearing loss, chronic renal failure, and drug-resistant microorganisms all occur as consequences of antibiotic therapy.

Question 30-4

Which of the following is characteristic of primary ciliary dyskinesia (immotile-cilia syndrome) but NOT CF?
A) Bronchiectasis.
B) Impaired mucociliary transport.
C) Diminished fertility.
D) Decreased nasal nitric oxide.
E) Recurrent sinopulmonary infections.

Discussion 30-4

The correct answer is "D." Nasal nitric oxide is a useful non-invasive screening test for primary ciliary dyskinesia (PCD), because patients with PCD have abnormally low exhaled nitric oxide. This is not true of patients with CF. Both CF and PCD predispose patients to bronchiectasis, abnormal mucociliary transport, decreased fertility, and recurrent sinopulmonary infections. The upper and lower respiratory tract epithelium is lined with small hairlike organelles called cilia. Cilia beat to help clear the airways (mucociliary clearance). In PCD, the person is born with defective cilia. Impaired sperm motility and ovum transit down the fallopian tubes can occur causing infertility. Both CF patients and those with PCD share the impaired ability to clear respiratory secretions; therefore, clinical manifestations overlap. But unlike patients with CF, those with PCD commonly present in the newborn period.

> **Helpful Tip**
>
> Kartagener syndrome, a subgroup of PCD, results in the triad of situs inversus, chronic sinusitis, and bronchiectasis.

Question 30-5

Which of the following is characteristic of CF but NOT primary ciliary dyskinesia?
A) Mutations are linked to a single gene.
B) Situs inversus.
C) Abnormal microtubule structure.
D) Susceptibility to hydrocephalus.
E) Hypochloremic metabolic acidosis.

Discussion 30-5

The correct answer is "A." CF is caused by mutations in a single gene (*CFTR*). PCD may be linked to hundreds of different genes that encode ciliary structures. PCD is associated with hydrocephalus and lateralization defects such as situs inversus (heart and abdominal organs are reversed, transposed, or duplicated). Patients with CF have chloride loss and are at increased risk of hypochloremic metabolic alkalosis.

QUICK QUIZ

Which of the following causes of pulmonary hypertension is most likely to be alleviated by nighttime ventilation?
A) Sickle cell disease.
B) Restrictive lung disease from thoracic deformity.
C) ANCA-positive vasculitis.
D) Eisenmenger syndrome.
E) Chronic thromboembolic disease.

Discussion

The correct answer is "B." Restrictive lung diseases caused by thoracic deformity can result in nighttime hypoventilation, which can then lead to pulmonary hypertension. The other diseases listed all can cause pulmonary hypertension, but do not have hypoventilation as a pathophysiologic mechanism.

QUICK QUIZ

Which of the following is most consistent with our current understanding of congenital airway malformations?
A) Potter sequence—arrest in the development of bronchial tree.

B) Extralobar pulmonary sequestration—accessory bud from the foregut gives rise to lung tissue not connected to the tracheobronchial tree and receives its blood supply from the systemic circulation.
C) Congenital pulmonary airway malformation—renal agenesis leads to oligohydramnios and pulmonary hypoplasia.
D) Congenital lobar emphysema—developing bronchus separates to form a noncommunicating cyst.
E) Bronchogenic cyst—partial bronchial obstruction, creating ball valve effect.

Discussion

The correct answer is "B." Pulmonary sequestrations do arise from accessory buds from the foregut. The Potter sequence arises from renal agenesis and oligohydramnios, causing pulmonary hypoplasia and flattened facies. Congenital pulmonary airway malformations (CCAM) are thought to occur due to arrested development of the bronchial tree. Congenital lobar emphysema develops as a result of partial obstruction, causing lobar hyperinflation. Bronchogenic cysts occur when a developing bronchus separates to form a cyst.

▶ CASE 31

A child who recently underwent surgery for congenital heart disease develops a left-sided pleural effusion. The color is white, the cell count is predominantly lymphocytes, and there is a high concentration of cholesterol.

Question 31-1

Why is there an effusion?
A) Transudative fluid movement due to elevated pulmonary venous pressure.
B) Transudative fluid movement due to protein-losing enteropathy.
C) Transudative fluid movement due to malnutrition.
D) Exudative process due to infection and capillary leak.
E) Chylous effusion due to injury of the thoracic duct.

Discussion 31-1

The correct answer is "E." The patient has a chylothorax, which is a common complication of surgery to repair congenital heart defects. The thoracic duct is injured, spilling lymph fluid (chyle) from the intestines into the chest. Chyle contains lymphocytes and is milky white from the high concentration of triglycerides. Test the fluid for triglycerides! Not allowing the patient to eat should decrease the effusion. If the patient is eating, the diet should be low fat and long-chain triglycerides (LCTs) should be excluded. Medium-chain triglycerides (MCTs), unlike LCTs, are directly absorbed in the bloodstream rather than transported by the lymphatics. Infant formulas high in MCTs and low in LCTs are commercially available; an alternative is to supplement with MCT oil.

⧖ QUICK QUIZ

All of the following are risk factors for sudden infant death syndrome (SIDS) EXCEPT:
A) Prematurity.
B) Smoke exposure.
C) Sleeping on a couch or in the parents' bed.
D) Sleeping in the supine position.
E) Cushioned pads lining the infant's crib.

Discussion

The correct answer is "D." SIDS is defined as the death of an infant that cannot be explained after examination of the death scene and autopsy. Since institution of "Back to Sleep" recommendations, the incidence of SIDS has decreased in the United States. Prematurity, smoke exposure, and unsafe sleep conditions have all been implicated as risk factors for infant death. Sleeping in baby slings, swings, and or car seats is not safe. Breastfeeding and pacifier use is protective. (Go, binkies!)

> **Helpful Tip**
> Sleeping supine to prevent SIDS does not increase the risk of choking and aspiration in infants, even those with gastroesophageal reflux. Elevation of the head of bed does not decrease reflux in infants and is not recommended.

▶ CASE 32

You are demonstrating pulmonary function tests to a group of medical students.

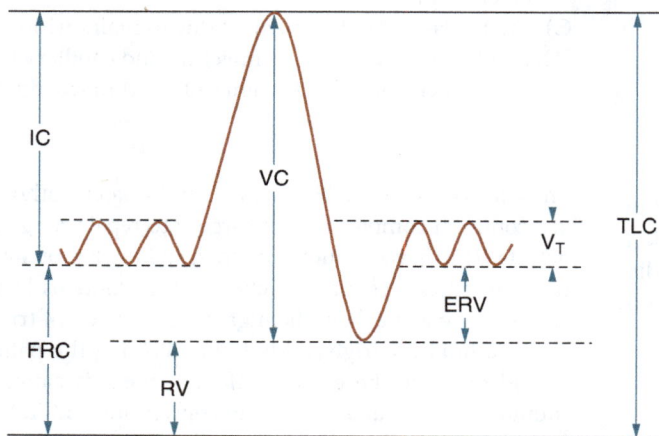

Question 32-1

A patient takes a full deep breath and exhales as quickly as possible until she can no longer exhale. The amount of gas exhaled is the:
A) Forced vital capacity.
B) Expiratory reserve volume.
C) Forced expiratory volume.
D) Functional residual capacity.
E) Total lung capacity.

Discussion 32-1

The correct answer is "A." Forced vital capacity (FVC) is the total volume of exhaled air. Spirometry measures flow and volume of air during a rapid, forceful, and maximum exhaled breath from total lung capacity (TLC) to residual volume (RV). These measurements are plotted to give a flow-volume loop. (See Figure 32–9.)

Question 32-2

After breathing comfortably, a patient inhales a full deep breath until he can no longer inhale. The amount of gas inhaled is the:
A) Inspiratory capacity.
B) Inspiratory reserve volume.
C) Peak inspiratory flow rate.
D) Tidal volume.
E) Total lung capacity.

Discussion 32-2

The correct answer is "A." Inspiratory capacity is the amount of air that can be inhaled after normal expiration.

Question 32-3

The amount of gas contained by the lungs and airways after exhalation during normal tidal breathing is the:

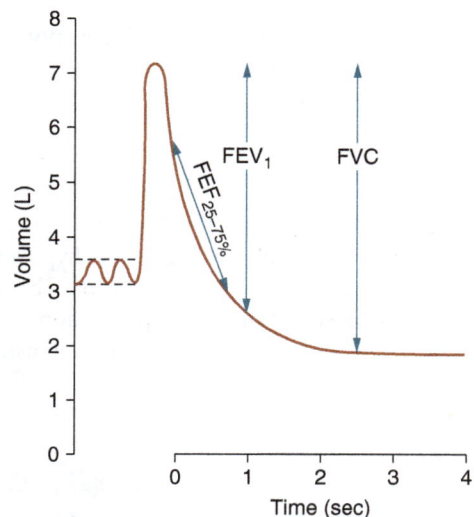

FIGURE 32–9. Pulmonary function tests. Pulmonary function tests. ERV, expiratory reserve volume; FEF 25–75%, forced expiratory flow measured during exhalation of 25% to 75% of the FVC; FEV$_1$, forced expiratory volume in 1 second; FRC, functional reserve capacity; FVC, forced vital capacity; IC, inspiratory capacity; RV, residual volume; TLC, total lung capacity; VC, vital capacity; V$_t$, tidal volume. (Reproduced with permission from Stern SDC, Cifu AS, Altkorn D, eds. *Symptom to Diagnosis: An Evidence-Based Guide.* 3rd ed. New York, NY: McGraw-Hill Education; 2015, Fig. 33-2.)

A) Residual volume.
B) Total lung capacity.
C) Functional residual capacity.
D) Expiratory reserve volume.
E) Peak expiratory flow rate.

Discussion 32-3

The correct answer is "C." Functional residual capacity (FRC) is the amount of air left in the lungs after exhaling a normal breath (tidal volume).

▶ CASE 33

A 15-year-old patient with CF has had progressive worsening of pulmonary function since age 8. Currently, FEV_1 is 60% of predicted and FVC 70% of predicted values.

Age	FEV_1 % Predicted	FVC % Predicted
8 years	100	100
15 years	60	70

Question 33-1

Why is the FVC diminished?
A) Weakness related to acute illness.
B) Chest wall deformity.
C) Air trapping from mucus plugs.
D) Fibrotic changes to lung parenchyma.
E) All of the above are possible; the mechanism cannot be determined with the information given.

Discussion 33-1

The correct answer is "E." Options "A" through "D" are all possible explanations for a decline in vital capacity. This patient is not exhaling a large ($\downarrow$FVC) or fast ($\downarrow FEV_1$) breath. To suck in a big breath then blow it out, you need strong respiratory muscles as well as a chest that expands normally. The air must be able to flow freely in and out. Finally, the volume is dependent on what the lungs can hold. Less lung tissue such as in fibrosis means less air volume.

Question 33-2

Which test would best distinguish between these possibilities?
A) Chest X-ray.
B) Whole body plethysmography.
C) Repeat spirometry following bronchodilator.
D) Arterial blood gas analysis.
E) Gas diffusion testing.

Discussion 33-2

The correct answer is "B." Whole body plethysmography would be most informative because it can distinguish between air trapping and restrictive changes. (See Table 32–7.) The entire child is placed in a plethysmograph or box that looks like a phone booth creating a closed system. Breathing through a mouth

TABLE 32-7 DIFFERENTIATING AIR TRAPPING FROM RESTRICTIVE CHANGES

Parameter	Restrictive Disease	Air Trapping (Obstructive)
TLC	Decreased	Normal or increased
FRC	Decreased	Increased
FVC	Decreased	Decreased

FRC, functional residual capacity; FVC, forced vital capacity; TLC, total lung capacity.

piece, the FRC is calculated. When air trapping occurs, gas diffusion underestimates the FRC.

▶ CASE 34

For Questions 34-1 through 34-5, refer to the figure below.

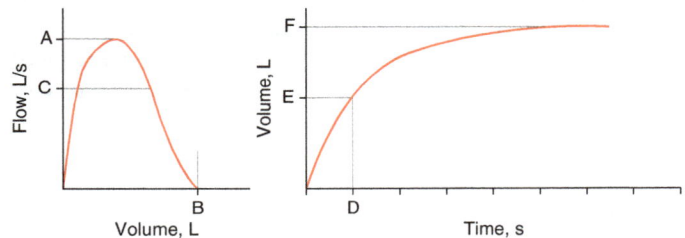

Question 34-1

Which of the following relationships is correct?
A) FEV_1 – C.
B) PEFR – E.
C) FVC – A.
D) FVC – F.
E) FEV_1 – D.

Discussion 34-1

The correct answer is "D." The volume that can be forcefully exhaled in a complete breath is the forced vital capacity (FVC). Option "A" is incorrect because point C is a flow, not a volume. Option "B" is incorrect because point E is a volume, not a flow. Option "C" is incorrect because point A is a flow, not a volume. Option "E" is incorrect because point D labels a time, not a volume.

> **Helpful Tip**
> If you are confused by pulmonary function tests, look at the units on figures to get helpful clues. Pulmonary function parameters that end in "capacity" or "volume" will have units of volume (L). Pulmonary function tests that end in "flow" or "flow rate" (eg, FEF_{50}, FEF_{75}, FEF_{25-75}, PEFR) will have units of volume divided by time, such as L/s.

Question 34-2

Which of the following points represents FVC?
A) Point A.
B) Point B.
C) Point C.
D) Point D.
E) Point E.

Discussion 34-2

The correct answer is "B." The maximum volume exhaled in one breath is the FVC.

Question 34-3

Which of the following points represents FEV_1?
A) Point A.
B) Point B.
C) Point C.
D) Point D.
E) Point E.

Discussion 34-3

The correct answer is "E." FEV_1 is the volume that can be forcefully exhaled in 1 second. Forced expiratory flow (FEF_{25-75}) measures airflow over the middle half of the FVC from 25% to 75% of the exhaled volume of air. Both FEV_1 and FEF_{25-75} are reduced in obstructive lung disorders, but FEF_{25-75} is a sensitive indicator of small airway obstruction.

Question 34-4

Which point is the PEFR?
A) Point A.
B) Point B.
C) Point C.
D) Point D.
E) Point E.

Discussion 34-4

The correct answer is "A." Point A is the maximum flow or peak expiratory flow rate (PEFR).

Question 34-5

Point F measures the same parameter as point:
A) Point A.
B) Point B.
C) Point C.
D) Point D.
E) Point E.

Discussion 34-5

The correct answer is "B." Points B and F are both representations of the FVC.

▶ CASE 35

A medical student draws the following graphic in an attempt to illustrate the relationships between several measures of lung function.

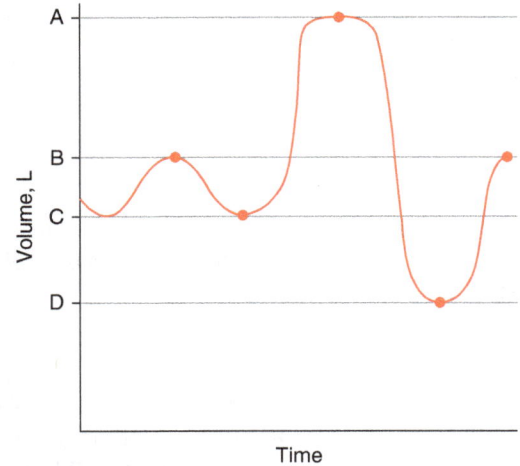

Question 35-1

Which of the lung volume relationships shown in the figure is INCORRECT?

	Parameter	Volume
A)	Functional residual capacity (FRC)	C
B)	Total lung capacity (TLC)	A
C)	Inspiratory capacity (IC)	A – C
D)	Forced vital capacity (FVC)	A – D
E)	Expiratory reserve volume (ERV)	B – D
F)	Residual volume (RV)	D
G)	Tidal volume (VT)	B – C

Discussion 35-1

The correct answer is "E." The expiratory reserve volume is the difference between FRC (point C, volume at the end of tidal exhalation) and RV (point D, the end of full exhalation) (see Figure 32–9, earlier.)

⧗ QUICK QUIZ

Which factor has the greatest effect on minute respiratory rate in normal individuals?
A) Hypoxemia.
B) Acidemia.
C) Fever.
D) Anemia.
E) Dietary carbon source.

Discussion

The correct answer is "B." Acidemia is the most powerful stimulator of ventilation in normal individuals.

▶ CASE 36

A 10-year-old has tachypnea (40 breaths per minute) with no cough, fever, or chest pain. He has no prior respiratory history. Lung fields are clear lung to auscultation and oxygen saturation is 99% on room air.

Question 36-1
Which test is best for evaluating his tachypnea?
A) Spirometry.
B) Chest radiography.
C) Lung volumes.
D) Capillary blood gas analysis.
E) Brain MRI.

Discussion 36-1
The correct answer is "D." The tachypnea is not accompanied by other respiratory symptoms. This suggests either that the tachypnea is either primary hyperventilation or is a compensation for underlying metabolic acidosis.

▶ CASE 37

A term newborn has cyanosis and tachypnea. You perform a hyperoxia test. After 10 minutes in a 100% oxygen tent, an arterial blood gas analysis is obtained, which shows pH 7.30, $Paco_2$ 35, Pao_2 98, and HCO_3^- 20.

Question 37-1
What is the likely etiology of the cyanosis?
A) Pneumonia.
B) Surfactant deficiency.
C) Right-to-left shunt.
D) Left-to-right shunt.
E) Hemoglobinopathy.

Discussion 37-1
The correct answer is "C." A hyperoxia test can help decide if cyanosis is a result of congenital cyanotic heart disease with right-to-left shunting. If not, the lungs or other pathology are to blame. The patient described has an abnormal hyperoxia test; the Pao_2 is low (< 150 mm Hg) despite 100% oxygen. Supplemental oxygen can correct hypoxemia related to diffusion, V/Q mismatch, and hypoventilation. It cannot correct hypoxemia caused by right-to-left shunt from cyanotic heart disease. Left-to-right shunt would not cause cyanosis. Abnormal hemoglobin could change the binding of oxygen by hemoglobin, but would not affect the Pao_2.

▶ CASE 38

A child is being treated for acute myeloid leukemia. After prescribing dapsone for chemoprophylaxis against *Pneumocystis jiroveci*, you note that he develops cyanosis. Arterial blood gas analysis shows that Pao_2 is 100 mm Hg on room air. Administering supplemental oxygen does not change his color.

Question 38-1
Why does the patient appear cyanotic?
A) Methemoglobinemia.
B) Anemia.
C) Hemolysis.
D) Pulmonary fibrosis due to doxorubicin.
E) Right-to-left shunting lesion.

Discussion 38-1
The correct answer is "A." This child has cyanosis that is unresponsive to oxygen and a normal arterial oxygen level. This strongly suggests methemoglobinemia acquired from dapsone. In methemoglobinemia, the iron molecule contained within hemoglobin is oxidized from a ferrous (Fe^{2+}) to a ferric (Fe^{3+}) state. Ferric iron cannot bind oxygen, so affected red blood cells are desaturated. The hemoglobin dissociation curve shifts to the left as the oxygenated red blood cells increase their affinity for oxygen. These processes result in decreased oxygen delivery to the tissues. Look for chocolate brown–colored blood. Pulse oximeters are not reliable when methemoglobin levels are elevated. Co-oximetry should be performed to confirm the presence of methemoglobin. Cyanosis becomes harder to detect in patients with anemia. Hemolysis is more likely to result in jaundice than cyanosis. Because the blood gas analysis shows a normal Pao_2 on room air, both pulmonary and shunting lesions are unlikely to explain the cyanosis. Doxorubicin causes cardiotoxicity. Bleomycin causes pulmonary toxicity.

▶ CASE 39

A patient is referred to you to evaluate digital clubbing.

Question 39-1
Which of the following diseases is associated with clubbing?
A) Liver disease.
B) Inflammatory bowel disease.
C) Cyanotic congenital heart disease.
D) Cystic fibrosis.
E) All of the above.

Discussion 39-1
The correct answer is "E." Clubbing is a nonspecific physical finding. Although it is common among patients with structural lung diseases, clubbing is observed in a wide variety of diseases. (See Figure 32–10.)

▶ CASE 40

A 4-month-old infant has respiratory distress with increased nasal secretions, bilateral wheezing, and crackles. She is feeding poorly and requires supplemental oxygen to maintain an Spo_2 greater than 92%.

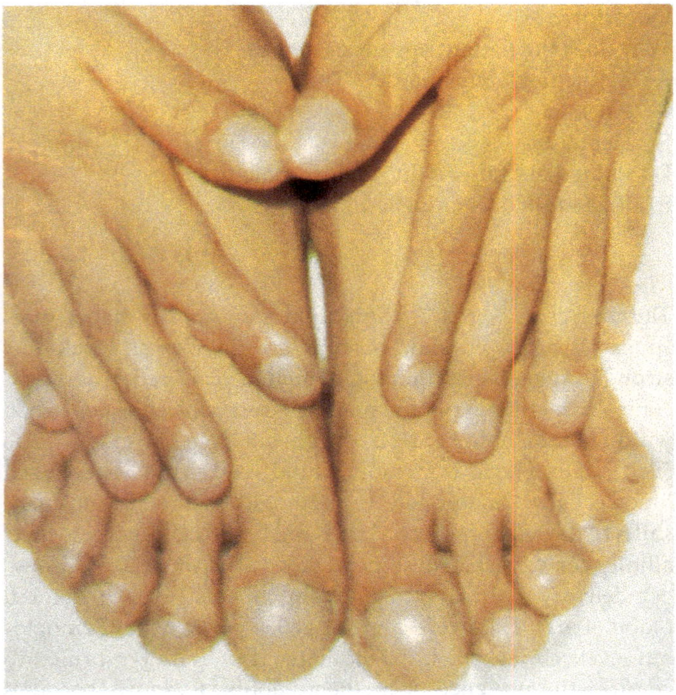

FIGURE 32–10. Clubbing of the fingers and toes. (Reproduced with permission from Fuster V, Walsh RA, Harrington RA, eds. *Hurst's The Heart.* 13th ed. New York, NY: McGraw-Hill Education; 2011, Fig. 14-1.)

Question 40-1

In addition to oxygen therapy, cost-effective evaluation and management should include:
A) RSV antigen testing.
B) Chest X-ray.
C) IV ampicillin.
D) Azithromycin.
E) Dexamethasone.
F) Suctioning as needed.

Discussion 40-1

The correct answer is "F." The infant described has bronchiolitis, a viral infection of the lungs affecting children younger than 2 years of age. Management is supportive, and may include suctioning, oxygen, and IV fluids. Respiratory syncytial virus (RSV) antigen testing is not cost-effective. Chest X-ray often leads to unnecessary antibiotic treatment due to confusion between atelectasis and pneumonia. Antibiotics and steroids are not necessary.

⧗ QUICK QUIZ

Which statement regarding the relationship between tracheostomy and aspiration is true?
A) Tracheostomy can impair deglutitive (swallowing) apnea.
B) Tracheostomy impairs superior movement of the larynx during swallowing.
C) Aspiration is increased in patients with tracheostomy.
D) Swallowing is delayed in patients with tracheostomy.
E) All of the above statements are true.

Discussion

The correct answer is "E." Tracheostomy can increase aspiration by all of the listed mechanisms.

▶ CASE 41

A 5-year-old boy has fever of 39°C (102.2°F), tachypnea (40 times per minute), respiratory distress, and hypoxemia. On examination, he has decreased right lower lung field sounds. He is diagnosed with pneumonia and hospital admission is arranged.

Question 41-1

Which of the following diagnostic tests has the strongest recommendation?
A) Urine antigen testing for pneumococcus.
B) Chest X-ray.
C) *Mycoplasma* serology.
D) Sputum culture.
E) C-reactive protein to assess whether the infection is bacterial.

Discussion 41-1

The correct answer is "B." This child has pneumonia based on history. The finding of decreased breath sounds rather than crackles is concerning. A chest X-ray is the only test of those listed that can determine if a complication of pneumonia such as pleural effusion or empyema is present. Therefore, it receives the strongest recommendation from the Infectious Disease Society of America. Urine antigen testing has poor specificity and is not recommended. *Mycoplasma* testing is weakly recommended in children with compatible clinical history. Sputum culture is weakly recommended in children who are able to produce sputum, but a 5-year-old is unlikely to produce sputum. C-reactive protein should not be relied upon to distinguish between viral and bacterial pneumonia. Since the child is being admitted, blood cultures should be obtained.

> **Helpful Tip**
> Children with pneumonia who do not require hospitalization can be started on antibiotics without testing or imaging, but with close follow-up.

> **Helpful Tip**
> A child who is being treated for pneumonia should improve after 48 hours of antibiotic therapy. If not, imaging should be obtained to look for complications such as effusion or empyema. Chest CT or ultrasound may be needed if the chest X-ray is inconclusive.

A chest X-ray is obtained and reveals a parapneumonic effusion.

Question 41-2

Which of the following are indications for chest tube drainage or video-assisted thoracoscopic surgery (VATS)?
  I. Effusion < 10 mm clinically stable.
 II. Effusion > 10 mm with empyema
III. Effusion > 10 mm with respiratory distress
 IV. Effusion opacifies over half of hemithorax and patient has respiratory distress
A) IV only.
B) II, III, and IV.
C) II and IV.
D) II and III.
E) All of the above.

Discussion 41-2

The correct answer is "B." Chest tube drainage should be completed if there is respiratory distress or empyema. Pneumonia complicated by small effusions (< 10 mm or one-fourth of thorax opacified) usually can be treated with antibiotics alone. Complicated pneumonia refers to the development of a loculated effusion. The pleural space becomes inflamed, forming a sterile effusion. Bacteria move into the fluid, forming pus and loculations—an empyema. Drainage options include VATS or a chest tube with fibrinolytic agents instilled into the chest. If chest tube drainage is unsuccessful, proceed to VATS. Infection spreads from the lung into the pleural space.

A diagnostic thoracentesis is performed on the patient, but only 1 mL of fluid is successfully aspirated.

Question 41-3

Which of the following tests on the pleural fluid is most important?
A) Lactate dehydrogenase.
B) Protein.
C) Cell count and differential.
D) Gram stain and culture.
E) pH.

Discussion 41-3

The correct answer is "D." Culture of pleural fluid gives a unique opportunity to determine the organism responsible for infection and tailor the antimicrobial therapy. Lactate dehydrogenase (LDH), protein, and pH of pleural fluid are unlikely to change management. The cell count and differential would potentially help if malignancy or atypical infection was in the differential diagnosis.

▶ CASE 42

A 3-year-old girl has had recurrent hospitalizations for pneumonia. Each illness was typified by fever, lethargy, hypoxemia, and focal crackles, and each illness affected different lung segments. She also has chronic otitis media, recurrent skin abscesses, and severe eczema.

Question 42-1

Which of the following is/are NOT included in your initial evaluation?
A) CBC with differential.
B) Quantitative immune globulins.
C) Pre- and postvaccination pneumococcal titers.
D) Bronchoscopy.
E) All of the above are important parts of the initial evaluation.

Discussion 42-1

The correct answer is "D." The case describes features of recurrent pneumonia related to immune deficiency, with severe, recurrent infections of both the skin and respiratory tract. Initial evaluation should focus on identifying the immune defect. It is not likely to arise from an airway abnormality, since different lung segments are affected.

▶ CASE 43

A 10-year-old boy is admitted to the general pediatric service with a diagnosis of community-acquired pneumonia. His condition worsens despite treatment with ceftriaxone and azithromycin. He is transferred to the intensive care unit with sepsis and respiratory failure. His initial X-ray shows interval development of abscess, and purulent secretions are aspirated with intubation.

Question 43-1

Which bacterial pathogen is most likely to be responsible?
A) *Streptococcus pyogenes.*
B) *Staphylococcus aureus.*
C) *Streptococcus pneumonia.*
D) *Haemophilus influenzae.*
E) *Mycoplasma pneumoniae.*

Discussion 43-1

The correct answer is "B." The patient has a necrotizing pneumonia, likely due to methicillin-resistant *S. aureus* (MRSA). All of the other options are covered well by ceftriaxone and azithromycin.

▶ CASE 44

A 4-year-old boy has had five hospitalizations for right middle lobe pneumonia since age 2. There were no respiratory symptoms prior to the initial pneumonia, and he has no history of recurrent otitis or other infections of the skin or soft tissues. On examination, his chest expands symmetrically, but there are crackles in the right middle lung fields.

Question 44-1

What is the most important test for evaluating his recurrent pneumonias?

A) Neutrophil oxidative burst assay.
B) Quantitative immune globulins.
C) Aeroallergen skin testing.
D) Bronchoscopy.
E) Diaphragm fluoroscopy.

Discussion 44-1

The correct answer is "D." Recurrent pneumonia in the same lobe suggests a localized anatomic obstruction, such as a retained foreign body. A neutrophil-killing defect or an antibody deficiency could result in pneumonia, but it would be unlikely to always infect the same lobe. One would also expect other infections such as otitis media to occur. Asthma can cause atelectasis and be confused with recurrent pneumonia, but the atelectasis tends to be migratory. Diaphragm fluoroscopy may be useful if there is asymmetry in chest expansion, suspected phrenic nerve injury, or both.

Question 44-2

Which of the following disorders is least likely to result in bronchiectasis?
A) Cystic fibrosis.
B) Primary ciliary dyskinesia.
C) Selective IgA deficiency.
D) Chronically retained foreign body.
E) Chronic granulomatous disease.

Question 44-2

The correct answer is "C." Selective IgA deficiency is often discovered incidentally and is rarely associated with bronchiectasis. All of the other disorders listed are associated with bronchiectasis.

► CASE 45

A child has a chest X-ray to evaluate cough and wheezing. (See the images below.)

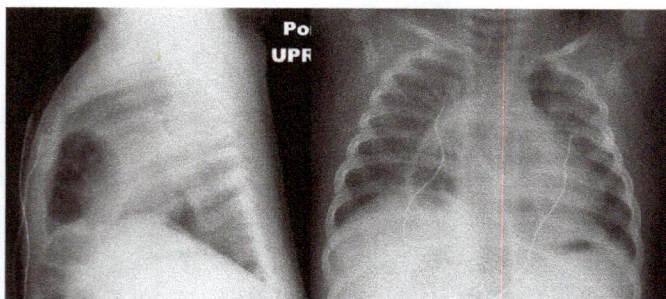

Question 45-1

What abnormality is identified by his X-ray?
A) Congenital hyperlucent lobe (congenital lobar emphysema).
B) Congenital bronchogenic cyst.
C) Anterior diaphragmatic hernia (Morgagni hernia).
D) Cardiomegaly.
E) Hiatal hernia.
F) Pneumomediastinum.

Discussion 45-1

The correct answer is "C." The patient has an anterior congenital diaphragmatic hernia, which was an incidental finding. The diaphragm fails to develop, leading to herniation of abdominal contents into the chest. Ninety percent of hernias are left sided. Symptomatic newborns have respiratory distress, unilateral decreased breath sounds, and a scaphoid abdomen. The lateral X-ray shows bowel contents in the anterior chest. The hyperlucency is bowel gas and does not fit the shape of a hyperlucent lobe.

> **Helpful Tip**
> Bochdalek hernias are on the left side. Think "Back and to the Left." Morgagni hernias are on the right side.

Question 45-2

Which of the following statements about congenital diaphragmatic hernia is true?
A) Symptoms vary depending on the size of the defect.
B) Pulmonary hyperplasia of varying degrees occurs.
C) Respiratory compliance is increased on the side of the diaphragm.
D) Less than 1% of patients with congenital diaphragmatic hernia are treated for pulmonary hypertension.
E) None of the above.

Discussion 45-2

The correct answer is "A." As in this case, diaphragmatic hernias may be asymptomatic. Congenital diaphragmatic hernia results in pulmonary hypoplasia. The more severe the defect, the worse oxygenation and ventilation become. The affected lung has decreased compliance. A recent large study shows approximately 30% of patients with congenital diaphragmatic hernias will receive some form of treatment for pulmonary hypertension.

► CASE 46

A 5-year-old boy is brought to your office because his asthma is poorly controlled. He has had worsening symptoms of shortness of breath with exertion and his albuterol inhaler does not seem to help. On physical examination you note distended neck veins, peripheral edema, an enlarged liver and a loud second heart sound (S2). You suspect that the child has been misdiagnosed and is actually suffering from pulmonary hypertension.

Question 46-1

Which of the following statements about pulmonary hypertension is false?
A) Mean pulmonary arterial pressure in most children and adolescents is less than 25 mm Hg.
B) Pulmonary arterial pressure may not be elevated in advanced pulmonary hypertension if right heart failure develops.

C) Pulmonary hypertension can develop in children with prolonged exposure to hypoxemia, including sleep apnea.

D) Exercise impairment is a late finding in pulmonary hypertension.

E) Patients with pulmonary hypertension cannot increase cardiac output sufficiently during exercise and illness, increasing their risk of syncope or sudden death.

Discussion 46-1

The correct answer is "D." Pulmonary hypertension often develops with few patient symptoms, but exercise impairment is usually the earliest sign. Patients are unable to increase their cardiac output in response to exercise because of high pulmonary vascular resistance. Normal children and adolescents have mean pulmonary arterial pressures between 10 and 16 mm Hg. As the right heart fails, pulmonary arterial pressures may not be elevated because the right heart is unable to overcome high pulmonary vascular resistance. This could result in peripheral edema and hepatomegaly.

Question 46-2

Which of the following factors is least likely to contribute to pulmonary hypertension in a premature infant?

A) High pulmonary vascular resistance in the fetal circulation.

B) Hypoxic vasoconstriction of pulmonary vasculature.

C) High pulmonary vasoreactivity.

D) Lower pulmonary arterial density due to incomplete lung development.

E) Patent foramen ovale.

Discussion 46-2

The correct answer is "E." It is unlikely that left-to-right atrial-level shunting could contribute to pulmonary hypertension in the newborn period unless the shunt is very large. Right-to-left atrial shunting through a patent foramen ovale could be protective by providing a "pop-off" valve to increase left heart filling during a pulmonary hypertensive crisis (blood not entering the lungs from the right side of the heart so less coming back to the left side). Options "A" through "D" are all factors that contribute to pulmonary hypertension in children born prematurely.

Question 46-3

Which of the following is true about chronic lung disease of prematurity (CLD)?

A) Despite changes in ventilation strategy, extensive fibroproliferative changes remain the principal histopathologic finding in CLD.

B) Airway hyperreactivity is uncommon in CLD.

C) Risk factors for CLD are highly interactive.

D) Intrauterine betamethasone exposure significantly reduces the incidence of CLD but has no effect on infant survival.

E) Higher $Paco_2$ in the first week of life and female sex are independent risk factors for CLD.

Discussion 46-3

The correct answer is "C." CLD, also known as bronchopulmonary dysplasia (BPD), is defined as a persistent oxygen need after 28 days of age. Risk factors for CLD include prematurity, surfactant deficiency, chorioamnionitis, sepsis, mechanical ventilation, and patent ductus arteriosus. Many of these risk factors coexist in individual patients. CLD has changed significantly over time, with fibroproliferative changes becoming less common. BPD formerly was associated with fibrotic changes from mechanical ventilation–induced barotrauma. This was before the days of pulmonary surfactant preparations. In the "new" BPD, fewer alveoli develop leading to decreased area for gas exchange. Airway hyperreactivity with wheezing is common in CLD. Low $Paco_2$ (related to increased mechanical ventilation) and male sex are independent risk factors for CLD. Intrauterine steroids confer survival benefit and decrease respiratory distress syndrome but do not reduce the incidence of CLD.

▶ CASE 47

You are caring for a former 24-week premature infant who is now 4 months old. She has CLD and requires ½ liter per minute of oxygen to maintain an Spo_2 greater than 92%.

Question 47-1

You recommend all of the following EXCEPT:

A) Regular immunizations.

B) Passive RSV immunoprophylaxis.

C) Avoidance of smoke exposure.

D) Initiation of lansoprazole.

E) Close monitoring of nutrition.

Discussion 47-1

The correct answer is "D." In the absence of symptoms of gastroesophageal reflux disease (GERD), acid suppression is unnecessary and may increase the risk of pulmonary infections in infants and young children. Treatment of children with CLD aims at promoting lung growth through nutrition, preventing lung injury related to infections or smoke exposure, and preventing complications such as pulmonary hypertension.

▶ CASE 48

An infant is evaluated in the emergency department for an apparent life-threatening event (ALTE).

Question 48-1

Which of the following findings on history and physical exam warrants admission for further evaluation?

A) Inconsistent histories.

B) Age younger than 2 weeks.

C) Repeated episodes of ALTE.

D) Stridor.

E) CPR administration by parent.

F) All of the above.

Discussion 48-1

The correct answer is "F." ALTE is a frightening event witnessed by a caregiver that involves some change in color, breathing, or tone. Basically, it presents as "my baby may have stopped breathing and it was scary." Most often, there is no identified cause of ALTE. The history and physical exam will guide what tests if any are ordered. Each of the findings listed in options "A" through "E" could suggest an underlying abnormality and warrants further evaluation. The first 2 weeks of infancy may be when congenital heart diseases, seizure disorders, infections, or metabolic disorders present. Stridor suggests an abnormal airway that would contribute to apnea. Inconsistent history raises the possibility of abuse. CPR administration and repeated episodes both increase the possibility for identifying an underlying disorder. The most important thing to remember is that ALTE and SIDS are not related.

▶ CASE 49

A 7-year-old boy has cough, shortness of breath, and hemoptysis. Lung examination reveals bilateral crackles. Spirometry shows decreased FVC and normal FEV_1/FVC. Diffusing capacity of the lung (DLCO) is increased. Lab studies show microcytic anemia with a hemoglobin of 9 mg/dL.

Question 49-1

Which of the following tests is consistent with a diagnosis of idiopathic pulmonary hemosiderosis?

A) Anti–glomerular basement membrane antibody.
B) Hemosiderin-laden macrophages on bronchoalveolar lavage.
C) c-ANCA (antinuclear cytoplasmic) antibody.
D) Endoglin mutations.
E) Chest CT revealing dilated bronchial arteries.

Discussion 49-1

The correct answer is "B." Idiopathic pulmonary hemosiderosis is a rare disorder (incidence of 1:1,000,000) that results in recurrent alveolar hemorrhage and pulmonary fibrosis. Some investigators have proposed an autoimmune or allergic basis to this disease, although this is not proven. Its diagnosis requires evidence of alveolar hemorrhage and the exclusion of other causes of pulmonary hemorrhage. Option "A" is consistent with Goodpasture disease, option "C" with granulomatosis–polyangiitis (formerly Wegener granulomatosis), option "D" with hereditary hemorrhagic telangiectasia syndrome, and option "E" with bronchial artery (not alveolar) hemorrhage.

BIBLIOGRAPHY

Bradley JS, Byington CL, Shah SS, et al; Pediatric Infectious Diseases Society, the Infectious Diseases Society of America. The management of community-acquired pneumonia in infants and children older than 3 months of age: Clinical practice guidelines by the Pediatric Infectious Diseases Society and the Infectious Diseases Society of America. *Clin Infect Dis.* 2011;53(7):e25–76.

Canani RB, Cirillo P, Roggero P, et al. Therapy with gastric acidity inhibitors increases the risk of acute gastroenteritis and community-acquired pneumonia in children. *Pediatrics.* 2006;117(5):e817–820.

Kleigman RM, Stanton BF, St. Geme JW, Schor NF, Behrman RE, eds. *Nelson Textbook of Pediatrics.* 19th ed. Philadelphia, PA: Saunders; 2011.

Manna A, Montella S, Maniscalco M, Maglione M, Santamaria F. Clinical application of nasal nitric oxide measurement in pediatric airway diseases. *Pediatr Pulmonol.* 2015;50(1):85–99.

Marcus CL, Brooks LJ, Draper KA, et al. Diagnosis and management of childhood obstructive sleep apnea syndrome. *Pediatrics.* 2012;130(3):e714–755.

Martins RHG, Hidalgo Ribeiro CB, Fernandes de Mello BMZ, Branco A, Tavares ELM. Dysphonia in children. *J Voice.* 2012; 26(5):674.e617–e620.

Wienberger M. Evaluation and initial management of chronic cough in children. First Consult. May 29, 2013.

Zaoutis LB, Chiang VW. *Comprehensive Pediatric Hospital Medicine.* Philadelphia, PA: Mosby; 2007.

Skin Disorders

33

Will Aughenbaugh and Lisa Muchard

► CASE 1

An 8-year-old boy presents with recurrent erythema, scale, and pruritus of the antecubital and popliteal fossae. His mother notes that his skin problems tend to flare in the winter months. Social history is notable for a pet cat. You suspect atopic dermatitis.

Question 1-1

What additional cutaneous finding supports your diagnosis?
A) Alopecia.
B) Erythema and scale of alar creases.
C) Keratosis pilaris.
D) Nail pits.
E) Scaling of elbows and knees.

Discussion 1-1

The correct answer is "C." The boy in this case has atopic dermatitis, which is associated with keratosis pilaris (KP). KP is an example of retention hyperkeratosis, characterized by adherent keratin at the apex of the hair follicle. KP has a rough, sandpaper texture and may be red in color. It is typically located on the extensor arms, thighs, cheeks, and buttocks. (See Figure 33–1.) Erythema and scale of the alar creases (creases near the tip of the nose) is more typical of seborrheic dermatitis. The scale is yellow, greasy, and concentrates on the scalp, postauricular sulci, brows, glabella, alar creases, nasolabial folds, mental crease, central chest, axillae, and groin. Nail pits (small depressions) and oil spots (yellow discoloration of the nail bed) as well as scaling of elbows and knees are classic for psoriasis. The terms *atopic dermatitis* and *eczema* may be used interchangeably. In addition to KP, eczema may present with additional cutaneous findings, including ichthyosis vulgaris (dry skin with fish-scale appearance), pityriasis alba (ill-defined hypopigmented patches of the face, trunk, and extremities), hyperlinear palms, Dennie-Morgan lines (extra skinfold under the eyes), and allergic salute (transverse nasal crease due to repeated rubbing of the nose). (See Figure 33–2.)

> **Helpful Tip**
> Pityriasis alba and vitiligo may be difficult to distinguish. Pityriasis is off-white in color and results from decreased pigment (hypopigmentation). (See Figure 33–3.) Vitiligo is milk white and results from absent pigment (depigmentation). Shining a Wood lamp on the skin accentuates depigmented skin and has no effect on hypopigmented skin, helping to differentiate the two conditions. (See Figure 33–4.)

You counsel the patient and his mother on dry skin care, including bathing daily to every other day, and applying bland emollients immediately after bathing.

Question 1-2

Which topical steroid is most appropriate for both acute and chronic management of the rash?
A) Clobetasol 0.05% cream.
B) Desonide 0.05% cream.
C) Hydrocortisone 1% cream.
D) Pimecrolimus 0.1% cream.
E) Triamcinolone 0.1% cream.

Discussion 1-2

The correct answer is "E." Triamcinolone 0.1% is a mid-potency steroid. It is a good starting point for rashes that occur on the trunk and extremities. Hydrocortisone and desonide are low-potency steroids. They may not be sufficiently potent to treat eczema of the trunk and extremities and are more appropriate for the face, groin, and skinfolds. Clobetasol is an ultra-potent steroid that must be used cautiously due to the risk of steroid-induced skin atrophy. Pimecrolimus (Elidel) cream is a topical calcineurin inhibitor. It carries a black box warning requiring it to be used second line and on a rotational basis. (See Table 33–1.)

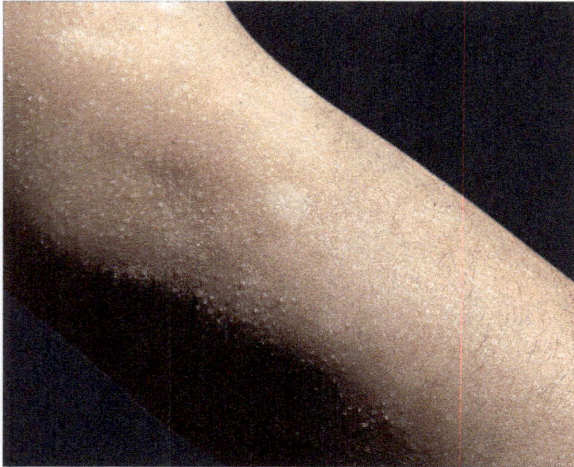

FIGURE 33–1. Keratosis pilaris is characterized by small papules with a sandpaper texture located on the extensor surfaces of proximal arms and thighs. Surrounding erythema may be present. It is associated with atopic dermatitis or eczema. (Reproduced with permission from Wolff K, Johnson RA, and Saavedra AP, eds. *Fitzpatrick's Color Atlas and Synopsis of Clinical Dermatology*, 7th ed. McGraw-Hill Education, Inc., 2013. Fig. 4-3.)

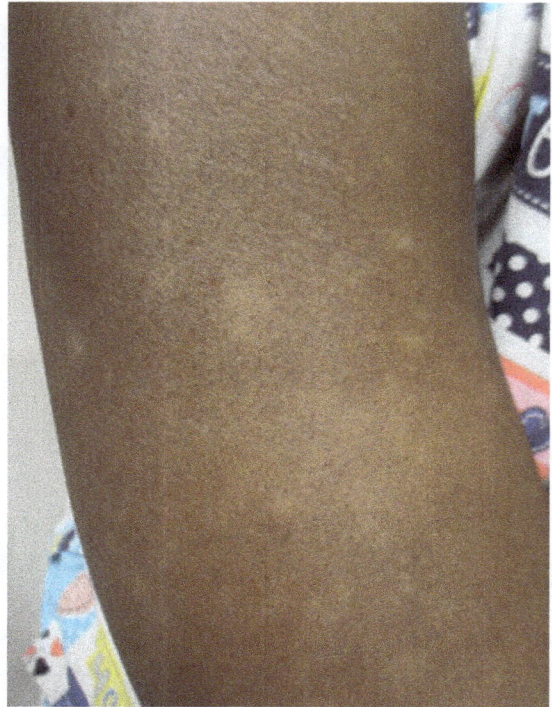

The boy and his mother return the next winter, as the rash has recurred. He resumed triamcinolone 0.1% cream twice daily but the symptoms have not improved. Itching is mild. You note fissures and serous drainage on exam.

Question 1-3

What is your next step?

A) Bacitracin.

B) Biopsy.

C) Bleach baths.

FIGURE 33–2. Atopic Dermatitis. The characteristics of atopic dermatitis or eczema vary by age. In childhood, lichenified erythematous plaques form on the flexor surfaces of the elbows and knees. Secondary excoriations may be present from pruritus. In infants with atopic dermatitis, the trunk and face may be involved but the diaper area is spared. (Used with permission from William Augehenbaugh, MD.)

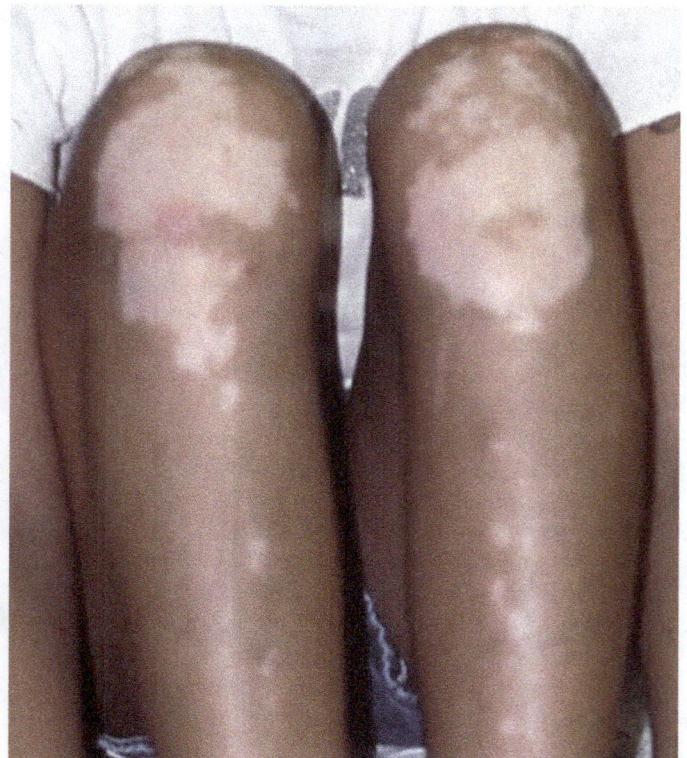

FIGURE 33–3. Pityriasis alba is characterized by ill-defined off-white–colored hypopigmented patches on the face, trunk, and extremities. Shining a Wood lamp on the skin does not change the lesions. (Used with permission from William Augehenbaugh, MD.)

FIGURE 33–4. Vitiligo is an autoimmune process that destroys the melanocytes, resulting in depigmented milky white–colored patches. Shining a Wood lamp on the skin accentuates the lesions. (Used with permission from William Augehenbaugh, MD.)

TABLE 33–1 TOPICAL STEROIDS USED IN THE MANAGEMENT OF ATOPIC DERMATITIS (ECZEMA)

Potency	Topical Corticosteroid	Location to Apply
Ultra potent	Betamethasone dipropionate 0.05%	Scalp
	Clobetasol propionate 0.05%	Palms and soles
Mid potency	Triamcinolone 0.1%	Trunk
		Extremities
Low potency	Betamethasone valerate 0.1%	Face
	Desonide 0.05%	Groin
	Hydrocortisone 1%	

D) Clobetasol 0.05% cream.
E) Oral prednisolone.

Discussion 1-3

The correct answer is "C." Atopic dermatitis (eczema) is characterized by a compromised skin barrier. It is not uncommon for the eczema plaques to become secondarily infected with *Staphylococcus aureus* (secondary impetiginization). (See Figure 33–5.) Adding ¼ cup of household bleach to the bathtub and bathing once or twice weekly may help treat eczema that fails to respond to standard therapy and prevent flares of eczema. Oral antibiotics are reserved for widespread infection or failure to respond to conservative therapy. Bacitracin has limited antibacterial properties and is associated with allergic contact dermatitis. Oral steroids may be added for severe flares once secondary infection has been addressed.

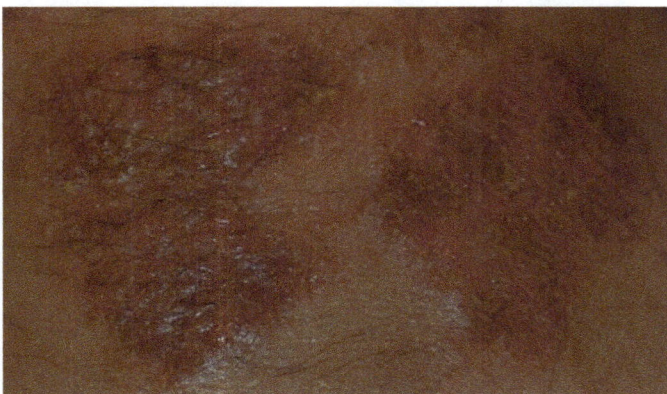

FIGURE 33–5. Impetiginized Atopic Dermatitis. Lesions of atopic dermatitis (eczema) may become acutely worse secondary to subsequent infection by *Staphylococcus aureus*, referred to as secondary impetiginization. The lesions become weepy, with serous drainage and crusting. (Used with permission from William Augehenbaugh, MD.)

QUICK QUIZ

Patients with atopic dermatitis are at risk for developing which disease?
A) Allergic contact dermatitis.
B) Allergic rhinitis.
C) Arthralgias.
D) Food allergy.
E) Psoriasis.

Discussion

The correct answer is "B." The atopic triad is comprised of asthma, allergic rhinitis, and atopic dermatitis (eczema). Patients may have one, two, or three of these elements of the triad. The association of food allergy and atopic dermatitis is a possible consideration in children younger than 2 years of age but does not typically occur in older children and adults.

Helpful Tip
Do not confuse bacitracin with mupirocin (Bactroban). Mupirocin is a topical antibiotic that treats staphylococcal infections, including impetigo. If secondarily infected eczema is focal, topical mupirocin may be a good choice for treatment. Bacitracin is a topical antibiotic that may cause allergic contact dermatitis.

Helpful Tip
Impetigo is a primary process whereby staphylococcal bacteria cause inflammation and honey-colored crusting of normal skin. Secondary impetiginization arises when staphylococcal bacteria settle into abraded skin and disrupt normal healing.

► CASE 2

A 14-year-old girl develops severe itching and linear erythema and blisters of her arms and legs after hiking in the woods. (See Figure 33–6.) She has a history of allergic rhinitis.

Question 2-1

What is the most likely cause of her rash?
A) Allergic contact dermatitis.
B) Atopic dermatitis.
C) Irritant contact dermatitis.
D) Factitious dermatitis.
E) Seborrheic dermatitis.

Discussion 2-1

The correct answer is "A." Rashes that are linear or geographic (square, triangular, etc) are commonly caused by agents that come in contact with the skin. Blisters arise from agents that elicit a severe inflammatory response. Blisters are common in

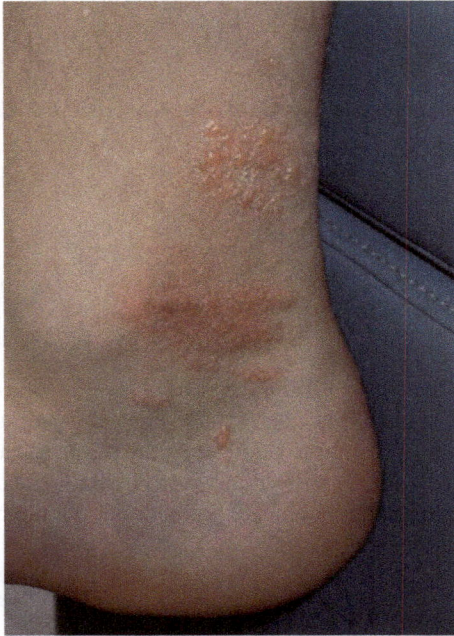

FIGURE 33–6. Allergic contact dermatitis is a delayed (type IV) hypersensitivity reaction to a particular allergen such as urushiol (found in poison ivy), as in this image. It is characterized by erythema and blisters in a linear pattern. In contrast, irritant contact dermatitis is a chemical or mechanical irritation of the skin that is not mediated by the immune system. (Used with permission from William Augehenbaugh, MD.)

allergic contact and irritant contact dermatitis, but would not be associated with atopic dermatitis, factitious (self-induced) dermatitis or seborrheic dermatitis.

> **Helpful Tip**
> Allergic contact dermatitis is unique to the individual who develops it. Therefore different people may or may not develop a reaction, and the degree of inflammation and itching may vary. Irritant contact dermatitis arises in *all* individuals, depending on the degree of exposure. For example, irritant hand dermatitis from repeated exposure to soap and water is most common in people who frequently wash their hands—bartenders, hair dressers, health care providers, etc.

You suspect she may have developed rhus dermatitis from exposure to poison ivy.

Question 2-2

How do you explain the etiology of allergic contact dermatitis?
A) Delayed-type hypersensitivity reaction, therefore the rash occurs with the first exposure.
B) Delayed-type hypersensitivity reaction, therefore the rash requires a sensitizing event.
C) Direct cellular cytotoxicity from a caustic agent.
D) Immediate-type hypersensitivity reaction, therefore the rash occurs with the first exposure.
E) Immediate-type hypersensitivity reaction, therefore the rash requires a sensitizing event.

Discussion 2-2

The correct answer is "B." (See Table 33–2.)

Question 2-3

Which treatment is NOT recommended in patients with rhus dermatitis?
A) Apply a high-potency topical steroid.
B) Avoid exposure to the offending plant.
C) Bathe pets that may have been exposed to plant material.
D) Prednisone 20 milligrams (mg) orally for 5 days.
E) Wash all clothing and gardening tools that were used.

Discussion 2-3

The correct answer is "D." Allergic contact dermatitis due to rhus allergens typically incites a severe inflammatory response. Patients are advised to avoid further exposure and wash the plant resin from clothing, pets, and tools with soap and water. High-potency topical steroids are typically required to provide relief from itching. Oral steroids (prednisone) should be dosed over a 3-week period, as shorter durations often result in a rebound phenomenon.

▶ CASE 3

A 15-year-old girl presents with redness and scaling of her eyebrows and alar creases. No itching is reported. She applies moisturizers without benefit.

TABLE 33–2 ETIOLOGIES OF DERMATITIS AND URTICARIA

	Pathogenesis	Timing	Degree of Exposure Required for Reaction
Allergic contact dermatitis	Delayed-type hypersensitivity (type IV)	Requires sensitizing event	First reaction occurs after at least 2 weeks of sustained exposure; subsequent reactions may occur with low-level exposures
Irritant contact dermatitis	Direct cellular toxicity (not immune mediated)	No sensitizing event necessary, so may occur on first exposure	Requires sufficient exposure to irritate the skin; dependent on the caustic nature of the irritant
Urticaria	Immediate-type hypersensitivity (type I)	No sensitizing event necessary	Low-level exposures

Question 3-1

What is the most likely diagnosis?
A) Allergic contact dermatitis.
B) Atopic dermatitis.
C) Irritant contact dermatitis.
D) Psoriasis.
E) Seborrheic dermatitis.

Discussion 3-1

The correct answer is "E." Seborrheic dermatitis may be present in infancy as "cradle cap." It is acquired at birth with exposure to yeast during vaginal delivery. The yeast remains part of the normal flora throughout life. Outbreaks of seborrheic dermatitis may reoccur at puberty and beyond. While most patients believe they have dry skin, the scale is typically yellow and moist in character. Commonly affected sites include scalp, postauricular sulci, eyebrows, glabella, alar creases, chin, chest, axillae, and groin. (See Figure 33–7.)

Question 3-2

What is your first-line treatment recommendation?
A) Clobetasol 0.05% cream.
B) Tacrolimus 0.1% ointment.
C) Terbinafine 1% cream.
D) Triamcinolone 0.1% cream.
E) Triamcinolone 0.1% ointment.

Discussion 3-2

The correct answer is "C." Seborrheic dermatitis typically responds well to topical treatment. Patients should be warned that seborrheic dermatitis is a recurrent condition. First-line treatments include topical antifungal agents or low-potency

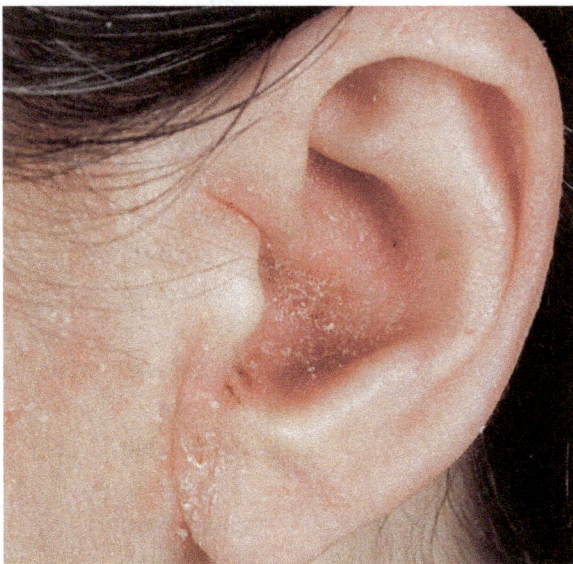

FIGURE 33–8. Guttate psoriasis is characterized by the abrupt onset of multiple small scaling plaques on the trunk and extremities. It is frequently triggered by *Streptococcus pyogenes* (group A streptococcal) pharyngitis. (Used with permission from William Augehenbaugh, MD.)

topical steroids, such as hydrocortisone 1% or 2.5% cream. The two may be combined if a single agent is ineffective. Treatment of the scalp includes antiseborrheic shampoos containing zinc, selenium sulfide, ketoconazole, or tar. The treatments should be initiated when redness and scale are present and stopped once skin changes resolve.

► CASE 4

An 18-year-old woman develops the acute onset of a mildly pruritic rash of the trunk and extremities. (See Figures 33–8 and 33–9.) She denies a history of atopy.

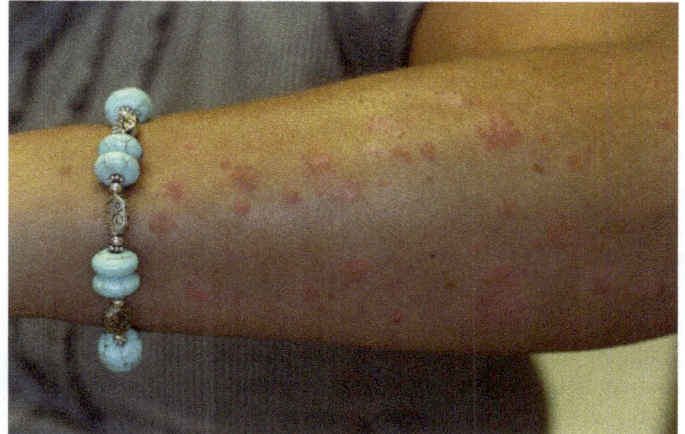

FIGURE 33–7. Seborrheic dermatitis is characterized by erythematous scaling with yellow greasy scales. (Reproduced with permission from Goldsmith LA, Katz SI, Gilchrest BA, Paller AS, Leffell DJ, Wolff K, eds. *Fitzpatrick's Dermatology in General Medicine.* 8th ed. New York, NY: McGraw-Hill Education; 2012, Fig. 22-4.)

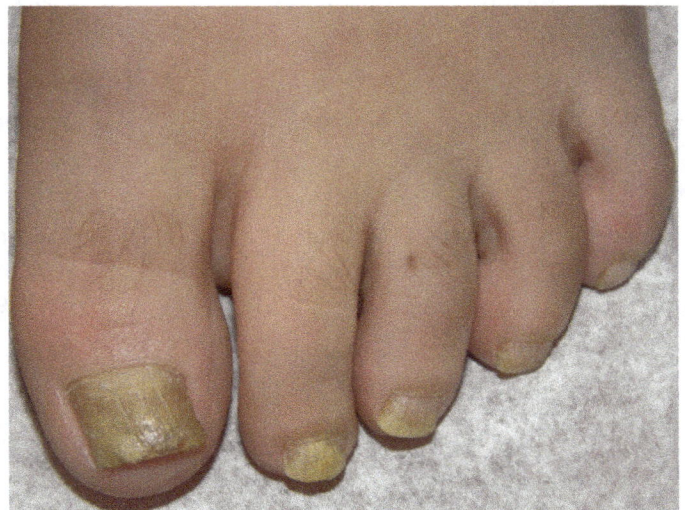

FIGURE 33–9. Psoriatic Nail Disease. The nails are thickened, discolored (yellow), and may be partially detached (onycholysis). Pitting may be seen. (Reproduced with permission from Goldsmith LA, Katz SI, Gilchrest BA, Paller AS, Leffell DJ, Wolff K, eds. *Fitzpatrick's Dermatology in General Medicine.* 8th ed. New York, NY: McGraw-Hill Education; 2012, Fig. 89-18.)

Question 4-1

What is the most likely diagnosis?

A) Atopic dermatitis.
B) Contact dermatitis.
C) Guttate psoriasis.
D) Plaque psoriasis.
E) Seborrheic dermatitis.

Discussion 4-1

The correct answer is "C." Psoriasis is characterized by sharply defined circular erythematous plaques with silver colored scales. Pinpoint bleeding may be seen with removal of the scale; this is known as the Auspitz sign. The fingernails or toenails may be involved. (See Figure 33–9.) Guttate psoriasis (*gutta* is the Greek word for droplet) typically affects patients younger than 30 years of age and is characterized by the abrupt onset of small pink, scaling plaques of the trunk and extremities. (See Figure 33–8.) Plaque psoriasis typically affects extensor surfaces (elbows and knees), scalp, and trunk. Atopic dermatitis (eczema) is characterized by ill-defined plaques that are extremely itchy, concentrating on flexural surfaces. Neonates may develop facial eczema, which is less common as the child grows older. (See Table 33–3.)

Question 4-2

What is the most likely associated symptom?

A) Abdominal pain.
B) Arthritis.
C) Cough.
D) Diarrhea.
E) Sore throat.

Discussion 4-2

The correct answer is "E." Guttate psoriasis is frequently triggered by streptococcal pharyngitis. Psoriatic arthritis affects 5% to 30% of patients and is most common with the plaque subtype.

⧖ QUICK QUIZ

Psoriasis may involve which of the following body areas?

A) Scalp.
B) Nails.
C) Perineum.
D) Elbows.
E) All of the above.

Discussion

The correct answer is "E." Psoriasis commonly involves the extensor surfaces of the elbows and knees, the back, and the scalp. Inverse psoriasis involves the intertriginous areas, including the inguinal, perineal, genital, intergluteal, and axillary areas. Think about psoriasis in an infant with recalcitrant diaper rash.

▶ CASE 5

A 15-year-old girl presents with mild acne vulgaris, predominantly characterized by comedones and rare inflammatory papules. (See Figure 33–10.)

TABLE 33-3 DIFFERENTIAL DIAGNOSIS OF SCALING DERMATITIS

	Age of Onset	Distribution	Clinical Features
Atopic dermatitis	Childhood	Face (infants), flexures	Erythema Scale Ill-defined borders
Contact dermatitis	Any age	Dependent on allergen	Erythema Scale Sharp borders
Seborrheic dermatitis	Childhood	Scalp, postauricular sulci, brows, glabella, alar creases, nasolabial folds, sternal chest, groin	Pink color Yellow, greasy scale Ill-defined borders
Guttate psoriasis	< 30 years	Trunk and extremities	Erythema Silver scale Small plaques Sharp borders
Plaque psoriasis	Any age Peaks at 20–30 years, and again at 50–60 years	Scalp, extensor extremities, trunk, penis, gluteal cleft	Erythema Silver scale Large plaques Sharp borders

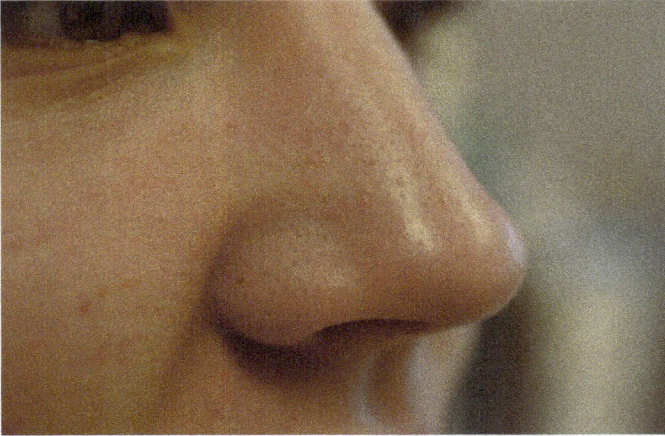

FIGURE 33–10. Acne Vulgaris. The girl in this photo has comedonal acne of her nose characterized by noninflammatory open and closed comedones, commonly referred to as blackheads and whiteheads. (Used with permission from William Augehenbaugh, MD.)

Question 5-1

Which agent is the most appropriate first-line therapy for this patient?
A) Adapalene gel twice daily to acne lesions.
B) Benzoyl peroxide gel once daily to the entire face.
C) Clindamycin gel once daily to acne.
D) Minocycline 100 mg once daily.
E) Tretinoin gel to the entire face at bedtime.

Discussion 5-1

The correct answer is "E." Topical retinoids are the primary first-line treatment for comedonal acne. Retinoids prevent formation of the microcomedone, a small blockage at the apex of the hair follicle, which is the first step in acne formation. Tretinoin (Retin A), adapalene (Differin), and tazarotene (Tazorac) are examples of topical retinoids. The primary side effect is irritation, so prescribing instructions include application of a pea-sized amount to the entire face at bedtime. Because they are used for acne prevention, they should be applied to the entire face. Topical antibiotics treat existing acne and provide anti-inflammatory effects. Therefore they are applied to individual inflamed acne lesions. Oral antibiotics are recommended for up to 3 months to reduce the burden of inflammatory acne.

Two years later, she notes a flare of acne, predominantly of the chin and jawline. She reports irregular periods but no increased facial hair. You start her on an estrogen-progestin oral contraceptive without improvement.

Question 5-2

What is your next step?
A) Oral doxycycline.
B) Oral isotretinoin.
C) Insertion of an intrauterine device to replace use of oral contraceptive pills.
D) Oral spironolactone.
E) Topical benzoyl peroxide.

Discussion 5-2

The correct answer is "D." The increase in androgens at puberty contributes to the development of acne. Estrogens, conversely, have an inhibitory effect on acne. The hallmark of a hormonal influence on acne in young women includes irregular menses, perimenstrual flares, and chin and jawline (beard) distribution of hair. Spironolactone is typically used in combination with oral contraceptive pills (OCPs). It competitively inhibits binding of androgens to androgen receptors, thereby reducing acne. Side effects include urinary frequency, headache, irregular menses or spotting, and feminization of a male fetus. Isotretinoin does not address the underlying hormonal influence and will not have a permanent effect on acne. Most OCPs that improve acne combine estrogen with low-androgenic progestins, such as drospirenone.

▶ CASE 6

A 17-year-old girl experiences a severe flare of acne. (See Figure 33–11.) She has not responded to topical benzoyl peroxide wash and oral minocycline. You are concerned about scarring potential and decide to start her on isotretinoin. You counsel her on the side effects of isotretinoin.

Question 6-1

Which of the following is NOT a side effect of isotretinoin?
A) Depression.
B) Headache and blurred vision (pseudotumor cerebri).
C) Hyperpigmentation.
D) Photosensitivity.
E) Teratogenicity.

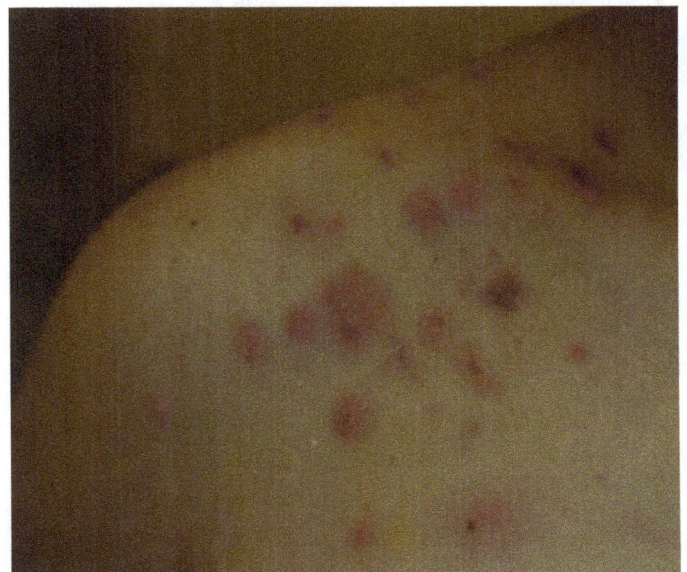

FIGURE 33–11. Inflammatory Acne. Acne may progress, causing inflammatory lesions that include papules, pustules, and nodules. (Used with permission from William Augehenbaugh, MD.)

Discussion 6-1

The correct answer is "C." Patients on isotretinoin should be counseled regarding the side effects of teratogenicity (female patients only), mood changes (controversial association with dysthymia, depression, suicidal ideation), dry skin, hyperlipidemia, arthralgias and myalgias, blurred vision, tinnitus, photosensitivity, and pseudotumor cerebri (leading to headache and blurred vision). (You decide which is worse—the side effect profile of isotretinoin or having acne?)

▶ CASE 7

A 15-year-old boy develops a single asymptomatic patch of alopecia. He was not concerned until multiple additional patches were noted. His mother has not witnessed him pulling his hair.

Question 7-1

What is the most likely diagnosis?
A) Alopecia areata.
B) Syphilis.
C) Telogen effluvium.
D) Tinea capitis.
E) Trichotillomania.

Discussion 7-1

The correct answer is "A." Alopecia areata is a common cause of nonscarring hair loss. It is characterized by the abrupt onset of patches of hair loss (focal alopecia areata; see Figure 33–12), complete loss of all scalp hair (alopecia totalis), or loss of all body hair (alopecia universalis). Alopecia tends to run a chronic

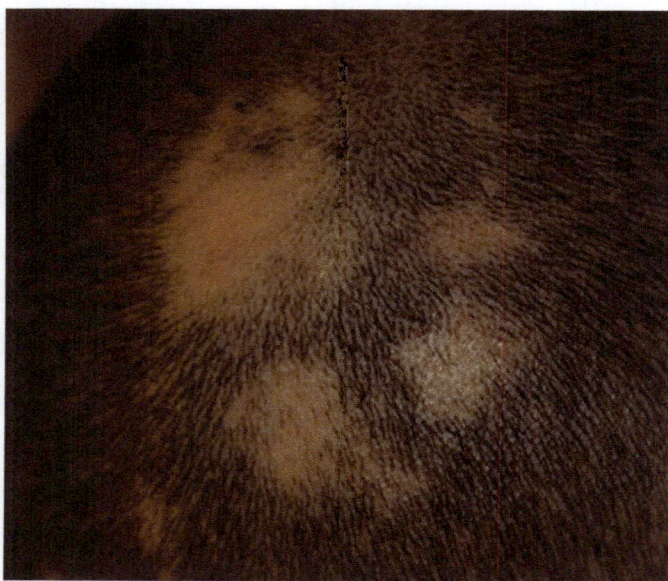

FIGURE 33–12. Alopecia areata typically affects the scalp, causing patches of complete hair loss. Notice the affected areas are smooth, circular, and well defined without scaling. (Used with permission from William Augehenbaugh, MD.)

and recurrent course, with the more severe variants being more resistant to treatment. Secondary syphilis is associated with a "moth-eaten" appearance of hair loss, coupled with scaling patches of the palms, trunk, or extremities. Telogen effluvium typically occurs following a physical or emotional stressor and involves the entire scalp. Patients note diffuse hair thinning, as opposed to discrete patches of hair loss. Tinea capitis is pruritic; examination demonstrates scale and broken hairs. A boggy, elevated lesion known as a kerion may develop. Trichotillomania is characterized by focal or widespread twisted and broken hairs, as a result of physical pulling and manipulation. (See Table 33–4.)

> **Helpful Tip**
> In trichotillomania, look for broken hairs of varying length in the patches of hair loss. In alopecia areata, look for "exclamation point hairs"—short broken-off hairs near the scalp.

Question 7-2

What additional physical exam finding supports your diagnosis of alopecia areata?
A) Hepatosplenomegaly.
B) Lymphadenopathy.
C) Nail thickening.
D) Rubbery nodule on the skin.
E) White patches of skin.

Discussion 7-2

The correct answer is "E." Alopecia areata is an autoimmune disease in which the immune system targets the hair bulb, resulting in miniaturization of the hair. It may be associated with vitiligo, characterized by bright white, nonscaling patches of depigmented skin with or without white hairs (poliosis). Hypothyroidism and pernicious anemia are additional associations. Nail pits, small depressions in the nail bed, may be seen as well. (See Table 33–4, earlier.)

Question 7-3

You recommend a high-potency topical steroid, applied twice daily to the affected area. The patient returns after 3 months, noting no response to therapy. What is your next step?
A) Intralesional steroid injection.
B) Oral methylprednisolone.
C) Topical minoxidil 5% solution.
D) Oral terbinafine.
E) Topical terbinafine.

Discussion 7-3

The correct answer is "A." Steroid injections are effective for the motivated patient as it delivers the medication to the appropriate depth. Serial injections spaced 4 to 8 weeks apart may be necessary to achieve effect. Methylprednisolone or other systemic immunosuppressants are rarely indicated and are most commonly used for rapid shedding seen in alopecia

TABLE 33–4 CONDITIONS ASSOCIATED WITH HAIR LOSS

	Alopecia Areata	Tinea Capitis	Telogen Effluvium	Trichotillomania
Etiology	Autoimmune process with inflammation around hair follicle	Fungal infection of hair shaft or scalp	Reaction to physical or emotional stress	Traumatic pulling of hairs
Clinical findings	Round patches Absence of scale Exclamation point (tapered) hairs Poliosis (white hair) Nail pits	Adherent white scale Black dots—ie, broken hairs at scalp Pustules and boggy plaque (kerion)	Thinning distributed across full scalp Hair pull test positive	Broken and twisted hairs Anxious demeanor
Associated diseases	Vitiligo Hypothyroidism Pernicious anemia	None	None	Psychiatric diseases
Comments	Often recurrent		Onset 2–3 months after physical or emotional stressor	
Treatment	Topical steroids Intralesional steroids Minoxidil (2nd line)	Terbinafine Griseofulvin	Eliminate the stressor Minoxidil	Behavioral modification Psychotherapy Psychotropic medications

totalis or universalis. Minoxidil solution is used for androgenetic alopecia, commonly referred to as male pattern baldness. It is occasionally used as an adjunctive therapy in alopecia areata to help minimize shedding. Since it does not have anti-inflammatory effects, it is minimally effective in alopecia areata. Topical and oral antifungal agents (terbinafine) are employed for tinea capitis.

QUICK QUIZ

What body site is most commonly affected in trichotillomania (nervous hair pulling)?
A) Beard.
B) Eyebrows.
C) Eyelashes.
D) Pubic hair.
E) Scalp.

Discussion

The correct answer is "E." Trichotillomania is most common among girls, with onset typically between the ages of 5 and 12 years. The scalp is most commonly affected. The *Diagnostic and Statistical Manual of Mental Disorders, Fifth Edition* (*DSM-V*) summarizes diagnostic criteria for this condition. (See Table 33–5.) There is no universally effective treatment for trichotillomania. Referral to a psychologist or psychiatrist may be helpful. Treatments include behavior modification, psychotherapy, and psychotropic medications.

> **Helpful Tip**
> Traction alopecia is hair loss resulting from chronic pulling on the hair, such as the tight hair braiding seen in certain cultural practices.

▶ CASE 8

A 6-year-old girl develops severe itching, erythema, and scale on the scalp. Physical exam does not reveal evidence of scarring. Her elbows, knees, and nails are clear. You initially diagnose seborrheic dermatitis, but she fails to respond to topical selenium sulfide shampoo.

TABLE 33–5 *DSM-V* CRITERIA FOR TRICHOTILLOMANIA

- Recurrent pulling out of one's hair, resulting in noticeable hair loss
- An increasing sense of tension immediately before pulling out hair or when attempting to resist the behavior
- Pleasure, gratification, or relief when pulling out hair
- The disturbance is not better accounted for by another mental disorder and is not due to a general medical condition
- The disturbance provokes clinically marked distress and/or impairment in occupational, social, or other areas of functioning

Question 8-1

What is your next step?

A) Bacterial culture.
B) Empiric treatment with a topical antifungal cream.
C) Scalp biopsy.
D) Scrape scalp and send scale for fungal culture.
E) Topical steroid solution to reduce inflammation.

Discussion 8-1

The correct answer is "D." Given the high incidence of tinea capitis among children, culture should be performed in those who do not respond to conservative treatment. (See Figure 33–13.) Tinea capitis presents with single or multiple areas of scaly, patchy hair loss that fluoresce when looked at with a Wood lamp. Seborrheic dermatitis occurs more commonly around the time of puberty and has additional involvement of the brows, glabella, and alar creases. Itching tends to be mild. Bacterial culture may be considered if honey-colored crusting, erosions, or pustules are present. Topical antifungal creams are typically not sufficient to penetrate past the hair and offer inadequate absorption. Although topical steroids may reduce inflammation, they do not address the underlying source of the problem. It is premature to obtain a scalp biopsy. Psoriasis may affect the scalp, but this child has no involvement of the skin or nails. That was a key historical clue snuck into the question.

> **Helpful Tip**
> Dermatophyte infections can be diagnosed by potassium hydroxide (KOH) exam of scrapings from the lesions or fungal culture. With scalp and foot infections, look for fluorescence under a Wood lamp.

Question 8-2

Which of the following is NOT a potential presentation of tinea capitis?

A) Black dots.
B) Boggy plaques.
C) Lymphadenopathy.
D) Pustules.
E) Twisted hairs.

Discussion 8-2

The correct answer is "E." Fungal scalp infections may be ectothrix or endothrix. Ectothrix (outside the hair shaft) infections occur with fungi that fail to penetrate the hair follicle and lead to an adherent white plaque on the scalp and hair follicles. Endothrix (inside the hair shaft) infections invade the hair follicle and lead to weakness of the hair shaft. Broken hairs are visible as black dots on the skin surface. Localized lymphadenopathy may be present. Boggy erythematous plaques and pustules, termed a *kerion*, arise from a severe inflammatory response to a more pathogenic fungus. Kerions may be complicated by permanent scarring. Twisted hairs, often in association with thinning of the eyebrows, are indicative of self-induced plucking of hairs (trichotillomania).

Question 8-3

What is the treatment of choice for tinea capitis?

A) Griseofulvin.
B) Itraconazole.
C) Ketoconazole.
D) Methylprednisolone.
E) Terbinafine.

Discussion 8-3

The correct answer is "E." Tinea capitis is treated with oral antifungal medication. Terbinafine has emerged as the treatment of choice for tinea capitis, as it demonstrates superior efficacy. Historically, griseofulvin was used. However, a longer treatment course is required and emerging resistance has made this a second-line therapy. Azole antifungals may be effective but have associated safety concerns, particularly with oral solutions.

⧗ QUICK QUIZ

Dermatophytes require what for growth?

A) Keratin.
B) Fibrin.
C) Elastin.
D) Collagen.
E) None of the above.

Discussion

The correct answer is "A." Dermatophytes are fungi that metabolize keratin for growth. The skin, nails, and hair are affected as keratin is the major protein of these structures.

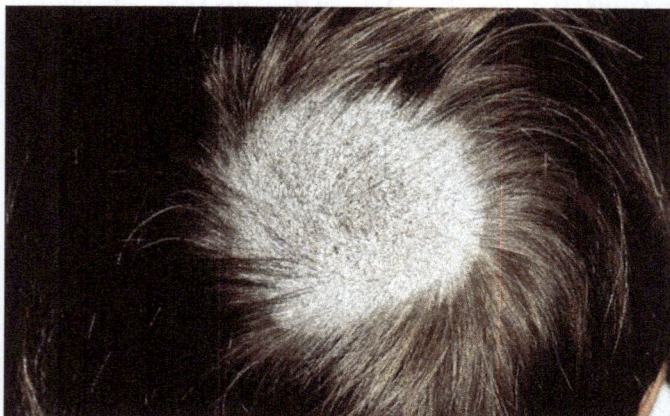

FIGURE 33–13. Tinea capitis is a fungal infection of the scalp that presents as single or multiple areas of scaling hair loss. Erythema, lymphadenopathy, and pruritus may occur. (Reproduced with permission from Wolff K, Johnson RA, and Saavedra AP, eds. *Fitzpatrick's Color Atlas and Synopsis of Clinical Dermatology*, 7th ed. McGraw-Hill Education, Inc., 2013. Fig. 26-43.)

> **Helpful Tip**
> Tinea infections may present with a generalized pruritic rash referred to as *autoeczematization reactions* or *id reactions*. Dermatophytid reactions can occur with tinea pedis, corporis, capitis, or cruris. Management involves treatment of the primary fungal infection.

► CASE 9

A 3-month-old girl presents with a rapidly growing bright red papule on the forehead. (See Figure 33–14.) It was first noted at 1 month of age.

Question 9-1

How do you counsel the family regarding the expected clinical course?
A) It will continue to grow until age 1, with spontaneous resolution by age 10.
B) It will continue to grow until age of 3, with spontaneous resolution by age 15.
C) The vascular lesion is replaced by prominent scarring in most cases.
D) Ulceration and bleeding are typical for the majority of hemangiomas.
E) It will not change.

Discussion 9-1

The correct answer is "A." Infantile (strawberry or capillary) hemangiomas occur in up to 10% of Caucasian infants, and are more common among female and premature infants. They may be superficial bright red papules or deep bluish compressible nodules or plaques. The majority are not visible at birth. They grow in the first 3 to 12 months of life, followed by slow resolution, with the majority resolving by age 9 or 10 years. Residual telangiectasias, scarring, or fibrofatty tissue changes may be left behind. Indications for treatment include potentially life-threatening locations (including airway hemangiomas), disfigurement (eg, lip, ear, or nose hemangiomas), obstruction of vision, ulceration, and psychosocial distress.

► CASE 10

A 2-month-old girl presents with a vascular plaque on the chin that has been present since birth. Parents report it has just started growing.

Question 10-1

What is your next step in management of this infantile hemangioma?
A) Otolaryngology consult.
B) Follow-up in 6 months.
C) Interferon.
D) Magnetic resonance imaging (MRI) to define the extent of the lesion.
E) Oral propranolol.

Discussion 10-1

The correct answer is "A." Hemangiomas in a 'beard' distribution (lower lip, chin, mandible or neck) may be a marker for potentially life threatening airway hemangiomas. Referral to otolaryngology (ENT) is essential. Symptoms of stridor, hoarseness, and cough typically occur in the first few months of life concurrent with growth of the lesion. Be aware, not all children with an airway hemangioma have cutaneous lesions. Lumbosacral hemangiomas may be a marker for spinal dysraphism and should be evaluated with MRI of the spine. Large segmental facial hemangiomas are associated with PHACES syndrome (**P**osterior fossa malformations, **H**emangioma, **A**rterial anomalies, **C**ardiac anomalies and aortic coarctation, **E**ye abnormalities, and **S**ternal clefting or supraumbilical abdominal raphe). Oral propranolol has replaced systemic corticosteroids and interferon for management of complicated hemangiomas. Ulcerated hemangiomas may be treated with pulsed dye laser and wound care. Topical beta-blockers are reserved for superficial infantile hemangiomas.

⧖ QUICK QUIZ

Which is NOT a potential side effect of propranolol therapy for hemangiomas?
A) Hypoglycemia.
B) Hypotension.
C) Bradycardia.
D) Bronchodilation.
E) All of the above.

Discussion

The correct answer is "D." Propranolol may cause bronchospasm. Oral propranolol peaks 1 to 3 hours after it is taken. Patients should be monitored during this time period when starting or increasing therapy.

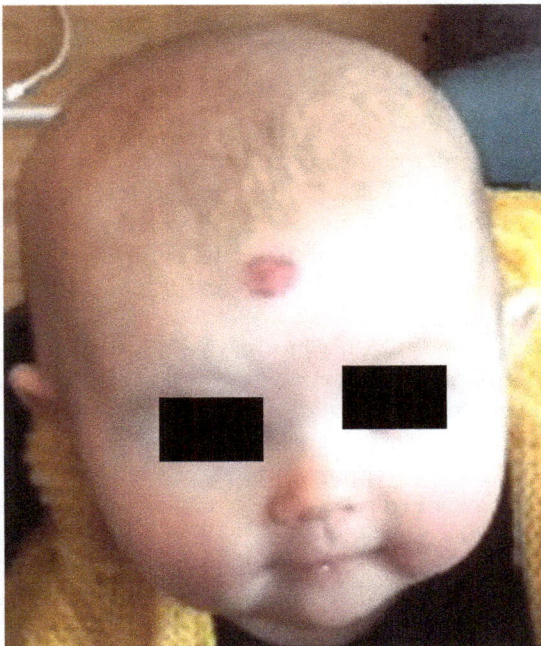

FIGURE 33–14. Infantile hemangiomas present after birth as superficial bright red raised lesions. Deep lesions have a bluish hue. (Used with permission from William Augehenbaugh, MD.)

> **Helpful Tip**
> Subglottic hemangiomas are often mistakenly diagnosed as croup (a viral infection) and treated with steroids. Because steroids treat the hemangioma, the patient improves temporarily.

► CASE 11

A 2-month-old girl presents with a dusky purple patch involving the right forehead, upper and lower eyelids, and cheek in a trigeminal nerve ophthalmic branch (V1) distribution.

Question 11-1

What is the appropriate workup for this infant?

A) Echocardiogram.
B) ENT evaluation.
C) Magnetic resonance angiogram (MRA) of the brain.
D) MRI of the brain and eye exam.
E) No workup is necessary as the birthmark will fade in the first few years of life.

Discussion 11-1

The correct answer is "D." Port-wine stains present at birth with pink to dark red coloration. When located in a V1 distribution, they may be associated with Sturge-Weber syndrome, characterized by glaucoma and leptomeningeal angiomatosis leading to risk of seizures. Ophthalmologic manifestations (glaucoma) occur in approximately 60% of patients with Sturge-Weber syndrome and 20% of those with an isolated port-wine stain; therefore, an eye exam is an important aspect of care for a patient with a port-wine stain in a V1 distribution. MRI is the preferred imaging modality to evaluate for leptomeningeal angiomatosis, and the findings are usually ipsilateral to the lesion. Treatment of uncomplicated lesions is not mandatory. Laser treatments may help reduce the purpura and progressive thickening that are expected over time.

> **Helpful Tip**
> Sturge-Weber syndrome is associated with a port-wine stain on the face in the distribution of the trigeminal nerve. (See Figure 33–15.)

► CASE 12

A 2-day-old healthy full-term Caucasian boy presents with papules and pustules and surrounding erythema on the face, trunk, and extremities. The parents report that the bumps were not present at birth.

Question 12-1

What is the most likely diagnosis?

A) Erythema toxicum neonatorum.
B) Neonatal acne.

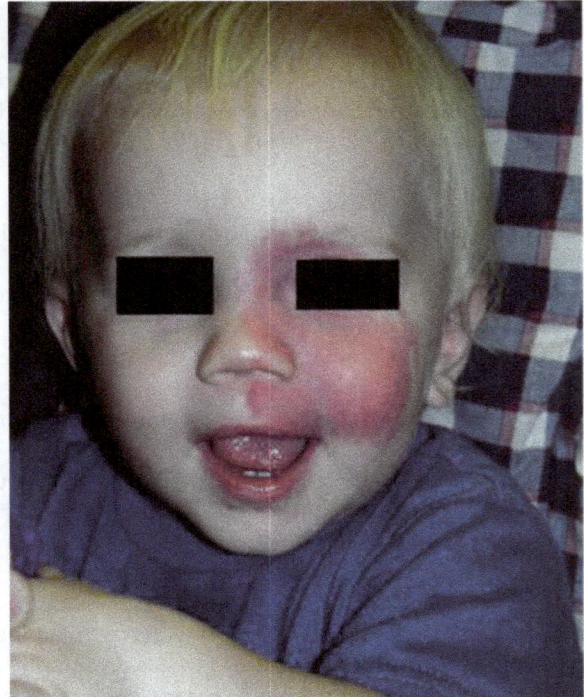

FIGURE 33–15. Sturge-Weber Syndrome. Port-wine stains in a distribution of cranial nerve V (trigeminal) warrant evaluation for Sturge-Weber syndrome or glaucoma, or both. This boy has Sturge-Weber syndrome with a port-wine stain involving V1 (ophthalmic branch) and V2 (maxillary branch). (Reproduced with permission from Brunicardi FC, Andersen DK, Billiar TR, et al, eds. *Schwartz's Principles of Surgery*, 10th ed. McGraw-Hill Education, Inc., 2015. Fig. 45-24B.)

C) Neonatal herpes.
D) Neonatal impetigo.
E) Transient neonatal pustular melanosis.

Discussion 12-1

The correct answer is "A." Erythema toxicum neonatorum is a common disorder, occurring in up to 70% of healthy full-term Caucasian newborns characterized by pustules on an erythematous base. Rarely present at birth, it occurs most commonly in the first 3 to 4 days of life, and can last up to approximately 2 weeks. The lesions may involve the trunk, extremities, or face but spare the palms and soles. (See Figure 33–16.) Transient neonatal pustular melanosis (TNPM) occurs in less than 1% of newborns, most commonly in black infants. It presents at birth with pustules that heal with a collarette of scale surrounding hyperpigmented macules. The palms and soles may be involved. This hyperpigmented macule resolves over weeks to months. (See Figure 33–17.) Neonatal acne, now referred to as neonatal cephalic pustulosis, is not due to androgen stimulation of the oil glands, as occurs in infantile acne (usually developing at 3 months of life). Papules and pustules are confined to the face and develop at age 3 weeks or older. Neonatal herpes is one not to miss. In utero infection with lesions at birth is rare. Typical onset is at 2 weeks of life with the development of weak vesicles on an erythematous base that

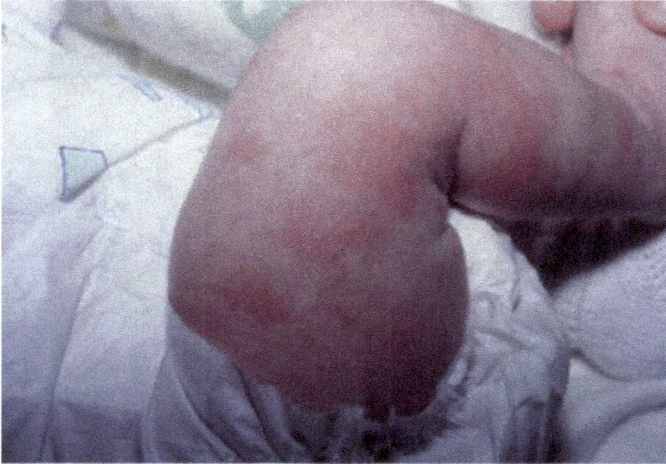

FIGURE 33–16. Erythema Toxicum Neonatorum. Erythema toxicum is a common benign newborn rash characterized by pustules on an erythematous base. Clues include sparing of the palms and soles, development after birth, and presence of eosinophils in lesions. (Reproduced with permission from Goldsmith LA, Katz SI, Gilchrest BA, Paller AS, Leffell DJ, Wolff K, eds. *Fitzpatrick's Dermatology in General Medicine.* 8th ed. New York, NY: McGraw-Hill Education; 2012, Fig. 107-3.)

cluster and coalesce. Neonatal impetigo is a superficial bacterial infection of the skin that can occur in the first few days to 2 weeks of life. It presents clinically as vesicles, pustules, or bullae on an erythematous base. These areas rupture easily and leave superficial erosions and crusting. Common locations of involvement are the skinfolds, such as the neck fold, axilla, and diaper regions.

QUICK QUIZ

A smear from a pustule of erythema toxicum stained with Giemsa would reveal:
A) Bacteria.
B) Eosinophils.
C) Lymphocytes.
D) Neutrophils.
E) Only cellular debris.

Discussion

The correct answer is "B." A smear from the pustular fluid, stained with Wright or Giemsa stain, will reveal eosinophils. In contrast, a smear from a pustule in TNPM shows neutrophils, cellular debris, and occasionally a few eosinophils. Why do you need to know this? For three reasons: (1) it may be on the board exam, (2) to confirm the diagnosis, and (3) to stump residents and medical students on rounds.

QUICK QUIZ

What is the most common cause of a gray patch of the lumbosacral region in an African-American neonate?
A) Congenital nevus.
B) Dermal melanocytosis.
C) Nevus of Ito.
D) Traumatic contusion.
E) Vascular hemangioma.

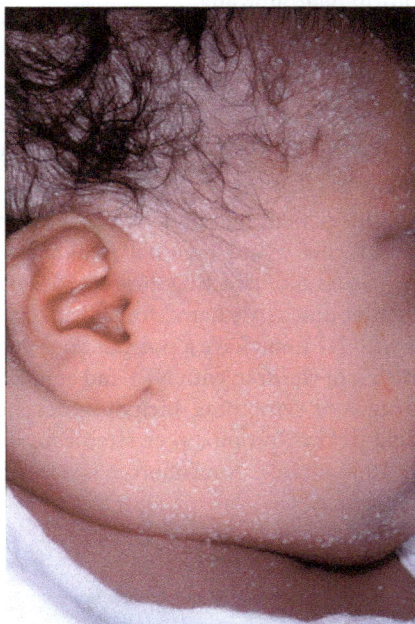
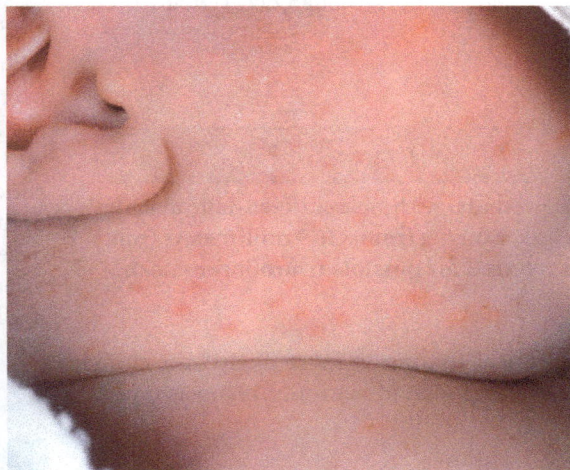

A   B

FIGURE 33–17. Transient neonatal pustular melanosis is a newborn rash characterized by pustules that rupture, leaving a hyperpigmented macule. Clues include presence at birth, involvement of the palms and soles, black race, and presence of neutrophils in lesions. (Reproduced with permission from Goldsmith LA, Katz SI, Gilchrest BA, Paller AS, Leffell DJ, Wolff K, eds. *Fitzpatrick's Dermatology in General Medicine.* 8th ed. New York, NY: McGraw-Hill Education; 2012, Fig 107-4A, B.)

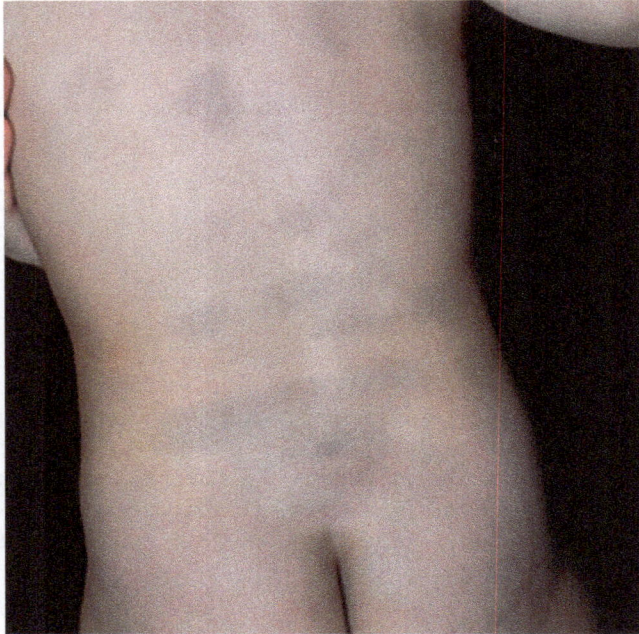

FIGURE 33–18. Dermal Melanocytosis. Multiple bluish plaques are present on the back and buttocks of this Asian child, consistent with dermal melanocytosis or mongolian spots. (Reproduced with permission from Goldsmith LA, Katz SI, Gilchrest BA, Paller AS, Leffell DJ, Wolff K, eds. *Fitzpatrick's Dermatology in General Medicine*. 8th ed. New York, NY: McGraw-Hill Education; 2012, Fig. 9-11.)

Discussion

The correct answer is "B." Dermal melanocytosis (mongolian spot) is a benign melanocytic lesion that occurs in more than 90% of African-American infants, more than 80% of Asian infants, 70% of Hispanic infants, and close to 10% of Caucasian infants. The lesions appear as gray, blue-black, or brown patches, most commonly over the lumbosacral back and buttocks. (See Figure 33–18.) Most are present at birth and fade in the first 2 to 3 years of life, although occasionally they persist into adulthood.

▶ CASE 13

A 5-year-old girl presents with five café-au-lait macules (CALMs) on the trunk, ranging from 5 to 9 millimeters (mm) in diameter. She is referred for possible neurofibromatosis.

Question 13-1

What additional physical finding is most likely in a child this age to support the diagnosis of neurofibromatosis type 1 (NF1)?
A) Axillary freckling.
B) Neurofibroma.
C) Lisch nodule.
D) Optic glioma.
E) None, as there are an insufficient number of CALMs for a diagnosis of NF1.

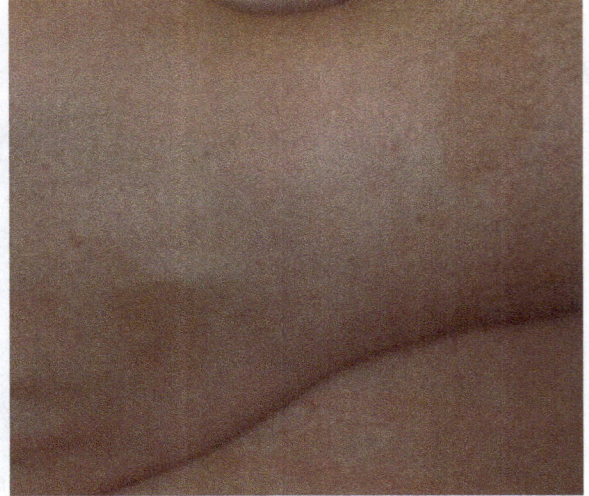

FIGURE 33–19. Café-au-Lait Macules. Two brown ovoid lesions consistent with café-au-lait macules are present on this child. Multiple lesions should raise the suspicion of neurofibromatosis type 1. (Used with permission from William Augehenbaugh, MD.)

Discussion 13-1

The correct answer is "A." Although NF1, also known as von Recklinghausen disease, is an autosomal dominant disorder, approximately 50% of cases are due to new mutations. In order to diagnose the disorder, the patient must have two or more of the following:

- Six CALMs 5 mm or larger in prepubescent patients and 1.5 centimeters (cm) or larger after puberty (see Figure 33–19)
- Axillary or inguinal freckling
- Plexiform neurofibroma
- Two or more dermal neurofibromas
- Two or more Lisch nodules
- Optic glioma
- Skeletal dysplasia (tibial or sphenoid wing dysplasia)
- First degree relative with NF1

Although this patient had only five CALMs, more can develop over time. Axillary and inguinal freckling usually occurs by age 3 to 5 years old, affecting 20% to 50% of individuals with NF1. Lisch nodules (iris hamartomas) affect more than 90% of patients with NF1 and have a postpubertal onset. Optic gliomas occur in 15% of children with NF1 and approximately one-third develop signs or symptoms, including decreased visual acuity, visual field defects, proptosis, or strabismus. Annual eye exam until age 10 is advised. Neurofibromas occur in later childhood and adolescence.

▶ CASE 14

A 10-year-old boy presents for treatment of shiny, pink papules on the face. They were noted at age 6 years. Neither pustules nor comedones are seen on physical exam. (See Figure 33–20.)

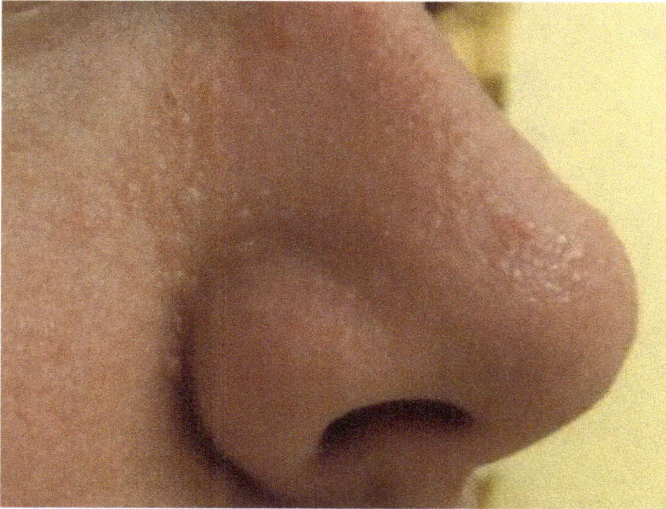

FIGURE 33–20. Angiofibromas looking like shiny, pink papules are present on the nose and malar region of this child with tuberous sclerosis. A clue is the lack of comedones. (Used with permission from William Augehenbaugh, MD.)

Question 14-1

What is your next step?
A) Topical benzoyl peroxide.
B) Oral isotretinoin.
C) Oral antibiotic.
D) Shave biopsy.
E) Topical metronidazole.

Discussion 14-1

The correct answer is "D." Angiofibromas may be mistaken for inflammatory acne papules. The shiny surface, onset between 2 and 6 years, and absence of comedones helps in distinguishing angiofibromas from acne.

You perform a biopsy due to your suspicion that the facial papules represent angiofibromas of tuberous sclerosis.

Question 14-2

What additional finding(s) on physical exam is/are expected with tuberous sclerosis in a child this age?
A) Dark macules of the iris.
B) Dental pits.
C) Hypopigmented macule of the trunk.
D) Skin-colored papule of the nail fold.
E) None of the above.

Discussion 14-2

The correct answer is "C." Hypopigmented macules, referred to as "ash-leaf spots," are usually present at birth. They may be lance-ovate resembling an ash leaf, small confetti-like, or oval in shape. (See Figure 33–21.) Use of a Wood lamp accentuates the lesions, which may be otherwise hard to

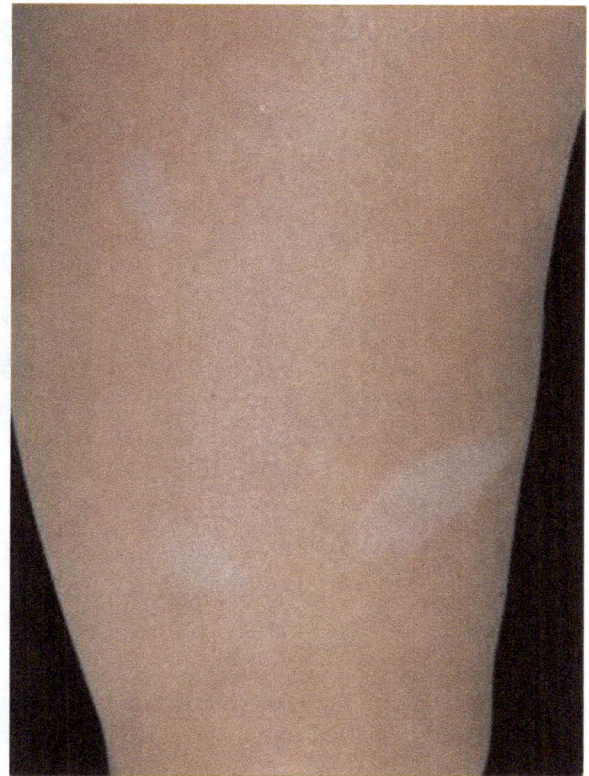

FIGURE 33–21. Ash-Leaf Spots. A hypopigmented ash-leaf macules are present on the skin of this child with tuberous sclerosis. (Reproduced with permission from Goldsmith LA, Katz SI, Gilchrest BA, Paller AS, Leffell DJ, Wolff K, eds. *Fitzpatrick's Dermatology in General Medicine*. 8th ed. New York, NY: McGraw-Hill Education; 2012, Fig. 16-2A.)

see. Collagenomas (Shagreen patches) typically present on the trunk during late childhood. They are flesh-colored subtle plaques with an "orange peel" surface. Periungual fibromas occur in or after puberty around the fingernails and toenails. Dental pits typically occur in adulthood. (See Figure 33–22.)

> **Helpful Tip**
> Systemic manifestations of tuberous sclerosis include seizures, cortical tubers, subependymal nodules or giant cell astrocytomas, cardiac rhabdomyomas, renal angiomyolipomas, multiple renal cysts, multiple retinal hamartomas, and lymphangioleiomyomatosis, among others.

▶ CASE 15

A 9-month-old boy presents with fevers of unknown origin. His parents report that he does not sweat with fevers or after exposure to hot weather. Physical examination reveals periorbital wrinkling, frontal bossing, a thick everted lip, and small low-set ears.

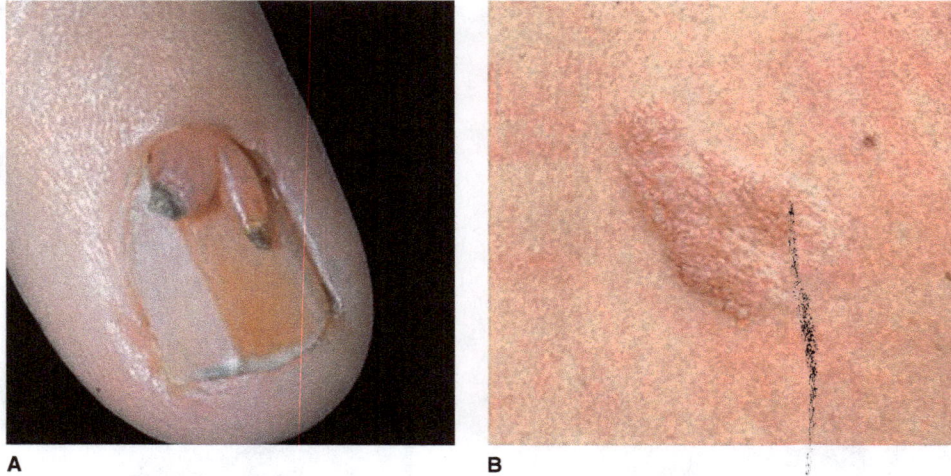

FIGURE 33–22. Cutaneous findings of tuberous sclerosis. (A) Periungual fibroma. (B) Shagreen patches are connective tissue nevi made of collagen that appear as skin-colored lesions with an orange peel texture. (Reproduced with permission from Goldsmith LA, Katz SI, Gilchrest BA, Paller AS, Leffell DJ, Wolff K, eds. *Fitzpatrick's Dermatology in General Medicine.* 8th ed. New York, NY: McGraw-Hill Education; 2012, Fig. 16-5A, B.)

Question 15-1

What additional feature supports your diagnosis of hypohidrotic ectodermal dysplasia?

A) Calcinosis cutis.
B) Nail dystrophy.
C) Numerous nevi.
D) Short sparse hair and abnormal dentition.
E) Thick, protuberant tongue.

Discussion 15-1

The correct answer is "D." This child has hypohidrotic (reduced sweating) ectodermal dysplasia, which is an X-linked recessive disorder affecting males. Patients have absent or reduced sweating, abnormal dentition, characteristic facies, and alopecia. The reduced or absent ability to sweat may cause fevers. Gastroesophageal reflux is common. A concurrent immunodeficiency may occur in some cases. Treatment is aimed at avoiding overheating and cooling the skin. Multidisciplinary care, including dentistry, is important. The most common form of hidrotic ectodermal dysplasia is characterized by the triad of sparse, brittle hair, nail dystrophy, and palmoplantar hyperkeratosis. It is inherited in an autosomal dominant fashion. This condition is associated with neither craniofacial abnormalities nor reduced sweating. Teeth are normal but are more likely to develop caries.

> **Helpful Tip**
> Ectodermal dysplasia is a group of disorders in which parts of the ectoderm, skin, teeth, hair, nails, sweat glands, or a combination of these, do not form correctly. The disorders are categorized as hypohidrotic/anhidrotic (no or reduced sweating) and hidrotic (normal sweating).

▶ CASE 16

A 14-year-old girl presents with a verrucous hairless plaque on the scalp. It was present at birth as a subtle yellow plaque that has gotten thicker over the past 1 to 2 years.

Question 16-1

What is the most likely diagnosis?

A) Aplasia cutis congenita.
B) Congenital nevus.
C) Nevus sebaceous.
D) Seborrheic keratosis.
E) Pilomatricoma.

Discussion 16-1

The correct answer is "C." Nevus sebaceous, a congenital hamartoma of the skin, usually presents at birth on the scalp or face and can be yellow or tan in color. It grows in proportion with the child and becomes thicker and more warty around puberty. Benign hyperplasia can occur within nevus sebaceous, but the risk of malignant growths is rare. (See Figure 33–23.) Aplasia cutis congenita affects the scalp. At birth, it is a circular open lesion that heals as a smooth, atrophic scar. Congenital nevi are typically pigmented with a cobbled surface. Pilomatricomas are hard, skin-colored to white nodules of the face and upper extremities. A nevus sebaceous is a warty, light-colored growth that appears stuck on the skin and occurs in adults.

▶ CASE 17

A 2-year-old boy presents with a 6-month history of multiple brown macules of the trunk. His mother notes that a wheal forms when the lesions are scratched.

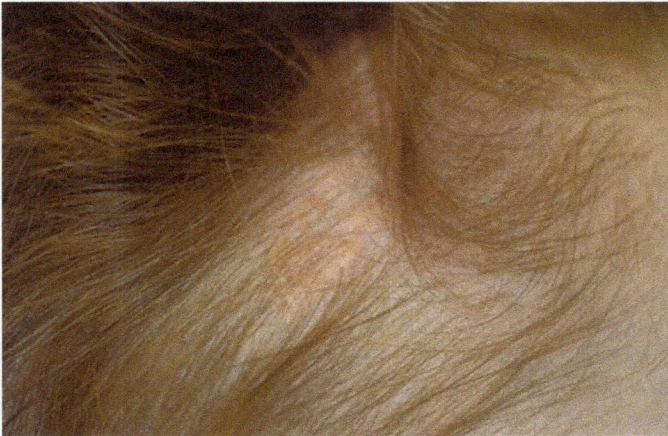

FIGURE 33–23. Nevus Sebaceous. On the scalp is a yellow, thickened, wartlike lesion consistent with a nevus sebaceous. (Used with permission from William Augehenbaugh, MD.)

Question 17-1

What additional symptom supports your diagnosis of mastocytosis?

A) Cough.
B) Diarrhea.
C) Headache.
D) Hematuria.
E) Hyperhidrosis.

Discussion 17-1

The correct answer is "B." Cutaneous mastocytosis refers to collections of mast cells in the skin. Solitary mastocytoma presents as a single tan plaque, whereas urticaria pigmentosa is characterized by multiple tan to brown macules or papules. (See Figure 33–24.) Bullae may occur with either condition. A positive Darier sign is expected with all subtypes of mastocytomas, whereby stroking the skin leads to erythema and urticaria of the lesion. Mast cells may also collect in the gut. When mast cells are stimulated to degranulate, histamine release leads to urticarial wheals or diarrhea, depending on where the cell are located. There is no cure for mastocytosis. Treatment is directed at symptomatic relief. Antihistamines are the mainstay of treatment. Topical or oral corticosteroids and phototherapy are rarely necessary.

⏳ QUICK QUIZ

Which is NOT a trigger of mast cell activation and degranulation?

A) Spicy foods.
B) Hot shower.
C) Acetaminophen.
D) Opioid medications.

Discussion

The correct answer is "C." In mastocytosis, disease triggers are non-IgE mediated, such as stress and temperature (hot showers). Patients severely affected by mastocytosis should avoid alcohol,

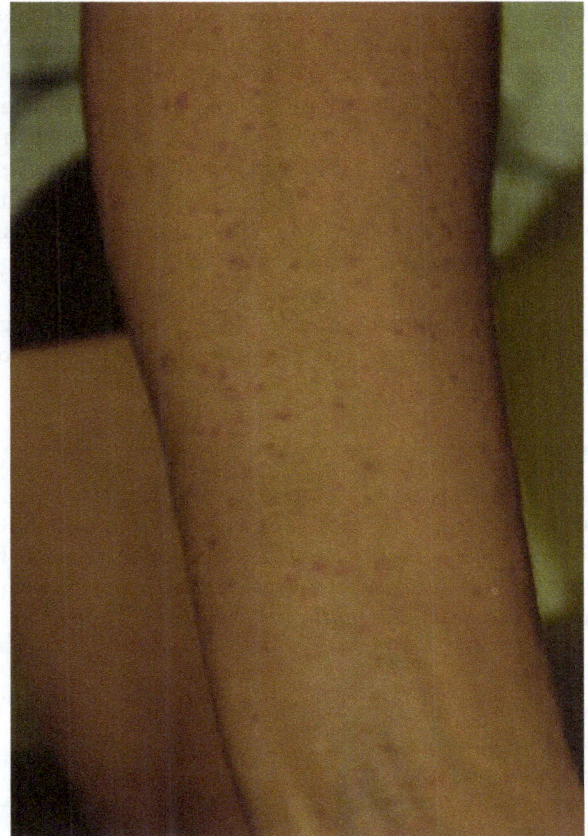

FIGURE 33–24. Cutaneous Mastocytosis. Mast cells collect in the skin to form brown to tan macules in mastocytosis. This patient has urticaria pigmentosa, with multiple mastocytomas present. (Used with permission from William Augehenbaugh, MD.)

aspirin, nonsteroidal anti-inflammatory drugs (NSAIDs), narcotics, egg whites, chocolate, strawberries, tomatoes, and citrus as these may stimulate mast cell degranulation.

▶ CASE 18

A newborn develops blisters and erosions in areas of trauma. No scarring is noted on physical exam. You suspect epidermolysis bullosa simplex.

Question 18-1

What is appropriate counseling for the family?

A) All types are associated with high mortality rate.
B) Basal cell carcinomas are a common complication.
C) Electron microscopy is required to subtype this disorder.
D) Epidermolysis bullosa simplex is likely to resolve spontaneously.
E) Scarring is common to all phenotypes of the disorder.

Discussion 18-1

The correct answer is "C." Epidermolysis bullosa is divided into three subtypes: simplex, junctional, and dystrophic. Each subtype has mild and severe phenotypes, depending on the defective or absent structure required to maintain cell-to-cell adhesion. Inheritance varies according to the different phenotypes. Most types show skin fragility leading to bullae and erosions in the newborn period. Additional findings may include growth retardation, nail dystrophy, milia, scarring, and oral erosions. In the more severe subtypes, scarring may lead to mitten hand deformities, joint contractures, and esophageal strictures. Electron microscopy and immunomapping are important for accurate diagnosis. In the recessive dystrophic subtype, squamous cell carcinoma occurs in 40% of patients by the age of 30 and can progress rapidly, resulting in death. Recent advances in gene therapy are revolutionizing treatment of epidermolysis bullosa.

▶ CASE 19

A full-term girl is born with vesicles in a linear distribution on the arm. She is otherwise well. Workup for neonatal herpes and bullous impetigo are negative. You make the diagnosis of incontinentia pigmenti.

Question 19-1

How do you counsel the family about how the lesions will appear into adulthood?
A) Atrophic plaques.
B) Hyperpigmented patches.
C) Hypopigmented patches.
D) Scars.
E) Verrucous papules.

Discussion 19-1

The correct answer is "C." Incontinentia pigmenti is an X-linked dominant disorder that is lethal in males, although rare cases in patients with Klinefelter syndrome and somatic mosaicism have been reported. Neonates present with erythematous macules and vesicles in a linear and whorled distribution, following developmental lines of Blaschko. After several days to weeks, the vesicles resolve and are replaced by verrucous papules. These papules resolve leaving behind hyperpigmented macules in a swirled pattern. Over time, the hyperpigmentation is replaced by hypopigmented macules. Ocular, skeletal, and neurologic abnormalities may occur.

> **Helpful Tip**
> The lines of Blaschko are usually not visible. In certain diseases of the skin and mucosa, they appear as whorls or wavelike shapes on the skin.

▶ CASE 20

A healthy 2-year-old boy presents with a 2 cm nodule on the midline nasal root. It was noted in infancy but has recently enlarged. You suspect a dermoid cyst. His parents request removal.

Question 20-1

What is your next step?
A) Incision and drainage.
B) MRI.
C) Oral antibiotics.
D) Punch biopsy.
E) Surgical excision.

Discussion 20-1

The correct answer is "B." Dermoid cysts are congenital lesions that arise along embryonic fusion planes. They may not become noticeable until later in childhood when they enlarge and become inflamed or infected. The lateral eyebrow is a common location; however, they may also be located on the midline nose, scalp, neck, back, and sternum. Lesions on the midline nose and midline scalp have higher risk of intracranial extension; therefore, imaging is required before any intervention is pursued.

▶ CASE 21

A 15-year-old boy presents with erythematous targetoid lesions of the arms. He has no active mucosal lesions. You elicit a history of herpes labialis 10 days prior to onset.

Question 21-1

What is the most likely diagnosis?
A) Erythema multiforme major.
B) Erythema multiforme minor.
C) Leukocytoclastic vasculitis.
D) Stevens-Johnson syndrome.
E) Toxic epidermal necrolysis.

Discussion 21-1

The correct answer is "B." Erythema multiforme is a self-limited eruption characterized by lesions that resemble a target. (See Figure 33–25.) The rash most commonly follows or occurs concurrently with a herpes simplex virus (HSV) infection. An alternative term is erythema multiforme minor (EM minor). The term *erythema multiforme major* (EM major) has been replaced by *Stevens-Johnson syndrome*. This syndrome is a severe inflammatory reaction to medication, infection, or underlying inflammatory disease. Stevens-Johnson syndrome and toxic epidermal necrolysis are variants of the same disease. Leukocytoclastic vasculitis may also arise from infection or medication and is a nonblanching, purpuric papule. This condition may lead to renal dysfunction, so close monitoring is imperative. (See Table 33–6.)

▶ CASE 22

A 12-year-old boy with epilepsy develops acute-onset malaise, fever, and painful skin 2 weeks after starting an anticonvulsant. The eruption starts on his trunk and then spreads to the entire body, resulting in widespread skin sloughing. You admit him to the hospital.

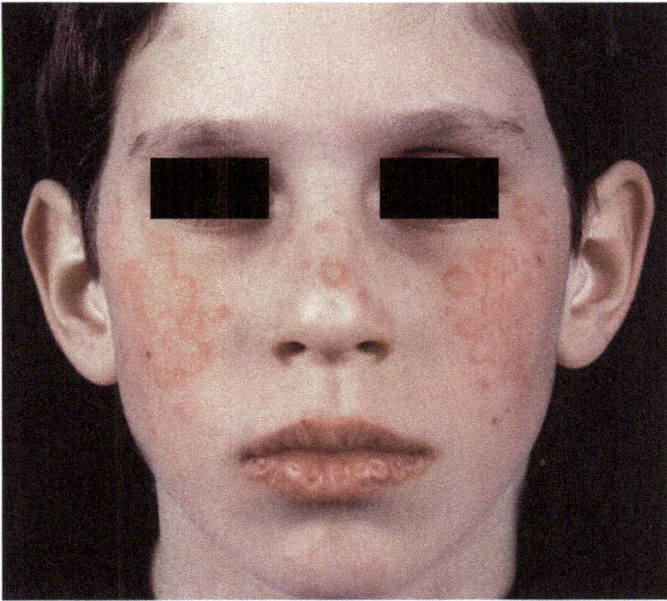

FIGURE 33-25. Erythema Multiforme Minor. Multiple, confluent, target-like papules on the face of a 12-year-old boy. The target morphology of the lesions is best seen on the lips. (Reproduced with permission from Wolff K, Johnson RA, Saavedra AP, eds. *Fitzpatrick's Color Atlas and Synopsis of Clinical Dermatology*. 7th ed. McGraw-Hill Education; 2013, Fig. 14-15.)

Question 22-1

What finding helps support your diagnosis of toxic epidermal necrolysis (TEN)?

A) Angioedema of the lips.
B) Facial edema.
C) Hemorrhagic crust on the lips.
D) Normal ocular conjunctivae.
E) Urticarial plaques.

Discussion 22-1

The correct answer is "C." Stevens-Johnson syndrome (SJS) and TEN result in a febrile illness with painful exanthems and mucosal erosions that may involve the mouth, eyes, gastrointestinal tract, respiratory tract, or urethra. (See Figures 33–26 and 33–27.) The epidermis becomes necrotic, with sloughing of the skin. Nikolsky sign (stroking of the skin causes blistering) may be positive. Both manifestations are considered part of the continuum of the same disorder. SJS is associated with less than 10% body surface area (BSA) involvement, SJS-TEN with 10% to 30% BSA involvement, and TEN with greater than 30% BSA involvement. (See Table 33–6, earlier.) The most common findings are the result of a severe reaction to medications (sulfa antibiotics, anticonvulsants, and allopurinol). *Mycoplasma pneumoniae* is a known trigger. SJS and TEN may be life threatening and require hospitalization.

TABLE 33–6 COMPARISONS OF ERYTHEMA MULTIFORME, STEVENS-JOHNSON SYNDROME, AND TOXIC EPIDERMAL NECROLYSIS

	Erythema Multiforme	Stevens-Johnson Syndrome	Toxic Epidermal Necrolysis
Synonym/Acronym	EM minor	EM major (outdated term) SJS	TEN
Etiology	Herpes simplex virus (50%) *Histoplasma*	Medications: NSAIDs, anticonvulsants, sulfonamide and penicillin antibiotics Infection: *Mycoplasma pneumoniae*, fungal infections, cytomegalovirus Inflammatory bowel disease	
Clinical findings	No systemic prodrome Targetoid lesions Oral erosions, typically mild	Prodrome Focal dusky red patches Hemorrhagic crust on lips Oral erosions, stomatitis Conjunctivitis Anogenital erosions Involved BSA < 10%	Prodrome Large dusky red patches Hemorrhagic crust on lips Oral erosions, stomatitis Conjunctivitis Anogenital erosions Involved BSA > 30%
Treatment	None required Suppressive oral antiviral for recurrent episodes	Discontinue offending drugs Admit to hospital (burn unit for TEN) Treat of infection if present Supportive care Ophthalmology consult	
Mortality		Up to 30%	25–50%

BSA, body surface area; NSAIDs, nonsteroidal anti-inflammatory medications.

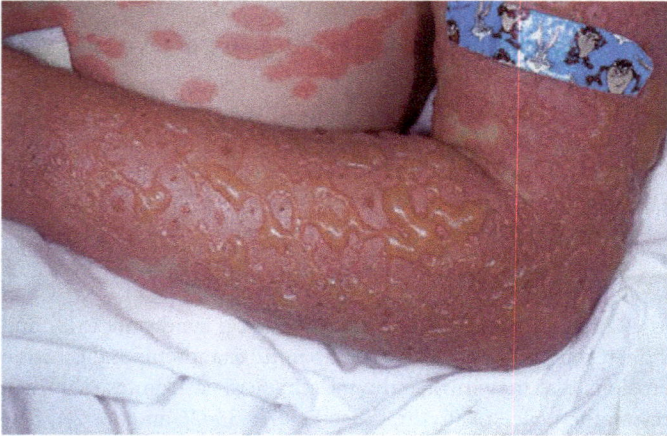

FIGURE 33–26. Stevens-Johnson Syndrome. The skin blisters and sloughs in Stevens-Johnson syndrome as a result of epidermal necrosis. (Reproduced with permission from Grippi MA, Elias JA, Fishman JA, Kotloff RM, Pack AI, Senior RM, eds. *Fishman's Pulmonary Disease and Disorders*. 5th ed. New York, NY: McGraw-Hill Education; 2015, Fig. 29-36.)

Helpful Tip

SJS and TEN are febrile exanthems (rashes) and enanthems (mucosal eruptions). Look for erythematous lesions with a dusky center that become bullae, coalesce, and rupture.

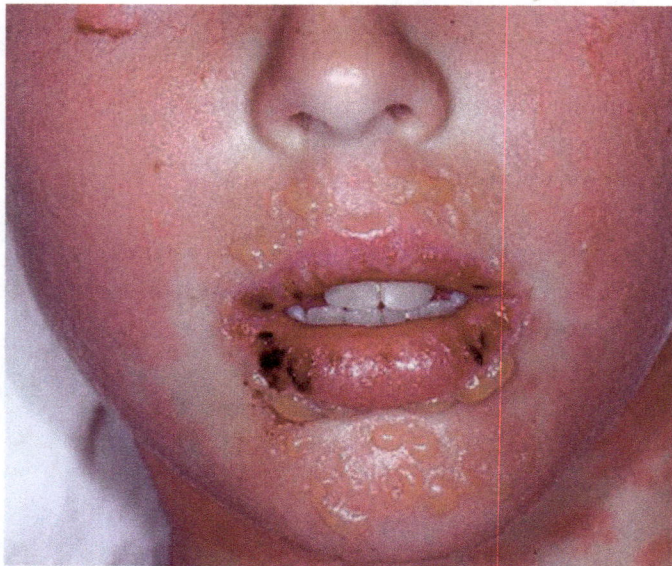

FIGURE 33–27. Mucositis and Stevens-Johnson Syndrome. In this patient with Stevens-Johnson syndrome, the oral mucosa and lips have painful hemorrhagic erosions. A gray-white membrane may cover the lesions. (Reproduced with permission from Grippi MA, Elias JA, Fishman JA, Kotloff RM, Pack AI, Senior RM, eds. *Fishman's Pulmonary Disease and Disorders*. 5th ed. New York, NY: McGraw-Hill Education; 2015, Fig. 29-37.)

► CASE 23

A 15-year-old healthy boy presents with crusting on the arm after falling off his skateboard 2 weeks earlier. (See Figure 33–28.) The erosion has not yet healed.

Question 23-1

Which test is most appropriate to confirm the diagnosis?
A) Bacterial culture.
B) Biopsy.
C) Fungal culture.
D) Tzanck preparation.
E) None of the above.

Discussion 23-1

The correct answer is "A." Impetigo is an infection of the epidermis primarily caused by *Staphylococcal aureus*. Primary impetigo results from bacterial invasion of normal skin and affects mainly toddlers. The face is a popular target, especially the chin and around the nose. Secondary impetigo commonly occurs following trauma, when the normal skin barrier is disrupted. Staphylococcal or streptococcal bacteria, or both, populate the wound base and impede healing. The classic appearance is a honey-colored crust. Lesions progress from papules to vesicles to pustules that rupture and become crusted. Although a bacterial culture may be performed, empiric treatment is common if the clinical appearance supports the diagnosis of impetigo. A KOH examination is used to diagnose a superficial fungal infection. Fungal culture is rarely necessary. A Tzanck preparation is used to diagnose herpes infections.

You confirm the diagnosis of impetigo based on physical exam.

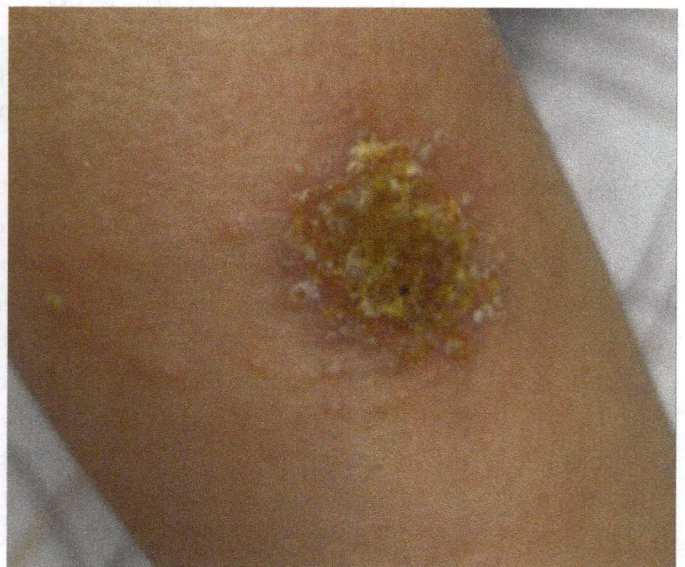

FIGURE 33–28. Impetigo is a superficial bacterial infection of the skin. In the nonbullous form, papules become vesicles that rupture, forming a honey-colored crust. Notice the thick honey-colored crust with surrounding erythematous pustules in this patient. (Used with permission from William Augehenbaugh, MD.)

Question 23-2

What is your recommended treatment?
A) Bacitracin ointment.
B) Cephalexin.
C) Dicloxacillin.
D) Erythromycin.
E) Mupirocin ointment.

Discussion 23-2

The correct answer is "E." Topical agents are most appropriate for nonbullous impetigo, which is a superficial infection. Mupirocin (Bactroban) is the treatment of choice. Oral antibiotics are typically reserved for bullous impetigo. Bacitracin provides little antibacterial effect and may be complicated by allergic contact dermatitis.

> **Helpful Tip**
> Impetigo lesions are very contagious. Remind family members to wash their hands and avoid touching the lesions.

⏳ QUICK QUIZ

Which of the following statements regarding impetigo is true?
A) Bullous impetigo is an infection of the dermis.
B) Bullous impetigo forms bullae on the skin.
C) Bullous impetigo is more common than nonbullous impetigo.
D) Bullous and nonbullous impetigo are characterized by a honey-colored crusting.
E) Bullous impetigo and nonbullous impetigo are more common in adults.

Discussion

The correct answer is "B." It seems intuitive that bullous impetigo forms bullae. Impetigo may be bullous or nonbullous, but both are epidermal infections that primarily affect young children. Nonbullous impetigo is the more common papulovesicular rash that forms a honey-colored crust. It can be caused by staphylococcal or streptococcal bacteria. In bullous impetigo, flaccid bullae form and rupture, leaving an erythematous base with a peeling rim and brown crust. (See Figure 33–29.) It is caused by toxin-producing *Staphylococcus aureus*.

▶ CASE 24

A 5-year-old previously healthy boy is hospitalized with a 3-day history of malaise, fever, and generalized erythema. He complains of skin pain. He was given acetaminophen (Tylenol) for the past 3 days without relief. Examination is notable for flaccid bullae and desquamation of the chest and

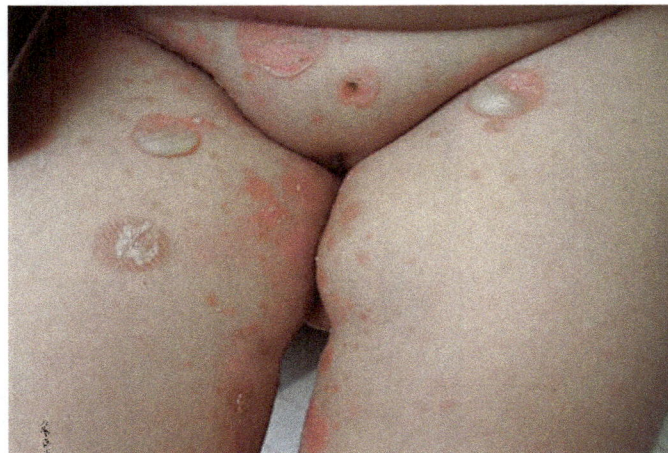

FIGURE 33–29. Bullous impetigo is less common that primary impetigo and affects mainly children. Flaccid bullae form and fill with cloudy fluid. The bullae rupture, leaving an erythematous base with peeling rim and brown crust. (Reproduced with permission from Goldsmith LA, Katz SI, Gilchrest BA, Paller AS, Leffell DJ, Wolff K, eds. *Fitzpatrick's Dermatology in General Medicine.* 8th ed. New York, NY: McGraw-Hill Education; 2012, Fig. 177-2.)

axillae. Oral, ocular, and genital mucosae are clear. Touching the skin causes it to slough.

Question 24-1

What is the most likely diagnosis?
A) Bullous impetigo.
B) Morbilliform drug eruption.
C) Pemphigus vulgaris.
D) Staphylococcal scalded skin syndrome.
E) Toxic epidermal necrolysis.

Discussion 24-1

The correct answer is "D." Staphylococcal scalded skin syndrome (SSSS) is caused by an exotoxin secreted by *Staphylococcus aureus*. This toxin targets the proteins that bind keratinocytes (epidermal skin cells) together. Disruption of these bonds leads to superficial sloughing of the skin. (See Figure 33–30.) Bullous impetigo arises as a single or multiple cutaneous erosions, as the blisters rupture easily. It has the same etiology as SSSS (toxin mediated) but is more localized and does not cause diffuse erythema. Morbilliform drug eruptions present as erythematous macules and papules that start on the trunk and spread to the extremities. Pemphigus vulgaris and toxic epidermal necrolysis (TEN) lead to blisters at the level of the dermoepidermal junction, resulting in higher morbidity and mortality. Both pemphigus vulgaris and TEN are associated with severe mucosal involvement.

> **Helpful Tip**
> Painful skin should always be taken seriously. Differential diagnosis of painful skin includes SSSS, Stevens-Johnson/TEN, pemphigus vulgaris, and thermal burns.

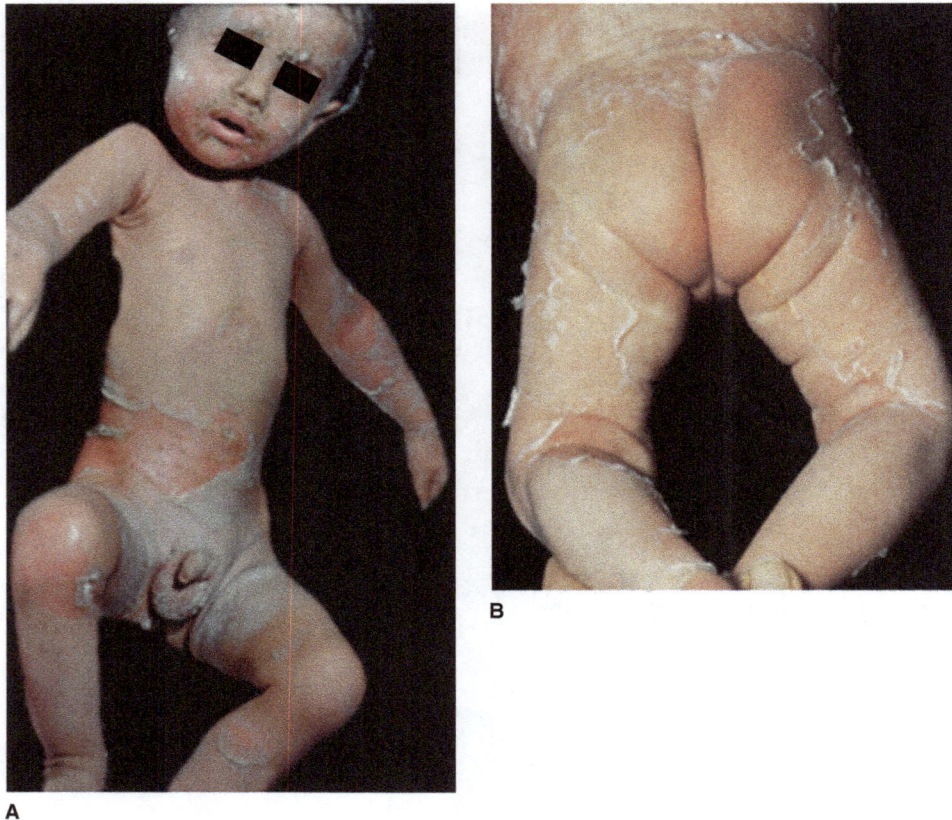

FIGURE 33–30. Staphylococcal Scalded Skin Syndrome. This infant developed staphylococcal scalded skin syndrome from perioral impetigo. The erythematous skin forms bullae and sloughs, leaving large areas of denuded skin. (Reproduced with permission from Goldsmith LA, Katz SI, Gilchrest BA, Paller AS, Leffell DJ, Wolff K, eds. *Fitzpatrick's Dermatology in General Medicine*. 8th ed. New York, NY: McGraw-Hill Education; 2012, Fig 25-40A, B.)

Question 24-2

Which test do you perform to confirm your suspicion of SSSS?

A) Biopsy.

B) Blood culture.

C) Culture of axillary vault.

D) Culture of a bullous lesion.

E) No tests are necessary as the diagnosis is made clinically.

Discussion 24-2

The correct answer is "E." Acute onset of painful skin, bullae, and skin sloughing is classic for SSSS. Imagine a really painful sunburn. SSSS typically affects neonates and children younger than 5 years of age. It starts with fever and diffuse tender erythema of the skin, especially around the mouth, eyes, axilla, and groin. Fissuring occurs around the eyes, nose, and mouth. The skin sloughs with gentle pressure (positive Nikolsky sign), forms bullae, and later desquamates. (See Figure 33–30, earlier.) Blood cultures are negative. Culture is of low yield, unless taken from the nares, nasopharynx, conjunctivae, or purulent material on the skin. Conversely, skin culture is typically high yield in bullous impetigo. Treatment of SSSS includes intravenous antibiotics, wound care, and supportive care.

Helpful Tip

Look for mucosal involvement to help differentiate staphylococcal scalded skin syndrome from Stevens-Johnson syndrome/toxic epidermal necrolysis. Mucositis is present in SJS and TEN but not SSSS.

QUICK QUIZ

The Nikolsky sign is positive in all of the following EXCEPT:

A) TEN.

B) Scarlet fever.

C) SSSS.

D) Pemphigus vulgaris.

E) Bullous impetigo.

Discussion

The correct answer is "B." The Nikolsky sign is not a perfect clinical test but it can be helpful. The test is positive when stroking the skin causes it to tear and wrinkle in a fashion similar to tissue paper. This indicates problems with the bonds between skin cells in the epidermis.

► CASE 25

A 17-year-old boy presents with discrete, pruritic papules of the arms and legs that have been present for 2 weeks. (See Figure 33–31.) No other family members are affected. You suggest a diagnosis of papular urticaria. The patient disagrees, noting "this has been going on too long to be bug bites."

Question 25-1

How do you counsel him?
A) Tell him all family members will eventually develop itchy bumps.
B) Tell him antihistamines are the treatment of choice.
C) Tell him insect bites may occur year round.
D) Tell him he is at risk for anaphylaxis.
E) Tell him permethrin is the treatment of choice.

Discussion 25-1

The correct answer is "C." The cutaneous reaction to arthropod (bug) bites is termed *papular urticaria*. Although most common in the summer and fall, insect bites may occur at any time of the year. Potential sources include outdoor exposure, pets, bird nests, and house plants, among others. Immediate reactions present as edematous wheals (eg, as in a mosquito bite). Delayed reactions are discrete, erythematous papules that may be clustered or widespread. Nodules and vesicles may occur. Recurrent or chronic papules may occur, especially in younger children. Because lesions may not appear immediately and insect bites may not have been noticed, convincing patients or families of this diagnosis can be a hard sell. Lesions arise from an immune reaction to allergens transmitted by the insect. The reaction is dependent on individual immunity, so a single family member may be the only one who reacts. Anaphylaxis is uncommon and is most frequently associated with bee, wasp, hornet, and ant bites. Treatment includes topical antipruritics (eg, menthol), mid- to high-potency topical steroids, intralesional steroid injections, and insect repellant. Permethrin is used for scabies treatment.

> **Helpful Tip**
> DEET is the most effective insect repellant. It may be applied directly to skin or clothing. The American Academy of Pediatrics suggests limiting DEET concentration to 10% to 30% in children older than 2 months of age. DEET should not be used on infants younger than 2 months of age.

► CASE 26

A 12-year-old girl returns home from summer camp noting severe itching, which is most pronounced at night. You note that papules and linear tracks are concentrated on her wrists and the web spaces of her hands.

Question 26-1

What is the most appropriate next step?
A) Biopsy to confirm diagnosis.
B) Empiric treatment with a topical steroid.
C) KOH examination.
D) Mineral oil preparation.
E) Tzanck preparation.

Discussion 26-1

The correct answer is "D." Pruritic rashes that concentrate in web spaces and display linear burrows are classic for scabies. (See Figure 33–32.) A mineral oil preparation (scabies prep) is used to confirm the diagnosis. (See Table 33–7.) Scabies mites infest the stratum corneum, so they are readily detected by skin scraping, application of a drop of mineral oil, and observation of mites, eggs, or scybala (feces) under the microscope. Biopsy is usually unnecessary to diagnose scabies. Not everyone has immediate access to a microscope, so it is reasonable to treat empirically for scabies.

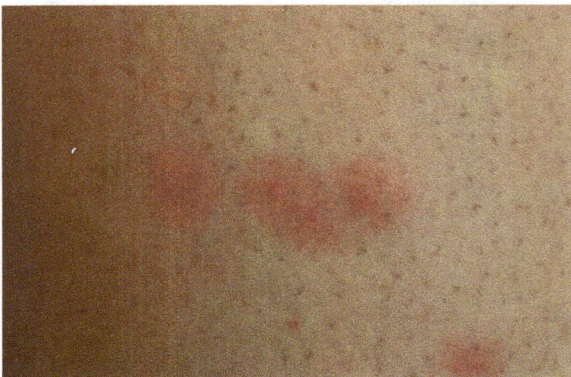

FIGURE 33–31. Papular urticaria is a delayed response to insect bites that presents as multiple erythematous, pruritic papules. (Used with permission from William Augehenbaugh, MD.)

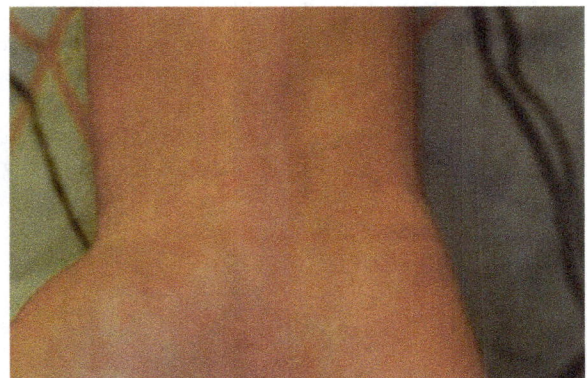

FIGURE 33–32. In scabies, look for small erythematous papules and burrows (thin red lines) in the skin, especially on the ventral surface of the wrist, finger webs, axilla, periumbilical area, buttocks, and feet. Excoriations may mask findings. (Used with permission from William Augehenbaugh, MD.)

TABLE 33–7 MICROSCOPIC DIAGNOSTIC SKIN TESTS

Diagnostic Skin Test	Associated Disease(s)	Location of Test	Microscopic Findings
Potassium hydroxide (KOH) examination	Tinea corporis, pedis, etc	Leading edge of scale	Septate hyphae
	Pityriasis versicolor	Any involved site	Hyphae and spores ("spaghetti and meatballs")
Tzanck preparation	Herpes simplex, zoster	Base of vesicle	Multinucleated giant cells
Mineral oil preparation	Scabies	Leading edge of burrow	Mites, eggs, scybala (feces)

Helpful Tip

Itching, especially at night, is the hallmark of scabies. Remember, scabies targets everyone, is very contagious, and is difficult to eradicate.

Question 26-2

What is your recommended treatment?
A) Ivermectin for the patient, only.
B) Ivermectin for the entire family.
C) Permethrin from the neck down overnight × 1 dose. Treat the entire family.
D) Permethrin from the neck down overnight × 1 dose. Treat the patient, only.
E) Permethrin from neck down overnight. Repeat in 1 week. Treat the entire family.

Discussion 26-2

The correct answer is "E." As scabies is transmitted through direct contact, all close contacts, including family members, should be treated. Permethrin is applied from the neck down, including finger and toe webs, left on overnight, and rinsed off in the morning. Scabies may infest the scalp and face of infants, so these areas should be treated. Scabies treatments kill live mites by paralyzing their breathing apparatus. Ivermectin is an oral medication that is reserved for widespread outbreaks or the emerging cases of permethrin resistance. The female fertilized mites lay eggs inside the skin—kind of like a gift that keeps on giving. Therefore, all scabies medications should be repeated in 1 week to kill any mites that hatched following the last treatment.

QUICK QUIZ

Which is NOT a clinical variant of scabies?
A) Urticarial scabies.
B) Nodular scabies.
C) Norwegian scabies.
D) Crusted scabies.

Discussion

The correct answer is "A." Nodular scabies presents as dome-shaped discrete nodules without visible burrows. This presentation is more common among infants. (See Figure 33–33.) Crusted (Norwegian) scabies presents as erythematous patches with thick, adherent scale. Patients then develop crusting and fissuring. This variant is often asymptomatic despite infestation with hundreds of thousands of mites. It is more common among immunosuppressed patients.

You discuss the importance of environmental controls to prevent reinfestation.

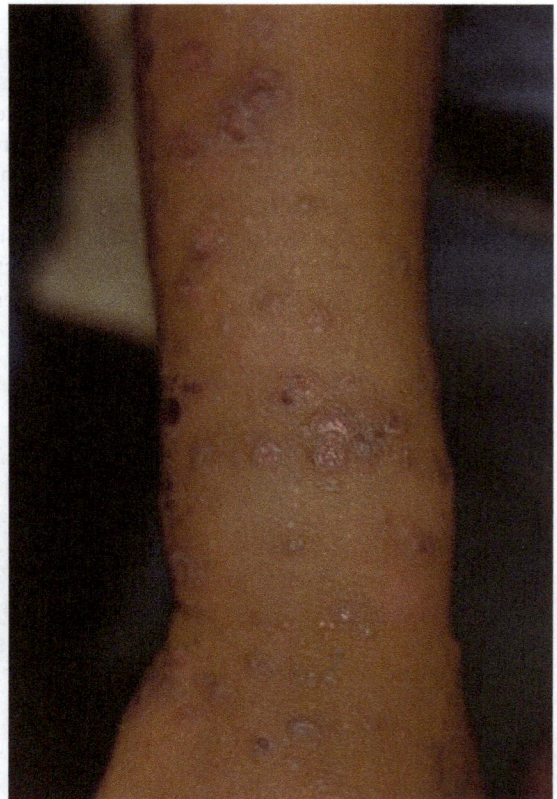

FIGURE 33–33. Nodular scabies presents as dome-shaped individual nodules without burrows. It is an atypical presentation of scabies. (Used with permission from William Augehenbaugh, MD.)

Question 26-3

What do you advise the family to do?

A) Call pest control.
B) Place clothing and bedding in a sealed bag for 24 hours.
C) Treat pets to prevent transmission.
D) Wash and dry all clothing and bedding.
E) Burn all stuffed animals.

Discussion 26-3

The correct answer is "D." Environmental controls are essential to preventing reinfestation. All clothing and bedding should be washed in hot water, placed in the dryer, and heated on high or sealed in bags for 72 hours, as the mites cannot live apart from a host for longer than 24 to 36 hours. Pets cannot harbor the human mites, so veterinary treatments are not necessary. Do not pull a Velveteen rabbit and burn beloved toys.

⏳ QUICK QUIZ

What causes the pruritus associated with scabies?

A) T-cell response.
B) Venom released from the mite.
C) Eggs deposited by the mite.
D) Disruption of the skin barrier.
E) Secondary bacterial infection of burrows.

Discussion

The correct answer is "A." The itching, which is worse at night, results from a type IV delayed hypersensitivity reaction to the mite, its feces, or eggs. The itching may persist even after treatment of the infestation. Antihistamines and topical steroids (once mites are gone) may be used.

▶ CASE 27

An 8-year-old girl develops round, scaling, pruritic patches on her arms.

Question 27-1

Which is the least likely cause of these skin patches?

A) Atopic dermatitis.
B) Contact dermatitis.
C) Granuloma annulare.
D) Plaque psoriasis.
E) Tinea corporis.

Discussion 27-1

The correct answer is "C." Eczematous dermatitis is a classification that encompasses a variety of conditions that mimic atopic dermatitis. They are characterized by red, scaly papules and plaques. Atopic dermatitis, contact dermatitis, plaque psoriasis, and tinea corporis are examples of such conditions. (See Figure 33–34.) Granuloma annulare, conversely, has an annular configuration (raised rim with central clearing), a pink

FIGURE 33–34. Tinea Corporis. The lesions of tinea corporis are annular with a raised scaly rim and central clearing. The presence of scaling differentiates it from granuloma annulare. (Used with permission from William Augehenbaugh, MD.)

quality, and absence of scale. It is often confused with tinea corporis. The etiology is unknown. Treatment includes topical or intralesional steroids and phototherapy.

A KOH exam confirms the presences of hyphae. (See Figure 33–35.)

Question 27-2

What is the first-line treatment for tinea corporis?

A) Bactroban ointment.
B) Ketoconazole tablets.
C) Nystatin cream.
D) Terbinafine cream.
E) Terbinafine tablets.

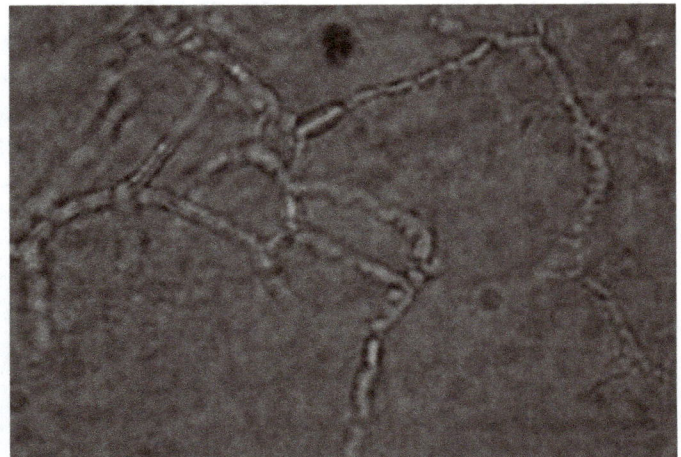

FIGURE 33–35. Microscopic examination of a KOH preparation of skin scrapings from a tinea lesion will show septate hyphae. (Used with permission from William Augehenbaugh, MD.)

Discussion 27-2

The correct answer is "D." Tinea infections are generally superficial and can be treated easily with topical agents. Dermatophyte infections respond to terbinafine, azole antifungals (eg, clotrimazole, ketoconazole, econazole), and ciclopirox. Mupirocin (Bactroban) is a topical antibiotic used for bacterial infections. Nystatin targets *Candida* yeast and is useful when treating diaper dermatitis.

⌛ QUICK QUIZ

Which is NOT a presentation of tinea pedis?
A) Moccasin tinea pedis.
B) Two foot–two hand tinea pedis.
C) Interdigital tinea pedis.
D) Bullous tinea pedis.
E) Pustular tinea pedis.

Discussion

The correct answer is "B." It is two foot–*one hand*, not two hand. Tinea pedis has variable presentations. Interdigital tinea pedis produces erythema, scale, and maceration of the web spaces. A moccasin distribution describes erythema and scale of the entire plantar foot and extension to the lateral aspects. Two foot–one hand tinea describes erythema and scale of the plantar feet with scaling of one palm (palmar involvement is an immune "id" reaction, not true infection). Bullous tinea pedis produces blisters. Pustular variants produce small pustules on an inflammatory background. Most types of tinea pedis may be treated with topical antifungals, as previously noted. Patients with severe inflammation and itch may require oral antifungals.

▶ CASE 28

A 17-year-old boy develops small, round, scaling, pink macules that are coalescent into a large patch on his back. The rash has grown steadily over the past 2 years. He lifts weights at the school weight room. He notes that the spots turn white in the summer.

Question 28-1

What is the most likely diagnosis?
A) Atopic dermatitis.
B) Pityriasis rosea.
C) Pityriasis versicolor.
D) Syphilis.
E) Tinea corporis.

Discussion 28-1

The correct answer is "C." Pityriasis (tinea) versicolor is caused by the yeast *Malassezia furfur*. The infection causes scaly patches that may be small and discrete or coalescent into large patches. The color is pink in individuals with fair skin. (See Figure 33–36.) The patches are hypopigmented when affecting those with dark skin or when the surrounding skin is tan. The eruption is often

FIGURE 33–36. Pityriasis versicolor is a yeast infection of the skin that presents with scaling pink patches on the trunk. (Used with permission from William Augehenbaugh, MD.)

chronic and recurrent. The yeast is spread by direct contact with an affected person or object, such as gym equipment. The KOH preparation has a "spaghetti and meatballs" appearance. Wood lamp examination may show fluorescence.

Question 28-2

Which is NOT a treatment option for pityriasis versicolor?
A) Topical ketoconazole.
B) Topical terbinafine.
C) Selenium sulfide shampoo.
D) Oral itraconazole.
E) All of the above.

Discussion 28-2

The correct answer is "E." Pityriasis versicolor typically responds well to antifungal agents. Topical antifungals (including terbinafine and azole antifungals) are preferred as they carry minimal risk. Oral antifungals may be added when the eruption is widespread and located on sites that are difficult to reach. Patients with recurrent pityriasis versicolor should be counseled to wash the skin once or twice a month with selenium sulfide shampoo (eg, Head and Shoulders or Selsun Blue). This decreases colonization with *Malassezia furfur* and reduces the risk of recurrent infections.

▶ CASE 29

A 1-year-old girl cries during diaper changes. Noting a rash in the inguinal folds and gluteal cleft, you diagnose diaper dermatitis.

Question 29-1

What clinical clue helps confirm cutaneous infection with *Candida*?
A) Bullae.
B) Erythema.
C) Satellite papules and pustules.
D) Scale.
E) White, adherent plaques.

Discussion 29-1

The correct answer is "C." *Candida* diaper dermatitis is described as confluent beefy red papules and pustules involving the skinfolds, with satellite lesions. (See Figure 33–37.) In contrast, irritant diaper dermatitis produces erythema but without satellite lesions and spares the skinfolds. Irritant diaper dermatitis is caused by wetness and contact with acidic stool, and may be complicated by secondary *Candida* infection. Consider an alternative cause or immunodeficiency if the diaper rash does not resolve, despite treatment.

> **Helpful Tip**
> Treatment tips for diaper dermatitis include:
> • Wash with soapless cleanser during diaper changes. Avoid baby wipes, which may contain irritants.
> • Dry the skin thoroughly. Avoid baby powder as they may abrade the skin.
> • Apply a topical anticandidal cream (eg, nystatin or azole antifungal).
> • Apply a barrier paste, such as zinc oxide paste.

> **Helpful Tip**
> Cutaneous candidiasis is also termed *intertrigo* (affects skinfolds). It commonly affects inframammary, abdominal pannus, and inguinal folds as the moist environment allows *Candida* yeast to grow.

► CASE 30

A 15-year-old boy presents for evaluation of multiple pink, scaling, thin plaques of the trunk. You suspect pityriasis rosea.

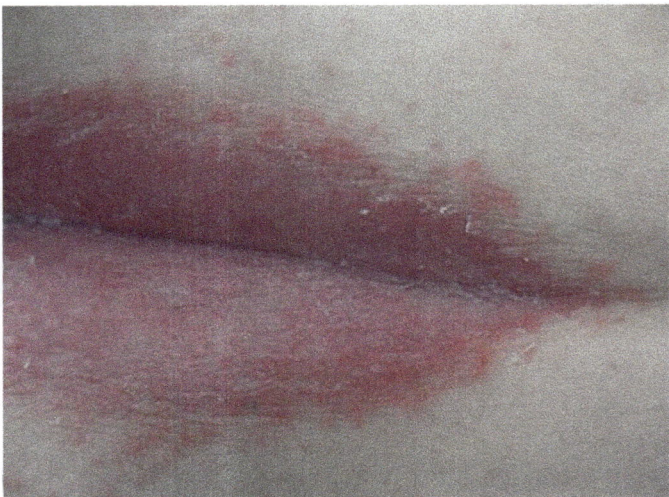

FIGURE 33–37. *Candida* Diaper Dermatitis. *Candida* infections are bright beefy red, involve the skinfolds, and have satellite lesions. (Used with permission from William Augehenbaugh, MD.)

Question 30-1

What additional clinical finding best supports your diagnosis?
A) Blunting of papillae on the tongue.
B) Erythematous plaque of the umbilicus.
C) Nail pits and oil spots.
D) Scalp erythema and scale.
E) Single large, scaling plaque that preceded the current lesions.

Discussion 30-1

The correct answer is "E." Pityriasis rosea starts with one large pink, scaling patch termed the *herald patch*. It is followed by the eruption of smaller patches in a "Christmas tree" distribution on the trunk. Psoriasis may present with geographic tongue (blunting of papillae on the tongue), nail pits and oil spots, and erythema and scale of the scalp, postauricular sulci, elbows, knees, umbilicus, and groin. (See Figure 33–38.)

Question 30-2

Which of the following is NOT recommended for patients with pityriasis rosea?
A) Observation.
B) Oral antihistamines.
C) Oral erythromycin.
D) Oral terbinafine.
E) Triamcinolone ointment.

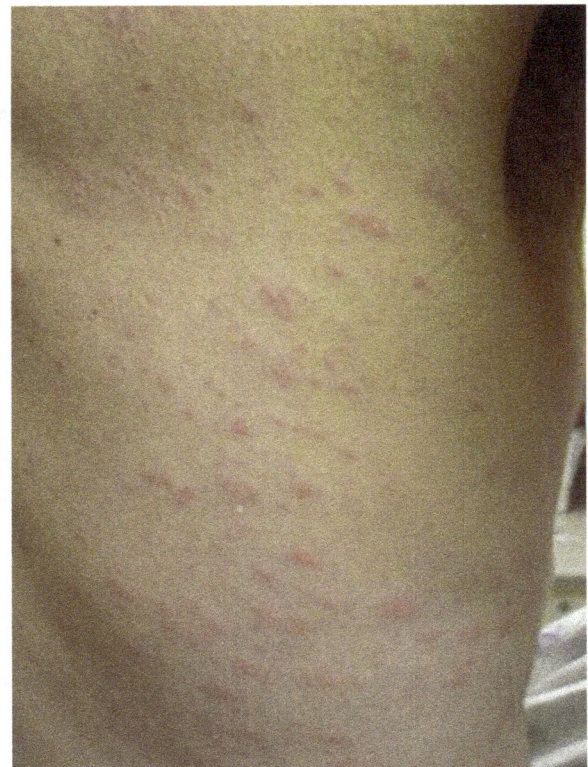

FIGURE 33–38. Pityriasis rosea presents as erythematous scaly ovals on the trunk in a "Christmas tree" pattern. The rash may be preceded by a single large lesion called a herald patch. (Used with permission from William Augehenbaugh, MD.)

Discussion 30-2

The correct answer is "D." Pityriasis rosea arises from infection with human herpesvirus-7 (HHV-7). The eruption typically runs a self-limited course and resolves spontaneously after several months. When associated with pruritus, oral antihistamines or mid-potency topical steroids may be added. Oral antibiotics, including erythromycin, have shown efficacy in shortening the duration of the rash. Oral and topical antifungal agents are not effective.

> ▶ **CASE 31**

A 5-year-old girl develops five skin-colored and pink papules on the trunk and extremities. She denies itching.

Question 31-1

What feature suggests a diagnosis of molluscum contagiosum?
A) Black dots.
B) Central dell.
C) Excoriations.
D) Pustule.
E) Yellow color.

Discussion 31-1

The correct answer is "B." Molluscum contagiosum is caused by a pox virus that produces chronic infection of a localized area of skin. The lesions are contagious, hence *contagiosum*, and can be spread to distal sites by autoinoculation. Papules are umbilicated, characterized by a central depression. (See Figure 33–39.) This may be more apparent when the lesion is treated with cryotherapy. Black dots (often called "roots" or "seeds" by patients) are seen in warts, resulting from thrombosis of blood vessels. (See Figure 33–40.)

Question 31-2

What is your first recommendation to the family?
A) Acyclovir.
B) Cantharidin.

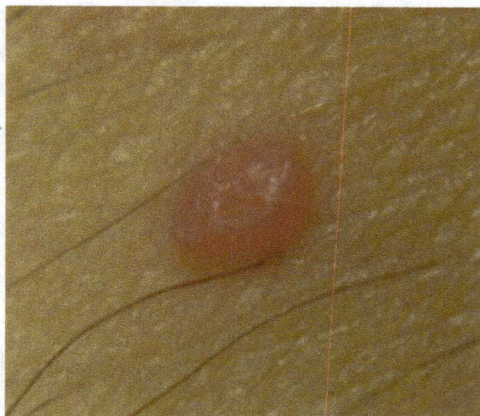

FIGURE 33–39. Molluscum Contagiosum. A single flesh-colored umbilicated papule is seen, consistent with molluscum contagiosum. (Used with permission from William Augehenbaugh, MD.)

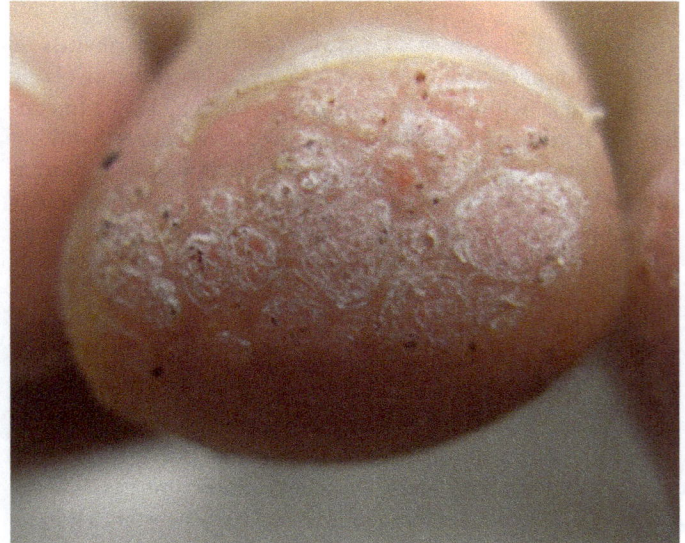

FIGURE 33–40. Wart (Verrucae). Warts have thrombosed capillaries that look like black dots. Warts also disrupt the skin lines. (Used with permission from William Augehenbaugh, MD.)

C) Cryotherapy.
D) Curettage.
E) Reassurance.

Discussion 31-2

The correct answer is "E." Most isolated papules of molluscum resolve spontaneously within 2 years. Indications for treatment include symptomatic, spreading, or cosmetically disfiguring lesions. Chemovesicants such as cantharidin (blister beetle extract) are painless with application, but must be rinsed off and carry the risks of dyspigmentation. Curettage (manual removal) and cryotherapy are painful and a good choice for older kids. Topical immunotherapy with tretinoin, imiquimod, or other irritants may be helpful. Oral antivirals are not effective in the treatment of molluscum.

> 🧍 **Helpful Tip**
> On exam, warts (verrucae) interrupt the skin lines and have thrombosed capillaries that look like black dots.

⏳ QUICK QUIZ

Which human papillomavirus (HPV) subtype is most commonly associated with condyloma acuminata?
A) HPV-1.
B) HPV-2.
C) HPV-6.
D) HPV-16.
E) HPV-31.

Discussion

The correct answer is "C." (See next quiz for discussion.)

QUICK QUIZ

Which HPV subtype is considered high risk for malignancy?
A) HPV-1.
B) HPV-2.
C) HPV-6.
D) HPV-11.
E) HPV-18.

Discussion

The correct answer is "E." More than 100 serotypes of HPV have been identified. HPV-1 and HPV-2 are most frequently associated with common warts and palmoplantar warts, respectively. Condyloma acuminata (anogenital warts) most commonly occur with HPV-6 and HPV-11, which have low oncogenic potential. HPV-16, -18, -31, and -33 are responsible for many cases of cervical, vulvar, penile, and anal cancers. The Centers for Disease Control and Prevention (CDC) recommends HPV vaccination for boys and girls at ages 11 or 12 years. The most commonly utilized option is a quadrivalent vaccine covering HPV-6, -11, -16, and -18.

CASE 32

A mother and her 5-year-old daughter rush to the clinic after they are notified of a lice outbreak at school. The mother saw her daughter scratching her head and found nits on examination.

Question 32-1

What is recommended as first-line treatment?
A) Ivermectin tablets.
B) Lindane 1% shampoo.
C) Malathion 0.5% lotion.
D) Permethrin 1% cream.
E) Petroleum jelly.

Discussion 32-1

The correct answer is "D." All topical pediculicides are neurotoxic to lice. Permethrin 1% cream is available over the counter. Increasing rates of resistance are reported throughout the world. Lindane is not recommended owing to risk of central nervous system toxicity. Malathion may have the best efficacy of a topical agent, but a longer contact time is required, making it a second-line option. Oral ivermectin is effective but is off-label for head lice. Occlusive products, such as petroleum jelly and oil, are not pesticidal (do not kill lice) and therefore not recommended for the treatment of head lice.

> **Helpful Tip**
> To diagnosis pediculosis capitis, a live louse must be seen. Nits (eggs) may persist for months after successful treatment.

You choose permethrin 1% cream and advise application to damp hair after shampooing, followed by rinsing after 10 minutes.

Question 32-2

How often should the medication be applied?
A) One application.
B) Once daily for 1 week.
C) Twice daily for 1 week.
D) Twice daily for 2 weeks.
E) Two applications 1 week apart.

Discussion 32-2

The correct answer is "E." Pediculosis capitis (head louse) is an obligate human parasite that cannot survive for more than 24 hours without a blood meal. The female louse lives for up to 30 days and lays 5 to 10 eggs per day. Eggs hatch 8 to 10 days later. After the initial application, treatment should be repeated in 7 to 10 days.

> **Helpful Tip**
> Pediculosis pubis (crab lice) may infest any region of body hair, including eyelashes, eyebrows, mustache, beard, axillae, and pubic areas. Phthirus pubis (the crab louse) may be more difficult to detect than head lice as they are skin colored. Slate gray macules of the trunk and thighs may be a clue to the diagnosis. Treatment of all hair-bearing areas is essential to ensure complete eradication. All close contacts should also be treated. Treatment is the same as described for pediculosis capitis.

CASE 33

A 2-month-old boy develops malaise, fussiness, and fever with edema and ill-defined erythema of the arm following an injury.

Question 33-1

Of the organisms listed below, which is the most likely to cause cellulitis in this patient?
A) *Escherichia coli*.
B) *Haemophilus influenzae*.
C) *Pseudomonas aeruginosa*.
D) *Streptococcus pyogenes*.
E) *Sporothrix schenckii*.
F) *Bartonella henselae*.

Discussion 33-1

The correct answer is "D." Cellulitis is most commonly caused by group A beta-hemolytic streptococci (*Streptococcus pyogenes*) and *Staphylococcus aureus*. Gram-positive cocci and gram-negative aerobes and anaerobes are more common among patients who are immunosuppressed. Cellulitis occurs following disruption of the skin barrier and is characterized by spreading erythema, indistinct borders, edema, and warmth.

> **Helpful Tip**
> Group A streptococcal infections may be complicated by sinusitis, mastoiditis, pneumonia, rheumatic fever, or acute glomerulonephritis.

▶ CASE 34

An 8-year-old boy develops cellulitis and is treated with empiric oral penicillin. He does not respond to therapy. He is febrile but hemodynamically stable. His leg is red, warm, and edematous.

Question 34-1

What is your next step to help direct therapy?
A) Blood culture.
B) MRI.
C) Tissue culture.
D) Ultrasound.
E) All of the above.

Discussion 34-1

The correct answer is "C." When a patient is not responding to treatment, stop and ask yourself the following questions: (1) Is the patient compliant? (2) Is the diagnosis correct? (3) Is the organism resistant to the current antibiotic? (4) Is the organism covered by the current antibiotic? (5) Has a complication developed (abscess)? (6) And, is this a "normal host" (ie, not immunosuppressed, or affected by chronic kidney disease)? Treatment is often empiric unless the organism is cultured. Blood cultures are positive in fewer than 5% of cases of cellulitis. Tissue culture has a higher yield of 20% to 40%. Culture of pus or fluid from an intact bullae may be helpful, if present on exam. Additionally, the patients antibiotics should be changed to provide coverage for methicillin-resistant *Staphylococcus aureus* (MRSA), and he may require admission for intravenous antibiotics.

⧗ QUIZ QUIZ

What is the most common cause of necrotizing fasciitis in young, immunocompetent patients?
A) *Escherichia coli*.
B) *Clostridium* spp.
C) *Streptococcus pyogenes*.
D) *Pseudomonas aeruginosa*.
E) *Staphylococcus aureus*.

Discussion

The correct answer is "C." Necrotizing fasciitis is increasing among young, previously healthy patients following penetrating or blunt injury. It is a rapidly progressive infection with a mortality rate of 20% to 40%. Polymicrobial infections are more common among diabetic and immunosuppressed patients. Necrotizing fasciitis is an infection of the deeper tissues, muscle fascia, and fat that progresses rapidly and may be fatal. The clinical presentation is a painful plaque resembling cellulitis. It evolves rapidly, becoming dusky to gray-blue within 36 hours of onset. Cutaneous necrosis develops with surrounding fibrosis. Patients must be managed aggressively with debridement of the tissue (including fascia), intravenous antibiotics, and supportive care.

> **Helpful Tip**
> Rapidly progressing "cellulitis" with pain out of proportion to exam is necrotizing fasciitis. Call a surgeon immediately for wound debridement.

▶ CASE 35

A 17-year-old girl returns to your office 5 days after excision of a mole. She reports swelling, redness, and purulent discharge.

Question 35-1

What is the most important step in management of this wound infection?
A) Apply topical antibiotics.
B) Culture purulent discharge.
C) Give ibuprofen to reduce swelling and treat pain.
D) Open the wound and drain pus.
E) Start oral antibiotics.

Discussion 35-1

The correct answer is "D." Most postoperative infections of the skin are caused by *Staphylococcus aureus*. The most important step is draining the abscess by removing some or all of the sutures and rinsing the base of the wound. The wound is then allowed to heal by secondary intention. Oral antibiotics may not be necessary if the infection is uncomplicated, without surrounding cellulitis. Routine culture is not required unless the wound fails to improve.

> **Helpful Tip**
> Abscesses are treated with incision and drainage. Systemic antibiotics are not always needed.

BIBLIOGRAPHY

Bolognia JL, Jorizzo JL, Rapini RP, eds. *Dermatology*. 3rd ed. Philadelphia, PA: Elsevier/Saunders; 2012.

Gupta D, Thappa DM. Mongolian spots. *Indian J Dermatol Venereol Leprol*. 2013;79(4):469–478.

Hirbe AC, Gutmann DH. Neurofibromatosis type 1: A multidisciplinary approach to care. *Lancet Neurol*. 2014;13(8):834–843.

Horn TM, Tidman MJ. The clinical spectrum of dystrophic epidermolysis bullosa. *Br J Dermatol*. 2002;146(2):267–274.

Metry DW, Hawrot A, Altman C, Frieden IJ. Association of solitary, segmental hemangiomas of the skin with visceral hemangiomatosis. *Arch Dermatol*. 2004;140(5):591–566.

O'Connor NR, McLaughlin MR, Ham P. Newborn skin: Part I. Common rashes. *Am Fam Physician*. 2008;77(1):47–52.

Thomas-Sohl KA, Vaslow DF, Maria BL. Weber syndrome: A review. *Pediatr Neurol*. 2004;30(5):303–310.

Sports Medicine and Physical Fitness 34

Andrew R. Peterson

▶ CASE 1

A teenage boy with one eye comes to your office for a preparticipation evaluation. He has a history of retinoblastoma that resulted in single enucleation. His remaining eye is healthy, with 20/20 vision. He has no other medical problems and no other concerns. He wants to play high school basketball.

Question 1-1

You advise him:

A) The risk of losing his remaining eye is too high for him to be allowed to play contact sports.
B) He can play basketball without protective eyewear if he is cleared by an ophthalmologist.
C) He can play basketball if he wears protective eyewear approved by the American National Standards Institute (ANSI).
D) He can play basketball if he wears a protective hard contact lens.
E) No restrictions.

Discussion 1-1

The correct answer is "C." This question is an example of a time when an athlete with a disability or medical condition can participate in sports with minor modifications. In this case, the loss of a paired organ does not preclude participation in basketball as long as the remaining eye is effectively protected. While a comprehensive review of every medical condition requiring accommodations is beyond this scope of this review, there are several common situations that are ripe for board questions. The next seven cases cover these situations. A rule of thumb is that if a player can compete safely, he or she should be allowed to.

▶ CASE 2

A high school basketball player was diagnosed with influenza yesterday. You see him in the athletic training room the next day. He is febrile to 38.9°C (102°F). He wants to play in tonight's playoff game.

Question 2-1

You tell him:

A) "No problem. Go get 'em."
B) "We can treat you with Tamiflu (oseltamivir) so that it's safe to play tonight."
C) "We can treat you with ibuprofen so that it's safe to play tonight."
D) "You shouldn't play tonight because of the risk of myocarditis."
E) "You shouldn't play tonight because of the risk of rhabdomyolysis."

Discussion 2-1

The correct answer is "D." The reasons are fuzzy, but playing with a fever increases risk of myocarditis and arrhythmia. There is a theoretical risk of rhabdomyolysis if an athlete plays when dehydrated and febrile, but acute illness has not been demonstrated to be an independent risk factor for muscle injury.

⏳ QUICK QUIZ

Which of the following is NOT a part of the standardized American Heart Association (AHA) preparticipation screening evaluation?

A) Electrocardiogram (ECG).
B) Blood pressure measurement.
C) Family history of unexplained death.
D) History of chest pain with exertion.
E) Cardiac auscultation.

Discussion

The correct answer is "A." This is *very* controversial, but the current American Academy of Pediatrics (AAP) recommendations for the preparticipation physical evaluation (PPE) do not include an ECG. The AAP endorses the AHA cardiac screening criteria, which involve obtaining a detailed history and basic cardiac examination. The PPE monograph changes frequently. You should make yourself familiar with the AAP endorsed PPE history and physical form (which is not reprinted here). But recognize that it is likely to change every few years as this controversial topic evolves.

► CASE 3

You are evaluating a high school football player who suffered a concussion 2 weeks ago. He says that he is completely back to normal. You use the Sideline Concussion Assessment Tool v.3 (SCAT3) in the office to evaluate for any lingering concussion symptoms. His symptom score is 0, but he does very poorly on the Balance Error Scoring System test and has trouble with tasks of attention and memory, including reverse order digits and months of the year in reverse.

Question 3-1

Right now, you wish you:
A) Had chosen a different career.
B) Knew how to score the SCAT3.
C) Had a computed tomography (CT) scanner in your office.
D) Knew the athlete's baseline neurocognitive abilities.
E) Could talk the school into banning football.

Discussion 3-1

The correct answer is "D." OK, you may have wished for any of the others as well. But it is always useful to know the baseline neurocognitive status of a contact or collision sport athlete. The first step in returning to sport after a concussion is to return to feeling and functioning normally. Some offices and schools use computer-based neurocognitive tests to help tell when an athlete has returned to his or her neurocognitive baseline. If such testing is not available, knowing how an athlete would be expected to perform on tasks of reaction time, memory, and attention is important if you are going to use any tests (including the SCAT3) to make a determination about return to play.

> **Helpful Tip**
> The SCAT3 is a standardized tool to evaluate an athlete 13 years of age or older for a concussion. Having a baseline score is helpful to interpret the child's score after an injury or for returning to play.

► CASE 4

An 8-year-old boy with trisomy 21 (Down syndrome) comes to the clinic with his parents because he wants to participate in Special Olympics wrestling.

Question 4-1

How do you respond?
A) Calmly explain that there is no Special Olympics wrestling.
B) Order flexion-extension cervical spine X-rays.
C) Discuss the risk of atlantoaxial instability in children with trisomy 21.

D) Encourage participation in sports with high dynamic or high static demands.
E) All of the above.

Discussion 4-1

The correct answer is "E." This is a poorly worded question. But it illustrates an important point. Athletes with trisomy 21 are at risk for atlantoaxial instability. For this reason, Special Olympics does not include any contact or collision sports or other activities that would put the athlete at risk for cervical spine injury. Obtaining flexion and extension cervical spine X-rays is an important part of screening in physically active children with trisomy 21. But they are also at risk for early cardiovascular disease, so participation in strenuous activities is still a good idea.

► CASE 5

A 15-year-old female swimmer has a long history of well-controlled epilepsy. She recently switched clubs and her new coach is uncomfortable with her continuing to compete as a swimmer. The patient is asking for a letter to her coach explaining that she should be allowed to swim whenever she likes.

Question 5-1

You respond by:
A) Telling her that unsupervised swimming is not recommended for an athlete with well-controlled epilepsy.
B) Advising that swimming increases risks of seizure and is not recommended for anyone with epilepsy.
C) Suggesting she consider a safer sport such as archery.
D) Handing her a pamphlet for your sky-diving school.
E) Telling her that she can compete as long as she wears an approved personal flotation. device, at all times, including in class and when she goes to the prom.

Discussion 5-1

The correct answer is "A." Swimming is permitted for athletes with epilepsy as long as it is supervised. It is a common misconception that swimming increases seizure risk. It does not. In fact, exercise of any type decreases seizure risk. There are sports that are not safe for patients with epilepsy, but they are all pretty obvious: archery, riflery, power lifting, sports involving heights, and so on.

► CASE 6

An 8-year-old with well-controlled type 1 diabetes mellitus is interested in playing tackle football. He currently uses an insulin pump.

Question 6-1

Which of the following is NOT true?
A) He may be able to continue to use his insulin pump while playing tackle football if he embeds it in a special pad.
B) He may be able to use a small dose of injectable insulin before practice and disconnect his pump while playing football.

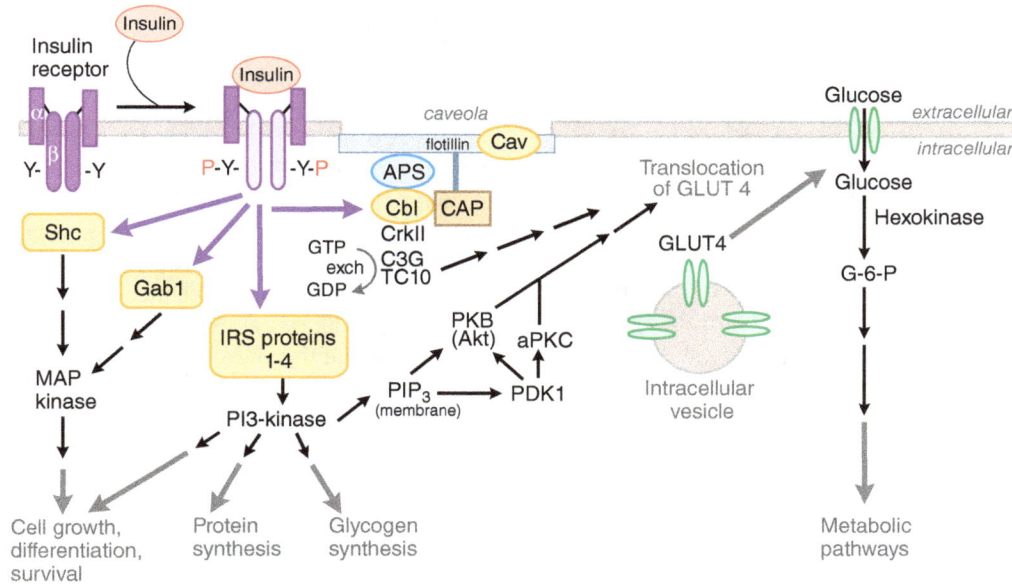

FIGURE 34–1. Insulin signal transduction in skeletal muscle. Skeletal muscle glucose receptors (GLUT4) can transport glucose into the cell without the need for insulin. CAP, Cbl-associated protein; IRS, insulin receptor substrate; PI-3-kinase, phosphatidylinositol 3-kinase. (Reproduced with permission from Brunton LL, Chabner BA, Knollman BC: Goodman & Gilman's: *The Pharmacological Basis of Therapeutics*, 12th ed. McGraw-Hill Education, Inc; 2011. Fig 43-4.)

C) His insulin needs will likely increase when he starts playing sports.

D) He may have more trouble with overnight lows as a result of playing sports.

E) His coaches or other team personnel should keep sugar-containing beverages or glucagon, or both, on the sideline.

Discussion 6-1

The correct answer is "C." Skeletal muscle glucose receptors can take up glucose without the aid of insulin, so insulin needs often go down when a patient with type 1 diabetes becomes more physically active. (See Figure 34–1.) There are many strategies for maintaining good glycemic control in the setting of contact sports. Athletes with diabetes should not be discouraged from playing any sport, but adjustments may need to be made in how and when they take their insulin, when they check their blood glucose, and when they eat.

> ▶ **CASE 7**

A 16-year-old comes for a preparticipation evaluation. She is tall, wears thick glasses, and has long tapered fingers. She has a murmur on exam.

Question 7-1

Which of the following is NOT a physical examination finding in her genetic syndrome?

A) Ectopia lentis.

B) Hyperopia.

C) Aortic dilation.

D) Arm span exceeding height.

E) Protrusio acetabuli.

Discussion 7-1

The correct answer is "B." People with Marfan syndrome are nearsighted (myopic). There are several diagnostic criteria that variably rely on genetic testing and family history. The most common findings are listed in Table 34–1.

⧗ QUICK QUIZ

True or False: Adolescents are at higher risk of injury from sports participation than any other age group.

A) True.

B) False.

Discussion

The correct answer is "A." Adolescents are indeed at increased risk of injury from sports participation, but it may be because of the types of sports they tend to play. For example, high school football is much more violent than youth football.

⧗ QUICK QUIZ

Which of the following measures has good evidence for preventing sports-related injuries?

A) Static stretching.

B) Ballistic stretching.

C) Neck strengthening to prevent concussions.

D) General conditioning to prevent all injuries.

E) Eccentric strengthening to prevent Achilles injuries.

TABLE 34–1 CHARACTERISTIC FINDINGS IN MARFAN SYNDROME

Trunk and limbs	Pectus carinatum, pectus excavatum, reduced upper-to-lower segment ratio, arm span-to-height ratio > 1.05, wrist and thumb sign, scoliosis, spondylolisthesis, reduced extension of elbow, pes planus, joint hypermobility
Head and face	Arched palate, crowding of teeth, dolichocephaly, malar hypoplasia, enophthalmos, retrognathia, downslanting palpebral fissures
Eyes	Ectopia lentis, abnormally flat corneas, increased axial length of globe, hypoplastic iris
Heart and vasculature	Dilation of ascending aorta, dissection of ascending aorta, mitral valve prolapse, dilation of main pulmonary artery
Lungs	Spontaneous pneumothorax, pulmonary apical blebs
Abdomen and torso	Stretch marks, hernia, lumbosacral dural ectasia
Genetics	Family history of Marfan syndrome, presence of *FBN1* mutation (fibrillin 1 gene)

Discussion

The correct answer is "D." Very few measures have actually been proven to prevent injuries, but general conditioning is one. The other options listed all represent common misconceptions. However, landing training does prevent anterior cruciate ligament (ACL) injuries, eccentric strengthening prevents hamstring injuries, and ankle proprioceptive drills prevent ankle sprains. And, in general, being in better shape prevents all kinds of injuries.

► CASE 8

Today is injury follow-up day in the training room. You dread having to explain to college athletes why they cannot return to play immediately. (*Rehabilitation* is not a word in their vocabulary.) You start thumbing through the charts to see how many physical therapy referrals you will be making today.

Question 8-1

Patients with which of the following injuries do NOT need to be rehabilitated before being allowed full return to sport?
A) Ankle sprain.
B) ACL tear after surgery.

C) Achilles tendon injury.
D) Clavicle fracture.
E) Quadriceps contusion.

Discussion 8-1

The correct answer is "D." Range of motion and proprioceptive training clearly prevents recurrent ankle sprains. ACL reconstruction requires a prolonged recovery course that focuses on muscular control of the reconstructed knee. Achilles tendon injuries respond well to eccentric training. Quadriceps contusions are less likely to develop heterotopic ossification (myositis ossificans) if they have early range of motion and activation therapy. However, patients who have clavicle fractures without any other associated injuries can return to sport when bony healing is adequate without any additional rehabilitation. In general, most injuries do better with a course of physical therapy.

> **Helpful Tip**
> Ankle proprioception drills decrease ankle sprains. To reduce all types of injuries, athletes must get in shape. Good physical conditioning is key.

► CASE 9

During a football game, a player is tackled. He was hit in the thigh by the other player's helmet, causing immediate pain and swelling. He is diagnosed with a quadriceps contusion and not allowed to return to play.

Question 9-1

Which of the following is NOT an appropriate treatment for a quadriceps contusion?
A) Early mobilization.
B) Immobilization in a fully flexed position.
C) Immobilization in a fully extended position.
D) Nonsteroidal anti-inflammatory drugs (NSAIDs).
E) Ice.

Discussion 9-1

The correct answer is "C." Quadriceps contusions are at high risk for developing heterotypic ossification (myositis ossificans). (See Figure 34–2.) Early mobilization, immobilization in a fully flexed position, NSAIDs, and ice have all been shown to decrease the risk of heterotypic ossification. Immobilization in a fully extended position clearly *increases* the risk of heterotopic ossification. Traditional knee immobilizers should be avoided at all costs.

► CASE 10

An obese 16-year-old high school football player becomes dizzy and nauseated at the end of a full-pads practice in the August heat. He is having painful cramps and attempts to opt out of end-of-practice conditioning. His coach, angry that the

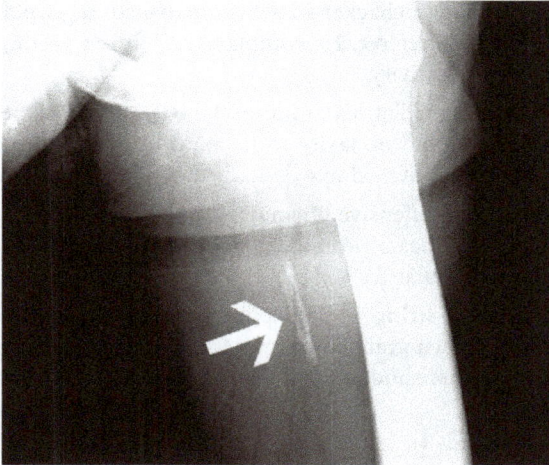

FIGURE 34–2. Myositis ossificans occurs most commonly in the lower extremity, especially the quadriceps. The muscle sustains a traumatic hematoma that heals like a fracture, forming bone. In the X-ray image, an area of ossification is seen in the hamstring (white arrow). (Reproduced with permission from Miller AE, Davis BA, Beckley OA, et al: Bilateral and recurrent myositis ossificans in an athlete: a case report and review of treatment options, *Arch Phys Med Rehabil.* 2006 Feb;87(2):286-290.))

TABLE 34–2 CHARACTERISTICS OF HEAT STROKE VERSUS HEAT EXHAUSTION	
Heat Stroke	**Heat Exhaustion**
Hot, dry skin	Hot, moist skin
Core body temperature > 40°C (104°F)	Core body temperature < 40°C (104°F)
Altered mental status— confusion, lethargy, or coma	Overwhelming fatigue
Rhabdomyolysis	Muscle cramps
Multiorgan system failure	

player is not training hard enough, punishes him by making him run additional cross-field sprints. The player collapses near mid-field. On initial evaluation, he is breathing, has a rapid pulse, has hot dry skin, and is unresponsive.

Question 10-1
Which of the following is/are associated with heat stroke?
A) Hot, dry skin.
B) Hot, moist skin.
C) Overwhelming fatigue.
D) Core temperature greater than 40°C (104°F).
E) Muscle cramps.
F) Confusion, lethargy, or coma.
G) Rhabdomyolysis.
H) Multiorgan failure.
I) Options A and D, only.
J) Options A, D, and F, only.
K) Options A, D, F, G, and H.

Discussion 10-1
The correct answer is "K." Athletes with heat stroke are at risk for death. They typically have hot, dry skin; a core temperature greater than 40°C, and profound mental status changes, and are at risk for muscle breakdown and organ failure.

Question 10-2
Which of the following is/are associated with heat exhaustion?
A) Hot, dry skin.
B) Hot, moist skin.
C) Overwhelming fatigue.
D) Core temperature greater than 40°C (104°F).
E) Muscle cramps.
F) Confusion, lethargy, or coma.
G) Rhabdomyolysis.
H) Multiorgan failure.
I) Options B and C, only.
J) Options B, C, and E.

Discussion 10-2
The correct answer is "J." Heat exhaustion, is much less severe than heat stroke. Athletes with heat exhaustion typically continue to sweat and maintain only a modestly elevated core temperature. Muscle cramps and overwhelming fatigue are common. (See Table 34–2.)

Question 10-3
Which of the following is the best way to cool the athlete?
A) Cold water immersion.
B) Cool water immersion.
C) Ice packs and a fan.
D) Helicopter downdraft (seriously, this has been studied).
E) Cool mist spray.

Discussion 10-3
The correct answer is "B." Believe it or not, all of these methods have been studied and nothing scrubs heat faster than cold water immersion. The more rapidly the athlete is cooled, the more likely he or she is to survive without significant long-term effects of the injury.

Question 10-4
Which of the following is/are acceptable as a method of measuring the temperature of the athlete suspected of having heat stroke?
A) Rectal thermistor with remote reader
B) Rectal thermometer
C) Axillary thermometer
D) Oral thermometer
E) Capsule thermistor
F) Options A and B, only.
G) Options A, B, and D.
H) Options A, B, and E.

Discussion 10-4

The correct answer is "H." Axillary, oral, temporal, and otic temperatures are remarkably inaccurate in the setting of heat stroke because peripheral perfusion is typically markedly compromised.

⏳ **QUICK QUIZ**

Which of the following is NOT a risk factor for heat illness?
A) Markedly thin body habitus.
B) Markedly obese body habits.
C) Young age (infants, toddlers).
D) Old age.
E) Stimulant use.

Discussion

The correct answer is "A." This seems pretty obvious, but people with thin body habitus scrub heat more effectively than those with a thicker body habitus. Infants scrub heat poorly because they generally have less surface area for their body volume/mass and do not sweat very effectively. The elderly are less efficient at all kinds of physiologic processes and although they can sweat and may be thin, they are also at greater risk for heat illness. Whether there is a link between stimulant use and heat illness is controversial. High doses of strong stimulants clearly raise core temperature and can impair sweating. Whether low-dose stimulants, such as methylphenidate for attention deficit hyperactivity disorder (ADHD), might increase risk of heat illness is somewhat controversial. You should not be asked about that on a board exam. But know that someone who is abusing potent stimulants is clearly at risk.

> **Helpful Tip**
> Heat stroke causes organ damage, rhabdomyolysis, and altered mental status. The skin is dry. Victims should be immersed in cold water immediately to lower the body temperature.

▶ **CASE 11**

You are the team physician for the Iowa State Cyclones. Following a game with the Iowa Hawkeyes, nearly all of your players are injured. The coaches have questions about when some of their key players might be able to return to play.

Questions 11-1 through 11-5

Pull out a piece of paper and outline your return-to-play recommendations for each of the following players:

11-1: Starting quarterback suffered a concussion in the first half. It is now the next morning and he feels completely normal.

11-2: Starting linebacker somehow managed to get poked in the eye by the referee. He complains of blurred vision, pain, and photosensitivity.

11-3: Starting tailback was hit on the outside of his knee and now has pain but no laxity with valgus load, at both neutral and 30 degrees of flexion.

11-4: Starting offensive lineman fell hard on the point of his shoulder and has a prominent bump and tenderness at his acromioclavicular (AC) joint.

11-5: Fourth-string backup punter suffered a neck sprain when the coach grabbed him by the facemask and told him to "get out there and put them in the ground."

Discussion 11-1 through 11-5

Your recommendations should include the following considerations:

11-1: There are several key points to return-to-play decision making in concussion management. First, a concussed athlete should not return to play on the same day as the injury. Some of the old guidelines were silent on this issue, but all modern concussion guidelines agree that this is a bad idea. There is a small risk of so-called second impact syndrome; this occurs when a concussed athlete suffers a second hit to the head and dies due to impaired vascular autoregulation, cerebral edema, and eventually brainstem herniation. This is thankfully a rare event. But it is very common for athletes to sustain a worse injury than they would have otherwise if they return to play too soon and suffer a second impact–type exposure. Second, a brief period of rest in the days following the injury is clearly beneficial. Athletes should rest and recover as much as possible for the first week after the injury, as long as they are symptomatic. What a symptomatic athlete should do after the first week of rest is controversial, so you probably won't be asked about that. Third, the athlete needs to return to normal before going back to play. This is largely for the reasons listed above. There are a lot of methods for ensuring this. A clinical history and examination are sufficient for most providers who are well-trained in concussion management. Sometimes clinicians use tools such as the SCAT3 or computer-based neurocognitive testing to help with this decision making. Fourth, the athlete should complete a graduated return to play program before going back to full contact sports. This usually involves a progression from easy aerobic exercise to more difficult aerobic exercise to strength and skill work to contact practice and finally to full contact play. This process typically takes 5 to 7 days. People tend to focus on the steps of graduated return to play, rather than the point. Remember, the reason for the program is to look for the reemergence of symptoms. If the athlete becomes symptomatic again, he or she is not ready for return to play and should stop progressing through the graduated return to play program. Finally, be ready for the next concussion. Be sure to have a good baseline neurologic and, ideally, neuropsychological examination. This will make future decisions about return to play much easier. Consider changes that could be made to the athlete's style of play or position that would decrease concussion risk. It is unlikely that any piece of equipment is beneficial for decreasing concussion risk.

> **Helpful Tip**
> Concussed children should not return to play the same day to avoid sustaining a more severe injury if hit again (sometimes called second impact syndrome). Before returning to play, the child must be back to normal and have successfully completed a graduated return to play program.

11-2: Many injuries can occur from a finger to the eye, but the two emergencies that are commonly encountered on the sideline are a hyphema and detached retina. A hyphema should be evident on physical examination as a pool of blood in the anterior chamber of the eye. (See Figure 34–3.) Although most hyphemas result in abnormal vision, not all do. However, in the absence of a hyphema, other severe eye injuries will cause abnormalities of vision. So, this athlete can return to play if he has no blood in the anterior chamber of his eye and normal vision. However, after the game, he should be further evaluated for other eye trauma (corneal abrasion, etc).

11-3: This athlete has a grade 1 medial collateral ligament (MCL) sprain. Grade 2 and 3 injuries are more severe and have laxity on examination. Athletes with these more severe injuries should be removed from play until they are healed

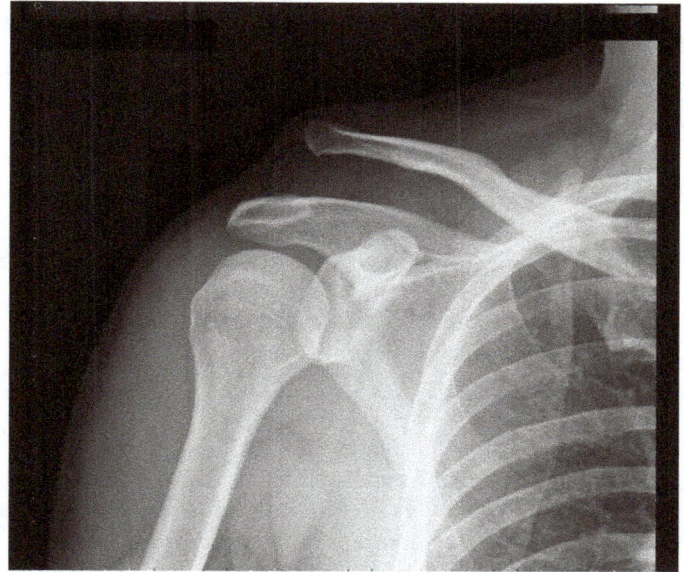

FIGURE 34–4. Acromioclavicular (AC) joint separation. The right AC joint is separated with displacement of the clavicle from the acromion. (Reproduced with permission from Maitin IB, Cruz E, eds. *Current Diagnosis and Treatment: Physical Medicine and Rehabilitation*. New York, NY: McGraw-Hill Education; 2015, Fig. 29-4.)

and rehabilitated. However, an athlete with grade 1 MCL injuries can return to play if he or she is able to run and cut at full speed on the injured knee. Remember, MCL injuries are often associated with ACL and medial meniscus injuries (the "terrible triad"). Do not forget to examine these other structures.

11-4: Acromioclavicular (AC) joint injuries are not dangerous, but they are painful. They rarely need to be repaired, and athletes can return to play when they can tolerate the pain of the injury. Football players can often pad the AC joint effectively, making return to play more tolerable. For the athlete described in this question, it would be a good idea to get a set of plain film X-rays to confirm the absence of associated fracture. (See Figure 34–4.)

11-5: Neck injuries are very common in football, but in general, injuries that don't have a violent mechanism of injury and don't result in any neurologic symptoms are benign. This athlete can return to play when his symptoms allow.

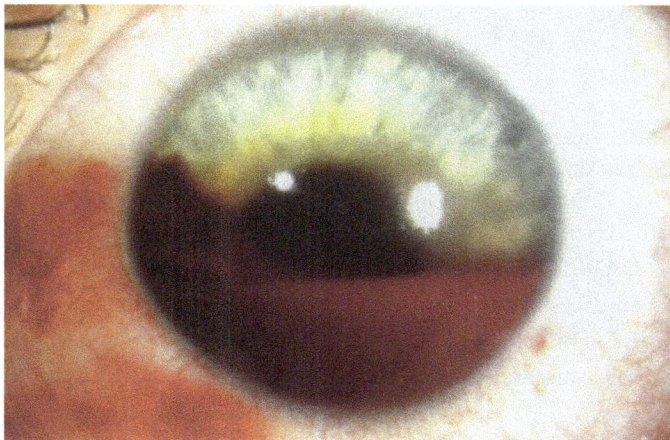

FIGURE 34–3. Posttraumatic hyphema and subconjunctival hemorrhage Layering blood is seen in the anterior chamber of eye consistent with a hyphema. Medially, a subconjunctival hemorrhage is present. (Reproduced with permission from Riordan-Eva P, Cunningham ET, eds. *Vaughan & Asbury's General Ophthalmology*. 18th ed. New York, NY: McGraw-Hill Education; 2011, Fig. 19-9.)

▶ CASE 12

A 14-year-old cross country runner comes to the clinic for evaluation of shin pain. She has tenderness at the medial border of the tibia but no pain with the hop test. X-rays are normal. She reports that she used to have regular periods, but has not had one in over a year. Her body mass index (BMI) is 20 kg/m².

Question 12-1

Which of the following statements is true?

A) Starting a birth control pill is an effective way to improve this patient's bone health.
B) The amenorrhea of the female athlete triad is due to ovarian failure.
C) Shin splints and tibial stress fractures are different gradations of the same injury.
D) Most athletes with the female athlete triad get adequate calcium and vitamin D from their diet.
E) This patient cannot have the female athlete triad because her BMI is in the normal range.

Discussion 12-1

The correct answer is "C." Shin splints and tibial stress fractures are different grades of the same injury. Shin splints is a mild bone stress injury that typically causes diffuse tenderness and pain at the medial border of the tibia (this is why it is called "medial tibial stress syndrome"). Stress fractures are more severe bone injuries that typically have more focal tenderness and more severe pain. If necessary, the two injuries can be differentiated on magnetic resonance imaging (MRI). Shin splints show only periosteal edema on T2-weighted images whereas stress fractures demonstrate edema in the cortex and marrow cavity of the bone. The female athlete triad comprises (1) disordered eating, (2) menstrual irregularities, and (3) impaired bone health. Note that low BMI is not necessary for the diagnosis. In fact it is common for particularly muscular female athletes with the female athlete triad to have normal or elevated BMI. The underlying problem is insufficient calories to sustain the level of activity. This causes impaired bone turnover and hypothalamic dysfunction that leads to menstrual irregularities (most commonly amenorrhea, but occasionally other patterns). The mainstay of treatment is increasing calories and decreasing exercise. Supplemental calcium and vitamin D is often necessary to meet dietary needs or make up for recent deficiencies. Supplemental estrogen in the form of oral contraceptive pills does not improve bone health. One note on terminology. Recently, there has been a movement to rename this condition "relative energy deficiency in sport" or "RED-S" to make it clear that males can also suffer from hypothalamic dysfunction and impaired bone health when they do not have adequate nutrition to fuel their exercise. However, it is unlikely that you will see this term on a board exam in the near future.

⏳ QUICK QUIZ

Which of the following statements is/are true about overuse injuries in children?

A) Bone injuries are more common than tendon injuries.
B) Tibial tubercle avulsion is a common complication of Osgood-Schlatter disease.
C) Sport specialization increases risk of overuse injuries.
D) Decreasing free play is important for preventing overuse injuries when children are participating in several hours of organized sports per week.
E) Some sports require early entry in order to reach the highest levels of success.
F) Options A and B, only.
G) Options A, B, and D.
H) Options A, C, and E.
I) Options A, C, D, and E.

Discussion

The correct answer is "H." Prior to skeletal maturity, tendon injuries are fairly rare because the tendon tissue is fairly robust and the surrounding bone is not. Tibial tubercle avulsion is typically a traumatic injury and does not occur as a complication of tibial tubercle apophysitis (Osgood-Schlatter disease). Early sport specialization does increase risk of overuse injuries. Children who play multiple sports or spend their time in free play have fewer injuries than those who spend most of their active time in a single sport. A good rule of thumb is that a child should not spend more hours per week playing a sport than years they are old (obviously, there are exceptions, but this is a good place to start and illustrates the point that diverse athletic exposures are beneficial). However, there are some sports that seem to require early entry in order to succeed at the highest levels. Tennis and gymnastics have the best data to support the need for early entry. It does not seem to make much difference in most team sports.

▶ CASE 13

A 7-year-old boy presents with heel pain. He no longer can play soccer. He does not remember falling or hurting his feet. On exam, he is tender on the underside of his heels.

Question 13-1

You suspect an apophysitis, but of which anatomic site?

A) Tibial tubercle.
B) Inferior pole of the patella.
C) Base of the fifth metatarsal.
D) Calcaneus.

Discussion 13-1

The correct answer is "D." He has Sever disease, an apophysitis of the calcaneus seen frequently in young athletic boys with heel pain. Other examples of apophysitis are listed below, with the site affected:

- Osgood-Schlatter disease: tibial tubercle (See Figure 34–5)
- Sinding-Larsen-Johansson disease: inferior pole of the patella
- Iselin disease: base of the fifth metatarsal
- Sever disease: calcaneus

Question 13-2

Which is NOT an effective treatment for Sever apophysitis?

A) Ice.
B) Gel heel cups.
C) Foot orthotics.
D) Rest.
E) Rehabilitation.

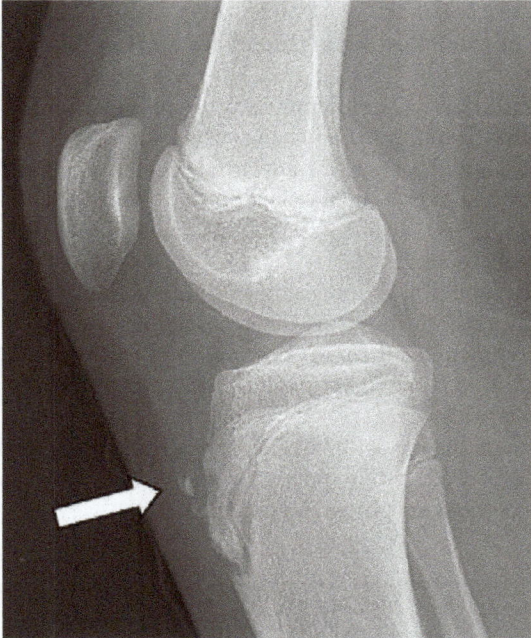

FIGURE 34–5. Osgood-Schlatter disease is an apophysitis of the proximal tibial tubercle at the insertion of the patella tendon. Lateral X-ray showing irregularity and fragmentation of the tubercle (white arrow). (Reproduced with permission from Davis KW: Imaging pediatric sports injuries: lower extremity, *Radiol Clin North Am.* 2010 Nov;48(6):1213-1235.)

Discussion 13-2

The correct answer is "E." Unfortunately rehabilitation does not make much difference for the treatment of most overuse apophysitis, including Sever. Ice makes the heel feel better, but does not fix the problem. Gel heel cups and foot orthotics decrease symptoms with activity. Rest does tend to improve the problem, but it commonly recurs with resumption of activity. Remember, apophysitis is not dangerous and does not cause long-term harm. There are not many conditions where it is okay to tell a 7-year-old to play through the pain, but Sever apophysitis is one of them.

▶ CASE 14

A 16-year-old girl was playing basketball when she stepped on another player's foot, rolling her ankle (inversion). She is diagnosed with a lateral ankle sprain.

Question 14-1

Which of the following is an expected finding in a lateral ankle sprain?
A) Inability to bear weight.
B) Tenderness at the posterior lateral malleolus.
C) Positive ankle drawer test.
D) Positive syndesmosis squeeze test.
E) Widened medial clear space on ankle X-rays.

TABLE 34–3 OTTAWA ANKLE RULES: IMAGING CRITERIA IN ACUTE ANKLE SPRAINS

Ankle X-rays Are Indicated:

Malleolar pain *and*	(1) Posterior tip of the lateral or medial malleolus tenderness
	or
	(2) Unable to bear weight
Midfoot pain *and*	(1) Base of the fifth metatarsal or navicular pain
	or
	(2) Unable to bear weight

Discussion 14-1

The correct answer is "C." Inability to bear weight and tenderness at the posterior lateral malleolus are concerning for distal fibular fracture (this is the crux of the Ottawa Ankle Rules for ruling out ankle fractures by history and physical exam in the emergency department). (See Table 34–3.) A positive ankle drawer test is seen with a grade 2 or 3 sprain of the anterior talofibular ligament, which is expected in more severe lateral ankle sprains. A positive syndesmosis squeeze test and widened medial clear space on ankle X-rays is concerning for a syndesmotic or "high" ankle sprain. This is a more severe injury that can lead to long-term ankle instability or arthritis, or both, and should be managed by someone with knowledge of the condition.

You explain to the girl that she sustained a grade 2 lateral ankle sprain involving the anterior talofibular ligament. She asks, "Is it completely torn"?

Question 14-2

Which of the following is true regarding a grade 2 ligament sprain?
A) The ligament is not torn.
B) The ligament has microscopic tears.
C) The ligament is completely torn.
D) The ligament is stretched.
E) The ligament is incompletely torn.

Discussion 14-2

The correct answer is "E." The three grades of ligament sprain are described as follows:

- Grade 1: Pain but no laxity. The ligament is only partially torn; there is internal disruption, but it is fully intact. The patient is able to bear weight and ambulate with minimal pain.
- Grade 2: Pain and mild laxity. The ligament is partially torn through, and there is more than just internal disruption. Weight bearing and ambulation are painful.
- Grade 3: Pain and laxity. The ligament is torn all the way through, causing significant instability and loss of motion. The patient is unable to bear weight or ambulate.

⧗ QUICK QUIZ

The acronym PRICE is commonly used in describing the treatment of common sprains.

What does PRICE stand for?
A) Protection, Rest, Ice, Compression, Elevation.
B) Pad, Rest, Ice, Compression, Elevation.
C) Protection, Rotate, Ice, Compression, Elevation.
D) Protection, Rest, Ice, Condition, Elevation.
E) Protection, Rest, Ice, Compression, Eversion.

Discussion

The correct answer is "A." Common sprains are treated with these five measures:

P – Protection

R – Rest

I – Ice

C – Compression

E – Elevation

▶ CASE 15

You overhear a medical student say that helmets prevent concussions in football players.

Question 15-1

You pull him aside and tell him what?
A) He is wrong.
B) He is really wrong.
C) He is dead wrong.
D) He needs to go home for the day.
E) All of the above.

Discussion 15-1

The correct answer is "E." It is well established that helmets do not prevent concussions in football players. Despite what you might hear, no helmet, helmet add-on, or other device prevents concussion in football. This includes mouthguards. The only thing that seems to make a difference is limiting hitting or changing hitting technique. Helmets do prevent many other dangerous injuries, including skull fracture, intracranial hemorrhage, and death. A mouthguard does an excellent job of preventing dental trauma. Athletes in collision sports should absolutely wear helmets and mouthguards.

▶ CASE 16

A teenage boy with one eye comes to your office for a preparticipation evaluation. He has a history of retinoblastoma that resulted in single enucleation and needs a form filled out for school. The school wants a list of "dos and don'ts" for one-eyed athletes.

Question 16-1

Which of the following is true about athletes who have lost an eye?
A) Due to their lack of depth perception, they should be prohibited from playing any ball sport.
B) They should wear ANSI-approved protective lenses for any sport that puts them at risk of being hit in the eye.
C) They should wear a full polycarbonate face shield when playing football.
D) They should have the vision in the remaining eye checked every 3 months to ensure that it has not suffered any damage.
E) It's funny to tell them to "keep your eye on the ball."

Discussion 16-1

The correct answer is "B." The buzzwords in this question are "ANSI approved." Every policy statement and article on this topic uses the same phrase. So don't forget it.

▶ CASE 17

A high school wrestler suffered a blow to his ear and now has a large auricular hematoma.

Question 17-1

Which of the following is NOT true about his risk of developing cauliflower ear?
A) Draining the hematoma will decrease the risk.
B) Using a pressure dressing over the drained ear will decrease the risk.
C) Protecting the ear with a headgear is sufficient to prevent most of these injuries.
D) Draining an auricular hematoma should only be done by an experienced provider because of the risk of infection.
E) Hearing is never affected by cauliflower ear.

Discussion 17-1

The correct answer is "D." Cauliflower ear is a permanent scarring of the auricle following an auricular hematoma. Draining the wound and applying pressure (with a dental caulking gun, sutured-in bolster, or just a pressure dressing) decreases the risk of scarring. Severe cauliflower ear can cause conductive hearing loss (obviously). Wrestling headgear is very effective in preventing auricular hematomas. Luckily, these injuries rarely become infected. In fact, many wrestlers drain each other's auricular hematomas in decidedly unsterile fashion with only very rare complications. The general pediatrician should feel comfortable draining an ear and applying a pressure dressing without fear of significant complications.

▶ CASE 18

You are back on the sideline covering the Iowa State Cyclones. This week they are playing the Merciful Blind Sisters of the Poor (some people call them "Illini"). Your starting tailback is hit hard 5 yards deep in the backfield and does not get up.

You rush onto the field and notice an open fracture of his lower leg. The player is not moving and does not respond to your verbal commands. He is breathing and does have a pulse.

Question 18-1

Which of the following is the first thing you should do while stabilizing this patient?
A) Remove the helmet and shoulder pads.
B) Remove the facemask of the helmet.
C) Splint the broken leg.
D) Confirm neurovascular status distal to the fracture site.
E) Stabilize the cervical spine.

Discussion 18-1

The correct answer is "E." It is easy to get distracted by the other injury in this setting, but do not forget than an unconscious athlete should be assumed to have a cervical spine injury until proven otherwise. It is a bad idea to remove the helmet and shoulder pads because the movement can exacerbate an unstable cervical spine injury. Removing the facemask might be important for the athlete because the movement can exacerbate The broken leg, while dramatic, is low priority in this setting.

It is now 2 weeks later, and the Cyclones are playing the Junior Varsity team from the Barron County Branch Campus of Stout State University (BCBCSSU). It is a close game. Your starting middle linebacker attempts to make a tackle and suffers an anterior dislocation of his shoulder.

Question 18-2

Which of the following is NOT true about first-time shoulder dislocations?
A) It is easier to reduce them on the field than to wait for the more controlled environment of the training room or emergency department.
B) Having the player reduce his own shoulder by clasping the hands around the knee and using the leg to provide a tractional load with the shoulder in 30 degrees of forward flexion is an effective way to safely reduce the shoulder.
C) Early surgical repair of any bony injury to the glenoid dramatically decreases risk of repeat dislocation.
D) It is important to check neurovascular status of the affected arm before attempting a reduction of an obvious shoulder dislocation.
E) The most common mechanism for shoulder dislocation is a fall on an outstretched hand.

Discussion 18-2

The correct answer is "E." Most shoulder dislocations are hyperabduction with external rotation injuries. (See Figure 34–6.) Rapid reduction (before there is much muscle spasm) is much easier than waiting until the player is off the field. There are many effective methods of shoulder reduction, some of which require two providers and some of which can be done by the patient. Surgical repair following a first-time shoulder dislocation is a very effective way of decreasing risk of future dislocation. The reason to check neurovascular status prior to

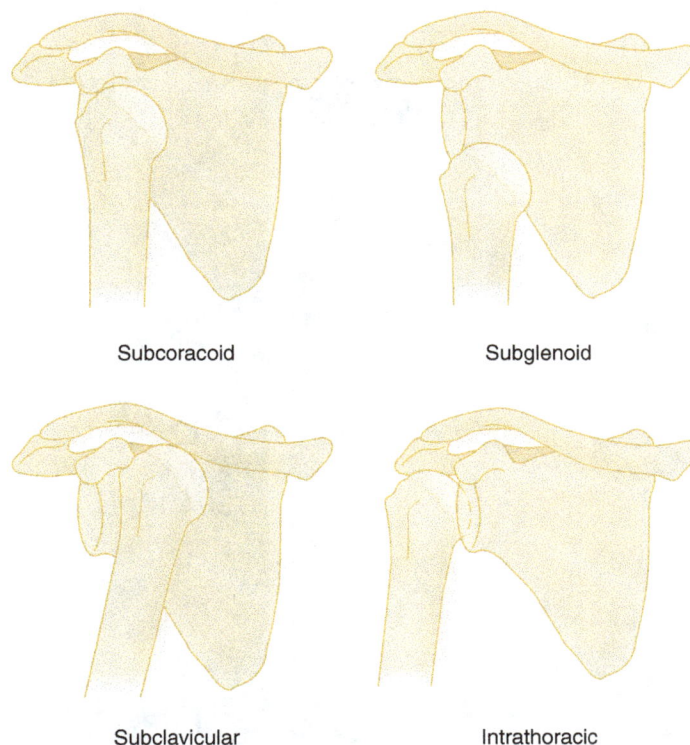

Subcoracoid

Subglenoid

Subclavicular

Intrathoracic

FIGURE 34–6. Types of anterior shoulder dislocation. (Reproduced with permission from Tintinalli JE, Stapczynski JS, Ma OJ, et al: *Tintinalli's Emergency Medicine: A Comprehensive Study Guide*, 8th ed. McGraw-Hill Education, Inc., 2016.)

attempting dislocation is twofold: First, you want to be sure that your intervention did not cause nerve or vessel injury. Second, if the neurovascular function of the limb is not intact, it is more likely that there is more to the injury than just a simple dislocation and urgent transport is warranted prior to attempting reduction on the field.

⏳ QUICK QUIZ

Children with trisomy 21 sometimes have atlantoaxial instability of the cervical spine.

Because of this, they should not be allowed to participate in which of the following sports:
A) Boxing.
B) Weight lifting.
C) Wrestling.
D) Football.
E) Swimming.
F) Options A and B, only.
G) Options A, C, and D.
H) All of the above.

Discussion

The correct answer is "G." Contact and collision sports are not permitted for children with trisomy 21. While some patients do not have atlantoaxial instability, the risk is high enough that it is prudent to restrict all children with trisomy 21 from participating in sports that put them at risk for cervical spine instability.

▶ CASE 19

A 17-year-old pankration athlete comes to your clinic because he suffered a dislocation of his elbow during a bout.

Question 19-1

Which of the following is true about this injury?
A) Elbow instability is very rare after a first dislocation.
B) Ulnar collateral ligament injury (UCL) is commonly the limiting factor for return to sport.
C) Reduction of the elbow involves placing the forearm in pronation and providing an axial load.
D) Fall on an outstretched hand is the most common mechanism of injury.
E) Prolonged immobilization in full flexion accelerates recovery and return to sport.

Discussion 19-1

The correct answer is "B." Elbow dislocations are dramatic events, but also fairly common in mixed martial arts fighting (pankration is a junior version of fighting; striking above the clavicle is typically prohibited in this style). Reduction involves placing a tractional load on the forearm in a supinated position. Following reduction, early mobilization speeds recovery and return to sport. Splinting in flexion can cause a severe flexion contracture that is very difficult to overcome with rehabilitation. UCL injuries are present in nearly all elbow dislocations and can be very slow to heal. Rarely, surgical reconstruction of the UCL is necessary for return to full activity. (See Figure 34–7.)

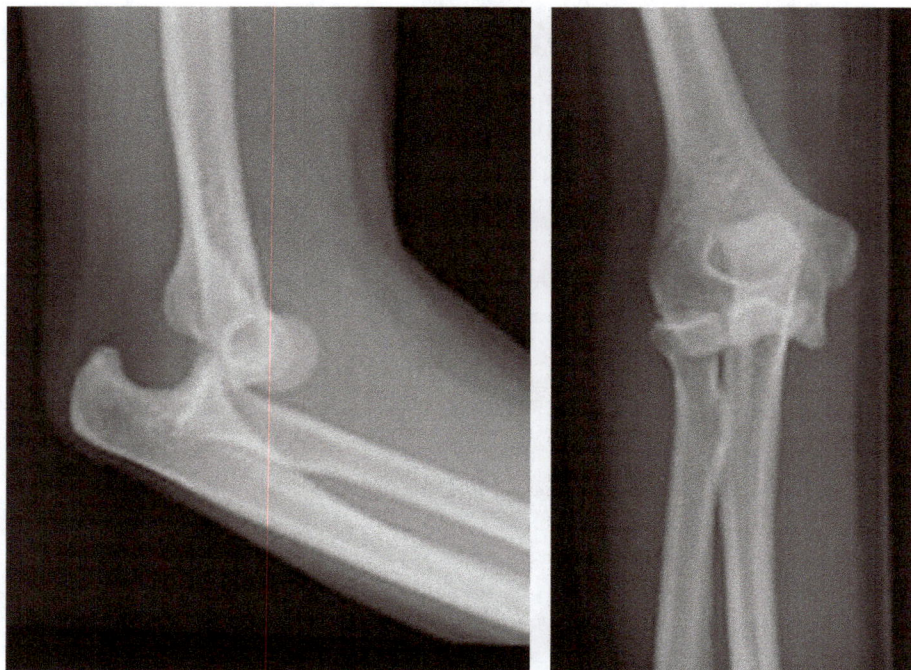

FIGURE 34–7. A posterior elbow dislocation is shown in these X-rays. (Reproduced with permission from Tintinalli JE, Stapczynski JS, Ma OJ, Yealy DM, Cline DM, Meckler GD, eds. *Tintinalli's Emergency Medicine: A Comprehensive Study Guide.* 8th ed. New York, NY: McGraw-Hill Education; 2016, Fig. 270-11.)

▶ CASE 20

A 12-year-old pitcher comes to the clinic to discuss pain and a "dead-arm" feeling he is getting with throwing. He plays on four teams in four different leagues, has an 80-mile-per hour (mph) fastball, and recently learned to throw a slider.

Question 20-1

Which of the following is NOT a risk factor for little league elbow?
A) Throwing in multiple leagues.
B) High-pitch velocity.
C) Less advanced skeletal maturity.
D) Throwing breaking pitches.
E) Throwing from an elevated pitcher's mound.

Discussion 20-1

The correct answer is "E." Little league elbow is a stress injury to the medial epicondylar physis in the throwing arm. Throwing more and throwing harder are by far the biggest risk factors for this injury. It tends to occur in younger throwers, and other medial elbow injuries begin to replace little league elbow as the thrower reaches skeletal maturity. Children who throw breaking pitches (curveballs, sliders, etc) are at higher risk of developing the injury, but this seems to be a confounder—only children who are really interested in pitching, throwing a lot, throwing harder, and throwing in more than one league tend to start throwing breaking pitches. So, you could think of both little league elbow and throwing breaking pitches as the result of throwing a lot. The risk of shoulder and elbow injuries is higher in pitchers who throw from an elevated pitching mound, but this association has not been made with little league elbow in younger throwers. Hence the choice of option "E" as the correct answer might be a bit controversial.

⏳ QUICK QUIZ

Which of the following statements regarding jersey and mallet fingers is false?
A) Distal finger flexion is lost with a jersey finger.
B) A jersey finger requires urgent surgical evaluation.
C) Distal finger extension is lost with a mallet finger.
D) A mallet finger requires urgent surgical evaluation.
E) None of the above.

Discussion

The correct answer is "D." Jersey finger is an injury to the flexor tendon as it inserts into the distal phalanx of a finger. It occurs when a player grabs a jersey as the opponent is pulling away, causing a hyperextension of the distal interphalangeal (DIP) joint while the proximal interphalangeal (PIP) is flexed and the flexor tendon is under extreme load. This causes a rupture of the flexor tendon and loss of finger flexion at the DIP joint. This is a surgically urgent injury because the tendon can

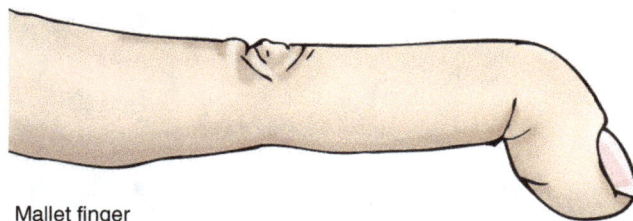

Mallet finger

FIGURE 34–8. Mallet Finger. Extension of the distal interphalangeal joint is lost due to rupture of the extensor tendon. (Reproduced with permission from Tintinalli JE, Stapczynski JS, Ma OJ, Yealy DM, Cline DM, Meckler GD, eds. *Tintinalli's Emergency Medicine: A Comprehensive Study Guide.* 8th ed. New York, NY: McGraw-Hill Education; 2016, Fig. 43-5 Part A.)

retract, making eventual repair and healing very difficult. Mallet finger is an injury to the extensor tendon as it inserts into the distal phalanx of a finger. (See Figure 34–8.) It occurs when a player is struck at the tip of the finger by a ball, forcing the DIP joint into hyperflexion. This causes rupture of the extensor tendon and loss of finger extension at the DIP joint. This is a fairly benign injury that responds to a brief period of splinting in full extension.

▶ CASE 21

A 19-year-old girl jammed her hand into her handlebars when she had to brake abruptly while riding her bike. On exam, she has pain in the anatomic snuff box.

Question 21-1

Which of the following is NOT true about this type of fracture?
A) Most scaphoid waist fractures heal without complications.
B) The scaphoid is the most common fractured carpal bone.
C) Fall on an outstretched hand is a common mechanism of injury.
D) Prolonged immobilization is required for proper healing.
E) None of the above.

Discussion 21-1

The correct answer is "E." This is another poorly worded question, but *none* of those answers are *not* true. Most scaphoid waist fractures (fractures of the distal third of the scaphoid) heal without complications. But enough do not heal well that vigilance is warranted. Check for pain to palpation in the anatomic snuffbox. The scaphoid waist is a vascular watershed area and nonunion fracture healing with eventual degenerative changes and collapse is not uncommon. (See Figure 34–9.) These injuries should be protected in a thumb spica cast for at least 6 weeks and monitored closely for healing. Any question of poor healing should prompt a referral to a hand surgeon to consider surgical fixation. The scaphoid is the most commonly fractured carpal bone, and a fall on an outstretched hand (FOOSH) injury is the most common mechanism.

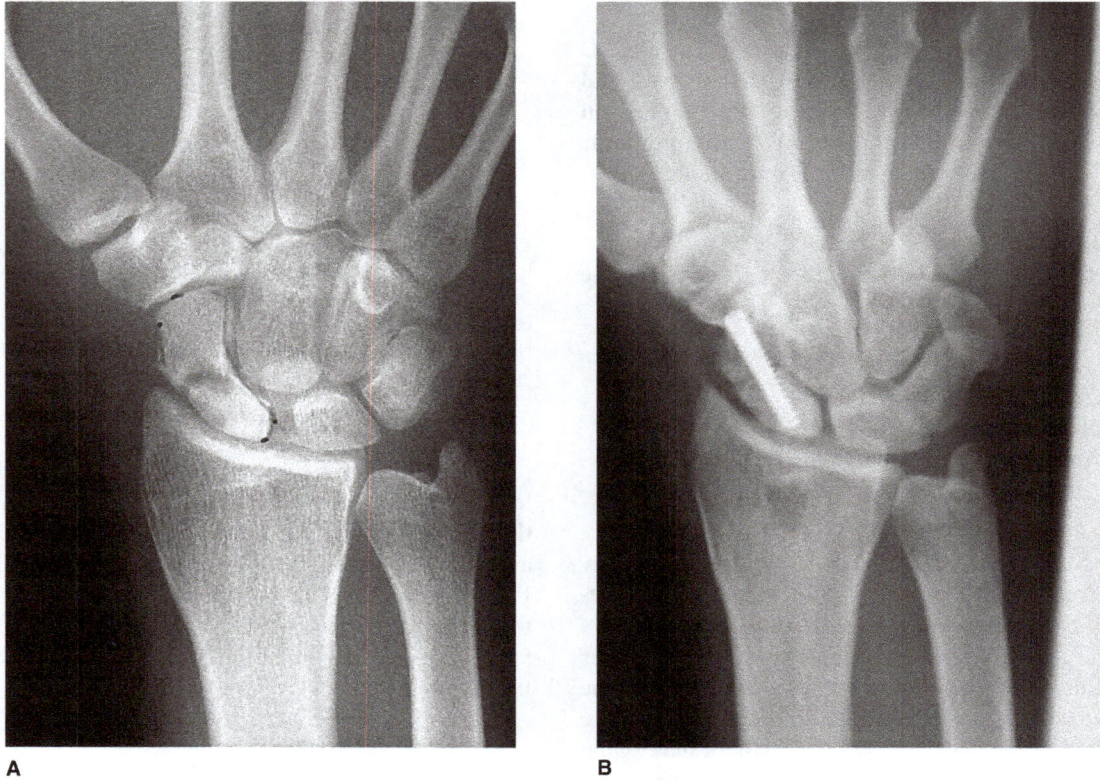

FIGURE 34–9. Scaphoid Fracture. A fracture of the scaphoid bone (outlined) is seen in this anteroposterior X-ray. (Reproduced with permission from Doherty GM, ed. *Current Diagnosis and Treatment: Surgery*. 14th ed. New York, NY: McGraw-Hill Education; 2015, Fig. 40-12A.)

> **Helpful Tip**
> Pain to palpation in the anatomic snuffbox is characteristic of a scaphoid fracture, which is an injury at high risk for poor healing.

▶ CASE 22

A 13-year-old female athlete presents for evaluation of anterior knee pain of several months' duration. She is a state champion in cross country running. Her pain is worse with running, which makes practice difficult, but she is able to "tough it out." Recently she felt her left knee buckle a few times. This scared her, prompting today's visit to your office.

Question 22-1
Which of the following knee tests is NOT useful for assessing a patient with patellofemoral stress syndrome (PFSS)?
A) Patellar compression test.
B) One-legged step-down test.
C) Patellar apprehension test.
D) Thessaly test.
E) Lachman test.
F) None of the above.

Discussion 22-1
The correct answer is "F." This is another poorly worded question, and somewhat of a trick question. All of the listed tests are useful, so let's review what each test reveals. The patellar compression test is typically positive in PFSS. The subpatellar space is tender, and pushing the patella hard against the trochlea should recreate the patient's pain. The one-legged step-down test commonly shows poor hip abduction control in PFSS. The typical finding is a valgus thrust of the knee as the patient steps down off a step. Patients with PFSS and poor hip abduction control typically respond well to physical therapy for treatment of their pain. The patellar apprehension test is usually positive in patellar dislocation or subluxation. The most common direction of instability is laterally. A positive patellar apprehension test occurs when the patient has a sense of apprehension (not pain) when the patella is pushed laterally. The Thessaly test is positive in a meniscus tear. The patient stands on one leg, bends the knee to 30 degrees of flexion, and twists back and forth. A painful click is highly suggestive of a meniscus tear, although it can also be positive in other injuries to the cartilage (eg, osteochondral defect or osteoarthritis). The Lachman test reveals laxity in the anterior-posterior direction when translating (sliding) the tibia on the femur. In a positive test there is increased translation, but also a soft end point when the tibia is translated anteriorly on the femur.

Helpful Tip

Keeping *valgus* versus *varus* straight can be difficult. These terms refer to the orientation of the extremity distal to the joint of interest.

- Varus: toward the midline (eg, genu varus = bowlegs)
- Valgus: away from the midline (eg, genu valgus = knock knees)

Question 22-2

Which of the following is NOT a risk factor for developing PFSS?

A) Hypermobility.
B) Female gender.
C) Tall stature.
D) Increased BMI.
E) Jumping sport.

Discussion 22-2

The correct answer is "C." All of the others are fairly strong risk factors for anterior knee pain.

▶ CASE 23

You will be serving as the team physician for a high school girls soccer team this year. You have been reading about the "epidemic" of knee injuries in girls and women's soccer and want to be sure you are ready for what you might see on the pitch.

Questions 23-1 through 23-4

Describe the characteristic physical findings of each of the following knee injuries. Be sure to comment on appearance, sites of maximal tenderness, range of motion, strength, laxity, and special tests that might be positive.

23-1: Anterior cruciate ligament (ACL) tear.
23-2: Posterior cruciate ligament (PCL) tear.
23-3: Medial meniscus tear.
23-4: Patellar dislocation.

Discussion 23-1 through 23-4

Your descriptions should include the following information:

23-1: The defining physical exam finding an ACL tear is anterior laxity. Mechanisms of injury include being hit on the lateral side of the knee when the foot is planted or sudden deceleration followed by a quick change in direction (cutting) or pivoting. Immediately following injury a large effusion is noted. (See Figure 34–10.) There may be tenderness at the femoral condyles or tibial plateau from bone bruising that occurs during the injury. (See Figure 34–11.) Strength is often limited by quadriceps inhibition, but there is no true muscular injury. There should be no laxity with varus or valgus

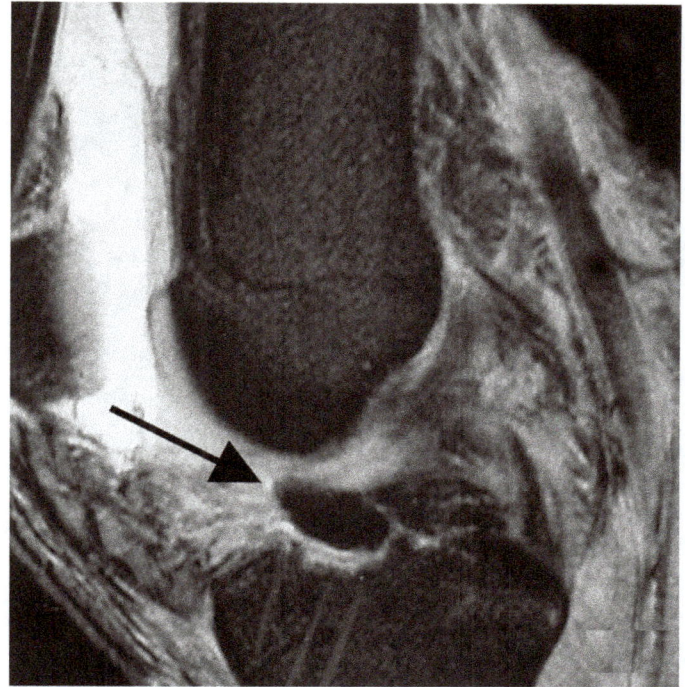

FIGURE 34–10. Anterior Cruciate Ligament (ACL) Tear. This sagittal T1-weighted MRI image demonstrates a rupture of the ACL (*arrow*) and a very large joint effusion. ACL tears bleed. A lot. A very large joint effusion just hours after the tear is characteristic of the injury. (Reproduced with permission from Doherty GM, ed. *Current Diagnosis and Treatment: Surgery.* 14th ed. New York, NY: McGraw-Hill Education; 2015, Fig. 40-30.)

stress unless there is an associated collateral ligament injury. It is somewhat common to have a medial meniscus or medial collateral ligament tear, or both, at the same time as an ACL injury. This combination is called a terrible triad. The Lachman and anterior drawer tests should be markedly positive. A positive Lachman and anterior drawer consist of both increased travel as the tibia is translated anteriorly on the femur but also a sensation of a soft anterior end point. (See Figure 34–12.)

23-2: The PCL injury is very similar to an ACL injury but much less common. The typical mechanism of injury is a hard blow to the anterior proximal tibia, causing a posterior translation on the tibia on the femur. The knee is commonly very swollen, with significant tenderness at the anterior proximal tibia. As in an ACL injury, there is laxity. However, this time it is in the posterior direction: the tibia sags posteriorly against the femur. (See Figure 34–13.) Associated collateral and meniscus injuries are much less common.

23-3: Patients with isolated medial meniscus tears (see Figure 34–14) commonly present with a small joint effusion and tenderness along the medial joint line. Certain meniscus tears can cause knee locking or other mechanical symptoms. A locked knee will have very little range of motion. Expect normal strength and normal tests of ligamentous laxity. McMurray test, which passively loads and shears the medial and lateral compartments of the knee, may demonstrate a

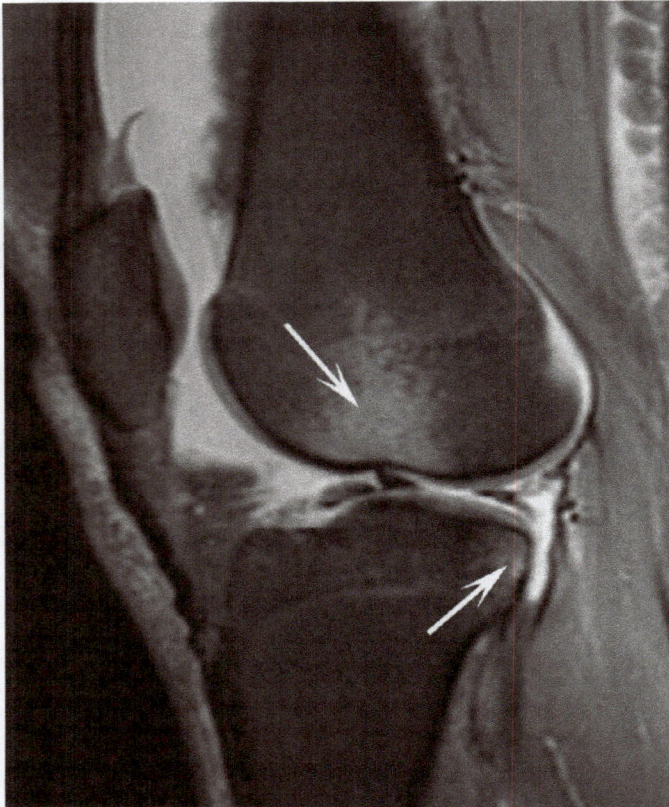

FIGURE 34–11. Bone Bruise after Anterior Cruciate Ligament (ACL) Tear. Sagittal MRI image of the knee in a patient with an ACL tear showing the classic associated bruising of the lateral femoral condyle and lateral tibial plateau (*arrows*). (Reproduced with permission from Chen MYM, Pope TL, Ott DJ, eds. *Basic Radiology*. 2nd ed. McGraw-Hill Education, Inc., 2011. Fig 7-21.)

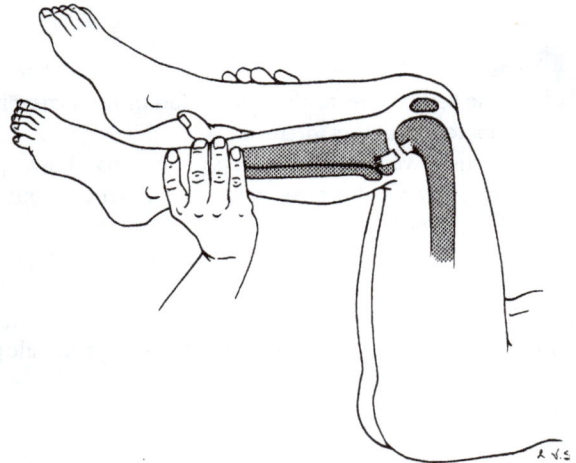

FIGURE 34–13. Posterior Cruciate Ligament (PCL) Sag. With a torn PCL, the tibia sags posteriorly below the femur when the leg is elevated and flexed at the hip and knee. (Reproduced with permission from Stone CK, Humphries RL, eds. *Current Diagnosis and Treatment: Emergency Medicine*. 7th ed. New York, NY: McGraw-Hill Education; 2011, Fig, 28-18.)

painful click felt along the medial joint line. In the Thessaly test, the patient stands on the affected leg with the knee bent, then actively rotates the knee internally and externally, producing a similar finding.

23-4: Most patellar dislocations reduce spontaneously when the patient first tries to extend the knee after the injury. A patella that is still dislocated is very obvious; the knee should be locked in flexion and the patella is easily palpated lateral to the expected position. However, most of the time you will see a

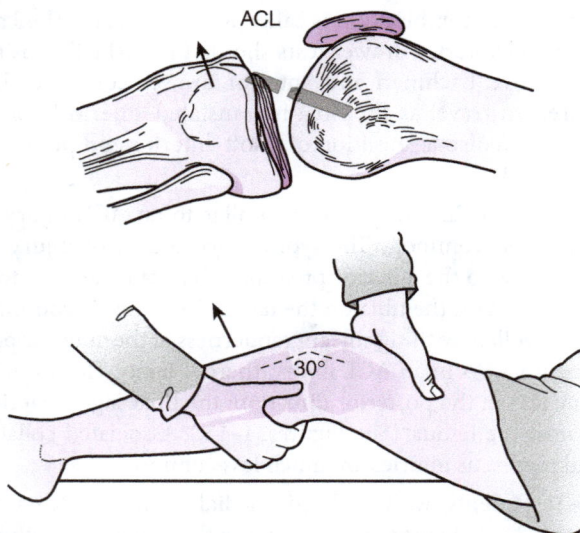

FIGURE 34–12. Lachman Test. The Lachman test is useful for diagnosing a tear of the anterior cruciate ligament. The knee is held in 30 degrees of flexion while the examiner pulls forward trying to anteriorly translate the tibia on the femur. Increased travel of the tibia forward indicates a positive test. (Reproduced with permission from Imboden JB, Hellmann DB, Stone JH, eds. *Current Diagnosis and Treatment: Rheumatology*. 3rd ed. New York, NY: McGraw-Hill Education; 2013, Fig. 12-2.)

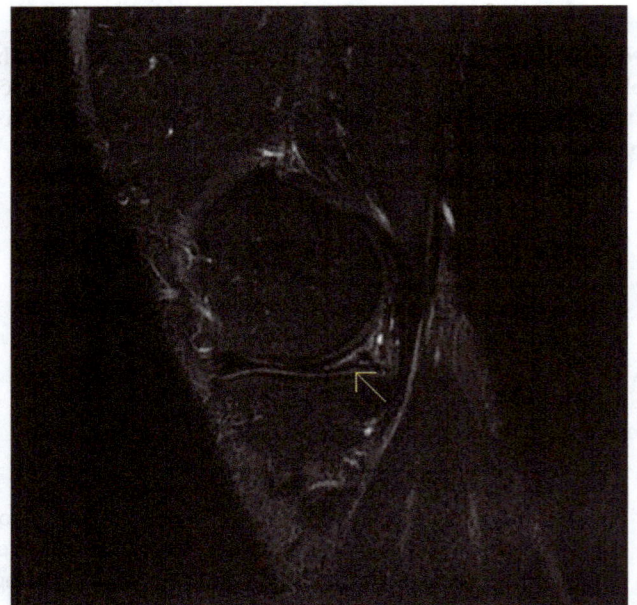

FIGURE 34–14. Medial Meniscus Tear. A tear in the posterior part of the medial meniscus (*arrow*) is shown in this sagittal MRI image of the knee. A normal meniscus should look like a "bow tie" on MRI. (Reproduced with permission from Maitin IB, Cruz E, eds. *Current Diagnosis and Treatment: Physical Medicine and Rehabilitation*. New York, NY: McGraw-Hill Education; 2015, Fig. 29-2.)

patellar dislocation after it is already reduced. The patient may have a small joint effusion, but it should not be as large as that seen in cruciate ligament injuries. There is typically exquisite tenderness at the medial pole of the patella and at the lateral femoral condyle. The patient demonstrates severe patellar apprehension when a lateralizing force is applied to the patella.

> **Helpful Tip**
> Tearing the ACL, medial meniscus, and medial collateral ligament at the same time is known as the terrible triad.

QUICK QUIZ

An osteochondral defect is most likely to be noticed at which common site in the knee?
A) Lateral aspect of the medial femoral condyle.
B) Medial aspect of the lateral femoral condyle.
C) Trochlea.
D) Medial patellar facet.
E) Tibial tubercle.

Discussion

The correct answer is "A." An osteochondral defect is most commonly seen at the lateral aspect of the medial femoral condyle. (See Figure 34–15.) For some reason, this is a commonly tested

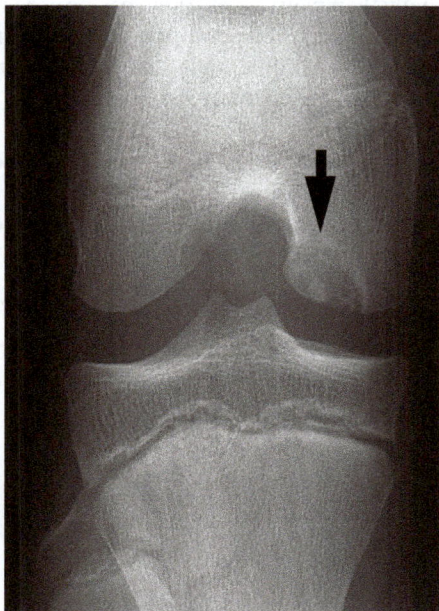

FIGURE 34–15. Osteochondral Defect (Osteochondritis Dissecans). An osteochondral defect is seen at the lateral aspect of the medial femoral condyle. It represents a separation of subchondral bone and articular cartilage from the underlying bone. (Reproduced with permission from Davis KW: Imaging pediatric sports injuries: lower extremity, *Radiol Clin North Am*. 2010 Nov;48(6):1213-1235.)

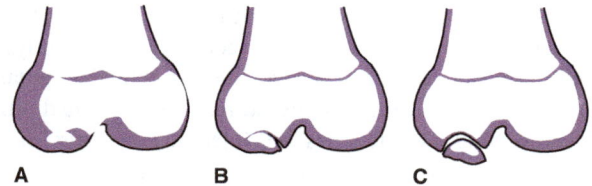

FIGURE 34–16. Forms of Osteochondral Defects (Osteochondritis Dissecans). Different forms of osteochondral defects seen in children include (A) an ossification center defect without cartilage defect, (B) a defect with a hinged flap, and (C) complete separation of bone and cartilage, which may cause a loose fragment in the knee. (Reproduced with permission from Skinner HB, McMahon PJ, eds. *Current Diagnosis and Treatment in Orthopedics*. 5th ed. New York, NY: McGraw-Hill Education; 2014, Fig. 10-27A–C.)

fact. The term *osteochondritis dissecans* is also sometimes used to describe the lesion. (See Figure 34–16.) Although occasionally caused by trauma, these lesions most often arise due to avascular necrosis of the subchondral bone, leaving the articular cartilage unsupported and prone to damage. Patients who have not yet reached skeletal maturity can be treated with a brief period of nonweightbearing to see if the lesion recovers. If it does not, or in older patients, surgical techniques such as osteochondral transfer procedures and microfracture procedures are useful. For the purpose of the pediatric boards, it is important to recognize the lesion on plain film X-rays and refer the patient to an orthopedic specialist.

▶ CASE 24

A 15-year-old wrestler presents with anterior knee pain and swelling. He denies feeling his knee lock or give way. No ligamentous instability is detected on exam. A large fluid collection is felt over the patella. It is mildly tender.

Question 24-1

Which of the following is NOT an effective treatment for prepatellar bursitis in a high school wrestler?
A) Drain the bursa and allow immediate return to wrestling.
B) Drain the bursa and compress and ice for 1 week before allowing return to wrestling.
C) Drain the bursa and inject a small dose of corticosteroids.
D) Drain the bursa and inject a small dose of doxycycline to act as a sclerosis agent.
E) Surgical bursectomy.

Discussion 24-1

The correct answer is "A." Prepatellar bursitis is very common in wrestlers. It results from trauma that causes irritation of the bursa sandwiched between the patella and skin. Draining the bursa works very well to decrease the pain and swelling; however, the swelling returns very quickly if nothing is done to prevent recurrence. Treating with ice and firm compression is usually effective. For resistant lesions, injecting a small dose of corticosteroids into the bursa after following draining can lower the risk of recurrence. Historically, difficult-to-control lesions have been treated with surgical bursectomy; but recently, use of sclerotic agents such as doxycycline has gained popularity. As a general pediatrician, you should feel comfortable draining and compressing these injuries, but injecting anything into the bursa should be performed by an orthopedic specialist.

> **Helpful Tip**
> Range of motion is usually not impaired with prepatellar bursitis as the swelling is outside the joint. In contrast, an acute knee effusion may cause limited flexion.

► CASE 25

You are seeing a 9-year-old tennis player who suffered an inversion ankle injury 1 hour before presentation. He is unable to bear weight and has exquisite tenderness on his distal fibula, approximately 1 cm from the distal tip. You obtain ankle X-rays, which show no abnormalities.

Question 25-1
Which of the following is an appropriate next step?
A) Ankle rehabilitation.
B) Weightbearing as tolerated.
C) Walking boot, but no crutches.
D) Cast and crutches.
E) Lace-up ankle brace.

Discussion 25-1
The correct answer is "D." Of the available choices, cast immobilization and nonweightbearing is the most appropriate. This 9-year-old is almost certainly skeletally immature. His inability to bear weight and the exquisite tenderness at the site of his distal fibular physis should make you very concerned for a Salter-Harris fracture. (See Figure 34–17.) His injury should be treated just like any other bony fracture. It is not uncommon to see no changes on plain film radiographs with either Salter-Harris I or Salter-Harris V injuries. If you are unsure if the patient has a Salter-Harris fracture, a brief period of immobilization and nonweightbearing with serial exams should clarify matters.

If the pain resolves over 1 to 2 weeks, it is unlikely to have been a fracture. While relatively benign at the distal fibula, the main concern with Salter-Harris fractures is the development of physeal bars and growth arrest.

> **Helpful Tip**
> The Salter-Harris classification system is used to describe physeal fractures that can cause premature closure of the physis. The higher the number classification correlates with higher risk for growth arrest. (See Figure 34–17.)

► CASE 26

You have been asked to speak at a convention for youth football coaches in Arizona. Your topic of education is fluid replacement during sports. Arizona seems like a fitting place to talk about fluids, heat, and dehydration.

Question 26-1
Which of the following is NOT true regarding fluid replacement during sports?
A) Athletes should never be restricted from consuming fluids during practice and competition. It does not make them tougher and does not train them to need less water.
B) Plain water is insufficient for maintaining hydration during short bouts of exercise and for rehydrating after exercise.
C) Sports drinks with carbohydrates and sodium are absorbed more rapidly than plain water. They may be used for exercise lasting longer than 1 hour in duration. There is no need to use a sports drink for fluid replacement after exercise.
D) For most athletes, using thirst as a guide for fluid intake it is adequate.
E) Dehydration resulting in loss of as little as 2% of body weight can significantly impair performance.
F) Dehydration can increase risk of heat illness when exercising in hot conditions.

Discussion 26-1
The correct answer is "B." Plain water is sufficient for maintaining hydration during short bouts of exercise and rehydrating

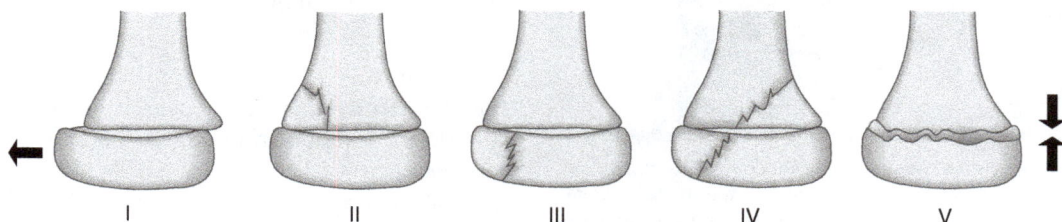

FIGURE 34–17. Salter-Harris classification of growth plate (physeal) injuries. *Salter I:* Fracture along the growth plate. *Salter II:* Fracture along the growth plate with extension into the metaphysis. *Salter III:* Fracture along the growth plate with extension into the epiphysis. *Salter IV:* Fracture across the growth plate with extension into the metaphysis and epiphysis. *Salter V:* Crush injury to the growth plate without obvious fracture. (Reproduced with permission from Doherty GM, ed. *Current Diagnosis and Treatment: Surgery.* 14th ed. New York, NY: McGraw-Hill Education; 2015, Fig. 40-22.)

after exercise. Had you read option "C" closely, you would have been able to spot the inaccuracy in option "B."

Your talk at the coach's convention was a success. Now you are asked to sit on a panel of experts for a question-and-answer session with parents of pee wee wrestlers at the national Take Down and Pin Palooza. A burly man asks if dehydration is an effective way for a wrestling athlete to make weight.

Question 26-2

You respond:

A) Yes, that is true.

B) No, that is false.

C) It depends on the age of the wrestler.

D) It depends on whether he or she will be wrestling in a single bout or tournament.

E) It is effective for heavier but not lighter weight wrestlers.

Discussion 26-2

The correct answer is "A." However, that does not mean that it is a good idea. Methods of rapid weight reduction typically impair performance. Some of these methods, such as exercising in very hot environments or severely restricting fluid intake, can be dangerous. Wrestling athletes should be reminded that dehydration can profoundly impair their ability to wrestle well. Most competitions require weigh-in only 1 hour prior to competition and that is not nearly enough time to rehydrate adequately. Similarly, using diuretics or laxatives to make weight should be discouraged. By far the safest and most effective method for making weight is slow gradual weight reduction focused on decreasing body fat as well as wrestling at a realistic body weight. A 200-pound child is never going to wrestle in the lightweight division.

A proud mother clad in a t-shirt bearing a picture of her sons dressed in singlets wants to know if her youngest son, with only 10% body fat, will be able to participate in high school wrestling when he gets older.

Question 26-3

Which of the following is true about weight control practices for high school wrestlers?

A) They are not allowed to compete at less than 12% body fat.

B) It takes a 3500-calorie deficit to lose 1 pound of body fat.

C) Impermeable rubber suits (sauna suits) are an allowed method of weight loss.

D) Laxatives are an allowed method of weight loss.

E) Less body fat does not provide a competitive advantage to the wrestler.

Discussion 26-3

The correct answer is "B." This is a favorite test question. It takes a fairly large calorie deficit to lose body fat. For this reason weight reduction should be done very gradually. High school wrestling has rules to prevent male wrestlers from competing at less than 7% body fat and female wrestlers from competing at less than 12% body fat. NCAA (National Collegiate Athletic Association) college wrestling permits body fat as low as 5%. Sauna suits and laxatives are both prohibited methods of rapid weight reduction. And clearly being less fat is a competitive advantage for weight-classified athletes.

Your next question relates to using anabolic steroids. A mother asks if her teenage son's recent flare of his acne and incredible moodiness is a sign he is taking steroids.

Question 26-4

Which of the following is true about the use of anabolic steroids in athletes?

A) Anabolic steroids do not provide a competitive advantage to male athletes with adequate testosterone levels.

B) Anabolic steroids do not provide a competitive advantage to female athletes because they do not have enough testosterone receptors.

C) The body efficiently aromatizes excess androgens into estrogens, preventing any unwanted virilization in women who take anabolic steroids.

D) Injectable anabolic steroids are generally safer than oral anabolic steroids.

E) Anabolic steroids do not provide any strength benefit to athletes who are not strength training.

Discussion 26-4

The correct answer is "D." This question addresses several of the misconceptions about anabolic steroids. Anabolic steroids are clearly effective for all athletes. Supraphysiologic doses of androgens improve muscle size and strength even in young man with normal testosterone production. Female athletes also see a large advantage from anabolic steroids and do have adequate testosterone receptors. One of the principal side effects seen in women who use anabolic steroids is virilization. However, some athletes who use anabolic steroids use aromatase inhibitors to prevent the estrogenic side effects and increase the effectiveness of the drugs. Contrary to popular belief, injectable anabolic steroids are generally safer than oral anabolic steroids because they bypass first-pass metabolism in the liver, resulting in less hepatocellular damage. But do not forget, these drugs are banned by most sport governing bodies and are mostly illegal. To answer the mother's question, steroids may cause acne and changes in personality but it is more likely her son is a normal moody teenager trying to get through puberty.

⌛ QUICK QUIZ

True or false: Most nutritional supplements used by athletes are effective for improving performance.

A) True.

B) False.

Discussion

The correct answer is "A." But it is a trick question. By far the most common nutritional supplements taken by athletes are calorie replacement beverages and food, which are obviously effective for fueling exercise. The next most common supplement is creatine, which is also safe and effective for increasing muscle strength and size in power athletes who weight train. However, there is a whole industry devoted to nutritional supplements that are ineffective and may be dangerous, depending on their ingredients. Athletes may come to you with questions about which supplements are safe, effective, and permitted. It is nearly impossible to know the entire supplement market, so each of these cases should be addressed individually. It may require a significant time investment to research and evaluate these products for the athlete. Also, many supplements are made on equipment that is used to produce other supplements or drugs, which may impair the purity of the product.

▶ CASE 27

You are caring for a high school football player who discloses to you that he is taking anabolic steroids. He asks you to do some laboratory tests to make sure that he is not harming himself with the drugs.

Question 27-1

Which of the following is NOT an appropriate response?
A) Since the drugs you are taking are illegal, it is illegal for me to provide you with medical care that makes the use of those drugs safer.
B) We will order a complete blood count because you might have an elevated level of red blood cells or platelets, or both.
C) We will check your cholesterol because elevated low-density lipoprotein (LDL) cholesterol and suppressed high-density lipoprotein (HDL) cholesterol is a common side effect of anabolic steroids.
D) We will check your follicle-stimulating hormone (FSH) and luteinizing hormone (LH) levels to confirm that you are really taking the drugs you think you are.
E) We will check your blood pressure because it can become dangerously high due to abuse of anabolic steroids.

Discussion 27-1
The correct answer is "A." This statement highlights a common misconception. It is illegal to provide the athlete with anabolic steroids, but it is legal and ethical to provide him with appropriate medical care. Options "B" through "E" address the most common side effects of anabolic steroid use. In steroid-abusing athletes, it is reasonable to monitor for erythrocytosis, thrombocytosis, dyslipidemia, gonadal axis suppression (which is expected, not really a side effect) and hypertension.

⏳ QUICK QUIZ

True or False: It is better to be fit than unfit.
A) True.
B) False.

Discussion
The correct answer is "A." This is an actual content area for the general pediatrics board exam. I'm not sure what type of question you could be asked about this, but there is almost no situation where it is better to be unfit. Maybe if you were getting ready for a movie role where you really needed to look doughy. Be aware that fitness and fatness are related, but not the same thing. Fit, but fat, adults have lower cardiovascular risk than the fat but unfit and there is some evidence that this tracks from childhood. That is, a fat but fit child may do better over the long term than if he or she was not fit.

BIBLIOGRAPHY

Bernhardt DT, Roberts WO, American Academy of Family Physicians, American Academy of Pediatrics. *PPE: Preparticipation physical evaluation.* 4th ed. Elk Grove Village, IL: American Academy of Pediatrics; 2010.

Peterson AR, Bernhardt DT. The preparticipation sports evaluation. *Pediatr Rev.* 2011;32(5):e53–65. doi: 10.1542/pir.32-5-e53.

Rice SG, American Academy of Pediatrics Council on Sports Medicine and Fitness. Medical conditions affecting sports participation. *Pediatrics*, 2008;121(4):841–848. doi: 10.1542/peds.2008-0080.

Substance Abuse

35

LaTisha L. Bader and Ross Mathiasen

Question 1

When scientists began to study addictive behaviors in _____, they believed that issues of morality or willpower were the reasons for dependence. Now, addiction is considered a chronic relapsing disease, with the brain being the affected organ.
A) 1920s.
B) 1940s.
C) 1910s.
D) 1930s.
E) 1950s.

Discussion 1

The correct answer is "D." Scientist began studying addiction in the 1930s, and over the intervening decades researchers have disproved a number of myths and misconceptions. Addiction is now considered a disease of both the brain and behavior. Drugs change the brain, both structurally and functionally. Biologic and environmental factors have been identified that cause the development and progression of the disease. The *Diagnostic and Statistical Manual of Mental Disorders, Fifth Edition* (*DSM-5*) characterizes addiction as compulsive drug seeking and use, despite harmful consequences.

Question 2

There are several ways to take drugs; however, the most addictive routes of administration are:
A) Ingested and smoked.
B) Smoked and orally.
C) Ingested and snorted.
D) Suppositories and intravenously.
E) Intravenously and smoked.

Discussion 2

The correct answer is "E." Drugs can be taken into the body in various ways, but when a drug is smoked or injected it begins to interact with the brain in seconds. When nicotine is smoked it begins to affect the brain in just 7 seconds—as fast as heroin.

Drugs interact with the pleasure pathway of the brain by flooding it with dopamine, producing an intense reaction. A drug's addiction potential increases when it produces this rush followed by a quick return to "normal," causing people to chase the "high."

Question 3

Addiction is a disease that has many variables, which include:
A) Biologic.
B) Environmental.
C) Neurologic.
D) Genetic.
E) All of the above.

Discussion 3

The correct answer is "E." Scientists estimate that 40% to 60% of a person's vulnerability to addiction is related to genetics, in addition to mental health, stage of development, and other medical conditions. How an individual responds to substance use and the thought patterns and beliefs that reinforce its use also help determine vulnerability. No one factor can predict an individual's risk for developing the disease of addiction. Rather, addiction is a collective influence of these factors that predispose and reinforce aspects of addiction.

Question 4

Individuals are _____ times more likely to suffer from dependence if one parent struggled with addiction himself or herself.
A) 2.
B) 3.
C) 4.
D) 5.
E) 6.

Discussion 4

The best answer is "C." The average rate of addiction in the population ranges from 8% to 15%. An individual with one parent

TABLE 35–1 RISK AND PROTECTIVE FACTORS FOR DRUG ABUSE AND ADDICTION

Risk Factors	Protective Factors
Aggressive behavior in childhood	Good self-control
Lack of parental supervision	Parental monitoring and support
Poor social skills	Positive relationships
Drug experimentation	Academic competence
Availability of drugs at school	School antidrug policies
Community poverty	Neighborhood pride

Reproduced with permission from National Institute on Drug Abuse. How science has revolutionized the understanding of drug addiction. In: *Drugs, Brains and Behavior: The Science of Addiction.* NIH Pub No. 14-5605. Bethesda, MD: National Institutes of Health; 2014 (original publication 2007).

who has struggled with addiction is four times more likely to become addicted. An individual with two biologic parents who have suffered from addiction is six times more likely to become addicted. (Some studies cite a two- to ninefold increased risk for developing alcoholism.) Genetic factors also influence receptors for drugs (eg, A1 allele, dopamine D_2 receptor gene), levels of tolerance, and withdrawal as well as our predisposition for reactions to substances. (See Table 35–1.)

Question 5

Consequences of adolescent drug use are vast and include medical, social, economic, and criminal justice costs such as:
A) Underachievement (declines in academics, dropout rates).
B) Delinquency, violence.
C) Unplanned pregnancies and infectious diseases.
D) Depression.
E) All of the above.

Discussion 5

The correct answer is "E." Alcohol and drug use increase the risk of all these factors in adolescents. Addiction develops from the interaction of social, cognitive, cultural, attitudinal, personality, and developmental factors. Temperament, hyperactivity, high novelty seeking, low harm avoidance, and early use of violent behavior are cited risk factors for adolescent drug use.

Question 6

The highest percentages of first-time substance users are between the ages of:
A) 21 and 25 years.
B) 18 and 20 years.
C) 16 and 17 years.
D) 14 and 15 years.
E) 12 and 13 years.

Discussion 6

The correct answer is "C." The age of first use is important because of the implications for ongoing brain development, particularly of the prefrontal cortex. The longer an individual delays the age of first use, the more prefrontal cortex advancement can occur. This part of the brain assesses situations, makes decisions, and modulates our emotions. Introducing drugs into our brains before they are fully developed can cause profound and long-lasting consequences.

Question 7

Once a patient has been identified with a substance use disorder and has been referred for and participated in treatment, it is important to reassess the disease on a frequent basis because addiction has a _____ rate of relapse.
A) 10% to 20%.
B) 30% to 50%.
C) 40% to 60%.
D) 50% to 70%.
E) 60% to 80%.

Discussion 7

The correct answer is "C." As with any other chronic, progressive disease (eg, hypertension, asthma, or diabetes), addiction has aspects of relapse within the disease model. It is important to remember that if an individual relapses following treatment, it does not mean that treatment failed. It may simply mean that the individual needs a higher level of care or return to effective means of coping with the disease. It is important to assess a person's recovery capital (supportive aspects they have around them: recovery community, financial support, access to services, etc) and how improvements can be made to provide adaptive coping. This is a lifelong disease and should be viewed as such.

You are evaluating a 14-year-old boy at a well-child visit. You have some suspicion that he has been using substances. His brother, who is 2 years older, has experimented with marijuana and tobacco, and an older cousin has been in trouble with the law.

Question 8

Which risk factors for use does this example illustrate?
A) Biologic.
B) Neurologic.
C) Environmental.
D) Genetic.
E) All of the above.

Discussion 8

The answer is "C." Home and family represent significant risks factors during childhood and increase the early use of substances. Individuals in the child's environment, such as parents or older family members, who abuse substances or engage in criminal behavior increase the risk for children to develop a substance problem. Additionally, influences such as peers and the school milieu represent other environmental factors. Peer influence—as well as academic failure or poor social skills—has a strong effect on the likelihood that a child will use.

Question 9

If you suspect that your adolescent patient may be struggling with substance use you may screen him or her using which of the following brief questionnaires?
A) CAGE.
B) SASSI-3.
C) CASA.
D) SADQ.
E) CRAFFT.

Discussion 9

The correct answer is "E." The CRAFFT is a behavioral health-screening tool for use with children younger than age 21 and is recommended by the American Academy of Pediatrics' Committee on Substance Abuse. It is printed on a pocket card and can be requested for clinical use. It has been translated into several languages. The screening questions are as follows:

C – Have you ever ridden in a CAR driven by someone (including yourself) who was "high" or had been using alcohol or drugs?

R – Do you ever use alcohol or drugs to RELAX, feel better about yourself, or fit in?

A – Do you ever use alcohol or drugs while you are by yourself, ALONE?

F – Do you ever FORGET things you did while using alcohol or drugs?

F – Do your family or FRIENDS ever tell you that you should cut down on your drinking or drug use?

T – Have you gotten in TROUBLE while you were using alcohol or drugs?

The DSM lists 11 criteria for substance use disorder. (See Table 35–2.)

Question 10

A child who smoked tobacco and drank is 65 times more likely to use _____ than a child who never used. A child who used marijuana is 104 times more likely to use _____ than peers who never used.
A) Marijuana; cocaine.
B) Hallucinogens; alcohol.
C) Nicotine; opiates.
D) Cocaine; stimulants.
E) Opiates; steroids.

Discussion 10

The correct answer is "A." Early use of substances places children on a deadly path. Research suggests that the earlier a substance is used, the greater the effect it can have on its user. In combination with early use, brain development, unstable relationships,

TABLE 35–2 SUMMARY OF *DSM-5* DIAGNOSTIC CRITERIA FOR SUBSTANCE USE DISORDER

1. Escalation of use–taking more of the substance or using it for longer periods of time.
2. Inability to quit or decrease use of the substance.
3. A lot of time is spent using, recovering from or seeking the substance.
4. Repeated attempts to quit or limit use
5. Neglected duties in order to use.
6. Continued use despite negative effects.
7. Giving up other activities to use.
8. Continuing to use despite self-identified hazards of use.
9. Physical or psychological problems related to use or made worse by use.
10. Tolerance to the substance.
11. Withdrawl symptoms occur when not using.

Notes:
Two or three symptoms = mild substance use disorder.
Four or five symptoms = moderate substance use disorder.
Six or more symptoms = severe substance use disorder.
Data from American Psychiatric Association. *Diagnostic and Statistical Manual of Mental Disorders*. 5th ed. Arlington, VA: American Psychiatric Association; 2013.

genetics, and exposure to violence can reinforce maladaptive substance use. Substance abuse is a complex issue with intertwined factors that pose daunting treatment challenges. Early prevention and focus on modifiable factors are good places to start.

Question 11

Physicians can best provide support to their patients, families, local schools, and community through:
A) Education regarding the disease of addiction.
B) Mandating treatment.
C) Frequent communication.
D) Both A and B.
E) Both A and C.

Discussion 11

The correct answer is "E." Although physicians are capable of mandating treatment according to law, they are often the most helpful when they share information with others about the facts of addiction and implications of substance use, and use open, honest communication to provide treatment options, referrals, medication, and encouragement. Educating others that this is a disease and not just a choice is important. It may help those close to the abuser gain understanding into his or her destructive patterns.

Question 12

You recognize symptoms of early adolescent drinking in one of your patients. You know this patient well enough to recognize that he responds better to education rather than fear tactics. As you begin to explain the physiological consequences of alcohol use, you emphasize that it results in damage to which of the following?

A) Brain.
B) Endocrine system.
C) Liver.
D) Growth.
E) All of the above.

Discussion 12

The correct answer is "E." Drinking can harm the liver, bones, heart, endocrine system, and brain, and interfere with growth. The brain is changing during adolescence, and when it is exposed to alcohol the effects can be lasting. Research suggests that adolescents may be less sensitive to some of the unpleasant effects of intoxication and more sensitive to alcohol's harmful effects on the brain. Elevated liver enzymes have been found in adolescents who drink, along with higher gamma glutamyl transpeptidase (GGT) and alanine aminotransferase (ALT). Moreover, young drinkers who also are overweight or obese exhibit elevated levels of serum ALT with even modest amounts of alcohol intake. Youth drinking has also been associated with early puberty, especially among females. Female teens are more sensitive to the consumption and long-term effects of alcohol than males. They also become more cognitively impaired, compared with males. Alcohol is one of the five most significant risk factors for diseases, with more than 60% of alcohol-related diseases being chronic conditions, including cancer, cirrhosis of the liver, diabetes, and cardiovascular disease.

Question 13

Parents report that the following behaviors are occurring in their child. You recognize they are all behavioral consequences of alcohol use EXCEPT:

A) Arguing with friends.
B) Academic problems.
C) Normal eating patterns.
D) Risky sexual behavior.
E) Sleep disruption.

Discussion 13

The correct answer is "C." When an adolescent begins drinking, the following behaviors can suggest difficulties: hangovers, academic problems, difficulties at work, arguing with friends and family, unwanted sexual activity, changes in eating patterns or weight, injuries, and damage to property.

Question 14

Primary care physicians play an important role in supporting recovery of their substance-using patients. They may be the first to assess a patient's substance use or to follow up with the patient during or after treatment by providing medically assisted treatment. If the patient has struggled with tobacco use, the provider may prescribe which of the following to help with cravings or relapse?

A) Buprenorphine.
B) Bupropion.
C) Acamprosate.
D) Naltrexone.
E) Disulfiram.

Discussion 14

The correct answer is "B." Medications used for tobacco addiction include nicotine replacement therapies (patch, inhaler, gum), bupropion, or varenicline. Medications for opioid addiction include methadone, buprenorphine, or naltrexone. Medications for alcohol and drug addiction include naltrexone, disulfiram, or acamprosate. These medications can interfere with triggers for stress and cues linked to substance use (such as people, places, things and moods) and maintain recovery. Be careful to know the best practices for prescribing these medications to patients younger than 18 years of age because some have not been systematically studied or are regulated differently by law.

The father of your 15-year-old male patient expresses concern that his son is using drugs and brought him in today, seeking to have him tested for drug use. You recognize that before ordering any tests, several issues must be addressed.

Question 15

Prior to testing for drugs of abuse, which of the following are important considerations that need to be discussed with the patient and family?

A) False-positive and false-negative test results.
B) Plan of action if the test results come back positive or negative.
C) Specific concerns that prompted the request for drug testing.
D) Consent of the patient.
E) Specimen collection method.
F) All of the above.

Discussion 15

The correct answer is "F." There are many issues related to testing for drugs of abuse that both physician and family should be aware of before the test is performed. This is one reason meeting with a health care professional is recommended over reliance on at-home or school-based testing. The plan of action after obtaining test results should be discussed before testing, including whether referral to a specialist will be made, and how the concerns that prompted the request (including physical, mental health, and behavioral changes) will be further addressed. The adolescent's consent for testing should be obtained. Consent may be waived in special circumstances, such as an emergency (eg, patient with unexplained altered mental status). Referral to a specialist should be performed if the patient declines consent and the provider has suspicion for drug use. False-positive and false-negative testing is very important to discuss prior to testing. The timing of drug use, cross-reactivity between other drugs (see Table 35–3), proper specimen collection, tampering or masking, and the laboratory panels, including the drug or

TABLE 35–3 EXAMPLES OF CROSS-REACTIVE SUBSTANCES IN DRUGS OF ABUSE LABORATORY TESTING

Drug of Abuse	May Cross-React With[a]
Phencyclidine (PCP)	Dextromethorphan
Cocaine	Amoxicillin
Opiates	Fluoroquinolones
Benzodiazepines	Sertraline
Cannabinoids	Ibuprofen, naproxen
Amphetamine	Fluoxetine, bupropion

[a]Substances may cause false-positive drug of abuse test.

metabolite tested for and cutoff values for a positive or negative test, all may affect the validity of the test. It is imperative that the clinician realize that drug testing is an adjunct to management of substance abuse disorders and does not preclude management of substance abuse.

Question 16

In the primary care setting, which of the following is the most common specimen type collected when testing for drugs of abuse?

A) Blood.
B) Breath.
C) Urine.
D) Saliva.
E) Hair.
F) Sweat.

Discussion 16

The correct answer is "C." Each type of specimen has benefits and limitations to its utility. The timing of the use as related to the specimen collection must be considered. For example, hair cannot be used to detect drug or alcohol use within the previous 7 to 10 days, whereas blood may be used to detect a substance used within the previous 12 hours. Obtaining a blood sample is invasive. Obtaining a urine sample is less invasive than blood sampling but is highly susceptible to tampering. Breath, saliva, and sweat testing are susceptible to tampering, and each has its own limitations in regard to timing of drug intake related to collection.

A 12-year-old girl presents with symptoms that include shortness of breath during exercise and a persistent cough. She has taken some over-the-counter (OTC) medicine for respiratory concerns. Because of the sudden onset of symptoms, your initial assessment includes the possibility that she might be using substances.

Question 17

What is considered a gateway drug for youth?

A) Alcohol.
B) Marijuana.
C) Stimulants.
D) Tobacco.
E) None of the above.

Discussion 17

The correct answer is "D." Tobacco use, specifically smoking, is the leading cause of preventable disease and mortality in the United States. The onset of tobacco use is usually during adolescence and thus should be a focus of identification and prevention. Longitudinal research suggests that there have been declines in lifetime tobacco use in youth, due to strong cohort effects and a decrease in supportive attitudes toward smoking. Information from self-reports suggests that smoking is a less attractive quality in a romantic partner than in previous survey years. It is surmised that external variables such as health campaigns, adverse publicity, and increases in federal tobacco taxes also make it less attractive for youth to purchase and use the substance. In some instances, as here, peer pressure can have positive effects, too.

> **Helpful Tip**
> Epidemiologic studies have shown that nicotine use is a gateway to the use of marijuana and cocaine.

Question 18

True or False: Campaigns for e-cigarettes target advertisements to youth smokers, in addition to current smokers as a means for smoking cessation.

A) True.
B) False.

Discussion 18

The correct answer is "A." Although many e-cigarette campaigns suggest that this form of smoking can help an individual with cessation effort, or provide a more polite way to smoke in public, the tobacco industry continues to spend a large portion of its marketing budget targeting young smokers. Many early tobacco campaigns included cartoon animals (eg, Camel) to entice young individuals to try their product, or used flavors to decrease the harsh smell and taste of tobacco. E-cigarettes are also following this trend with flavored cartridges, such as bubble gum, and starter packs that are being sold in kiosks at shopping malls. The health risks of long-term use of e-cigarettes are not yet known, and they can be used to smoke illicit drugs.

Question 19

Which of the following remains the leading cause of preventable disease and death in the United States?

A) Drunk driving.
B) Alcohol poisoning.
C) Cigarette smoking.
D) Smokeless tobacco.
E) Cocaine use.

Discussion 19

The correct answer is "C." This is a test of whether you are paying attention. Of course the answer is cigarettes—you learned that earlier. There are many reasons for this continued cause of mortality. Nicotine is highly addictive and works to change the mind and mood in an average of 7 seconds (which is similar to heroin). Although studies suggest that lifetime prevalence of cigarette use is on the decline, adolescents continue to make up a large portion of new users. Taxes are one way the government has attempted to decrease the use of tobacco, especially in teens; and health campaigns support education to increase disapproval rates. Because of its fast-acting nature, ability to change the mind and mood, easy access, and affordability, the use of nicotine is often seen in individuals who experience trauma or have mental health conditions.

Question 20

Which of the following is also indicated as a risk factor for early initiation of substance use, especially tobacco?
A) Socioeconomic status.
B) Race or ethnicity.
C) Early puberty.
D) Gender.
E) Living in an urban setting.

Discussion 20

The correct answer is "C." Studies recognize several risk factors that influence an individual's chances of using substances. Early maturation seems to exacerbate a number of factors, such as peer influence, appearance of being older (access to substance), and even within the youth population tobacco has reportedly been used to offset weight gain, especially in young girls. Remember that early substance use has been associated with several negative outcomes, such as early pregnancy and criminal convictions. Each year that an individual can delay the onset of use decreases the likelihood of developing a lifetime substance use disorder.

> **Helpful Tip**
> A longitudinal study in children who were followed over a period 15 years (ages 11 to 26 years) suggested that individuals who struggled with being overweight or obese had the highest likelihood of being regular smokers.

An 11-year-old boy presents to your office for a sports physical. During the review of symptoms and last year's history, his parents report a concern about changes in his behavior and a slight drop in his grades. He has started hanging out with different friends on the weekends and is being slightly secretive about belongings, such as his backpack.

Question 21

What substance is the most widely used by youth?
A) Tobacco.
B) Alcohol.
C) Marijuana.
D) Stimulants.
E) Synthetic marijuana.

Discussion 21

The correct answer is "B." Alcohol remains the most widely used substance by youth. Although declines in use have been reported over the years, consumption remains high, with approximately 3 in 10 children having consumed alcohol by the end of eight grade, and 7 in 10 students (68%) having consumed alcohol by the end of high school. Half of these individuals reporting being drunk at least once.

> **Helpful Tip**
> A longitudinal study suggested that heavy episodic binge drinking predicted the potential for driving while intoxicated (DWI) and riding with impaired drivers. The study concluded that parental monitoring, especially by fathers over mothers, was a protective factor against DWI.

Question 22

Marijuana can be taken in what forms?
A) Orally.
B) Mixed with food.
C) Smoked.
D) As hash oil in e-cigarettes.
E) All of the above.

Discussion 22

The correct answer is "E." Recreational use in the United States continues to be defined by smoking cannabis in rolled cigarettes ("joints"), in pipes or water pipes, or hollowed out cigarettes ("blunts"). With the recent advent and commercialization of e-cigarettes, hashish oil can also be smoked or "vaped" using these devices. Individuals can also engage in "dabbing," which is the consumption of a more concentrated version of cannabis that is placed on a heated surface and then inhaled as vapors. Increases in illicit drug use usually fluctuates due to the changing beliefs and use of cannabis. The recent legalization of recreational marijuana use in the states of Colorado and Washington (2014), serves to illustrate the changing beliefs of the overall population regarding this mind- and mood-altering substance. The longitudinal studies reveal that the perceived risk associated with marijuana use, as well as its disapproval rating, continues to decline in youth surveys, suggesting changing beliefs regarding its negative consequences. A recent study surveyed youth's attitudes about the legalization of cannabis; it reported that 10% of non–cannabis-using students reported intent to initiate use if legal. Additionally, 18% of lifetime users reported intent to use more often if marijuana was legal. Legalization appears to place an already high-risk group (males, white, cigarette smokers) at increased risk for continued use, and to position low-risk groups (noncigarette smokers, religious individuals, with friends who disapprove) as a new group of users. Interestingly, the odds of using are reduced when friends disapprove.

Question 23

How many 12th graders say they can get marijuana fairly easily or very easily if they want?
A) 81% to 90%.
B) 75% to 82%.
C) 50% to 60%.
D) 65% to 75%.
E) 85% to 90%.

Discussion 23

The correct answer is "A." Marijuana is believed to be a readily accessible substance for youth. Research suggests that as far back as 1975, 81% to 90% of 12th graders each year said that they could get marijuana fairly or very easily if they wanted it. There are also synthetic versions of the drug, originally sold over the counter as Spice and K2. Synthetic cannabis was advertised as a herbal material that has been sprayed with one or more synthesized chemicals that fall in the cannabinoid family. In March 2011, the Drug Enforcement Agency (DEA) made this substance illegal. In 2013, youth statistics suggested that synthetic marijuana was the second most widely used illicit drug after marijuana among 12th graders. For 8th graders, it was the third, behind marijuana and inhalants.

Question 24

Numerous physiologic consequences are associated with cannabis use. They include short-term and long-term effects. Which is not a short-term effect of cannabis use?
A) Altered senses.
B) Decreased heart rate.
C) Impaired body movement.
D) Difficulty with thinking and problem solving.
E) Changes in mood.

Discussion 24

The correct answer is "B." The highest density of cannabinoid receptors is found in parts of the brain that influence pleasure, memory, thinking, concentration, sensory and time perception, and coordinated movement. Marijuana overactivates the endocannabinoid system, causing the "high" and other effects that users experience. These effects include altered perceptions and mood, altered sense of time, impaired coordination, difficulty with thinking and problem solving, and disrupted learning and memory. Reported physical effects include breathing problems (daily coughing, phlegm, and higher risks of lung infections), increased heart rate (raising heart rate for up to 3 hours after smoking, increased change of heart attack), and problems with child development during and after pregnancy (brain and behavioral problems in infants; and problems with attention, memory, and problem solving in children). Additionally, research suggests that a loss of mental stability is one significant side effect from recreational use. Temporary hallucinations and paranoia have been reported, as well as strong links between cannabis use and later development of and vulnerability to psychosis. Long-term use is associated with physiological consequences that include impaired memory and loss of an average of eight IQ points.

Question 25

You are trying to identify some common behavioral consequences of cannabis use and come across a list in a scientific journal. All of the following sequelae are listed EXCEPT:
A) Increased tardiness.
B) Delayed development of social skills.
C) Decreased academic performance.
D) Improved ability to shift attention.
E) Increased accidents.

Discussion 25

The correct answer is "D." Cannabis compromises the ability to learn and remember information, thus affecting the ability to perform at work, home, and in social settings. Individuals fall behind in acquiring social skills, job training, and intelligence. Students are likely to attain lower grades and are less likely to graduate. They struggled with attention, memory, and learning. Cannabis users are more likely to have problems on the job, increased absences, tardiness, accidents, and to spend time on personal matters or daydreaming rather than on academics or work.

Question 26

When an illicit drug first appears, its alleged benefits and consequences are not fully known. This period of time is called:
A) Generational forgetting.
B) Grace period.
C) Trending.
D) Legalization.
E) Popularization.

Discussion 26

The correct answer is "B." The benefits of using a drug spread much faster than its adverse consequences, giving it a "grace period" before individuals receive an informed message about its benefits and dangers. Broadcasting of alleged benefits requires only a couple testimonials or rumors, usually spread by word of mouth, social media, or the Internet, whereas the adverse consequences (overdose, deaths, disease, and addiction) take much longer to disseminate. The positives of drug use, or euphoric recall, persist among that generation of users until they are matched with enough negative outcomes or "war stories." When the negatives begin to outweigh the benefits, use begins to decline (as seen recently with bath salts). What is unfortunate is that out-of-favor drugs often make a comeback once enough people in a particular age group have not been directly affected by the negative consequences of use, or during periods when public campaigns are targeting other substances. This leads to "generational forgetting," in which an older drug is rediscovered by a younger generation. For example, LSD and methamphetamine made a comeback in the 1990s, after decreased use in the 1960s. Currently, heroin use is spiking, after a period of decline.

Your 14-year-old patient suffered a compound fracture in his right arm approximately 8 weeks ago when he fell while hiking. It was treated appropriately with reduction and immobilization. He continues to report intense pain, and you have ruled out pathology related to the injury. He requests additional opiates for his symptoms. You have some concern that he might be misusing the prescription. You begin to investigate signs of possible misuse of the drug.

Question 27

Which of the following is NOT typical of the opiate toxidrome?

A) Lacrimation.
B) Respiratory depression.
C) Central nervous system depression.
D) Pinpoint pupils.
E) Bradycardia.

Discussion 27

The correct answer is "A." When deciphering whether or not someone could be suffering from opioid intoxication, it is helpful to think of opioids as "something that slows things down." In addition to those listed above, symptoms may include hypotension, muscle flaccidity, and hypothermia. Lacrimation would be viewed as an increase in tear production, not a decrease.

Question 28

What is the antidote to opioids?

A) Physostigmine.
B) 2-PAM.
C) Naloxone.
D) Atropine.
E) N-acetylcysteine.

Discussion 28

The correct answer is "C." Atropine and pralidoxime (2-PAM) are used in organophosphate poisoning. N-acetylcysteine is used in acetaminophen toxicity. Physostigmine is sometimes used with benzodiazepines as the treatment for anticholinergic toxicity.

Question 29

If ingested, which of the following is associated with the opiate toxidrome?

A) Methadone.
B) Heroin.
C) Dextromethorphan.
D) All of the above.

Discussion 29

The correct answer is "D." Methadone is a prescription opiate medication. Heroin, an illicit drug, is a synthetic opiate. Dextromethorphan is structurally related to a synthetic opioid agonist and may cause symptoms of opiate ingestion, depending on the amount ingested.

During your shift in the emergency department, you are evaluating a 17-year-old boy with acute psychosis that developed while attending a party. In addition to hypertension and tachycardia, you note rotary nystagmus on examination of his eyes.

Question 30

Which of the following hallucinogens do you suspect the patient ingested?

A) Lysergic acid diethylamide (LSD).
B) Phencyclidine (PCP).
C) Mescaline.
D) Dextromethorphan.

Discussion 30

The correct answer is "B." All options are hallucinogens—substances that alter how a person feels, thinks, or senses. In addition to the effects of the other hallucinogens listed (which include tachycardia, hypertension, hyperthermia, acute psychosis, and hallucinations), PCP is known to cause vertical or rotary nystagmus. Repetitive hallucinogen abuse is related to the euphoric effects provided, as most hallucinogens do not cause physiologic addiction.

Question 31

Which of the following is contraindicated in management of patients under the influence of hallucinogens?

A) Administration of benzodiazepines.
B) Placing the patient in a low stimulation environment.
C) Placing the patient in physical restraints.
D) Administration of intravenous normal saline.
E) Administration of antihypertensive medications.

Discussion 31

The correct answer is "C." Physical restraints may increase agitation. The hypertension, hyperthermia, and tachycardia are secondary to the agitation. Calming the patient with a low stimulation environment and pharmaceutically with benzodiazepines are often enough to control these symptoms. In extreme cases of hyperthermia and hypertension, cooling measures such as use of intravenous fluids and antihypertensive medications may be necessary.

Question 32

Typical users of hallucinogens fit the following profile:

A) Young; male; employed.
B) Young; female; legal problems.
C) Young; male; unemployed.
D) Young; male; legal problems; unemployed
E) Young; female; unemployed; legal problems.

Discussion 32

The correct answer is "D." The twenty-first century synthetic drugs (eg, bath salts) are finding company with previous generations of hallucinogens, thanks in part to "generational forgetting." When a generation becomes numb to the effects of a drug, lacking exposure to education and prevention campaigns, as well as decreased peer pressure, it is common for a class of drugs to make a resurgence. The typical users of these substances are young and male, with similar education levels, unemployment, and legal problems, while differing in ethnicity and race identity.

You are evaluating another 17-year-old boy who presents to the emergency department with agitation and hallucinations, which developed while he was attending a party. His friend states that your patient also had a nosebleed earlier in the night. You astutely suspect cocaine intoxication, a sympathomimetic toxidrome, as the cause of his symptoms.

Question 33

Which of the following is NOT consistent with a sympathomimetic toxidrome?

A) Tachycardia.
B) Dry skin.
C) Muscular rigidity.
D) Mydriasis.

Discussion 33

The correct answer is "B." Hallmarks of the sympathomimetic toxidrome include agitation, hyperthermia, tachycardia, hypertension, mydriasis (dilated pupils), and diaphoresis. Distinguishing sympathomimetic from anticholinergic toxidromes (eg, diphenhydramine ingestion) is often difficult due to overlapping features, including tachycardia and pupillary dilation.

> **Helpful Tip**
> Intoxication with either sympathomimetics or anticholinergics causes tachycardia, hyperthermia, mydriasis (dilated pupils), and hallucinations, but:
>
> Sympathomimetic = diaphoresis (wet skin) and hyperactive bowel sounds.
>
> Anticholinergic = dry skin ("dry as a bone") and hypoactive bowel sounds.

You now know that your patient has ingested cocaine. Snorting cocaine is associated with nosebleeds and, with chronic use, nasal septum perforation due to its vasoconstrictive effects. He is now complaining of chest pain, and you order an electrocardiogram (ECG) to evaluate the cardiac rhythm and look for ischemic changes, as dysrhythmias and ischemia are associated with cocaine-related chest pain.

Question 34

Which of the following medications is contraindicated in patients who have ingested cocaine?

A) Beta-blockers.
B) Aspirin.
C) Benzodiazepines.
D) Nitroglycerin.
E) Sodium bicarbonate.

Discussion 34

The correct answer is "A." Beta-blockers should be avoided in patients who have ingested cocaine due to concern of unopposed alpha-receptor stimulation. Aspirin and nitroglycerin

are safe for use. Along with supportive cares, benzodiazepines may be utilized for sedation, hyperthermia, tachycardia, seizures, and muscular rigidity. Sodium bicarbonate is the treatment for wide-complex dysrhythmias associated with cocaine intoxication.

> **Helpful Tip**
> A binge pattern of cocaine use is more commonly associated with smoking and injecting due to faster absorption and shorter duration of action with these routes than with intranasal use.

A 13-year-old girl presents to the emergency department seizing. Her parents found an empty bottle of methylphenidate next to her.

Question 35

Which medication is the best choice for treatment of her seizure?

A) Lorazepam.
B) Phenytoin.
C) Haloperidol.
D) Phenobarbital.
E) Options A and B are equally efficacious.

Discussion 35

The correct answer is "A." Benzodiazepines are the treatment of choice for amphetamine-induced seizures. Other anticonvulsant medications, including phenytoin and phenobarbital, are generally not indicated for toxicologic-induced seizures. Amphetamines may be used medically, for example, in treatment of narcolepsy and attention deficit hyperactivity disorder (ADHD), as in this case. These prescription medications are sometimes used for recreational purposes, as amphetamines increase norepinephrine and dopamine release, causing a feeling of pleasure, self-confidence, and well-being.

Question 36

MDMA (also known as ecstasy or Molly) is an amphetamine that is used recreationally. If a patient who is known to have used MDMA presents seizing, what electrolyte abnormality is most likely to be present?

A) Hypokalemia.
B) Hyperkalemia.
C) Hypernatremia.
D) Hyponatremia.

Discussion 36

The correct answer is "D." Similar to cocaine, amphetamines cause tachycardia, hypertension, hyperthermia, and diaphoresis. In addition, MDMA is associated with hyponatremia due to increased release of vasopressin (antidiuretic hormone). MDMA is known for being used recreationally at dance parties or "raves." Isotonic fluid loss due to sweating while dancing and fluid replacement with oral free water compound the risk for hyponatremia.

Methamphetamine (meth, crank, ice) can be used orally, intravenously, or inhaled. The symptoms and medical treatment of amphetamine ingestion are similar to those for cocaine. Supportive care includes cooling if needed and intravenous hydration, and benzodiazepines are the mainstay of treatment.

You are the treating physician on call when a group of intoxicated adolescents are brought into the emergency department. The teens have all been at a party together and give you conflicting reports about the substances available there. A friend who arrives with them reports it was a "pharm" party. You quickly review the classes of over-the-counter medication and prescriptions and notice the symptoms observed best fit with stimulant intoxication.

Question 37

Symptoms of intoxication following stimulant use include:

A) Inappropriate aggressive behavior, mood lability, slurred speech, nystagmus, and stupor.
B) Drowsiness, slurred speech, impaired attention, psychomotor agitation, and pupillary constriction.
C) Dizziness, incoordination, unsteady gait, depressed reflexes, general muscle weakness, and belligerence.
D) Affective blunting, changes in sociability, hypervigilance, interpersonal sensitivity, chills, and pupillary dilation.

Discussion 37

The correct answer is "D." The symptoms listed in option "A" suggest sedative, hypnotic, and anxiolytic intoxication such as occurs with benzodiazepines. Option "B" suggests opioid intoxication. Option "C" suggests inhalant intoxication. After marijuana, prescription medications are the most common drugs abused by adolescents. In contrast to several previously described drugs, stimulants are often used to help teens study. Adolescents misuse stimulants prescribed to themselves or to others, such as Adderall (amphetamine and dextroamphetamine), as performance enhancers. Casually referred to as the "midterm drug," stimulants are used in both academic and sports settings to increase a person's competitive edge. Individuals exposed to stimulants or amphetamine-type stimulants can develop disordered use as rapidly as 1 week later. Studies suggest that approximately 1 in every 6 high school seniors has had exposure to prescription stimulants, for medical or nonmedical reasons. Researchers went on to clarify that 59.3% of high school seniors had used prescription stimulants for medical reasons only, 22.9% reported medical use followed by nonmedical use, and 17.8% reported nonmedical use before medical use.

A 12-year-old boy is brought to the emergency department by emergency medical services (EMS) after his parents found him in his room with altered mental status. His parents report he seemed normal at dinner 20 minutes before they found him in his room. EMS reports he was lethargic with a pulse of 40 beats per minute. In the emergency department, you are evaluating him 30 minutes after EMS arrived on scene. He is now acting normally and has normal vital signs.

Question 38

What is the most likely cause of this patient's presentation?

A) LSD ingestion.
B) Hydrocarbon inhalation.
C) Concussion.
D) Calcium channel blocker overdose.
E) Beta-blocker overdose.

Discussion 38

The correct answer is "B." Hydrocarbons are a type of inhaled substance used for their euphoric effects. Inhalants are gases or fumes that can be inhaled for the purpose of getting high. Most are found as inexpensive household items and can be purchased and possessed legally by youth (glue, nail polish remover, gasoline, solvents, etc). Sometimes referred to as "kids drugs," this class of drugs differs from other drugs of abuse because it is most commonly used by younger adolescents, and then use declines as they age. The risk associated with use was well communicated in the mid-1990s by Partnership for a Drug-Free America, which educated youth and improved the accurate perception of risk. Currently, over 80% of adolescents would disapprove of using inhalants. Inhalants have a rapid onset and their effects usually last no more than 30 minutes. The euphoric effect may be followed by depressive symptoms, including bradycardia and lethargy, followed by return to baseline. Management is supportive, including exposure to fresh air. Prolonged symptoms suggest an alternate etiology. Long-term use of inhalants is associated with fatal dysrhythmias, sometimes termed "sudden sniffing death," due to increased sensitivity of the heart to catecholamines.

> **Helpful Tip**
> Glue sniffer's rash is a perioral dermatitis caused by the drying effects of inhalants.

Question 39

Which of the following is ingested for its euphoric effect and is found in many over-the-counter cough and cold medications?

A) Salicylic acid.
B) Red dye #40.
C) Dextromethorphan.
D) Guaifenesin.

Discussion 39

The correct answer is "C." Dextromethorphan is ingested recreationally for its euphoric effect, and is dose dependent. At lower doses, a stimulant effect may be noted, while at higher doses its effects are similar to phencyclidine (PCP), including hallucination and dissociation. Salicylic acid ingestion can lead to salicylic intoxication, in which clinically the patient will have metabolic acidosis and compensatory respiratory alkalosis. Red dye #40 is a coloring agent. Guaifenesin is an expectorant found in many dextromethorphan-containing medications, its side effects include nausea and vomiting.

BIBLIOGRAPHY

American Psychiatric Association. *Diagnostic and Statistical Manual of Mental Disorders.* 5th ed. Arlington, VA: American Psychiatric Association; 2013.

Blok BK, Cheung DS, Platts-Mills TF. *First Aid for the Emergency Medicine Boards.* New York, NY: McGraw-Hill; 2009.

Johnston LD, O'Malley PM, Miech RA, Bachman JG, Schulenberg JE. *Monitoring the Future National Survey Results on Drug Use: 1975–2013: Overview Key Findings on Adolescent Drug Use.* Ann Arbor, MI: Institute for Social Research, University of Michigan; 2014.

Kandel ER, Kandel DB. A molecular basis for nicotine as a gateway drug. *New Engl J Med.* 2014;371:932–943.

Lanza HI, Grella CE, Chung PJ. Does adolescent weight status predict problematic substance use patterns? *Am J Health Behav.* 2014;38(5):708–716.

Lee JS, McCarty CA, Ahrens K, King KM, Stoep AV, McCauley EA. Pubertal timing and adolescent substance initiation. *J Social Work Pract Addict.* 2014;14(3):286–307.

Levy S, Siqueira LM, Committee on Substance Abuse. Testing for drugs of abuse in children and adolescents. *Pediatrics.* 2014;133(6):1798–1807.

Li K, Simons-Morton BG, Brooks-Russell A, Ehsani J, Hingson R. Drinking and parenting practices as predictors of impaired driving behaviors among US adolescents. *J Stud Alcohol Drugs.* 2014;75(1):5–15.

Maxwell JC. Psychoactive substances—some new, some old: A scan of the situation in the US. *Drug Alcohol Depend.* 2014;134:71–77.

McCabe SE, West BT. Medical and nonmedical use of prescription stimulants: Results from a national multi-cohort study. *J Am Acad Child Adolesc Psychiatry.* 2013;52(12):1272–1280.

Meier MH, Caspi A, Ambler A, et al. Persistent cannabis users show neuropsychological decline from childhood to midlife. *Proc Natl Acad Sci.* 2012;109(40):E2657–E2664.

National Institute on Drug Abuse. How science has revolutionized the understanding of drug addiction. In: *Drugs, Brains and Behavior: The Science of Addiction.* NIH Pub No. 14-5605. Bethesda, MD: National Institutes of Health; 2014 (original publication 2007).

National Institute on Drug Abuse. Is there a link between marijuana use and mental illness? *Research Report Series.* NIH Pub No. 15-3859. Bethesda, MD: National Institutes of Health; 2012.

Palamar JJ, Ompad DC, Petkova E. Correlates of intentions to use cannabis among US high school seniors in the case of cannabis legalization: *Int J Drug Policy.* 2014;25(3):424–435.

Final Exam

Answer key is on page 807. Discussion of the concept being tested can be found on the page number listed in bold text after each question.

1. A teenage boy asks how tall he can expect to be as a full-grown adult. His mother is 160 cm tall and his father is 180 cm tall. He is healthy and has had normal growth and development. His full-grown brother is 182 cm tall. You tell him that his approximate expected adult height is: **(1)**

   A) 180 cm
   B) 160 cm
   C) 182 cm
   D) 176.5 cm
   E) 163.5 cm

2. Which of the following is the most effective method of preventing unwanted pregnancy? **(15)**

   A) Rhythm method
   B) Male condom
   C) Female condom
   D) Implantable etonogestrel rod
   E) Oral contraceptive pills

3. Which of the following is a characteristic of middle adolescence? **(20)**

   A) Appearance of acne and body odor
   B) Mainly interested in same-sex relationships
   C) Desires privacy from parents
   D) Physically mature
   E) Becomes less influenced by peers

4. Which of the following is true of a typical adolescent girl's first few menstrual cycles? **(21)**

   A) Anovulation is rare
   B) Age of first menses is usually around 10 years in healthy well-nourished Americans

C) Typically precedes thelarche by 1 to 2 years
D) Occurs at regular 30-day intervals
E) Typical menstrual product use is 3 to 6 pads or tampons per day

5. Which of the following is more characteristic of T-cell immunodeficiencies than of other types of immunodeficiencies? **(25–27)**

   A) Vaccines tend not to produce an immune response
   B) Live virus vaccines may lead to active infection in the patient
   C) Skin abscesses are common
   D) Overwhelming infections occur with common bacterial pathogens
   E) Oral corticosteroids can provide effective treatment

6. Which of the following is a characteristic of mild persistent asthma? **(39)**

   A) Has symptoms that wake from sleep 3 to 4 times per month
   B) Requires a short-acting beta-agonist daily for symptom control
   C) FEV_1 is less than 80% of predicted
   D) Never requires systemic corticosteroids for symptom control
   E) Has daytime symptoms less than 2 days per week.

7. Which of the following is appropriate treatment for an adolescent with intermittent asthma? **(41)**

   A) Short-acting beta-agonists as needed
   B) Low-dose inhaled corticosteroids
   C) Medium-dose inhaled corticosteroids
   D) Inhaled corticosteroids plus long-acting beta-agonist
   E) Inhaled corticosteroids plus leukotriene receptor antagonist

8. Which of the following is the most effective long-term controller medication for young children with asthma? **(42)**

    A) Short-acting beta-agonists
    B) Long-acting beta-agonists
    C) Inhaled corticosteroids
    D) Leukotriene receptor antagonists
    E) Mast cell stabilizers

9. Which of the following is the most common cause of food allergy in childhood? **(45)**

    A) Soy
    B) Wheat
    C) Shellfish
    D) Peanut
    E) Milk

10. Which of the following is NOT a marker of toilet training readiness? **(52–53)**

    A) Has sibling who was toilet trained at the same age
    B) Can walk to the toilet
    C) Can follow simple commands
    D) Wants to please caregivers
    E) Seems distressed or bothered by dirty diapers

11. Which is NOT an appropriate intervention for managing a tantrum? **(54)**

    A) Ignore the behavior until the child stops
    B) Time-out
    C) Place the child in a safe area to prevent injury
    D) Immediately give in to the child's demand so the tantrum does not escalate
    E) Offer to help the child after he or she calms down

12. Which of the following is a characteristic of good sleep hygiene? **(58)**

    A) Go to bed when tired
    B) No naps during the day
    C) No electronic devices or gadgets in the bedroom
    D) Start planning for the child's bedtime when the parents become tired
    E) Set out pajamas in the morning so they will be ready for the child at bedtime

13. Which of the following is true about excessive infant crying (colic)? **(59)**

    A) Typically starts around 2 weeks of age
    B) Typically resolves by 12 to 16 weeks of age
    C) Is defined by crying more than 3 hours per day, more than 3 days per week, and more than 3 weeks in duration
    D) Is equally common in breastfed and formula-fed babies
    E) All of the above

14. Which of the following is NOT an anxiety disorder? **(64)**

    A) Social phobia
    B) Obsessive compulsive disorder
    C) Specific phobia
    D) Panic disorder
    E) Separation anxiety disorder

15. Which of the following laboratory values is consistent with iron deficiency anemia? **(73)**

    A) Elevated hemoglobin
    B) Low mean corpuscular volume
    C) Elevated ferritin
    D) Elevated haptoglobin
    E) Absent reticulocytes

16. Which of the following is associated with painless hematuria? **(75–76)**

    A) Wilms tumor
    B) Pyelonephritis
    C) Nephrocalcinosis
    D) Rhabdomyolysis
    E) Urethral stricture

17. Which of the following is an appropriate first-line treatment for immune thrombocytopenia (ITP)? **(77)**

    A) Observation
    B) Intravenous immunoglobulin (IVIG)
    C) Anti-D immune globulin
    D) Systemic corticosteroids
    E) All of the above

18. Which of the following laboratory findings is common in acute tumor lysis syndrome? **(91)**

    A) Hyperkalemia
    B) Hypophosphatemia
    C) Hypercalcemia
    D) Hypouricemia
    E) Hypernatremia

19. Which of the following is true regarding the treatment of sickle cell disease? **(102)**

    A) Penicillin prophylaxis should be started at birth
    B) Once the spleen involutes, patients with sickle cell disease are at increased risk for infections with viruses
    C) Treatment with hydroxyurea decreases risk of ischemic stroke by increasing the production of fetal hemoglobin (HbF)
    D) Siblings of the affected child have at least a 75% chance of being affected as well
    E) The standard 13-valent pneumococcal vaccine (PCV-13) should be given before age 1

20. Which of the following cardiac conditions will cause a holosystolic murmur? **(112, 114)**

    A) Atrial septal defect
    B) Ventricular septal defect
    C) Hypertrophic cardiomyopathy
    D) Patent ductus arteriosus
    E) All of the above

21. Which of the following arrhythmias will present with the fastest ventricular rate? **(122, 125)**

    A) Atrial fibrillation
    B) Supraventricular tachycardia
    C) Sinus tachycardia
    D) Third-degree heart block
    E) Pulseless electrical activity

22. Which of the following heart conditions is associated with Turner syndrome? **(127)**

    A) Coarctation of the aorta
    B) Dilated aorta
    C) Bicuspid aortic valve
    D) Partial anomalous pulmonary venous return
    E) All of the above

23. Which of the following is true about tetralogy of Fallot? **(127–128)**

    A) The murmur is due to the large ventricular septal defect (VSD)
    B) The murmur is due to pulmonary stenosis
    C) Oxygen therapy can reverse the left-to-right shut across the VSD during a "Tet" spell
    D) Ketamine may improve oxygenation by decreasing systemic vascular resistance during a "Tet" spell
    E) The condition is autosomal dominant

24. When evaluating a newborn with persistent cyanosis, which of the following conditions is UNLIKELY to be the cause? **(129)**

    A) Truncus arteriosus
    B) Transposition of the great arteries (DTGA)
    C) Tricuspid atresia
    D) Ebstein anomaly
    E) Peripheral pulmonary stenosis

25. Which of the following is an early symptom of autism spectrum disorders? **(133)**

    A) Attachment disorder
    B) Failure to roll over by 6 months of age
    C) Limited babbling
    D) Excessive imaginary play
    E) Higher activity level

26. Initial screening for autism spectrum disorders should occur at what age? **(134)**

    A) < 6 months
    B) 6–12 months
    C) 12–18 months
    D) 18–24 months
    E) 24–30 months

27. Which receptive language skill is matched with the correct age of normal acquisition? **(137)**

    A) Alerts or quiets to sound—birth
    B) Responds to own name—12 months
    C) Stops when told "no"—18 months
    D) Follows simple commands—24 months
    E) Answers simple questions—4 years

28. Which expressive language skill is NOT matched with the correct age of normal acquisition? **(138)**

    A) Cooing—2 months
    B) Babbling—6 months
    C) Pointing—6 months
    D) Two-word phrases—18 months
    E) Able to tell or retell a familiar story—36 months

29. Which of the following is NOT required by law? **(144–146)**

    A) An individual education plan (IEP) for a student with dyslexia
    B) Continuing academic modifications for a student with a 504 plan who will attend college
    C) Braille education for a blind child
    D) Wheelchair access at a public elementary school
    E) An IEP for a student with a concussion who is unable to complete classwork now but is expected to make a full recovery

30. Which of the following is NOT a common laboratory finding in systemic lupus erythematosus (SLE)? **(152)**

    A) Leukocytosis
    B) Lymphopenia
    C) Anemia
    D) Decreased C3 and C4 complement levels
    E) Hematuria

31. Which of the following is NOT a major manifestation of acute rheumatic fever? **(153)**

    A) Polyarthritis
    B) Erythema migrans
    C) Chorea
    D) Carditis
    E) Subcutaneous nodules

32. Which of the following is a late manifestation of Henoch-Schönlein purpura? **(154)**

    A) End-stage kidney disease
    B) Chronic abdominal pain
    C) Scarring of the skin on the buttocks and lower extremities
    D) Chronic headaches
    E) Chronic arthritis

33. Which of the following accurately describes systemic onset juvenile idiopathic arthritis (JIA)? **(157)**

    A) Gradual onset
    B) Girls affected more than boys
    C) Diffuse lymphadenopathy
    D) More than four joints involved
    E) HLA-B27 positive

34. Which of the following is NOT seen in juvenile dermatomyositis (JDM)? **(159)**

    A) Gottron papules
    B) Periungual telangiectases
    C) Distal muscle weakness
    D) Heliotrope rash
    E) Photosensitivity

35. What is the appropriate size of cuffed endotracheal tube for a 4-year-old? **(168)**

    A) 2.0
    B) 3.0
    C) 4.0
    D) 5.0
    E) 6.0

36. Which of the following substances can cause hepatic failure in overdose? **(168)**

    A) Acetaminophen
    B) Ibuprofen
    C) Phenylephrine
    D) Diphenhydramine
    E) All of the above

37. What is the most appropriate place to check for a pulse in an infant who has become unresponsive? **(169)**

    A) Carotid artery
    B) Chest wall (point of maximal impulse)
    C) Brachial artery
    D) Radial artery
    E) Femoral artery

38. What is the appropriate first treatment for a patient with ventricular tachycardia with a pulse and poor perfusion? **(170)**

    A) Adenosine 0.1 mg/kg IV
    B) Synchronized cardioversion at 0.5 J/kg

    C) Nonsynchronized defibrillation at 2 J/kg
    D) Epinephrine 0.01 mg/kg IV
    E) Application of ice to the face

39. What is the most common bacterial cause of acute otitis media? **(180)**

    A) *Streptococcus pneumoniae*
    B) Nontypeable *Haemophilus influenzae*
    C) *Moraxella catarrhalis*
    D) *Staphylococcus aureus*
    E) *Pseudomonas aeruginosa*

40. Which is NOT a complication of acute bacterial sinusitis? **(188)**

    A) Subdural abscess
    B) Cavernous sinus thrombosis
    C) Meningitis
    D) Orbital cellulitis
    E) Tonsillitis

41. What is the most common complication of a tonsillectomy and adenoidectomy? **(191)**

    A) Aspiration pneumonia
    B) Bleeding
    C) Dental trauma
    D) Dehydration
    E) Velopharyngeal insufficiency

42. What is the most common midline neck mass in children? **(196)**

    A) Cystic hygroma
    B) Brachial cleft cyst
    C) Thyroglossal duct cyst
    D) Lymphoma
    E) Thyroid nodule

43. Which of the following detects sensorineural hearing loss? **(197–198)**

    A) Evoked otoacoustic emissions
    B) Tympanometry
    C) Pneumatic otoscopy
    D) Automated brainstem response
    E) Magnetic resonance imaging

44. Which is NOT a part of the evaluation of a febrile neonate? **(204)**

    A) Blood culture
    B) Urine culture
    C) Sputum culture
    D) Cerebrospinal fluid culture
    E) Chest X-ray (if respiratory symptoms present)

45. Tetanus immunization is indicated in all of the following EXCEPT: **(206)**

    A) Patient with simple, clean wound and unknown vaccination history
    B) Patient with contaminated wound and unknown vaccination history
    C) Patient with a simple, clean wound who has received < 3 doses of the tetanus vaccine
    D) Patient with a simple, clean wound who has received ≥ 3 doses of the tetanus, vaccine with the last dose received 5 years earlier
    E) Patient with a contaminated wound who has received ≥ 3 doses of the tetanus vaccine, with the last dose received 6 years earlier

46. Which is NOT a sign of a pediatric skull fracture? **(211)**

    A) Scalp hematoma
    B) Posttraumatic clear rhinorrhea
    C) Bruising behind the ear
    D) Palpable step-off or crepitus
    E) Forehead contusion

47. Which is a late sign of compartment syndrome complicating a tibia fracture? **(218)**

    A) Pulselessness
    B) Pain
    C) Pallor
    D) Paresthesia
    E) Poikilothermia

48. In classic congenital adrenal hyperplasia due to 21-hydroxlyase deficiency, which of the following adrenal steroids is NOT elevated? **(219–221)**

    A) Androstenedione
    B) Aldosterone
    C) Testosterone
    D) 17-Hydroxyprogesterone
    E) Dehydroepiandrosterone

49. Which is NOT a cause of tall stature in childhood? **(226)**

    A) Hypothyroidism
    B) Overnutrition
    C) Growth hormone excess
    D) Precious puberty
    E) Familial tall stature

50. Which is an example of precious puberty? **(226–228)**

    A) 8-year-old girl with breast buds
    B) 11-year-old boy with pubic hair
    C) 12-year-old girl with menarche
    D) 7-year-old girl with breast buds
    E) 9-year-old boy with testicle enlargement

51. Which laboratory value is NOT characteristic of Graves disease? **(231)**

    A) Low thyroid-stimulating hormone (TSH)
    B) Elevated free T_4
    C) Elevated T_3
    D) Elevated thyroid peroxidase antibodies
    E) Elevated thyroid-simulating immunoglobulins

52. Which laboratory value is NOT characteristic of acquired primary adrenal insufficiency (Addison disease)? **(232)**

    A) Hyponatremia
    B) Elevated adrenocorticotropic hormone (ACTH)
    C) Hypokalemia
    D) Low cortisol
    E) Hypoglycemia

53. Which hormone is NOT made by the anterior pituitary gland? **(234)**

    A) Adrenocorticotropic hormone (ACTH)
    B) Antidiuretic hormone (ADH)
    C) Thyroid-stimulating hormone (TSH)
    D) Growth hormone (GH)
    E) Follicle-stimulating hormone (FSH)

54. Which of the following positively correlates with improved treatment adherence by patients? **(242)**

    A) Physician's specialty
    B) Physician's years of experience
    C) Physician's knowledge
    D) Effective communication of the health care team
    E) Ethics consultation

55. Which of the following is NOT true? **(247–251)**

    A) In the setting of an emergency and parental refusal of treatment, treatment may be provided to a child without a court order overriding the parents' refusal
    B) A pediatrician may treat his or her own children or the children of family members for minor conditions, emergencies, and in underserved areas where no other physician capable of providing pediatric care is available
    C) Expensive gifts from patients should not be accepted, as they could seem to influence the pediatrician's professional judgment
    D) Genetic testing for carrier status of conditions in childhood is not recommended if medical management during childhood does not change
    E) Parental consent is always needed to treat adolescents for contraception, sexually transmitted diseases, and mental illness

56. A 3-day-old newborn has acute onset of bilateral eyelid swelling, conjunctival chemosis and hyperemia, purulent drainage, and fever. What is the most likely cause of infection? **(257)**

    A) Respiratory syncytial virus
    B) *Neisseria gonorrhea*
    C) *Chlamydia trachomatis*
    D) Herpes simplex virus
    E) *Streptococcus agalactiae*

57. Which of the following signs or symptoms distinguishes orbital cellulitis from preseptal cellulitis? **(260)**

    A) Painful extraocular movements
    B) Vision changes
    C) Proptosis
    D) Ophthalmoplegia
    E) All of the above

58. Chronic inflammation of an obstructed meibomian gland in the eyelid is known as: **(262)**

    A) Chalazion
    B) Hordeolum
    C) Molluscum contagiosum
    D) Stye
    E) Blepharitis

59. The triad of epiphora, blepharospasm, and photophobia with corneal clouding on exam is consistent with what pediatric ophthalmologic emergency? **(265–267)**

    A) Congenital nasolacrimal duct obstruction
    B) Orbital cellulitis
    C) Primary congenital glaucoma
    D) Endemic keratoconjunctivitis
    E) Congenital Horner syndrome

60. What is the most common cause of amblyopia? **(270)**

    A) Uncorrected refractive error
    B) Cataract
    C) Eyelid hemangioma
    D) Strabismus
    E) Ptosis

61. Which is NOT a sign of neonatal hypoglycemia? **(283)**

    A. Hypothermia
    B. Respiratory distress
    C. Strong suck
    D. Lethargy
    E. Exaggerated Moro reflex

62. Which is NOT a risk factor for developing severe neonatal hyperbilirubinemia? **(286)**

    A) Exclusive breastfeeding with weight loss
    B) East Asian race

C) ABO incompatibility
D) Discharge after 72 hours of age
E) Cephalohematoma

63. An ultrasound of the head in a premature infant shows hemorrhage involving the ventricles without extension of the bleeding to the cerebral cortex or ventricle dilation. What grade of intraventricular hemorrhage (IVH) is present? **(290)**

    A) Grade I
    B) Grade II
    C) Grade III
    D) Grade IV
    E) Grade V

64. A 29-week gestational age infant has respiratory distress and hypoxia after delivery. A chest X-ray shows decreased lung expansion and diffuse ground glass opacities. This is consistent with what condition? **(291–292)**

    A) Transient tachypnea of the newborn
    B) Neonatal pneumonia
    C) Persistent pulmonary hypertension
    D) Meconium aspiration syndrome
    E) Respiratory distress syndrome

65. Premature infants are at risk for which of the following? **(292–293)**

    A) Respiratory distress syndrome
    B) Necrotizing enterocolitis
    C) Sepsis
    D) Apnea
    E) All of the above

66. A newborn is unable to move his right arm. The arm is adducted, internally rotated, and extended. The forearm is pronated and the wrist flexed. This is most consistent with an injury to which of the following nerves? **(294)**

    A) C5, C6, and C7
    B) C5 and C6
    C) C7, C8, and T1
    D) C8 and T1
    E) C5, C6, C7, C8, and T1

67. Sunken eyes, parched skin, anuria, and altered mental status are associated with what percentage of dehydration in a 3-year-old child? **(301)**

    A) 3%
    B) 6%
    C) 9%
    D) 10%
    E) 15%

68. Which is NOT a cause of hypocalcemia? **(304)**

    A) Vitamin D deficiency
    B) Hypoparathyroidism
    C) Hypermagnesemia
    D) Pancreatitis
    E) Hyperphosphatemia

69. What metabolic derangement is seen in dehydrated infants with pyloric stenosis? **(305)**

    A) Hypochloremic metabolic alkalosis
    B) Hyperchloremic metabolic acidosis
    C) Hyperkalemia
    D) Hyponatremia
    E) Hypophosphatemia

70. Which is NOT a treatment of hyperkalemia? **(308–309)**

    A) Albuterol
    B) Insulin and intravenous (IV) dextrose
    C) Calcium gluconate
    D) Sodium polystyrene sulfonate
    E) Normal saline IV fluid bolus

71. Which is NOT a cause of an anion-gap metabolic acidosis? **(314)**

    A) Isoniazid
    B) Diabetic ketoacidosis
    C) Salicylate ingestion
    D) Diarrhea
    E) Uremia

72. A blood gas measurement is obtained, revealing the following: pH 7.39, PCO_2 28, HCO_3 18. This is consistent with what metabolic derangement? **(315)**

    A) Compensated metabolic acidosis
    B) Uncompensated respiratory acidosis
    C) Uncompensated respiratory alkalosis
    D) Compensated respiratory alkalosis
    E) Partially compensated respiratory acidosis

73. Which of the following causes of acute abdominal pain is common in infants and adolescents, but not school-aged children? **(324)**

    A) Appendicitis
    B) Intussusception
    C) Ovarian torsion
    D) Gastroenteritis
    E) Pyelonephritis

74. Which is NOT a common symptom of acute appendicitis? **(324)**

    A) Pain
    B) Anorexia
    C) Nausea

D) Fever
E) Flatulence

75. Which of the following is the most common cause of acute pancreatitis? **(326)**

    A) Viral infections
    B) Hyperlipidemia
    C) Cholelithiasis
    D) Medications
    E) Scorpion bites

76. At what age does malrotation typically become symptomatic? **(327)**

    A) First month of life
    B) 1 month to 3 months
    C) 3 months to 3 years
    D) 3 years to puberty
    E) After puberty

77. At what ages does intestinal intussusception most commonly occur? **(328)**

    A) First month of life
    B) 1 month to 3 months
    C) 3 months to 3 years
    D) 3 years to puberty
    E) After puberty

78. Which of the following pathogens is most likely to cause "pseudoappendicitis," in which severe abdominal pain occurs before the onset of diarrhea? **(337)**

    A) *Campylobacter*
    B) *Escherichia coli*
    C) *Clostridium difficile*
    D) Epstein-Barr virus
    E) *Salmonella*

79. Which of the following conditions is more common in children with trisomy 21? **(363)**

    A) Leukemia
    B) Duodenal atresia
    C) Atlantoaxial instability
    D) Celiac disease
    E) All of the above

80. Which of the following is NOT a feature of 22q11.2 deletion syndrome? **(365)**

    A) Abnormal facies
    B) Cardiac defects
    C) Thymus hypoplasia
    D) Cleft palate
    E) Hyperparathyroidism

81. A pregnant woman is a known carrier of Duchenne muscular dystrophy. What is the chance that her child will be affected? **(373)**

    A) 100%
    B) 50%
    C) 25%
    D) 3%
    E) 0%

82. Which pathogen is the most common cause of urinary tract infection in otherwise healthy children? **(378)**

    A) *Escherichia coli*
    B) *Pseudomonas aeruginosa*
    C) *Enterococcus faecalis*
    D) *Streptococcus pneumonia*
    E) *Streptococcus viridans*

83. Which of the following is true when using DDAVP in the treatment of nocturnal enuresis? **(385)**

    A) It may cause hypernatremia if given at too high a dose
    B) The intranasal solution is considered safer than oral tablets
    C) An ECG should be obtained before starting treatment
    D) The dose may need to be titrated over time to achieve all-night dryness
    E) It may make the child more difficult to awaken in the morning

84. The "blue dot sign" is indicative of what condition? **(389)**

    A) Torsion of the testicular appendage
    B) Testicular torsion
    C) Henoch-Schönlein purpura
    D) Congenital adrenal hyperplasia
    E) Solitary testicle

85. What is the most common type of kidney stone? **(395)**

    A) Calcium oxalate dihydrate
    B) Calcium phosphate
    C) Uric acid
    D) Ammonium acid urate
    E) Struvite

86. Which of the following testicular masses is associated with precocious puberty? **(397)**

    A) Testicular hamartoma
    B) Epidermoid cyst
    C) Teratoma
    D) Leydig cell tumor
    E) Yolk-sac tumor

87. Which of the following is NOT a complication of craniosynostosis? **(408)**

    A) Facial asymmetry
    B) Intracranial hypotension

C) Hydrocephalus
D) Strabismus
E) Dental malocclusion

88. What is expected average daily weight gain for a 1-month-old infant? **(410)**

    A) ≥ 100 g/day
    B) ≥ 60 g/day
    C) ≥ 20 g/day
    D) ≥ 10 g/day
    E) ≥ 7 g/day

89. "Symmetric" failure to thrive refers to: **(411)**

    A) Low weight but otherwise normal growth
    B) Low weight, followed by decreased linear growth
    C) Low weight, followed by decreased head growth
    D) Low weight, with decreased linear growth and head growth
    E) Shortened lower and upper extremities

90. A 12-year-old boy weighs 75 kg and is 150 cm tall. What are his body mass index (BMI) and body weight classification? **(412)**

    A) 22.2—healthy
    B) 22.2—overweight
    C) 22.2—obese
    D) 33.3—healthy
    E) 33.3—obese

91. Which of the following infant reflexes will not be preset at day of life 7? **(414)**

    A) Palmar grasp
    B) Parachute
    C) Moro
    D) Tonic neck
    E) Rooting

92. Which of the following would be considered normal speech development for an 18-month-old? **(416)**

    A) Two-word sentences
    B) Speech 50% understandable by a stranger
    C) Vocabulary of 10 to 50 words
    D) Use of plurals
    E) Able to name seven body parts

93. Which infectious disease is a contraindication to breast-feeding in the United States? **(424)**

    A) Latent tuberculosis
    B) Group B streptococcus
    C) Cytomegalovirus
    D) Hepatitis B (in the setting of cracked nipples)
    E) Herpes simplex virus with active labial and genital lesions

94. Which mother received adequate intrapartum antibiotic prophylaxis for prevention of group B streptococcus (GBS) transmission? **(424–425)**

    A) Term infant, mother GBS positive, mother received IV penicillin 4 hours prior to delivery
    B) Premature infant, mother GBS unknown, mother received no antibiotics prior to delivery
    C) Premature infant, mother GBS unknown, mother received IV clindamycin 2 hours prior to delivery
    D) Term infant, mother GBS negative but history of prior infant with GBS pneumonia, mother received no antibiotics prior to delivery
    E) All of the above

95. Erythema migrans is the hallmark rash of which infectious agent? **(430)**

    A) *Ixodes scapularis*
    B) *Borrelia burgdorferi*
    C) Epstein-Barr virus
    D) *Streptococcus pyogenes*
    E) Human immunodeficiency virus

96. Which of the following viruses is characterized by airborne (as opposed to contact or droplet) transmission? **(432)**

    A) Mumps
    B) Measles
    C) Influenza
    D) Adenovirus
    E) Human metapneumovirus

97. Which of the following is NOT associated with measles infection? **(449–450)**

    A) Fever
    B) Cough
    C) Coryza
    D) Conjunctivitis
    E) Morbilliform rash that spreads from the extremities to the trunk

98. Which of the following types of inborn errors of metabolism can be effectively managed by avoiding fasting? **(460)**

    A) Glycogen storage diseases
    B) Aminoacidurias
    C) Organic acidemias
    D) Urea cycle defects
    E) Mitochondrial myopathies

99. Which of the following conditions is NOT associated with elevated ammonia? **(460)**

    A) Phenylketonuria
    B) Maple syrup urine disease
    C) Propionic acidemia
    D) Ornithine transcarbamylase deficiency
    E) Tay-Sachs disease

100. Which of the following is associated with ketotic hypoglycemia? **(464)**

    A) Infant of a diabetic mother
    B) Exogenous insulin
    C) Fatty acid oxidation disorder
    D) Fasting/starvation
    E) Nesidioblastosis

101. Which of the following causes of ketotic hypoglycemia will NOT respond to a glucagon test? **(464)**

    A) Panhypopituitarism
    B) Adrenal insufficiency
    C) Organic acidemia
    D) Hereditary fructose intolerance
    E) Mitochondrial defects

102. Which of the following is NOT a potential complication of phenylketonuria (PKU)? **(475)**

    A) Seizures
    B) Cardiomyopathy
    C) Hypopigmentation of the hair and skin
    D) Microcephaly
    E) Eczema

103. Which is NOT a finding in congenital clubfoot (talipes equinovarus)? **(484)**

    A) Metatarsus adductus
    B) Hindfoot valgus
    C) Rigid equinus
    D) Cavus foot
    E) Full range of motion in the hip and knee

104. Which of the following is true of supracondylar humerus fractures in children? **(495)**

    A) Traction injuries are the most common mechanism
    B) They are often associated with child abuse
    C) The median nerve is the most commonly injured nerve
    D) Vascular insufficiency to the forearm almost always occurs immediately, and delayed vascular complications are rare
    E) The presence of a posterior elbow fat pad can be normal, and comparison views should be obtained if one is seen on X-ray

105. Legg-Calvé-Perthes disease is defined as: **(501)**

    A) Idiopathic osteonecrosis of the femoral head
    B) Avascular necrosis of the femoral head
    C) Physeal fracture involving the proximal femoral physis
    D) Avascular necrosis of the medial aspect of the lateral femoral condyle
    E) Insufficiency fracture of the mid-shaft of the femur

106. Spondylolysis may be seen on which of the following types of images? (504–506)

    A) X-ray (especially oblique views of the lumbar spine)
    B) CT scan
    C) MRI
    D) Bone scan
    E) All of the above

107. Which of the following is an indication for brain MRI when evaluating a child with headaches? (511–512)

    A) Focal neurologic symptoms (weakness, numbness)
    B) Headache worse later in the day
    C) Presence of aura prior to onset of headache
    D) Presence of rebound headaches when over-the-counter analgesics wear off
    E) Age greater than 6 years

108. Which is associated with central, rather than peripheral, hypotonia in children? (514)

    A) Normal mental status
    B) Absent reflexes
    C) Presence of seizures
    D) Muscle fasciculations
    E) Weak cough

109. Which is the most common cause of fatal meningitis infection among college students? (515)

    A) *Streptococcus pneumoniae*
    B) *Escherichia coli*
    C) *Listeria monocytogenes*
    D) *Neisseria meningitidis*
    E) Enterovirus

110. Which is a characteristic of spinal fluid in acute bacterial meningitis? (516)

    A) Elevated glucose
    B) Low protein
    C) Elevated white blood cell (WBC) count with eosinophilic predominance
    D) Elevated WBC count with lymphocytic predominance
    E) Elevated WBC count with neutrophilic predominance

111. Which of the following is associated with complex partial seizures? (522)

    A) Impaired level of consciousness
    B) Induced by hyperventilation
    C) Clusters upon awakening
    D) Absence of a postictal period
    E) Presence of hypsarrhythmia on EEG

112. Which of the following is NOT a benefit of exclusive breast milk feeding? (542)

    A) Decreased respiratory tract infections
    B) Increased diarrheal infections

    C) Decreased likelihood of atopic disease
    D) Decreased risk of obesity
    E) Decreased risk of sudden infant death syndrome (SIDS)

113. Which is NOT an indication for soy formula? (543)

    A) Galactosemia
    B) Congenital lactase deficiency
    C) Family wanting a vegetarian diet
    D) Prematurity
    E) All of the above

114. Which disease is NOT paired with its correct vitamin deficiency? (545–548)

    A) Scurvy and vitamin C (ascorbic acid) deficiency
    B) Beriberi and vitamin B_1 (thiamine) deficiency
    C) Pellagra and vitamin B_3 (niacin) deficiency
    D) Severe measles infection and vitamin A deficiency
    E) Night blindness and vitamin E deficiency

115. Which is NOT a clinical feature of rickets? (549)

    A) Tall stature
    B) Genu valgus
    C) Craniotabes
    D) Kyphoscoliosis
    E) Physeal widening

116. Which of the following has been shown to be the most common contributor to medical errors and sentinel events? (563)

    A) Poor communication
    B) Inadequate staffing
    C) Computerized physician order entry
    D) Incomplete documentation
    E) Lack of proper education for staff

117. Harm that reaches the patient in the absence of medical error is classified as which of the following? (562)

    A) Lapse
    B) Sentinel event
    C) Nonpreventable adverse event
    D) Preventable adverse event
    E) Near-miss event

118. Successful quality improvement projects utilize repeated PDSA cycles until change is achieved. Which is NOT part of the PDSA acronym? (564)

    A) Perform
    B) Study
    C) Do
    D) Act
    E) Plan

119. Which of the following describes the best approach for identifying the top few factors causing the majority of events? (566)

    A) Key driver diagram
    B) Pareto chart
    C) Run chart
    D) Statistical process control chart
    E) Shewhart chart

120. A healthy person starts taking a prescribed medication twice daily that has a half-life of 10 hours. How long will it take for the medication to reach a steady-state concentration? (574)

    A) 50 hours
    B) 24 hours
    C) 72 hours
    D) 36 hours
    E) 96 hours

121. The fraction of an administered dose of unchanged drug that reaches the systemic circulation is known as what? (575)

    A) Half-life
    B) Bioavailability
    C) Steady-state concentration
    D) Peak concentration
    E) Clearance

122. What type of adverse drug effect results from altered drug metabolism based on racial background? (577)

    A) Pharmacokinetic
    B) Pharmacodynamic
    C) Pharmacogenomic
    D) Idiosyncratic
    E) Allergic

123. Which is NOT an adverse effect of systemic glucocorticoid use? (579)

    A) Immunosuppression
    B) Adrenal suppression
    C) Short stature
    D) Osteoporosis
    E) Hypoglycemia

124. Which is NOT an adverse effect of stimulant medications? (583)

    A) Hallucinations
    B) Hypertension
    C) Blurry vision
    D) Hyperphagia
    E) Insomnia

125. For a nonemergent procedure requiring sedation, what is the minimum recommended time between ingestion of infant formula and administration of a sedative? (589–590)

    A) 2 hours
    B) 3 hours
    C) 4 hours
    D) 6 hours
    E) 8 hours

126. What monitoring is necessary when performing moderate or deep sedation? (591–592)

    A) Continuous pulse oximetry
    B) Continuous cardiorespiratory monitoring
    C) Frequent blood pressure monitoring
    D) Licensed provider whose sole responsibility is to monitor the patient
    E) All of the above

127. Which is NOT a treatment for salicylate poisoning? (597–598)

    A) Intravenous sodium bicarbonate
    B) Hemodialysis
    C) Activated charcoal
    D) *N*-acetylcysteine
    E) Urine alkalization

128. In acute acetaminophen ingestions with known time of ingestion, when should the acetaminophen level first be drawn? (601)

    A) 2 hours postingestion
    B) 4 hours postingestion
    C) 6 hours postingestion
    D) 8 hours postingestion
    E) 12 hours postingestion

129. Right upper quadrant pain, oliguria, and rising values for liver function tests are characteristic of which phase of acetaminophen toxicity? (600)

    A) Phase 1
    B) Phase 2
    C) Phase 3
    D) Phase 4
    E) Phase 5

130. Which is NOT a sign or symptom of opioid ingestion? (603)

    A) Altered mental status
    B) Hypotension
    C) Tachypnea
    D) Miosis
    E) Seizures

131. Which is NOT a symptom of anticholinergic toxicity? **(603)**

    A) Hypothermia
    B) Urinary retention
    C) Mydriasis
    D) Hallucinations
    E) Flushed skin

132. Which is NOT an ECG finding seen with tricyclic antidepressant toxicity? **(606)**

    A) Prolonged QRS
    B) Sinus tachycardia
    C) Ventricular tachycardia
    D) Right bundle branch block
    E) Shortened PR interval

133. A 3-year-old presents after ingesting a liquid. Laboratory testing shows an anion-gap metabolic acidosis, elevated serum osmolar gap, elevated creatinine, and hypocalcaemia. This is consistent with ingestion of which of the following? **(608–609)**

    A) Ethanol
    B) Methanol
    C) Isopropyl alcohol
    D) Ethylene glycol
    E) Salicylate

134. At what lead level should chelation therapy be initiated? **(616)**

    A) 10 mcg/dL
    B) 15 mcg/dL
    C) 25 mcg/dL
    D) 30 mcg/dL
    E) 45 mcg/dL

135. Which is NOT an indication for endoscopic removal of a foreign body? **(618)**

    A) Disc battery in the esophagus
    B) Coin in the proximal esophagus with dysphagia
    C) Coin in the stomach for 24 hours
    D) Coin in the esophagus for 36 hours
    E) Multiple magnets in the stomach

136. Which is NOT a contraindication to the live attenuated influenza virus vaccine? **(625)**

    A) Age less than 2 years old
    B) Immunosuppression
    C) Pregnancy
    D) Egg allergy
    E) History of wheezing as an infant

137. Which is NOT a contraindication to the single antigen varicella vaccine? **(628–629)**

    A) Pregnant woman
    B) Child with severe combined immunodeficiency

    C) Child with human immunodeficiency virus (HIV)
    D) Child with history of anaphylaxis to neomycin
    E) Child with leukemia

138. Which of the following regarding water safety is FALSE? **(635–637)**

    A) Vest- or horseshoe-style personal floatation devices are appropriate for children who are weak swimmers
    B) Bath rings should not be used in place of close supervision during bath time
    C) Swimming pools should be surrounded by a four-sided fence with a latching gate
    D) Children should begin swimming lessons at 1 year of age
    E) Five-gallon buckets full of water should not be left unattended around young children

139. Which of the following regarding sun safety is FALSE? **(635)**

    A) Sunscreens should provide sun protective factor (SPF) 45 or higher
    B) Peak sun hours should be avoided
    C) Sunscreen should be reapplied every 2 hours or after swimming or sweating
    D) Young infants should be kept in the shade
    E) Children should wear sunglasses, a hat, and tightly woven clothing when in the sun

140. Which of the following is an adverse risk of secondhand smoke exposure? **(640)**

    A) Increased risk of sudden infant death syndrome (SIDS)
    B) Increased number of viral respiratory tract infections
    C) Increased number of ear infections
    D) Increased number of asthma exacerbations
    E) All of the above

141. Which of the following is not one of Elisabeth Kübler-Ross's stages of loss and grief? **(644)**

    A) Denial and isolation
    B) Anger
    C) Bargaining
    D) Anxiety
    E) Acceptance

142. Which of the following statistics about foster care in the United States is true? **(647)**

    A) There are approximately 750,000 children in foster care
    B) There are approximately 75,000 children in foster care
    C) Each year, approximately 5,000 children "age out" of the foster care system
    D) Each year, approximately 100,000 children "age out" of the foster care system
    E) Only approximately 10% of foster children are placed with foster families due to child abuse or denial of critical care

143. Which is NOT a risk factor for vulnerable child syndrome? **(648)**

   A) Child's life was at risk during pregnancy
   B) Prematurity
   C) Excessive reassurance from physician
   D) Maternal history of multiple spontaneous abortions
   E) Mother had postpartum depression

144. Which of the following is NOT an injury suggestive of child abuse? **(653)**

   A) Rib fractures
   B) Femur fracture in nonambulatory child
   C) Tibia fracture in ambulatory child
   D) Sternum fracture
   E) Bilateral long-bone fracture

145. Which of the following sites of bruising is most concerning for child abuse? **(655)**

   A) Knees
   B) Abdomen
   C) Shins
   D) Forehead
   E) Forearms

146. Which of the following characteristics is most concerning for fabricated childhood illness (Munchausen syndrome by proxy)? **(658)**

   A) Father brings the child to medical appointments
   B) Parent is overly attentive to the child
   C) Family has minimal or no knowledge of medicine
   D) Family is reassured when a diagnosis is ruled out
   E) Seeks care at only one facility or with one provider

147. Of the following, which is considered the highest level of evidence? **(661)**

   A) Cross-sectional study
   B) Randomized controlled trial
   C) Prospective cohort
   D) Case-control study
   E) Animal research

148. Which of the following is a characteristic of a case-control study? **(662–663)**

   A) Controls for all variables
   B) Prospective
   C) Retrospective
   D) Does not involve a control group
   E) All of the above

149. What is the difference between statistical and clinical significance? **(667)**

   A) Clinical but not statistical significance can be determined by the *P* value

   B) A result can be clinically significant but not statistically significant
   C) A result can be statistically significant but not clinically significant
   D) A statistically significant result is always clinically significant
   E) None of the above

150. The "P" in PICO question stands for: **(667)**

   A) Pilot
   B) Preliminary
   C) Pathologic
   D) Premature
   E) Patient

151. Which of the following is the most common cause of recurrent, painless gross hematuria? **(672)**

   A) Kidney stones
   B) Urinary tract infection
   C) IgA nephropathy
   D) Hemolytic uremic syndrome
   E) Minimal change disease

152. How is the urine in myoglobinuria different from that in hematuria? **(673)**

   A) Dipstick urinalysis will not show blood
   B) Urine color will be dark yellow instead of pink, red, or brown
   C) Red blood cells (RBCs) will be more fragile and lyse soon after collection
   D) There will be no RBCs on microscopy
   E) It only becomes evident after IVF rehydration

153. Which of the following medications is NOT generally considered to be nephrotoxic? **(676)**

   A) Acetaminophen
   B) Acyclovir
   C) Penicillin
   D) Ibuprofen
   E) Tacrolimus

154. Which of the following is the equation to calculate the free water deficit for a patient with hypernatremia? **(680)**

   A) Free water deficit (liters) = Weight (kg) × (Actual Na − Goal Na)/Goal Na
   B) Free water deficit (liters) = 0.6 × Weight (kg) × (Goal Na − Actual Na)/Actual Na
   C) Free water deficit (liters) = 0.6 × Weight (kg) × (Actual Na − Goal Na)/Goal Na
   D) Free water deficit (liters) = 0.6 × Weight (kg) × (Goal Na − Actual Na)/Goal Na
   E) Free water deficit (liters) = Weight (kg) × (Goal Na − Actual Na)/Actual Na

155. Bright red blood in the urine is most commonly seen with: **(682)**

    A) Lower urinary tract pathology
    B) Upper urinary tract pathology
    C) Muscle breakdown
    D) Toxin ingestion
    E) Urethral stricture

156. What is the classic radiographic finding in croup? **(698)**

    A) Thumb sign
    B) Widened retropharyngeal space
    C) Radiopaque circle
    D) Steeple sign
    E) Subcutaneous emphysema

157. Which of the following causes expiratory stridor (instead of inspiratory or biphasic stridor)? **(699)**

    A) Laryngomalacia
    B) Croup
    C) Epiglottitis
    D) Vascular ring
    E) Vocal cord paralysis

158. The normal respiratory rate for an infant (in breaths per minute) is: **(709)**

    A) 30–60
    B) 60–80
    C) 20–40
    D) 12–30
    E) 12–16

159. Clubbing of the digits can be associated with which of the following types of illnesses? **(721)**

    A) Lung disease
    B) Cyanotic heart disease
    C) Inflammatory bowel disease
    D) Liver disease
    E) All of the above

160. Which of the following is the most common organism in necrotizing pneumonia of a child? **(723)**

    A) *Streptococcus pyogenes*
    B) *Staphylococcus aureus*
    C) *Streptococcus pneumoniae*
    D) *Haemophilus influenza*
    E) *Mycoplasma pneumoniae*

161. Which of the following is true about vitiligo? **(727–728)**

    A) It is autoimmune
    B) It is made worse by trauma
    C) Shining a Wood lamp on the skin does not accentuate the lesions

    D) It can result in hyperpigmentation of the involved skin
    E) All of the above

162. Which of the following body regions is least likely to be affected by psoriasis? **(732)**

    A) Scalp
    B) Nails
    C) Elbow
    D) Perineum
    E) Face

163. Which of the following is the most common cause of erythema multiforme? **(745)**

    A) Herpes simples virus
    B) Nonsteroidal anti-inflammatory drugs (NSAIDs)
    C) Fungal infections
    D) Cytomegalovirus
    E) Inflammatory bowel disease

164. Which of the following is the most effective method of treating a skin abscess? **(756)**

    A) Topical antibiotics
    B) Oral antibiotics
    C) Oral corticosteroids
    D) IV antibiotics
    E) Incision and drainage

165. Which of the following is a routine part of the sports pre-participation physical evaluation? **(759)**

    A) Echocardiogram
    B) Electrocardiogram
    C) Baseline concussion testing
    D) Detailed physical examination of each major joint
    E) None of the above

166. Which of the following is true regarding glucose metabolism in skeletal muscle? **(761)**

    A) The insulin receptor is only necessary for restoring glycogen stores
    B) Insulin can act directly on GLUT4
    C) GLUT4 can transport glucose into the cell without the need for insulin when a muscle is exercising
    D) The insulin receptor can transport glucose into the cell without the need for insulin when the muscle is exercising
    E) Skeletal muscles do not have insulin receptors

167. Which of the following sports should an athlete with trisomy 21 be allowed to participate in? **(770)**

    A) Boxing
    B) Wrestling
    C) Football
    D) Weight lifting
    E) None of the above

168. Which of the following physical examination maneuvers is used to test for an anterior cruciate ligament injury? **(774)**

    A) Lachman
    B) Posterior sag
    C) McMurray
    D) Valgus stress
    E) Varus stress

169. Which of the following is the most common specimen type to use when testing for drugs of abuse? **(783)**

    A) Blood
    B) Breath
    C) Urine
    D) Saliva
    E) Hair

170. Which of the following is the leading cause of preventable death and disease in the United States? **(783)**

    A) Drunk driving
    B) Alcohol poisoning
    C) Cocaine
    D) Heroin
    E) Cigarettes

171. Which of the following medications is contraindicated in patients who have ingested cocaine? **(787)**

    A) Beta-blockers
    B) Aspirin
    C) Benzodiazepines
    D) Nitroglycerin
    E) Sodium bicarbonate

Answer Key

1. D	33. C	65. E
2. D	34. C	66. A
3. A	35. D	67. C
4. E	36. A	68. C
5. B	37. C	69. A
6. A	38. B	70. E
7. A	39. A	71. D
8. C	40. E	72. D
9. E	41. B	73. C
10. A	42. C	74. E
11. D	43. D	75. A
12. C	44. C	76. A
13. E	45. D	77. C
14. B	46. E	78. A
15. B	47. A	79. E
16. A	48. B	80. E
17. E	49. A	81. C
18. A	50. D	82. A
19. E	51. D	83. D
20. B	52. C	84. A
21. B	53. B	85. A
22. E	54. D	86. D
23. B	55. E	87. B
24. E	56. B	88. C
25. C	57. E	89. D
26. D	58. A	90. E
27. A	59. C	91. B
28. C	60. D	92. C
29. B	61. C	93. D
30. A	62. D	94. A
31. B	63. B	95. B
32. A	64. E	96. B

97. E	122. C	147. B
98. A	123. E	148. C
99. E	124. D	149. C
100. D	125. D	150. E
101. D	126. E	151. C
102. B	127. D	152. D
103. B	128. B	153. A
104. C	129. B	154. C
105. A	130. C	155. A
106. E	131. A	156. D
107. A	132. E	157. D
108. C	133. D	158. A
109. D	134. E	159. E
110. E	135. C	160. B
111. A	136. E	161. A
112. B	137. C	162. E
113. D	138. D	163. A
114. E	139. A	164. E
115. A	140. E	165. E
116. A	141. D	166. C
117. C	142. A	167. D
118. A	143. C	168. A
119. B	144. C	169. C
120. A	145. B	170. E
121. B	146. B	171. A

Index

Note: Page numbers followed by f refer to figures; those followed by t refer to tables.